NATIONAL LEAGUE FOR NURSING

Official Guide to

Undergraduate and Graduate

NURSING PROGRAMS

SECOND EDITION

JONES AND BARTLETT PUBLISHERS

Sudbury, Massachusetts

BOSTON   TORONTO   LONDON   SINGAPORE

World Headquarters
Jones and Bartlett Publishers
40 Tall Pine Drive
Sudbury, MA 01776
978-443-5000
info@jbpub.com
www.jbpub.com

Jones and Bartlett Publishers Canada
2406 Nikanna Road
Mississauga, ON L5C 2W6
CANADA

Jones and Bartlett Publishers International
Barb House, Barb Mews
London W6 7PA
UK

Copyright © 2004 by the National League for Nursing

Cover Photo © Ablestock

Library of Congress Cataloging-in-Publication Data
Official guide to undergraduate and graduate nursing programs / National League for
Nursing.
   p. cm.
Includes bibliographical references and index.
   ISBN 0-7637-1807-6 (pbk.)
   1. Nursing schools—United States—Directories.   2. Nursing students—United States
Directories. 3. Nursing—Vocational guidance—Directories. 4. Schools, Nursing—United States—
Directory.   I. National League for Nursing.
   RT73.034 2003
   610.73'071'173—dc21

            2003040077

The program information presented in the *Official Guide to Undergraduate and Graduate Nursing Programs, Second Edition,* has been derived from data provided by the National League for Nursing (NLN). The Publisher has made every effort to ensure that the information presented is as complete and accurate as is possible. For questions and comments, please contact the NLN at 1-800-669-1656 or Tbreymei@mmcweb.com.

Production Manager: Amy Rose
Production Assistant: Tracey Chapman
Editorial Assistant: Amy Sibley
Marketing Associate: Elizabeth Waterfall
Production Coordination: Jennifer Bagdigian
Cover Design: Anne Spencer
Composition: Northeast Compositors
Manufacturing Buyer: Amy Bacus
Printing and Binding: Courier Stoughton
Cover Printing: Courier Stoughton

Printed in the United States of America
07 06 05 04 03   10 9 8 7 6 5 4 3 2 1

Preface

It is with great pride that the National League for Nursing (NLN) publishes this revised edition of the comprehensive directory of undergraduate and graduate nursing programs. More than 75 years ago, the NLN's predecessor—the National League for Nursing Education—initiated a comprehensive database about all nursing programs in the United States and its territories. This is the only database of its kind. We have been diligent about maintaining an accurate source of data about nursing programs, and we are particularly proud to present this updated compilation of information to you. Such a publication continues the NLN's tradition of excellence and contributes to our Mission: *To advance quality nursing education that prepares the nursing workforce to meet the needs of diverse populations in an ever-changing healthcare environment.*

We are confident that you will find this guide extremely helpful. It provides a great deal of information about the vast majority of nursing programs, and allows you to make comparisons between schools. As such, this guide is an excellent resource to individuals who are making decisions about entering the nursing profession or advancing their preparation in the field, as well as to individuals who want to know more about the preparation of nurses today.

Nursing is a profession that demands intellectual rigor, compassion, technological skill, a commitment to quality, and passion. It offers the clinician an opportunity to be involved in people's lives at their most vulnerable times, to improve the health of communities, and to influence the development of policies related to health and health care. Additionally, with graduate preparation, nursing provides career options in advanced practice, education, administration, case management, research, and informatics, among other roles. This reference guide introduces you to many of those options and provides information on how to explore these opportunities on your own.

We welcome you to the world of nursing education and encourage you to consider pursuing or advancing your career in nursing. Your feedback about this resource would be appreciated.

Ruth D. Corcoran, EdD, RN
Chief Executive Officer
National League for Nursing

Theresa M. Valiga, EdD, RN, FAAN
Chief Program Officer
National League for Nursing

Contributors

Diane M. Billings, EdD, RN, FAAN
Professor of Nursing and Associate Dean for Teaching, Learning, and Information Resources
Indiana University School of Nursing

Jane Lithgow, MN, RN
Coordinator of Professional Initiatives
National League for Nursing

Contents

Section 1

A Career in Nursing

What You'll Find in This Book

The *Official Guide to Undergraduate and Graduate Nursing Programs* was designed to help you compare many fine programs based on criteria that are important to students. Selecting the right nursing school is not an easy task. Many variables need to be considered. This guide is designed to serve as your road map as you consider a career in nursing and the schools at which you can get your education.

Organization of the Guide

This volume is divided into three main parts: an introductory section (Section 1), school profiles (Sections 2 and 3), and expanded school profiles (Section 4). Also included are two indexes, one listing schools by specialty programs at the graduate level, the other listing schools in alphabetical order (Section 5).

The introductory section contains separate sections on pursuing and advancing your career in nursing, distance learning, financial support for your nursing education, and scholarships and loans specifically for nursing students. All of these sections will help you decide which nursing program best meets your needs, and will also provide you with information on how to finance your education.

Nursing School Profiles

At the heart of this book are the school entries, which profile over 2000 schools of nursing in the United States. The schools are organized by program type, associate degree, diploma, baccalaureate, BSN for RNs, master's, and doctorate. Within the program type, individual schools are organized alphabetically within their respective state.

We have carefully designed the layout of each school's information for you. Focus groups were conducted with nursing students, high school students, and guidance counselors to find out which pieces of information were most important to students selecting a nursing program. The design of this guide reflects this research and the feedback we received. We were told that the design should be consistent across schools and should make school-to-school comparisons easy. An attractive design was important to keep things interesting and to make the search process quicker. Prospective students didn't want to be flooded with details immediately, so we have limited the design to the top facts on every school.

The guide profiles are organized into the sections listed below and are clearly identified with the accompanying icon. Each profile is organized in a consistent manner to make information retrieval as easy as possible.

Research Procedures

The NLN has been gathering extensive statistics on nursing schools for over 40 years. The data contained in this guide was based on information gathered during the 2001–2002 academic year. Questionnaires were sent to all schools in the US. All the information in this edition was submitted by the schools themselves. All information that was received in time for publication has been included in the guide. When specific information was not available from a particular school, this is indicated with the notation *Not Provided*. Individuals should check directly with the school they are applying to at the time of application to verify that school-specific information has not changed since the publication of this guide.

Basic School Information

Each profile begins with basic school information: name, address, phone number, and a key contact name. A school's Web site address may also appear here. Indicators will appear at the end of the profiles for schools that have reader reply numbers for further information and/or in-depth profiles in this guide.

GENERAL INFORMATION

This section aims to give students a general idea about the entire college or university of which the nursing school is a part.

Type of School: possible options are public, private (independent), private (religious)

Total enrollment: total number of students in all academic areas including nursing

Accreditation: Regional accreditation awarded to the entire institution. Colleges and universities themselves seek accreditation from a regional accrediting body (e.g., New England Association of Schools and Colleges). This involves self-analysis and critical review by peers from outside the university. While regional accreditation does not address specifics of any particular program offered by the college or university (e.g., Nursing), it does indicate that the institution as a whole has met predetermined standards.

PROGRAM INFORMATION

This section provides information about the specifics of the nursing school, including programs offered.

Accreditation: Schools of nursing that prepare students for beginning practice roles (as LPNs or RNs) must be approved by their state's Board of Nursing. In addition to this basic approval to offer a program, schools may choose to pursue accreditation of their programs. Accreditation is a voluntary process in which a school provides evidence of how it meets predetermined standards or criteria and then engages in a rigorous review by colleagues from similar schools. If the result of this self-analysis and external peer review reveals that the school has met the established standards, the school is granted accreditation.

In nursing, LPN, diploma, associate degree, baccalaureate, and master's programs may seek accreditation through the National League for Nursing Accrediting Commission (NLNAC), a body that is recognized by the U.S. Department of Education. Baccalaureate and master's programs also may seek accreditation through the Commission on Collegiate Nursing Education (CCNE). The accreditation status of each program in 2001–2002 is noted in this guide.

Areas of Study with Specialization (for graduate programs only):

Nurse Anesthetist

Case Management

Clinical Nurse Specialist: possible options are Acute Care, Adult, Community/Home Health, Critical Care, Family, Gerontology, Neonatology, Oncology, Pediatrics, Perinatology, Psychiatric/Mental Health, School Nursing, Women's Health, and Other

CNS–NP

Health Policy

Nursing Administration/Management: possible options are Administration/Executive—Community Health, Administration/Executive—General, Management/Administrative/Executive—Other, Mid-level Nursing Management, and MSN/MBA

Nursing Education: possible options are Academic Role, General, and Staff Development

Nurse-Midwifery

Nurse Practitioner: possible options are Acute Care, Adult, Critical Care, Family, Gerontology, Neonatology, Pediatrics, Perinatology, Psychiatric/Mental Health, Rural Health, Women's Health, and Other

NURSING STUDENT PROFILE

This section provides an idea of the size of the nursing program.

(Undergraduate section)

Total Nursing Enrollment: combined number of students pursuing a degree or diploma in nursing

Full-Time Enrollment

Part-Time Enrollment

Female Enrollment

Male Enrollment

Total Graduates: total number of students graduating in a given year

(Graduate section)

Total Nursing Enrollment: combined number of students pursuing graduate degrees in nursing

Full-Time Enrollment

Part-Time Enrollment

Female Enrollment

Male Enrollment

Total Graduates: total number of students graduating in a given year

FINANCES

This section answers the question of how much it will cost to attend a specific school.

Resident Annual Tuition

Non-Resident Annual Tuition

General Institution Fees, Annually

Additional Nursing Student Fees, Annually

Expanded School Profiles

All nursing schools were given the opportunity to provide additional information concerning their programs to interested students. The profiles of schools that have elected to do so appear in this section. As with the Nursing School profiles, all of the information that appears in this section was provided directly by the schools.

Schools Included in the Guide

This guide contains all associate, baccalaureate, BSN for RNs, diploma, masters, and doctoral programs in the U.S. that submitted an annual survey to the National League for Nursing in 2001–2002. For your convenience, graduate specialty area listings, by state, can be found in the Specialty Index in Section 5.

Contact Schools Directly for More Information

A large number of the schools in this guide will be happy to send you more information directly. If a reader reply card number appears in a school's profile simply circle the number on the card in the back of the book. You may circle as many schools as you like. Complete the necessary fields of information and send in the card. In a few weeks you will receive information directly from the selected school or schools.

Glossary/Abbreviations

Accreditation: A voluntary, peer review process in which a school provides evidence regarding how it meets pre-determined standards or criteria and then engages in a rigorous review by colleagues from similar schools (See Introduction for further explanation)

AD: Associate Degree

ADN: Associate Degree in Nursing

ANP: Adult Nurse Practitioner

APN/APRN: Advanced Practice Registered Nurse

Articulation: A process in which a nurse who has one credential may advance to a higher level in nursing without duplication or repetition

Associate Degree Program: A two-year program primarily affiliated with junior and community colleges

Baccalaureate Program: A four-year program affiliated with a university or senior college

Baccalaureate Programs for RNs: Programs in senior colleges or universities designed solely for individuals already licensed as RNs

Basic Student: An individual who enters a collegiate program directly from high school. This individual typically is in the 18–22 year old age range, has no previous college credits or professional preparation, and often enrolls on a full-time basis

BSN: Bachelor of Science in Nursing

CCNE: Commission on Collegiate Nursing Education

Diploma program: A nursing program that is hospital based, and takes 2–3 years to complete

DNS/DNSc: Doctor of Nursing Science

EdD: Doctor of Education

FAAN: Fellow in the American Academy of Nursing

FAF: Financial Aid Form

FAFSA: Free Application for Federal Student Aid

GPA (Grade Point Average): The translation of a student's letter grades into a numeric system reflecting academic performance. The most common system counts four points for an "A," three points for a "B," two points for a "C," one point for a "D," and no points for an "E" or "F"

GRE (Graduate Record Examination): A standard battery of general and subject exams for college graduates interested in applying to graduate school; administered by the Educational Testing Service

LPN: Licensed Practical Nurse

LVN: Licensed Vocational Nurse

MAT: Miller Analogies Test

MBA: Master of Business Administration

MSN: Master of Science in Nursing

ND: Doctor of Nursing/Nurse Doctorate

NLN: National League for Nursing

NLNAC: National League for Nursing Accrediting Commission

Non-traditional student: An individual who does not enroll in a collegiate program immediately after completing high school or who re-enters a collegiate program after a hiatus. This individual typically is older than the traditional 18–22 year old college student, may work while attending school, and may have earned college credits previously

NP: Nurse Practitioner

Pell Grant: A gift-aid program sponsored by the federal government

Perkins Loan: A program of federally funded, college-administered loans available to students from low-income families

PhD: Doctor of Philosophy

RN: Registered Nurse

Semester system: A calendar in which the academic year is divided into two units of roughly 16 weeks each

Introduction

Making decisions about your education is one of the most important processes in which you can engage. As your education forms the basis for your future work, it also provides for your entrée to certain arenas of endeavor, and sets the stage for fulfillment in critical aspects of your life. The National League for Nursing has been dedicated, since its inception over 100 years ago, to fostering the educational development of nurses and nursing, and to providing assistance to individual nurses and the profession as we plan for our individual and collective future. This resource book is one approach to assuring nurses and future nurses of the many opportunities and options they have to fulfill their dreams. A career in nursing is exciting and extraordinarily diverse. The ways in which men and women can prepare to be nurses is only equaled by the array of options left open to nurses once they have achieved their basic nursing education.

Neither our profession, nor our society, has ever needed well prepared and thoughtful nurses to provide the services our citizens need for good health more than is needed today. This resource book can be thought of as a map to that world. It provides outstanding resources from which interested individuals can discover learning opportunities and paths to realize their dreams.

The world of nursing is eager to welcome you, and the National League for Nursing is eager to serve you as you enter or advance in a nursing career. As an organization dedicated to nursing education, it is only fitting that these educational pathways be illuminated through our work.

My sincerest wish is that your nursing career is as rewarding and fulfilling to you as mine has been to me.

Joyce P. Murray

Joyce P. Murray, EdD, RN, FAAN
President
National League for Nursing

Pursuing a Career in Nursing

Since the beginning of time, people have been caring for one another, particularly during times of need and crisis. Caring for others has been part of the "calling" for those in religious orders, part of the responsibility of those in the military, and part of the fabric of daily life for ordinary citizens around the world. The essence of nursing—caring—therefore, is as old as time itself, and it is not unique to those who put RN, LPN, or APRN after their names. However, there **is** something very unique about the caring that nurses provide.

One of the features that distinguishes "nursing care" from "basic human care" is that the care nurses provide is based on a strong foundation of knowledge, and nursing, therefore, is as much an intellectual undertaking as is it a physical one. In their educational programs, nurses learn about the structure and functioning of the human body (anatomy and physiology), how to prevent or minimize negative consequences of the transmission of microorganisms (microbiology), what it means to be human (psychology), how families function (family dynamics), social phenomena (sociology), disruptions in normal human functioning (pathophysiology), and, among other things, how medications affect human functioning (pharmacology). Like students in many other fields, they also learn about the history of our country and the world, the influence of the arts in our lives, how to communicate effectively, how to find and use information, how to make precise calculations, how to make decisions in uncertainty, and how to be productive citizens. In nursing, therefore, caring about others is critical, but it is not enough. Practice must be knowledge-based.

Another way in which "nursing care" differs from "basic human care" relates to the recipient of care. In addition to caring for individuals, nurses care for families, groups, and entire communities. They care for these individuals when they are ill and when they are well. Thus, nurses focus on promoting health and preventing disease, as well as on helping individuals recover from illness.

Nurses also differ in their approach to caring by the holistic perspective they bring to any care situation. In other words, while nurses are concerned with the treatment of an illness, they are even more concerned with what that illness means to the individual and his/her family. They help individuals manage dietary, activity, and other lifestyle changes that may be needed as a result of a disease or its treatment. They help individuals gain access to resources that will help them manage changes that may be needed in their home environment, job changes that may be needed, or changes in family responsibilities. They also teach individuals, families, and communities how to care for themselves and how to create new life situations that may be required as a result of an illness or to maintain a healthy lifestyle.

Finally, nurses have a unique opportunity to become intimately involved in the lives of strangers, particularly as they face major crises in their lives. Nurses are there when deformed babies are born. They are there when someone suffers a stroke or debilitating heart attack. They are there to care for burn victims or accident victims. They are there to help people with cancer or AIDS live full lives. And they are there when people breathe their last breath. No other profession offers its members the privilege of caring for people when they are at their most vulnerable moments and touching people at the most critical moments of their lives.

Pursuing a career in nursing provides an almost unlimited number of choices regarding one's work. You can work with pregnant families and newborns, being there at the very beginning of life. You can work with well children in schools or ill children in hospitals and rehabilitation centers. You can work with young adults in need of psychiatric intervention or individuals who are struggling with addictions. You can work with the incarcerated in prisons. You can work with adults undergoing major surgery, invasive diagnostic procedures, or extensive and long-term treatment of a chronic illness. You can work with cancer patients throughout the diagnostic process, the difficult treatment times, the good times when they are in remission, and the times when they need to talk with their families about the impact of their illness. You can work with the elderly in community-based senior centers, long term care facilities, skilled nursing facilities, or their homes. Or you can work with entire communities through public health departments or community centers. These are only some of the many opportunities for nurses in today's healthcare arena, and many more options await the nurse of tomorrow.

Career Opportunities

Nursing has been identified as one of the fastest-growing fields in our nation and one where employment opportunities are almost unlimited. The number of available positions for Registered Nurses (RNs) is expected to continue to grow at least through 2020, and the nature of those positions is quite varied.

In addition to practicing in hospitals (where approximately 60% work), RNs also practice in many other settings: homes, schools, rehabilitation centers, long term care facilities, insurance companies, clinics, psychiatric facilities, prisons, college campuses, skilled nursing facilities, public health departments, reservations, rural communities, and birthing centers, among others. In these settings, nurses fulfill any number of roles, including direct care provider, manager, patient educator, or staff educator, and they implement these roles in collaboration with members of many other health professions (physicians, pharmacists, physical therapists, social workers, speech therapists, and so on).

Nurses with graduate preparation have additional career opportunities available to them. They may function as educators in schools of nursing, administrators of nursing services, nurse practitioners, nurse anesthetists, nurse midwives, clinical specialists, public policy makers, consultants, researchers, writers, professional association staff, or entrepreneurs who manage their own creative businesses. This advanced educational preparation helps nurses develop specialized knowledge that is balanced with a broad professional perspective, research, and information management skills, as well as the skills needed to provide leadership on a national level and on interdisciplinary teams.

Nurses Make a Difference

Many people think that nurses do little more than "soothe fevered brows" or hold the hand of those undergoing difficult procedures. Nurses do, indeed, play these very significant roles that serve to ease someone's anxiety or provide emotional support to individuals. But the care that nurses give has other significant results.

In a series of studies conducted since 2000, results such as the following have been documented:

- When there are more RNs involved in giving care, patients experience fewer instances of urinary tract infections, upper gastrointestinal bleeding, pneumonia, and shock or cardiac arrest.
- When there are more RNs involved in giving care, medical patients experience a shorter length of stay in the hospital.
- When there are more RNs involved in giving care, there are fewer medication errors.
- The level of patient satisfaction with their care is linked directly to the quality of nursing care they receive.
- Primary care delivered by advanced practice nurses is of similar quality to that provided by physicians, and it is of lower cost.

Evidence is mounting, therefore, that nurses have a positive impact on the health and safety of patients, as well as on the cost of health care. Nurses do, indeed, make a significant difference, and pursuing a career in nursing is rewarding in many ways.

Types of Nursing Programs that Prepare Registered Nurses

Individuals wishing to prepare as a Registered Nurse (RN) can accomplish that goal through one of five routes. Graduates of each type of program are eligible to take the licensing examination (NCLEX-RN®) that allows them to practice as an RN.

Associate Degree Programs. Associate degree (AD) nursing programs have been in existence since the 1950s, and in 2002, there were approximately 875 such programs in existence. They are offered in community or junior colleges, and most are two years in length. AD programs provide students with foundational courses in the liberal arts and sciences, nursing courses, and clinical experiences in local hospitals, long term care facilities, and community-based agencies. Most students in associate degree programs are from the local community in which the school is located, many are older, and many plan to work in the same community in which they were educated. Graduates of these types of programs earn an Associate Degree in Nursing (ADN) or an Associate Degree with a major in nursing.

Hospital Diploma Programs. Hospital diploma programs have been preparing RNs since the late 1800s. While they had been the mainstay of nursing education for many years, today there are only about 70 such programs in existence. Typically, they are three years in length and include courses in the sciences (often taken at a local community or junior college) and nursing. While students may have clinical experiences in any number of agencies, many of those experiences take place within the sponsoring healthcare system's hospitals, clinics, long term care facilities, and/or home care agencies. Individuals who graduate from these types of programs earn a diploma in nursing, but they may also earn an Associate Degree in Science, depending on the design of the program and the number of credits they complete through the local community or junior college.

Baccalaureate Programs. Graduates of baccalaureate programs earn a BSN (Bachelor of Science in Nursing) degree, or a BA (Bachelor of Arts) or BS (Bachelor of Science) degree with a major in nursing, upon program completion. Such programs are four years in length and incorporate an extensive general education component, including english, psychology, sociology, mathematics, arts, literature, political science, chemistry, and other sciences. Students' clinical experiences are in varied settings, including hospitals, home care agencies, communities, schools, out-patient clinics, long term care facilities, and nurse-managed clinics. The number of baccalaureate programs in nursing in 2002 was approximately 550, with an additional 150 or so that limit their admissions to individuals who are already licensed as RNs (through completion of an associate degree or hospital diploma program) and wish to earn the baccalaureate degree. They typically are "housed" in senior colleges and universities.

Generic Master's Programs. A relatively new phenomenon in nursing education is the generic master's degree program, which combines baccalaureate-level preparation and advanced, specialty master's-level preparation. Typically these types of programs are designed for individuals who hold a bachelor's degree in a field outside nursing and who complete the nursing requirements in a concentrated, intensive sequence of learning experiences. Students often complete science pre-requisites prior to beginning the intensive program, complete all baccalaureate-level requirements in a year's time, and sit for the licensing examination while they continue to complete master's-level courses in their chosen specialty. Completion of the master's degree often is done within two years of completion of baccalaureate-level requirements.

Nurse Doctorate Programs. Another relatively new phenomenon is the nurse doctorate (ND) program. Like a generic master's program, the ND program combines baccalaureate-level preparation with preparation in an advanced clinical practice area and/or research. Again, these types of programs typically are designed for individuals who hold a bachelor's degree in a field outside nursing and who complete science pre-requisites prior to beginning the intensive program, complete all baccalaureate-level requirements in (generally) a year's time, sit for the licensing examination while they continue to complete master's-level courses in their chosen specialty, and complete a research project. Completion of the ND degree often is done within three or four years.

Criteria for Selection of a Nursing Program

Individuals seeking to pursue educational preparation as a nurse often ask the National League for Nursing (NLN) about which school or program is "the best." Because the criteria used to judge "the best" school or program are so varied and individualized, the NLN does not provide such rankings. However, it is important for you to think about the criteria that are important to you before making your selection of a program. The following criteria should be considered:

The Curriculum. What kinds of courses are required in the program? What kinds of opportunities will you have to study with individuals in other fields and learn from faculty who are experts in fields outside nursing? How much clinical experience will you have in the program, and where will those experiences take place? How innovative is the program, and how well does it prepare graduates for twenty-first century nursing practice?

The Faculty. What is the level of preparation of the faculty in terms of their academic degrees? Have they received those degrees from a variety of institutions? What kinds of personal clinical nursing experiences do faculty bring to the teaching/learning experience? How well prepared are faculty for their teaching roles? How many faculty are there, and what kind of student to teacher ratio does that allow for in the classroom and in the clinical setting? How important do faculty think student advising and counseling are? How many faculty are actively involved in professional associations, research, ongoing clinical practice, and other professional activities?

The Students. How involved are students in the life of the nursing program (do they participate on committees and take part in decision making)? How diverse is the student body? What kinds of opportunities are there for students to work together and learn from one another? What kinds of policies and support systems are in place regarding students' progression from one point in the program to the next? What percentage of students complete the program in the usual timeframe (2 years, 3 years, 4 years)? What percentage of graduating students pass the licensing examination on the first attempt? How many graduates are offered the kind of nursing positions they were seeking? In the eyes of employers, how do graduates of this program compare with graduates of other programs?

The Teaching/Learning Environment. How do faculty and students describe the teaching/learning environment? Is there mutual respect between and among students and teachers? Do students feel free to express their ideas and disagree with faculty? Is there a sense of "wonder" and a "spirit of inquiry" among the students and faculty? Do faculty use innovative approaches to facilitate learning? To what extent is instruction individualized?

Other. What kind of tutoring, counseling, and remedial services are available through the school? Is there an active student nursing organization through which students can develop professional and leadership skills? What is the tuition? What kind of financial assistance programs are available? Is there on-campus housing? What kind of additional fees are there for nursing students? Where is the campus located? How do students get to the clinical agencies where they have clinical experiences? What are the relationships like between the school and the agencies used for students' clinical experiences? Are classrooms well-equipped with state-of-the-art technology? Is there a nursing practice laboratory with state-of-the-art equipment?

It is clear that there are many criteria to consider when selecting a nursing program. You need to decide which of these criteria are most important to you and make your selection of programs based on how they fare in relation to those criteria.

You may find answers to many of these questions in the school's catalogue, on their Web site, or in videos they send. But you also will find answers by visiting the school, talking with faculty and students, and sitting in on some classes. Choosing the program that is right for you is a most important decision, and it is not always an easy task. You should begin your search early, explore programs in depth, ask as many questions as you need to ask, and consider all answers seriously. By doing so, you are more likely to find the program that is best in helping you achieve your career goals.

Advancing in Your Nursing Career

Although the direct care of patients and families is exciting and rewarding, many nurses reach a point in their career when they look for new opportunities and challenges. Such opportunities can be found by moving to another unit in your institution (transferring to critical care or ambulatory clinics), or by moving to another institution altogether. New opportunities may also be found, however, by changing your career direction, and that often requires advanced educational preparation.

Nurses with graduate preparation (master's or doctoral) have an exciting array of career options available to them and are prepared to assume a number of unique positions. Those career options include advanced clinical practice, administration, education, research, public policy, informatics, consultation, and professional association work, among others. In each of these roles, the nurse builds on or draws from the knowledge and skills developed in basic education to create new ways to contribute to the profession. Each of these role categories will be discussed here, as will the nature of master's, post-master's, doctoral, and post-doctoral education.

Types of Graduate Programs

Master's Education. There are more than 350 master's programs in nursing today, and they are located in small liberal arts colleges, comprehensive universities, academic health science centers, and research-intensive universities. The particular degree awarded by a school may vary, but the core or essence of most master's programs is similar. Among the degrees awarded upon completion of a master's program with a "major" in nursing are the MA (Master of Arts), MS or MSc (Master of Science), MSN (Master of Science in Nursing), MEd (Master of Education), or MPH (Master of Public Health).

Nearly all master's programs have a "core" of courses that students take, regardless of the specialty they plan to pursue. This core may include courses in theory or nursing science, research, healthcare issues and trends, public policy development, clinical concepts, leadership, ethics, care of vulnerable populations, and so on. The specifics of the core are determined by standards for master's education in nursing and the unique emphasis of a particular program.

If a school offers only clinical specialty areas as the focus of study, the core may also include advanced-level courses in physiology, health assessment, pathophysiology, and pharmacology. If such courses are not included in the core for all students, they typically are core for all students pursuing clinical specializations.

In addition to these core courses, graduate programs in nursing include courses that are designed to help the student develop expertise in a particular area (advanced practice, nursing education, etc.). These specialty courses may be offered in or outside the nursing program, and they typically blend theoretical learning and application of that knowledge in practicum courses. Practica are individually designed by the student and faculty, and students are quite independent in these experiences, where learning is guided by faculty and experts who are implementing the role in their own settings.

Master's programs in nursing range from 30 to 60 post-baccalaureate credits, with most schools requiring between 36 and 45 credits for program completion. Many master's students study on a part-time basis while they continue to work as RNs, and most programs are designed to accommodate this kind of flexibility.

Although the requirements for admission differ from one school to the next, there are some commonalities among most schools. Students typically are required to hold a baccalaureate degree in nursing, although more master's programs are providing "generic master's" program options designed for individuals who hold a baccalaureate degree in a field outside nursing. In these programs, students complete selected baccalaureate-level courses, then continue with their graduate courses while they sit for the RN licensing examination. Upon completion of the generic master's program, the graduate will be licensed as an RN and earn the master's degree, but she/he may not earn a baccalaureate degree in nursing.

Admission requirements may also include a minimum of one year experience as an RN (although more and more programs are changing this requirement as a way to encourage nurses to pursue and attain their master's degree very early in their career). Most programs will specify a minimum undergraduate GPA as an admission requirement, and most also require that applicants attain a specified minimum score on a standardized test (GRE or MAT). Finally, references from professionals who are in a position to comment on the applicant's abilities and potential to succeed in graduate school are usually required. Some schools may require applicants to participate in an admission interview, and some may ask for samples of papers or articles the applicant has written.

Post-Master's Certificate Programs. Many schools of nursing now offer post-master's certificate programs in a variety of areas. A common program of this type allows master's prepared clinical nurse specialists or nurse administrators to prepare as nurse practitioners. Students enrolled in a post-master's program enroll only in those courses that are specific to the new specialty (they usually do not re-take core courses), and they complete all theory and practicum courses related to that specialty. Upon completion of this sequence of courses, the individual is awarded a certificate (not a degree), receives a transcript that documents the courses completed, and is eligible to sit for any certifying or licensing examinations associated with the specialty.

Doctoral Programs. At present there are nearly 80 doctoral programs in nursing. As is true at the master's level, doctoral programs may award any one of a number of degrees including the PhD (Doctor of Philosophy), the EdD (Doctor of Education), or the DNS or DNSc (Doctor of Nursing Science). Recent research has indicated that while each of these programs is thought to be different on a conceptual level (the PhD is a research degree and the DNSc is a clinical degree), there are many similarities among them.

All doctoral programs aim to prepare scholars, so there is a heavy emphasis on research. These pro-

grams are also designed to prepare leaders in the field, so many include courses or mentoring experiences in leadership, policy development, and the like. Finally, many programs include courses or other individually-designed learning experiences in one's area of focus (education, policy development, research).

Most doctoral programs are very flexible so that each student can design it to meet her/his individual needs and goals. In many instances, a student works in a mentoring relationship with a faculty member, and those experiences take the place of formal courses. In all instances, however, students are expected to demonstrate their scholarly ability by completing a dissertation that is presented and "defended" to a panel of faculty experts. This is the culminating experience in the doctoral program, and it signifies that the individual has demonstrated skills of scholarship, has a broad understanding of the field, and has developed a specific area of expertise within the field.

Admission requirements for doctoral programs are quite rigorous and include a review of master's-level work, an interview, references, a personal statement, and writing samples. In addition, some doctoral programs ask the applicant to outline the type of research question(s) she/he would be interested in pursuing throughout the program.

Post-Doctoral Experiences. Many graduates of doctoral programs desire to further develop their research skills, and they apply for post-doctoral fellowships to help them do this. A "post-doc" usually is offered through a research-intensive university, and it allows the fellow to work with an experienced researcher (or team of researchers), thereby refining her/his research skills and strengthening her/his area of expertise.

Other. You may have heard about Nurse Doctorate (ND) programs that are offered by a few schools today. The ND is considered both the first professional degree for nurses (much as the MD is the first professional degree for physicians) and an advanced degree. Students with baccalaureate degrees in other fields enter the ND program and complete selected baccalaureate-level nursing program requirements. This provides them with the basics of nursing practice and allows them to sit for the NCLEX-RN® licensing examination. They then continue with selected master's courses through which they develop an area of specialization. In some programs, these students then continue on to complete a series of research courses. Since these programs are so unique, you should talk with the faculty in the schools where they are offered to learn more about admission requirements, program expectations, and graduates' employment opportunities.

Career Opportunities Available with Advanced Education

Advanced Practice. The role of an advanced practice nurse (APN) is the most direct extension of the clinical practice role an individual probably assumed as a Registered Nurse (RN). In most instances, this role requires preparation at the master's level, with specialization in a clinical area. Advanced practice roles typically include nurse practitioners, nurse midwives, nurse anesthetists, and clinical nurse specialists.

Nurse Practitioners. Nurse practitioners have played a role in health care since the early 1970s. At that time, any RN who completed a prescribed course of study and earned a certificate for that preparation could call her/himself a nurse practitioner (NP) and practice in that role. The "certificate program" consisted of anywhere from 3 months to 18 months of study, and the role most often was focused on primary care. The first NPs conducted physical assessments (which was not a typical activity of nurses at the time), collaborated with physicians to determine a client's health needs, and focused on helping clients stay well. There was no special licensure as an NP, and the number of nurses fulfilling these roles was rather limited.

In more recent years, the role of the NP has expanded, and preparation for that role has moved into graduate programs. NPs carry an additional license and/or certification that allows them to practice, and the number of NPs involved in healthcare delivery has grown enormously. NPs have been shown to provide care that is of high quality and lower cost.

Today, one can practice as an NP in any number of specialty areas including family (FNP), pediatrics (PNP), women's health (WHNP), psych (PyNP), gerontology (GNP), and adult (ANP). They focus on primary care or acute care, and practice in community settings, schools, physician practices and hospitals, among other settings.

Preparation for an NP role occurs in a master's program and integrates courses in core nursing areas (theory development, research, broad healthcare issues and trends, leadership, etc.) and advanced clinical (pharmacology, pathophysiology, family health, women's health, etc.). These programs combine theory courses and extensive clinical experiences, the latter of which occur under the guidance of an NP preceptor. Upon completion, graduates are eligible to be licensed as an APN and to sit for an examination that will certify them as experts in a chosen area, such as gerontology.

Upon graduation, NPs function relatively independently, contributing to the interdisciplinary healthcare team and referring clients to physicians or other NPs as needed. In most instances, they receive direct reimbursement from insurers for their services.

Nurse Midwives. Midwives have been a part of the world's history for centuries, but the role of *nurse* midwife is a more recent one. Like NPs, nurse midwives have been in practice for a number of years, but their original preparation was in post-RN certificate programs. Today, nurse midwives are prepared in graduate programs that combine clinical courses with nursing theory and research, community concepts, family theory, and other knowledge that is relevant to the role.

Nurse midwives function independently as they care for women during the pre-natal phase. They deliver babies in hospitals or birthing centers, and they provide follow-up care to the new mother and baby. In addition, nurse midwives address the needs of the father and other children in the family throughout the pregnancy, birth, and post-natal periods. During all phases of conception, pregnancy, birth, post-natal, and newborn care, the nurse midwife refers difficult or complicated cases to a physician as appropriate, and these health professionals collaborate to ensure that high quality, holistic care is delivered to the mother, baby, and entire family.

Nurse Anesthetists. CRNAs (Certified Registered Nurse Anesthetists) have been providing anesthesia care in the United States for more than 100 years. They provide anesthetics to patients in collaboration with surgeons, anesthesiologists, dentists, podiatrists, and other qualified healthcare professionals, but they are the sole anesthesia providers in nearly 50% of all hospitals and more than 65% of rural hospitals, enabling these healthcare facilities to provide obstetrical, surgical, and trauma stabilization services. They practice in every setting in which anesthesia is delivered: hospital surgical suites and obstetrical delivery rooms, ambulatory surgical centers, and the offices of dentists, podiatrists, ophthalmologists, and plastic surgeons.

Nurse anesthesia programs are 24–36 months in length, and they include extensive clinical training as well as theoretical knowledge in anesthesia and core nursing content. Upon completion of this program, graduates are eligible to sit for the certification examination that allows them to practice in this role.

Clinical Nurse Specialists. Clinical nurse specialists (CNSs) are prepared at the graduate level to assume clinical leadership roles in a variety of settings. Their program of study focuses on developing knowledge and skill in a particular area of clinical practice, such as oncology or chronic illness, patient/family teaching, consultation, research, and core nursing concepts.

In the clinical arena, CNSs often serve as resources to other nursing staff members as they plan and deliver care to patients with complex health needs. In these instances, the CNS is "tapped" for her/his clinical expertise, knowledge of relevant research, and ability to help others learn how to design and implement effective plans of care. They often are the key nursing "voice" on interdisciplinary care teams, and they are sought out as consultants.

Graduate preparation has been required for a CNS role for many, many years. Such a program integrates core nursing courses with extensive study in one's specialty area and research skills.

Nursing Administration.
The nurse "administrator" may hold the title of nurse manager, director of nursing, vice president for nursing, vice president for patient care services, or something similar. Whatever the title, individuals in this role are responsible for creating environments that support excellent nursing practice. They do this by designing appropriate policies, managing the finances for the institution's nursing services, hiring and supervising qualified individuals, and ensuring that quality care is provided and the institution's goals are met.

The nurse administrator is often the "official voice for nursing" in an institution. As such, she/he must be visionary and well aware of issues currently facing nurses and the nursing profession, the resources needed to meet patient care needs, future trends in nursing practice and healthcare delivery, and current research that affects nursing practice and patient care. The nurse administrator also must be skilled in financial management, organizational psychology, strategic planning, conflict management, and orchestrating change.

Graduate programs that prepare nurse administrators incorporate learning experiences in all these areas. In addition, many draw from courses in a university's business school so that students can blend their nursing expertise with sound business principles. Some schools require students to complete clinical courses as part of their graduate program, but since the impact of this role on patient care is more indirect, rather than as a direct care provider, clinically-focused learning experiences often explore broad trends and issues in practice. Students, therefore, usually do not develop a narrow clinical specialty, as is the case in other types of programs.

Nurse Educator. While most nurses engage in patient teaching activities, those who prepare for and assume the role of nurse educator have a very different scope of responsibility. Nurse educators may teach in schools of nursing (in a faculty role) or in healthcare agencies (in a staff development role). They are responsible for designing curricula, using a variety of strategies with groups of students to facilitate their learning, evaluating what students have learned, and documenting the outcomes of a program of study.

Most staff development educators work in acute care hospitals, but they also may work in long term care facilities, community health or home care agencies, or ambulatory services. They often are responsible for planning the orientation of new staff, providing programs that help nurses remain current, and creating environments that encourage continuous professional growth.

Academic educators may work in technical schools, community colleges, hospital-based schools, or senior colleges and universities. They are responsible for classroom teaching, teaching in the clinical setting, advising students, and participating in the governance of their institution. In addition, faculty in senior colleges and universities typically are expected to engage in scholarly activities, publish, be actively involved in their communities and/or professional associations, make presentations at professional conferences, write grant proposals, maintain their clinical competence, and serve as consultants in the field.

Faculty who teach in associate degree and baccalaureate programs are required to hold a minimum of a master's degree in nursing. This level of preparation also is expected in most hospital diploma programs and many practical nurse programs. Individuals who wish to teach in master's programs typically are required to hold a doctoral degree, and in many universities, the doctorate is required for tenure and for promotion to the higher ranks.

Researcher. Many nurses currently function in the role of researcher in hospitals or other health care agencies, with drug companies that are conducting clinical trials, in professional associations, or in schools of nursing. In many instances, this individual is one of a team of researchers, and she/he may have responsibility for designing studies, collecting data, analyzing data, writing reports of the study, and presenting the study to professional colleagues. Preparation for the researcher role typically requires an earned doctorate and extensive experience with research.

Public Policy Development. Many nurses participate in activities that influence the development of public policy, but for some nurses, this is their primary role. Such individuals are usually master's prepared, and most hold an earned doctorate. They understand how laws are made and policy is developed, are politically astute, are excellent communicators, know how to influence change, can mobilize people to take action, have a very broad perspective on health care issues, and understand the myriad of factors that influence decision making. Nurses whose primary role is public policy may work for professional associations, federal or state governments, or independent organizations, and they bring their nursing knowledge and expertise to bear on issues that affect the health of the public and the good of society.

Informatics. Nursing informatics is one of the newest specialties in professional nursing, and it is an area of specialization for nurses that continues to grow. The term "informatics" was defined in 1983 as computer science plus information science. Used in conjunction with the name of a discipline, it denotes an application of computer science and information science to the management and processing of data, information, and knowledge in that discipline. Thus nursing informatics is a combination of computer science, information science, and nursing science designed to assist in the management and processing of nursing data, information, and knowledge to support the practice of nursing and the delivery of nursing care. Nurses who are experts in informatics may work in educational programs, healthcare facilities, or independent organizations. They usually have graduate preparation and are technologically proficient, knowledgeable about a wide range of implementation issues, and visionary.

Consultants. There are many opportunities for nurses to work as consultants once they have developed and been acknowledged for their expertise in a particular area. Nurses are consultants to healthcare and governmental institutions regarding practice environments, staffing issues, finance, policy development, ethics, and other areas. Consultants also assist educational institutions in areas related to curriculum innovation, faculty development, program outcomes assessment, student retention, new teaching/ learning strategies, critical thinking, and so on. In most instances, consultants are prepared at the master's or doctoral level, and they function independently (with many owning their own businesses).

Professional Association Roles. While graduate preparation is not necessarily required for leadership roles in professional associations, it usually is preferred. As the spokespersons for an organization, association leaders must be visionary, have a broad perspective, be articulate, have effective political skills, be financially competent, and be knowledgeable about issues that affect nursing, health care, and association management. Working in a professional association provides a nurse with an opportunity to influence change at a state, regional, or national level. It also helps her/him develop professional networks, exercise leadership, and create new futures for the profession as a whole.

Summary

There are innumerable opportunities available for nurses who hold graduate preparation at the master's or doctoral level, and you are encouraged to explore these opportunities and pursue completion of a graduate degree in nursing. The vast majority of leaders in our field are those individuals who hold master's or doctoral degrees. We hope this book will help you pursue your goal of graduate preparation to become one of these leaders in nursing.

Distance Learning

Diane M. Billings, EdD, RN, FAAN
Professor of Nursing and Associate Dean for Teaching, Learning, and Information Resources
Center for Teaching and Lifelong Learning
Indiana University School of Nursing
Indianapolis, IN

Although most nursing courses and academic degree programs are still offered in traditional ways in classrooms and on college campuses, many nursing programs now seek to make education available to students in ways that are accessible and convenient. One way nursing schools do this is through *distance learning* options. If you are considering enrolling in any of these courses or programs, you should familiarize yourself with these options to determine if they are right for you.

What is Distance Learning?

Distance learning refers to courses in which the faculty member and the student are separated in space and often in time, as well. This is accomplished when the course is offered in a way that allows you to participate from a site (home, clinical agency, library) that is at a distance from the site where the course originates. Distance learning courses involve using educational technology such as the telephone (audio conferencing), television (video conferencing), the Internet (Web-based courses), or a combination of all of these. When courses are offered in a way that requires faculty and students to participate at the same time, for example, in an audio conference, video conference, or Internet "chat," the course is referred to as being "synchronous." If the course does not require same-time participation, such as a discussion board on the Internet, the course is referred to as being "asynchronous."

Distance learning also refers to the use of educational technology to support and enhance teaching and learning, particularly through Web-based tools such as discussion or chat rooms, bulletin boards, and testing tools. These tools promote active learning, offer possibilities for rich and rapid feedback, provide opportunities for increased interaction among the faculty and learners, support diverse ways of learning, and give greater access to resources. Nursing courses are referred to as "technology-enhanced" or "technology-supported" when such resources are used.

Schools may use combinations of on-campus and distance learning approaches. For example, courses that provide foundational knowledge (anatomy and physiology) may be offered by distance learning, while clinical nursing courses are offered "face-to-face" or in the clinical setting.

Are Distance Learning Courses Effective?
Nursing faculty develop distance learning courses with the same attention to learning outcomes, interactive teaching and learning strategies, and methods of assessing learning as their on-campus counterparts. Evaluation results of distance learning courses and programs indicate that the learning outcomes of distance learning courses are similar to those in traditionally taught courses. While most students find that distance learning courses are accessible and convenient, they often miss being able to interact with the faculty and their classmates. Also, because distance learning involves the use of technology, students and faculty must become adept at using the particular technology that is used to support the teaching and learning for the course.

The quality of distance learning courses is judged using the same criteria used for judging the quality of nursing programs in general. Indicators of quality of both campus-based programs and distance learning programs include factors such as the qualifications of the faculty, student-to-faculty ratios, resources to support the program, and the design and sequence of courses in the curriculum. Academic nursing programs with distance learning options must meet the same accreditation standards as those that are offered on a college campus.

Is Distance Learning Right For You? Distance learning options appeal to students who are not able to participate in traditional courses and programs because of distance, family or work commitments, or other factors. Other students like these courses because they are more flexible and convenient for their schedules. Still other students choose distance learning because it affords them an opportunity to work with a particular faculty member or to enroll in a course or academic program that will help them meet their career goals.

If you choose to enroll in distance learning courses or degree programs, you need to be aware that these courses are designed to involve active learning and high levels of participation. You must plan to spend time on the course, complete course requirements, write papers, participate in learning activities, take exams, and attain course outcomes. Students who are successful in distance learning courses are self-directed, are flexible in their learning styles, can work independently, can use a wide network of resources, and are able to collaborate with faculty and classmates to achieve the course and their own learning goals. They also are comfortable using technology and tools that support the course.

As a student in nursing programs now and in the future, you will find that nursing courses and academic programs will be attentive to your learning and career goals, and increasingly will use distance learning strategies, tools, and resources to support your learning needs. You can prepare to take advantage of the options made possible by distance learning by becoming a competent information-age learner.

Financial Support for Your Nursing Education

Nursing is an exciting career with many different opportunities for those who have acquired the necessary education and skills. The decision to begin or continue your nursing education is a big one, and determining how you will finance your studies is part of that decision.

You should not be discouraged in pursuing your goals by lack of funds. Public sources for financial aid include federal and state scholarships and loans, as well as work study programs. In addition, many schools and universities have their own financial aid packages. Finally, all sorts of community groups and membership organizations offer scholarships and loans for a variety of special purposes and for specific constituencies.

You are more likely to be successful financing your education if you start applying early and if you put time and effort into the search. Start by choosing the schools in which you are interested. Most financial aid comes through the schools themselves, which administer state and federal funds as well as school or university scholarships and loans.

Financial aid may be based on need (financial), merit (academic achievement), or a combination of the two. The group or organization awarding a grant, scholarship, or loan outlines the criteria for the award, and it is your responsibility as an applicant to demonstrate that you meet each of those criteria.

You can demonstrate that you meet criteria by following the requirements or processes specified by the group or organization giving the award. You may be required to complete a financial aid form, write an essay, and/or participate in an interview. Whatever the requirements, you are expected to meet **all** of them and complete **all** steps of the application process in order to be eligible for consideration. Incomplete applications that are poorly presented (spelling errors, grammatical errors, or incorrect calculations) are often not reviewed as positively as those that are neat, correct, and well-presented.

In many instances, students who are seeking financial aid (including loans) are required to complete a need-analysis form, which is a means of estimating your need for financial assistance to meet educational expenses. The analysis determines how much money you or your family can contribute to your total educational expenses and how much additional funding is needed. The smaller your income, the smaller your individual contribution would need to be. Financial aid, as determined by this method, is based only on need, and your accomplishments or "merit" are not taken into consideration. An excellent description of need analysis, including advice for those who do not automatically qualify for need-based assistance, is given in a book called *Don't Miss Out* by Robert and Anna Leider.

The schools to which you apply will usually send you a need-analysis form (called the Free Application for Federal Student Aid, or FAFSA) even before you are notified of acceptance. Since many schools use and require this form, you can complete it once and send copies to various schools. Be sure to read all forms thoroughly because they are complicated, and they will be returned to you for correction if you make any errors or leave out information. This may slow the approval process, and you may miss out on opportunities to receive aid. You should fill out and submit the forms as soon as you and your family have collected financial records for the current tax year because the amount of aid available at each school is limited.

If you are applying to a basic nursing program, you should request that one copy of your FAFSA be sent to the Department of Education for consideration for a Pell Grant. The Pell Grant program is the largest of the federal aid programs and is designed for undergraduate students only. About six weeks after you have sent in the form for analysis, you will receive a Student Aid Report, which will include an estimate of the amount you and your family would be expected to contribute toward your college expenses. For a fee, you can have copies of this Student Aid Report sent to each of the schools to which you have applied for admission.

Once the amount you and your family can contribute to your education is computed by the need analysis, it will remain the same regardless of which schools you apply to or what their tuition and fees are. For example, the need analysis may determine that your income will allow you to pay $2,000 a year toward your educational costs. In this case, your family or individual contribution will always be $2,000, whether the school you wish to attend has an annual tuition and fees of $4,000 or $20,000.

What will vary is your remaining need and the financial assistance that different schools offer you. The amount offered is determined by the school's resources, the number of applicants being considered, and how early an application is received. The variation in these "financial aid packages," as they are called, is one reason many students apply to several schools.

The Financial Aid Package

A school will compute a financial aid package for you only after you have been accepted for admission. Admission to a school, however, does not commit you to attend, so you can make your decision after you have compared the financial aid offer you receive from each school.

The school's financial aid office will try to make up the difference between your family or individual contribution (as determined by the need analysis) and the cost of the nursing program for a year. The financial aid package you are offered is drawn from federal and state sources available to the school and from the school's own resources. It will often include grants, loans, and work-study support.

Federal Sources of Financial Assistance

All federal sources of educational assistance depend on congressional appropriations. Therefore, funding amounts may differ greatly from one year to the next, and the amount of federal aid available to students in one year may not be available in future years.

Nursing programs that are accredited by the NLNAC (National League for Nursing Accrediting Commission) are eligible to participate in all of the federal aid programs. You should consult the catalogues of the schools in which you are interested to learn about their accreditation status, and you should

consult the schools' financial aid offices for information about the federal aid programs available there.

Pell Grants. This major federal program for education is designed to assist students with a demonstrated need for financial assistance to study in a **basic** nursing program (or in other fields of undergraduate study). The size of the award calculated for a Pell Grant depends on your need for assistance, the cost of tuition and fees at the school, and other factors. This amount is then incorporated into the financial aid package offered by a school, provided that school is eligible to participate in the Pell Grant program. You must complete the need-analysis form each year in order to continue to receive a Pell Grant, but there is **no** need to repay these grants. You may request a free copy of *The Student Guide: Financial Aid* from the Federal Student Financial Aid Information Center, P.O. Box 84, Washington, DC, 20044. Telephone (800) 4-FED-AID.

Supplemental Education Opportunity Grants (SEOG). Students enrolled in **basic** nursing programs (or other fields of undergraduate study) at schools that participate in the SEOG program are eligible for these grants if they study at least on a half-time basis as a regular student. You must be a U.S. citizen or an eligible non-citizen. Unlike some other programs, only students of **exceptional** financial need are eligible for these grants, which award up to $4,000 per year and which require no payback. Schools that participate in the SEOG program have a set amount of funds to distribute among students, so they determine the specific amount of each award. Since these funds typically are quite limited at each school, it is important to apply early.

College Work-Study Programs. This federal program provides funds to students who have demonstrated financial need and are enrolled in colleges and universities that participate in the program. These funds support part-time employment, on or off campus, for public or nonprofit organizations, and at a salary that is equal to or higher than the current minimum wage. You must submit an application to your school early each calendar year, and the financial aid office will make the award. The school then arranges the job and sets the number of hours you may work.

Nursing Student Loan Program of the U.S. Department of Health and Human Services. Loans of up to $2,500 per academic year for freshmen and sophomores and up to $4,000 for juniors and seniors are available for **basic** or **non-traditional** students who demonstrate financial need, and who are studying in nursing schools located in participating colleges and universities. Repayment of these low-interest loans begins nine months after you graduate (or leave school), and you are allowed up to ten years to repay the entire loan. In many instances, applications are made through the school of nursing.

Perkins Loans (formerly National Direct Student Loans). These loans are available to students in basic RN preparation programs, RN students in undergraduate programs, or graduate students. Participating schools act as the lenders for these loans, which are funded by the federal government, and since there are limited funds, students must demonstrate exceptional need. Repayment begins nine months after you graduate (or leave school). All Perkins loans are subsidized, with the school paying the interest while the student is enrolled.

Stafford Loans. Students who are new borrowers and demonstrate financial need are eligible for Stafford Loans. These loans must be arranged privately through banks, credit unions, savings and loan associations, or other commercial lenders who are guarantee agencies. Repayment can be deferred until after you graduate (or leave school), and there is a liberal amount of time in which to repay the loan. Stafford loans have variable interest rates.

PLUS Loans. The PLUS Loan program (Parents Loan for Undergraduate Students) is for parents with dependent children who are students. These loans are not dependent on financial need, but they may be limited to those with an approved credit rating.

State Sources of Financial Assistance

All states have need-based grants for education, and some of them allow grants for study outside the state. The financial aid office will include this source in creating your financial aid package.

State programs can be an important source of assistance for nursing students. Since each state has a different financial aid program, you can learn about your state's program by writing the appropriate education agency in your state (State Department of Education or Department of Health) or by contacting the financial aid office in state colleges and universities.

Other Sources of Financial Assistance

Alumni funds often are available to provide loans and scholarships for students in need of financial assistance. The financial aid office or the school catalogue will inform you about whether a school has its own sources of need-based aid.

Some students are eligible for United Student Aid Funds. This private, not-for-profit corporation guarantees loans made to students by commercial lenders when students are unable to get loans from other sources. You can contact them at 800-824-7044 or *www.usagroup.com*.

Scholarships and Loans Specifically for Nursing Students

The sources of financial aid specifically for students in nursing programs are many and varied. Some are open to applications from any nursing student; others are designed for study in a particular nursing specialty or at a specific level of nursing education. Some that offer support for nursing students are also broader in scope and are available to students in other health profession fields as well. Many of these scholarships and grants are for licensed RNs who want to continue their education.

Since specifics about these sources of financial aid change frequently, this guide does not provide extensive details about any of them. Instead, it lists the sources of funds, indicates whether they are available to support beginning RN study (noted by a 1), completion of the baccalaureate degree by an RN (noted by a 2), advanced clinical study for RNs (noted by a 3), graduate study, master's, or doctoral (noted by a 4), or doctoral study only (noted by a 5). Special grants, research, traineeships, or funds to support post-doctoral work are designated by a 6.

Air Force ROTC Nursing Scholarship (1, 2, 3)

www.airforce.com

Alpha Tau Delta, National Fraternity for Professional Nurses (1, 2, 3, 4)

National Awards Committee Chairperson, Alpha Tau Delta, 5207 Mesada Street, Alta Loma, CA 91737
909-980-3536

American Association of Critical Care Nurses (AACN) (3, 4, 6)

AACN Research Department, 101 Columbia, Aliso Viejo, CA 92656-1491
800-899-AACN
www.aacn.org

American Association of Nurse Anesthetists (AANA) (3, 6)

Finance Director, American Association of Nurse Anesthetists, 222 Prospect Avenue, Park Ridge, IL 60068-5790
847-692-7050
www.aana.com

American Association of Occupational Health Nurses, Inc. (AAOHN) (2, 3, 4, 6)

AAOHN, Inc. Suite 1000, 2920 Brandywine Road, Atlanta, GA 30341
770-455-7757
www.aaohn.org

American Cancer Society (4, 5, 6)

American Cancer Society, Extramural Grant Department, 1599 Clifton Road NE, Atlanta, GA 30329-4251
404-329-7558
www.cancer.org
grants@cancer.org

American Holistic Nurses' Association (AHNA) (2, 4)

American Holistic Nurses' Association, P.O. Box 2130 Flagstaff, AZ 86003-2130
800-278-2462, x14
www.anha.org
AHNA-Admin#@flaglink.com

American Legion (2, 3, 4)

The American Legion Education Program, Box 1055, Indianapolis, IN 46206, Attention: Eight and Forty Scholarships
317-630-1323
www.legion.org

American Nephrology Nurses' Association (ANNA) (2, 4)

American Nephrology Nurses' Association National Office, East Holly Avenue, Pitman, NJ 08071-0056
856-256-2320
www.annanurse.org

Army ROTC (1, 2)

QUEST Center, P.O. Box 3279, Warminster, PA 18974-0128
800-872-7682 (800-USA-ROTC)
www.armyrotc.com

Association of Operating Room Nurses (AORN) (2, 4)

AORN Scholarship Committee, AORN Inc., 2170 S. Parker Road #300, Denver, CO 80231-5711
303-755-6300, x366
www.aorn.org

Association of Women's Health, Obstetric, and Neonatal Nurses (AWHONN) (3, 4, 5, 6)

AWHONN, 2000 L Street, NW, Suite 740, Washington, DC 20036
800-673-8499
www.awhonn.org

Business and Professional Women's Foundation (1, 2, 3, 4)

Scholarships, Business and Professional Women's Foundation, 2012 Massachusetts Avenue, NW, Washington, DC 20036
202-293-1200, x169
www.bpwusa.org

Commissioned Officer Student Training and Extern Program, Public Health Services, U.S. Department of Health and Human Services (1, 3)

U.S. Public Health Service Recruitment, 8201 Greensboro Drive, Suite 600, McLean, VA 22102
800-279-1605

The Commonwealth Fund

The Commonwealth Fund does **not** provide funding for individuals.
One East 75th Street, New York, NY 10021-2692
212-606-3500
www.cmwf.org

Department of Defense, United States Navy (1, 2, 6)

Contact the medical programs officer at a Navy Recruiting District near your home or school.
800-327-6289 (800-USA-NAVY)
www.navyjobs.com

Department of Veterans Affairs, Health Professional Scholarship Program

Funding has been discontinued.

Emergency Nurses Association (ENA) Foundation (2, 3, 4, 6)

ENA Foundation, 915 Lee Street, Des Plains, IL 60016-6569
800-900-9659
www.ena.org

Foundation of the National Student Nurses' Association (NSNA) (1, 2, 3, 4)

The Foundation of The National Student Nurses' Association, Inc., 45 Main Street, Suite 606, Brooklyn, NY 11201
718-210-0705
www.nsna.org

Health Canada's National Health Research and Development Program (NHRDP) Personnel Awards (Master's, Doctorate, Post-Doctorate, and Scholar Levels)

The NHRDP **no longer offers personal awards.** Please refer to the Canadian Institute of Health Research (CIHR), *www.cihr.ca*, for information about funding.

Marine Corps Scholarship Foundation, Inc. (1, 2, 6)

Marine Corps Scholarship Foundation, Inc., P.O. Box 3008, Princeton, NJ 08543-3008
800-292-7777
www.marine-scholars.org

Massachusetts Nurses Foundation (1, 2, 4)

781-830-5745
www.mass-nurses-foundation.org

Maternity Center Association Foundation (2, 3, 4, 6)

Maternity Center Association Foundation, 281 Park Avenue South, 5th floor, New York, NY 10010
212-777-5000
www.maternity.org

National Association of Orthopaedic Nurses (NAON) Foundation (3, 4, 5, 6, 7)

National Association of Orthopaedic Nurses Foundation, East Holly Avenue, Box 56, Pitman, NJ 08071-0056
856-256-2310
www.naon.inurse.com

National Association of Pediatric Nurse Associates and Practitioners (NAPNAP) (3, 4)

National Association of Pediatric Nurse Associates and Practitioners, 1101 Kings Highway North, Suite # 206, Cherry Hill, NJ 08034
856-667-1773
www.napnap.org
74224.51@compuserve.com

National Certification Board: Perioperative Nursing, Inc. (NCB:PNI) Scholarship (2, 4)

AORN Scholarships Board, c/o AORN Headquarters, 2170 South Parker Road, Suite 300, Denver, CO 80231-5711
800-755-2676, x366
www.aorn.org

National Foundation for Infectious Diseases (4, 6)

National Foundation for Infectious Diseases, 4733 Bethesda Avenue, Suite 750, Bethesda, MD 20814
301-656-0003

National Health Service Corps (Bureau of Primary Health Care) Loan Repayment Program (6)

NHSC Loan Repayment Program, 2070 Chain Bridge Road, Suite 450, Vienna, VA 22182
800-221-9393

National Institute of Nursing Research, National Institute of Health, U.S. Department of Health and Human Services (5, 6)

Office of Information and Legislation, National Institute of Nursing Research, National Institute of Health, Building 31, Room 5B03, Bethesda MD 20892
301-496-0207
Extramural Outreach and Information Resources, Office of Extramural Research, National Institute of Health, 6701 Rockledge Drive, Suite 6095, Bethesda, MD 20892-2178
301-435-0714
www.nih.gov/ninr
asknih@odrockm1.od.nih.gov

National Society of the Daughters of the American Revolution (1, 2)

National Society, Daughters of the American Revolution, Office of the Committees-Scholarships, 1776 D Street, NW, Washington, DC 20006-5392 (NOTE: All written inquiries must be accompanied by a self-addressed, stamped envelope).
202-879-3292
www.nsdar.org

Nurse Anesthetist Traineeship, Division of Nursing, Bureau Of Health Professions, U.S. Department of Health and Human Services (4)

Division of Nursing, Bureau of Health Professions, Health Resources and Services Administration, Room 9-36, Parklawn Building, Nursing Education/Practice Resources Branch, 5600 Fishers Lane, Rockville, MD 20857

301-443-5736

Nurses' Educational Fund, Inc. (4)

Nurses Educational Fund, Inc. 555 West 57th Street, New York, NY 10019

212-399-1428

www.N-E-F.org

BBNEF@aol.com

Nursing Education Loan Repayment Program (2, 4)

NELRP, 4350 East-West Highway, 10th Floor, Bethesda, MD 20814

800-435-6464

DSLR@HRSA.GOV

Oncology Nursing Foundation (2, 4, 6)

Oncology Nursing Foundation, 501 Holiday Drive, Pittsburgh, PA 15220-2749

412-921-7373, x278

www.ons.org

Partnerships for Training

This program does not directly support individuals. Association for Academic Health Centers, 1400 Sixteenth Street, NW, Suite 720, Washington, DC 20036

202-483-8896

www.achnet.org

Professional Nurse Traineeships, Division of Nursing, Bureau of Health Professions, U.S. Department of Health and Human Services (4)

Traineeship applications must be made directly to the school in which you are enrolled, not to the Division of Nursing.

Division of Nursing, Bureau of Health Professions, Health Resources and Services Administration, Room 9-36, Parklawn Building, Rockville, MD 20857

301-443-5763

Rehabilitation Nursing Certification Board (2)

Scholarship Program, Association of Rehabilitation Nurses, 4700 West Lake Avenue, Glenview, IL 60025

800-229-7530 or 847-375-4710

www.arn.org

Sigma Theta Tau International, Honor Society of Nursing (5, 6)

Sigma Theta Tau International, Honor Society of Nursing, 550 West North Street, Indianapolis, IN 46202

888-634-7575

www.nursingsociety.org or *research@stti.iupui.edu*

Western Regional Graduate Program (4)

Western Regional Graduate Program, WICHE, P.O. Box 9752, Boulder, CO 80301-9752

303-541-0210

www.wiche.edu

Wound, Ostomy, and Continence Nurses Society (WOCN) (2, 4)

Wound, Ostomy, and Continence Nurses Society (WOCN), 1550 South Coast Highway, Suite 201, Laguna Beach, CA 92615

888-224-WOCN

www.wocn.org

Scholarships for Minority Students

In addition to all the resources previously identified, there also are a number of scholarships that are awarded specifically to minority students who wish to pursue a career in nursing and, in some cases, healthcare related fields. While some of the scholarships listed below are available to non-minority students as well, the number of awards granted to such non-minority applicants is very small because funds for aid are always limited.

There also are many sources of aid for minority students that are not specifically related to nursing. Two books in particular—*Directory of Special Programs for Minority Group Members* and *Financial Aid for Minorities in Health Fields*—list both general and specialty programs that target members of minority groups, as well as highlight general programs that may have special provisions or emphasis for minority students. In addition to the aid mentioned here for American Indian students, many states and tribes have special programs. Listings are available from the Indian Fellowship Program, U.S. Department of Education, Office of Elementary and Secondary Education, Washington, DC 20202.

American Indian Graduate Center (4)

American Indian Graduate Center, 4520 Montgomery Boulevard, NE, Albuquerque, NM 87109

American Nurses' Association Clinical Training Program Fellowships (5, 6)

American Nurses' Association, Ethnic/Racial Minority Fellowship Programs, 600 Maryland Avenue SW, Suite 100W, Washington, DC 20024
202-651-7244
www.ana.org

Career Advancement Scholarship Program for Women (1, 2, 3)

Business and Professional Women's Foundation, Scholarships and Loans, 2012 Massachusetts Avenue, NW, Washington, DC 20036
Enclose a #10 business-size, self-addressed, double-stamped envelope.
202-293-1200, x169
www.bpwusa.org

Foundation of the National Student Nurses' Association (NSNA) (1, 2, 4)

Foundation of the National Student Nurses' Association, 45 Main Street, Suite 606, Brooklyn, NY 11201
718-210-0705
www.nsna.org

Health Resources and Services Administration: Nursing Education Opportunities for the Disadvantaged

This program does not award funds to individual students.
Division of Nursing, Health Resources and Services Administration, 5600 Fishers Lane, Parklawn Building, Room 9-36, Rockville, MD 20857
301-443-6193 or 301-443-6880

Higher Education Grant Program For Indians (1, 2, 4)

Contact your tribe or agency/area education office. If you do not have this information, contact the Branch of Post-Secondary Education, Office of Indian Education Programs, 1849 C Street, NW—MS-3512-MB, Washington, DC 20240
202-219-1127

Indian Health Service Scholarship Program, DHHS, PHS, Indian Health Service, U.S. Department of Health and Human Services (1, 2, 4)

The IHS Scholarship Program, Twinbrook Metro Plaza Building, Suite 100A, 12300 Twinbrook Parkway, Rockville, MD 20852

301-443-6197

www.ihs.gov/jobcareerDevelopment

National Association of Hispanic Nurses (1, 2, 4)

National Association of Hispanic Nurses, 1501 16th Street, NW, Washington, DC 20036

www.thehispanicnurses.org

National Black Nurses' Association (1, 2, 4)

National Black Nurses' Association, 8360 Fenton Street, Suite 300, Silver Springs, MD 20910-3803 Enclose a self-addressed, business size envelope with double first class postage for application processing.

301-589-3200

www.nbna.org

National Caucus and Center on Black Aged Long-Term Care Minority Training and Development Program (6)

Minority Training and Development Program, National Caucus and Center on Black Aged, 1424 K Street, NW, Suite 500, Washington, DC 20005

202-637-8400

National Institute of Mental Health (4, 6)

Director, Division of Neuroscience and Behavioral Science, National Institute of Mental Health, 5600 Fishers Lane, Parklawn Building, Rockville, MD 20857

302-443-3563

Director, Division of Clinical and Treatment Research, National Institute of Mental Health, 5600 Fishers Lane, Parklawn Building, Rockville, MD 20857

301-443-3264

gniedere@nih.gov, gopher.nih.gov, www.nih.gov

National Society of the Colonial Dames of America (1, 2)

The National Society of the Colonial Dames of America, Indian Nurse Scholarship Awards, Consultant, 3064 Luvan Boulevard, deBordieu, Georgetown, SC 29440

www.nscda.org

Nurses' Educational Fund, Inc. (4, 5)

Nurses Education Fund, Inc., 555 West 57th Street, New York, NY 10019

Scholarship kits are $5.00 to cover the cost of postage and handling.

Oncology Nursing Foundation (2, 3, 4)

Oncology Nursing Foundation, 501 Holiday Drive, Pittsburgh, PA 15220-2749

412-921-7373, x278

www.ons.org

United Negro College Fund (1, 2, 4)

The College Fund/UNCF Program Services, 8260 Willow Oaks Corporate Drive, Fairfax, VA 22031

800-331-2244

www.uncf.org

William Randolph Hearst Foundations (3, 7)

Grants are not provided to individuals.

William Randolph Hearst Foundations, 888 Seventh Avenue, 45th Floor, New York, NY 10106-0057

Women of the Evangelical Lutheran Church in America (1, 2)

Women of the Evangelical Lutheran Church in America, 8765 West Higgins Road, Chicago, IL 60631

773-380-2747

www.elca.org

Special Awards, Post-Doctoral Study, and Research Grants

In addition to the resources previously noted, there are additional sources of financial support for nurses pursuing studies at or beyond the doctoral level, or outside a formal academic course of study. These consist largely of grants, traineeships, and fellowships for post-doctoral study, advanced nursing research, or other special projects.

Agency for Healthcare Research and Quality (AHRQ), (formerly the Agency for HealthCare Policy and Research, AHCPR) Public Health Service

AHRQ Publications Clearinghouse, P.O. Box 8547, Silver Spring, MD 20907-8547
800-358-9295
www.ahcpr.gov

American Association of Critical-Care Nurses (AACN)

American Association of Critical Care Nurses, Research Department 101 Columbia, Aliso Viejo, CA 92656-1491
800-899-AACN
www.aacn.org

American Association of Occupational Health Nurses, Inc. (AAOHN)

American Association of Occupational Health Nursing, Inc., Suite 100, 2920 Brandywine Road, Atlanta, GA 30341
770-455-7757
www.aohn.org/fund_grants_2003.htm

American Association of University Women Educational Foundation

American Association of University Women Educational Foundation, 40 Customer Service Center, 2201 North Dodge Street, Department 177, Iowa City, IA 52243-4030
319-337-1716, x177
www.aauw.org

American Cancer Society

800-ACS-2345

American Lung Association

American Lung Association, Medical Affairs Division, 1740 Broadway, New York, NY 10019-4374
212-315-8700
www.lungusa.org

American Nephrology Nurses' Association

Chairperson, Awards Committee, American Nephrology Nurses' Association, East Holly Avenue, Box 56, Pitman, NJ 08071-0056
856-256-2320
www.anna.inurse.com

American Nurses' Foundation, Nursing Research Grants Program

American Nurses' Foundation, Nursing Research Grant, 600 Maryland Avenue, SW, Suite 100W, Washington, DC 20024
202-651-7298
www.nursingworld.org/anf/

American Society for Parental and Enteral Nutrition Research Grants

Director, American Society for Parental and Enteral Nutrition, Research Grants, 8630 Fenton Street, Suite 412, Silver Springs, MD 20910
800-727-4567
www.clinnutr.org

Arthritis Foundation

Arthritis Foundation Research Department, 1330 West Peachtree Street, Atlanta, GA 30309
404-965-7537
www.arthritis.org/StartingPoints/research_grants.asp

Association of University Programs in Health Administration (Investing in the Future of Health Management Leaders)

Association of University Programs in Health Administration, 730 11ᵗʰ Street NW, 4ᵗʰ Floor, Washington, DC 20001-4510
202-638-1448
www.aupha.org

Health Resources and Services Administration (HRSA)

Grants Manager Branch, Health Resources and Services Administration, Bureau of Health Professions, Parklawn Building, Room 8C26, 5600 Fishers Lane, Rockville, MD 20857
301-443-6193
www.hrsa.gov/grants.htm

Canadian Nurses Foundation

Canadian Nurses Foundation, 50 Driveway, Ottawa ON K2P IE2, Canada
613-237-2133

Canadian Nurses Respiratory Society (The Lung Association of Canada)

The Lung Association, 300 Raymond Street, Suite 300, Ottawa, ON KIR IA3, Canada
613-569-6411
www.info@lung.ca

Epilepsy Foundation of America

The Epilepsy Foundation, Research Department, 4351 Barden City Drive, Landover, MD 20785
301-459-3700
www.epilepsyfoundation.org

Geriatric Mental Health Academic Awards

The National Institute of Health, National Institute on Aging, 5600 Fisher Lane, Parklawn Building, Rockville, MD 20587
www.nih.gov/nia

Lillian Sholtis Brunner Summer Fellowship for Historical Research in Nursing

Center Director, The Center for the Study of the History of Nursing, School of Nursing, University of Pennsylvania, 307 Nursing Education Building, Philadelphia, PA 19104-6906
215-898-4502
history@pobox.upenn.edu or *www.upenn.edu/nursing/*

Michigan Nurses Association, Conduct and Utilization of Research in Nursing (CURN) Award

Michigan Nurses Association, 2310 Jolly Oak, Okemos, MI 48864
www.minurses.org

National Cancer Institute Cancer Prevention and Control Research Small Grants Programs

Division of Cancer Prevention and Control, National Cancer Institute, 6130 Executive Boulevard, Executive Plaza N, Bethesda, MD 20892
301-496-8520 or 301-402-2221
www.nih.nci.gov or *gopher.nih.gov*

National Cancer Institute National Research Service Award—Individual Pre-Doctoral Research Fellowship for Oncology Nurses

Program Director, Cancer Training Branch, CTP, DCTDC, EPN520, National Cancer Institute, Bethesda, MD 20892
301-496-8580
www.nci.nih.gov

National Foundation for Infectious Diseases—Young Investigator Matching Grants

Grants Manager, The National Foundation for Infectious Diseases, 4733 Bethesda Avenue, Suite 750, Bethesda, MD 20814
301-656-0003
www.nifd.org

National Heart, Lung, and Blood Institute Short-Term Training Grants

Special research training programs are available **for minority and disabled** pre-doctoral students.

Division of Extramural Affairs, National Heart, Lung and Blood Institute, Two Rockledge Center, Suite 7100, 6701 Rockledge Drive MSC 7902, Bethesda, MD 20892-7902
301-435-0222
www.nhlbi.gov

National Institute of Environmental Health Sciences

The National Institute of Environmental Health Sciences, P.O. Box 12233, Research Triangle Park, NC 27709
919-541-7628
www.niehs.nih.gov

National Institute on Aging

National Institute on Aging, 7201 Wisconsin Avenue, Gateway Building, Bethesda, MD 20892
301-496-1472
Biology of Aging, 301-496-4996
Geriatrics and Clinical Research, 301-496-6761
Behavioral and Social Research, 301-496-3136
Neuroscience and Neuropsychology of Aging Research, 301-496-9350
Small Business Innovation Research, 301-496-9322

National Institute of Child Health and Human Development Breastfeeding and Human Milk Research Grants

National Institute of Child Health and Human Development, 31 Center Drive, Building 31, Room 2A32, MSC 2425, Bethesda, MD 20892
301-496-1848
www.nih.gov/nichd

National Institute of Mental Health

Division of Clinical Research, National Institute of Mental Health, 5600 Fishers Lane, Parklawn Building, Rockville, MD 20857
301-443-9700
www.nih.gov/nimh

National Institute of Nursing Research, National Institute of Health, U.S. Department of Health and Human Services

National Institute of Nursing Research, 45 Center Dr., Natcher Building, Bethesda, MD 20892
301-594-6869

National League for Nursing, Nursing Education Research Grants Program

Chief Program Officer, National League for Nursing, 61 Broadway, 33rd Floor, New York, NY 10006
212-812-0383
www.nln.org

Oncology Nursing Society/Oncology Nursing Foundation

The Oncology Nursing Society/The Oncology Nursing Foundation, 501 Holiday Drive, Pittsburgh, PA 15220-2749
412-921-7373
www.ons.org

Pan American Sanitary Bureau Fellowships

The U.S. and Canadian governments do not participate in this program, and their citizens, therefore, are not eligible for these fellowships.

Pan American Sanitary Bureau Fellowships, Pan American Health Organization, 525 23rd Street, NW, Washington, DC 20037
202-974-3000
www.paho.org

Rehabilitation Nursing Foundation

Rehabilitation Nursing Foundation, 4700 West Lake Avenue, Glenview, IL 60025
800-229-7530 or 847-375-4710
www.rehabnurse.org

Small Business Innovation Research (SBIR) Nursing Research Grants

PHS/SBIR/STTR Solicitation Office, 13687 Baltimore Avenue, Laurel, MD 20707-5096

301-206-9385

www.nih.gov/grants/funding/sbir.htm or *a2y@cu.nih.gov*

Substance Abuse and Mental Health Services Administration (SAMHSA), Department of Health and Human Services

Division of Grants Management, SAMHSA, Rockwall II, 6th Floor, 5600 Fishers Lane, Rockville, MD 20857

301-443-9777

www.samhsa.gov

United States Pharmacopeia Fellowship Program

United States Pharmacopeia, Office of External Affairs, 12601 Twinbrook Parkway, Rockville, MD 20852

800-822-8772

www.usp.org

Resources

Much of the financial aid described in this guide is specific for nursing education and research. Many other sources exist, and the references listed below will guide you in finding them. The inexpensive pamphlets, *Don't Miss Out* and *Need a Lift?*, will open your eyes to the myriad organizations and agencies that give money for education. The more expensive publications listed here are reference books and should be available in public or school libraries.

If you are serious in your ambition to advance your nursing career educationally or by conducting research, and if you are willing to put time and effort into exploring available sources, you are likely to find ways to help finance your goal!

Annual Register of Grant Support: A Directory of Funding Sources
R.R. Bowker, a Division of Reed Elsevier, 121 Chanlon Road, New Providence, NJ 07974; 908-464-6800. $199.95. More than 3,200 listings of grants, fellowships, and awards in various fields.

The A's and B's of Academic Scholarships
Octameron Associates, P.O. Box 2748, Alexandria, VA 22301. Updated annually. $9.00 (postpaid). Listings of academic scholarships from individual colleges and universities and some other sources. For undergraduate studies only.

The Big Book of Minority Opportunities
Edited by Willis L. Johnson. Garrett Park Press, Garrett Park, MD 20896. $39.00 plus $3.00 for shipping and handling. Lists more than 2,900 general programs of interest to minority group members, including national, regional, and area scholarship programs, employment services, special academic programs, and job banks, plus federal programs and aid offered by individual colleges and universities.

Chronicle Financial Aid Guide
Chronicle Guidance Publications, Inc., 66 Aurora Street, P.O. Box 1190, Moravia, NY 13118-1190. Revised annually. $22.47 plus $2.50 for shipping and handling. Information on more than 1,600 financial aid programs for high school seniors, college undergraduates, and adult learners from private corporations, labor unions, federal government, and state education agencies. A subject index gives easy access to programs by majors for which students may be eligible.

The College Blue Book: Scholarships, Fellowships, Grants, and Loans
Macmillan Library Reference, 1633 Broadway, 5th Floor, New York, NY 10019-6785. $48.00. This volume of *The College Blue Book* is arranged by area of interest and includes 80 separate nursing scholarships.

The College Cost Book
College Board Publications, Box 886, New York, NY 10101. Annual. $16.95. A step-by-step guide for determining college costs (including worksheets) and applying for financial aid. Outlines major aid programs and lists current costs at more than 3,100 institutions.

College Financial Aid for Dummies
Dr. Herm Davis and Joyce Lain Kennedy. IDG Books Worldwide, 919 E. Hillsdale Boulevard, Suite 400, Foster City, CA 94404. Internet: *www.dummies.com*. $16.95. A how-to book with scholarships for both traditional and non-traditional (adults, part-timers, distance education, international) students, as well as U.S. students studying abroad.

The College Financial Aid Emergency Kit

Joyce Lain Kennedy and Dr. Herm Davis. Sun Features, Inc., Box 368, Cardiff, CA 92007. $6.40 plus $0.55 for postage. Comprehensive pocket guide to applying for financial aid.

Directory of Biomedical and Health Care Grants

An important resource in tracking large grant-making institutional awards to individuals, universities, colleges, nonprofit organizations, hospitals, and other healthcare-related institutions. This resource is commonly found in public, college, and university libraries.

Directory of Financial Aid for Minorities

Reference Service Press, 1100 Industrial Road, Suite 9, San Carlos, CA 94070. $47.50 plus $4.50 for shipping and handling. A thorough source for available financial aid for minorities that describes more than 2,000 funding opportunities.

Directory of Financial Aid for Women

Gail A. Schlachter, Reference Service Press, 5000 Windplay Drive, Suite 4, El Dorado Hills, CA 95762. $45 plus $4.50 for shipping. Identifies more than 1,800 scholarships, fellowships, grants, loans, awards, and internships set aside for women and women's organizations.

Don't Miss Out: The Ambitious Student's Guide to Financial Aid

Robert Leider and Anna Leider. Octameron Associates, Inc., P.O. Box 2748, Alexandria, VA 22301. Updated annually, $9.00 (postpaid). Explains how to calculate college costs and family contribution, and offers advice on different routes to explore for assistance depending on your abilities and interests. Section on aid for health careers, minorities, and women.

Encyclopedia of Associations: International Organizations

Gale Research, Inc., 835 Penobscot Building, Detroit, MI 48226. $550.00. Reference guide to more than 19,400 multinational and national organizations in more than 200 countries. On-line data offered. 800-877-GALE.

Encyclopedia of Associations: National Organizations of the U.S.

Gale Research, 835 Penobscot Building, Detroit, MI 48226. 32nd edition. Reference source for comprehensive listings and descriptions of national organizations, nonprofit groups, fraternal organizations, and other groups in three volumes: Volume 1: *National Organizations of the U.S.*, $460; Volume 2: *Geographic and Executive Indexes*, $355; Volume 3: *Supplement*, $390. On-line data offered. 800-877-GALE.

Encyclopedia of Associations: Regional, State, and Local Organizations

Gale Research, Inc., 835 Penobscot Building, Detroit, MI 48226. Reference guide to non-profit membership organizations with interstate, state, intrastate, city, or local scope and interest. Five volumes at $30 per volume; $125 for entire set. On-line data offered. 800-877-GALE.

Financial Advice for Minority Students Seeking an Education in the Health Professions

Health Professions Career Opportunity Program, 1600 Ninth Street, Room 441, Sacramento, CA 95814. An informative brochure for minority students. Free.

Financial Aid for Minorities in Health Fields

Garret Park Press, P.O. Box 190F, Garret Park, MD 20896. Published annually. $5.90 per booklet plus $1.50 for shipping and handling. Summary of employment outlook and the number of minority members in each field, directory of several hundred financial aid programs, list of associations or organizations in each field, and resources for supplementary information.

Foundation Grants to Individuals

Foundation Center, 79 Fifth Avenue, New York, NY 10003. $65.00 plus $4.50 for shipping. An important source for independent and corporate foundations that awards grants to individuals. It is also an important source for undergraduate and graduate scholarships, fellowships, research grants, residencies, internships, and grants offered by U.S. foundations; includes company-sponsored aid.

Health Professions Education Directory
American Medical Association, 515 North State Street, Chicago, IL 60610. $54.95 plus $11.95 for shipping and handling. Provides information on nearly 5,000 health education programs sponsored by more than 2,200 institutions. Covers 41 health careers, including dental-related, dietetic, and audiology/speech language pathology occupations. Also includes data on enrollment, graduation, and attrition for most occupations. 800-621-8335.

Loans and Grants from Uncle Sam: Am I Eligible and for How Much?
Octameron Associates, P.O. Box 2748, Alexandria, VA 22301. Updated annually, $6.00 (postpaid). Explains whether you are eligible for federal grants and loans, as well as how to decide which of the many forms of loans from the federal government are appropriate for you.

National Guide to Funding in Health
An important resource in tracking large grant-making institutional awards to individuals, universities, colleges, nonprofit organizations, and other health-care-related institutions. This resource is commonly found in public, college, and university libraries.

Need a Lift?
Emblem Sales, P.O. Box 1050, Indianapolis, IN 46206. Published annually. $3.00 (prepaid). Lists sources of aid for all students, including federal and state programs, private sources, and student employment and cooperative education programs, as well as aid offered by The American Legion and sources for assistance for veterans and their dependents.

Scholarship Directory: Minority Guide to Scholarships and Financial Aid
Tinsley Communications, Inc., 100 Bridge Street, Suite A-3, Hampton, VA 23669 $7.00 plus $0.98 for shipping. A valuable directory to scholarships and financial aid for minorities.

Scholarships, Fellowships and Loans
Gale Research, 835 Penobscot Building, 645 Griswold, Detroit, MI 48226. $155.00. Contains listings of information about financial aid for students at all levels of study in the United States and Canada, cross referenced by vocational goals, field of study, legal residence, place of study, special recipient, and organization and award indexes. Includes many national and state sources for nursing. 800-877-GALE.

A Selected List of Fellowship Opportunities and Aids to Advanced Education for United States Citizens and Foreign Nationals
National Science Foundation, Publications Office, 1800 G Street, NW, Room 232, Washington, DC 20550. Free. Lists more than 100 fellowships for advanced study in various fields.

Sources of Financial Aid Available to American Indian Students
Indian Resource Development, New Mexico State University, Box 30001, Department 3 IRD, Las Cruces, NM 88003. $4.00. A helpful guide to current financial aid awards available to American Indian students.

Additional NLN Resources Available Through Jones and Bartlett Publishers

Carpenter, D.R. and Hudacek, S. 1996. *On Doctoral Education in Nursing: The Voice of the Student.* $27.95. Doctoral candidates in nursing face a range of confusing choices. Choosing the best program that meets your particular criteria can be a harrowing experience. This book helps you learn from the mistakes and successes of the diverse range of doctoral students and educators in PhD, EdD, and DNSc programs. It also introduces you to the challenges these students have faced and overcome, such as economic difficulties, family responsibilities, and long hours. This book is essential for anyone considering pursuing a doctoral degree in nursing.

Fondiller, S.H. and Nerone, B.J. 1993. *Nursing: The Career of a Lifetime.* $19.95. An all-inclusive guide to nursing as a life-long career. Professional options are thoroughly explored for all levels of nursing students and licensed practitioners.

Henderson, F.C. and McGettigan, B.O. 1994. *Managing Your Career in Nursing* (2nd edition). $25.95. A "mentor-in-print" for any nurse who wants to take a practical, self-directed approach to lifelong career management. Community nursing, self-employment, informatics, nursing research, education and administration, and new nursing roles are covered. Perfect for new graduates or current professionals.

Vogel, G. and Doleysh, N. 1988. *Entrepreneuring: A Nurse's Guide to Starting a Business* (2nd edition). $24.95. A practical guide to career enhancement through entrepreneuring in health care, including ventures in clinical practices, consulting, home care, product support, and much more.

Winstead-Fry, P. 1990. *Career Planning: A Nurse's Guide to Career Advancement.* $16.50. A revealing text for career development courses, as an aid in recruitment, and as a self-help manual for nurses interested in pursuing careers outside of the traditional hospital setting.

Section 2

ASSOCIATE DEGREE PROGRAMS

UNIVERSITY OF ALASKA—ANCHORAGE

Address: 3211 Providence Drive, Anchorage, AK 99508-8030
Phone: 907-786-4571
Fax: 907-786-4558
Contact: Tina D. DeLapp, EdD, RN, Director
Email: aftdd@uaa.alaska.edu

GENERAL INFORMATION

Type of School: *4-Year College or University, Public* • Accreditation: *Northwestern Association of Schools and Colleges* • Total Enrollment: *17000*

PROGRAM INFORMATION

LPN/LVN Exit: *No* • NLNAC Accreditation: *Yes*

NURSING STUDENT PROFILE

Total Nursing Enrollment: *62* • Full-Time Enrollment: *8* • Part-Time Enrollment: *54* • Female Enrollment: *59* • Male Enrollment: *3* • Total New Admissions Who Enrolled for Fall: *28* • Total Graduates: *18*

FINANCES

Residential Annual Tuition: *$2,800–3,264* • Non-Residential Annual Tuition: *$9,376–9,554* • General Institution Fees: *$352* • Additional Nursing Fees: *$200*

ALABAMA SOUTHERN COMMUNITY COLLEGE

Address: P.O. Box 2000, Monroeville, AL 36461
Phone: 251-575-3156
Fax: 251-575-5356
Contact: Phyllis Waits, EdD, MSN, Director
Email: pwaits@ascc.edu

GENERAL INFORMATION

Type of School: *2-Year College or University, Public* • Accreditation: *Southern Association of Colleges and Schools* • Total Enrollment: *1201*

PROGRAM INFORMATION

LPN/LVN Exit: *No* • NLNAC Accreditation: *Not Reported*

NURSING STUDENT PROFILE

Total Nursing Enrollment: *31* • Full-Time Enrollment: *30* • Part-Time Enrollment: *1* • Female Enrollment: *31* • Male Enrollment: *0* • Total New Admissions Who Enrolled for Fall: *15* • Total Graduates: *10*

FINANCES

Residential Annual Tuition: *$2,100* • Non-Residential Annual Tuition: *$4,200* • General Institution Fees: *$280* • Additional Nursing Fees: *$115*

BEVILL STATE COMMUNITY COLLEGE

Address: P.O. Box 9 Highway 78 South, Hamilton, AL
           35570
Phone: 800-648-3271
Fax: Not Reported
Contact: Alice Roberts, MSN, RN, Assistant Dean
Email: Not Reported

GENERAL INFORMATION

Type of School: *2-Year College or University, Public* •
Accreditation: *Southern Association of Colleges and Schools* •
Total Enrollment: *3554*

PROGRAM INFORMATION

LPN/LVN Exit: *Not Reported* • NLNAC Accreditation: *Yes*

NURSING STUDENT PROFILE

Total Nursing Enrollment: *146* • Full-Time Enrollment: *Not Reported* • Part-Time Enrollment: *Not Reported* • Female Enrollment: *Not Reported* • Male Enrollment: *Not Reported* • Total New Admissions Who Enrolled for Fall: *Not Reported* • Total Graduates: *109*

FINANCES

Residential Annual Tuition: *$2,688* • Non-Residential Annual Tuition: *$4,420* • General Institution Fees: *$30* • Additional Nursing Fees: *$45*

BISHOP STATE COMMUNITY COLLEGE

Address: 1365 Dr. Martin L King Avenue, Mobile, AL
           36603
Phone: 334-405-4495
Fax: Not Reported
Contact: Linda P. Shepherd, MSN, RN, Director
Email: lshepherd@bscc.cc.al.us

GENERAL INFORMATION

Type of School: *2-Year College or University, Public* •
Accreditation: *Southern Association of Colleges and Schools* •
Total Enrollment: *4000*

PROGRAM INFORMATION

LPN/LVN Exit: *No* • NLNAC Accreditation: *Yes*

NURSING STUDENT PROFILE

Total Nursing Enrollment: *392* • Full-Time Enrollment: *392* • Part-Time Enrollment: *0* • Female Enrollment: *Not Reported* • Male Enrollment: *Not Reported* • Total New Admissions Who Enrolled for Fall: *80* • Total Graduates: *Not Reported*

FINANCES

Residential Annual Tuition: *$2,688* • Non-Residential Annual Tuition: *$5,376* • General Institution Fees: *$16* • Additional Nursing Fees: *$120*

CHATTAHOOCHEE VALLEY COMMUNITY COLLEGE

Address: 2602 College Drive, Phenix City, AL 36869
Phone: 334-291-4925
Fax: 334-214-4812
Contact: Dixie Peterson, MSN, BSN, AS, Division Chairperson
Email: dixie.peterson@cvcc.cc.al.us

GENERAL INFORMATION

Type of School: *2-Year College or University, Public* •
Accreditation: *Southern Association of Colleges and Schools* •
Total Enrollment: *1896*

PROGRAM INFORMATION

LPN/LVN Exit: *Yes* • NLNAC Accreditation: *Yes*

NURSING STUDENT PROFILE

Total Nursing Enrollment: *32* • Full-Time Enrollment: *32* •
Part-Time Enrollment: *0* • Female Enrollment: *28* • Male
Enrollment: *4* • Total New Admissions Who Enrolled for
Fall: *0* • Total Graduates: *19*

FINANCES

Residential Annual Tuition: *$2,240* • Non-Residential
Annual Tuition: *$4,160* • General Institution Fees: *Not
Reported* • Additional Nursing Fees: *$561*

GADSDEN STATE COMMUNITY COLLEGE

Address: P.O. Box 227, Gadsden, AL 35902-0227
Phone: 256-549-8321
Fax: 256-549-8458
Contact: Connie W. Meloun, MSN, RN, Division Chair, Health Sciences
Email: cmeloun@gadsdenst.cc.al.us

GENERAL INFORMATION

Type of School: *2-Year College or University, Public* •
Accreditation: *Southern Association of Colleges and Schools* •
Total Enrollment: *4680*

PROGRAM INFORMATION

LPN/LVN Exit: *No* • NLNAC Accreditation: *Yes*

NURSING STUDENT PROFILE

Total Nursing Enrollment: *154* • Full-Time Enrollment: *92* •
Part-Time Enrollment: *62* • Female Enrollment: *133* • Male
Enrollment: *21* • Total New Admissions Who Enrolled for
Fall: *75* • Total Graduates: *47*

FINANCES

Residential Annual Tuition: *$2,688* • Non-Residential
Annual Tuition: *$4,864* • General Institution Fees: *$120* •
Additional Nursing Fees: *$86*

JEFFERSON DAVIS COMMUNITY COLLEGE

Address: P.O.Box 958, Brewton, AL 36427
Phone: 334-809-1618
Fax: 334-809-1527
Contact: Ann H. Mantel, MSN, RN, Division Chair and
            Director
Email: amantel@acet.net

GENERAL INFORMATION

Type of School: *2-Year College or University, Public* •
Accreditation: *Southern Association of Colleges and Schools* •
Total Enrollment: *1200*

PROGRAM INFORMATION

LPN/LVN Exit: *No* • NLNAC Accreditation: *Yes*

NURSING STUDENT PROFILE

Total Nursing Enrollment: *104* • Full-Time Enrollment: *73* •
Part-Time Enrollment: *31* • Female Enrollment: *104* • Male
Enrollment: *0* • Total New Admissions Who Enrolled for
Fall: *27* • Total Graduates: *45*

FINANCES

Residential Annual Tuition: *$2,816* • Non-Residential
Annual Tuition: *$5,612* • General Institution Fees: *$100* •
Additional Nursing Fees: *$39*

JF DRAKE STATE TECHNICAL COLLEGE

Address: 3421 Meridian Street North, Huntsvillle, AL
            35811
Phone: 205-856-6022
Fax: 205-856-7725
Contact: Janice S. Pyle, MSN, RN, BSN, Chair, Division
            of Health Sciences/Director of
Email: jspyle@jscc.cc.al.us

GENERAL INFORMATION

Type of School: *Other, Public* • Accreditation: *None* • Total
Enrollment: *700*

PROGRAM INFORMATION

LPN/LVN Exit: *No* • NLNAC Accreditation: *Yes*

NURSING STUDENT PROFILE

Total Nursing Enrollment: *129* • Full-Time Enrollment:
129 • Part-Time Enrollment: *0* • Female Enrollment: *118* •
Male Enrollment: *11* • Total New Admissions Who Enrolled
for Fall: *39* • Total Graduates: *59*

FINANCES

Residential Annual Tuition: *$2,688* • Non-Residential
Annual Tuition: *$5,376* • General Institution Fees: *$0* •
Additional Nursing Fees: *$500*

JOHN C. CALHOUN COMMUNITY COLLEGE

Address: P. O. Box 2216, Decatur, AL 35609
Phone: 256-306-2795
Fax: 256-306-2525
Contact: Jan J. Peek, MSN, RN, Chairperson
Email: jpk@calhoun.cc.al.us

GENERAL INFORMATION

Type of School: *Other, Public* • Accreditation: *Southern Association of Colleges and Schools* • Total Enrollment: *7974*

PROGRAM INFORMATION

LPN/LVN Exit: *No* • NLNAC Accreditation: *Yes*

NURSING STUDENT PROFILE

Total Nursing Enrollment: *177* • Full-Time Enrollment: *177* • Part-Time Enrollment: *0* • Female Enrollment: *Not Reported* • Male Enrollment: *Not Reported* • Total New Admissions Who Enrolled for Fall: *98* • Total Graduates: *82*

FINANCES

Residential Annual Tuition: *$2,688* • Non-Residential Annual Tuition: *$4,864* • General Institution Fees: *$150* • Additional Nursing Fees: *$300*

LAWSON STATE COMMUNITY COLLEGE

Address: 3060 Wilson Road, Birmingham, AL 35221
Phone: 205-929-6437
Fax: 205-929-6440
Contact: Sheila P. Marable, MSN, DSN, RN(c), Chairperson
Email: smarable@cougar.ls.cc.al.us

GENERAL INFORMATION

Type of School: *2-Year College or University, Public* • Accreditation: *Southern Association of Colleges and Schools* • Total Enrollment: *1800*

PROGRAM INFORMATION

LPN/LVN Exit: *No* • NLNAC Accreditation: *Yes*

NURSING STUDENT PROFILE

Total Nursing Enrollment: *94* • Full-Time Enrollment: *94* • Part-Time Enrollment: *0* • Female Enrollment: *91* • Male Enrollment: *3* • Total New Admissions Who Enrolled for Fall: *58* • Total Graduates: *18*

FINANCES

Residential Annual Tuition: *$2,176* • Non-Residential Annual Tuition: *$4,352* • General Institution Fees: *$34* • Additional Nursing Fees: *$113*

NORTHEAST ALABAMA COMMUNITY COLLEGE

Address: P.O. Box 159, 138 Highway 35 West, Rainsville,
           AL 35986
Phone: 256-228-6001
Fax: 256-228-6861
Contact: Cindy Jones, EdD, RN, Director
Email: jonesc@nacc.edu

GENERAL INFORMATION

Type of School: *2-Year College or University, Public* •
Accreditation: *Southern Association of Colleges and Schools* •
Total Enrollment: *1657*

PROGRAM INFORMATION

LPN/LVN Exit: *No* • NLNAC Accreditation: *Yes*

NURSING STUDENT PROFILE

Total Nursing Enrollment: *130* • Full-Time Enrollment: *36* •
Part-Time Enrollment: *94* • Female Enrollment: *125* • Male
Enrollment: *5* • Total New Admissions Who Enrolled for
Fall: *78* • Total Graduates: *47*

FINANCES

Residential Annual Tuition: *$2,432* • Non-Residential
Annual Tuition: *$4,480* • General Institution Fees: *$0* •
Additional Nursing Fees: *$177*

NORTHWEST SHOALS COMMUNITY COLLEGE

Address: NWSCC 2080 College Road, Phil Campbell, AL
           35581
Phone: 256-331-6237
Fax: 256-331-6272
Contact: Anita Rhodes, MSN, RN, Chair Health Studies
Email: rhodes@nwscc.cc.al.us

GENERAL INFORMATION

Type of School: *2-Year College or University, Public* •
Accreditation: *Southern Association of Colleges and Schools* •
Total Enrollment: *5200*

PROGRAM INFORMATION

LPN/LVN Exit: *No* • NLNAC Accreditation: *Yes*

NURSING STUDENT PROFILE

Total Nursing Enrollment: *168* • Full-Time Enrollment:
119 • Part-Time Enrollment: *49* • Female Enrollment: *152* •
Male Enrollment: *16* • Total New Admissions Who Enrolled
for Fall: *96* • Total Graduates: *45*

FINANCES

Residential Annual Tuition: *$2,688* • Non-Residential
Annual Tuition: *$4,096* • General Institution Fees: *$240* •
Additional Nursing Fees: *$0*

OAKWOOD COLLEGE

Address: Oakwood Road, North West, Huntsville, AL
          35896
Phone: 256-726-7287
Fax: 256-726-8338
Contact: Carol Easley Allen, PhD, RN, Chair
Email: callen@oakwood.edu

GENERAL INFORMATION

Type of School: *Not Reported* • Accreditation: *Not Reported* •
Total Enrollment: *Not Reported*

PROGRAM INFORMATION

LPN/LVN Exit: *No* • NLNAC Accreditation: *Not Reported*

NURSING STUDENT PROFILE

Total Nursing Enrollment: *30* • Full-Time Enrollment: *30* •
Part-Time Enrollment: *0* • Female Enrollment: *28* • Male
Enrollment: *2* • Total New Admissions Who Enrolled for
Fall: *0* • Total Graduates: *6*

FINANCES

Annual Tuition: *$6,519* • General Institution Fees: *$104* •
Additional Nursing Fees: *$15*

SHELTON STATE COMMUNITY COLLEGE

Address: 9500 Old Greensboro Road, Tuscaloosa, AL
          35405
Phone: 205-391-2448
Fax: 205-391-2448
Contact: Gladys D Hill, MSN, BSN, Director of Nursing
          Programs
Email: ghill@shelton.cc.as.us

GENERAL INFORMATION

Type of School: *2-Year College or University, Public* •
Accreditation: *Southern Association of Colleges and Schools* •
Total Enrollment: *6800*

PROGRAM INFORMATION

LPN/LVN Exit: *No* • NLNAC Accreditation: *Yes*

NURSING STUDENT PROFILE

Total Nursing Enrollment: *86* • Full-Time Enrollment: *86* •
Part-Time Enrollment: *Not Reported* • Female Enrollment:
79 • Male Enrollment: *7* • Total New Admissions Who
Enrolled for Fall: *53* • Total Graduates: *29*

FINANCES

Residential Annual Tuition: *$2,432* • Non-Residential
Annual Tuition: *$4,352* • General Institution Fees: *$26* •
Additional Nursing Fees: *Not reported*

SOUTHERN UNION STATE COMMUNITY COLLEGE

Address: 1701 LaFayette Parkway, Opelika, AL 36801
Phone: 334-745-6437
Fax: 334-745-6342
Contact: Lynn Harris, MSN, RN, Chair, Department of Nursing
Email: lharris@suscc.cc.al.us

GENERAL INFORMATION

Type of School: *2-Year College or University, Public* •
Accreditation: *Southern Association of Colleges and Schools* •
Total Enrollment: *5000*

PROGRAM INFORMATION

LPN/LVN Exit: *No* • NLNAC Accreditation: *Yes*

NURSING STUDENT PROFILE

Total Nursing Enrollment: *148* • Full-Time Enrollment: *148* • Part-Time Enrollment: *Not Reported* • Female Enrollment: *136* • Male Enrollment: *12* • Total New Admissions Who Enrolled for Fall: *38* • Total Graduates: *45*

FINANCES

Residential Annual Tuition: *$2,640* • Non-Residential Annual Tuition: *$5,280* • General Institution Fees: *$704* • Additional Nursing Fees: *$15*

TROY STATE UNIVERSITY

Address: 400 Pell Avenue, Troy, AL 36082
Phone: 334-241-8655
Fax: 334-241-8627
Contact: Donna H. Bedsole, EdD, RN, ASN Program Director
Email: dbedsole@troyst.edu

GENERAL INFORMATION

Type of School: *4-Year College or University, Public* •
Accreditation: *Southern Association of Colleges and Schools* •
Total Enrollment: *6777*

PROGRAM INFORMATION

LPN/LVN Exit: *No* • NLNAC Accreditation: *Yes*

NURSING STUDENT PROFILE

Total Nursing Enrollment: *166* • Full-Time Enrollment: *54* • Part-Time Enrollment: *112* • Female Enrollment: *147* • Male Enrollment: *19* • Total New Admissions Who Enrolled for Fall: *71* • Total Graduates: *39*

FINANCES

Residential Annual Tuition: *$1,766* • Non-Residential Annual Tuition: *$3,376* • General Institution Fees: *$426* • Additional Nursing Fees: *$300*

UNIVERSITY OF MOBILE

Address: P.O. Box 13220, Mobile, AL 36663
Phone: 251-442-2227
Fax: 251-442-2520
Contact: Rosemarie Adams, PhD, RN, Dean
Email: Not Reported

GENERAL INFORMATION

Type of School: *Not Reported* • Accreditation: *None* • Total Enrollment: *Not Reported*

PROGRAM INFORMATION

LPN/LVN Exit: *Not Reported* • NLNAC Accreditation: *Not Reported*

NURSING STUDENT PROFILE

Total Nursing Enrollment: *Not Reported* • Full-Time Enrollment: *Not Reported* • Part-Time Enrollment: *Not Reported* • Female Enrollment: *Not Reported* • Male Enrollment: *Not Reported* • Total New Admissions Who Enrolled for Fall: *Not Reported* • Total Graduates: *Not Reported*

FINANCES

Residential Annual Tuition: *Not Reported* • Non-Residential Annual Tuition: *Not Reported* • General Institution Fees: *Not Reported* • Additional Nursing Fees: *Not Reported*

UNIVERSITY OF WEST ALABAMA

Address: Station # 28, Livingston, AL 35470
Phone: 205-652-3517
Fax: 205-652-3778
Contact: Sylvia B. Homan, MSN, RN, MSCE,
            Chairperson Division of Nursing
Email: shoman@uwa.edu

GENERAL INFORMATION

Type of School: *4-Year College or University, Public* • Accreditation: *Southern Association of Colleges and Schools* • Total Enrollment: *1800*

PROGRAM INFORMATION

LPN/LVN Exit: *No* • NLNAC Accreditation: *Yes*

NURSING STUDENT PROFILE

Total Nursing Enrollment: *82* • Full-Time Enrollment: *82* • Part-Time Enrollment: *0* • Female Enrollment: *74* • Male Enrollment: *8* • Total New Admissions Who Enrolled for Fall: *51* • Total Graduates: *42*

FINANCES

Residential Annual Tuition: *$3,060* • Non-Residential Annual Tuition: *$7,120* • General Institution Fees: *$370* • Additional Nursing Fees: *$150*

WALLACE COMMUNITY COLLEGE-DOTHAN

Address: 1141 Wallace Drive, Dothan, AL 36303
Phone: 334-983-3521
Fax: 334-983-3600
Contact: Jackie Spivey, MSN, RN, Division Director,
            Associate Degree Nursing
Email: jspivey@wallace.edu

GENERAL INFORMATION

Type of School: *2-Year College or University, Public* •
Accreditation: *Southern Association of Colleges and Schools* •
Total Enrollment: *4065*

PROGRAM INFORMATION

LPN/LVN Exit: *Not Reported* • NLNAC Accreditation: *Yes*

NURSING STUDENT PROFILE

Total Nursing Enrollment: *187* • Full-Time Enrollment: *42* •
Part-Time Enrollment: *145* • Female Enrollment: *171* • Male
Enrollment: *16* • Total New Admissions Who Enrolled for
Fall: *54* • Total Graduates: *44*

FINANCES

Residential Annual Tuition: *$2,176* • Non-Residential
Annual Tuition: *$4,096* • General Institution Fees: *$312* •
Additional Nursing Fees: *$53*

WALLACE COMMUNITY COLLEGE-SELMA

Address: 3000 Earl Goodwin Parkway, Selma, AL 36702
Phone: 334-876-9271
Fax: 334-876-9332
Contact: Becky Casey, MSN, RN, ADN Director
Email: Not Reported

GENERAL INFORMATION

Type of School: *2-Year College or University, Public* •
Accreditation: *Southern Association of Colleges and Schools* •
Total Enrollment: *1579*

PROGRAM INFORMATION

LPN/LVN Exit: *No* • NLNAC Accreditation: *Yes*

NURSING STUDENT PROFILE

Total Nursing Enrollment: *110* • Full-Time Enrollment: *95* •
Part-Time Enrollment: *15* • Female Enrollment: *106* • Male
Enrollment: *4* • Total New Admissions Who Enrolled for
Fall: *34* • Total Graduates: *35*

FINANCES

Residential Annual Tuition: *$1,440* • Non-Residential
Annual Tuition: *$2,880* • General Institution Fees: *$112* •
Additional Nursing Fees: *$190*

WALLACE STATE COMMUNITY COLLEGE

Address: P.O.Box 2000, Hanceville, AL 35077
Phone: 256-352-8198
Fax: 256-352-8206
Contact: Denise H. Elliott, MSN, RN, Director
Email: deniseelliott@wallacestate.org

GENERAL INFORMATION

Type of School: *2-Year College or University, Public* •
Accreditation: *Southern Association of Colleges and Schools* •
Total Enrollment: *4775*

PROGRAM INFORMATION

LPN/LVN Exit: *No* • NLNAC Accreditation: *Yes*

NURSING STUDENT PROFILE

Total Nursing Enrollment: *168* • Full-Time Enrollment: *Not Reported* • Part-Time Enrollment: *Not Reported* • Female Enrollment: *148* • Male Enrollment: *20* • Total New Admissions Who Enrolled for Fall: *131* • Total Graduates: *67*

FINANCES

Residential Annual Tuition: *$1,200* • Non-Residential Annual Tuition: *$2,400* • General Institution Fees: *$4* • Additional Nursing Fees: *$31*

AMERICAN SAMOA COMMUNITY COLLEGE

Address: American Samoa Community College, P.O.Box 2609, AM 96799
Phone: 684-699-9155
Fax: 684-699-2062
Contact: Lele Mageo, RN, BSN, Chairperson
Email: leleahmumageo@yahoo.com

GENERAL INFORMATION

Type of School: *2-Year College or University, Public* •
Accreditation: *Western Association of Schools and Colleges* •
Total Enrollment: *1180*

PROGRAM INFORMATION

LPN/LVN Exit: *No* • NLNAC Accreditation: *Not Reported*

NURSING STUDENT PROFILE

Total Nursing Enrollment: *6* • Full-Time Enrollment: *6* • Part-Time Enrollment: *0* • Female Enrollment: *6* • Male Enrollment: *0* • Total New Admissions Who Enrolled for Fall: *6* • Total Graduates: *4*

FINANCES

Residential Annual Tuition: *$45* • Non-Residential Annual Tuition: *$60* • General Institution Fees: *$70* • Additional Nursing Fees: *$80*

ARIZONA WESTERN COLLEGE

Address: 9500 South Avenue 8E, Yuma, AZ 85366-0929
Phone: 520-344-7798
Fax: 520-317-6119
Contact: Patti Nicks, MSN, RN, Director of Nursing and
             Allied Health
Email: pnicks@awc.cc.az.us

GENERAL INFORMATION

Type of School: *2-Year College or University, Public* •
Accreditation: *North Central Association of Colleges and
Schools* • Total Enrollment: *Not Reported*

PROGRAM INFORMATION

LPN/LVN Exit: *Yes* • NLNAC Accreditation: *Yes*

NURSING STUDENT PROFILE

Total Nursing Enrollment: *73* • Full-Time Enrollment: *73* •
Part-Time Enrollment: *0* • Female Enrollment: *66* • Male
Enrollment: *7* • Total New Admissions Who Enrolled for
Fall: *40* • Total Graduates: *33*

FINANCES

Residential Annual Tuition: *$930* • Non-Residential Annual
Tuition: *$5,298* • General Institution Fees: *$0* • Additional
Nursing Fees: *$260*

CENTRAL ARIZONA COLLEGE

Address: 8470 North Overfeld Road, Coolidge, AZ 85228
Phone: 520-426-4331
Fax: 520-426-4580
Contact: Eleanor L. Strang, PhD, RN, BS, MS, Director
Email: ellie_strang@python.cac.cc.az.us

GENERAL INFORMATION

Type of School: *2-Year College or University, Public* •
Accreditation: *North Central Association of Colleges and
Schools* • Total Enrollment: *4538*

PROGRAM INFORMATION

LPN/LVN Exit: *Yes* • NLNAC Accreditation: *Yes*

NURSING STUDENT PROFILE

Total Nursing Enrollment: *36* • Full-Time Enrollment: *35* •
Part-Time Enrollment: *1* • Female Enrollment: *31* • Male
Enrollment: *5* • Total New Admissions Who Enrolled for
Fall: *14* • Total Graduates: *18*

FINANCES

Residential Annual Tuition: *$1,120* • Non-Residential
Annual Tuition: *$5,992* • General Institution Fees: *$12* •
Additional Nursing Fees: *$20*

COCHISE COLLEGE

Address: 4190 West Highway 80, Douglas, AZ 85607-
             9724
Phone: 520-417-4016
Fax: 520-417-4061
Contact: Susan L. Macdonald, RN, BSN, MSN, MBA,
             Director
Email: sumac@cochise.cc.az.us

GENERAL INFORMATION

Type of School: *2-Year College or University, Public* •
Accreditation: *North Central Association of Colleges and
Schools* • Total Enrollment: *4500*

PROGRAM INFORMATION

LPN/LVN Exit: *Yes* • NLNAC Accreditation: *Yes*

NURSING STUDENT PROFILE

Total Nursing Enrollment: *92* • Full-Time Enrollment: *47* •
Part-Time Enrollment: *45* • Female Enrollment: *76* • Male
Enrollment: *16* • Total New Admissions Who Enrolled for
Fall: *56* • Total Graduates: *34*

FINANCES

Residential Annual Tuition: *$1,216* • Non-Residential
Annual Tuition: *$4,980* • General Institution Fees: *$60* •
Additional Nursing Fees: *$344*

EASTERN ARIZONA COLLEGE

Address: 3714 West Church Street, Thatcher, AZ 85552
Phone: 520-428-8389
Fax: 520-428-8462
Contact: Mayuree Sozanski, DNS, RNc, Director
Email: sozanski@eac.cc.az.uz

GENERAL INFORMATION

Type of School: *2-Year College or University, Public* •
Accreditation: *North Central Association of Colleges and
Schools* • Total Enrollment: *1469*

PROGRAM INFORMATION

LPN/LVN Exit: *No* • NLNAC Accreditation: *Not Reported*

NURSING STUDENT PROFILE

Total Nursing Enrollment: *40* • Full-Time Enrollment: *40* •
Part-Time Enrollment: *0* • Female Enrollment: *36* • Male
Enrollment: *4* • Total New Admissions Who Enrolled for
Fall: *20* • Total Graduates: *14*

FINANCES

Residential Annual Tuition: *$810* • Non-Residential Annual
Tuition: *$4,980* • General Institution Fees: *$0* • Additional
Nursing Fees: *$110*

GATEWAY COMMUNITY COLLEGE

Address: 108 North 40th Street, Phoenix, AZ 85034
Phone: 602-392-5099
Fax: 602-392-5004
Contact: Cathy Lucius, RN, MS, Director, Nursing
             Division
Email: c.lucius@gwmail.maricopa.edu

GENERAL INFORMATION

Type of School: *Not Reported* • Accreditation: *Not Reported* •
Total Enrollment: *Not Reported*

PROGRAM INFORMATION

LPN/LVN Exit: *Yes* • NLNAC Accreditation: *Yes*

NURSING STUDENT PROFILE

Total Nursing Enrollment: *235* • Full-Time Enrollment:
103 • Part-Time Enrollment: *132* • Female Enrollment:
212 • Male Enrollment: *23* • Total New Admissions Who
Enrolled for Fall: *53* • Total Graduates: *58*

FINANCES

Residential Annual Tuition: *$1,230* • Non-Residential
Annual Tuition: *$5,310* • General Institution Fees: *$5* •
Additional Nursing Fees: *$50*

MARICOPA COMMUNITY COLLEGE

Address: 6000 W Olive Ave, Glendale, AZ 85302
Phone: 623-845-3209
Fax: Not Reported
Contact: Lucy Flaaten, EdD, RN, MS, Chair
Email: lucy.flaaten@gcmail.maricopa.edu

GENERAL INFORMATION

Type of School: *Not Reported* • Accreditation: *Not Reported* •
Total Enrollment: *Not Reported*

PROGRAM INFORMATION

LPN/LVN Exit: *Not Reported* • NLNAC Accreditation: *Yes*

NURSING STUDENT PROFILE

Total Nursing Enrollment: *73* • Full-Time Enrollment: *73* •
Part-Time Enrollment: *0* • Female Enrollment: *64* • Male
Enrollment: *9* • Total New Admissions Who Enrolled for
Fall: *Not Reported* • Total Graduates: *56*

FINANCES

Residential Annual Tuition: *$1,472* • Non-Residential
Annual Tuition: *Not Reported* • General Institution Fees: *$5* •
Additional Nursing Fees: *$25*

MARICOPA SKILL CENTER

Address: Pima and Chapparral Road, Scottsdale, AZ
             85266-2699
Phone: 602-423-6225
Fax: Not Reported
Contact: Nellie Nelson
Email: Not Reported

GENERAL INFORMATION

Type of School: *Not Reported* • Accreditation: *Not Reported* •
Total Enrollment: *Not Reported*

PROGRAM INFORMATION

LPN/LVN Exit: *Yes* • NLNAC Accreditation: *Not Reported*

NURSING STUDENT PROFILE

Total Nursing Enrollment: *107* • Full-Time Enrollment: *40* •
Part-Time Enrollment: *67* • Female Enrollment: *Not
Reported* • Male Enrollment: *Not Reported* • Total New
Admissions Who Enrolled for Fall: *Not Reported* • Total
Graduates: *Not Reported*

FINANCES

Residential Annual Tuition: *Not Reported* • Non-Residential
Annual Tuition: *Not Reported* • General Institution Fees:
$230 • Additional Nursing Fees: *Not Reported*

MOHAVE COMMUNITY COLLEGE

Address: 1971 Jagerson Avenue, Kingman, AZ 86401
Phone: 520-757-0863
Fax: 520-757-0875
Contact: Lynn Young, MSN, RN, Associate Dean of
             Health Occupational Services
Email: lynyou@et.mohave.cc.az.us

GENERAL INFORMATION

Type of School: *Not Reported* • Accreditation: *Not Reported* •
Total Enrollment: *Not Reported*

PROGRAM INFORMATION

LPN/LVN Exit: *Not Reported* • NLNAC Accreditation: *Not
Reported*

NURSING STUDENT PROFILE

Total Nursing Enrollment: *85* • Full-Time Enrollment: *Not
Reported* • Part-Time Enrollment: *Not Reported* • Female
Enrollment: *Not Reported* • Male Enrollment: *Not Reported* •
Total New Admissions Who Enrolled for Fall: *25* • Total
Graduates: *Not Reported*

FINANCES

Residential Annual Tuition: *$840* • Non-Residential Annual
Tuition: *$4,840* • General Institution Fees: *Not Reported* •
Additional Nursing Fees: *Not Reported*

NORTH WEST ARKANSAS COMMUNITY COLLEGE

Address: One College Drive, Bentonville, AZ 72712
Phone: Not Reported
Fax: Not Reported
Contact: Ann Garriquez, MSN, RN, Director
Email: Not Reported

NORTHLAND PIONEER COLLEGE

Address: P.O. Box 610, Holbrook, AZ 86025-0610
Phone: 520-537-2976
Fax: 520-524-2227
Contact: Karen Jones, MSN, RN, Director
Email: Not Reported

GENERAL INFORMATION

Type of School: *Not Reported* • Accreditation: *Not Reported* •
Total Enrollment: *Not Reported*

GENERAL INFORMATION

Type of School: *2-Year College or University, Public* •
Accreditation: *North Central Association of Colleges and
Schools* • Total Enrollment: *51*

PROGRAM INFORMATION

LPN/LVN Exit: *Not Reported* • NLNAC Accreditation: *Not
Reported*

PROGRAM INFORMATION

LPN/LVN Exit: *Not Reported* • NLNAC Accreditation: *Not
Reported*

NURSING STUDENT PROFILE

Total Nursing Enrollment: *Not Reported* • Full-Time
Enrollment: *Not Reported* • Part-Time Enrollment: *Not
Reported* • Female Enrollment: *Not Reported* • Male
Enrollment: *Not Reported* • Total New Admissions Who
Enrolled for Fall: *Not Reported* • Total Graduates: *Not
Reported*

NURSING STUDENT PROFILE

Total Nursing Enrollment: *51* • Full-Time Enrollment: *51* •
Part-Time Enrollment: *0* • Female Enrollment: *46* • Male
Enrollment: *5* • Total New Admissions Who Enrolled for
Fall: *Not Reported* • Total Graduates: *33*

FINANCES

Residential Annual Tuition: *$1,472* • Non-Residential
Annual Tuition: *$3,744* • General Institution Fees: *Not
Reported* • Additional Nursing Fees: *Not Reported*

FINANCES

Residential Annual Tuition: *$720* • Non-Residential Annual
Tuition: *$3,210* • General Institution Fees: *$350* •
Additional Nursing Fees: *$30*

PHOENIX COLLEGE

Address: 2411 West 14th Street, Tempe, AZ 85281-6942
Phone: 602-285-7133
Fax: 602-285-7775
Contact: Margaret Souders, RNC, MS, CNS, Chair
Email: margaret.souders@pcmail.maricopa.edu

PIMA COMMUNITY COLLEGE

Address: 2202 Ankland Road, Tucson, AZ 85709-0275
Phone: 520-206-6661
Fax: Not Reported
Contact: Vernone Erickson, RN, MS, Director
Email: verickson@pimacc.pima.edu

GENERAL INFORMATION

Type of School: *2-Year College or University, Public* •
Accreditation: *North Central Association of Colleges and Schools* • Total Enrollment: *264000*

GENERAL INFORMATION

Type of School: *Not Reported* • Accreditation: *Not Reported* • Total Enrollment: *Not Reported*

PROGRAM INFORMATION

LPN/LVN Exit: *Yes* • NLNAC Accreditation: *Not Reported*

PROGRAM INFORMATION

LPN/LVN Exit: *No* • NLNAC Accreditation: *Yes*

NURSING STUDENT PROFILE

Total Nursing Enrollment: *72* • Full-Time Enrollment: *72* •
Part-Time Enrollment: *0* • Female Enrollment: *64* • Male
Enrollment: *8* • Total New Admissions Who Enrolled for
Fall: *29* • Total Graduates: *74*

NURSING STUDENT PROFILE

Total Nursing Enrollment: *260* • Full-Time Enrollment: *260* • Part-Time Enrollment: *0* • Female Enrollment: *Not Reported* • Male Enrollment: *Not Reported* • Total New Admissions Who Enrolled for Fall: *60* • Total Graduates: *125*

FINANCES

Residential Annual Tuition: *$1,230* • Non-Residential
Annual Tuition: *$5,340* • General Institution Fees: *$5* •
Additional Nursing Fees: *$25*

FINANCES

Residential Annual Tuition: *$1,092* • Non-Residential Annual Tuition: *$6,500* • General Institution Fees: *Not Reported* • Additional Nursing Fees: *Not Reported*

UNIVERSITY OF ARIZONA

Address: 1305 North Martin, P.O. Box 210203, Tucson, AZ 85721-0203
Phone: 501-569-8000
Fax: 501-371-7546
Contact: Ann B. Schlumberger, EdD, MSN, Chairperson
Email: abschlumberg@ualr.edu

GENERAL INFORMATION

Type of School: *4-Year College or University, Public* • Accreditation: *North Central Association of Colleges and Schools* • Total Enrollment: *34300*

PROGRAM INFORMATION

LPN/LVN Exit: *No* • NLNAC Accreditation: *Yes*

NURSING STUDENT PROFILE

Total Nursing Enrollment: *178* • Full-Time Enrollment: *96* • Part-Time Enrollment: *82* • Female Enrollment: *158* • Male Enrollment: *20* • Total New Admissions Who Enrolled for Fall: *100* • Total Graduates: *61*

FINANCES

Residential Annual Tuition: *$3,300* • Non-Residential Annual Tuition: *$6,180* • General Institution Fees: *$41* • Additional Nursing Fees: *$49*

YAVAPAI COLLEGE

Address: 1100 East Sheldon, Prescott, AZ 86301
Phone: 520-776-2246
Fax: 520-776-2394
Contact: Lynn Nugent, PhD, RN, Division Chair
Email: lynn_nugent@yavapai.cc.az.us

GENERAL INFORMATION

Type of School: *2-Year College or University, Public* • Accreditation: *North Central Association of Colleges and Schools* • Total Enrollment: *7947*

PROGRAM INFORMATION

LPN/LVN Exit: *Yes* • NLNAC Accreditation: *Yes*

NURSING STUDENT PROFILE

Total Nursing Enrollment: *96* • Full-Time Enrollment: *96* • Part-Time Enrollment: *0* • Female Enrollment: *89* • Male Enrollment: *7* • Total New Admissions Who Enrolled for Fall: *54* • Total Graduates: *47*

FINANCES

Residential Annual Tuition: *$930* • Non-Residential Annual Tuition: *$1,230* • General Institution Fees: *Not Reported* • Additional Nursing Fees: *$84*

ARKANSAS STATE UNIVERSITY

Address: P.O.Box 910, State University, AR 72467
Phone: 870-972-3074
Fax: 870-972-2954
Contact: Bonnie Deuter, MNSc, RNP, Program Director
Email: bdeuter@crow.astate.edu

GENERAL INFORMATION

Type of School: *4-Year College or University, Public* • Accreditation: *North Central Association of Colleges and Schools* • Total Enrollment: *10000*

PROGRAM INFORMATION

LPN/LVN Exit: *No* • NLNAC Accreditation: *Yes*

NURSING STUDENT PROFILE

Total Nursing Enrollment: *111* • Full-Time Enrollment: *111* • Part-Time Enrollment: *0* • Female Enrollment: *101* • Male Enrollment: *10* • Total New Admissions Who Enrolled for Fall: *66* • Total Graduates: *75*

FINANCES

Residential Annual Tuition: *$2,520* • Non-Residential Annual Tuition: *$6,456* • General Institution Fees: *$180* • Additional Nursing Fees: *$20*

EAST ARKANSAS COMMUNITY COLLEGE

Address: 1700 New Castle Road, Forrest City, AR 72335-2204
Phone: 870-633-4480
Fax: 870-633-7222
Contact: Barbara Wende, EdD, RN, Chairperson
Email: bwende@eacc.cc.ar.us

GENERAL INFORMATION

Type of School: *2-Year College or University, Public* • Accreditation: *North Central Association of Colleges and Schools* • Total Enrollment: *1358*

PROGRAM INFORMATION

LPN/LVN Exit: *No* • NLNAC Accreditation: *Yes*

NURSING STUDENT PROFILE

Total Nursing Enrollment: *36* • Full-Time Enrollment: *33* • Part-Time Enrollment: *3* • Female Enrollment: *35* • Male Enrollment: *1* • Total New Admissions Who Enrolled for Fall: *13* • Total Graduates: *52*

FINANCES

Residential Annual Tuition: *$568* • Non-Residential Annual Tuition: *$1,140* • General Institution Fees: *$72* • Additional Nursing Fees: *$120*

GARLAND COUNTY COMMUNITY COLLEGE

Address: 101 College Drive, Hot Springs, AR 71913
Phone: 501-760-4288
Fax: 501-760-4183
Contact: Linda Castaldi, RN, MNSc, Division Chair and
             Director
Email: lcastaldi@admin.gccc.cc.ar.us

GENERAL INFORMATION

Type of School: *2-Year College or University, Public* •
Accreditation: *North Central Association of Colleges and
Schools* • Total Enrollment: *2400*

PROGRAM INFORMATION

LPN/LVN Exit: *No* • NLNAC Accreditation: *Yes*

NURSING STUDENT PROFILE

Total Nursing Enrollment: *94* • Full-Time Enrollment: *44* •
Part-Time Enrollment: *50* • Female Enrollment: *84* • Male
Enrollment: *10* • Total New Admissions Who Enrolled for
Fall: *65* • Total Graduates: *45*

FINANCES

Residential Annual Tuition: *$1,008* • Non-Residential
Annual Tuition: *$2,760* • General Institution Fees: *$20* •
Additional Nursing Fees: *$55*

MISSISSIPPI COUNTY COMMUNITY COLLEGE

Address: P.O.Box 1109, Blytheville, AR 72316-1109
Phone: 870-383-2911
Fax: 870-780-6382
Contact: Sharon Fulling, RN, BSN, MSN, Assistant Dean
             and Director of Nursing and HPER
Email: sfulling@mccc.cc.ar.us

GENERAL INFORMATION

Type of School: *2-Year College or University, Public* •
Accreditation: *North Central Association of Colleges and
Schools* • Total Enrollment: *2000*

PROGRAM INFORMATION

LPN/LVN Exit: *No* • NLNAC Accreditation: *Yes*

NURSING STUDENT PROFILE

Total Nursing Enrollment: *79* • Full-Time Enrollment: *60* •
Part-Time Enrollment: *19* • Female Enrollment: *77* • Male
Enrollment: *2* • Total New Admissions Who Enrolled for
Fall: *49* • Total Graduates: *19*

FINANCES

Residential Annual Tuition: *$912* • Non-Residential Annual
Tuition: *$2,352* • General Institution Fees: *$37* • Additional
Nursing Fees: *$30*

NORTH ARKANSAS COLLEGE

Address: 1515 Pioneer Drive, Harrison, AR 72601
Phone: 870-743-3000
Fax: 870-391-3354
Contact: Elizabeth Robinson, MSN, RN, Chair
Email: brobinson@northark.cc.ar.us

GENERAL INFORMATION

Type of School: *2-Year College or University, Public* • Accreditation: *North Central Association of Colleges and Schools* • Total Enrollment: *1817*

PROGRAM INFORMATION

LPN/LVN Exit: *No* • NLNAC Accreditation: *Yes*

NURSING STUDENT PROFILE

Total Nursing Enrollment: *59* • Full-Time Enrollment: *36* • Part-Time Enrollment: *23* • Female Enrollment: *54* • Male Enrollment: *5* • Total New Admissions Who Enrolled for Fall: *26* • Total Graduates: *27*

FINANCES

Residential Annual Tuition: *$1,176* • Non-Residential Annual Tuition: *$2,376* • General Institution Fees: *$162* • Additional Nursing Fees: *$51*

PHILLIPS COMMUNITY COLLEGE

Address: 1000 Campus Drive, P.O. Box 785, Helena, AR 72342
Phone: 870-338-6474
Fax: 870-338-7542
Contact: Amy Hudson, MSN, RN, Dean of Allied Health
Email: ahudson@pccua.edu

GENERAL INFORMATION

Type of School: *2-Year College or University, Public* • Accreditation: *North Central Association of Colleges and Schools* • Total Enrollment: *2267*

PROGRAM INFORMATION

LPN/LVN Exit: *No* • NLNAC Accreditation: *Yes*

NURSING STUDENT PROFILE

Total Nursing Enrollment: *72* • Full-Time Enrollment: *72* • Part-Time Enrollment: *0* • Female Enrollment: *70* • Male Enrollment: *2* • Total New Admissions Who Enrolled for Fall: *37* • Total Graduates: *22*

FINANCES

Residential Annual Tuition: *$492* • Non-Residential Annual Tuition: *$600* • General Institution Fees: *$58* • Additional Nursing Fees: *$1,300*

SOUTHEAST ARKANSAS COLLEGE

Address: 1900 Hazel Street, Pine Bluff, AR 71603
Phone: 870-543-5929
Fax: 870-543-5912
Contact: Diann W. Williams, MSN, RN, Dean, Nursing
            and Allied Health
Email: dwilliams@seark.edu

GENERAL INFORMATION

Type of School: *2-Year College or University, Public* •
Accreditation: *North Central Association of Colleges and
Schools* • Total Enrollment: *Not Reported*

PROGRAM INFORMATION

LPN/LVN Exit: *No* • NLNAC Accreditation: *Not Reported*

NURSING STUDENT PROFILE

Total Nursing Enrollment: *15* • Full-Time Enrollment: *15* •
Part-Time Enrollment: *0* • Female Enrollment: *14* • Male
Enrollment: *1* • Total New Admissions Who Enrolled for
Fall: *16* • Total Graduates: *14*

FINANCES

Residential Annual Tuition: *$495* • Non-Residential Annual
Tuition: *$990* • General Institution Fees: *$20* • Additional
Nursing Fees: *$45*

SOUTHERN ARKANSAS UNIVERSITY

Address: 100 East University, Magnolia, AR 71754
Phone: 870-235-4331
Fax: 870-235-5058
Contact: Joyce Taylor, DSN, RN, Chairperson
Email: hjtaylor@saumag.edu

GENERAL INFORMATION

Type of School: *4-Year College or University, Public* •
Accreditation: *North Central Association of Colleges and
Schools* • Total Enrollment: *3127*

PROGRAM INFORMATION

LPN/LVN Exit: *No* • NLNAC Accreditation: *Yes*

NURSING STUDENT PROFILE

Total Nursing Enrollment: *101* • Full-Time Enrollment:
101 • Part-Time Enrollment: *0* • Female Enrollment: *95* •
Male Enrollment: *6* • Total New Admissions Who Enrolled
for Fall: *55* • Total Graduates: *39*

FINANCES

Residential Annual Tuition: *$1,248* • Non-Residential
Annual Tuition: *$1,920* • General Institution Fees: *$75* •
Additional Nursing Fees: *$180*

UNIVERSITY OF ARKANSAS COMMUNITY COLLEGE

Address: P.O. Box 3350, 1 Bruce St., Morrilton, AR
           72110
Phone: 870-612-2070
Fax: Not Reported
Contact: Dawn Stueve, RN, APN, MNSc, Division Chair
Email: dstueve@uaccb.cc.ar.us

GENERAL INFORMATION

Type of School: *2-Year College or University, Public* •
Accreditation: *North Central Association of Colleges and
Schools* • Total Enrollment: *Not Reported*

PROGRAM INFORMATION

LPN/LVN Exit: *No* • NLNAC Accreditation: *Yes*

NURSING STUDENT PROFILE

Total Nursing Enrollment: *25* • Full-Time Enrollment: *25* •
Part-Time Enrollment: *Not Reported* • Female Enrollment:
24 • Male Enrollment: *1* • Total New Admissions Who
Enrolled for Fall: *25* • Total Graduates: *25*

FINANCES

Residential Annual Tuition: *$1,560* • Non-Residential
Annual Tuition: *$3,420* • General Institution Fees: *$10* •
Additional Nursing Fees: *$280*

UNIVERSITY OF ARKANSAS COMM. COLLEGE-BATESVILLE

Address: P.O. Box 3350, Batesville, AR 72503
Phone: 870-612-2070
Fax: Not Reported
Contact: Dawn Stueve, RN, APM, MNSc, Division Chair
Email: dstueve@uaccb.cc.ar.us

GENERAL INFORMATION

Type of School: *2-Year College or University, Public* •
Accreditation: *North Central Association of Colleges and
Schools* • Total Enrollment: *1056*

PROGRAM INFORMATION

LPN/LVN Exit: *No* • NLNAC Accreditation: *Yes*

NURSING STUDENT PROFILE

Total Nursing Enrollment: *25* • Full-Time Enrollment: *25* •
Part-Time Enrollment: *0* • Female Enrollment: *24* • Male
Enrollment: *1* • Total New Admissions Who Enrolled for
Fall: *25* • Total Graduates: *25*

FINANCES

Residential Annual Tuition: *$960* • Non-Residential Annual
Tuition: *$1,200* • General Institution Fees: *$960* •
Additional Nursing Fees: *$50*

UNIVERSITY OF ARKANSAS— LITTLE ROCK

Address: 2801 South University Avenue, Little Rock, AR
             72204
Phone: 501-569-8081
Fax: 501-371-7546
Contact: Ann B. Schlumberger, EdD, MSN, Chairperson
Email: abschlumberg@ualr.edu

GENERAL INFORMATION

Type of School: *4-Year College or University, Public* •
Accreditation: *North Central Association of Colleges and
Schools* • Total Enrollment: *11000*

PROGRAM INFORMATION

LPN/LVN Exit: *No* • NLNAC Accreditation: *Yes*

NURSING STUDENT PROFILE

Total Nursing Enrollment: *178* • Full-Time Enrollment: *96* •
Part-Time Enrollment: *82* • Female Enrollment: *158* • Male
Enrollment: *20* • Total New Admissions Who Enrolled for
Fall: *100* • Total Graduates: *61*

FINANCES

Residential Annual Tuition: *$4,064* • Non-Residential
Annual Tuition: *$11,264* • General Institution Fees: *$110* •
Additional Nursing Fees: *$49*

WESTARK COLLEGE

Address: P.O.Box 364, Fort Smith, AR 72913-3649
Phone: 501-788-7371
Fax: 501-788-7869
Contact: Jo Alice Dobbs, MSN, RN, Director
Email: jdobbs@pipeline.westark.edu

GENERAL INFORMATION

Type of School: *2-Year College or University, Public* •
Accreditation: *North Central Association of Colleges and
Schools* • Total Enrollment: *Not Reported*

PROGRAM INFORMATION

LPN/LVN Exit: *No* • NLNAC Accreditation: *Yes*

NURSING STUDENT PROFILE

Total Nursing Enrollment: *129* • Full-Time Enrollment:
129 • Part-Time Enrollment: *0* • Female Enrollment: *109* •
Male Enrollment: *20* • Total New Admissions Who Enrolled
for Fall: *26* • Total Graduates: *66*

FINANCES

Residential Annual Tuition: *$1,170* • Non-Residential
Annual Tuition: *$2,880* • General Institution Fees: *$20* •
Additional Nursing Fees: *$50*

ALLAN HANCOCK COLLEGE

Address: 800 South College Drive, Santa Maria, CA
            93454
Phone: 805-922-6966
Fax: 805-922-1403
Contact: Dorothy L. Phillips, RN, MN, Associate Dean
            for Health Occupations
Email: drdotty@sbceo.org

GENERAL INFORMATION

Type of School: *Not Reported* • Accreditation: *None* • Total
Enrollment: *Not Reported*

PROGRAM INFORMATION

LPN/LVN Exit: *Yes* • NLNAC Accreditation: *Yes*

NURSING STUDENT PROFILE

Total Nursing Enrollment: *25* • Full-Time Enrollment: *25* •
Part-Time Enrollment: *0* • Female Enrollment: *23* • Male
Enrollment: *2* • Total New Admissions Who Enrolled for
Fall: *27* • Total Graduates: *Not Reported*

FINANCES

Residential Annual Tuition: *$576* • Non-Residential Annual
Tuition: *$4,768* • General Institution Fees: *Not Reported* •
Additional Nursing Fees: *Not Reported*

AMERICAN RIVER COLLEGE

Address: 4700 College Oak Drive, Sacramento, CA 95841
Phone: 916-484-8335
Fax: Not Reported
Contact: Lucille Rybka, EdD, RN, Director
Email: Not Reported

GENERAL INFORMATION

Type of School: *Not Reported* • Accreditation: *Not Reported* •
Total Enrollment: *Not Reported*

PROGRAM INFORMATION

LPN/LVN Exit: *No* • NLNAC Accreditation: *Not Reported*

NURSING STUDENT PROFILE

Total Nursing Enrollment: *60* • Full-Time Enrollment: *60* •
Part-Time Enrollment: *0* • Female Enrollment: *55* • Male
Enrollment: *5* • Total New Admissions Who Enrolled for
Fall: *30* • Total Graduates: *60*

FINANCES

Residential Annual Tuition: *$360* • Non-Residential Annual
Tuition: *$4,500* • General Institution Fees: *$100* •
Additional Nursing Fees: *$15*

ANTELOPE VALLEY COLLEGE

Address: 3041 West Avenue K, Lancaster, CA 93551
Phone: 661-722-6402
Fax: 661-722-6403
Contact: Karen Cowell, PhD, RN, C, Dean and Director
Email: KCowell@avc.edu

GENERAL INFORMATION

Type of School: *2-Year College or University, Public* •
Accreditation: *Western Association of Schools and Colleges* •
Total Enrollment: *11442*

PROGRAM INFORMATION

LPN/LVN Exit: *No* • NLNAC Accreditation: *Not Reported*

NURSING STUDENT PROFILE

Total Nursing Enrollment: *120* • Full-Time Enrollment: *73* •
Part-Time Enrollment: *47* • Female Enrollment: *103* • Male
Enrollment: *17* • Total New Admissions Who Enrolled for
Fall: *44* • Total Graduates: *55*

FINANCES

Residential Annual Tuition: *$576* • Non-Residential Annual
Tuition: *$4,768* • General Institution Fees: *$2* • Additional
Nursing Fees: *$15*

BAKERSFIELD COLLEGE

Address: 1801 Panorama Drive, Bakersfield, CA 93305
Phone: 661-395-4281
Fax: 661-395-4295
Contact: Sheran DeLeon, MEd, RN, Director
Email: Not Reported

GENERAL INFORMATION

Type of School: *2-Year College or University, Public* •
Accreditation: *Western Association of Schools and Colleges* •
Total Enrollment: *12000*

PROGRAM INFORMATION

LPN/LVN Exit: *No* • NLNAC Accreditation: *Not Reported*

NURSING STUDENT PROFILE

Total Nursing Enrollment: *150* • Full-Time Enrollment:
150 • Part-Time Enrollment: *0* • Female Enrollment: *148* •
Male Enrollment: *2* • Total New Admissions Who Enrolled
for Fall: *Not Reported* • Total Graduates: *Not Reported*

FINANCES

Residential Annual Tuition: *$576* • Non-Residential Annual
Tuition: *$4,768* • General Institution Fees: *Not Reported* •
Additional Nursing Fees: *Not Reported*

BUTTE COLLEGE

Address: 3536 Butte Campus, Oroville, CA 95965
Phone: 508-895-2329
Fax: 508-895-2329
Contact: Lynn Phillips, MSN, RN, Chair
Email: Not Reported

GENERAL INFORMATION

Type of School: *Not Reported* • Accreditation: *Not Reported* •
Total Enrollment: *Not Reported*

PROGRAM INFORMATION

LPN/LVN Exit: *Not Reported* • NLNAC Accreditation: *Not Reported*

NURSING STUDENT PROFILE

Total Nursing Enrollment: *Not Reported* • Full-Time
Enrollment: *Not Reported* • Part-Time Enrollment: *Not Reported* • Female Enrollment: *Not Reported* • Male
Enrollment: *Not Reported* • Total New Admissions Who
Enrolled for Fall: *Not Reported* • Total Graduates: *Not Reported*

FINANCES

Residential Annual Tuition: *$352* • Non-Residential Annual
Tuition: *$5,088* • General Institution Fees: *Not Reported* •
Additional Nursing Fees: *Not Reported*

CABRILLO COLLEGE

Address: 6500 Soquel Drive, Aptos, CA 95003
Phone: 831-479-6455
Fax: 831-479-5748
Contact: Kathleen S. Welch, PhD, RN, Director
Email: kawelch@cabrillo.cc.ca.us

GENERAL INFORMATION

Type of School: *Not Reported* • Accreditation: *None* • Total
Enrollment: *Not Reported*

PROGRAM INFORMATION

LPN/LVN Exit: *No* • NLNAC Accreditation: *Not Reported*

NURSING STUDENT PROFILE

Total Nursing Enrollment: *76* • Full-Time Enrollment: *76* •
Part-Time Enrollment: *0* • Female Enrollment: *67* • Male
Enrollment: *9* • Total New Admissions Who Enrolled for
Fall: *42* • Total Graduates: *37*

FINANCES

Residential Annual Tuition: *$330* • Non-Residential Annual
Tuition: *$400* • General Institution Fees: *$0* • Additional
Nursing Fees: *$0*

CALIFORNIA STATE UNIVERSITY-LOS ANGELES

Address: 5151 State University Drive, Los Angeles, CA
            90032-4226
Phone: 323-343-4727
Fax: 323-343-6454
Contact: Judith Papenhausen, PhD, RN, Director
Email: jpapenh@calstatela.edu

GENERAL INFORMATION

Type of School: *Not Reported* • Accreditation: *Not Reported* •
Total Enrollment: *Not Reported*

PROGRAM INFORMATION

LPN/LVN Exit: *Not Reported* • NLNAC Accreditation: *Not Reported*

NURSING STUDENT PROFILE

Total Nursing Enrollment: *Not Reported* • Full-Time
Enrollment: *Not Reported* • Part-Time Enrollment: *Not Reported* • Female Enrollment: *Not Reported* • Male
Enrollment: *Not Reported* • Total New Admissions Who
Enrolled for Fall: *Not Reported* • Total Graduates: *Not Reported*

FINANCES

Residential Annual Tuition: *$1,629.50* • Non-Residential
Annual Tuition: *$6,830.75* • General Institution Fees: *Not Reported* • Additional Nursing Fees: *Not Reported*

CERRITOS COLLEGE

Address: 11110 East Alondra Boulevard, Norwalk, CA
            90650-6298
Phone: 562-860-2451
Fax: 561-467-5005
Contact: D Harristla, MSN, RN
Email: Not Reported

GENERAL INFORMATION

Type of School: *Not Reported* • Accreditation: *Not Reported* •
Total Enrollment: *Not Reported*

PROGRAM INFORMATION

LPN/LVN Exit: *Not Reported* • NLNAC Accreditation: *Yes*

NURSING STUDENT PROFILE

Total Nursing Enrollment: *161* • Full-Time Enrollment: *80* •
Part-Time Enrollment: *81* • Female Enrollment: *Not Reported* • Male Enrollment: *Not Reported* • Total New
Admissions Who Enrolled for Fall: *Not Reported* • Total
Graduates: *60*

FINANCES

Residential Annual Tuition: *$352* • Non-Residential Annual
Tuition: *$4,768* • General Institution Fees: *Not Reported* •
Additional Nursing Fees: *Not Reported*

CHAFFEY COLLEGE

Address: 5885 Haven Avenue, Rancho Cucamonga, CA
           91737
Phone: 909-941-2694
Fax: 909-466-2887
Contact: Marcha Talton, MSN, RN, ADN Director
Email: mtalton@chaffey.cc.ca.us

GENERAL INFORMATION

Type of School: *2-Year College or University, Public* •
Accreditation: *Western Association of Schools and Colleges* •
Total Enrollment: *16500*

PROGRAM INFORMATION

LPN/LVN Exit: *Not Reported* • NLNAC Accreditation: *Yes*

NURSING STUDENT PROFILE

Total Nursing Enrollment: *130* • Full-Time Enrollment:
113 • Part-Time Enrollment: *17* • Female Enrollment: *119* •
Male Enrollment: *11* • Total New Admissions Who Enrolled
for Fall: *30* • Total Graduates: *43*

FINANCES

Residential Annual Tuition: *$330* • Non-Residential Annual
Tuition: *$4,650* • General Institution Fees: *$100* •
Additional Nursing Fees: *$100*

CITY COLLEGE OF SAN FRANCISO

Address: 50 Phelan Avenue, San Francisco, CA 94112
Phone: Not Reported
Fax: Not Reported
Contact: Cecile Dawydisk, MSN, RN, Chairperson
Email: Not Reported

GENERAL INFORMATION

Type of School: *Not Reported* • Accreditation: *Not Reported* •
Total Enrollment: *Not Reported*

PROGRAM INFORMATION

LPN/LVN Exit: *Not Reported* • NLNAC Accreditation: *Not
Reported*

NURSING STUDENT PROFILE

Total Nursing Enrollment: *180* • Full-Time Enrollment:
100 • Part-Time Enrollment: *80* • Female Enrollment: *Not
Reported* • Male Enrollment: *Not Reported* • Total New
Admissions Who Enrolled for Fall: *Not Reported* • Total
Graduates: *72*

FINANCES

Residential Annual Tuition: *$576* • Non-Residential Annual
Tuition: *$5,184* • General Institution Fees: *Not Reported* •
Additional Nursing Fees: *Not Reported*

COLLEGE OF MARIN

Address: 835 College Avenue, Kentfield, CA 94904
Phone: 415-485-9326
Fax: 415-456-5086
Contact: Rosalind Hartman, MSN, RN, Director of Health Services
Email: hartman@marin.cc.ca.us

GENERAL INFORMATION

Type of School: *2-Year College or University, Public* •
Accreditation: *Western Association of Schools and Colleges* •
Total Enrollment: *7828*

PROGRAM INFORMATION

LPN/LVN Exit: *No* • NLNAC Accreditation: *Yes*

NURSING STUDENT PROFILE

Total Nursing Enrollment: *90* • Full-Time Enrollment: *90* •
Part-Time Enrollment: *0* • Female Enrollment: *75* • Male
Enrollment: *15* • Total New Admissions Who Enrolled for
Fall: *44* • Total Graduates: *34*

FINANCES

Residential Annual Tuition: *$330* • Non-Residential Annual
Tuition: *$4,650* • General Institution Fees: *$116* •
Additional Nursing Fees: *$150*

COLLEGE OF SAN MATEO

Address: 1700 West Hillsdale Boulevard, San Mateo, CA 94402
Phone: 650-574-6218
Fax: 650-574-6503
Contact: Ruth McCracken, MSN, RNEd, Director
Email: mccracken@smccd.net

GENERAL INFORMATION

Type of School: *2-Year College or University, Public* •
Accreditation: *Western Association of Schools and Colleges* •
Total Enrollment: *20000*

PROGRAM INFORMATION

LPN/LVN Exit: *No* • NLNAC Accreditation: *Not Reported*

NURSING STUDENT PROFILE

Total Nursing Enrollment: *96* • Full-Time Enrollment: *96* •
Part-Time Enrollment: *0* • Female Enrollment: *87* • Male
Enrollment: *9* • Total New Admissions Who Enrolled for
Fall: *48* • Total Graduates: *34*

FINANCES

Residential Annual Tuition: *$264* • Non-Residential Annual
Tuition: *$5,976* • General Institution Fees: *$36* • Additional
Nursing Fees: *$400*

COLLEGE OF THE DESERT

Address: 43-500 Monterey Avenue, Palm Desert, CA
           92260
Phone: 760-773-2580
Fax: 760-776-7414
Contact: Sandi Emerson, MSN, RN, Chairperson and
           Director, Nursing Programs
Email: semerson@dccd.cc.ca.us

GENERAL INFORMATION

Type of School: *Not Reported* • Accreditation: *Not Reported* •
Total Enrollment: *Not Reported*

PROGRAM INFORMATION

LPN/LVN Exit: *No* • NLNAC Accreditation: *Yes*

NURSING STUDENT PROFILE

Total Nursing Enrollment: *104* • Full-Time Enrollment:
104 • Part-Time Enrollment: *0* • Female Enrollment: *82* •
Male Enrollment: *22* • Total New Admissions Who Enrolled
for Fall: *30* • Total Graduates: *51*

FINANCES

Residential Annual Tuition: *$584* • Non-Residential Annual
Tuition: *$5,128* • General Institution Fees: *$82* • Additional
Nursing Fees: *$15*

COLLEGE OF THE SEQUOIAS

Address: 915 South Mooney Road, Visalia, CA 93227
Phone: 559-730-3732
Fax: Not Reported
Contact: Cherie Rector, PhD, RNc, Director
Email: cherier@giant.sequoias.cc.ca.us

GENERAL INFORMATION

Type of School: *Not Reported* • Accreditation: *Not Reported* •
Total Enrollment: *Not Reported*

PROGRAM INFORMATION

LPN/LVN Exit: *Not Reported* • NLNAC Accreditation: *Not
Reported*

NURSING STUDENT PROFILE

Total Nursing Enrollment: *Not Reported* • Full-Time
Enrollment: *Not Reported* • Part-Time Enrollment: *Not
Reported* • Female Enrollment: *Not Reported* • Male
Enrollment: *Not Reported* • Total New Admissions Who
Enrolled for Fall: *Not Reported* • Total Graduates: *Not
Reported*

FINANCES

Residential Annual Tuition: *$576* • Non-Residential Annual
Tuition: *$5,536* • General Institution Fees: *Not Reported* •
Additional Nursing Fees: *Not Reported*

COMPTON COMMUNITY COLLEGE

Address: 1111 East Artesia Boulevard, Compton, CA 90221
Phone: 310-900-1600
Fax: Not Reported
Contact: Roberta West, MSN, RN, Dean of Human Services and Nursing
Email: Not Reported

GENERAL INFORMATION

Type of School: *2-Year College or University, Public* •
Accreditation: *Western Association of Schools and Colleges* •
Total Enrollment: *6500*

PROGRAM INFORMATION

LPN/LVN Exit: *No* • NLNAC Accreditation: *Not Reported*

NURSING STUDENT PROFILE

Total Nursing Enrollment: *22* • Full-Time Enrollment: *22* •
Part-Time Enrollment: *0* • Female Enrollment: *20* • Male
Enrollment: *2* • Total New Admissions Who Enrolled for
Fall: *16* • Total Graduates: *44*

FINANCES

Residential Annual Tuition: *$360* • Non-Residential Annual
Tuition: *$3,480* • General Institution Fees: *$88* • Additional
Nursing Fees: *$225*

CONTRA COSTA COLLEGE

Address: 2600 Mission Bell Drive, San Pablo, CA 94806
Phone: 510-235-7800
Fax: Not Reported
Contact: Roseanne Packard, RN, MS, JD, Primary Administrator
Email: Not Reported

GENERAL INFORMATION

Type of School: *2-Year College or University, Public* •
Accreditation: *Western Association of Schools and Colleges* •
Total Enrollment: *6000*

PROGRAM INFORMATION

LPN/LVN Exit: *No* • NLNAC Accreditation: *Not Reported*

NURSING STUDENT PROFILE

Total Nursing Enrollment: *100* • Full-Time Enrollment:
100 • Part-Time Enrollment: *0* • Female Enrollment: *85* •
Male Enrollment: *15* • Total New Admissions Who Enrolled
for Fall: *51* • Total Graduates: *33*

FINANCES

Residential Annual Tuition: *$330* • Non-Residential Annual
Tuition: *$4,410* • General Institution Fees: *$2* • Additional
Nursing Fees: *$75*

CUESTA COLLEGE

Address: P.O. Box 8106, San Luis Obispo, CA 93405
Phone: 805-546-3119
Fax: 805-596-3961
Contact: Mary N. Parker, EdD, RN, BSN, MN, Director
Email: Not Reported

GENERAL INFORMATION

Type of School: *2-Year College or University, Public* •
Accreditation: *Western Association of Schools and Colleges* •
Total Enrollment: *10000*

PROGRAM INFORMATION

LPN/LVN Exit: *No* • NLNAC Accreditation: *Not Reported*

NURSING STUDENT PROFILE

Total Nursing Enrollment: *84* • Full-Time Enrollment: *84* •
Part-Time Enrollment: *0* • Female Enrollment: *77* • Male
Enrollment: *7* • Total New Admissions Who Enrolled for
Fall: *45* • Total Graduates: *34*

FINANCES

Residential Annual Tuition: *$352* • Non-Residential Annual
Tuition: *$5,728* • General Institution Fees: *Not Reported* •
Additional Nursing Fees: *$800*

CYPRESS COLLEGE

Address: 9200 Valley View, Cypress, CA 90630
Phone: 714-484-7283
Fax: 714-527-2175
Contact: Andrea L. Hannon, MSN, RN, Director of
Nursing
Email: ahannon@cypress.cc.ca.us

GENERAL INFORMATION

Type of School: *2-Year College or University, Public* •
Accreditation: *Western Association of Schools and Colleges* •
Total Enrollment: *15000*

PROGRAM INFORMATION

LPN/LVN Exit: *No* • NLNAC Accreditation: *Yes*

NURSING STUDENT PROFILE

Total Nursing Enrollment: *138* • Full-Time Enrollment:
138 • Part-Time Enrollment: *0* • Female Enrollment: *117* •
Male Enrollment: *21* • Total New Admissions Who Enrolled
for Fall: *40* • Total Graduates: *67*

FINANCES

Residential Annual Tuition: *$264* • Non-Residential Annual
Tuition: *$3,120* • General Institution Fees: *$27* • Additional
Nursing Fees: *$60*

DE ANZA COLLEGE

Address: 21250 Stevens Creek Boulevard, Cupertino, CA
             95014-5793
Phone: 619-279-4500
Fax: 619-279-4885
Contact: Beverly Peterson, PhD, RN, Director
Email: Not Reported

GENERAL INFORMATION

Type of School: *Not Reported* • Accreditation: *None* • Total
Enrollment: *Not Reported*

PROGRAM INFORMATION

LPN/LVN Exit: *Not Reported* • NLNAC Accreditation: *Not
Reported*

NURSING STUDENT PROFILE

Total Nursing Enrollment: *154* • Full-Time Enrollment:
154 • Part-Time Enrollment: *0* • Female Enrollment: *Not
Reported* • Male Enrollment: *Not Reported* • Total New
Admissions Who Enrolled for Fall: *Not Reported* • Total
Graduates: *125*

FINANCES

Residential Annual Tuition: *$384* • Non-Residential Annual
Tuition: *$4,000* • General Institution Fees: *Not Reported* •
Additional Nursing Fees: *Not Reported*

EAST LOS ANGELES COLLEGE

Address: 1301 Avenida Cesar Chavez, Montery Park, CA
             91754
Phone: 323-265-8114
Fax: Not Reported
Contact: Lurelean B. Gaines, MSN, RN, Chair
Email: lurelean_b._gaines@laccd.cc.ca.us

GENERAL INFORMATION

Type of School: *Not Reported* • Accreditation: *Not Reported* •
Total Enrollment: *Not Reported*

PROGRAM INFORMATION

LPN/LVN Exit: *Not Reported* • NLNAC Accreditation: *Not
Reported*

NURSING STUDENT PROFILE

Total Nursing Enrollment: *165* • Full-Time Enrollment:
165 • Part-Time Enrollment: *0* • Female Enrollment: *Not
Reported* • Male Enrollment: *Not Reported* • Total New
Admissions Who Enrolled for Fall: *60* • Total Graduates: *60*

FINANCES

Residential Annual Tuition: *$384* • Non-Residential Annual
Tuition: *$4,928* • General Institution Fees: *Not Reported* •
Additional Nursing Fees: *Not Reported*

EL CAMINO COMMUNITY COLLEGE

Address: 16007 Crenshaw Boulevard, Torrance, CA 90506
Phone: 310-660-3282
Fax: 310-660-3439
Contact: Katherine Townsend, EdD, MS, BSN, Director of Nursing
Email: ktownsend@elcamino.cc.ca.us

GENERAL INFORMATION

Type of School: *2-Year College or University, Public* •
Accreditation: *Western Association of Schools and Colleges* •
Total Enrollment: *23785*

PROGRAM INFORMATION

LPN/LVN Exit: *No* • NLNAC Accreditation: *Yes*

NURSING STUDENT PROFILE

Total Nursing Enrollment: *188* • Full-Time Enrollment: *188* • Part-Time Enrollment: *0* • Female Enrollment: *164* • Male Enrollment: *24* • Total New Admissions Who Enrolled for Fall: *92* • Total Graduates: *62*

FINANCES

Residential Annual Tuition: *$330* • Non-Residential Annual Tuition: *$3,630* • General Institution Fees: *$20* • Additional Nursing Fees: *$50*

FRESNO CITY COLLEGE

Address: 1101 East University Avenue, Fresno, CA 93741
Phone: 559-244-2695
Fax: 559-244-2626
Contact: Dianne S. Moore, PhD, RN, CNM, MN, MPH, Director of Nursing
Email: dianne.moore@scccd.com

GENERAL INFORMATION

Type of School: *2-Year College or University, Public* •
Accreditation: *Western Association of Schools and Colleges* •
Total Enrollment: *25000*

PROGRAM INFORMATION

LPN/LVN Exit: *No* • NLNAC Accreditation: *Not Reported*

NURSING STUDENT PROFILE

Total Nursing Enrollment: *252* • Full-Time Enrollment: *252* • Part-Time Enrollment: *0* • Female Enrollment: *213* • Male Enrollment: *39* • Total New Admissions Who Enrolled for Fall: *145* • Total Graduates: *127*

FINANCES

Residential Annual Tuition: *$330* • Non-Residential Annual Tuition: *$330* • General Institution Fees: *$264* • Additional Nursing Fees: *Not Reported*

GAVILAN COLLEGE

Address:　5055 Santa Teresa Boulevard, Gilroy, CA 95020
Phone:　　408-848-4883
Fax:　　　408-848-4769
Contact:　K Bedell, MSN, RN, Director
Email:　　Not Reported

GLENDALE COMMUNITY COLLEGE

Address:　1500 North Verdugo Road, Glendale, CA 91208
Phone:　　818-551-5270
Fax:　　　818-551-5271
Contact:　Sharon M. Hall, EdD, RN, MN, Associate
　　　　　Dean, Allied Health
Email:　　shall@glendale.edu

GENERAL INFORMATION

Type of School: *Not Reported* • Accreditation: *Western Association of Schools and Colleges* • Total Enrollment: *4500*

GENERAL INFORMATION

Type of School: *2-Year College or University, Public* • Accreditation: *Northwestern Association of Schools and Colleges* • Total Enrollment: *15000*

PROGRAM INFORMATION

LPN/LVN Exit: *Not Reported* • NLNAC Accreditation: *Not Reported*

PROGRAM INFORMATION

LPN/LVN Exit: *No* • NLNAC Accreditation: *Not Reported*

NURSING STUDENT PROFILE

Total Nursing Enrollment: *164* • Full-Time Enrollment: *Not Reported* • Part-Time Enrollment: *Not Reported* • Female Enrollment: *Not Reported* • Male Enrollment: *Not Reported* • Total New Admissions Who Enrolled for Fall: *36* • Total Graduates: *57*

NURSING STUDENT PROFILE

Total Nursing Enrollment: *103* • Full-Time Enrollment: *100* • Part-Time Enrollment: *3* • Female Enrollment: *88* • Male Enrollment: *15* • Total New Admissions Who Enrolled for Fall: *35* • Total Graduates: *47*

FINANCES

Residential Annual Tuition: *$352* • Non-Residential Annual Tuition: *$5,536* • General Institution Fees: *Not Reported* • Additional Nursing Fees: *Not Reported*

FINANCES

Residential Annual Tuition: *$352* • Non-Residential Annual Tuition: *$4,832* • General Institution Fees: *$75* • Additional Nursing Fees: *$53*

GOLDEN WEST COLLEGE

Address: 15744 Golden West Street, P.O. Box 2748,
           Huntington Beach, CA 92647
Phone: 714-895-8157
Fax: 714-895-8166
Contact: Linda Stevens, MSN, RN, Dean, Math, Sciences
           and Health Professions
Email: lstevens@gwc.cccd.edu

GENERAL INFORMATION

Type of School: *2-Year College or University, Public* •
Accreditation: *Western Association of Schools and Colleges* •
Total Enrollment: *13000*

PROGRAM INFORMATION

LPN/LVN Exit: *Not Reported* • NLNAC Accreditation: *Yes*

NURSING STUDENT PROFILE

Total Nursing Enrollment: *194* • Full-Time Enrollment:
194 • Part-Time Enrollment: *0* • Female Enrollment: *175* •
Male Enrollment: *19* • Total New Admissions Who Enrolled
for Fall: *53* • Total Graduates: *72*

FINANCES

Residential Annual Tuition: *$352* • Non-Residential Annual
Tuition: *$4,224* • General Institution Fees: *$93* • Additional
Nursing Fees: *$125*

GROSSMONT COLLEGE

Address: 8800 Grossmont College Drive, El Cajon, CA
           92020
Phone: 619-644-7815
Fax: 619-644-7961
Contact: Elisabeth Hamel, EdD, RN, Associate Dean of
           Health Professions
Email: elisabeth.hamel@gcccd.net

GENERAL INFORMATION

Type of School: *2-Year College or University, Private
(Independent)* • Accreditation: *Western Association of Schools
and Colleges* • Total Enrollment: *16000*

PROGRAM INFORMATION

LPN/LVN Exit: *No* • NLNAC Accreditation: *Yes*

NURSING STUDENT PROFILE

Total Nursing Enrollment: *151* • Full-Time Enrollment:
151 • Part-Time Enrollment: *0* • Female Enrollment: *130* •
Male Enrollment: *21* • Total New Admissions Who Enrolled
for Fall: *93* • Total Graduates: *74*

FINANCES

Residential Annual Tuition: *$250* • Non-Residential Annual
Tuition: *$3,120* • General Institution Fees: *$36* • Additional
Nursing Fees: *$90*

HARTNELL COLLEGE

Address: 156 Homestead Avenue, Salinas, CA 93901
Phone: Not Reported
Fax: Not Reported
Contact: Chris Eaton, PhD, RN, Not Provided
Email: Not Reported

HUMBOLDT STATE UNIVERSITY

Address: 1 Harpst Street, Arcata, CA 95521
Phone: Not Reported
Fax: Not Reported
Contact: Judith Paperhausen, PhD, RN, Chairperson
Email: Not Reported

GENERAL INFORMATION

Type of School: *2-Year College or University, Public* •
Accreditation: *None* • Total Enrollment: *8300*

GENERAL INFORMATION

Type of School: *4-Year College or University, Public* •
Accreditation: *Western Association of Schools and Colleges* •
Total Enrollment: *7500*

PROGRAM INFORMATION

LPN/LVN Exit: *Not Reported* • NLNAC Accreditation: *Not Reported*

PROGRAM INFORMATION

LPN/LVN Exit: *Not Reported* • NLNAC Accreditation: *Not Reported*

NURSING STUDENT PROFILE

Total Nursing Enrollment: *59* • Full-Time Enrollment: *59* •
Part-Time Enrollment: *0* • Female Enrollment: *Not Reported* • Male Enrollment: *Not Reported* • Total New Admissions Who Enrolled for Fall: *Not Reported* • Total Graduates: *69*

NURSING STUDENT PROFILE

Total Nursing Enrollment: *Not Reported* • Full-Time Enrollment: *Not Reported* • Part-Time Enrollment: *Not Reported* • Female Enrollment: *Not Reported* • Male Enrollment: *Not Reported* • Total New Admissions Who Enrolled for Fall: *Not Reported* • Total Graduates: *Not Reported*

FINANCES

Residential Annual Tuition: *$352* • Non-Residential Annual Tuition: *$4,864* • General Institution Fees: *Not Reported* • Additional Nursing Fees: *Not Reported*

FINANCES

Residential Annual Tuition: *$1,832* • Non-Residential Annual Tuition: *$9,024* • General Institution Fees: *Not Reported* • Additional Nursing Fees: *Not Reported*

IMPERIAL VALLEY COLLEGE

Address: P. O. Box 158, Imperial, CA 92251
Phone: 760-355-6348
Fax: Not Reported
Contact: Kathy Berry, RN,MSN, Interim Director
Email: Kathyb@imperial.cc.ca.us

GENERAL INFORMATION

Type of School: *Not Reported* • Accreditation: *None* • Total Enrollment: *Not Reported*

PROGRAM INFORMATION

LPN/LVN Exit: *Not Reported* • NLNAC Accreditation: *Not Reported*

NURSING STUDENT PROFILE

Total Nursing Enrollment: *72* • Full-Time Enrollment: *72* • Part-Time Enrollment: *0* • Female Enrollment: *Not Reported* • Male Enrollment: *Not Reported* • Total New Admissions Who Enrolled for Fall: *20* • Total Graduates: *35*

FINANCES

Residential Annual Tuition: *$352* • Non-Residential Annual Tuition: *$4,640* • General Institution Fees: *Not Reported* • Additional Nursing Fees: *Not Reported*

LOMA LINDA UNIVERSITY

Address: 11234 Anderson Street, Loma Linda, CA 92350
Phone: 909-558-4517
Fax: 909-558-4134
Contact: Helen Emori King, PhD, RN, Dean
Email: hking@sn.llu.edu

GENERAL INFORMATION

Type of School: *4-Year College or University, Private (Religious)* • Accreditation: *Western Association of Schools and Colleges* • Total Enrollment: *3338*

PROGRAM INFORMATION

LPN/LVN Exit: *Not Reported* • NLNAC Accreditation: *Not Reported*

NURSING STUDENT PROFILE

Total Nursing Enrollment: *Not Reported* • Full-Time Enrollment: *Not Reported* • Part-Time Enrollment: *Not Reported* • Female Enrollment: *Not Reported* • Male Enrollment: *Not Reported* • Total New Admissions Who Enrolled for Fall: *Not Reported* • Total Graduates: *Not Reported*

FINANCES

Residential Annual Tuition: *$17,640* • Non-Residential Annual Tuition: *Not Reported* • General Institution Fees: *Not Reported* • Additional Nursing Fees: *Not Reported*

LONG BEACH CITY COLLEGE

Address: 4901-East Carson Street, Los Angeles, CA 90056
Phone: 562-938-4172
Fax: 562-938-4191
Contact: Brenda McCane Harrell, MSN, RN, EdD,
          Program Director
Email: bharrell@lbcc.cc.ca.us

GENERAL INFORMATION

Type of School: *2-Year College or University, Public* •
Accreditation: *Western Association of Schools and Colleges* •
Total Enrollment: *27000*

PROGRAM INFORMATION

LPN/LVN Exit: *Yes* • NLNAC Accreditation: *Yes*

NURSING STUDENT PROFILE

Total Nursing Enrollment: *202* • Full-Time Enrollment:
202 • Part-Time Enrollment: *0* • Female Enrollment: *171* •
Male Enrollment: *31* • Total New Admissions Who Enrolled
for Fall: *63* • Total Graduates: *83*

FINANCES

Residential Annual Tuition: *$264* • Non-Residential Annual
Tuition: *$3,096* • General Institution Fees: *$110* •
Additional Nursing Fees: *$44*

LOS ANGELES COMMUNITY COLLEGE OF NURSING AND ALLIED HEALTH

Address: 1200 N State St Muir Hall 114, Los Angeles, CA
          90033
Phone: 323-226-4911
Fax: 323-226-5835
Contact: Nancy Miller, MSN, RN, Director and Dean
Email: Not Reported

GENERAL INFORMATION

Type of School: *Not Reported* • Accreditation: *Not Reported* •
Total Enrollment: *Not Reported*

PROGRAM INFORMATION

LPN/LVN Exit: *Not Reported* • NLNAC Accreditation: *Not
Reported*

NURSING STUDENT PROFILE

Total Nursing Enrollment: *152* • Full-Time Enrollment: *18* •
Part-Time Enrollment: *134* • Female Enrollment: *120* • Male
Enrollment: *32* • Total New Admissions Who Enrolled for
Fall: *Not Reported* • Total Graduates: *75*

FINANCES

Residential Annual Tuition: *$2,400* • Non-Residential
Annual Tuition: *$2,400* • General Institution Fees: *$125* •
Additional Nursing Fees: *Not Reported*

LOS ANGELES HARBOR COLLEGE

Address: 1111 Figueroa Place, Wilmington, CA 90744
Phone: 310-522-8341
Fax: 310-522-8440
Contact: Wendy W. Hollis, RN, MN, Chairperson
Email: hollisww@lahc.cc.ca.us

GENERAL INFORMATION

Type of School: *2-Year College or University, Public* •
Accreditation: *Western Association of Schools and Colleges* •
Total Enrollment: *5800*

PROGRAM INFORMATION

LPN/LVN Exit: *No* • NLNAC Accreditation: *Yes*

NURSING STUDENT PROFILE

Total Nursing Enrollment: *148* • Full-Time Enrollment:
148 • Part-Time Enrollment: *0* • Female Enrollment: *134* •
Male Enrollment: *14* • Total New Admissions Who Enrolled
for Fall: *56* • Total Graduates: *42*

FINANCES

Residential Annual Tuition: *$576* • Non-Residential Annual
Tuition: *$5,088* • General Institution Fees: *$22* • Additional
Nursing Fees: *$50*

LOS ANGELES PIERCE COLLEGE

Address: Los Angeles Pierce College, Woodlands Hills, CA
           91371
Phone: 818-710-2963
Fax: 818-710-4386
Contact: Marcia Solomon, EdD, RN, Director and
           Chairperson
Email: solomonms@pierce.laccd.edu

GENERAL INFORMATION

Type of School: *2-Year College or University, Public* •
Accreditation: *Western Association of Schools and Colleges* •
Total Enrollment: *18000*

PROGRAM INFORMATION

LPN/LVN Exit: *No* • NLNAC Accreditation: *Yes*

NURSING STUDENT PROFILE

Total Nursing Enrollment: *136* • Full-Time Enrollment:
136 • Part-Time Enrollment: *0* • Female Enrollment: *130* •
Male Enrollment: *6* • Total New Admissions Who Enrolled
for Fall: *46* • Total Graduates: *60*

FINANCES

Residential Annual Tuition: *$576* • Non-Residential Annual
Tuition: *$5,344* • General Institution Fees: *$0* • Additional
Nursing Fees: *$0*

LOS ANGELES SOUTHWEST COLLEGE

Address: 1600 West Imperial Highway, Los Angeles, CA
            90047
Phone: 323-241-5461
Fax: 323-241-5405
Contact: Jo Ann Williams, MN, RN, Department
            Chairperson and Director
Email: Williajt@lasc.cc.ca.us

GENERAL INFORMATION

Type of School: *Other* • Accreditation: *Western Association of Schools and Colleges* • Total Enrollment: *7029*

PROGRAM INFORMATION

LPN/LVN Exit: *No* • NLNAC Accreditation: *Not Reported*

NURSING STUDENT PROFILE

Total Nursing Enrollment: *180* • Full-Time Enrollment: *180* • Part-Time Enrollment: *0* • Female Enrollment: *161* • Male Enrollment: *19* • Total New Admissions Who Enrolled for Fall: *44* • Total Graduates: *70*

FINANCES

Residential Annual Tuition: *$352* • Non-Residential Annual Tuition: *$4,864* • General Institution Fees: *Not Reported* • Additional Nursing Fees: *$25*

LOS ANGELES TRADE-TECHNICAL COLLEGE

Address: 400 West Washington Boulevard, Los Angeles,
            CA 90015
Phone: 213-744-9453
Fax: 213-748-7334
Contact: Gladys Smith, RN, MN, Associate Dean
Email: gladysgsmith@laccd.cc.ca.us

GENERAL INFORMATION

Type of School: *2-Year College or University, Public* • Accreditation: *Western Association of Schools and Colleges* • Total Enrollment: *14000*

PROGRAM INFORMATION

LPN/LVN Exit: *Yes* • NLNAC Accreditation: *Yes*

NURSING STUDENT PROFILE

Total Nursing Enrollment: *119* • Full-Time Enrollment: *119* • Part-Time Enrollment: *0* • Female Enrollment: *102* • Male Enrollment: *17* • Total New Admissions Who Enrolled for Fall: *36* • Total Graduates: *36*

FINANCES

Residential Annual Tuition: *$240* • Non-Residential Annual Tuition: *$3,000* • General Institution Fees: *$33* • Additional Nursing Fees: *$100*

LOS ANGELES VALLEY COLLEGE

Address: 5800 Fulton Avenue, Van Nuys, CA 91401-4062
Phone: 818-947-2847
Fax: 818-947-2850
Contact: Gina M. Aguirre, MSN, RN, Chair and Director, Nursing Program
Email: gina_m._aguirre@laccd.cc.ca.us

GENERAL INFORMATION

Type of School: *2-Year College or University, Public* •
Accreditation: *Western Association of Schools and Colleges* •
Total Enrollment: *17000*

PROGRAM INFORMATION

LPN/LVN Exit: *No* • NLNAC Accreditation: *Yes*

NURSING STUDENT PROFILE

Total Nursing Enrollment: *160* • Full-Time Enrollment: *160* • Part-Time Enrollment: *0* • Female Enrollment: *136* • Male Enrollment: *24* • Total New Admissions Who Enrolled for Fall: *85* • Total Graduates: *85*

FINANCES

Residential Annual Tuition: *$330* • Non-Residential Annual Tuition: *$4,290* • General Institution Fees: *Not Reported* • Additional Nursing Fees: *$1,500*

LOS MEDANOS COLLEGE

Address: 2700 East Leland Road, Pittsburg, CA 94565
Phone: 925-439-2181
Fax: 925-439-5649
Contact: Elisabeth V. Coats, MSN, RN, ADN Director
Email: ecoats@losmedanos.net

GENERAL INFORMATION

Type of School: *2-Year College or University, Public* •
Accreditation: *Western Association of Schools and Colleges* •
Total Enrollment: *9800*

PROGRAM INFORMATION

LPN/LVN Exit: *No* • NLNAC Accreditation: *Yes*

NURSING STUDENT PROFILE

Total Nursing Enrollment: *81* • Full-Time Enrollment: *81* • Part-Time Enrollment: *0* • Female Enrollment: *71* • Male Enrollment: *10* • Total New Admissions Who Enrolled for Fall: *33* • Total Graduates: *39*

FINANCES

Residential Annual Tuition: *$330* • Non-Residential Annual Tuition: *$4,020* • General Institution Fees: *Not Reported* • Additional Nursing Fees: *$18*

MERCED COLLEGE

Address: 3600 M Street, Merced, CA 95348-2898
Phone: 209-384-6133
Fax: Not Reported
Contact: Mary Ann Duncan, MSN, RN, RN Program
   Director
Email: duncanm@merced.cc.ca.us

GENERAL INFORMATION

Type of School: *2-Year College or University, Public* •
Accreditation: *Western Association of Schools and Colleges* •
Total Enrollment: *6000*

PROGRAM INFORMATION

LPN/LVN Exit: *No* • NLNAC Accreditation: *Not Reported*

NURSING STUDENT PROFILE

Total Nursing Enrollment: *46* • Full-Time Enrollment: *46* •
Part-Time Enrollment: *0* • Female Enrollment: *42* • Male
Enrollment: *4* • Total New Admissions Who Enrolled for
Fall: *34* • Total Graduates: *17*

FINANCES

Residential Annual Tuition: *$576* • Non-Residential Annual
Tuition: *$6,176* • General Institution Fees: *$40* • Additional
Nursing Fees: *$15*

MERRITT COLLEGE

Address: 12500 Campus Drive, Oakland, CA 94619
Phone: 510-436-2433
Fax: Not Reported
Contact: Patricia A Dudley, MS, BS, RN, Director
Email: pdudley@concentric.net

GENERAL INFORMATION

Type of School: *2-Year College or University, Public* •
Accreditation: *Western Association of Schools and Colleges* •
Total Enrollment: *6000*

PROGRAM INFORMATION

LPN/LVN Exit: *Not Reported* • NLNAC Accreditation: *Not
Reported*

NURSING STUDENT PROFILE

Total Nursing Enrollment: *Not Reported* • Full-Time
Enrollment: *Not Reported* • Part-Time Enrollment: *Not
Reported* • Female Enrollment: *Not Reported* • Male
Enrollment: *Not Reported* • Total New Admissions Who
Enrolled for Fall: *Not Reported* • Total Graduates: *Not
Reported*

FINANCES

Residential Annual Tuition: *Not Reported* • Non-Residential
Annual Tuition: *Not Reported* • General Institution Fees: *Not
Reported* • Additional Nursing Fees: *Not Reported*

MODESTO JUNIOR COLLEGE

Address: 435 Colege Avenue, Modesto, CA 95350-9977
Phone: 209-575-6384
Fax: 209-575-6593
Contact: Teryl M. Ward, MSN, RN, Interim Director of
           Nursing
Email: wardt@yosemite.cc.ca.us

GENERAL INFORMATION

Type of School: *2-Year College or University, Public* •
Accreditation: *Western Association of Schools and Colleges* •
Total Enrollment: *15000*

PROGRAM INFORMATION

LPN/LVN Exit: *No* • NLNAC Accreditation: *Not Reported*

NURSING STUDENT PROFILE

Total Nursing Enrollment: *147* • Full-Time Enrollment:
147 • Part-Time Enrollment: *0* • Female Enrollment: *123* •
Male Enrollment: *24* • Total New Admissions Who Enrolled
for Fall: *49* • Total Graduates: *84*

FINANCES

Residential Annual Tuition: *$330* • Non-Residential Annual
Tuition: *$4,020* • General Institution Fees: *Not Reported* •
Additional Nursing Fees: *Not Reported*

MONTEREY PENINSULA COLLEGE

Address: 980 Fremont Street, Monterey, CA 93940
Phone: 831-646-4258
Fax: 831-645-1325
Contact: Debra Schulte, MSN, RN, Director
Email: debra_schulte@mpc.cc.ca.us

GENERAL INFORMATION

Type of School: *2-Year College or University, Public* •
Accreditation: *Western Association of Schools and Colleges* •
Total Enrollment: *6500*

PROGRAM INFORMATION

LPN/LVN Exit: *No* • NLNAC Accreditation: *Yes*

NURSING STUDENT PROFILE

Total Nursing Enrollment: *94* • Full-Time Enrollment: *94* •
Part-Time Enrollment: *0* • Female Enrollment: *79* • Male
Enrollment: *15* • Total New Admissions Who Enrolled for
Fall: *48* • Total Graduates: *34*

FINANCES

Residential Annual Tuition: *$216* • Non-Residential Annual
Tuition: *$2,160* • General Institution Fees: *$44* • Additional
Nursing Fees: *$0*

MOORPARK COLLEGE

Address: 7075 Campus Drive, Moorpark, CA 93021
Phone: 805-378-1433
Fax: 805-378-1548
Contact: Denise J. Byrne, RN, BSN, MSN, Coordinator
            of Health Sciences
Email: dbyrne@vcccd.net

GENERAL INFORMATION

Type of School: *2-Year College or University, Public* •
Accreditation: *Western Association of Schools and Colleges* •
Total Enrollment: *12849*

PROGRAM INFORMATION

LPN/LVN Exit: *No* • NLNAC Accreditation: *Yes*

NURSING STUDENT PROFILE

Total Nursing Enrollment: *115* • Full-Time Enrollment:
115 • Part-Time Enrollment: *0* • Female Enrollment: *106* •
Male Enrollment: *9* • Total New Admissions Who Enrolled
for Fall: *33* • Total Graduates: *Not Reported*

FINANCES

Residential Annual Tuition: *$576* • Non-Residential Annual
Tuition: *$5,344*• General Institution Fees: *Not Reported* •
Additional Nursing Fees: *Not Reported*

MOUNT SAN JACINTO COLLEGE

Address: 28237 La Piedra Road, Menifee, CA 92584
Phone: 909-672-6752
Fax: 909-672-6954
Contact: Wayne Boyer, MSN, RN, Director
Email: wboyer@msjc.cc.ca.us

GENERAL INFORMATION

Type of School: *2-Year College or University, Public* •
Accreditation: *Western Association of Schools and Colleges* •
Total Enrollment: *10000*

PROGRAM INFORMATION

LPN/LVN Exit: *No* • NLNAC Accreditation: *Not Reported*

NURSING STUDENT PROFILE

Total Nursing Enrollment: *61* • Full-Time Enrollment: *61* •
Part-Time Enrollment: *0* • Female Enrollment: *56* • Male
Enrollment: *5* • Total New Admissions Who Enrolled for
Fall: *12* • Total Graduates: *16*

FINANCES

Residential Annual Tuition: *$352* • Non-Residential Annual
Tuition: *$4,480* • General Institution Fees: *$0* • Additional
Nursing Fees: *$0*

MT. SAN ANTONIO COLLEGE

Address: 1100 Grand Avenue, Walnut, CA 91789
Phone: 909-594-5611
Fax: Not Reported
Contact: Genene Arvidson-Perkins, MSN, RN, PHN,
             Chair and Director
Email: garvidso@ibm.mtsac.edu

GENERAL INFORMATION

Type of School: *2-Year College or University, Public* •
Accreditation: *Western Association of Schools and Colleges* •
Total Enrollment: *23619*

PROGRAM INFORMATION

LPN/LVN Exit: *No* • NLNAC Accreditation: *Not Reported*

NURSING STUDENT PROFILE

Total Nursing Enrollment: *117* • Full-Time Enrollment:
117 • Part-Time Enrollment: *0* • Female Enrollment: *103* •
Male Enrollment: *14* • Total New Admissions Who Enrolled
for Fall: *40* • Total Graduates: *38*

FINANCES

Residential Annual Tuition: *$144* • Non-Residential Annual
Tuition: *$1,500* • General Institution Fees: *$12* • Additional
Nursing Fees: *$143*

NAPA VALLEY COLLEGE

Address: 2277 Napa/Vallejo Highway, Napa, CA 94558
Phone: 707-253-3142
Fax: 707-259-8933
Contact: Margaret M. Craig, RN, MS, Assistant Dean
Email: mcraig@campus.nvc.cc.ca.us

GENERAL INFORMATION

Type of School: *2-Year College or University, Public* •
Accreditation: *Western Association of Schools and Colleges* •
Total Enrollment: *9000*

PROGRAM INFORMATION

LPN/LVN Exit: *No* • NLNAC Accreditation: *Not Reported*

NURSING STUDENT PROFILE

Total Nursing Enrollment: *93* • Full-Time Enrollment: *93* •
Part-Time Enrollment: *0* • Female Enrollment: *81* • Male
Enrollment: *12* • Total New Admissions Who Enrolled for
Fall: *55* • Total Graduates: *43*

FINANCES

Residential Annual Tuition: *$330* • Non-Residential Annual
Tuition: *$3,960* • General Institution Fees: *$1* • Additional
Nursing Fees: *$120*

OHLONE COLLEGE

Address: 43600 Mission Boulevard, Fremont, CA 94538
Phone: 510-659-6030
Fax: 510-659-6070
Contact: Sharlene Limon, MN, RN, Dean
Email: slimon@ahlone.cc.ca.us

GENERAL INFORMATION

Type of School: *2-Year College or University, Public* •
Accreditation: *Western Association of Schools and Colleges* •
Total Enrollment: *Not Reported*

PROGRAM INFORMATION

LPN/LVN Exit: *No* • NLNAC Accreditation: *Yes*

NURSING STUDENT PROFILE

Total Nursing Enrollment: *79* • Full-Time Enrollment: *79* •
Part-Time Enrollment: *0* • Female Enrollment: *68* • Male
Enrollment: *11* • Total New Admissions Who Enrolled for
Fall: *22* • Total Graduates: *40*

FINANCES

Residential Annual Tuition: *$330* • Non-Residential Annual
Tuition: *$4,320* • General Institution Fees: *$0* • Additional
Nursing Fees: *$0*

PACIFIC UNION COLLEGE

Address: One Angwin Avenue, Angwin, CA 94508
Phone: 707-965-7262
Fax: 707-965-6499
Contact: Julia L. Pearce, PhD, Chair, Department of
          Nursing
Email: jlpearce@puc.edu

GENERAL INFORMATION

Type of School: *Not Reported* • Accreditation: *None* • Total
Enrollment: *Not Reported*

PROGRAM INFORMATION

LPN/LVN Exit: *Not Reported* • NLNAC Accreditation: *Yes*

NURSING STUDENT PROFILE

Total Nursing Enrollment: *138* • Full-Time Enrollment:
136 • Part-Time Enrollment: *2* • Female Enrollment: *116* •
Male Enrollment: *22* • Total New Admissions Who Enrolled
for Fall: *74* • Total Graduates: *58*

FINANCES

Residential Annual Tuition: *$14,105* • Non-Residential
Annual Tuition: *$14,105* • General Institution Fees: *$150* •
Additional Nursing Fees: *Not Reported*

PALOMAR COLLEGE

Address: 1140 West Mission Road, San Marcos, CA
92069-1487
Phone: 760-744-1150
Fax: 760-744-8123
Contact: Kathleen G. Clyne, RN, MR, Chairperson/
Associate Professor
Email: kclyne@palomar.edu

GENERAL INFORMATION

Type of School: *Not Reported* • Accreditation: *Western Association of Schools and Colleges* • Total Enrollment: *27904*

PROGRAM INFORMATION

LPN/LVN Exit: *No* • NLNAC Accreditation: *Yes*

NURSING STUDENT PROFILE

Total Nursing Enrollment: *115* • Full-Time Enrollment: *115* • Part-Time Enrollment: *0* • Female Enrollment: *104* • Male Enrollment: *11* • Total New Admissions Who Enrolled for Fall: *37* • Total Graduates: *54*

FINANCES

Residential Annual Tuition: *$991* • Non-Residential Annual Tuition: *$1,595* • General Institution Fees: *$0* • Additional Nursing Fees: *$15*

PASADENA CITY COLLEGE

Address: 1570 East Colorado Boulevard, Pasadena, CA
91106-2003
Phone: 626-484-7324
Fax: 626-585-7977
Contact: Kathryn Meglitsch-Tate, MSN, RN, ADN
Program Director
Email: Kameglitsch-Tate@paccd.cc.ca.us

GENERAL INFORMATION

Type of School: *2-Year College or University, Public* • Accreditation: *Western Association of Schools and Colleges* • Total Enrollment: *29000*

PROGRAM INFORMATION

LPN/LVN Exit: *No* • NLNAC Accreditation: *Yes*

NURSING STUDENT PROFILE

Total Nursing Enrollment: *201* • Full-Time Enrollment: *201* • Part-Time Enrollment: *0* • Female Enrollment: *163* • Male Enrollment: *38* • Total New Admissions Who Enrolled for Fall: *64* • Total Graduates: *67*

FINANCES

Residential Annual Tuition: *$264* • Non-Residential Annual Tuition: *$3,120* • General Institution Fees: *$152* • Additional Nursing Fees: *$415*

RIO HONDO COLLEGE

Address: 3600 Workman Mill Road, Whittier, CA 90601
Phone: 562-692-0921
Fax: 562-699-4110
Contact: Marcia McCormick, MEd, MSN, RN, Director
Email: mmccormick@rh.cc.ca.us

RIVERSIDE COMMUNITY COLLEGE

Address: 4800 Magnolia Avenue, Riverside, CA 92506-1299
Phone: 909-222-8408
Fax: 909-222-8745
Contact: Donna Schutte, DNSc, RN, Dean and Director
Email: dschutte@rccd.cc.ca.us

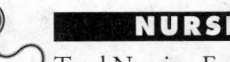

GENERAL INFORMATION

Type of School: *2-Year College or University, Public* •
Accreditation: *Western Association of Schools and Colleges* •
Total Enrollment: *15000*

GENERAL INFORMATION

Type of School: *2-Year College or University, Public* •
Accreditation: *Western Association of Schools and Colleges* •
Total Enrollment: *27406*

PROGRAM INFORMATION

LPN/LVN Exit: *No* • NLNAC Accreditation: *Not Reported*

PROGRAM INFORMATION

LPN/LVN Exit: *No* • NLNAC Accreditation: *Yes*

NURSING STUDENT PROFILE

Total Nursing Enrollment: *92* • Full-Time Enrollment: *92* •
Part-Time Enrollment: *0* • Female Enrollment: *72* • Male
Enrollment: *20* • Total New Admissions Who Enrolled for
Fall: *44* • Total Graduates: *46*

NURSING STUDENT PROFILE

Total Nursing Enrollment: *209* • Full-Time Enrollment:
209 • Part-Time Enrollment: *0* • Female Enrollment: *179* •
Male Enrollment: *30* • Total New Admissions Who Enrolled
for Fall: *87* • Total Graduates: *110*

FINANCES

Residential Annual Tuition: *$330* • Non-Residential Annual
Tuition: *$3,750* • General Institution Fees: *$24* • Additional
Nursing Fees: *$0*

FINANCES

Residential Annual Tuition: *$352* • Non-Residential Annual
Tuition: *$4,288* • General Institution Fees: *$120* •
Additional Nursing Fees: *$0*

SACRAMENTO CITY COLLEGE

Address: 3835 Freeport Boulevard, Sacramento, CA
95822
Phone: 916-558-2275
Fax: Not Reported
Contact: Diane D. Welch, MSN, RN, Director
Email: welchd@mail.xcc.losrios.cc.ca.us

GENERAL INFORMATION

Type of School: *2-Year College or University, Public* •
Accreditation: *Western Association of Schools and Colleges* •
Total Enrollment: *2500*

PROGRAM INFORMATION

LPN/LVN Exit: *No* • NLNAC Accreditation: *Not Reported*

NURSING STUDENT PROFILE

Total Nursing Enrollment: *114* • Full-Time Enrollment:
114 • Part-Time Enrollment: *0* • Female Enrollment: *95* •
Male Enrollment: *19* • Total New Admissions Who Enrolled
for Fall: *30* • Total Graduates: *49*

FINANCES

Residential Annual Tuition: *$121* • Non-Residential Annual
Tuition: *$1,375* • General Institution Fees: *$0* • Additional
Nursing Fees: *$25*

SADDLEBACK COLLEGE

Address: 28000 Marguerite Parkway, Mission Viejo, CA
92692
Phone: 949-582-7324
Fax: 949-347-1533
Contact: Julie Bright, MSN, RN, Dean and Director
Email: jbright@saddleback.cc.ca.us

GENERAL INFORMATION

Type of School: *2-Year College or University, Public* •
Accreditation: *Western Association of Schools and Colleges* •
Total Enrollment: *23135*

PROGRAM INFORMATION

LPN/LVN Exit: *No* • NLNAC Accreditation: *Yes*

NURSING STUDENT PROFILE

Total Nursing Enrollment: *175* • Full-Time Enrollment:
173 • Part-Time Enrollment: *2* • Female Enrollment: *159* •
Male Enrollment: *16* • Total New Admissions Who Enrolled
for Fall: *55* • Total Graduates: *97*

FINANCES

Residential Annual Tuition: *$352* • Non-Residential Annual
Tuition: *$4,000* • General Institution Fees: *$31* • Additional
Nursing Fees: *$100*

SAN BERNARDINO VALLEY COLLEGE

Address: 701 Mount Vernon Avenue, San Bernardino, CA 92410
Phone: 909-888-6511
Fax: 909-885-7312
Contact: Arlene H. Johnson, MS, RN, Dean
Email: ajohnson@sbccd.cc.ca.us

GENERAL INFORMATION

Type of School: *2-Year College or University, Public* •
Accreditation: *Western Association of Schools and Colleges* •
Total Enrollment: *12000*

PROGRAM INFORMATION

LPN/LVN Exit: *No* • NLNAC Accreditation: *Yes*

NURSING STUDENT PROFILE

Total Nursing Enrollment: *195* • Full-Time Enrollment:
195 • Part-Time Enrollment: *0* • Female Enrollment: *158* •
Male Enrollment: *37* • Total New Admissions Who Enrolled
for Fall: *39* • Total Graduates: *66*

FINANCES

Residential Annual Tuition: *$231* • Non-Residential Annual
Tuition: *$2,961* • General Institution Fees: *$33* • Additional
Nursing Fees: *$33*

SAN DIEGO CITY COLLEGE

Address: 1313-12th Avenue, San Diego, CA 92101
Phone: 619-388-3439
Fax: 619-388-3821
Contact: Jo-Ann L. Rossitto, DNS, RNc, Associate Dean
          and Director
Email: jrossitt@sdccd.net

GENERAL INFORMATION

Type of School: *2-Year College or University, Public* •
Accreditation: *Western Association of Schools and Colleges* •
Total Enrollment: *14135*

PROGRAM INFORMATION

LPN/LVN Exit: *Not Reported* • NLNAC Accreditation: *Yes*

NURSING STUDENT PROFILE

Total Nursing Enrollment: *103* • Full-Time Enrollment:
103 • Part-Time Enrollment: *0* • Female Enrollment: *79* •
Male Enrollment: *24* • Total New Admissions Who Enrolled
for Fall: *50* • Total Graduates: *46*

FINANCES

Residential Annual Tuition: *$132* • Non-Residential Annual
Tuition: *$1,440* • General Institution Fees: *$74* • Additional
Nursing Fees: *$126*

Circle 107 on reader card   **See in-depth profile for more information**

SAN JOAQUIN DELTA COLLEGE

Address: 5151 Pacific Avenue, Stokton, CA 95207
Phone: 209-954-5516
Fax: 209-954-5514
Contact: Debra Lewis, MSN, RN, Director of Health
           Sciences
Email: dlewis@deltacollege.org

GENERAL INFORMATION

Type of School: *2-Year College or University, Public* •
Accreditation: *Western Association of Schools and Colleges* •
Total Enrollment: *18546*

PROGRAM INFORMATION

LPN/LVN Exit: *No* • NLNAC Accreditation: *Yes*

NURSING STUDENT PROFILE

Total Nursing Enrollment: *181* • Full-Time Enrollment:
181 • Part-Time Enrollment: *0* • Female Enrollment: *158* •
Male Enrollment: *23* • Total New Admissions Who Enrolled
for Fall: *61* • Total Graduates: *81*

FINANCES

Residential Annual Tuition: *$402* • Non-Residential Annual
Tuition: *$5,439* • General Institution Fees: *$0* • Additional
Nursing Fees: *$250*

SAN JOSE/EVERGREEN COMMUNITY COLLEGE DISTRICT

Address: 3095 Yerba Buena Road, San Jose, CA 95135
Phone: 408-270-6448
Fax: 408-528-1267
Contact: LaZelle Westbrook, MA, RN, Interim Director,
           Nursing Education
Email: lazelle.westbrook@sjeccd.cc.ca.us

GENERAL INFORMATION

Type of School: *2-Year College or University, Public* •
Accreditation: *Western Association of Schools and Colleges* •
Total Enrollment: *10500*

PROGRAM INFORMATION

LPN/LVN Exit: *No* • NLNAC Accreditation: *Yes*

NURSING STUDENT PROFILE

Total Nursing Enrollment: *100* • Full-Time Enrollment:
100 • Part-Time Enrollment: *0* • Female Enrollment: *92* •
Male Enrollment: *8* • Total New Admissions Who Enrolled
for Fall: *60* • Total Graduates: *34*

FINANCES

Residential Annual Tuition: *$330* • Non-Residential Annual
Tuition: *$4,080* • General Institution Fees: *$10* • Additional
Nursing Fees: *$30*

SANTA ANA COLLEGE

Address: 1530 West 17th Street, Santa Ana, CA 92706
Phone: 714-564-6839
Fax: 714-564-6344
Contact: Carol Comeau, MSN, RN, Director
Email: comeau_carol@rsccd.org

GENERAL INFORMATION

Type of School: *2-Year College or University, Public* •
Accreditation: *Western Association of Schools and Colleges* •
Total Enrollment: *17000*

PROGRAM INFORMATION

LPN/LVN Exit: *No* • NLNAC Accreditation: *Yes*

NURSING STUDENT PROFILE

Total Nursing Enrollment: *137* • Full-Time Enrollment: *137* • Part-Time Enrollment: *0* • Female Enrollment: *105* • Male Enrollment: *32* • Total New Admissions Who Enrolled for Fall: *36* • Total Graduates: *71*

FINANCES

Residential Annual Tuition: *$352* • Non-Residential Annual Tuition: *$1,600* • General Institution Fees: *$15* • Additional Nursing Fees: *$30*

SANTA BARBARA CITY COLLEGE

Address: 721 Clif Drive, Santa Barbara, CA 93109-2312
Phone: 805-965-0581
Fax: 805-963-7222
Contact: Jan Anderson, RN, BSN, MSN, Director
Email: adersoj@sbcc.net

GENERAL INFORMATION

Type of School: *2-Year College or University, Public* •
Accreditation: *Western Association of Schools and Colleges* •
Total Enrollment: *14957*

PROGRAM INFORMATION

LPN/LVN Exit: *No* • NLNAC Accreditation: *Yes*

NURSING STUDENT PROFILE

Total Nursing Enrollment: *102* • Full-Time Enrollment: *102* • Part-Time Enrollment: *0* • Female Enrollment: *92* • Male Enrollment: *10* • Total New Admissions Who Enrolled for Fall: *42* • Total Graduates: *29*

FINANCES

Residential Annual Tuition: *$264* • Non-Residential Annual Tuition: *$3,000* • General Institution Fees: *$24* • Additional Nursing Fees: *$132*

SANTA CLARITA COMMUNITY COLLEGE DISTRICT—COLLEGE OF THE CANYONS

Address: 26455 Rockwell Canyon Road, Santa Clarita, CA 91355
Phone: 661-255-7438
Fax: 661-255-7438
Contact: Sue Albert, MSN, RN, MHA, Assistant Dean of Allied Health
Email: albert_a@mail.coc.cc.ca.us

GENERAL INFORMATION

Type of School: *2-Year College or University, Public* •
Accreditation: *Western Association of Schools and Colleges* •
Total Enrollment: *1200*

PROGRAM INFORMATION

LPN/LVN Exit: *Yes* • NLNAC Accreditation: *Yes*

NURSING STUDENT PROFILE

Total Nursing Enrollment: *75* • Full-Time Enrollment: *75* •
Part-Time Enrollment: *0* • Female Enrollment: *68* • Male
Enrollment: *7* • Total New Admissions Who Enrolled for
Fall: *24* • Total Graduates: *45*

FINANCES

Residential Annual Tuition: *$268* • Non-Residential Annual
Tuition: *$3,000* • General Institution Fees: *$0* • Additional
Nursing Fees: *$0*

SANTA MONICA COLLEGE

Address: 1900 Pico Boulevard, Santa Monica, CA 90405
Phone: 310-434-3452
Fax: 310-434-3469
Contact: Marilyn J. Humphrey, MA, MPA, RN, Assistant Dean
Email: humphrey_marilyn@smc.edu

GENERAL INFORMATION

Type of School: *2-Year College or University, Public* •
Accreditation: *Western Association of Schools and Colleges* •
Total Enrollment: *30000*

PROGRAM INFORMATION

LPN/LVN Exit: *Yes* • NLNAC Accreditation: *Yes*

NURSING STUDENT PROFILE

Total Nursing Enrollment: *107* • Full-Time Enrollment:
107 • Part-Time Enrollment: *0* • Female Enrollment: *88* •
Male Enrollment: *19* • Total New Admissions Who Enrolled
for Fall: *30* • Total Graduates: *54*

FINANCES

Residential Annual Tuition: *$256* • Non-Residential Annual
Tuition: *$2,556* • General Institution Fees: *$150* •
Additional Nursing Fees: *$207*

SANTA ROSA JUNIOR COLLEGE

Address: 1501 Mendocino Drive, Santa Rosa, CA 95401
Phone: 707-527-4527
Fax: Not Reported
Contact: Marian O'Laughlin, MSN, RN, Director
Email: Not Reported

GENERAL INFORMATION

Type of School: *Other, Public* • Accreditation: *None* • Total Enrollment: *34000*

PROGRAM INFORMATION

LPN/LVN Exit: *Not Reported* • NLNAC Accreditation: *Not Reported*

NURSING STUDENT PROFILE

Total Nursing Enrollment: *Not Reported* • Full-Time Enrollment: *Not Reported* • Part-Time Enrollment: *Not Reported* • Female Enrollment: *Not Reported* • Male Enrollment: *Not Reported* • Total New Admissions Who Enrolled for Fall: *Not Reported* • Total Graduates: *Not Reported*

FINANCES

Residential Annual Tuition: *$576* • Non-Residential Annual Tuition: *$5,536* • General Institution Fees: *Not Reported* • Additional Nursing Fees: *Not Reported*

SHASTA COLLEGE

Address: 11555 Old Oregon Trail, Redding, CA 96049-6006
Phone: 530-225-4725
Fax: 530-225-4780
Contact: Jan Dinkel, MSN, RN, Dean, Center for Human Development
Email: jdinkel@shastacollege.edu

GENERAL INFORMATION

Type of School: *2-Year College or University, Public* • Accreditation: *Western Association of Schools and Colleges* • Total Enrollment: *14000*

PROGRAM INFORMATION

LPN/LVN Exit: *No* • NLNAC Accreditation: *Not Reported*

NURSING STUDENT PROFILE

Total Nursing Enrollment: *50* • Full-Time Enrollment: *50* • Part-Time Enrollment: *0* • Female Enrollment: *35* • Male Enrollment: *15* • Total New Admissions Who Enrolled for Fall: *20* • Total Graduates: *50*

FINANCES

Residential Annual Tuition: *$330* • Non-Residential Annual Tuition: *$4,230* • General Institution Fees: *$48* • Additional Nursing Fees: *$950*

SIERRA COLLEGE

Address: Sierra College, Rocklin, CA 95677
Phone: 916-781-6221
Fax: Not Reported
Contact: Margaret White, MSN, RN, Associate Dean
Email: mwhite@scmail.sierra.cc.ca.us

GENERAL INFORMATION

Type of School: *2-Year College or University, Public* •
Accreditation: *Western Association of Schools and Colleges* •
Total Enrollment: *17000*

PROGRAM INFORMATION

LPN/LVN Exit: *No* • NLNAC Accreditation: *Not Reported*

NURSING STUDENT PROFILE

Total Nursing Enrollment: *85* • Full-Time Enrollment: *67* •
Part-Time Enrollment: *18* • Female Enrollment: *74* • Male
Enrollment: *11* • Total New Admissions Who Enrolled for
Fall: *40* • Total Graduates: *Not Reported*

FINANCES

Residential Annual Tuition: *$576* • Non-Residential Annual
Tuition: *$4,768* • General Institution Fees: *Not Reported* •
Additional Nursing Fees: *Not Reported*

SOLANO COMMUNITY COLLEGE

Address: 4000 Suisun Valley Road, Suisun, CA 94585-
            3197
Phone: 707-864-7000
Fax: 707-863-7803
Contact: Faith Zobel, MSN, RN, Dean
Email: fzobel@solano.cc.ca.us

GENERAL INFORMATION

Type of School: *2-Year College or University, Public* •
Accreditation: *Western Association of Schools and Colleges* •
Total Enrollment: *11000*

PROGRAM INFORMATION

LPN/LVN Exit: *Yes* • NLNAC Accreditation: *Not Reported*

NURSING STUDENT PROFILE

Total Nursing Enrollment: *78* • Full-Time Enrollment: *78* •
Part-Time Enrollment: *0* • Female Enrollment: *75* • Male
Enrollment: *3* • Total New Admissions Who Enrolled for
Fall: *78* • Total Graduates: *43*

FINANCES

Residential Annual Tuition: *$330* • Non-Residential Annual
Tuition: *$660* • General Institution Fees: *$11* • Additional
Nursing Fees: *$800*

SOUTH COUNTY COMMUNITY COLLEGE DISTRICT

Address: 7011 Koll Center Parkway, Suite 200, Pleasanton, CA 94566
Phone: 510-723-6871
Fax: 510-782-9315
Contact: Nancy Cowan, MSN, RN, EdD, Director
Email: ncowan@wpgate.clpccd.cc.ca.us

GENERAL INFORMATION

Type of School: *2-Year College or University, Public* •
Accreditation: *Western Association of Schools and Colleges* •
Total Enrollment: *22000*

PROGRAM INFORMATION

LPN/LVN Exit: *No* • NLNAC Accreditation: *Not Reported*

NURSING STUDENT PROFILE

Total Nursing Enrollment: *68* • Full-Time Enrollment: *68* •
Part-Time Enrollment: *0* • Female Enrollment: *60* • Male
Enrollment: *8* • Total New Admissions Who Enrolled for
Fall: *30* • Total Graduates: *25*

FINANCES

Residential Annual Tuition: *$264* • Non-Residential Annual
Tuition: *$3,408* • General Institution Fees: *$16* • Additional
Nursing Fees: *$50*

SOUTHWESTERN COLLEGE

Address: 900 Otay Lakes Road, Chula Vista, CA 91910-7299
Phone: 619-421-6700
Fax: 619-482-6439
Contact: Sandra A. Comstock, MSN, CNM, RNP, Director
Email: scomstock@swc.cc.ca.us

GENERAL INFORMATION

Type of School: *2-Year College or University, Public* •
Accreditation: *Western Association of Schools and Colleges* •
Total Enrollment: *19538*

PROGRAM INFORMATION

LPN/LVN Exit: *No* • NLNAC Accreditation: *Yes*

NURSING STUDENT PROFILE

Total Nursing Enrollment: *70* • Full-Time Enrollment: *0* •
Part-Time Enrollment: *70* • Female Enrollment: *57* • Male
Enrollment: *13* • Total New Admissions Who Enrolled for
Fall: *31* • Total Graduates: *26*

FINANCES

Residential Annual Tuition: *$215* • Non-Residential Annual
Tuition: *$2,827* • General Institution Fees: *$42* • Additional
Nursing Fees: *$182*

VENTURA COLLEGE

Address: 4667 Telegraph Road, Ventura, CA 93003
Phone: 805-654-6342
Fax: 805-654-6395
Contact: Joan Beem, MSN, RN, MSHS, Coordinator, Health Sciences
Email: jbeem@vcccd.net

GENERAL INFORMATION

Type of School: *Not Reported* • Accreditation: *Not Reported* • Total Enrollment: *Not Reported*

PROGRAM INFORMATION

LPN/LVN Exit: *No* • NLNAC Accreditation: *Not Reported*

NURSING STUDENT PROFILE

Total Nursing Enrollment: *158* • Full-Time Enrollment: *158* • Part-Time Enrollment: *0* • Female Enrollment: *143* • Male Enrollment: *15* • Total New Admissions Who Enrolled for Fall: *48* • Total Graduates: *67*

FINANCES

Residential Annual Tuition: *$330* • Non-Residential Annual Tuition: *$3,900* • General Institution Fees: *Not Reported* • Additional Nursing Fees: *Not Reported*

VICTOR VALLEY COLLEGE

Address: 18422 Bear Valley Road, Victorville, CA 92392
Phone: 760-245-4271
Fax: 760-951-5861
Contact: Patricia E. Green, MSN, RN, MA, Director of Nursing
Email: pgreen@victor.cc.ca.us

GENERAL INFORMATION

Type of School: *2-Year College or University, Public* • Accreditation: *Western Association of Schools and Colleges* • Total Enrollment: *11000*

PROGRAM INFORMATION

LPN/LVN Exit: *No* • NLNAC Accreditation: *Yes*

NURSING STUDENT PROFILE

Total Nursing Enrollment: *110* • Full-Time Enrollment: *110* • Part-Time Enrollment: *0* • Female Enrollment: *95* • Male Enrollment: *15* • Total New Admissions Who Enrolled for Fall: *35* • Total Graduates: *49*

FINANCES

Residential Annual Tuition: *$330* • Non-Residential Annual Tuition: *$3,900* • General Institution Fees: *$40* • Additional Nursing Fees: *$12*

YUBA COLLEGE

Address: 2088 North Beale Road, Marysville, CA 95901
Phone: 530-741-6785
Fax: Not Reported
Contact: Betty G Bonner, MSN, RN, Director of Nursing
Email: bbonner@ms.yuba.cc.ca.us

GENERAL INFORMATION

Type of School: *Not Reported* • Accreditation: *None* • Total Enrollment: *Not Reported*

PROGRAM INFORMATION

LPN/LVN Exit: *No* • NLNAC Accreditation: *Not Reported*

NURSING STUDENT PROFILE

Total Nursing Enrollment: *80* • Full-Time Enrollment: *80* • Part-Time Enrollment: *0* • Female Enrollment: *Not Reported* • Male Enrollment: *Not Reported* • Total New Admissions Who Enrolled for Fall: *50* • Total Graduates: *26*

FINANCES

Residential Annual Tuition: *$352* • Non-Residential Annual Tuition: *$5,088* • General Institution Fees: *Not Reported* • Additional Nursing Fees: *Not Reported*

ARAPAHOE COMMUNITY COLLEGE

Address: 5900 South Santa Fe Drive, Littleton, CO 80120
Phone: 303-797-5896
Fax: 303-797-5842
Contact: Linda Stroup, MScN, RN, Director, Nursing Program
Email: lstroup@arapahoe.edu

GENERAL INFORMATION

Type of School: *2-Year College or University, Public* • Accreditation: *North Central Association of Colleges and Schools* • Total Enrollment: *Not Reported*

PROGRAM INFORMATION

LPN/LVN Exit: *No* • NLNAC Accreditation: *Not Reported*

NURSING STUDENT PROFILE

Total Nursing Enrollment: *121* • Full-Time Enrollment: *121* • Part-Time Enrollment: *0* • Female Enrollment: *116* • Male Enrollment: *5* • Total New Admissions Who Enrolled for Fall: *62* • Total Graduates: *59*

FINANCES

Residential Annual Tuition: *$1,584* • Non-Residential Annual Tuition: *$7,068* • General Institution Fees: *$90* • Additional Nursing Fees: *$270*

COLORADO MOUNTAIN COLLEGE

Address: 3000 County Road 14, Glenwood Springs, CO 81601
Phone: 970-947-8251
Fax: 970-945-1227
Contact: Nancy Kuhrik, PhD, RN, Director of Nursing Program
Email: nkuhrik@coloradomtn.edu

GENERAL INFORMATION

Type of School: *2-Year College or University, Public* • Accreditation: *North Central Association of Colleges and Schools* • Total Enrollment: *20000*

PROGRAM INFORMATION

LPN/LVN Exit: *No* • NLNAC Accreditation: *Not Reported*

NURSING STUDENT PROFILE

Total Nursing Enrollment: *13* • Full-Time Enrollment: *13* • Part-Time Enrollment: *0* • Female Enrollment: *11* • Male Enrollment: *2* • Total New Admissions Who Enrolled for Fall: *13* • Total Graduates: *14*

FINANCES

Residential Annual Tuition: *$1,980* • Non-Residential Annual Tuition: *$6,450* • General Institution Fees: *$130* • Additional Nursing Fees: *$200*

COMMUNITY COLLEGE OF DENVER

Address: 1070 Yosemite Street, Denver, CO 80230
Phone: 303-365-8367
Fax: 303-365-8396
Contact: Vicki Earnest, RN, MS, Nursing Coordinator
Email: vicki.earnest@ccd.cccoes.edu

GENERAL INFORMATION

Type of School: *2-Year College or University, Public* • Accreditation: *North Central Association of Colleges and Schools* • Total Enrollment: *5452*

PROGRAM INFORMATION

LPN/LVN Exit: *Yes* • NLNAC Accreditation: *Not Reported*

NURSING STUDENT PROFILE

Total Nursing Enrollment: *138* • Full-Time Enrollment: *117* • Part-Time Enrollment: *21* • Female Enrollment: *115* • Male Enrollment: *23* • Total New Admissions Who Enrolled for Fall: *36* • Total Graduates: *39*

FINANCES

Residential Annual Tuition: *$1,862* • Non-Residential Annual Tuition: *$8,014* • General Institution Fees: *Not Reported* • Additional Nursing Fees: *$15*

FRONT RANGE COMMUNITY COLLEGE- FORT COLLINS

Address: 4616 South Fields, Fort Collins, CO 80526
Phone: 303-404-5202
Fax: Not Reported
Contact: Alma Mueller, RN, MED, Chair of Nursing
Email: Not Reported

GENERAL INFORMATION

Type of School: *Not Reported* • Accreditation: *Not Reported* •
Total Enrollment: *Not Reported*

PROGRAM INFORMATION

LPN/LVN Exit: *Yes* • NLNAC Accreditation: *Not Reported*

NURSING STUDENT PROFILE

Total Nursing Enrollment: *216* • Full-Time Enrollment:
206 • Part-Time Enrollment: *10* • Female Enrollment: *199* •
Male Enrollment: *17* • Total New Admissions Who Enrolled
for Fall: *75* • Total Graduates: *99*

FINANCES

Residential Annual Tuition: *$801* • Non-Residential Annual
Tuition: *$3,577* • General Institution Fees: *Not Reported* •
Additional Nursing Fees: *$200*

FRONT RANGE COMMUNITY COLLEGE- WESTMINSTER

Address: 3645 West 112th Avenue, Westiminster, CO
80031
Phone: 303-404-5202
Fax: Not Reported
Contact: Alma L. Mueller, MeD, RN, Program Chair
Email: fr_alma@ccs.ccoes.edu

GENERAL INFORMATION

Type of School: *2-Year College or University, Public* •
Accreditation: *North Central Association of Colleges and
Schools* • Total Enrollment: *13073*

PROGRAM INFORMATION

LPN/LVN Exit: *Yes* • NLNAC Accreditation: *Not Reported*

NURSING STUDENT PROFILE

Total Nursing Enrollment: *215* • Full-Time Enrollment:
202 • Part-Time Enrollment: *13* • Female Enrollment: *193* •
Male Enrollment: *22* • Total New Admissions Who Enrolled
for Fall: *75* • Total Graduates: *96*

FINANCES

Residential Annual Tuition: *$676* • Non-Residential Annual
Tuition: *$3,202* • General Institution Fees: *$73* • Additional
Nursing Fees: *$119*

MORGAN COMMUNITY COLLEGE—NORTHEASTERN JUNIOR COLLEGE

Address: 17800 Road South, Fort Morgan, CO 80701
Phone: 970-542-3235
Fax: Not Reported
Contact: Sheryl George, MSN, RN, Nursing Program
Coordinator
Email: sherylgeorge@mcc.cccoes.edu

GENERAL INFORMATION

Type of School: *2-Year College or University, Public* •
Accreditation: *North Central Association of Colleges and
Schools* • Total Enrollment: *1600*

PROGRAM INFORMATION

LPN/LVN Exit: *Not Reported* • NLNAC Accreditation: *Not
Reported*

NURSING STUDENT PROFILE

Total Nursing Enrollment: *11* • Full-Time Enrollment: *11* •
Part-Time Enrollment: *0* • Female Enrollment: *9* • Male
Enrollment: *2* • Total New Admissions Who Enrolled for
Fall: *13* • Total Graduates: *13*

FINANCES

Residential Annual Tuition: *$1,650* • Non-Residential
Annual Tuition: *$7,830* • General Institution Fees: *$200* •
Additional Nursing Fees: *$20*

OTERO JUNIOR COLLEGE

Address: 18th and Colorado, La Junta, CO 81050
Phone: 719-384-6894
Fax: Not Reported
Contact: Denise Root, RN, ADN, BSN, MSN,
Department Director
Email: denise.root@ojc.cccoes.edu

GENERAL INFORMATION

Type of School: *2-Year College or University, Public* •
Accreditation: *North Central Association of Colleges and
Schools* • Total Enrollment: *Not Reported*

PROGRAM INFORMATION

LPN/LVN Exit: *No* • NLNAC Accreditation: *Yes*

NURSING STUDENT PROFILE

Total Nursing Enrollment: *36* • Full-Time Enrollment: *34* •
Part-Time Enrollment: *2* • Female Enrollment: *32* • Male
Enrollment: *4* • Total New Admissions Who Enrolled for
Fall: *20* • Total Graduates: *23*

FINANCES

Residential Annual Tuition: *$1,553* • Non-Residential
Annual Tuition: *$6,659* • General Institution Fees: *$28* •
Additional Nursing Fees: *$70*

PIKES PEAK COMMUNITY COLLEGE

Address: 11195 Highway 83W-209, Colorado Springs, CO 80919
Phone: 719-538-5417
Fax: 719-538-5439
Contact: Mary Ann Wermers, MSN, RN, Nursing Program Coordinator
Email: mary-ann.wermers@ppcc.cccoes.edu

GENERAL INFORMATION

Type of School: *Other, Public* • Accreditation: *North Central Association of Colleges and Schools* • Total Enrollment: *Not Reported*

PROGRAM INFORMATION

LPN/LVN Exit: *Yes* • NLNAC Accreditation: *Not Reported*

NURSING STUDENT PROFILE

Total Nursing Enrollment: *108* • Full-Time Enrollment: *108* • Part-Time Enrollment: *0* • Female Enrollment: *Not Reported* • Male Enrollment: *Not Reported* • Total New Admissions Who Enrolled for Fall: *Not Reported* • Total Graduates: *Not Reported*

FINANCES

Residential Annual Tuition: *$2,113.60* • Non-Residential Annual Tuition: *$11,044.80* • General Institution Fees: *Not Reported* • Additional Nursing Fees: *Not Reported*

PUEBLO COMMUNITY COLLEGE

Address: 415 Harrison, Pueblo, CO 81004-1499
Phone: 719-549-3479
Fax: 719-549-3491
Contact: C.R. Dagnillo, RN, MS, CNS, Chair Nursing Department
Email: charles.dagnillo@pcc.cccoes.edu

GENERAL INFORMATION

Type of School: *2-Year College or University, Public* • Accreditation: *North Central Association of Colleges and Schools* • Total Enrollment: *787*

PROGRAM INFORMATION

LPN/LVN Exit: *Yes* • NLNAC Accreditation: *Yes*

NURSING STUDENT PROFILE

Total Nursing Enrollment: *64* • Full-Time Enrollment: *46* • Part-Time Enrollment: *18* • Female Enrollment: *55* • Male Enrollment: *9* • Total New Admissions Who Enrolled for Fall: *64* • Total Graduates: *46*

FINANCES

Residential Annual Tuition: *$2,013* • Non-Residential Annual Tuition: *$8,032* • General Institution Fees: *$59* • Additional Nursing Fees: *$3,666*

TRINDAD STATE JUNIOR COLLEGE

Address: 600 Prospect St., Box 150, Trinidad, CO 81082
Phone: 800-937-6884
Fax: Not Reported
Contact: Judie Stichel, MSN, RN, Coordinator
Email: Not Reported

GENERAL INFORMATION

Type of School: *Not Reported* • Accreditation: *Not Reported* • Total Enrollment: *Not Reported*

PROGRAM INFORMATION

LPN/LVN Exit: *Not Reported* • NLNAC Accreditation: *Not Reported*

NURSING STUDENT PROFILE

Total Nursing Enrollment: *Not Reported* • Full-Time Enrollment: *Not Reported* • Part-Time Enrollment: *Not Reported* • Female Enrollment: *Not Reported* • Male Enrollment: *Not Reported* • Total New Admissions Who Enrolled for Fall: *Not Reported* • Total Graduates: *Not Reported*

FINANCES

Residential Annual Tuition: *Not Reported* • Non-Residential Annual Tuition: *Not Reported* • General Institution Fees: *Not Reported* • Additional Nursing Fees: *Not Reported*

CAPITAL COMMUNITY-TECHNICAL COLLEGE

Address: 61 Woodland Street, Hartford, CT 06105
Phone: 860-906-5151
Fax: Not Reported
Contact: Cindy Adams, MSN, RN, Director, Division of Nursing and Health Careers
Email: cadams@ccc.commnet.edu

GENERAL INFORMATION

Type of School: *2-Year College or University, Public* • Accreditation: *New England Association of Schools and Colleges* • Total Enrollment: *2850*

PROGRAM INFORMATION

LPN/LVN Exit: *Not Reported* • NLNAC Accreditation: *Yes*

NURSING STUDENT PROFILE

Total Nursing Enrollment: *Not Reported* • Full-Time Enrollment: *Not Reported* • Part-Time Enrollment: *Not Reported* • Female Enrollment: *Not Reported* • Male Enrollment: *Not Reported* • Total New Admissions Who Enrolled for Fall: *Not Reported* • Total Graduates: *Not Reported*

FINANCES

Residential Annual Tuition: *$2,704* • Non-Residential Annual Tuition: *$8,112* • General Institution Fees: *Not Reported* • Additional Nursing Fees: *Not Reported*

NAUGATUCK VALLEY COMMUNITY COLLEGE

Address: 750 Chase Parkway, Waterbury, CT 06708
Phone: 203-575-8057
Fax: 203-575-8146
Contact: Patricia C. Bouffard, DNSc, RN, Director
Email: nv_bouffard@commnet.edu

GENERAL INFORMATION

Type of School: *2-Year College or University, Public* •
Accreditation: *New England Association of Schools and
Colleges* • Total Enrollment: *5054*

PROGRAM INFORMATION

LPN/LVN Exit: *No* • NLNAC Accreditation: *Yes*

NURSING STUDENT PROFILE

Total Nursing Enrollment: *148* • Full-Time Enrollment: *3* •
Part-Time Enrollment: *145* • Female Enrollment: *129* • Male
Enrollment: *19* • Total New Admissions Who Enrolled for
Fall: *79* • Total Graduates: *58*

FINANCES

Residential Annual Tuition: *$1,608* • Non-Residential
Annual Tuition: *$5,232* • General Institution Fees: *$103* •
Additional Nursing Fees: *Not Reported*

NORWALK COMMUNITY COLLEGE

Address: 188 Richards Ave., Norwalk, CT 06854
Phone: 203-857-7123
Fax: 203-857-3364
Contact: Mary E. Schuler, EdD, RN, Director of Nursing
             and Allied Health
Email: nk_schuler@commnet.edu

GENERAL INFORMATION

Type of School: *Not Reported* • Accreditation: *None* • Total
Enrollment: *Not Reported*

PROGRAM INFORMATION

LPN/LVN Exit: *No* • NLNAC Accreditation: *Yes*

NURSING STUDENT PROFILE

Total Nursing Enrollment: *82* • Full-Time Enrollment: *30* •
Part-Time Enrollment: *52* • Female Enrollment: *77* • Male
Enrollment: *5* • Total New Admissions Who Enrolled for
Fall: *55* • Total Graduates: *27*

FINANCES

Residential Annual Tuition: *$1,888* • Non-Residential
Annual Tuition: *$5,816* • General Institution Fees: *Not
Reported* • Additional Nursing Fees: *$60*

SAINT VINCENT'S COLLEGE

Address: 2800 Main Street, Bridgeport, CT 06606
Phone: 203-576-5556
Fax: 203-581-6533
Contact: Joanne R. Wolfertz, EdD, RN, Professor and Chair, Nursing
Email: jwolfertz@stvincentscollege.edu

GENERAL INFORMATION

Type of School: *2-Year College or University, Private (Religious)* • Accreditation: *New England Association of Schools and Colleges* • Total Enrollment: *317*

PROGRAM INFORMATION

LPN/LVN Exit: *No* • NLNAC Accreditation: *Yes*

NURSING STUDENT PROFILE

Total Nursing Enrollment: *144* • Full-Time Enrollment: *28* • Part-Time Enrollment: *116* • Female Enrollment: *131* • Male Enrollment: *13* • Total New Admissions Who Enrolled for Fall: *36* • Total Graduates: *38*

FINANCES

Residential Annual Tuition: *$8,990* • Non-Residential Annual Tuition: *Not Reported* • General Institution Fees: *$420* • Additional Nursing Fees: *Not Reported*

THREE RIVERS COMMUNITY COLLEGE

Address: Mohegan Campus, Mahan Drive, Norwich, CT 06360
Phone: 860-383-5241
Fax: 860-383-5271
Contact: Ann Branchini, MSN, RN, Director of Nursing and Allied Health
Email: abranchini@trcc.commnet.edu

GENERAL INFORMATION

Type of School: *2-Year College or University, Public* • Accreditation: *New England Association of Schools and Colleges* • Total Enrollment: *3507*

PROGRAM INFORMATION

LPN/LVN Exit: *No* • NLNAC Accreditation: *Yes*

NURSING STUDENT PROFILE

Total Nursing Enrollment: *117* • Full-Time Enrollment: *117* • Part-Time Enrollment: *0* • Female Enrollment: *108* • Male Enrollment: *9* • Total New Admissions Who Enrolled for Fall: *64* • Total Graduates: *30*

FINANCES

Residential Annual Tuition: *$1,680* • Non-Residential Annual Tuition: *$5,232* • General Institution Fees: *$208* • Additional Nursing Fees: *Not Reported*

DELAWARE TECHNICAL & COMMUNITY COLLEGE— OWENS CAMPUS

Address:　P. O. Box 610, Georgetown, DE 19947
Phone:　302-855-1614
Fax:　302-858-5460
Contact:　June S. Turansky, MSN, RN, Nursing Department Chairperson
Email:　jturansk@outland.dtcc.edu

GENERAL INFORMATION

Type of School: *2-Year College or University, Public* • Accreditation: *Middle States Association of Colleges and Schools* • Total Enrollment: *3300*

PROGRAM INFORMATION

LPN/LVN Exit: *Yes* • NLNAC Accreditation: *Yes*

NURSING STUDENT PROFILE

Total Nursing Enrollment: *105* • Full-Time Enrollment: *105* • Part-Time Enrollment: *0* • Female Enrollment: *97* • Male Enrollment: *8* • Total New Admissions Who Enrolled for Fall: *40* • Total Graduates: *48*

FINANCES

Residential Annual Tuition: *$1,584* • Non-Residential Annual Tuition: *$3,960* • General Institution Fees: *$30* • Additional Nursing Fees: *$58*

DELAWARE TECHNICAL & COMMUNITY COLLEGE— STANTON CAMPUS

Address:　400 Staton Christiana Road, Newark, DE 19713-2111
Phone:　302-454-3948
Fax:　302-368-6620
Contact:　Nancy W. Snyder, MSN, RN, Chairperson
Email:　nsnyder@college.dtcc.edu

GENERAL INFORMATION

Type of School: *2-Year College or University, Public* • Accreditation: *Middle States Association of Colleges and Schools* • Total Enrollment: *3515*

PROGRAM INFORMATION

LPN/LVN Exit: *No* • NLNAC Accreditation: *Yes*

NURSING STUDENT PROFILE

Total Nursing Enrollment: *191* • Full-Time Enrollment: *156* • Part-Time Enrollment: *35* • Female Enrollment: *180* • Male Enrollment: *11* • Total New Admissions Who Enrolled for Fall: *65* • Total Graduates: *71*

FINANCES

Residential Annual Tuition: *$1,584* • Non-Residential Annual Tuition: *$3,960* • General Institution Fees: *$126* • Additional Nursing Fees: *$195*

DELAWARE TECHNICAL & COMMUNITY COLLEGE—TERRY CAMPUS

Address: 100 Campus Drive, Dover, DE 19904
Phone: 302-857-1300
Fax: 302-857-1398
Contact: Ruth C. Yanos, MSN, RN, Nursing Department
       Chairman
Email: ryanos@outland.dtcc.edu

GENERAL INFORMATION

Type of School: *2-Year College or University, Public* •
Accreditation: *Middle States Association of Colleges and Schools* • Total Enrollment: *1900*

PROGRAM INFORMATION

LPN/LVN Exit: *Yes* • NLNAC Accreditation: *Yes*

NURSING STUDENT PROFILE

Total Nursing Enrollment: *34* • Full-Time Enrollment: *34* •
Part-Time Enrollment: *0* • Female Enrollment: *33* • Male
Enrollment: *1* • Total New Admissions Who Enrolled for
Fall: *16* • Total Graduates: *12*

FINANCES

Residential Annual Tuition: *$3,960* • Non-Residential
Annual Tuition: *$9,900* • General Institution Fees: *$363* •
Additional Nursing Fees: *$600*

WESLEY COLLEGE

Address: 120 North State Street, Dover, DE 19901
Phone: 302-736-2550
Fax: 302-736-2548
Contact: Nancy D. Rubino, EdD, RN, C, Program
       Director
Email: rubina@mail.wesley.edu

GENERAL INFORMATION

Type of School: *4-Year College or University, Private
(Religious)* • Accreditation: *Middle States Association of
Colleges and Schools* • Total Enrollment: *2150*

PROGRAM INFORMATION

LPN/LVN Exit: *Not Reported* • NLNAC Accreditation: *Yes*

NURSING STUDENT PROFILE

Total Nursing Enrollment: *53* • Full-Time Enrollment: *49* •
Part-Time Enrollment: *4* • Female Enrollment: *49* • Male
Enrollment: *4* • Total New Admissions Who Enrolled for
Fall: *26* • Total Graduates: *13*

FINANCES

Residential Annual Tuition: *$11,314* • Non-Residential
Annual Tuition: *$11,314* • General Institution Fees: *$705* •
Additional Nursing Fees: *$96*

HOWARD UNIVERSITY

Address: 501 Bryant Street North West, Washington, DC
            20059
Phone: 202-806-5431
Fax: Not Reported
Contact: Pedro Lecca, PhD, RN, Dean
Email: plecca@howard.edu

GENERAL INFORMATION

Type of School: *4-Year College or University, Private
(Independent)* • Accreditation: *Middle States Association of
Colleges and Schools* • Total Enrollment: *10000*

PROGRAM INFORMATION

LPN/LVN Exit: *Not Reported* • NLNAC Accreditation: *No*

NURSING STUDENT PROFILE

Total Nursing Enrollment: *Not Reported* • Full-Time
Enrollment: *Not Reported* • Part-Time Enrollment: *Not
Reported* • Female Enrollment: *Not Reported* • Male
Enrollment: *Not Reported* • Total New Admissions Who
Enrolled for Fall: *Not Reported* • Total Graduates: *Not
Reported*

FINANCES

Residential Annual Tuition: *Not Reported* • Non-Residential
Annual Tuition: *Not Reported* • General Institution Fees: *Not
Reported* • Additional Nursing Fees: *Not Reported*

UNIVERSITY OF THE DISTRICT OF COLUMBIA

Address: 4200 Connecticut Avenue, NW, Building 44,
            Washington, DC 20008
Phone: 202-274-5899
Fax: 202-274-5952
Contact: Connie M Webster, MSN, BSN, DNSc, RN,
            Chairperson, Department of Nursing and Allied
            Health and Director of Nursing
Email: cwebster@udc.edu

GENERAL INFORMATION

Type of School: *Not Reported* • Accreditation: *None* • Total
Enrollment: *Not Reported*

PROGRAM INFORMATION

LPN/LVN Exit: *Not Reported* • NLNAC Accreditation: *No*

NURSING STUDENT PROFILE

Total Nursing Enrollment: *178* • Full-Time Enrollment:
106 • Part-Time Enrollment: *72* • Female Enrollment: *164* •
Male Enrollment: *14* • Total New Admissions Who Enrolled
for Fall: *45* • Total Graduates: *72*

FINANCES

Residential Annual Tuition: *$2,070* • Non-Residential
Annual Tuition: *$4,710* • General Institution Fees: *$135* •
Additional Nursing Fees: *$50*

BREVARD COMMUNITY COLLEGE

Address: 1519 Clearlake Road, Cocoa, FL 32922
Phone: 321-632-1111
Fax: 321-634-3731
Contact: Constance Bobik, RN, BSN, MSN, Chair
Email: bobikc@brevardcc.edu

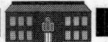

GENERAL INFORMATION

Type of School: *2-Year College or University, Public* •
Accreditation: *Southern Association of Colleges and Schools* •
Total Enrollment: *14000*

PROGRAM INFORMATION

LPN/LVN Exit: *No* • NLNAC Accreditation: *Not Reported*

NURSING STUDENT PROFILE

Total Nursing Enrollment: *131* • Full-Time Enrollment:
131 • Part-Time Enrollment: *0* • Female Enrollment: *119* •
Male Enrollment: *12* • Total New Admissions Who Enrolled
for Fall: *60* • Total Graduates: *81*

FINANCES

Residential Annual Tuition: *$1,508* • Non-Residential
Annual Tuition: *$5,389* • General Institution Fees: *$1,000* •
Additional Nursing Fees: *$200*

BROWARD COMMUNITY COLLEGE

Address: 3501 SW Davie Road, Davie, FL 33314
Phone: 954-475-6851
Fax: 954-473-9037
Contact: Diane Whitehead, EdD, RN, Department Head
Email: dwhitehe@broward.edu

GENERAL INFORMATION

Type of School: *Not Reported* • Accreditation: *Not Reported* •
Total Enrollment: *Not Reported*

PROGRAM INFORMATION

LPN/LVN Exit: *No* • NLNAC Accreditation: *Yes*

NURSING STUDENT PROFILE

Total Nursing Enrollment: *793* • Full-Time Enrollment:
793 • Part-Time Enrollment: *0* • Female Enrollment: *708* •
Male Enrollment: *85* • Total New Admissions Who Enrolled
for Fall: *225* • Total Graduates: *330*

FINANCES

Residential Annual Tuition: *$1,449* • Non-Residential
Annual Tuition: *$5,796* • General Institution Fees: *$234* •
Additional Nursing Fees: *$500*

CENTRAL FLORIDA COMMUNITY COLLEGE

Address: 3001 College Road/ P. O. Box 1388, Ocala, FL
           34478
Phone: 352-854-2322
Fax: 352-873-5889
Contact: Gwen Lapham-Alcorn, PhD, RN, Associate
           Dean, Health Occupations
Email: alcorng@cfcc.cc.fl.us

CHIPOLA JUNIOR COLLEGE

Address: 3094 Indian Circle, Marianna, FL 32446
Phone: 850-718-2495
Fax: 850-718-2495
Contact: Kathy G Wheeler, ARNP, MSN, Director
Email: wheelerk@chipola.cc.fl.us

GENERAL INFORMATION

Type of School: *2-Year College or University, Public* •
Accreditation: *Southern Association of Colleges and Schools* •
Total Enrollment: *5708*

GENERAL INFORMATION

Type of School: *2-Year College or University, Public* •
Accreditation: *Southern Association of Colleges and Schools* •
Total Enrollment: *Not Reported*

PROGRAM INFORMATION

LPN/LVN Exit: *No* • NLNAC Accreditation: *Yes*

PROGRAM INFORMATION

LPN/LVN Exit: *No* • NLNAC Accreditation: *Not Reported*

NURSING STUDENT PROFILE

Total Nursing Enrollment: *143* • Full-Time Enrollment:
143 • Part-Time Enrollment: *0* • Female Enrollment: *125* •
Male Enrollment: *18* • Total New Admissions Who Enrolled
for Fall: *34* • Total Graduates: *66*

NURSING STUDENT PROFILE

Total Nursing Enrollment: *70* • Full-Time Enrollment: *70* •
Part-Time Enrollment: *0* • Female Enrollment: *Not
Reported* • Male Enrollment: *Not Reported* • Total New
Admissions Who Enrolled for Fall: *33* • Total Graduates: *29*

FINANCES

Residential Annual Tuition: *$1,831* • Non-Residential
Annual Tuition: *$6,795* • General Institution Fees: *Not
Reported* • Additional Nursing Fees: *$1,092*

FINANCES

Residential Annual Tuition: *$1,840* • Non-Residential
Annual Tuition: *$5,616* • General Institution Fees: *Not
Reported* • Additional Nursing Fees: *Not Reported*

DAYTONA BEACH COMMUNITY COLLEGE

Address: 1200 West International Speedway Boulevard, Daytona Beach, FL 32120
Phone: 386-255-8131
Fax: 386-947-3181
Contact: Linda Miles, MSN, RN, Chair, Department of Nursing
Email: miles1@dbcc.cc.fl.us

GENERAL INFORMATION

Type of School: *2-Year College or University, Public* •
Accreditation: *Southern Association of Colleges and Schools* •
Total Enrollment: *10000*

PROGRAM INFORMATION

LPN/LVN Exit: *No* • NLNAC Accreditation: *Yes*

NURSING STUDENT PROFILE

Total Nursing Enrollment: *196* • Full-Time Enrollment: *196* • Part-Time Enrollment: *0* • Female Enrollment: *191* • Male Enrollment: *5* • Total New Admissions Who Enrolled for Fall: *96* • Total Graduates: *56*

FINANCES

Residential Annual Tuition: *$52* • Non-Residential Annual Tuition: *$195* • General Institution Fees: *Not Reported* • Additional Nursing Fees: *$280*

EDISON COMMUNITY COLLEGE

Address: 8099 College Parkway, Fort Myers, FL 33919
Phone: 941-489-9239
Fax: 941-985-8352
Contact: Shirley Ruder, RN, MS, MSN, EdD, Director of Nursing
Email: sruder@edison.edu

GENERAL INFORMATION

Type of School: *2-Year College or University, Public* •
Accreditation: *Southern Association of Colleges and Schools* •
Total Enrollment: *8922*

PROGRAM INFORMATION

LPN/LVN Exit: *No* • NLNAC Accreditation: *Yes*

NURSING STUDENT PROFILE

Total Nursing Enrollment: *220* • Full-Time Enrollment: *140* • Part-Time Enrollment: *80* • Female Enrollment: *205* • Male Enrollment: *15* • Total New Admissions Who Enrolled for Fall: *74* • Total Graduates: *109*

FINANCES

Residential Annual Tuition: *$1,449* • Non-Residential Annual Tuition: *$5,370* • General Institution Fees: *Not Reported* • Additional Nursing Fees: *$108*

FLORIDA COMMUNITY COLLEGE-JACKSONVILLE

Address: 4501 Capper Road, Jacksonville, FL 32218
Phone: 904-766-6550
Fax: 904-713-4859
Contact: June M. Chandler, BSN, MSN, EdD, Director
          of Nursing
Email: jmchandl@fccj.org

GENERAL INFORMATION

Type of School: *2-Year College or University, Public* •
Accreditation: *Southern Association of Colleges and Schools* •
Total Enrollment: *85000*

PROGRAM INFORMATION

LPN/LVN Exit: *No* • NLNAC Accreditation: *Yes*

NURSING STUDENT PROFILE

Total Nursing Enrollment: *383* • Full-Time Enrollment:
383 • Part-Time Enrollment: *0* • Female Enrollment: *355* •
Male Enrollment: *28* • Total New Admissions Who Enrolled
for Fall: *132* • Total Graduates: *Not Reported*

FINANCES

Residential Annual Tuition: *$1,853* • Non-Residential
Annual Tuition: *$6,912* • General Institution Fees: *Not
Reported* • Additional Nursing Fees: *Not Reported*

FLORIDA HOSPITAL COLLEGE OF HEALTH SCIENCES

Address: 795 Lake Estelle Drive, Orlando, FL 32803
Phone: 407-303-5764
Fax: 407-303-1872
Contact: Vicki McDonald, MS, ARNP, Associate Professor
Email: vicki_mcdonald@fhchs.edu

GENERAL INFORMATION

Type of School: *4-Year College or University, Private
(Religious)* • Accreditation: *Southern Association of Colleges
and Schools* • Total Enrollment: *Not Reported*

PROGRAM INFORMATION

LPN/LVN Exit: *No* • NLNAC Accreditation: *Yes*

NURSING STUDENT PROFILE

Total Nursing Enrollment: *121* • Full-Time Enrollment:
121 • Part-Time Enrollment: *0* • Female Enrollment: *99* •
Male Enrollment: *22* • Total New Admissions Who Enrolled
for Fall: *78* • Total Graduates: *44*

FINANCES

Residential Annual Tuition: *$4,200* • Non-Residential
Annual Tuition: *Not Reported* • General Institution Fees:
$90 • Additional Nursing Fees: *$175*

FLORIDA KEYS COMMUNITY COLLEGE

Address: 5901 College Road, Key West, FL 33040
Phone: 305-296-9081
Fax: 305-292-5155
Contact: Coleen Dooley, MSN, RN, CS, Director
Nursing and Allied Health
Email: dooley_c@fkcc.edu

GENERAL INFORMATION

Type of School: *2-Year College or University, Public* •
Accreditation: *Southern Association of Colleges and Schools* •
Total Enrollment: *58*

PROGRAM INFORMATION

LPN/LVN Exit: *No* • NLNAC Accreditation: *Not Reported*

NURSING STUDENT PROFILE

Total Nursing Enrollment: *58* • Full-Time Enrollment: *58* •
Part-Time Enrollment: *0* • Female Enrollment: *52* • Male
Enrollment: *6* • Total New Admissions Who Enrolled for
Fall: *26* • Total Graduates: *22*

FINANCES

Residential Annual Tuition: *$3,000* • Non-Residential
Annual Tuition: *$8,000* • General Institution Fees: *$20* •
Additional Nursing Fees: *$100*

GULF COAST COMMUNITY COLLEGE

Address: 5230 West Highway 98, Panama City, FL
32401-1058
Phone: 850-913-3317
Fax: 850-747-3246
Contact: Cindy O'Bryon, MSN, RN, Coordinator,
Nursing
Email: cobryon@mail.gc.cc.fl.us

GENERAL INFORMATION

Type of School: *2-Year College or University, Public* •
Accreditation: *Southern Association of Colleges and Schools* •
Total Enrollment: *5930*

PROGRAM INFORMATION

LPN/LVN Exit: *No* • NLNAC Accreditation: *Yes*

NURSING STUDENT PROFILE

Total Nursing Enrollment: *130* • Full-Time Enrollment:
130 • Part-Time Enrollment: *0* • Female Enrollment: *108* •
Male Enrollment: *22* • Total New Admissions Who Enrolled
for Fall: *40* • Total Graduates: *53*

FINANCES

Residential Annual Tuition: *$1,473* • Non-Residential
Annual Tuition: *$5,482* • General Institution Fees: *Not
Reported* • Additional Nursing Fees: *$30*

Circle 55 on reader card   See in-depth profile for more information

HILLSBOROUGH COMMUNITY COLLEGE

Address: P. O. Box 300030, Tampa, FL 33630-3030
Phone: 813-253-7370
Fax: 813-253-7491
Contact: Bonnie Hesselberg, EdD, ARNP, Dean
Email: bhesselberg@hcc.cc.fl.us

INDIAN RIVER COMMUNITY COLLEGE

Address: 3209 Virginia Avenue, Fort Pierce, FL 34981
Phone: 772-462-4778
Fax: 772-462-4900
Contact: Jane P. Cebelak, RN, MS, Director of Nursing
Email: jcebelak@ircc.cc.fl.us

GENERAL INFORMATION

Type of School: *2-Year College or University, Public* •
Accreditation: *Southern Association of Colleges and Schools* •
Total Enrollment: *43000*

GENERAL INFORMATION

Type of School: *2-Year College or University, Public* •
Accreditation: *Southern Association of Colleges and Schools* •
Total Enrollment: *3800*

PROGRAM INFORMATION

LPN/LVN Exit: *No* • NLNAC Accreditation: *Yes*

PROGRAM INFORMATION

LPN/LVN Exit: *No* • NLNAC Accreditation: *Yes*

NURSING STUDENT PROFILE

Total Nursing Enrollment: *512* • Full-Time Enrollment: *96* •
Part-Time Enrollment: *416* • Female Enrollment: *463* • Male
Enrollment: *49* • Total New Admissions Who Enrolled for
Fall: *163* • Total Graduates: *165*

NURSING STUDENT PROFILE

Total Nursing Enrollment: *205* • Full-Time Enrollment:
205 • Part-Time Enrollment: *0* • Female Enrollment: *182* •
Male Enrollment: *23* • Total New Admissions Who Enrolled
for Fall: *64* • Total Graduates: *58*

FINANCES

Residential Annual Tuition: *$1,440* • Non-Residential
Annual Tuition: *$5,310* • General Institution Fees: *Not
Reported* • Additional Nursing Fees: *$25*

FINANCES

Residential Annual Tuition: *$50* • Non-Residential Annual
Tuition: *$180* • General Institution Fees: *$0* • Additional
Nursing Fees: *$286*

LAKE CITY COMMUNITY COLLEGE

Address: Route 19, Box 1030, Lake City, FL 32025
Phone: 386-754-4304
Fax: 386-754-4579
Contact: Robbie Smith, MSN, RN, Coordinator of Nursing Programs
Email: smithr@mail.lakecity.cc.fl.us

GENERAL INFORMATION

Type of School: *2-Year College or University, Public* •
Accreditation: *Southern Association of Colleges and Schools* •
Total Enrollment: *2143*

PROGRAM INFORMATION

LPN/LVN Exit: *Not Reported* • NLNAC Accreditation: *Yes*

NURSING STUDENT PROFILE

Total Nursing Enrollment: *96* • Full-Time Enrollment: *24* •
Part-Time Enrollment: *72* • Female Enrollment: *84* • Male
Enrollment: *12* • Total New Admissions Who Enrolled for
Fall: *50* • Total Graduates: *36*

FINANCES

Residential Annual Tuition: *$1,684* • Non-Residential
Annual Tuition: *$6,267* • General Institution Fees: *$30* •
Additional Nursing Fees: *$397*

LAKE- SUMTER COMMUNITY COLLEGE

Address: 9501 US Highway 441, Leesburg, FL 34788-8751
Phone: 352-365-3519
Fax: 352-365-3508
Contact: Susan Pennacchia, ARNP, MSN, Nursing Program Director
Email: pennaccs@lscc.cc.fl.us

GENERAL INFORMATION

Type of School: *2-Year College or University, Public* •
Accreditation: *Southern Association of Colleges and Schools* •
Total Enrollment: *2881*

PROGRAM INFORMATION

LPN/LVN Exit: *No* • NLNAC Accreditation: *Not Reported*

NURSING STUDENT PROFILE

Total Nursing Enrollment: *99* • Full-Time Enrollment: *99* •
Part-Time Enrollment: *0* • Female Enrollment: *85* • Male
Enrollment: *14* • Total New Admissions Who Enrolled for
Fall: *42* • Total Graduates: *52*

FINANCES

Residential Annual Tuition: *$1,530* • Non-Residential
Annual Tuition: *$5,730* • General Institution Fees: *$0* •
Additional Nursing Fees: *$214*

MANATEE COMMUNITY COLLEGE

Address: 5840 26th Street West, Bradenton, FL 34207
Phone: 941-752-5526
Fax: 941-727-8304
Contact: Carol Singer, BSN, MS, EdD, RN, Associate
            Dean, Health Sciences
Email: singerc@mcc.cc.fl.us

GENERAL INFORMATION

Type of School: *2-Year College or University, Public* •
Accreditation: *Southern Association of Colleges and Schools* •
Total Enrollment: *7200*

PROGRAM INFORMATION

LPN/LVN Exit: *No* • NLNAC Accreditation: *Yes*

NURSING STUDENT PROFILE

Total Nursing Enrollment: *188* • Full-Time Enrollment: *25* •
Part-Time Enrollment: *163* • Female Enrollment: *158* • Male
Enrollment: *30* • Total New Admissions Who Enrolled for
Fall: *76* • Total Graduates: *86*

FINANCES

Residential Annual Tuition: *$3,782* • Non-Residential
Annual Tuition: *$14,126* • General Institution Fees: *$20* •
Additional Nursing Fees: *$117*

MIAMI–DADE COMMUNITY COLLEGE

Address: 950 North West 20th Street, Miami, FL 33127
Phone: 305-237-4039
Fax: 305-237-4119
Contact: Frances Aronovitz, PhD, ARNP, Director, School
            of Nursing
Email: faronovi@mdcc.edu

GENERAL INFORMATION

Type of School: *2-Year College or University, Public* •
Accreditation: *Southern Association of Colleges and Schools* •
Total Enrollment: *53486*

PROGRAM INFORMATION

LPN/LVN Exit: *No* • NLNAC Accreditation: *Yes*

NURSING STUDENT PROFILE

Total Nursing Enrollment: *876* • Full-Time Enrollment:
652 • Part-Time Enrollment: *224* • Female Enrollment:
715 • Male Enrollment: *161* • Total New Admissions Who
Enrolled for Fall: *270* • Total Graduates: *327*

FINANCES

Residential Annual Tuition: *$51* • Non-Residential Annual
Tuition: *$179* • General Institution Fees: *$270* • Additional
Nursing Fees: *$270*

PALM BEACH COMMUNITY COLLEGE

Address: 4200 Congress Avenue, Lake Worth, FL 33461
Phone: 561-439-8091
Fax: 561-434-5186
Contact: Selma Ann Verse, RN, MEd, Associate Dean of Academic Affairs
Email: verses@pbcc.cc.fl.us

GENERAL INFORMATION

Type of School: *2-Year College or University, Public* • Accreditation: *Southern Association of Colleges and Schools* • Total Enrollment: *18000*

PROGRAM INFORMATION

LPN/LVN Exit: *Yes* • NLNAC Accreditation: *Yes*

NURSING STUDENT PROFILE

Total Nursing Enrollment: *262* • Full-Time Enrollment: *262* • Part-Time Enrollment: *0* • Female Enrollment: *236* • Male Enrollment: *26* • Total New Admissions Who Enrolled for Fall: *77* • Total Graduates: *156*

FINANCES

Residential Annual Tuition: *$1,830* • Non-Residential Annual Tuition: *$5,100* • General Institution Fees: *$30* • Additional Nursing Fees: *$60*

PASCO–HERNANDO COMMUNITY COLLEGE

Address: 10230 Ridge Road, New Port Richey, FL 34654
Phone: 727-816-3280
Fax: 727-816-3309
Contact: Karen H. Richardson, MS, ARNP, Director of Nursing
Email: karen_richardson@pasco-hernandocc.com

GENERAL INFORMATION

Type of School: *2-Year College or University, Public* • Accreditation: *Southern Association of Colleges and Schools* • Total Enrollment: *6000*

PROGRAM INFORMATION

LPN/LVN Exit: *Not Reported* • NLNAC Accreditation: *Yes*

NURSING STUDENT PROFILE

Total Nursing Enrollment: *166* • Full-Time Enrollment: *166* • Part-Time Enrollment: *0* • Female Enrollment: *145* • Male Enrollment: *21* • Total New Admissions Who Enrolled for Fall: *84* • Total Graduates: *85*

FINANCES

Residential Annual Tuition: *$1,440* • Non-Residential Annual Tuition: *$5,370* • General Institution Fees: *Not Reported* • Additional Nursing Fees: *$240*

PENSACOLA JUNIOR COLLEGE

Address: 5555 West Highway 98, Pensacola, FL 32507
Phone: 850-484-2253
Fax: 850-484-2326
Contact: Claudette Coleman, EdD, MSN, Department
            Head, Nursing
Email: ccoleman@pjc.cc.fl.us

GENERAL INFORMATION

Type of School: *2-Year College or University, Public* •
Accreditation: *Southern Association of Colleges and Schools* •
Total Enrollment: *30742*

PROGRAM INFORMATION

LPN/LVN Exit: *No* • NLNAC Accreditation: *Not Reported*

NURSING STUDENT PROFILE

Total Nursing Enrollment: *201* • Full-Time Enrollment:
118 • Part-Time Enrollment: *83* • Female Enrollment: *179* •
Male Enrollment: *22* • Total New Admissions Who Enrolled
for Fall: *65* • Total Graduates: *78*

FINANCES

Residential Annual Tuition: *$3,492* • Non-Residential
Annual Tuition: *$13,021* • General Institution Fees: *$49* •
Additional Nursing Fees: *$810*

POLK COMMUNITY COLLEGE

Address: 999 Ave H NE, Winter Haven, FL 33881
Phone: Not Reported
Fax: Not Reported
Contact: Sharon Davis, MSN, RN, Director
Email: Not Reported

GENERAL INFORMATION

Type of School: *Not Reported* • Accreditation: *Not Reported* •
Total Enrollment: *Not Reported*

PROGRAM INFORMATION

LPN/LVN Exit: *Not Reported* • NLNAC Accreditation: *Yes*

NURSING STUDENT PROFILE

Total Nursing Enrollment: *Not Reported* • Full-Time
Enrollment: *Not Reported* • Part-Time Enrollment: *Not
Reported* • Female Enrollment: *Not Reported* • Male
Enrollment: *Not Reported* • Total New Admissions Who
Enrolled for Fall: *Not Reported* • Total Graduates: *Not
Reported*

FINANCES

Residential Annual Tuition: *Not Reported* • Non-Residential
Annual Tuition: *Not Reported* • General Institution Fees: *Not
Reported* • Additional Nursing Fees: *Not Reported*

SAINT JOHNS RIVER COMMUNITY COLLEGE

Address: 5001 Saint John's Avenue, Palatka, FL 32177-3898
Phone: 386-312-4176
Fax: 386-312-4191
Contact: Virginia E. McColm, MSN, RN, Director of Nursing Education
Email: mccolm_v@hotmail.com

GENERAL INFORMATION

Type of School: *2-Year College or University, Public* •
Accreditation: *Southern Association of Colleges and Schools* •
Total Enrollment: *Not Reported*

PROGRAM INFORMATION

LPN/LVN Exit: *No* • NLNAC Accreditation: *Not Reported*

NURSING STUDENT PROFILE

Total Nursing Enrollment: *36* • Full-Time Enrollment: *36* •
Part-Time Enrollment: *0* • Female Enrollment: *35* • Male
Enrollment: *1* • Total New Admissions Who Enrolled for
Fall: *36* • Total Graduates: *Not Reported*

FINANCES

Residential Annual Tuition: *$1,135* • Non-Residential
Annual Tuition: *$4,265* • General Institution Fees: *$20* •
Additional Nursing Fees: *$118*

SANTA FE COMMUNITY COLLEGE

Address: 3000 North West 83rd Street, W-201, Gainesville, FL 32606
Phone: 352-395-5731
Fax: 352-395-5711
Contact: Rita Sutherland, ARNP, MSN, Director, Nursing Programs
Email: rita.sutherland@santafe.cc.fl.us

GENERAL INFORMATION

Type of School: *2-Year College or University, Public* •
Accreditation: *Southern Association of Colleges and Schools* •
Total Enrollment: *12000*

PROGRAM INFORMATION

LPN/LVN Exit: *No* • NLNAC Accreditation: *Yes*

NURSING STUDENT PROFILE

Total Nursing Enrollment: *206* • Full-Time Enrollment:
206 • Part-Time Enrollment: *0* • Female Enrollment: *159* •
Male Enrollment: *47* • Total New Admissions Who Enrolled
for Fall: *100* • Total Graduates: *95*

FINANCES

Residential Annual Tuition: *$3,484* • Non-Residential
Annual Tuition: *$13,014* • General Institution Fees: *$200* •
Additional Nursing Fees: *Not Reported*

SEMINOLE COMMUNITY COLLEGE

Address: 100 Weldon Boulevard, Sanford, FL 32773
Phone: 407-328-2013
Fax: 407-328-2277
Contact: Laura Aromado, MSN, RN, Department Chair
Email: aromanol@scc-fl.com

GENERAL INFORMATION

Type of School: *2-Year College or University, Public* •
Accreditation: *Southern Association of Colleges and Schools* •
Total Enrollment: *30000*

PROGRAM INFORMATION

LPN/LVN Exit: *Not Reported* • NLNAC Accreditation: *Yes*

NURSING STUDENT PROFILE

Total Nursing Enrollment: *Not Reported* • Full-Time
Enrollment: *Not Reported* • Part-Time Enrollment: *Not
Reported* • Female Enrollment: *Not Reported* • Male
Enrollment: *Not Reported* • Total New Admissions Who
Enrolled for Fall: *Not Reported* • Total Graduates: *Not
Reported*

FINANCES

Residential Annual Tuition: *$1,535* • Non-Residential
Annual Tuition: *$4,665* • General Institution Fees: *Not
Reported* • Additional Nursing Fees: *Not Reported*

SOUTH FLORIDA COMMUNITY COLLEGE

Address: 600 West College Drive, Avon Park, FL 33825
Phone: 863-784-7118
Fax: Not Reported
Contact: Mary Ann Fritz, PhD, RN, Chair, Nursing
            Education
Email: fritma5671@sfcc.cc.fl.us

GENERAL INFORMATION

Type of School: *2-Year College or University, Public* •
Accreditation: *Southern Association of Colleges and Schools* •
Total Enrollment: *2500*

PROGRAM INFORMATION

LPN/LVN Exit: *Not Reported* • NLNAC Accreditation: *Not
Reported*

NURSING STUDENT PROFILE

Total Nursing Enrollment: *24* • Full-Time Enrollment: *24* •
Part-Time Enrollment: *0* • Female Enrollment: *23* • Male
Enrollment: *1* • Total New Admissions Who Enrolled for
Fall: *14* • Total Graduates: *21*

FINANCES

Residential Annual Tuition: *$1,400* • Non-Residential
Annual Tuition: *$5,000* • General Institution Fees: *Not
Reported* • Additional Nursing Fees: *$220*

ST. PETERSBURG COLLEGE

Address: P.O. Box 13489, Saint Petersburg, FL 33733
Phone: 727-345-7752
Fax: 727-341-3646
Contact: Verine J. Parks-Doyle, MSN, EdD, BSN, RN,
          Director of Nursing
Email: parksj@spjc.edu
Web: www.spjc.edu

GENERAL INFORMATION

Type of School: *4-Year College or University, Public* •
Accreditation: *Southern Association of Colleges and Schools* •
Total Enrollment: *58,000*

PROGRAM INFORMATION

LPN/LVN Exit: *No* • NLNAC Accreditation: *Yes*

NURSING STUDENT PROFILE

Total Nursing Enrollment: *362* • Full-Time Enrollment:
362 • Part-Time Enrollment: *0* • Female Enrollment: *335* •
Male Enrollment: *27* • Total New Admissions Who Enrolled
for Fall: *105* • Total Graduates: *233*

FINANCES

Residential Annual Tuition: *$1,511* • Non-Residential
Annual Tuition: *$5,580* • General Institution Fees: *Not
Reported* • Additional Nursing Fees: *$267*

TALLAHASSEE COMMUNITY COLLEGE

Address: 444 Appleyard Drive, Tallahassee, FL 32304
Phone: 850-201-8333
Fax: Not Reported
Contact: Carolann Gegenheimer, MSN, RN, Chair
Email: gegenhec@tcc.cc.fl.us

GENERAL INFORMATION

Type of School: *2-Year College or University, Public* •
Accreditation: *Southern Association of Colleges and Schools* •
Total Enrollment: *10000*

PROGRAM INFORMATION

LPN/LVN Exit: *Not Reported* • NLNAC Accreditation: *Not
Reported*

NURSING STUDENT PROFILE

Total Nursing Enrollment: *71* • Full-Time Enrollment: *71* •
Part-Time Enrollment: *0* • Female Enrollment: *61* • Male
Enrollment: *10* • Total New Admissions Who Enrolled for
Fall: *40* • Total Graduates: *29*

FINANCES

Residential Annual Tuition: *$1,600* • Non-Residential
Annual Tuition: *$5,984* • General Institution Fees: *Not
Reported* • Additional Nursing Fees: *Not Reported*

Circle 113 on reader card   See in-depth profile for more information

UNIVERSITY OF CENTRAL FLORIDA

Address: 4000 Central Florida Boulevard, Orlando, FL 32816
Phone: Not Reported
Fax: Not Reported
Contact: Elizabeth Stullenbarger, PhD, RN, Director of Nursing
Email: Not Reported

GENERAL INFORMATION

Type of School: *4-Year College or University, Public* • Accreditation: *Southern Association of Colleges and Schools* • Total Enrollment: *36000*

PROGRAM INFORMATION

LPN/LVN Exit: *Not Reported* • NLNAC Accreditation: *Not Reported*

NURSING STUDENT PROFILE

Total Nursing Enrollment: *Not Reported* • Full-Time Enrollment: *Not Reported* • Part-Time Enrollment: *Not Reported* • Female Enrollment: *Not Reported* • Male Enrollment: *Not Reported* • Total New Admissions Who Enrolled for Fall: *Not Reported* • Total Graduates: *Not Reported*

FINANCES

Residential Annual Tuition: *$2,029* • Non-Residential Annual Tuition: *$11,203* • General Institution Fees: *Not Reported* • Additional Nursing Fees: *Not Reported*

VALENCIA COMMUNITY COLLEGE

Address: 1800 S Kirkman Rd, Orlando, FL 32811
Phone: 407-299-5000
Fax: 407-292-2730
Contact: Ann Miller Quida, MSN, RN, Director
Email: Not Reported

GENERAL INFORMATION

Type of School: *Not Reported* • Accreditation: *Not Reported* • Total Enrollment: *Not Reported*

PROGRAM INFORMATION

LPN/LVN Exit: *Not Reported* • NLNAC Accreditation: *Yes*

NURSING STUDENT PROFILE

Total Nursing Enrollment: *Not Reported* • Full-Time Enrollment: *Not Reported* • Part-Time Enrollment: *Not Reported* • Female Enrollment: *Not Reported* • Male Enrollment: *Not Reported* • Total New Admissions Who Enrolled for Fall: *Not Reported* • Total Graduates: *Not Reported*

FINANCES

Residential Annual Tuition: *$1,593* • Non-Residential Annual Tuition: *$4,780* • General Institution Fees: *Not Reported* • Additional Nursing Fees: *Not Reported*

ABRAHAM BALDWIN AGRICULTURAL COLLEGE

Address: 2802 Moore Highway, Tifton, GA 31794
Phone: 229-386-3937
Fax: 229-391-6862
Contact: Wanda Golden, MSN, RN, CCRN, Chair
Email: wgolden@abac.edu

GENERAL INFORMATION

Type of School: *2-Year College or University, Public* •
Accreditation: *Southern Association of Colleges and Schools* •
Total Enrollment: *2625*

PROGRAM INFORMATION

LPN/LVN Exit: *No* • NLNAC Accreditation: *Yes*

NURSING STUDENT PROFILE

Total Nursing Enrollment: *106* • Full-Time Enrollment:
106 • Part-Time Enrollment: *0* • Female Enrollment: *90* •
Male Enrollment: *16* • Total New Admissions Who Enrolled
for Fall: *46* • Total Graduates: *43*

FINANCES

Residential Annual Tuition: *$640* • Non-Residential Annual
Tuition: *$2,560* • General Institution Fees: *$192* •
Additional Nursing Fees: *$690*

ATHENS TECHNICAL COLLEGE

Address: 800 US Highway 29 North, Athens, GA 30601
Phone: 706-355-5047
Fax: 706-355-5181
Contact: Gloria L. Buck, PhD, MSN, RN, Program
Director, ADN
Email: buck@aati.edu

GENERAL INFORMATION

Type of School: *2-Year College or University, Public* •
Accreditation: *Southern Association of Colleges and Schools* •
Total Enrollment: *2739*

PROGRAM INFORMATION

LPN/LVN Exit: *No* • NLNAC Accreditation: *Yes*

NURSING STUDENT PROFILE

Total Nursing Enrollment: *74* • Full-Time Enrollment: *29* •
Part-Time Enrollment: *45* • Female Enrollment: *66* • Male
Enrollment: *8* • Total New Admissions Who Enrolled for
Fall: *37* • Total Graduates: *33*

FINANCES

Residential Annual Tuition: *$1,152* • Non-Residential
Annual Tuition: *$2,304* • General Institution Fees: *$140* •
Additional Nursing Fees: *$15*

AUGUSTA STATE UNIVERSITY

Address: 2500 Walton Way, Augusta, GA 30904
Phone: 706-737-1725
Fax: 706-667-4116
Contact: Letha M. Lierman, PhD, RN, Professor and
            Chair
Email: llierman@aug.edu

GENERAL INFORMATION

Type of School: *4-Year College or University, Public* •
Accreditation: *Southern Association of Colleges and Schools* •
Total Enrollment: *5090*

PROGRAM INFORMATION

LPN/LVN Exit: *Not Reported* • NLNAC Accreditation: *Yes*

NURSING STUDENT PROFILE

Total Nursing Enrollment: *55* • Full-Time Enrollment: *12* •
Part-Time Enrollment: *43* • Female Enrollment: *50* • Male
Enrollment: *5* • Total New Admissions Who Enrolled for
Fall: *31* • Total Graduates: *25*

FINANCES

Residential Annual Tuition: *$966* • Non-Residential Annual
Tuition: *$3,864* • General Institution Fees: *$175* •
Additional Nursing Fees: *$30*

COASTAL GEORGIA COMMUNITY COLLEGE

Address: 3700 Altama Ave, Brunswick, GA 315203644
Phone: 912-262-3340
Fax: 912-261-3970
Contact: Donna R Post, MSN, RN, Department Head
Email: Not Reported

GENERAL INFORMATION

Type of School: *Not Reported* • Accreditation: *Not Reported* •
Total Enrollment: *Not Reported*

PROGRAM INFORMATION

LPN/LVN Exit: *Not Reported* • NLNAC Accreditation: *Not
Reported*

NURSING STUDENT PROFILE

Total Nursing Enrollment: *Not Reported* • Full-Time
Enrollment: *Not Reported* • Part-Time Enrollment: *Not
Reported* • Female Enrollment: *Not Reported* • Male
Enrollment: *Not Reported* • Total New Admissions Who
Enrolled for Fall: *Not Reported* • Total Graduates: *Not
Reported*

FINANCES

Residential Annual Tuition: *$666* • Non-Residential Annual
Tuition: *$2,664* • General Institution Fees: *Not Reported* •
Additional Nursing Fees: *Not Reported*

COLUMBUS STATE UNIVERSITY

Address: 4225 University Avenue, Columbus, GA 31907
Phone: 706-568-2413
Fax: 706-569-3101
Contact: Peggy H. Batastini, RNC, MEd, MSN, Director, ASN Program
Email: batastini_peggy@colstate.edu

GENERAL INFORMATION

Type of School: *4-Year College or University, Public* • Accreditation: *Southern Association of Colleges and Schools* • Total Enrollment: *5522*

PROGRAM INFORMATION

LPN/LVN Exit: *No* • NLNAC Accreditation: *Yes*

NURSING STUDENT PROFILE

Total Nursing Enrollment: *9* • Full-Time Enrollment: *5* • Part-Time Enrollment: *4* • Female Enrollment: *6* • Male Enrollment: *3* • Total New Admissions Who Enrolled for Fall: *Not Reported* • Total Graduates: *17*

FINANCES

Residential Annual Tuition: *$1,876* • Non-Residential Annual Tuition: *$5,628* • General Institution Fees: *$197* • Additional Nursing Fees: *$0*

COOSA VALLEY TECHNICAL INSTITUTE

Address: 1151 Route 53 Alternate, Calhoun, GA 30701
Phone: 256-378-5576
Fax: 256-378-5281
Contact: Melenie C. Bolton, PhD, RN, Associate Dean
Email: mbolcvsn@corel.wwisp.net

GENERAL INFORMATION

Type of School: *Not Reported* • Accreditation: *None* • Total Enrollment: *Not Reported*

PROGRAM INFORMATION

LPN/LVN Exit: *Not Reported* • NLNAC Accreditation: *Not Reported*

NURSING STUDENT PROFILE

Total Nursing Enrollment: *Not Reported* • Full-Time Enrollment: *Not Reported* • Part-Time Enrollment: *Not Reported* • Female Enrollment: *Not Reported* • Male Enrollment: *Not Reported* • Total New Admissions Who Enrolled for Fall: *Not Reported* • Total Graduates: *Not Reported*

FINANCES

Residential Annual Tuition: *$2,200* • Non-Residential Annual Tuition: *Not Reported* • General Institution Fees: *Not Reported* • Additional Nursing Fees: *$1,805*

DALTON STATE COLLEGE

Address: 213 North College Drive, Dalton, GA 30720
Phone: 706-272-2463
Fax: 706-272-2533
Contact: Trudy Swilling, BS, MSN, Division Chair and
             Associate Professor
Email: tswilling@em.daltonstate.edu

GENERAL INFORMATION

Type of School: *2-Year College or University, Public* •
Accreditation: *Southern Association of Colleges and Schools* •
Total Enrollment: *3655*

PROGRAM INFORMATION

LPN/LVN Exit: *No* • NLNAC Accreditation: *Yes*

NURSING STUDENT PROFILE

Total Nursing Enrollment: *88* • Full-Time Enrollment: *40* •
Part-Time Enrollment: *48* • Female Enrollment: *83* • Male
Enrollment: *5* • Total New Admissions Who Enrolled for
Fall: *53* • Total Graduates: *38*

FINANCES

Residential Annual Tuition: *$2,091* • Non-Residential
Annual Tuition: *$3,069* • General Institution Fees: *$15* •
Additional Nursing Fees: *$0*

DARTON COLLEGE

Address: 2400 Gillionville Road, Albany, GA 31707
Phone: 229-430-6900
Fax: 229-430-6818
Contact: Joan Darden, MSN, PhD, RN, Chairman,
             Nursing and Allied Health
Email: dardenj@mail.dartnet.peachnet.edu

GENERAL INFORMATION

Type of School: *2-Year College or University, Public* •
Accreditation: *Southern Association of Colleges and Schools* •
Total Enrollment: *3179*

PROGRAM INFORMATION

LPN/LVN Exit: *Not Reported* • NLNAC Accreditation: *Yes*

NURSING STUDENT PROFILE

Total Nursing Enrollment: *227* • Full-Time Enrollment: *77* •
Part-Time Enrollment: *150* • Female Enrollment: *205* • Male
Enrollment: *22* • Total New Admissions Who Enrolled for
Fall: *75* • Total Graduates: *47*

FINANCES

Residential Annual Tuition: *$636* • Non-Residential Annual
Tuition: *$2,556* • General Institution Fees: *$112* •
Additional Nursing Fees: *$35*

FLOYD COLLEGE

Address: PO Box 1864, Rome, GA 30162-1864
Phone: 706-295-6321
Fax: 706-295-6732
Contact: Barbara B. Rees, DSN, RN, Nursing Program
Director
Email: brees@mail.fc.peachnet.edu

GENERAL INFORMATION

Type of School: *2-Year College or University, Public* •
Accreditation: *Southern Association of Colleges and Schools* •
Total Enrollment: *2091*

PROGRAM INFORMATION

LPN/LVN Exit: *No* • NLNAC Accreditation: *Yes*

NURSING STUDENT PROFILE

Total Nursing Enrollment: *104* • Full-Time Enrollment: *27* •
Part-Time Enrollment: *77* • Female Enrollment: *96* • Male
Enrollment: *8* • Total New Admissions Who Enrolled for
Fall: *53* • Total Graduates: *42*

FINANCES

Residential Annual Tuition: *$1,280* • Non-Residential
Annual Tuition: *$5,120* • General Institution Fees: *$342* •
Additional Nursing Fees: *$2,500*

GEORGIA PERIMETER COLLEGE

Address: 555 N Indian Creek Dr, Clarkston, GA 30021-
2361
Phone: 404-299-4179
Fax: 404-298-3945
Contact: Elizabeth F. Mistretta, PhD, RN, Interim Chair
Email: jmistret@gpc.peachnet.edu

GENERAL INFORMATION

Type of School: *2-Year College or University, Public* •
Accreditation: *Southern Association of Colleges and Schools* •
Total Enrollment: *14091*

PROGRAM INFORMATION

LPN/LVN Exit: *Yes* • NLNAC Accreditation: *Yes*

NURSING STUDENT PROFILE

Total Nursing Enrollment: *241* • Full-Time Enrollment:
241 • Part-Time Enrollment: *0* • Female Enrollment: *224* •
Male Enrollment: *17* • Total New Admissions Who Enrolled
for Fall: *147* • Total Graduates: *99*

FINANCES

Residential Annual Tuition: *$1,280* • Non-Residential
Annual Tuition: *$5,180* • General Institution Fees: *$103* •
Additional Nursing Fees: *$56*

GEORGIA SOUTHWESTERN STATE UNIVERSITY

Address:　800 Wheatley Street, Americus, GA 31709
Phone:　229-931-2275
Fax:　229-931-2288
Contact:　Patricia C. Cook, RN, MN, Department Chair
Email:　pcc@canes.gsw.edu

GENERAL INFORMATION

Type of School: *4-Year College or University, Public* •
Accreditation: *Southern Association of Colleges and Schools* •
Total Enrollment: *2622*

PROGRAM INFORMATION

LPN/LVN Exit: *No* • NLNAC Accreditation: *Yes*

NURSING STUDENT PROFILE

Total Nursing Enrollment: *26* • Full-Time Enrollment: *11* •
Part-Time Enrollment: *15* • Female Enrollment: *26* • Male
Enrollment: *0* • Total New Admissions Who Enrolled for
Fall: *0* • Total Graduates: *27*

FINANCES

Residential Annual Tuition: *$3,752* • Non-Residential
Annual Tuition: *$15,012* • General Institution Fees: *$268* •
Additional Nursing Fees: *$80*

GORDON COLLEGE

Address:　419 College Drive, Barnesville, GA 30204
Phone:　770-358-5085
Fax:　770-358-5064
Contact:　Pamela V. O'Neal, PhD, RN, CCRN, Director,
　　　　　Division of Nursing and Health Sciences
Email:　poneal@falcon.gdn.peachnet.edu

GENERAL INFORMATION

Type of School: *2-Year College or University, Public* •
Accreditation: *Southern Association of Colleges and Schools* •
Total Enrollment: *2805*

PROGRAM INFORMATION

LPN/LVN Exit: *Not Reported* • NLNAC Accreditation: *Yes*

NURSING STUDENT PROFILE

Total Nursing Enrollment: *138* • Full-Time Enrollment:
138 • Part-Time Enrollment: *0* • Female Enrollment: *132* •
Male Enrollment: *6* • Total New Admissions Who Enrolled
for Fall: *130* • Total Graduates: *50*

FINANCES

Residential Annual Tuition: *$710* • Non-Residential Annual
Tuition: *$2,676* • General Institution Fees: *$70* • Additional
Nursing Fees: *$25*

MACON STATE COLLEGE

Address: 100 College Station Drive, Macon, GA 31206-5144
Phone: 478-471-2761
Fax: 478-471-2983
Contact: Diane M. Craine, PhD, RN, Professor and Chair, Division of Nursing
Email: dcraine@mail.maconstate.edu

GENERAL INFORMATION

Type of School: *4-Year College or University, Public* • Accreditation: *Southern Association of Colleges and Schools* • Total Enrollment: *4485*

PROGRAM INFORMATION

LPN/LVN Exit: *No* • NLNAC Accreditation: *Yes*

NURSING STUDENT PROFILE

Total Nursing Enrollment: *137* • Full-Time Enrollment: *137* • Part-Time Enrollment: *0* • Female Enrollment: *126* • Male Enrollment: *11* • Total New Admissions Who Enrolled for Fall: *58* • Total Graduates: *51*

FINANCES

Residential Annual Tuition: *$640* • Non-Residential Annual Tuition: *$2,560* • General Institution Fees: *$79* • Additional Nursing Fees: *$34*

MIDDLE GEORGIA COLLEGE

Address: 1100 Second Street SE, Cochran, GA 31014
Phone: 478-934-3414
Fax: 478-934-3418
Contact: Debbie Greene, MSN, RN, Nursing Program Director
Email: dgreene@warrior.mgc.peachnet.edu

GENERAL INFORMATION

Type of School: *Governmental Agency, Public* • Accreditation: *Southern Association of Colleges and Schools* • Total Enrollment: *2000*

PROGRAM INFORMATION

LPN/LVN Exit: *No* • NLNAC Accreditation: *Yes*

NURSING STUDENT PROFILE

Total Nursing Enrollment: *78* • Full-Time Enrollment: *78* • Part-Time Enrollment: *0* • Female Enrollment: *74* • Male Enrollment: *4* • Total New Admissions Who Enrolled for Fall: *57* • Total Graduates: *24*

FINANCES

Residential Annual Tuition: *$1,772* • Non-Residential Annual Tuition: *$5,612* • General Institution Fees: *$231* • Additional Nursing Fees: *$15*

NORTH GEORGIA COLLEGE AND STATE UNIVERSITY

Address: Rt. 60, Dahlonega, GA 30597
Phone: 706-864-1930
Fax: 706-864-1845
Contact: Jill Hayes, PhD, RN, Department Head
Email: jhayes@ngcsu.edu

GENERAL INFORMATION

Type of School: *4-Year College or University, Public* •
Accreditation: *Southern Association of Colleges and Schools* •
Total Enrollment: *3400*

PROGRAM INFORMATION

LPN/LVN Exit: *No* • NLNAC Accreditation: *Yes*

NURSING STUDENT PROFILE

Total Nursing Enrollment: *129* • Full-Time Enrollment: *97* •
Part-Time Enrollment: *32* • Female Enrollment: *122* • Male
Enrollment: *7* • Total New Admissions Who Enrolled for
Fall: *74* • Total Graduates: *46*

FINANCES

Residential Annual Tuition: *$1,876* • Non-Residential
Annual Tuition: *$8,840* • General Institution Fees: *$239* •
Additional Nursing Fees: *$92*

SOUTH GEORGIA COLLEGE

Address: 100 W. College Park Drive, Douglas, GA 31533
Phone: 912-389-4503
Fax: 912-389-4631
Contact: Carol Hurst, MSN, RN, FNP-C, Chair, Division
           of Nursing
Email: churst@mail.sgc.peachnet.edu

GENERAL INFORMATION

Type of School: *2-Year College or University, Public* •
Accreditation: *Southern Association of Colleges and Schools* •
Total Enrollment: *1250*

PROGRAM INFORMATION

LPN/LVN Exit: *No* • NLNAC Accreditation: *Yes*

NURSING STUDENT PROFILE

Total Nursing Enrollment: *109* • Full-Time Enrollment: *50* •
Part-Time Enrollment: *59* • Female Enrollment: *101* • Male
Enrollment: *8* • Total New Admissions Who Enrolled for
Fall: *56* • Total Graduates: *52*

FINANCES

Residential Annual Tuition: *$1,280* • Non-Residential
Annual Tuition: *$3,840* • General Institution Fees: *$124* •
Additional Nursing Fees: *$15*

STATE UNIVERSITY OF WEST GEORGIA

Address: 1601 Maple St, Carrollton, GA 30118-4500
Phone: 770-836-6552
Fax: 770-836-4409
Contact: Jeanette C Bernnardt, Ph.D., RN, Chair
Email: jcb@westga.edu

GENERAL INFORMATION

Type of School: *4-Year College or University, Public* •
Accreditation: *Southern Association of Colleges and Schools* •
Total Enrollment: *8978*

PROGRAM INFORMATION

LPN/LVN Exit: *No* • NLNAC Accreditation: *Not Reported*

NURSING STUDENT PROFILE

Total Nursing Enrollment: *Not Reported* • Full-Time
Enrollment: *Not Reported* • Part-Time Enrollment: *Not
Reported* • Female Enrollment: *Not Reported* • Male
Enrollment: *Not Reported* • Total New Admissions Who
Enrolled for Fall: *Not Reported* • Total Graduates: *Not
Reported*

FINANCES

Residential Annual Tuition: *Not Reported* • Non-Residential
Annual Tuition: *Not Reported* • General Institution Fees: *Not
Reported* • Additional Nursing Fees: *Not Reported*

HAWAII COMMUNITY COLLEGE

Address: 523 West Lanikaula Street, Hilo, HI 96720
Phone: 808-974-7560
Fax: Not Reported
Contact: Elizabeth Ojala, PhD, RN, Director of Nursing
Program
Email: ojala@hawaii.edu

GENERAL INFORMATION

Type of School: *2-Year College or University, Public* •
Accreditation: *Western Association of Schools and Colleges* •
Total Enrollment: *1564*

PROGRAM INFORMATION

LPN/LVN Exit: *No* • NLNAC Accreditation: *Yes*

NURSING STUDENT PROFILE

Total Nursing Enrollment: *30* • Full-Time Enrollment: *27* •
Part-Time Enrollment: *3* • Female Enrollment: *26* • Male
Enrollment: *4* • Total New Admissions Who Enrolled for
Fall: *20* • Total Graduates: *17*

FINANCES

Residential Annual Tuition: *$1,032* • Non-Residential
Annual Tuition: *$5,808* • General Institution Fees: *$50* •
Additional Nursing Fees: *$40*

KAPIOLANI COMMUNITY COLLEGE

Address: 4303 Diamond Head Road, Honolulu, HI 96816-4421
Phone: 808-734-9302
Fax: Not Reported
Contact: Donna J. DeMello, MSN, RN, Program Director
Email: mellode@hawaii.edu

GENERAL INFORMATION

Type of School: *Other, Public* • Accreditation: *Western Association of Schools and Colleges* • Total Enrollment: *6800*

PROGRAM INFORMATION

LPN/LVN Exit: *Yes* • NLNAC Accreditation: *Yes*

NURSING STUDENT PROFILE

Total Nursing Enrollment: *109* • Full-Time Enrollment: *109* • Part-Time Enrollment: *0* • Female Enrollment: *88* • Male Enrollment: *21* • Total New Admissions Who Enrolled for Fall: *Not Reported* • Total Graduates: *Not Reported*

FINANCES

Residential Annual Tuition: *$1,440* • Non-Residential Annual Tuition: *$7,744* • General Institution Fees: *Not Reported* • Additional Nursing Fees: *Not Reported*

MAUI COMMUNITY COLLEGE

Address: 310 Kaahumanu Avenue, Kahului, HI 96732
Phone: 808-984-3250
Fax: 808-249-2175
Contact: Nancy Johnson, RN, MSN, FNP, Program Coordinator
Email: Nancy.Johnson@maui.cc.hawaii.edu

GENERAL INFORMATION

Type of School: *Other, Public* • Accreditation: *Western Association of Schools and Colleges* • Total Enrollment: *25000*

PROGRAM INFORMATION

LPN/LVN Exit: *Not Reported* • NLNAC Accreditation: *Yes*

NURSING STUDENT PROFILE

Total Nursing Enrollment: *70* • Full-Time Enrollment: *70* • Part-Time Enrollment: *0* • Female Enrollment: *61* • Male Enrollment: *9* • Total New Admissions Who Enrolled for Fall: *43* • Total Graduates: *23*

FINANCES

Residential Annual Tuition: *$1,575* • Non-Residential Annual Tuition: *Not Reported* • General Institution Fees: *$10* • Additional Nursing Fees: *$80*

UNIVERSITY OF HAWAII KAUAI COMMUNITY COLLEGE

Address: 3-1901 Kaumualii Highway, Lihue, HI 96766
Phone: 808-245-8255
Fax: Not Reported
Contact: Richard W. Carmichael, APRN, MS, MPN,
           Director of Nursing
Email: rickc@aloha.net

GENERAL INFORMATION

Type of School: *2-Year College or University, Public •* Accreditation: *Western Association of Schools and Colleges •* Total Enrollment: *1200*

PROGRAM INFORMATION

LPN/LVN Exit: *Yes •* NLNAC Accreditation: *Yes*

NURSING STUDENT PROFILE

Total Nursing Enrollment: *12 •* Full-Time Enrollment: *6 •* Part-Time Enrollment: *6 •* Female Enrollment: *11 •* Male Enrollment: *1 •* Total New Admissions Who Enrolled for Fall: *12 •* Total Graduates: *17*

FINANCES

Residential Annual Tuition: *$1,042 •* Non-Residential Annual Tuition: *$5,818 •* General Institution Fees: *$5 •* Additional Nursing Fees: *Not Reported*

BOISE STATE UNIVERSITY

Address: 1910 University Drive, Boise, ID 83725-1840
Phone: 208-426-3600
Fax: 208-426-1370
Contact: Pam Springer, PhD, RN, Director
Email: pspringer@boisestate.edu

GENERAL INFORMATION

Type of School: *4-Year College or University, Public •* Accreditation: *Northwestern Association of Schools and Colleges •* Total Enrollment: *16300*

PROGRAM INFORMATION

LPN/LVN Exit: *No •* NLNAC Accreditation: *Yes*

NURSING STUDENT PROFILE

Total Nursing Enrollment: *93 •* Full-Time Enrollment: *93 •* Part-Time Enrollment: *0 •* Female Enrollment: *81 •* Male Enrollment: *12 •* Total New Admissions Who Enrolled for Fall: *44 •* Total Graduates: *48*

FINANCES

Residential Annual Tuition: *$6,000 •* Non-Residential Annual Tuition: *$6,000 •* General Institution Fees: *$1,423 •* Additional Nursing Fees: *$125*

BRIGHAM YOUNG UNIVERSITY—IDAHO

Address: 175 Clarke, Rexburg, ID 834600620
Phone: 208-356-1328
Fax: 208-356-1474
Contact: Kim Vanwagoner, MA, MSN, RN, Chair of Nursing
Email: vanwagonerk@ricks.edu

GENERAL INFORMATION

Type of School: *Not Reported* • Accreditation: *None* • Total Enrollment: *Not Reported*

PROGRAM INFORMATION

LPN/LVN Exit: *Not Reported* • NLNAC Accreditation: *Yes*

NURSING STUDENT PROFILE

Total Nursing Enrollment: *152* • Full-Time Enrollment: *130* • Part-Time Enrollment: *22* • Female Enrollment: *126* • Male Enrollment: *26* • Total New Admissions Who Enrolled for Fall: *88* • Total Graduates: *84*

FINANCES

Residential Annual Tuition: *$2,100* • Non-Residential Annual Tuition: *$3,120* • General Institution Fees: *Not Reported* • Additional Nursing Fees: *$80*

COLLEGE OF SOUTHERN IDAHO

Address: P.O. Box 1238, Twin Falls, ID 83303
Phone: 208-733-9554
Fax: 208-736-4743
Contact: Claudeen R. Buettner, RN, EdD, Chairperson
Email: cbuettner@csi.edu

GENERAL INFORMATION

Type of School: *2-Year College or University, Public* • Accreditation: *Northwestern Association of Schools and Colleges* • Total Enrollment: *7000*

PROGRAM INFORMATION

LPN/LVN Exit: *No* • NLNAC Accreditation: *Yes*

NURSING STUDENT PROFILE

Total Nursing Enrollment: *116* • Full-Time Enrollment: *116* • Part-Time Enrollment: *0* • Female Enrollment: *100* • Male Enrollment: *16* • Total New Admissions Who Enrolled for Fall: *55* • Total Graduates: *41*

FINANCES

Residential Annual Tuition: *$1,400* • Non-Residential Annual Tuition: *$2,800* • General Institution Fees: *Not Reported* • Additional Nursing Fees: *$125*

NORTH IDAHO COLLEGE

Address: 1000 West Garden, Coeur D'Alene, ID 83814
Phone: 208-769-3484
Fax: 208-769-7774
Contact: Beverly J. Hatrock, MS, BS, RN, Interim Director
Email: bjhatroc@nic.edu

GENERAL INFORMATION

Type of School: *2-Year College or University, Public* • Accreditation: *Northwestern Association of Schools and Colleges* • Total Enrollment: *4049*

PROGRAM INFORMATION

LPN/LVN Exit: *No* • NLNAC Accreditation: *Yes*

NURSING STUDENT PROFILE

Total Nursing Enrollment: *71* • Full-Time Enrollment: *71* • Part-Time Enrollment: *0* • Female Enrollment: *61* • Male Enrollment: *10* • Total New Admissions Who Enrolled for Fall: *33* • Total Graduates: *35*

FINANCES

Residential Annual Tuition: *$1,296* • Non-Residential Annual Tuition: *$4,456* • General Institution Fees: *Not Reported* • Additional Nursing Fees: *$170*

RICKS COLLEGE

Address: 175 Clarke Building, Roxburg, ID 83460
Phone: 208-356-1326
Fax: 208-356-1474
Contact: Kim Vanwagoner, MA, MSN, RN, Chair of Nursing
Email: vanwagonerk@ricks.edu

GENERAL INFORMATION

Type of School: *Other, Private (Religious)* • Accreditation: *Northwestern Association of Schools and Colleges* • Total Enrollment: *9200*

PROGRAM INFORMATION

LPN/LVN Exit: *Yes* • NLNAC Accreditation: *Yes*

NURSING STUDENT PROFILE

Total Nursing Enrollment: *152* • Full-Time Enrollment: *130* • Part-Time Enrollment: *22* • Female Enrollment: *126* • Male Enrollment: *26* • Total New Admissions Who Enrolled for Fall: *88* • Total Graduates: *84*

FINANCES

Residential Annual Tuition: *$2,100* • Non-Residential Annual Tuition: *$3,120* • General Institution Fees: *$0* • Additional Nursing Fees: *$80*

ADVOCATE NORTH SIDE KUTSCH

Address: 2318 W Irving Park Rd Building C, Chicago, IL
             60618
Phone: 773-866-6921
Fax: 773-866-6952
Contact: Phyllis D. Thomson, MS, RN, Executive Dean
Email: pthomson@rhmc.com

BLACK HAWK COLLEGE

Address: 6600 34th Ave, Moline, IL 61265
Phone: 309-796-5363
Fax: 309-792-3418
Contact: Cheryl Hardison, MSN, RN, Department
             Chairperson and Professor
Email: hardisonc@bhcl.bhc.edu

GENERAL INFORMATION

Type of School: *Other, Private (Independent)* • Accreditation:
North Central Association of Colleges and Schools • Total
Enrollment: *75*

GENERAL INFORMATION

Type of School: *2-Year College or University, Public* •
Accreditation: *North Central Association of Colleges and
Schools* • Total Enrollment: *5100*

PROGRAM INFORMATION

LPN/LVN Exit: *No* • NLNAC Accreditation: *Not Reported*

PROGRAM INFORMATION

LPN/LVN Exit: *No* • NLNAC Accreditation: *Yes*

NURSING STUDENT PROFILE

Total Nursing Enrollment: *70* • Full-Time Enrollment: *70* •
Part-Time Enrollment: *0* • Female Enrollment: *61* • Male
Enrollment: *9* • Total New Admissions Who Enrolled for
Fall: *26* • Total Graduates: *47*

NURSING STUDENT PROFILE

Total Nursing Enrollment: *93* • Full-Time Enrollment: *74* •
Part-Time Enrollment: *19* • Female Enrollment: *91* • Male
Enrollment: *2* • Total New Admissions Who Enrolled for
Fall: *29* • Total Graduates: *34*

FINANCES

Residential Annual Tuition: *$7,488* • Non-Residential
Annual Tuition: *$7,488* • General Institution Fees: *$514* •
Additional Nursing Fees: *$0*

FINANCES

Residential Annual Tuition: *$1,836* • Non-Residential
Annual Tuition: *$9,324* • General Institution Fees: *$140* •
Additional Nursing Fees: *$700*

CARL SANDBURG COLLEGE

Address: 2400 Tom L. Wilson Blvd., Galesburg, IL
            61401-9574
Phone: 309-341-5292
Fax: 309-341-5429
Contact: Doris K. Kowalski, MA, RN, Coordinator of
            Nursing Programs
Email: dkowalski@csc.cc.il.us

GENERAL INFORMATION

Type of School: *2-Year College or University, Public* •
Accreditation: *North Central Association of Colleges and
Schools* • Total Enrollment: *3500*

PROGRAM INFORMATION

LPN/LVN Exit: *No* • NLNAC Accreditation: *Not Reported*

NURSING STUDENT PROFILE

Total Nursing Enrollment: *47* • Full-Time Enrollment: *47* •
Part-Time Enrollment: *0* • Female Enrollment: *47* • Male
Enrollment: *0* • Total New Admissions Who Enrolled for
Fall: *24* • Total Graduates: *22*

FINANCES

Residential Annual Tuition: *$1,272* • Non-Residential
Annual Tuition: *$3,900* • General Institution Fees: *$192* •
Additional Nursing Fees: *Not Reported*

COLLEGE OF DUPAGE

Address: 425 22nd St, Glen Ellyn, IL 60137-6784
Phone: 630-942-2652
Fax: 630-858-5409
Contact: Ellen L. Davel, EdD, RN, Coordinator
Email: davele@cdnet.cod.edu

GENERAL INFORMATION

Type of School: *2-Year College or University, Public* •
Accreditation: *North Central Association of Colleges and
Schools* • Total Enrollment: *34000*

PROGRAM INFORMATION

LPN/LVN Exit: *No* • NLNAC Accreditation: *Yes*

NURSING STUDENT PROFILE

Total Nursing Enrollment: *159* • Full-Time Enrollment: *57* •
Part-Time Enrollment: *102* • Female Enrollment: *147* • Male
Enrollment: *12* • Total New Admissions Who Enrolled for
Fall: *89* • Total Graduates: *69*

FINANCES

Residential Annual Tuition: *$840* • Non-Residential Annual
Tuition: *$4,000* • General Institution Fees: *Not Reported* •
Additional Nursing Fees: *$137*

COLLEGE OF LAKE COUNTY

Address: 19351 West Washington Street, Lakes County, IL
            33215
Phone: 847-543-2339
Fax: Not Reported
Contact: Delores M. Swan, RN, MEd, Director of
            Nursing Education
Email: hur093@clc.cc.il.us

GENERAL INFORMATION

Type of School: *2-Year College or University, Public* •
Accreditation: *North Central Association of Colleges and
Schools* • Total Enrollment: *16000*

PROGRAM INFORMATION

LPN/LVN Exit: *No* • NLNAC Accreditation: *Yes*

NURSING STUDENT PROFILE

Total Nursing Enrollment: *183* • Full-Time Enrollment: *0* •
Part-Time Enrollment: *183* • Female Enrollment: *68* • Male
Enrollment: *115* • Total New Admissions Who Enrolled for
Fall: *Not Reported* • Total Graduates: *Not Reported*

FINANCES

Residential Annual Tuition: *$1,632* • Non-Residential
Annual Tuition: *$5,664* • General Institution Fees: *Not
Reported* • Additional Nursing Fees: *Not Reported*

DANVILLE AREA COMMUNITY COLLEGE

Address: 200 East Main Street, Danville, IL 61832
Phone: 217-443-8814
Fax: Not Reported
Contact: Ann Wogle, MS, RN, Director, School of
            Nursing
Email: awogle@dccc.cc.il.us

GENERAL INFORMATION

Type of School: *Not Reported* • Accreditation: *Not Reported* •
Total Enrollment: *Not Reported*

PROGRAM INFORMATION

LPN/LVN Exit: *Not Reported* • NLNAC Accreditation: *Not
Reported*

NURSING STUDENT PROFILE

Total Nursing Enrollment: *Not Reported* • Full-Time
Enrollment: *Not Reported* • Part-Time Enrollment: *Not
Reported* • Female Enrollment: *Not Reported* • Male
Enrollment: *Not Reported* • Total New Admissions Who
Enrolled for Fall: *Not Reported* • Total Graduates: *Not
Reported*

FINANCES

Residential Annual Tuition: *$1,500* • Non-Residential
Annual Tuition: *$6,000* • General Institution Fees: *Not
Reported* • Additional Nursing Fees: *Not Reported*

ELGIN COMMUNITY COLLEGE

Address: 1700 Spartan Dr., Elgin, IL 60123
Phone: 847-214-7326
Fax: 847-214-7527
Contact: Maryann K. Vaca, RN, MA, MEd, Associate Dean, Health Professions
Email: mvaca@elgin.edu

GENERAL INFORMATION

Type of School: *2-Year College or University, Public* • Accreditation: *North Central Association of Colleges and Schools* • Total Enrollment: *11973*

PROGRAM INFORMATION

LPN/LVN Exit: *Yes* • NLNAC Accreditation: *Yes*

NURSING STUDENT PROFILE

Total Nursing Enrollment: *134* • Full-Time Enrollment: *134* • Part-Time Enrollment: *0* • Female Enrollment: *124* • Male Enrollment: *10* • Total New Admissions Who Enrolled for Fall: *52* • Total Graduates: *61*

FINANCES

Residential Annual Tuition: *$1,984* • Non-Residential Annual Tuition: *$10,092* • General Institution Fees: *$0* • Additional Nursing Fees: *$550*

HEARTLAND COMMUNITY COLLEGE

Address: 1500 West Raab Rd., Normal, IL 61761
Phone: 309-268-8608
Fax: 309-268-7991
Contact: Catherine Miller, MSN, RN, Division Chair, Human Services
Email: catherine.miller@hcc.cc.il.us

GENERAL INFORMATION

Type of School: *2-Year College or University, Public* • Accreditation: *North Central Association of Colleges and Schools* • Total Enrollment: *4000*

PROGRAM INFORMATION

LPN/LVN Exit: *Yes* • NLNAC Accreditation: *Yes*

NURSING STUDENT PROFILE

Total Nursing Enrollment: *60* • Full-Time Enrollment: *9* • Part-Time Enrollment: *51* • Female Enrollment: *52* • Male Enrollment: *8* • Total New Admissions Who Enrolled for Fall: *37* • Total Graduates: *23*

FINANCES

Residential Annual Tuition: *$1,056* • Non-Residential Annual Tuition: *$2,112* • General Institution Fees: *$98* • Additional Nursing Fees: *$360*

HIGHLAND COMMUNITY COLLEGE

Address:　　2998 Pearl City Rd, Freeport, IL 61032
Phone:　　　Not Reported
Fax:　　　　Not Reported
Contact:　　Alice Nied, MSN, RN, Director
Email:　　　Not Reported

GENERAL INFORMATION

Type of School: *Not Reported* • Accreditation: *Not Reported* • Total Enrollment: *Not Reported*

PROGRAM INFORMATION

LPN/LVN Exit: *Not Reported* • NLNAC Accreditation: *Not Reported*

NURSING STUDENT PROFILE

Total Nursing Enrollment: *Not Reported* • Full-Time Enrollment: *Not Reported* • Part-Time Enrollment: *Not Reported* • Female Enrollment: *Not Reported* • Male Enrollment: *Not Reported* • Total New Admissions Who Enrolled for Fall: *Not Reported* • Total Graduates: *Not Reported*

FINANCES

Residential Annual Tuition: *Not Reported* • Non-Residential Annual Tuition: *Not Reported* • General Institution Fees: *Not Reported* • Additional Nursing Fees: *Not Reported*

ILLINOIS CENTRAL COLLEGE

Address:　　201 SW Adams, Peoria, IL 61625
Phone:　　　309-999-4655
Fax:　　　　309-673-9626
Contact:　　Mary Beth Kiefner, RN, MS, Program Supervisor
Email:　　　mkiefner@icc.cc.il.us

GENERAL INFORMATION

Type of School: *2-Year College or University, Public* • Accreditation: *North Central Association of Colleges and Schools* • Total Enrollment: *11740*

PROGRAM INFORMATION

LPN/LVN Exit: *No* • NLNAC Accreditation: *Yes*

NURSING STUDENT PROFILE

Total Nursing Enrollment: *112* • Full-Time Enrollment: *40* • Part-Time Enrollment: *72* • Female Enrollment: *108* • Male Enrollment: *4* • Total New Admissions Who Enrolled for Fall: *70* • Total Graduates: *41*

FINANCES

Residential Annual Tuition: *$50* • Non-Residential Annual Tuition: *$110* • General Institution Fees: *$1,200* • Additional Nursing Fees: *$300*

ILLINOIS EASTERN COMMUNITY COLLEGES

Address: District 529, Onley Central College, 305 N West
            Street, Olney, IL 391430
Phone: 618-395-7777
Fax: 618-395-4200
Contact: Donna C. Henry, RN, MS, CHIP, Associate
            Dean of Nursing and Allied Health
Email: henryd@iecc.cc.il.us

GENERAL INFORMATION

Type of School: *2-Year College or University, Public* •
Accreditation: *North Central Association of Colleges and
Schools* • Total Enrollment: *1400*

PROGRAM INFORMATION

LPN/LVN Exit: *Yes* • NLNAC Accreditation: *Yes*

NURSING STUDENT PROFILE

Total Nursing Enrollment: *110* • Full-Time Enrollment: *69* •
Part-Time Enrollment: *41* • Female Enrollment: *98* • Male
Enrollment: *12* • Total New Admissions Who Enrolled for
Fall: *110* • Total Graduates: *56*

FINANCES

Residential Annual Tuition: *$960* • Non-Residential Annual
Tuition: *$3,500* • General Institution Fees: *$16* • Additional
Nursing Fees: *$61*

ILLINOIS VALLEY COMMUNITY COLLEGE

Address: 2578 350th Rd., Oglesby, IL 61348
Phone: 815-224-0485
Fax: 815-224-3033
Contact: Gloria Bouxsein, MSN, RN, Director of Nursing
Email: bouxsein@ivcc.edu

GENERAL INFORMATION

Type of School: *2-Year College or University, Public* •
Accreditation: *North Central Association of Colleges and
Schools* • Total Enrollment: *4100*

PROGRAM INFORMATION

LPN/LVN Exit: *Yes* • NLNAC Accreditation: *Yes*

NURSING STUDENT PROFILE

Total Nursing Enrollment: *93* • Full-Time Enrollment: *93* •
Part-Time Enrollment: *0* • Female Enrollment: *90* • Male
Enrollment: *3* • Total New Admissions Who Enrolled for
Fall: *44* • Total Graduates: *40*

FINANCES

Residential Annual Tuition: *$1,344* • Non-Residential
Annual Tuition: *$4,488* • General Institution Fees: *Not
Reported* • Additional Nursing Fees: *Not Reported*

JOHN A. LOGAN COLLEGE

Address: 700 Logan College Rd., Building G, Carterville, IL 62918
Phone: 618-985-3741
Fax: 618-985-9181
Contact: Marilyn J. Murphy, MSN, RN, CNA, Director of Nursing
Email: marilyn.murphy@jal.cc.il.us

GENERAL INFORMATION

Type of School: *2-Year College or University, Public* •
Accreditation: *North Central Association of Colleges and Schools* • Total Enrollment: *40*

PROGRAM INFORMATION

LPN/LVN Exit: *Yes* • NLNAC Accreditation: *Not Reported*

NURSING STUDENT PROFILE

Total Nursing Enrollment: *53* • Full-Time Enrollment: *30* •
Part-Time Enrollment: *23* • Female Enrollment: *48* • Male
Enrollment: *5* • Total New Admissions Who Enrolled for
Fall: *40* • Total Graduates: *Not Reported*

FINANCES

Residential Annual Tuition: *Not Reported* • Non-Residential
Annual Tuition: *Not Reported* • General Institution Fees: *Not
Reported* • Additional Nursing Fees: *Not Reported*

JOHN WOOD COMMUNITY COLLEGE

Address: 150 South 48th St., Quincy, IL 62302
Phone: 217-224-6564
Fax: 217-224-4208
Contact: Julie Barry, PhD, RNC, Director of Health Services
Email: barry@jwcc.edu

GENERAL INFORMATION

Type of School: *2-Year College or University, Public* •
Accreditation: *North Central Association of Colleges and Schools* • Total Enrollment: *2500*

PROGRAM INFORMATION

LPN/LVN Exit: *No* • NLNAC Accreditation: *Not Reported*

NURSING STUDENT PROFILE

Total Nursing Enrollment: *54* • Full-Time Enrollment: *54* •
Part-Time Enrollment: *0* • Female Enrollment: *54* • Male
Enrollment: *0* • Total New Admissions Who Enrolled for
Fall: *20* • Total Graduates: *28*

FINANCES

Residential Annual Tuition: *$1,730* • Non-Residential
Annual Tuition: *Not Reported* • General Institution Fees: *Not
Reported* • Additional Nursing Fees: *$120*

JOLIET JUNIOR COLLEGE

Address: 1215 Houbolt Rd., Joliet, IL 60431
Phone: 815-280-2560
Fax: 815-280-6710
Contact: Judith M. Kachel, EdD, RN, Chairperson
Email: jkachel@jjc.cc.il.us

GENERAL INFORMATION

Type of School: *2-Year College or University, Public* •
Accreditation: *North Central Association of Colleges and Schools* • Total Enrollment: *12000*

PROGRAM INFORMATION

LPN/LVN Exit: *No* • NLNAC Accreditation: *Yes*

NURSING STUDENT PROFILE

Total Nursing Enrollment: *211* • Full-Time Enrollment: *211* • Part-Time Enrollment: *0* • Female Enrollment: *198* • Male Enrollment: *13* • Total New Admissions Who Enrolled for Fall: *50* • Total Graduates: *91*

FINANCES

Residential Annual Tuition: *$1,176* • Non-Residential Annual Tuition: *$5,328* • General Institution Fees: *$187* • Additional Nursing Fees: *Not Reported*

KANKAKEE COMMUNITY COLLEGE

Address: Box 888 River Rd, Kankakee, IL 60901
Phone: 815-933-0295
Fax: Not Reported
Contact: Phyllis Nichols, MSN, RN, Director of Nursing
Email: pnichols@kankahee.edu

GENERAL INFORMATION

Type of School: *Other* • Accreditation: *None* • Total Enrollment: *Not Reported*

PROGRAM INFORMATION

LPN/LVN Exit: *Not Reported* • NLNAC Accreditation: *Not Reported*

NURSING STUDENT PROFILE

Total Nursing Enrollment: *Not Reported* • Full-Time Enrollment: *Not Reported* • Part-Time Enrollment: *Not Reported* • Female Enrollment: *Not Reported* • Male Enrollment: *Not Reported* • Total New Admissions Who Enrolled for Fall: *Not Reported* • Total Graduates: *Not Reported*

FINANCES

Residential Annual Tuition: *$1,760* • Non-Residential Annual Tuition: *$5,132.80* • General Institution Fees: *Not Reported* • Additional Nursing Fees: *Not Reported*

KASKASKIA COLLEGE

Address: 27210 College Rd., Centralia, IL 62801
Phone: 618-545-3331
Fax: 618-532-2365
Contact: Mary Lou Whitten, MSN, RN, Director of
             Nursing Education Programs
Email: mwhitten@kc.cc.il.us

GENERAL INFORMATION

Type of School: *2-Year College or University, Public* •
Accreditation: *North Central Association of Colleges and
Schools* • Total Enrollment: *2677*

PROGRAM INFORMATION

LPN/LVN Exit: *No* • NLNAC Accreditation: *Yes*

NURSING STUDENT PROFILE

Total Nursing Enrollment: *136* • Full-Time Enrollment: *90* •
Part-Time Enrollment: *46* • Female Enrollment: *123* • Male
Enrollment: *13* • Total New Admissions Who Enrolled for
Fall: *46* • Total Graduates: *74*

FINANCES

Residential Annual Tuition: *$1,504* • Non-Residential
Annual Tuition: *$8,184* • General Institution Fees: *$12* •
Additional Nursing Fees: *$80*

KENNEDY-KING COLLEGE-CHICAGO CITY COLLEGES

Address: 6800 S. Wentworth Ave., Chicago, IL 60621
Phone: 773-602-5221
Fax: 773-602-5216
Contact: Stephanie Fisher-Lanfair, MSN, RN,
             Chairperson, Department of Nursing
Email: slanfair@ccc.edu

GENERAL INFORMATION

Type of School: *2-Year College or University, Public* •
Accreditation: *North Central Association of Colleges and
Schools* • Total Enrollment: *2458*

PROGRAM INFORMATION

LPN/LVN Exit: *No* • NLNAC Accreditation: *Yes*

NURSING STUDENT PROFILE

Total Nursing Enrollment: *65* • Full-Time Enrollment: *65* •
Part-Time Enrollment: *0* • Female Enrollment: *60* • Male
Enrollment: *5* • Total New Admissions Who Enrolled for
Fall: *23* • Total Graduates: *41*

FINANCES

Residential Annual Tuition: *$1,664* • Non-Residential
Annual Tuition: *$6,472* • General Institution Fees: *$117* •
Additional Nursing Fees: *$100*

KISHWAUKEE COLLEGE

Address: 21193 Malta Rd., Malta, IL 60150
Phone: 815-826-2086
Fax: Not Reported
Contact: Heather Peters, RN, MS, MBA, Director of
             Nursing
Email: Not Reported

GENERAL INFORMATION

Type of School: *2-Year College or University, Public* •
Accreditation: *None* • Total Enrollment: *Not Reported*

PROGRAM INFORMATION

LPN/LVN Exit: *Not Reported* • NLNAC Accreditation: *Not
Reported*

NURSING STUDENT PROFILE

Total Nursing Enrollment: *Not Reported* • Full-Time
Enrollment: *Not Reported* • Part-Time Enrollment: *Not
Reported* • Female Enrollment: *Not Reported* • Male
Enrollment: *Not Reported* • Total New Admissions Who
Enrolled for Fall: *Not Reported* • Total Graduates: *Not
Reported*

FINANCES

Residential Annual Tuition: *$1,792* • Non-Residential
Annual Tuition: *$8,011* • General Institution Fees: *Not
Reported* • Additional Nursing Fees: *Not Reported*

LAKE LAND COLLEGE

Address: 5001 Lake Land Blvd., Matton, IL 61938
Phone: 217-234-5452
Fax: 217-234-5463
Contact: Kathleen M. Doehring, RN, BS, MS, Director
Email: kdoehring@lakeland.cc.il.us

GENERAL INFORMATION

Type of School: *2-Year College or University, Public* •
Accreditation: *North Central Association of Colleges and
Schools* • Total Enrollment: *4676*

PROGRAM INFORMATION

LPN/LVN Exit: *Not Reported* • NLNAC Accreditation: *Yes*

NURSING STUDENT PROFILE

Total Nursing Enrollment: *65* • Full-Time Enrollment: *65* •
Part-Time Enrollment: *0* • Female Enrollment: *56* • Male
Enrollment: *9* • Total New Admissions Who Enrolled for
Fall: *61* • Total Graduates: *17*

FINANCES

Residential Annual Tuition: *$1,800* • Non-Residential
Annual Tuition: *$9,000* • General Institution Fees: *$360* •
Additional Nursing Fees: *$100*

LEWIS & CLARK COMMUNITY COLLEGE

Address: 5800 Godfrey Rd., Godfrey, IL 62035
Phone: 618-468-4436
Fax: 618-468-2252
Contact: Donna Meyer, MSN, RN, Nursing Program
            Coordinator
Email: dmever@lc.edu

LINCOLN LAND COMMUNITY COLLEGE

Address: 5250 Shepherd Rd., PO Box 19256, Springfield,
            IL 62703
Phone: 217-786-2436
Fax: 217-786-2776
Contact: Joan Lewis, MSN, CNP, Department Chair
Email: joan.lewis@llcc.cc.us

GENERAL INFORMATION

Type of School: *2-Year College or University, Public* •
Accreditation: *North Central Association of Colleges and
Schools* • Total Enrollment: *6950*

GENERAL INFORMATION

Type of School: *2-Year College or University, Public* •
Accreditation: *North Central Association of Colleges and
Schools* • Total Enrollment: *8000*

PROGRAM INFORMATION

LPN/LVN Exit: *No* • NLNAC Accreditation: *Yes*

PROGRAM INFORMATION

LPN/LVN Exit: *No* • NLNAC Accreditation: *Yes*

NURSING STUDENT PROFILE

Total Nursing Enrollment: *116* • Full-Time Enrollment: *95* •
Part-Time Enrollment: *21* • Female Enrollment: *110* • Male
Enrollment: *6* • Total New Admissions Who Enrolled for
Fall: *23* • Total Graduates: *39*

NURSING STUDENT PROFILE

Total Nursing Enrollment: *127* • Full-Time Enrollment:
127 • Part-Time Enrollment: *0* • Female Enrollment: *122* •
Male Enrollment: *5* • Total New Admissions Who Enrolled
for Fall: *40* • Total Graduates: *76*

FINANCES

Residential Annual Tuition: *$1,248* • Non-Residential
Annual Tuition: *$4,656* • General Institution Fees: *$12* •
Additional Nursing Fees: *$213*

FINANCES

Residential Annual Tuition: *$1,260* • Non-Residential
Annual Tuition: *$3,700* • General Institution Fees: *$15* •
Additional Nursing Fees: *$0*

MALCOLM X COLLEGE

Address: 1900 W. Van Buren, Chicago, IL 60612
Phone: 773-850-7145
Fax: Not Reported
Contact: Beverly Anderson, RN, MS, Chairperson
Email: banderson@ccc.edu

GENERAL INFORMATION

Type of School: *2-Year College or University, Public* •
Accreditation: *North Central Association of Colleges and Schools* • Total Enrollment: *2129*

PROGRAM INFORMATION

LPN/LVN Exit: *Not Reported* • NLNAC Accreditation: *Yes*

NURSING STUDENT PROFILE

Total Nursing Enrollment: *33* • Full-Time Enrollment: *33* • Part-Time Enrollment: *0* • Female Enrollment: *30* • Male Enrollment: *3* • Total New Admissions Who Enrolled for Fall: *23* • Total Graduates: *Not Reported*

FINANCES

Residential Annual Tuition: *$1,140* • Non-Residential Annual Tuition: *$5,050* • General Institution Fees: *$115* • Additional Nursing Fees: *$100*

MORAINE VALLEY COMMUNITY COLLEGE

Address: 10900 South 88th St., Palos Hills, IL 60465
Phone: 708-974-5303
Fax: 708-974-0185
Contact: Gloria A. Victoria, MSN, RN, Department Chair, Nursing
Email: victoria@morainevalley.edu

GENERAL INFORMATION

Type of School: *2-Year College or University, Public* •
Accreditation: *North Central Association of Colleges and Schools* • Total Enrollment: *14500*

PROGRAM INFORMATION

LPN/LVN Exit: *No* • NLNAC Accreditation: *Yes*

NURSING STUDENT PROFILE

Total Nursing Enrollment: *172* • Full-Time Enrollment: *172* • Part-Time Enrollment: *0* • Female Enrollment: *157* • Male Enrollment: *15* • Total New Admissions Who Enrolled for Fall: *Not Reported* • Total Graduates: *Not Reported*

FINANCES

Residential Annual Tuition: *$1,696* • Non-Residential Annual Tuition: *$7,616* • General Institution Fees: *Not Reported* • Additional Nursing Fees: *Not Reported*

MORTON COLLEGE

Address: 3801 S. Central Ave., Cicero, IL 60804
Phone: 708-656-8000
Fax: 708-656-3197
Contact: Aline Tupa, MSN, ED, Coordinator of Nursing
Email: tupaa@morton.cc.il.us

GENERAL INFORMATION

Type of School: *2-Year College or University, Public* •
Accreditation: *North Central Association of Colleges and Schools* • Total Enrollment: *5000*

PROGRAM INFORMATION

LPN/LVN Exit: *Yes* • NLNAC Accreditation: *Not Reported*

NURSING STUDENT PROFILE

Total Nursing Enrollment: *133* • Full-Time Enrollment: *133* • Part-Time Enrollment: *0* • Female Enrollment: *120* • Male Enrollment: *13* • Total New Admissions Who Enrolled for Fall: *75* • Total Graduates: *43*

FINANCES

Residential Annual Tuition: *$1,128* • Non-Residential Annual Tuition: *$4,704* • General Institution Fees: *$1,668* • Additional Nursing Fees: *$75*

OAKTON COMMUNITY COLLEGE

Address: 1600 E. Golf Rd., Des Plaines, IL 60016
Phone: 847-635-1720
Fax: 847-635-1764
Contact: Marilou Wasseluk, MS, MPA, RN, Chairperson
Email: wasseluk@oakton.edu

GENERAL INFORMATION

Type of School: *2-Year College or University, Public* •
Accreditation: *North Central Association of Colleges and Schools* • Total Enrollment: *10000*

PROGRAM INFORMATION

LPN/LVN Exit: *Not Reported* • NLNAC Accreditation: *Yes*

NURSING STUDENT PROFILE

Total Nursing Enrollment: *122* • Full-Time Enrollment: *122* • Part-Time Enrollment: *0* • Female Enrollment: *107* • Male Enrollment: *15* • Total New Admissions Who Enrolled for Fall: *61* • Total Graduates: *46*

FINANCES

Residential Annual Tuition: *$1,856* • Non-Residential Annual Tuition: *$7,424* • General Institution Fees: *Not Reported* • Additional Nursing Fees: *$85*

OLIVE-HARVEY COLLEGE

Address: 10001 S Woodlawn Ave, Chicago, IL 60628
Phone: 773-850-7145
Fax: Not Reported
Contact: Marilou Wassaluk, RN, MPA, Chairperson
Email: bsnderson@ccc.edu

PARKLAND COLLEGE

Address: 2400 W. Bradley, Champaign, IL 61821
Phone: 217-373-3750
Fax: 217-373-3830
Contact: Hope R. Wolfe, MSN, RNC, CS, Nursing
          Program Director
Email: hwolfe@parkland.cc.il.us

GENERAL INFORMATION

Type of School: *Not Reported* • Accreditation: *Not Reported* •
Total Enrollment: *Not Reported*

GENERAL INFORMATION

Type of School: *2-Year College or University, Public* •
Accreditation: *North Central Association of Colleges and
Schools* • Total Enrollment: *10000*

PROGRAM INFORMATION

LPN/LVN Exit: *Not Reported* • NLNAC Accreditation: *Yes*

PROGRAM INFORMATION

LPN/LVN Exit: *Not Reported* • NLNAC Accreditation: *Yes*

NURSING STUDENT PROFILE

Total Nursing Enrollment: *Not Reported* • Full-Time
Enrollment: *Not Reported* • Part-Time Enrollment: *Not
Reported* • Female Enrollment: *Not Reported* • Male
Enrollment: *Not Reported* • Total New Admissions Who
Enrolled for Fall: *Not Reported* • Total Graduates: *Not
Reported*

NURSING STUDENT PROFILE

Total Nursing Enrollment: *155* • Full-Time Enrollment: *30* •
Part-Time Enrollment: *125* • Female Enrollment: *145* • Male
Enrollment: *10* • Total New Admissions Who Enrolled for
Fall: *47* • Total Graduates: *51*

FINANCES

Residential Annual Tuition: *$1,664* • Non-Residential
Annual Tuition: *$6,473* • General Institution Fees: *Not
Reported* • Additional Nursing Fees: *Not Reported*

FINANCES

Residential Annual Tuition: *$1,272* • Non-Residential
Annual Tuition: *$4,512* • General Institution Fees: *Not
Reported* • Additional Nursing Fees: *Not Reported*

PRAIRIE STATE COLLEGE

Address: 202 South Halsted St., Chicago Heights, IL
            60144
Phone: 708-709-3766
Fax: Not Reported
Contact: Gwen M. Dean, MA, RN, Nursing Program
            Coordinator
Email: gdean@prairie.cc.il.us

GENERAL INFORMATION

Type of School: *2-Year College or University, Public* •
Accreditation: *North Central Association of Colleges and
Schools* • Total Enrollment: *2500*

PROGRAM INFORMATION

LPN/LVN Exit: *No* • NLNAC Accreditation: *Yes*

NURSING STUDENT PROFILE

Total Nursing Enrollment: *99* • Full-Time Enrollment: *99* •
Part-Time Enrollment: *0* • Female Enrollment: *94* • Male
Enrollment: *5* • Total New Admissions Who Enrolled for
Fall: *75* • Total Graduates: *33*

FINANCES

Residential Annual Tuition: *$1,224* • Non-Residential
Annual Tuition: *$5,216* • General Institution Fees: *$100* •
Additional Nursing Fees: *$70*

REND LAKE COLLEGE

Address: 468 N. Ken Gray Parkway, Ina, IL 62846
Phone: Not Reported
Fax: Not Reported
Contact: Wilanna Patton, MSN, RN, Chair
Email: Not Reported

GENERAL INFORMATION

Type of School: *Not Reported* • Accreditation: *Not Reported* •
Total Enrollment: *Not Reported*

PROGRAM INFORMATION

LPN/LVN Exit: *Not Reported* • NLNAC Accreditation: *Not
Reported*

NURSING STUDENT PROFILE

Total Nursing Enrollment: *Not Reported* • Full-Time
Enrollment: *Not Reported* • Part-Time Enrollment: *Not
Reported* • Female Enrollment: *Not Reported* • Male
Enrollment: *Not Reported* • Total New Admissions Who
Enrolled for Fall: *Not Reported* • Total Graduates: *Not
Reported*

FINANCES

Residential Annual Tuition: *$1,536* • Non-Residential
Annual Tuition: *$4,860* • General Institution Fees: *Not
Reported* • Additional Nursing Fees: *Not Reported*

RICHARD J. DALEY COLLEGE

Address: 7500 S. Pulaski, Chcago, IL 60652
Phone: 773-838-7681
Fax: 773-838-7424
Contact: Genevieve A. Harris, MSN, RN,
           Chairperson/Director
Email: gharris@ccc.edu

GENERAL INFORMATION

Type of School: *2-Year College or University, Public* •
Accreditation: *North Central Association of Colleges and
Schools* • Total Enrollment: *3700*

PROGRAM INFORMATION

LPN/LVN Exit: *Not Reported* • NLNAC Accreditation: *Yes*

NURSING STUDENT PROFILE

Total Nursing Enrollment: *113* • Full-Time Enrollment:
100 • Part-Time Enrollment: *13* • Female Enrollment: *99* •
Male Enrollment: *14* • Total New Admissions Who Enrolled
for Fall: *60* • Total Graduates: *26*

FINANCES

Residential Annual Tuition: *$1,400* • Non-Residential
Annual Tuition: *$5,600* • General Institution Fees: *$125* •
Additional Nursing Fees: *$0*

RICHLAND COMMUNITY COLLEGE

Address: 1 College Park Dr., Decatur, IL 62521
Phone: 217-875-7200
Fax: 217-875-6965
Contact: Carol A. Wood, MSN, RN, CNS, Nursing
           Program Coordinator
Email: cwood@richland.cc.il.us

GENERAL INFORMATION

Type of School: *2-Year College or University, Public* •
Accreditation: *North Central Association of Colleges and
Schools* • Total Enrollment: *3674*

PROGRAM INFORMATION

LPN/LVN Exit: *No* • NLNAC Accreditation: *Yes*

NURSING STUDENT PROFILE

Total Nursing Enrollment: *47* • Full-Time Enrollment: *47* •
Part-Time Enrollment: *0* • Female Enrollment: *47* • Male
Enrollment: *0* • Total New Admissions Who Enrolled for
Fall: *25* • Total Graduates: *18*

FINANCES

Residential Annual Tuition: *$1,116* • Non-Residential
Annual Tuition: *$4,800* • General Institution Fees: *$20* •
Additional Nursing Fees: *Not Reported*

ROCK VALLEY COLLEGE

Address: 3301 Northmulford Rd., Rockford, IL 61114
Phone: 815-654-4410
Fax: 815-654-4408
Contact: Cynthia R. Luxton, MS, RN, Director of Nursing and Allied Health
Email: fahsicl@ruc.cc.il.us

GENERAL INFORMATION

Type of School: *2-Year College or University, Public* • Accreditation: *North Central Association of Colleges and Schools* • Total Enrollment: *13000*

PROGRAM INFORMATION

LPN/LVN Exit: *No* • NLNAC Accreditation: *Not Reported*

NURSING STUDENT PROFILE

Total Nursing Enrollment: *71* • Full-Time Enrollment: *71* • Part-Time Enrollment: *0* • Female Enrollment: *69* • Male Enrollment: *2* • Total New Admissions Who Enrolled for Fall: *22* • Total Graduates: *31*

FINANCES

Residential Annual Tuition: *$1,312* • Non-Residential Annual Tuition: *$4,972* • General Institution Fees: *Not Reported* • Additional Nursing Fees: *$31*

SAUK VALLEY COMMUNITY COLLEGE

Address: 173 Illinois RTE #2, Dixon, IL 61021
Phone: 815-288-5511
Fax: 815-288-1880
Contact: Rosemary Johnson, RN, MS, Director of Health Careers Education
Email: johnsonr@svcc.edu

GENERAL INFORMATION

Type of School: *2-Year College or University, Public* • Accreditation: *North Central Association of Colleges and Schools* • Total Enrollment: *2962*

PROGRAM INFORMATION

LPN/LVN Exit: *No* • NLNAC Accreditation: *Not Reported*

NURSING STUDENT PROFILE

Total Nursing Enrollment: *44* • Full-Time Enrollment: *44* • Part-Time Enrollment: *0* • Female Enrollment: *43* • Male Enrollment: *1* • Total New Admissions Who Enrolled for Fall: *31* • Total Graduates: *17*

FINANCES

Residential Annual Tuition: *$1,224* • Non-Residential Annual Tuition: *$6,384* • General Institution Fees: *$24* • Additional Nursing Fees: *$35*

SHAWNEE COMMUNITY COLLEGE

Address: 8364 Shawnee College Rd, Ullin, IL 62992
Phone: Not Reported
Fax: Not Reported
Contact: J Hayduk, PhD, RN, Director
Email: Not Reported

GENERAL INFORMATION

Type of School: *Not Reported* • Accreditation: *Not Reported* • Total Enrollment: *Not Reported*

PROGRAM INFORMATION

LPN/LVN Exit: *Not Reported* • NLNAC Accreditation: *Not Reported*

NURSING STUDENT PROFILE

Total Nursing Enrollment: *Not Reported* • Full-Time Enrollment: *Not Reported* • Part-Time Enrollment: *Not Reported* • Female Enrollment: *Not Reported* • Male Enrollment: *Not Reported* • Total New Admissions Who Enrolled for Fall: *Not Reported* • Total Graduates: *Not Reported*

FINANCES

Residential Annual Tuition: *Not Reported* • Non-Residential Annual Tuition: *Not Reported* • General Institution Fees: *Not Reported* • Additional Nursing Fees: *Not Reported*

SOUTH SUBURBAN COLLEGE

Address: 15800 S. State St., South Holland, IL 604723
Phone: 708-569-2000
Fax: 708-225-5831
Contact: Judith Coglianese, RN, MS, Associate Dean of Nursing and Allied Health
Email: jcoglianese@ssc.cc.il.us

GENERAL INFORMATION

Type of School: *2-Year College or University, Public* • Accreditation: *North Central Association of Colleges and Schools* • Total Enrollment: *9500*

PROGRAM INFORMATION

LPN/LVN Exit: *No* • NLNAC Accreditation: *Yes*

NURSING STUDENT PROFILE

Total Nursing Enrollment: *172* • Full-Time Enrollment: *172* • Part-Time Enrollment: *0* • Female Enrollment: *165* • Male Enrollment: *7* • Total New Admissions Who Enrolled for Fall: *64* • Total Graduates: *69*

FINANCES

Residential Annual Tuition: *$1,272* • Non-Residential Annual Tuition: *$7,232* • General Institution Fees: *$25* • Additional Nursing Fees: *$50*

SOUTHEASTERN ILLINOIS COLLEGE

Address: 3575 College Rd, Harrisburg, IL 62946
Phone: 773-866-6921
Fax: 773-866-6952
Contact: Phyllis D Thomson, MS, RN, Executive Dean
Email: pthomson@rhmc.com

GENERAL INFORMATION

Type of School: *Other* • Accreditation: *None* • Total Enrollment: *Not Reported*

PROGRAM INFORMATION

LPN/LVN Exit: *Not Reported* • NLNAC Accreditation: *Not Reported*

NURSING STUDENT PROFILE

Total Nursing Enrollment: *Not Reported* • Full-Time Enrollment: *Not Reported* • Part-Time Enrollment: *Not Reported* • Female Enrollment: *Not Reported* • Male Enrollment: *Not Reported* • Total New Admissions Who Enrolled for Fall: *Not Reported* • Total Graduates: *Not Reported*

FINANCES

Residential Annual Tuition: *$1,664* • Non-Residential Annual Tuition: *$2,784* • General Institution Fees: *Not Reported* • Additional Nursing Fees: *Not Reported*

SOUTHWESTERN ILLINOIS COLLEGE

Address: 2500 Carlyle, Belleville, IL 62221
Phone: 618-235-2700
Fax: 618-235-2052
Contact: Carol Eckert, MSN, RN, Director Nursing Education
Email: carol.eckert@southwestern.cc.il.us

GENERAL INFORMATION

Type of School: *2-Year College or University, Public* • Accreditation: *North Central Association of Colleges and Schools* • Total Enrollment: *13500*

PROGRAM INFORMATION

LPN/LVN Exit: *No* • NLNAC Accreditation: *Yes*

NURSING STUDENT PROFILE

Total Nursing Enrollment: *107* • Full-Time Enrollment: *102* • Part-Time Enrollment: *5* • Female Enrollment: *103* • Male Enrollment: *4* • Total New Admissions Who Enrolled for Fall: *73* • Total Graduates: *29*

FINANCES

Residential Annual Tuition: *$1,128* • Non-Residential Annual Tuition: *$4,872* • General Institution Fees: *$10* • Additional Nursing Fees: *$125*

SPOON RIVER COLLEGE

Address: 23235 N Co. 22, Canton, IL 61520
Phone: 309-649-6333
Fax: 309-649-6238
Contact: Katherine Walls, RN, MS, Assistant Dean of
            Nursing and Allied Health
Email: kwalls@src.cc.il.us

GENERAL INFORMATION

Type of School: *2-Year College or University, Public* •
Accreditation: *North Central Association of Colleges and
Schools* • Total Enrollment: *1909*

PROGRAM INFORMATION

LPN/LVN Exit: *Yes* • NLNAC Accreditation: *Not Reported*

NURSING STUDENT PROFILE

Total Nursing Enrollment: *25* • Full-Time Enrollment: *17* •
Part-Time Enrollment: *8* • Female Enrollment: *24* • Male
Enrollment: *1* • Total New Admissions Who Enrolled for
Fall: *29* • Total Graduates: *25*

FINANCES

Residential Annual Tuition: *$1,920* • Non-Residential
Annual Tuition: *$4,464* • General Institution Fees: *Not
Reported* • Additional Nursing Fees: *Not Reported*

TRINITY COLLEGE OF NURSING

Address: 555 6th St., STE 300, Moline, IL 61265
Phone: 309-757-2630
Fax: Not Reported
Contact: Sanora Bellinger, MSN, RN, Academic Dean
Email: bellingers@trinityqc.com

GENERAL INFORMATION

Type of School: *Hospital, Private (Independent)* •
Accreditation: *North Central Association of Colleges and
Schools* • Total Enrollment: *75*

PROGRAM INFORMATION

LPN/LVN Exit: *No* • NLNAC Accreditation: *Not Reported*

NURSING STUDENT PROFILE

Total Nursing Enrollment: *75* • Full-Time Enrollment: *64* •
Part-Time Enrollment: *11* • Female Enrollment: *75* • Male
Enrollment: *0* • Total New Admissions Who Enrolled for
Fall: *59* • Total Graduates: *28*

FINANCES

Residential Annual Tuition: *$3,998* • Non-Residential
Annual Tuition: *$3,998* • General Institution Fees: *$100* •
Additional Nursing Fees: *$30*

TRITON COMMUNITY COLLEGE

Address: 2000 5th Ave., River Grove, IL 60171
Phone: 708-456-0300
Fax: 708-583-3336
Contact: Joan Libner, MSN, RN, C, Chairperson
Email: jlibner@triton.cc.il.us

GENERAL INFORMATION

Type of School: *2-Year College or University, Public* •
Accreditation: *North Central Association of Colleges and
Schools* • Total Enrollment: *19374*

PROGRAM INFORMATION

LPN/LVN Exit: *Yes* • NLNAC Accreditation: *Yes*

NURSING STUDENT PROFILE

Total Nursing Enrollment: *199* • Full-Time Enrollment: *0* •
Part-Time Enrollment: *199* • Female Enrollment: *189* • Male
Enrollment: *10* • Total New Admissions Who Enrolled for
Fall: *49* • Total Graduates: *96*

FINANCES

Residential Annual Tuition: *$1,032* • Non-Residential
Annual Tuition: *$3,600* • General Institution Fees: *Not
Reported* • Additional Nursing Fees: *$389*

TRUMAN COLLEGE

Address: 1145 W Wilson Ave, Chicago, IL 60640
Phone: 773-907-4641
Fax: 773-907-4645
Contact: Jim Weiner, Chair
Email: Not Reported

GENERAL INFORMATION

Type of School: *Not Reported* • Accreditation: *Not Reported* •
Total Enrollment: *Not Reported*

PROGRAM INFORMATION

LPN/LVN Exit: *Not Reported* • NLNAC Accreditation: *Not
Reported*

NURSING STUDENT PROFILE

Total Nursing Enrollment: *145* • Full-Time Enrollment: *Not
Reported* • Part-Time Enrollment: *Not Reported* • Female
Enrollment: *Not Reported* • Male Enrollment: *Not Reported* •
Total New Admissions Who Enrolled for Fall: *69* • Total
Graduates: *63*

FINANCES

Residential Annual Tuition: *$1,664* • Non-Residential
Annual Tuition: *$6,473* • General Institution Fees: *Not
Reported* • Additional Nursing Fees: *Not Reported*

UNIVERSITY OF ST. FRANCIS—JOLIET

Address: 290 N. Springfield Ave., Joliet, IL 60435
Phone: 260-434-7610
Fax: 260-434-7404
Contact: Margaret Griffin, MS, RN, ASN Program Director
Email: mgriffin@sf.edu

GENERAL INFORMATION

Type of School: *4-Year College or University, Private (Religious)* • Accreditation: *North Central Association of Colleges and Schools* • Total Enrollment: *1650*

PROGRAM INFORMATION

LPN/LVN Exit: *No* • NLNAC Accreditation: *Yes*

NURSING STUDENT PROFILE

Total Nursing Enrollment: *204* • Full-Time Enrollment: *104* • Part-Time Enrollment: *100* • Female Enrollment: *197* • Male Enrollment: *7* • Total New Admissions Who Enrolled for Fall: *60* • Total Graduates: *70*

FINANCES

Residential Annual Tuition: *$13,100* • Non-Residential Annual Tuition: *$13,100* • General Institution Fees: *$470* • Additional Nursing Fees: *$200*

WAUBONSEE COMMUNITY COLLEGE

Address: RTE 47, Waubonsee Dr., Suger Grove, IL 60554
Phone: 630-466-2350
Fax: 630-466-4119
Contact: Patricia Brown, MS, RN, CCRN, Associate Dean, Health and Life Sciences
Email: pbrown@mail.wcc.cc.il

GENERAL INFORMATION

Type of School: *2-Year College or University, Public* • Accreditation: *North Central Association of Colleges and Schools* • Total Enrollment: *51000*

PROGRAM INFORMATION

LPN/LVN Exit: *Not Reported* • NLNAC Accreditation: *Not Reported*

NURSING STUDENT PROFILE

Total Nursing Enrollment: *82* • Full-Time Enrollment: *82* • Part-Time Enrollment: *0* • Female Enrollment: *74* • Male Enrollment: *8* • Total New Admissions Who Enrolled for Fall: *41* • Total Graduates: *32*

FINANCES

Residential Annual Tuition: *$5,772.48* • Non-Residential Annual Tuition: *$6,956.68* • General Institution Fees: *$160* • Additional Nursing Fees: *$100*

WILLIAM RAINEY HARPER COLLEGE

Address: 1200 W. Algonquin, Palatine, IL 60067
Phone: 847-925-6533
Fax: 847-925-6047
Contact: Cheryl H Kisunzu, MSN, RN, Assistant Dean
            and Director of Nursing
Email: cwandamb@harper.cc.il.us

GENERAL INFORMATION

Type of School: *2-Year College or University, Public* •
Accreditation: *North Central Association of Colleges and
Schools* • Total Enrollment: *24000*

PROGRAM INFORMATION

LPN/LVN Exit: *Yes* • NLNAC Accreditation: *Yes*

NURSING STUDENT PROFILE

Total Nursing Enrollment: *200* • Full-Time Enrollment:
200 • Part-Time Enrollment: *0* • Female Enrollment: *190* •
Male Enrollment: *10* • Total New Admissions Who Enrolled
for Fall: *123* • Total Graduates: *109*

FINANCES

Residential Annual Tuition: *$1,296* • Non-Residential
Annual Tuition: *$6,312* • General Institution Fees: *$16* •
Additional Nursing Fees: *$110*

BALL STATE UNIVERSITY

Address: 2000 University Blvd, Muncie, IN 47306
Phone: 765-285-8718
Fax: 765-285-2169
Contact: Linda L. Siktberg, PhD, RN, Associate Director
Email: lsiktber@bsu.edu

GENERAL INFORMATION

Type of School: *4-Year College or University, Public* •
Accreditation: *North Central Association of Colleges and
Schools* • Total Enrollment: *18000*

PROGRAM INFORMATION

LPN/LVN Exit: *Not Reported* • NLNAC Accreditation: *Yes*

NURSING STUDENT PROFILE

Total Nursing Enrollment: *16* • Full-Time Enrollment: *16* •
Part-Time Enrollment: *0* • Female Enrollment: *14* • Male
Enrollment: *2* • Total New Admissions Who Enrolled for
Fall: *Not Reported* • Total Graduates: *10*

FINANCES

Residential Annual Tuition: *$3,576* • Non-Residential
Annual Tuition: *$9,736* • General Institution Fees: *$110* •
Additional Nursing Fees: *$83*

| Circle 9 on reader card | See in-depth profile for more information |

INDIANA STATE UNIVERSITY

Address: 210 N. 7th Street, Terre Haute, IN 47809
Phone: 812-237-7600
Fax: 812-237-4300
Contact: Kathleen Pickrell, MSN, RN, Associate Professor
Email: k-pickrell@indstate.edu

GENERAL INFORMATION

Type of School: *4-Year College or University, Public* •
Accreditation: *North Central Association of Colleges and Schools* • Total Enrollment: *11321*

PROGRAM INFORMATION

LPN/LVN Exit: *No* • NLNAC Accreditation: *Yes*

NURSING STUDENT PROFILE

Total Nursing Enrollment: *156* • Full-Time Enrollment: *82* • Part-Time Enrollment: *74* • Female Enrollment: *141* • Male Enrollment: *15* • Total New Admissions Who Enrolled for Fall: *21* • Total Graduates: *94*

FINANCES

Residential Annual Tuition: *$3,744* • Non-Residential Annual Tuition: *$4,673* • General Institution Fees: *$3,744* • Additional Nursing Fees: *$766*

INDIANA UNIVERSITY EAST

Address: 2325 Chester Boulevard, Richmond, IN 47374
Phone: 765-973-8257
Fax: 765-973-8220
Contact: Joanne Rains, DNS, RN, Dean
Email: jrains@indiana.edu

GENERAL INFORMATION

Type of School: *4-Year College or University, Public* •
Accreditation: *North Central Association of Colleges and Schools* • Total Enrollment: *2600*

PROGRAM INFORMATION

LPN/LVN Exit: *No* • NLNAC Accreditation: *Yes*

NURSING STUDENT PROFILE

Total Nursing Enrollment: *74* • Full-Time Enrollment: *23* • Part-Time Enrollment: *51* • Female Enrollment: *72* • Male Enrollment: *2* • Total New Admissions Who Enrolled for Fall: *23* • Total Graduates: *19*

FINANCES

Residential Annual Tuition: *$4,432* • Non-Residential Annual Tuition: *$10,382* • General Institution Fees: *$112* • Additional Nursing Fees: *$145*

INDIANA UNIVERSITY— KOKOMO

Address: PO Box 9003, Bloomington, IN 46904-9003
Phone: 765-455-9288
Fax: 765-455-9421
Contact: Penny S. Cass, PhD, RN, Dean, School of Nursing
Email: pcass@iuk.edu

GENERAL INFORMATION

Type of School: *4-Year College or University, Public* •
Accreditation: *North Central Association of Colleges and Schools* • Total Enrollment: *37963*

PROGRAM INFORMATION

LPN/LVN Exit: *No* • NLNAC Accreditation: *Yes*

NURSING STUDENT PROFILE

Total Nursing Enrollment: *109* • Full-Time Enrollment: *30* • Part-Time Enrollment: *79* • Female Enrollment: *103* • Male Enrollment: *6* • Total New Admissions Who Enrolled for Fall: *87* • Total Graduates: *Not Reported*

FINANCES

Residential Annual Tuition: *$4,462* • Non-Residential Annual Tuition: *$10,413* • General Institution Fees: *Not Reported* • Additional Nursing Fees: *Not Reported*

INDIANA UNIVERSITY— NORTHWEST

Address: 3400 Broadway, Gary, IN 46408
Phone: 219-980-6604
Fax: 219-980-6578
Contact: Linda A. Rooda, PhD, RN, Professor and Dean
Email: lrooda@iun.edu

GENERAL INFORMATION

Type of School: *4-Year College or University, Public* •
Accreditation: *North Central Association of Colleges and Schools* • Total Enrollment: *4649*

PROGRAM INFORMATION

LPN/LVN Exit: *No* • NLNAC Accreditation: *Yes*

NURSING STUDENT PROFILE

Total Nursing Enrollment: *96* • Full-Time Enrollment: *57* • Part-Time Enrollment: *39* • Female Enrollment: *91* • Male Enrollment: *5* • Total New Admissions Who Enrolled for Fall: *49* • Total Graduates: *34*

FINANCES

Residential Annual Tuition: *$4,537* • Non-Residential Annual Tuition: *$10,487* • General Institution Fees: *$230* • Additional Nursing Fees: *$266*

INDIANA UNIVERSITY— PURDUE UNIVERSITY

Address: 355 Lansing Street, Indianapolis, IN 46202-2896
Phone: 317-274-8010
Fax: 317-274-2996
Contact: Donna L. Boland, PhD, RN, Associate Dean for Undergraduate Programs
Email: dboland@iupui.edu

GENERAL INFORMATION

Type of School: *4-Year College or University, Public* • Accreditation: *North Central Association of Colleges and Schools* • Total Enrollment: *27500*

PROGRAM INFORMATION

LPN/LVN Exit: *No* • NLNAC Accreditation: *Yes*

NURSING STUDENT PROFILE

Total Nursing Enrollment: *176* • Full-Time Enrollment: *72* • Part-Time Enrollment: *104* • Female Enrollment: *163* • Male Enrollment: *13* • Total New Admissions Who Enrolled for Fall: *40* • Total Graduates: *76*

FINANCES

Residential Annual Tuition: *$5,703* • Non-Residential Annual Tuition: *$14,886* • General Institution Fees: *$350* • Additional Nursing Fees: *$650*

INDIANA UNIVERSITY— PURDUE UNIVERSITY — FORT WAYNE

Address: 2101 E Coliseum Blvd, Fort Wayne, IN 46805-1445
Phone: 219-481-6816
Fax: 219-481-5767
Contact: Linda Meyer, PhD, RN, Director, Undergraduate Nursing
Email: meyer@ipfw.edu

GENERAL INFORMATION

Type of School: *4-Year College or University, Public* • Accreditation: *North Central Association of Colleges and Schools* • Total Enrollment: *11129*

PROGRAM INFORMATION

LPN/LVN Exit: *No* • NLNAC Accreditation: *Yes*

NURSING STUDENT PROFILE

Total Nursing Enrollment: *265* • Full-Time Enrollment: *111* • Part-Time Enrollment: *154* • Female Enrollment: *243* • Male Enrollment: *22* • Total New Admissions Who Enrolled for Fall: *90* • Total Graduates: *72*

FINANCES

Residential Annual Tuition: *$1,480* • Non-Residential Annual Tuition: *$3,404* • General Institution Fees: *$103* • Additional Nursing Fees: *Not Reported*

INDIANA UNIVERSITY— SOUTH BEND

Address: 1700 Mishawaka Ave, South Bend, IN 46634
Phone: 219-237-4207
Fax: Not Reported
Contact: Marian M Pettengill, PhD., RN, Dean
Email: mpetteng@iusb.edu

GENERAL INFORMATION

Type of School: *4-Year College or University, Public* •
Accreditation: *North Central Association of Colleges and
Schools* • Total Enrollment: *7000*

PROGRAM INFORMATION

LPN/LVN Exit: *Not Reported* • NLNAC Accreditation: *Yes*

NURSING STUDENT PROFILE

Total Nursing Enrollment: *Not Reported* • Full-Time
Enrollment: *Not Reported* • Part-Time Enrollment: *Not
Reported* • Female Enrollment: *Not Reported* • Male
Enrollment: *Not Reported* • Total New Admissions Who
Enrolled for Fall: *Not Reported* • Total Graduates: *Not
Reported*

FINANCES

Residential Annual Tuition: *$4,570* • Non-Residential
Annual Tuition: *$11,163* • General Institution Fees: *Not
Reported* • Additional Nursing Fees: *Not Reported*

INDIANA VOCATIONAL TECH COLLEGE REG 11

Address: Highway 62 and Ivy Tech Drive, Madison, IN
            47250
Phone: 812-265-2580
Fax: Not Reported
Contact: Gene Ann Shapinsky, MSN, RN, Nursing
            Department Chair
Email: gshapins@ivy.tec.in.us

GENERAL INFORMATION

Type of School: *Not Reported* • Accreditation: *Not Reported* •
Total Enrollment: *Not Reported*

PROGRAM INFORMATION

LPN/LVN Exit: *No* • NLNAC Accreditation: *Not Reported*

NURSING STUDENT PROFILE

Total Nursing Enrollment: *32* • Full-Time Enrollment: *32* •
Part-Time Enrollment: *0* • Female Enrollment: *32* • Male
Enrollment: *0* • Total New Admissions Who Enrolled for
Fall: *36* • Total Graduates: *30*

FINANCES

Residential Annual Tuition: *$3,366* • Non-Residential
Annual Tuition: *$5,406* • General Institution Fees: *$132* •
Additional Nursing Fees: *$0*

IVY TECH STATE COLLEGE

Address: 2401 Valley Drive, Valparaiso, IN 46383
Phone: 765-966-2656
Fax: 765-939-2641
Contact: Jillene K. Anderson, MSN, RN, Department of Nursing Chair
Email: janderso@ivy.tec.in.us

GENERAL INFORMATION

Type of School: *Other, Public* • Accreditation: *North Central Association of Colleges and Schools* • Total Enrollment: *48000*

PROGRAM INFORMATION

LPN/LVN Exit: *No* • NLNAC Accreditation: *Yes*

NURSING STUDENT PROFILE

Total Nursing Enrollment: *28* • Full-Time Enrollment: *28* • Part-Time Enrollment: *0* • Female Enrollment: *27* • Male Enrollment: *1* • Total New Admissions Who Enrolled for Fall: *28* • Total Graduates: *26*

FINANCES

Residential Annual Tuition: *$1,655* • Non-Residential Annual Tuition: *$3,227* • General Institution Fees: *$0* • Additional Nursing Fees: *$99*

IVY TECH STATE COLLEGE— REGION 10

Address: 3116 Canterbury Ct., Bloomington, IN 47401
Phone: 812-332-1559
Fax: 812-332-1782
Contact: Vera Cline, MSN, RN, TC, AS, Program Chair and Assistant Professor
Email: vcline@ivy.tec.in.us

GENERAL INFORMATION

Type of School: *Not Reported* • Accreditation: *Not Reported* • Total Enrollment: *Not Reported*

PROGRAM INFORMATION

LPN/LVN Exit: *No* • NLNAC Accreditation: *Yes*

NURSING STUDENT PROFILE

Total Nursing Enrollment: *67* • Full-Time Enrollment: *67* • Part-Time Enrollment: *0* • Female Enrollment: *66* • Male Enrollment: *1* • Total New Admissions Who Enrolled for Fall: *34* • Total Graduates: *34*

FINANCES

Residential Annual Tuition: *$1,986* • Non-Residential Annual Tuition: *$3,705* • General Institution Fees: *$0* • Additional Nursing Fees: *$200*

IVY TECH STATE COLLEGE— REGION 12

Address: 3501 First Avenue, Evansville, IN 47710
Phone: 812-429-1496
Fax: 812-429-1483
Contact: Judith A. McCutchan, MSN, RN, Professor and Program Chair
Email: jmccutch@ivy.tec.in.us

GENERAL INFORMATION

Type of School: *2-Year College or University, Public* • Accreditation: *North Central Association of Colleges and Schools* • Total Enrollment: *Not Reported*

PROGRAM INFORMATION

LPN/LVN Exit: *No* • NLNAC Accreditation: *Yes*

NURSING STUDENT PROFILE

Total Nursing Enrollment: *66* • Full-Time Enrollment: *66* • Part-Time Enrollment: *0* • Female Enrollment: *62* • Male Enrollment: *4* • Total New Admissions Who Enrolled for Fall: *38* • Total Graduates: *26*

FINANCES

Residential Annual Tuition: *$2,359* • Non-Residential Annual Tuition: *$4,597* • General Institution Fees: *$0* • Additional Nursing Fees: *$2,596*

IVY TECH STATE COLLEGE— REGION 2

Address: 220 Dean Johnson Boulevard, South Bend, IN 46601
Phone: 219-289-7001
Fax: 219-236-7166
Contact: Mary Wcisel, MSN, RN, ASN Program Chair
Email: mwcisel@ivy.tec.in.us

GENERAL INFORMATION

Type of School: *Not Reported* • Accreditation: *Not Reported* • Total Enrollment: *Not Reported*

PROGRAM INFORMATION

LPN/LVN Exit: *No* • NLNAC Accreditation: *Yes*

NURSING STUDENT PROFILE

Total Nursing Enrollment: *79* • Full-Time Enrollment: *5* • Part-Time Enrollment: *74* • Female Enrollment: *72* • Male Enrollment: *7* • Total New Admissions Who Enrolled for Fall: *37* • Total Graduates: *38*

FINANCES

Residential Annual Tuition: *$1,584* • Non-Residential Annual Tuition: *$1,584* • General Institution Fees: *Not Reported* • Additional Nursing Fees: *Not Reported*

IVY TECH STATE COLLEGE—REGION 4

Address: 3101 S. Creasy Lane, P.O. Box 6299, Lafayette, IN 47903
Phone: 765-772-9237
Fax: 765-772-9248
Contact: Karen L. Dolk, MSN, RN, Chair, ASN Program
Email: kdolk@ivy.tech.in.us

GENERAL INFORMATION

Type of School: *Vocational/Technical School, Public* • Accreditation: *North Central Association of Colleges and Schools* • Total Enrollment: *3300*

PROGRAM INFORMATION

LPN/LVN Exit: *No* • NLNAC Accreditation: *Yes*

NURSING STUDENT PROFILE

Total Nursing Enrollment: *85* • Full-Time Enrollment: *85* • Part-Time Enrollment: *0* • Female Enrollment: *82* • Male Enrollment: *3* • Total New Admissions Who Enrolled for Fall: *30* • Total Graduates: *40*

FINANCES

Residential Annual Tuition: *$1,584* • Non-Residential Annual Tuition: *$3,096* • General Institution Fees: *$0* • Additional Nursing Fees: *$100*

IVY TECH STATE COLLEGE—REGION 8

Address: One West 26th Street, Indianapolis, IN 46208
Phone: 317-927-7176
Fax: 317-927-0242
Contact: Janet Kramer, MSN, RN, ASN Program Chair
Email: jkramer@ivy.tec.in.us

GENERAL INFORMATION

Type of School: *2-Year College or University, Public* • Accreditation: *North Central Association of Colleges and Schools* • Total Enrollment: *Not Reported*

PROGRAM INFORMATION

LPN/LVN Exit: *No* • NLNAC Accreditation: *Yes*

NURSING STUDENT PROFILE

Total Nursing Enrollment: *101* • Full-Time Enrollment: *101* • Part-Time Enrollment: *0* • Female Enrollment: *94* • Male Enrollment: *7* • Total New Admissions Who Enrolled for Fall: *47* • Total Graduates: *35*

FINANCES

Residential Annual Tuition: *$1,584* • Non-Residential Annual Tuition: *$2,964* • General Institution Fees: *Not Reported* • Additional Nursing Fees: *$150*

MARIAN COLLEGE

Address: 3200 Cold Spring Rd, Indianapolis, IN 46222
Phone: 317-955-6155
Fax: 317-955-6135
Contact: Marian Pettengill, PhD, RN, Professor and Chair
Email: mpettengill@marian.edu

GENERAL INFORMATION

Type of School: *4-Year College or University, Private (Religious)* • Accreditation: *North Central Association of Colleges and Schools* • Total Enrollment: *1260*

PROGRAM INFORMATION

LPN/LVN Exit: *No* • NLNAC Accreditation: *Yes*

NURSING STUDENT PROFILE

Total Nursing Enrollment: *87* • Full-Time Enrollment: *44* • Part-Time Enrollment: *43* • Female Enrollment: *84* • Male Enrollment: *3* • Total New Admissions Who Enrolled for Fall: *30* • Total Graduates: *38*

FINANCES

Residential Annual Tuition: *$14,499* • Non-Residential Annual Tuition: *$14,499* • General Institution Fees: *$100* • Additional Nursing Fees: *$950*

PURDUE UNIVERSITY— CALUMET CAMPUS

Address: 2200 169th Street, Hammond, IN 46323
Phone: 219-989-2814
Fax: 219-989-2848
Contact: Gail D. Wegner, RN, MS, Coordinator
           Undergraduate Program
Email: wegner@calumet.purdue.edu

GENERAL INFORMATION

Type of School: *4-Year College or University, Public* • Accreditation: *North Central Association of Colleges and Schools* • Total Enrollment: *9100*

PROGRAM INFORMATION

LPN/LVN Exit: *No* • NLNAC Accreditation: *Yes*

NURSING STUDENT PROFILE

Total Nursing Enrollment: *93* • Full-Time Enrollment: *45* • Part-Time Enrollment: *48* • Female Enrollment: *85* • Male Enrollment: *8* • Total New Admissions Who Enrolled for Fall: *29* • Total Graduates: *67*

FINANCES

Residential Annual Tuition: *$3,450* • Non-Residential Annual Tuition: *$8,674* • General Institution Fees: *$25* • Additional Nursing Fees: *$200*

PURDUE UNIVERSITY— NORTH CENTRAL

Address: 1401 S. US 421, Westville, IN 46391
Phone: 219-785-5246
Fax: 219-785-5495
Contact: Marilyn J. Asteriads, MSN, RN, Chair
Email: mja@purduenc.edu

GENERAL INFORMATION

Type of School: *4-Year College or University, Public* •
Accreditation: *North Central Association of Colleges and Schools* • Total Enrollment: *3500*

PROGRAM INFORMATION

LPN/LVN Exit: *No* • NLNAC Accreditation: *Yes*

NURSING STUDENT PROFILE

Total Nursing Enrollment: *151* • Full-Time Enrollment: *102* • Part-Time Enrollment: *49* • Female Enrollment: *146* • Male Enrollment: *5* • Total New Admissions Who Enrolled for Fall: *32* • Total Graduates: *51*

FINANCES

Residential Annual Tuition: *$4,900* • Non-Residential Annual Tuition: *$10,750* • General Institution Fees: *Not Reported* • Additional Nursing Fees: *$135*

UNIVERSITY OF INDIANAPOLIS

Address: 1400 E Hanna Ave, Indianapolis, IN 46227-3630
Phone: 317-788-3206
Fax: 317-788-3542
Contact: Sharon Isaac, EdD, RN, Dean
Email: isaac@vindy.edu

GENERAL INFORMATION

Type of School: *4-Year College or University, Private (Religious)* • Accreditation: *North Central Association of Colleges and Schools* • Total Enrollment: *2839*

PROGRAM INFORMATION

LPN/LVN Exit: *No* • NLNAC Accreditation: *Yes*

NURSING STUDENT PROFILE

Total Nursing Enrollment: *52* • Full-Time Enrollment: *3* • Part-Time Enrollment: *49* • Female Enrollment: *49* • Male Enrollment: *3* • Total New Admissions Who Enrolled for Fall: *28* • Total Graduates: *18*

FINANCES

Residential Annual Tuition: *$14,630* • Non-Residential Annual Tuition: *$14,630* • General Institution Fees: *$0* • Additional Nursing Fees: *$90*

VINCENNES UNIVERSITY

Address: 1002 North First Street, Vincennes, IN 47591
Phone: 812-888-4406
Fax: 812-888-4550
Contact: Julie A. Herrold, MSN, RN, Chair
Email: jherrold@indian.vinu.edu

DES MOINES AREA COMMUNITY COLLEGE

Address: 1800 Grand, Des Moines, IA 50021
Phone: 800-362-2127
Fax: 515-433-5033
Contact: Connie Booth, MSN, RN, Nursing Program Chair
Email: cjbooth@dmacc.cc.ia.us

GENERAL INFORMATION

Type of School: *2-Year College or University, Public* • Accreditation: *North Central Association of Colleges and Schools* • Total Enrollment: *4755*

GENERAL INFORMATION

Type of School: *Other* • Accreditation: *None* • Total Enrollment: *Not Reported*

PROGRAM INFORMATION

LPN/LVN Exit: *Not Reported* • NLNAC Accreditation: *Yes*

PROGRAM INFORMATION

LPN/LVN Exit: *Yes* • NLNAC Accreditation: *Yes*

NURSING STUDENT PROFILE

Total Nursing Enrollment: *89* • Full-Time Enrollment: *80* • Part-Time Enrollment: *9* • Female Enrollment: *81* • Male Enrollment: *8* • Total New Admissions Who Enrolled for Fall: *61* • Total Graduates: *44*

NURSING STUDENT PROFILE

Total Nursing Enrollment: *25* • Full-Time Enrollment: *22* • Part-Time Enrollment: *3* • Female Enrollment: *23* • Male Enrollment: *2* • Total New Admissions Who Enrolled for Fall: *30* • Total Graduates: *18*

FINANCES

Residential Annual Tuition: *$3,000* • Non-Residential Annual Tuition: *$7,200* • General Institution Fees: *$40* • Additional Nursing Fees: *$172*

FINANCES

Residential Annual Tuition: *$1,830* • Non-Residential Annual Tuition: *$3,660* • General Institution Fees: *$126* • Additional Nursing Fees: *Not Reported*

DES MOINES AREA COMMUNITY COLLEGE— ANKENY

Address: 2006 South Ankeny Blvd, Ankeny, IA 50021
Phone: 515-964-6466
Fax: 515-964-6440
Contact: Virginia Wangerin, MSN, RN, Nursing Program Chair
Email: vwangerin@dmacc.cc.ia.us

GENERAL INFORMATION

Type of School: *Not Reported* • Accreditation: *Not Reported* • Total Enrollment: *Not Reported*

PROGRAM INFORMATION

LPN/LVN Exit: *Yes* • NLNAC Accreditation: *Yes*

NURSING STUDENT PROFILE

Total Nursing Enrollment: *30* • Full-Time Enrollment: *30* • Part-Time Enrollment: *0* • Female Enrollment: *29* • Male Enrollment: *1* • Total New Admissions Who Enrolled for Fall: *30* • Total Graduates: *54*

FINANCES

Residential Annual Tuition: *$2,412* • Non-Residential Annual Tuition: *$4,572* • General Institution Fees: *$126* • Additional Nursing Fees: *Not Reported*

DES MOINES AREA COMMUNITY COLLEGE— CARROLL

Address: 906 North Grant Rd, Carroll, IA 51401
Phone: 800-622-3334
Fax: 712-792-6358
Contact: Lou Blanchfield, MSN, RN, Nursing Program Chair
Email: slblanchfield@dmacc.cc.ia.us

GENERAL INFORMATION

Type of School: *Not Reported* • Accreditation: *Not Reported* • Total Enrollment: *Not Reported*

PROGRAM INFORMATION

LPN/LVN Exit: *Yes* • NLNAC Accreditation: *Yes*

NURSING STUDENT PROFILE

Total Nursing Enrollment: *Not Reported* • Full-Time Enrollment: *Not Reported* • Part-Time Enrollment: *Not Reported* • Female Enrollment: *Not Reported* • Male Enrollment: *Not Reported* • Total New Admissions Who Enrolled for Fall: *Not Reported* • Total Graduates: *5*

FINANCES

Residential Annual Tuition: *$2,669* • Non-Residential Annual Tuition: *Not Reported* • General Institution Fees: *$126* • Additional Nursing Fees: *Not Reported*

EASTERN IOWA COMMUNITY COLLEGE

Address: 306 West River Drive, Davenport, IA 52801-1221
Phone: 563-441-4256
Fax: 563-441-4154
Contact: Ruth Sueverkruebbe, RN, BSN, MS, Coordinator
Email: rsueverkruebbe@eiccd.cc.ia.us

GENERAL INFORMATION

Type of School: *Not Reported* • Accreditation: *Not Reported* • Total Enrollment: *Not Reported*

PROGRAM INFORMATION

LPN/LVN Exit: *Not Reported* • NLNAC Accreditation: *Not Reported*

NURSING STUDENT PROFILE

Total Nursing Enrollment: *213* • Full-Time Enrollment: *213* • Part-Time Enrollment: *0* • Female Enrollment: *204* • Male Enrollment: *9* • Total New Admissions Who Enrolled for Fall: *110* • Total Graduates: *76*

FINANCES

Residential Annual Tuition: *$1,280* • Non-Residential Annual Tuition: *$1,920* • General Institution Fees: *Not Reported* • Additional Nursing Fees: *Not Reported*

ELLSWORTH COMMUNITY COLLEGE/IOWA VALLEY COMMUNITY COLLEGE DISTRICT

Address: 1100 College Ave, Iowa Falls, IA 50126
Phone: 515-648-4611
Fax: 515-648-3128
Contact: Mavis A Hunt, MSN, RN, Coordinator
Email: Not Reported

GENERAL INFORMATION

Type of School: *Not Reported* • Accreditation: *Not Reported* • Total Enrollment: *Not Reported*

PROGRAM INFORMATION

LPN/LVN Exit: *Yes* • NLNAC Accreditation: *Not Reported*

NURSING STUDENT PROFILE

Total Nursing Enrollment: *13* • Full-Time Enrollment: *11* • Part-Time Enrollment: *2* • Female Enrollment: *Not Reported* • Male Enrollment: *Not Reported* • Total New Admissions Who Enrolled for Fall: *13* • Total Graduates: *14*

FINANCES

Residential Annual Tuition: *$2,592* • Non-Residential Annual Tuition: *$3,888* • General Institution Fees: *Not Reported* • Additional Nursing Fees: *Not Reported*

HAWKEYE COMMUNITY COLLEGE

Address: 1501 E Orange Rd Box 8015, Waterloo, IA
             50704-8015
Phone: 319-296-2320
Fax: Not Reported
Contact: Brenda Hempen, MSN, RN, Coordinator,
             Nursing Program
Email: bhempen@hawkeye.cc.ia.us

GENERAL INFORMATION

Type of School: *2-Year College or University, Public* •
Accreditation: *North Central Association of Colleges and
Schools* • Total Enrollment: *Not Reported*

PROGRAM INFORMATION

LPN/LVN Exit: *Yes* • NLNAC Accreditation: *Not Reported*

NURSING STUDENT PROFILE

Total Nursing Enrollment: *69* • Full-Time Enrollment: *60* •
Part-Time Enrollment: *9* • Female Enrollment: *66* • Male
Enrollment: *3* • Total New Admissions Who Enrolled for
Fall: *25* • Total Graduates: *69*

FINANCES

Residential Annual Tuition: *Not Reported* • Non-Residential
Annual Tuition: *Not Reported* • General Institution Fees:
$850 • Additional Nursing Fees: *$382*

INDIAN HILLS COMMUNITY COLLEGE

Address: 525 Grandview, Ottumwa, IA 52501
Phone: 515-583-5162
Fax: 515-683-5184
Contact: Ann Aulwes, MSN, RN, Department Chair
Email: Not Reported

GENERAL INFORMATION

Type of School: *2-Year College or University, Public* •
Accreditation: *North Central Association of Colleges and
Schools* • Total Enrollment: *3294*

PROGRAM INFORMATION

LPN/LVN Exit: *Not Reported* • NLNAC Accreditation: *Not
Reported*

NURSING STUDENT PROFILE

Total Nursing Enrollment: *Not Reported* • Full-Time
Enrollment: *Not Reported* • Part-Time Enrollment: *Not
Reported* • Female Enrollment: *Not Reported* • Male
Enrollment: *Not Reported* • Total New Admissions Who
Enrolled for Fall: *Not Reported* • Total Graduates: *Not
Reported*

FINANCES

Residential Annual Tuition: *$2,528* • Non-Residential
Annual Tuition: *$3,808* • General Institution Fees: *Not
Reported* • Additional Nursing Fees: *Not Reported*

IOWA CENTRAL COMMUNITY COLLEGE

Address: 330 Ave M, Fort Dodge, IA 50501
Phone: 515-576-0099
Fax: 515-576-5656
Contact: Connie K. Boyd, MSN, RN, Director of Health Sciences
Email: boyd@triton.iccc.cc.ia.us

IOWA CENTRAL COMMUNITY COLLEGE— WEBSTER CITY

Address: 1725 Beach St, Webster City, IA 50595
Phone: 515-576-0099
Fax: 515-576-5656
Contact: Connie K Boyd, MSN, RN, Director of Health Sciences
Email: boyd@triton.iccc.cc.ia.us

GENERAL INFORMATION

Type of School: *2-Year College or University, Public* • Accreditation: *North Central Association of Colleges and Schools* • Total Enrollment: *4567*

GENERAL INFORMATION

Type of School: *Not Reported* • Accreditation: *Not Reported* • Total Enrollment: *Not Reported*

PROGRAM INFORMATION

LPN/LVN Exit: *No* • NLNAC Accreditation: *Yes*

PROGRAM INFORMATION

LPN/LVN Exit: *No* • NLNAC Accreditation: *Yes*

NURSING STUDENT PROFILE

Total Nursing Enrollment: *192* • Full-Time Enrollment: *171* • Part-Time Enrollment: *21* • Female Enrollment: *185* • Male Enrollment: *7* • Total New Admissions Who Enrolled for Fall: *68* • Total Graduates: *39*

NURSING STUDENT PROFILE

Total Nursing Enrollment: *33* • Full-Time Enrollment: *14* • Part-Time Enrollment: *19* • Female Enrollment: *30* • Male Enrollment: *3* • Total New Admissions Who Enrolled for Fall: *26* • Total Graduates: *14*

FINANCES

Residential Annual Tuition: *$2,070* • Non-Residential Annual Tuition: *$3,105* • General Institution Fees: *$8* • Additional Nursing Fees: *$0*

FINANCES

Residential Annual Tuition: *None* • Non-Residential Annual Tuition: *$2,250* • General Institution Fees: *Not Reported* • Additional Nursing Fees: *Not Reported*

IOWA CENTRAL COMMUNITY COLLEGE—WEBSTER CITY

Address: 610 West 4th Street, Box 2020, Storm Lake, IA 50588
Phone: 515-576-0099 x2378
Fax: 515-576-7206
Contact: Connie K Boyd, MSN, RN, Director of Health Sciences
Email: boerner@triton.iccc.cc.ia.us

GENERAL INFORMATION

Type of School: *2 Year, Public* • Accreditation: *North Central Association of Colleges* • Total Enrollment: *4295*

PROGRAM INFORMATION

LPN/LVN Exit: *No* • NLNAC Accreditation: *Yes*

NURSING STUDENT PROFILE

Total Nursing Enrollment: *42* • Full-Time Enrollment: *30* • Part-Time Enrollment: *12* • Female Enrollment: *41* • Male Enrollment: *1* • Total New Admissions Who Enrolled for Fall: *27* • Total Graduates: *14*

FINANCES

Residential Annual Tuition: *None* • Non-Residential Annual Tuition: *$2,250* • General Institution Fees: *Not Reported* • Additional Nursing Fees: *Not Reported*

IOWA LAKES COMMUNITY COLLEGE

Address: 3200 College Dr, Emmetsburg, IA 50536
Phone: 712-852-5285
Fax: 712-852-2152
Contact: Judi Donahue, MSN, RN, Director of Nursing Education
Email: jdonahue@ilcc.cc.ia

GENERAL INFORMATION

Type of School: *2-Year College or University, Public* • Accreditation: *North Central Association of Colleges and Schools* • Total Enrollment: *3500*

PROGRAM INFORMATION

LPN/LVN Exit: *Yes* • NLNAC Accreditation: *Not Reported*

NURSING STUDENT PROFILE

Total Nursing Enrollment: *Not Reported* • Full-Time Enrollment: *Not Reported* • Part-Time Enrollment: *Not Reported* • Female Enrollment: *Not Reported* • Male Enrollment: *Not Reported* • Total New Admissions Who Enrolled for Fall: *Not Reported* • Total Graduates: *Not Reported*

FINANCES

Residential Annual Tuition: *$2,880* • Non-Residential Annual Tuition: *$2,944* • General Institution Fees: *Not Reported* • Additional Nursing Fees: *Not Reported*

IOWA VALLEY COMMUNITY COLLEGE DISTRICT

Address: 3700 South Center Street, Marshalltown, IA
            50158
Phone: 641-752-7106
Fax: Not Reported
Contact: Mavis A Hunt, RN, MS, Coordinator Nursing
            Education
Email: mahunt@iavally.cc.ia.us

GENERAL INFORMATION

Type of School: *Not Reported* • Accreditation: *None* • Total
Enrollment: *Not Reported*

PROGRAM INFORMATION

LPN/LVN Exit: *Yes* • NLNAC Accreditation: *Not Reported*

NURSING STUDENT PROFILE

Total Nursing Enrollment: *37* • Full-Time Enrollment: *33* •
Part-Time Enrollment: *4* • Female Enrollment: *Not
Reported* • Male Enrollment: *Not Reported* • Total New
Admissions Who Enrolled for Fall: *41* • Total Graduates: *Not
Reported*

FINANCES

Residential Annual Tuition: *$2,592* • Non-Residential
Annual Tuition: *$3,888* • General Institution Fees: *Not
Reported* • Additional Nursing Fees: *Not Reported*

IOWA WESTERN COMMUNITY COLLEGE

Address: 2712 12th St, Harlan, IA 51537
Phone: Not Reported
Fax: Not Reported
Contact: Carol Maxwell, MSN, RN, Coordinator
Email: Not Reported

GENERAL INFORMATION

Type of School: *2-Year College or University, Public* •
Accreditation: *North Central Association of Colleges and
Schools* • Total Enrollment: *Not Reported*

PROGRAM INFORMATION

LPN/LVN Exit: *Not Reported* • NLNAC Accreditation: *Not
Reported*

NURSING STUDENT PROFILE

Total Nursing Enrollment: *Not Reported* • Full-Time
Enrollment: *Not Reported* • Part-Time Enrollment: *Not
Reported* • Female Enrollment: *Not Reported* • Male
Enrollment: *Not Reported* • Total New Admissions Who
Enrolled for Fall: *Not Reported* • Total Graduates: *Not
Reported*

FINANCES

Residential Annual Tuition: *$2,912* • Non-Residential
Annual Tuition: *$4,368* • General Institution Fees: *Not
Reported* • Additional Nursing Fees: *Not Reported*

KIRKWOOD COMMUNITY COLLEGE

Address: 6301 Kirkwood Blvd., Box 2068, Cedar Rapids, IA 52406
Phone: 319-398-5566
Fax: 319-398-1293
Contact: Linda Kalb Schwartz, MSN, RN, Department Coordinator
Email: lschwar@kirkwood.cc.ia.us

GENERAL INFORMATION

Type of School: *2-Year College or University, Public* • Accreditation: *North Central Association of Colleges and Schools* • Total Enrollment: *11500*

PROGRAM INFORMATION

LPN/LVN Exit: *Yes* • NLNAC Accreditation: *Not Reported*

NURSING STUDENT PROFILE

Total Nursing Enrollment: *156* • Full-Time Enrollment: *156* • Part-Time Enrollment: *0* • Female Enrollment: *129* • Male Enrollment: *27* • Total New Admissions Who Enrolled for Fall: *48* • Total Graduates: *64*

FINANCES

Residential Annual Tuition: *$1,560* • Non-Residential Annual Tuition: *$3,120* • General Institution Fees: *$0* • Additional Nursing Fees: *$0*

MERCY COLLEGE OF HEALTH SCIENCES

Address: 928 6th Ave, Des Moines, IA 50309
Phone: 515-643-6615
Fax: 515-643-6698
Contact: Mary Kelly, PhD, RN, Chair, Division of Nursing
Email: mkelly@mercydesmoines.org

GENERAL INFORMATION

Type of School: *4-Year College or University, Private (Religious)* • Accreditation: *North Central Association of Colleges and Schools* • Total Enrollment: *420*

PROGRAM INFORMATION

LPN/LVN Exit: *No* • NLNAC Accreditation: *Yes*

NURSING STUDENT PROFILE

Total Nursing Enrollment: *191* • Full-Time Enrollment: *161* • Part-Time Enrollment: *30* • Female Enrollment: *181* • Male Enrollment: *10* • Total New Admissions Who Enrolled for Fall: *57* • Total Graduates: *66*

FINANCES

Residential Annual Tuition: *$7,800* • Non-Residential Annual Tuition: *$7,800* • General Institution Fees: *$0* • Additional Nursing Fees: *$0*

NORTH IOWA AREA

Address: 500 College Dr, Mason City, IA 50401
Phone: 641-422-4216
Fax: 641-422-4115
Contact: Donna J. Orton, MSN, RN, Chairperson,
           Health Division
Email: ortondon@miacc.cc.ia.us

GENERAL INFORMATION

Type of School: *2-Year College or University, Public* •
Accreditation: *North Central Association of Colleges and
Schools* • Total Enrollment: *Not Reported*

PROGRAM INFORMATION

LPN/LVN Exit: *No* • NLNAC Accreditation: *Yes*

NURSING STUDENT PROFILE

Total Nursing Enrollment: *60* • Full-Time Enrollment: *46* •
Part-Time Enrollment: *14* • Female Enrollment: *58* • Male
Enrollment: *2* • Total New Admissions Who Enrolled for
Fall: *34* • Total Graduates: *24*

FINANCES

Residential Annual Tuition: *$1,920* • Non-Residential
Annual Tuition: *$2,880* • General Institution Fees: *$17* •
Additional Nursing Fees: *$80*

NORTHEAST IOWA COMMUNITY COLLEGE

Address: 10250 Sundown Rd, Peosta, IA 52068
Phone: 319-562-4357
Fax: 319-562-4357
Contact: Betty Helgerson, RN, BSN, MAN, Dean of
           Health and Assistant Head of Nursing
Email: helgersb@nicc.cc.ia.us

GENERAL INFORMATION

Type of School: *2-Year College or University, Public* •
Accreditation: *North Central Association of Colleges and
Schools* • Total Enrollment: *3621*

PROGRAM INFORMATION

LPN/LVN Exit: *Yes* • NLNAC Accreditation: *No*

NURSING STUDENT PROFILE

Total Nursing Enrollment: *18* • Full-Time Enrollment: *18* •
Part-Time Enrollment: *0* • Female Enrollment: *13* • Male
Enrollment: *5* • Total New Admissions Who Enrolled for
Fall: *18* • Total Graduates: *28*

FINANCES

Residential Annual Tuition: *Not Reported* • Non-Residential
Annual Tuition: *Not Reported* • General Institution Fees:
$12 • Additional Nursing Fees: *$30*

NORTHEAST IOWA COMMUNITY COLLEGE— CALMAR

Address: Box 400 Hwy 150 South, Calmar, IA 52132
Phone: 319-562-4357
Fax: 319-562-4357
Contact: Betty Helgerson, RN, BSN, MSN, Dean of Health, Assistant Head of Nursing
Email: helbersb@nicc.cc.ia.us

GENERAL INFORMATION

Type of School: *2-Year College or University, Public* • Accreditation: *North Central Association of Colleges and Schools* • Total Enrollment: *Not Reported*

PROGRAM INFORMATION

LPN/LVN Exit: *Not Reported* • NLNAC Accreditation: *Not Reported*

NURSING STUDENT PROFILE

Total Nursing Enrollment: *18* • Full-Time Enrollment: *18* • Part-Time Enrollment: *0* • Female Enrollment: *13* • Male Enrollment: *5* • Total New Admissions Who Enrolled for Fall: *18* • Total Graduates: *28*

FINANCES

Residential Annual Tuition: *$1,500* • Non-Residential Annual Tuition: *$3,000* • General Institution Fees: *Not Reported* • Additional Nursing Fees: *Not Reported*

SOUTHWESTERN COMMUNITY COLLEGE

Address: 1501 W Townline St, Creston, IA 50801
Phone: 641-782-7081
Fax: 641-782-3312
Contact: Loretta A. Eckels, RN, BS, MS, Chairperson, Nursing Education
Email: eckels@swcc.cc.ia.us

GENERAL INFORMATION

Type of School: *2-Year College or University, Public* • Accreditation: *North Central Association of Colleges and Schools* • Total Enrollment: *1200*

PROGRAM INFORMATION

LPN/LVN Exit: *Yes* • NLNAC Accreditation: *Not Reported*

NURSING STUDENT PROFILE

Total Nursing Enrollment: *49* • Full-Time Enrollment: *48* • Part-Time Enrollment: *1* • Female Enrollment: *47* • Male Enrollment: *2* • Total New Admissions Who Enrolled for Fall: *46* • Total Graduates: *42*

FINANCES

Residential Annual Tuition: *$1,776* • Non-Residential Annual Tuition: *$2,520* • General Institution Fees: *Not Reported* • Additional Nursing Fees: *$15*

ST. LUKE'S COLLEGE—IOWA

Address: 2720 Stone Park Blvd., Sioux City, IA 51104
Phone: 712-279-7969
Fax: 712-279-3155
Contact: JoAnn Breyfogle, RN, MS, Dean of Academic
          Services and Nursing Program
Email: breyfojf@stlukes.org

GENERAL INFORMATION

Type of School: *Hospital, Private (Independent)* •
Accreditation: *North Central Association of Colleges and
Schools* • Total Enrollment: *110*

PROGRAM INFORMATION

LPN/LVN Exit: *Not Reported* • NLNAC Accreditation: *Not
Reported*

NURSING STUDENT PROFILE

Total Nursing Enrollment: *80* • Full-Time Enrollment: *61* •
Part-Time Enrollment: *19* • Female Enrollment: *74* • Male
Enrollment: *6* • Total New Admissions Who Enrolled for
Fall: *48* • Total Graduates: *27*

FINANCES

Residential Annual Tuition: *$8,698* • Non-Residential
Annual Tuition: *$8,698* • General Institution Fees: *$516* •
Additional Nursing Fees: *$0*

WESTERN IOWA TECH

Address: 4647 Stone Ave PO Box 265, Sioux City, IA
          51102
Phone: 712-274-8733
Fax: 712-274-6412
Contact: Gloria Stewart, MSN, RN, EdD, Department
          Chair, Nursing
Email: stewarg@witcc.com

GENERAL INFORMATION

Type of School: *2-Year College or University, Public* •
Accreditation: *North Central Association of Colleges and
Schools* • Total Enrollment: *29000*

PROGRAM INFORMATION

LPN/LVN Exit: *Yes* • NLNAC Accreditation: *Yes*

NURSING STUDENT PROFILE

Total Nursing Enrollment: *101* • Full-Time Enrollment:
101 • Part-Time Enrollment: *0* • Female Enrollment: *96* •
Male Enrollment: *5* • Total New Admissions Who Enrolled
for Fall: *66* • Total Graduates: *93*

FINANCES

Residential Annual Tuition: *$756* • Non-Residential Annual
Tuition: *$3,024* • General Institution Fees: *$48* • Additional
Nursing Fees: *$130*

BARTON COUNTY COMMUNITY COLLEGE

Address: 245 North East 30th Road, Great Bend, KS 67530
Phone: 316-792-9355
Fax: 316-786-1166
Contact: Cheryl A. Berg, MSN, CNS, Director of Nursing Education
Email: berg@barton.cc.ks.us

GENERAL INFORMATION

Type of School: *2-Year College or University, Public* • Accreditation: *North Central Association of Colleges and Schools* • Total Enrollment: *4201*

PROGRAM INFORMATION

LPN/LVN Exit: *Yes* • NLNAC Accreditation: *Yes*

NURSING STUDENT PROFILE

Total Nursing Enrollment: *46* • Full-Time Enrollment: *46* • Part-Time Enrollment: *0* • Female Enrollment: *43* • Male Enrollment: *3* • Total New Admissions Who Enrolled for Fall: *34* • Total Graduates: *17*

FINANCES

Residential Annual Tuition: *$672* • Non-Residential Annual Tuition: *$672* • General Institution Fees: *$18* • Additional Nursing Fees: *$132*

BETHEL COLLEGE

Address: 300 East 27th, North Newton, KS 67117
Phone: 215-257-2594
Fax: 219-257-3326
Contact: Ruth Davidhizar, DNS, RN, CS, FAAN, Dean of Nursing
Email: Davidhr@Bethelcollege.edu

GENERAL INFORMATION

Type of School: *4-Year College or University, Private (Religious)* • Accreditation: *North Central Association of Colleges and Schools* • Total Enrollment: *502*

PROGRAM INFORMATION

LPN/LVN Exit: *No* • NLNAC Accreditation: *No*

NURSING STUDENT PROFILE

Total Nursing Enrollment: *29* • Full-Time Enrollment: *29* • Part-Time Enrollment: *0* • Female Enrollment: *27* • Male Enrollment: *2* • Total New Admissions Who Enrolled for Fall: *18* • Total Graduates: *11*

FINANCES

Residential Annual Tuition: *$6,650* • Non-Residential Annual Tuition: *$6,650* • General Institution Fees: *$75* • Additional Nursing Fees: *$280*

CLOUD COUNTY COMMUNITY COLLEGE

Address: P.O. Box 507, Beloit, KS 67420
Phone: 785-738-9025
Fax: 785-738-2903
Contact: Vera Streit, MN, RN, Nursing Program Director
Email: vstreit@ncktc.tec.ks.us

COLBY COMMUNITY COLLEGE

Address: 1255 South Range, Colby, KS 67701
Phone: 785-462-3984
Fax: Not Reported
Contact: Tracey Stark, MSN, ARNP, Director of Nursing
Email: tracey@colby.cc.ks.us

GENERAL INFORMATION

Type of School: *2-Year College or University, Public* • Accreditation: *North Central Association of Colleges and Schools* • Total Enrollment: *Not Reported*

GENERAL INFORMATION

Type of School: *Not Reported* • Accreditation: *None* • Total Enrollment: *Not Reported*

PROGRAM INFORMATION

LPN/LVN Exit: *Yes* • NLNAC Accreditation: *Yes*

PROGRAM INFORMATION

LPN/LVN Exit: *Yes* • NLNAC Accreditation: *Yes*

NURSING STUDENT PROFILE

Total Nursing Enrollment: *28* • Full-Time Enrollment: *28* • Part-Time Enrollment: *0* • Female Enrollment: *28* • Male Enrollment: *0* • Total New Admissions Who Enrolled for Fall: *28* • Total Graduates: *34*

NURSING STUDENT PROFILE

Total Nursing Enrollment: *Not Reported* • Full-Time Enrollment: *Not Reported* • Part-Time Enrollment: *Not Reported* • Female Enrollment: *Not Reported* • Male Enrollment: *Not Reported* • Total New Admissions Who Enrolled for Fall: *Not Reported* • Total Graduates: *Not Reported*

FINANCES

Residential Annual Tuition: *$1,984* • Non-Residential Annual Tuition: *$2,592* • General Institution Fees: *Not Reported* • Additional Nursing Fees: *Not Reported*

FINANCES

Residential Annual Tuition: *$1,280* • Non-Residential Annual Tuition: *$2,528* • General Institution Fees: *Not Reported* • Additional Nursing Fees: *Not Reported*

DODGE CITY COMMUNITY COLLEGE

Address: 501 North 14 Street, Dodge City, KS 67801
Phone: 316-227-9226
Fax: 316-227-9319
Contact: Linda Sanko, MS, MN, RN, Director of Nursing Education
Email: lsanko@dccc.cc.ks.us

FORT SCOTT COMMUNITY COLLEGE

Address: 2108 South Horton, Fort Scott, KS 66701
Phone: 316-223-2700
Fax: 316-223-4927
Contact: Jo Ann Thomas, MN, ARNP, CNAA, Director of Nursing and Allied Health
Email: joannt@fsccax.ftscott.cc.ks.us

GENERAL INFORMATION

Type of School: *2-Year College or University, Public* • Accreditation: *North Central Association of Colleges and Schools* • Total Enrollment: *2002*

GENERAL INFORMATION

Type of School: *2-Year College or University, Public* • Accreditation: *North Central Association of Colleges and Schools* • Total Enrollment: *1677*

PROGRAM INFORMATION

LPN/LVN Exit: *Yes* • NLNAC Accreditation: *Yes*

PROGRAM INFORMATION

LPN/LVN Exit: *No* • NLNAC Accreditation: *Yes*

NURSING STUDENT PROFILE

Total Nursing Enrollment: *25* • Full-Time Enrollment: *17* • Part-Time Enrollment: *8* • Female Enrollment: *23* • Male Enrollment: *2* • Total New Admissions Who Enrolled for Fall: *27* • Total Graduates: *17*

NURSING STUDENT PROFILE

Total Nursing Enrollment: *38* • Full-Time Enrollment: *38* • Part-Time Enrollment: *0* • Female Enrollment: *31* • Male Enrollment: *7* • Total New Admissions Who Enrolled for Fall: *11* • Total Graduates: *33*

FINANCES

Residential Annual Tuition: *$1,280* • Non-Residential Annual Tuition: *$2,280* • General Institution Fees: *$28* • Additional Nursing Fees: *$200*

FINANCES

Residential Annual Tuition: *$744* • Non-Residential Annual Tuition: *$2,088* • General Institution Fees: *$28* • Additional Nursing Fees: *$100*

GARDEN CITY COMMUNITY COLLEGE

Address: 801 Campus Dr., Garden City, KS 67846
Phone: 316-276-9560
Fax: 316-276-9569
Contact: Evelyn Bowman, PhD, RN, Director of Nursing
            and Allied Health Education
Email: ebowman@gccc.cc.ks.us

GENERAL INFORMATION

Type of School: *2-Year College or University, Public* •
Accreditation: *North Central Association of Colleges and
Schools* • Total Enrollment: *2355*

PROGRAM INFORMATION

LPN/LVN Exit: *No* • NLNAC Accreditation: *Yes*

NURSING STUDENT PROFILE

Total Nursing Enrollment: *54* • Full-Time Enrollment: *54* •
Part-Time Enrollment: *0* • Female Enrollment: *47* • Male
Enrollment: *7* • Total New Admissions Who Enrolled for
Fall: *36* • Total Graduates: *26*

FINANCES

Residential Annual Tuition: *$744* • Non-Residential Annual
Tuition: *$1,560* • General Institution Fees: *$13* • Additional
Nursing Fees: *$145*

HESSTON COLLEGE

Address: P.O. Box 3000, Hesston, KS 67062
Phone: 620-327-8140
Fax: 620-327-8300
Contact: Bonnie K. Sowers, RN, MS, Director,
            Department of Nursing
Email: bonnies@hesston.edu

GENERAL INFORMATION

Type of School: *2-Year College or University, Private
(Religious)* • Accreditation: *North Central Association of
Colleges and Schools* • Total Enrollment: *445*

PROGRAM INFORMATION

LPN/LVN Exit: *No* • NLNAC Accreditation: *Yes*

NURSING STUDENT PROFILE

Total Nursing Enrollment: *59* • Full-Time Enrollment: *41* •
Part-Time Enrollment: *18* • Female Enrollment: *56* • Male
Enrollment: *3* • Total New Admissions Who Enrolled for
Fall: *39* • Total Graduates: *25*

FINANCES

Residential Annual Tuition: *$11,996* • Non-Residential
Annual Tuition: *$11,996* • General Institution Fees: *$200* •
Additional Nursing Fees: *$1,470*

HUTCHINSON COMMUNITY COLLEGE

Address: 815 North Walnut, Hutchinson, KS 67501
Phone: 316-665-4930
Fax: 316-665-4988
Contact: Debra J. Hackler, MSN, RN, Director
Email: hacklerd@hutchh.edu

GENERAL INFORMATION

Type of School: *2-Year College or University, Public* • Accreditation: *North Central Association of Colleges and Schools* • Total Enrollment: *4000*

PROGRAM INFORMATION

LPN/LVN Exit: *No* • NLNAC Accreditation: *Yes*

NURSING STUDENT PROFILE

Total Nursing Enrollment: *74* • Full-Time Enrollment: *32* • Part-Time Enrollment: *42* • Female Enrollment: *68* • Male Enrollment: *6* • Total New Admissions Who Enrolled for Fall: *45* • Total Graduates: *30*

FINANCES

Residential Annual Tuition: *$864* • Non-Residential Annual Tuition: *$2,352* • General Institution Fees: *$33* • Additional Nursing Fees: *$100*

JOHNSON COUNTY COMMUNITY COLLEGE

Address: 10000 West 75th North Street, Suite 241, Merriam, KS 66204
Phone: 913-469-8500
Fax: 913-469-2504
Contact: Jeanne Walsh, MSN, RN, Academic Director, Nursing
Email: jwalsh@jccc.net

GENERAL INFORMATION

Type of School: *2-Year College or University, Public* • Accreditation: *North Central Association of Colleges and Schools* • Total Enrollment: *32000*

PROGRAM INFORMATION

LPN/LVN Exit: *Not Reported* • NLNAC Accreditation: *Yes*

NURSING STUDENT PROFILE

Total Nursing Enrollment: *120* • Full-Time Enrollment: *75* • Part-Time Enrollment: *45* • Female Enrollment: *108* • Male Enrollment: *12* • Total New Admissions Who Enrolled for Fall: *65* • Total Graduates: *59*

FINANCES

Residential Annual Tuition: *$1,856* • Non-Residential Annual Tuition: *$4,448* • General Institution Fees: *Not Reported* • Additional Nursing Fees: *Not Reported*

KANSAS CITY KANSAS COMMUNITY COLLEGE

Address: 7250 State Ave, Kansas City, KS 66112
Phone: 913-288-7126
Fax: 919-288-7649
Contact: Shirley Wendel, PhD, RN, Dean of Nursing and Allied Health
Email: swendel@toto.net

GENERAL INFORMATION

Type of School: *2-Year College or University, Public* • Accreditation: *North Central Association of Colleges and Schools* • Total Enrollment: *Not Reported*

PROGRAM INFORMATION

LPN/LVN Exit: *No* • NLNAC Accreditation: *Yes*

NURSING STUDENT PROFILE

Total Nursing Enrollment: *153* • Full-Time Enrollment: *Not Reported* • Part-Time Enrollment: *Not Reported* • Female Enrollment: *142* • Male Enrollment: *11* • Total New Admissions Who Enrolled for Fall: *43* • Total Graduates: *76*

FINANCES

Residential Annual Tuition: *$1,080* • Non-Residential Annual Tuition: *$2,760* • General Institution Fees: *$144* • Additional Nursing Fees: *$200*

KANSAS WESLEYAN UNIVERSITY

Address: 100 East Claflin Avenue, Salina, KS 67401
Phone: 785-827-5541
Fax: 785-827-0927
Contact: Patricia D. Kissell, PhD, RN, Chair
Email: pkissell@kwu.edu

GENERAL INFORMATION

Type of School: *4-Year College or University, Private (Religious)* • Accreditation: *North Central Association of Colleges and Schools* • Total Enrollment: *755*

PROGRAM INFORMATION

LPN/LVN Exit: *No* • NLNAC Accreditation: *Yes*

NURSING STUDENT PROFILE

Total Nursing Enrollment: *47* • Full-Time Enrollment: *36* • Part-Time Enrollment: *11* • Female Enrollment: *43* • Male Enrollment: *4* • Total New Admissions Who Enrolled for Fall: *30* • Total Graduates: *21*

FINANCES

Residential Annual Tuition: *$14,200* • General Institution Fees: *Not Reported* • Additional Nursing Fees: *Not Reported*

LABETTE COMMUNITY COLLEGE

Address: 200 S. 14th, Parsons, KS 67357
Phone: 620-820-1263
Fax: 620-421-1539
Contact: Patricia R. Thompson, MSN, RN, Director of Nursing Education
Email: patt@labette.cc.ks.us

GENERAL INFORMATION

Type of School: *2-Year College or University, Public •* Accreditation: *North Central Association of Colleges and Schools •* Total Enrollment: *Not Reported*

PROGRAM INFORMATION

LPN/LVN Exit: *Yes •* NLNAC Accreditation: *Yes*

NURSING STUDENT PROFILE

Total Nursing Enrollment: *72 •* Full-Time Enrollment: *0 •* Part-Time Enrollment: *72 •* Female Enrollment: *66 •* Male Enrollment: *6 •* Total New Admissions Who Enrolled for Fall: *49 •* Total Graduates: *29*

FINANCES

Residential Annual Tuition: *$369 •* Non-Residential Annual Tuition: *$1,056 •* General Institution Fees: *$144 •* Additional Nursing Fees: *$175*

MANHATTAN AREA TECHNICAL COLLEGE

Address: 3136 Dickens Avenue, Manhattan, KS 66503
Phone: 785-587-2800
Fax: 785-587-2804
Contact: Myrna J Bartel, MS, RN, Coordinator
Email: mbartel@matc.net

GENERAL INFORMATION

Type of School: *Other, Public •* Accreditation: *None •* Total Enrollment: *289*

PROGRAM INFORMATION

LPN/LVN Exit: *No •* NLNAC Accreditation: *No*

NURSING STUDENT PROFILE

Total Nursing Enrollment: *21 •* Full-Time Enrollment: *21 •* Part-Time Enrollment: *0 •* Female Enrollment: *19 •* Male Enrollment: *2 •* Total New Admissions Who Enrolled for Fall: *22 •* Total Graduates: *15*

FINANCES

Residential Annual Tuition: *$1,700 •* Non-Residential Annual Tuition: *Not Reported •* General Institution Fees: *Not Reported •* Additional Nursing Fees: *$80*

NEOSHO COUNTY COMMUNITY COLLEGE

Address: 800 West 14th Street, Chanute, KS 66720
Phone: 316-431-2820
Fax: 316-431-0082
Contact: Carol J. Fox, MN, MA, RN, Director of Nursing Education
Email: cfox@neosho.cc.ks.us

GENERAL INFORMATION

Type of School: *2-Year College or University, Public* •
Accreditation: *North Central Association of Colleges and Schools* • Total Enrollment: *Not Reported*

PROGRAM INFORMATION

LPN/LVN Exit: *Yes* • NLNAC Accreditation: *Yes*

NURSING STUDENT PROFILE

Total Nursing Enrollment: *85* • Full-Time Enrollment: *85* •
Part-Time Enrollment: *0* • Female Enrollment: *82* • Male
Enrollment: *3* • Total New Admissions Who Enrolled for
Fall: *34* • Total Graduates: *60*

FINANCES

Residential Annual Tuition: *$990* • Non-Residential Annual
Tuition: *$1,485* • General Institution Fees: *$240* •
Additional Nursing Fees: *$100*

NORTH CENTRAL KANSAS TECHNICAL COLLEGE

Address: 2205 Wheatland, Hays, KS 67601
Phone: 785-625-2437
Fax: 785-623-6157
Contact: Sandra M. Gottschalk, MSN, RN, Director of Nursing Education
Email: sgottschalk@ncktc.tec.ks.us

GENERAL INFORMATION

Type of School: *Vocational/Technical School, Public* •
Accreditation: *North Central Association of Colleges and Schools* • Total Enrollment: *449*

PROGRAM INFORMATION

LPN/LVN Exit: *Yes* • NLNAC Accreditation: *Yes*

NURSING STUDENT PROFILE

Total Nursing Enrollment: *18* • Full-Time Enrollment: *18* •
Part-Time Enrollment: *0* • Female Enrollment: *15* • Male
Enrollment: *3* • Total New Admissions Who Enrolled for
Fall: *20* • Total Graduates: *15*

FINANCES

Residential Annual Tuition: *$1,597* • Non-Residential
Annual Tuition: *Not Reported* • General Institution Fees:
$20 • Additional Nursing Fees: *$950*

PRATT COMMUNITY COLLEGE & AREA VO-TECH SCHOOL NURSING DEPARTMENT

Address: 348 NE S.R. 61, Pratt, KS 67124
Phone: 620-672-5641
Fax: 620-672-5288
Contact: Diane Okeson, EdD, RN, ARNP, CNS, Dean of Nursing and Allied Health
Email: dianeo@pcc.cc.ks.us

GENERAL INFORMATION

Type of School: *2-Year College or University, Public* • Accreditation: *North Central Association of Colleges and Schools* • Total Enrollment: *13502*

PROGRAM INFORMATION

LPN/LVN Exit: *Not Reported* • NLNAC Accreditation: *Yes*

NURSING STUDENT PROFILE

Total Nursing Enrollment: *57* • Full-Time Enrollment: *57* • Part-Time Enrollment: *0* • Female Enrollment: *51* • Male Enrollment: *6* • Total New Admissions Who Enrolled for Fall: *36* • Total Graduates: *25*

FINANCES

Residential Annual Tuition: *$696* • Non-Residential Annual Tuition: *$796* • General Institution Fees: *$18* • Additional Nursing Fees: *$186*

SEWARD COUNTY COMMUNITY COLLEGE

Address: PO Box 1137, Liberal, KS 67901
Phone: 316-626-3026
Fax: 316-626-3040
Contact: Steve Hecox, MSN, RN, Director of Nursing
Email: shecox@sccc.net

GENERAL INFORMATION

Type of School: *2-Year College or University, Public* • Accreditation: *North Central Association of Colleges and Schools* • Total Enrollment: *1688*

PROGRAM INFORMATION

LPN/LVN Exit: *Yes* • NLNAC Accreditation: *Yes*

NURSING STUDENT PROFILE

Total Nursing Enrollment: *27* • Full-Time Enrollment: *27* • Part-Time Enrollment: *0* • Female Enrollment: *25* • Male Enrollment: *2* • Total New Admissions Who Enrolled for Fall: *27* • Total Graduates: *19*

FINANCES

Residential Annual Tuition: *$960* • Non-Residential Annual Tuition: *$1,650* • General Institution Fees: *$36* • Additional Nursing Fees: *$55*

ASHLAND COMMUNITY COLLEGE

Address: 1400 College Drive, Ashland, KY 41101
Phone: 606-326-2087
Fax: 606-326-2115
Contact: Janie R. Kitchen, MSN, MHEd, RN, Associate
             Degree Nursing Coordinator
Email: janie.kitchen@kctcs.edu

GENERAL INFORMATION

Type of School: *2-Year College or University, Public* •
Accreditation: *Southern Association of Colleges and Schools* •
Total Enrollment: *2200*

PROGRAM INFORMATION

LPN/LVN Exit: *No* • NLNAC Accreditation: *Yes*

NURSING STUDENT PROFILE

Total Nursing Enrollment: *123* • Full-Time Enrollment: *60* •
Part-Time Enrollment: *63* • Female Enrollment: *114* • Male
Enrollment: *9* • Total New Admissions Who Enrolled for
Fall: *78* • Total Graduates: *45*

FINANCES

Residential Annual Tuition: *$700* • Non-Residential Annual
Tuition: *$2,175* • General Institution Fees: *$0* • Additional
Nursing Fees: *$12*

EASTERN KENTUCKY UNIVERSITY

Address: Rowlett Bldg, RM 220, Richmond, KY 40475
Phone: 606-622-1942
Fax: Not Reported
Contact: Pat A. Holden, DSN, RN, Professor and Chair
Email: adnholde@acs.eku.edu

GENERAL INFORMATION

Type of School: *4-Year College or University, Public* •
Accreditation: *Southern Association of Colleges and Schools* •
Total Enrollment: *14997*

PROGRAM INFORMATION

LPN/LVN Exit: *No* • NLNAC Accreditation: *Yes*

NURSING STUDENT PROFILE

Total Nursing Enrollment: *303* • Full-Time Enrollment:
130 • Part-Time Enrollment: *173* • Female Enrollment:
274 • Male Enrollment: *29* • Total New Admissions Who
Enrolled for Fall: *77* • Total Graduates: *142*

FINANCES

Residential Annual Tuition: *$2,390* • Non-Residential
Annual Tuition: *$6,430* • General Institution Fees: *$30* •
Additional Nursing Fees: *$17*

ELIZABETHTOWN COMMUNITY COLLEGE

Address: 600 College Street Road, Elizabethtown, KY 42701
Phone: 270-769-2371
Fax: 270-769-0736
Contact: Middy L. Judd, RN, BSN, MSN, Coordinator, ADN
Email: middy.judd@kctcs.edu

GENERAL INFORMATION

Type of School: *2-Year College or University, Public* • Accreditation: *Southern Association of Colleges and Schools* • Total Enrollment: *Not Reported*

PROGRAM INFORMATION

LPN/LVN Exit: *No* • NLNAC Accreditation: *Yes*

NURSING STUDENT PROFILE

Total Nursing Enrollment: *105* • Full-Time Enrollment: *66* • Part-Time Enrollment: *39* • Female Enrollment: *101* • Male Enrollment: *4* • Total New Admissions Who Enrolled for Fall: *33* • Total Graduates: *51*

FINANCES

Residential Annual Tuition: *$725* • Non-Residential Annual Tuition: *$2,175* • General Institution Fees: *$0* • Additional Nursing Fees: *$0*

HAZARD COMMUNITY COLLEGE

Address: One Community College Drive, Hazard, KY 41701
Phone: 606-436-5721
Fax: Not Reported
Contact: Gwen Collins, RN, Coordinator
Email: Gwen.Collins@kctcs.net

GENERAL INFORMATION

Type of School: *Not Reported* • Accreditation: *None* • Total Enrollment: *Not Reported*

PROGRAM INFORMATION

LPN/LVN Exit: *Not Reported* • NLNAC Accreditation: *No*

NURSING STUDENT PROFILE

Total Nursing Enrollment: *130* • Full-Time Enrollment: *79* • Part-Time Enrollment: *51* • Female Enrollment: *Not Reported* • Male Enrollment: *Not Reported* • Total New Admissions Who Enrolled for Fall: *45* • Total Graduates: *50*

FINANCES

Residential Annual Tuition: *Not Reported* • Non-Residential Annual Tuition: *Not Reported* • General Institution Fees: *Not Reported* • Additional Nursing Fees: *Not Reported*

HENDERSON COMMUNITY COLLEGE

Address: 2660 South Green Street, Henderson, KY 42420
Phone: 270-830-5310
Fax: 270-830-5355
Contact: Mary Gail Wilder, DSN, RN, Coordinator AD
           Nursing Program and Chair, BioSciences
Email: mary.wilder@kctcs.edu

GENERAL INFORMATION

Type of School: *2-Year College or University, Public* •
Accreditation: *Southern Association of Colleges and Schools* •
Total Enrollment: *93*

PROGRAM INFORMATION

LPN/LVN Exit: *Not Reported* • NLNAC Accreditation: *Yes*

NURSING STUDENT PROFILE

Total Nursing Enrollment: *93* • Full-Time Enrollment: *42* •
Part-Time Enrollment: *51* • Female Enrollment: *90* • Male
Enrollment: *3* • Total New Admissions Who Enrolled for
Fall: *39* • Total Graduates: *34*

FINANCES

Residential Annual Tuition: *$2,370* • Non-Residential
Annual Tuition: *$7,110* • General Institution Fees: *$0* •
Additional Nursing Fees: *$136*

HOPKINSVILLE COMMUNITY COLLEGE

Address: PO Box 2100, Hopkinsville, KY 42241
Phone: 270-886-3921
Fax: 270-885-7993
Contact: Elwanda Adams, MSN, RN, Nursing Program
           Coordinator
Email: elwanda.adams.@kctcs.edu

GENERAL INFORMATION

Type of School: *2-Year College or University, Public* •
Accreditation: *Southern Association of Colleges and Schools* •
Total Enrollment: *2249*

PROGRAM INFORMATION

LPN/LVN Exit: *No* • NLNAC Accreditation: *Yes*

NURSING STUDENT PROFILE

Total Nursing Enrollment: *91* • Full-Time Enrollment: *57* •
Part-Time Enrollment: *34* • Female Enrollment: *84* • Male
Enrollment: *7* • Total New Admissions Who Enrolled for
Fall: *51* • Total Graduates: *37*

FINANCES

Residential Annual Tuition: *$2,370* • Non-Residential
Annual Tuition: *$7,110* • General Institution Fees: *$0* •
Additional Nursing Fees: *$150*

KENTUCKY STATE UNIVERSITY

Address: 400 East Main Street, Frankfort, KY 40601
Phone: 502-597-5957
Fax: 502-597-5818
Contact: Sheila P. Patros, MSN, RN, Acting Chairperson
Email: spatros@gwmail.kysu.edu

GENERAL INFORMATION

Type of School: *4-Year College or University, Public* •
Accreditation: *Southern Association of Colleges and Schools* •
Total Enrollment: *2000*

PROGRAM INFORMATION

LPN/LVN Exit: *No* • NLNAC Accreditation: *Yes*

NURSING STUDENT PROFILE

Total Nursing Enrollment: *67* • Full-Time Enrollment: *Not Reported* • Part-Time Enrollment: *Not Reported* • Female Enrollment: *62* • Male Enrollment: *5* • Total New Admissions Who Enrolled for Fall: *37* • Total Graduates: *31*

FINANCES

Residential Annual Tuition: *$2,100* • Non-Residential Annual Tuition: *$6,300* • General Institution Fees: *$340* • Additional Nursing Fees: *$35*

KENTUCKY WESLEYAN COLLEGE

Address: 3000 Frederica Street, Owensboro, KY 42302-1039
Phone: 270-923-3111
Fax: Not Reported
Contact: D.L. Wilkey, PhD, RN, Chair
Email: Not Reported

GENERAL INFORMATION

Type of School: *4-Year College or University, Private (Religious)* • Accreditation: *Southern Association of Colleges and Schools* • Total Enrollment: *685*

PROGRAM INFORMATION

LPN/LVN Exit: *Not Reported* • NLNAC Accreditation: *No*

NURSING STUDENT PROFILE

Total Nursing Enrollment: *Not Reported* • Full-Time Enrollment: *Not Reported* • Part-Time Enrollment: *Not Reported* • Female Enrollment: *Not Reported* • Male Enrollment: *Not Reported* • Total New Admissions Who Enrolled for Fall: *Not Reported* • Total Graduates: *17*

FINANCES

Residential Annual Tuition: *Not Reported* • Non-Residential Annual Tuition: *Not Reported* • General Institution Fees: *Not Reported* • Additional Nursing Fees: *Not Reported*

LEXINGTON COMMUNITY COLLEGE

Address: 303 D Oswald Bldg, Copper Drive, Lexington,
           KY 40506
Phone: 859-257-4872
Fax: 859-257-9581
Contact: Linda Yonts, RN, MSN, Acting Coordinator
Email: lmyont0@uky.edu

GENERAL INFORMATION

Type of School: *2-Year College or University, Public* •
Accreditation: *Southern Association of Colleges and Schools* •
Total Enrollment: *Not Reported*

PROGRAM INFORMATION

LPN/LVN Exit: *Yes* • NLNAC Accreditation: *Yes*

NURSING STUDENT PROFILE

Total Nursing Enrollment: *159* • Full-Time Enrollment: *Not
Reported* • Part-Time Enrollment: *Not Reported* • Female
Enrollment: *149* • Male Enrollment: *10* • Total New
Admissions Who Enrolled for Fall: *107* • Total Graduates: *57*

FINANCES

Residential Annual Tuition: *$1,043* • Non-Residential
Annual Tuition: *$2,918* • General Institution Fees: *$0* •
Additional Nursing Fees: *$1,000*

MADISONVILLE COMMUNITY COLLEGE

Address: 750 North Laffoon St., Madisonville, KY 42431
Phone: 502-821-2250
Fax: 502-825-8553
Contact: Linda Thomas, MSN, RN, Nursing Program
           Coordinator
Email: ljthoma@pop/vky.edu

GENERAL INFORMATION

Type of School: *Vocational/Technical School, Public* •
Accreditation: *None* • Total Enrollment: *500*

PROGRAM INFORMATION

LPN/LVN Exit: *Not Reported* • NLNAC Accreditation: *Yes*

NURSING STUDENT PROFILE

Total Nursing Enrollment: *133* • Full-Time Enrollment: *55* •
Part-Time Enrollment: *78* • Female Enrollment: *124* • Male
Enrollment: *9* • Total New Admissions Who Enrolled for
Fall: *Not Reported* • Total Graduates: *69*

FINANCES

Residential Annual Tuition: *$1,080* • Non-Residential
Annual Tuition: *$3,240* • General Institution Fees: *$80* •
Additional Nursing Fees: *Not Reported*

MAYSVILLE COMMUNITY COLLEGE

Address: 1755 US 68, Maysville, KY 41056
Phone: 606-759-7141
Fax: 606-759-7176
Contact: Linda K. Dunaway, MSN, RN, Coordinator, Associate Degree Nursing Program
Email: Linda.Dunaway@kctcs.net

GENERAL INFORMATION

Type of School: *Other, Public* • Accreditation: *Southern Association of Colleges and Schools* • Total Enrollment: *1393*

PROGRAM INFORMATION

LPN/LVN Exit: *No* • NLNAC Accreditation: *No*

NURSING STUDENT PROFILE

Total Nursing Enrollment: *49* • Full-Time Enrollment: *7* • Part-Time Enrollment: *42* • Female Enrollment: *46* • Male Enrollment: *3* • Total New Admissions Who Enrolled for Fall: *26* • Total Graduates: *17*

FINANCES

Residential Annual Tuition: *$725* • Non-Residential Annual Tuition: *$2,175* • General Institution Fees: *$0* • Additional Nursing Fees: *$102*

MIDWAY COLLEGE

Address: 512 E. Stephens St., Midway, KY 40347
Phone: 859-846-5335
Fax: 859-846-5876
Contact: Diana Weaver, DNS, RN, FAAN, Chair
Email: dweaver@midway.edu

GENERAL INFORMATION

Type of School: *Independent, Private (Religious)* • Accreditation: *Southern Association of Colleges and Schools* • Total Enrollment: *900*

PROGRAM INFORMATION

LPN/LVN Exit: *No* • NLNAC Accreditation: *Yes*

NURSING STUDENT PROFILE

Total Nursing Enrollment: *103* • Full-Time Enrollment: *103* • Part-Time Enrollment: *0* • Female Enrollment: *100* • Male Enrollment: *3* • Total New Admissions Who Enrolled for Fall: *48* • Total Graduates: *48*

FINANCES

Residential Annual Tuition: *$10,200* • Non-Residential Annual Tuition: *$10,200* • General Institution Fees: *Not Reported* • Additional Nursing Fees: *$35*

MOREHEAD STATE UNIVERSITY

Address: 150 University Blvd., Morehead, KY 40351
Phone: 606-783-2297
Fax: 606-783-9104
Contact: Donna J. Corley, MSN, RN, MEd, Coordinator
Email: d.corley@moreheadstate.edu

GENERAL INFORMATION

Type of School: *4-Year College or University, Public* •
Accreditation: *Southern Association of Colleges and Schools* •
Total Enrollment: *8500*

PROGRAM INFORMATION

LPN/LVN Exit: *No* • NLNAC Accreditation: *Yes*

NURSING STUDENT PROFILE

Total Nursing Enrollment: *60* • Full-Time Enrollment: *60* •
Part-Time Enrollment: *0* • Female Enrollment: *55* • Male
Enrollment: *5* • Total New Admissions Who Enrolled for
Fall: *33* • Total Graduates: *21*

FINANCES

Residential Annual Tuition: *$1,463* • Non-Residential
Annual Tuition: *$3,602* • General Institution Fees: *$250* •
Additional Nursing Fees: *$76*

NORTHERN KENTUCKY UNIVERSITY

Address: Nunn Drive.AHC 303, Highland Heights, KY
          41099
Phone: 859-572-5247
Fax: 859-572-6098
Contact: Sarah H. Dessner, MSN, RN, OCN, Director
Email: dessner@nku.edu

GENERAL INFORMATION

Type of School: *4-Year College or University, Public* •
Accreditation: *Southern Association of Colleges and Schools* •
Total Enrollment: *12000*

PROGRAM INFORMATION

LPN/LVN Exit: *No* • NLNAC Accreditation: *Yes*

NURSING STUDENT PROFILE

Total Nursing Enrollment: *188* • Full-Time Enrollment:
134 • Part-Time Enrollment: *54* • Female Enrollment: *178* •
Male Enrollment: *10* • Total New Admissions Who Enrolled
for Fall: *115* • Total Graduates: *60*

FINANCES

Residential Annual Tuition: *$2,256* • Non-Residential
Annual Tuition: *$6,504* • General Institution Fees: *$30* •
Additional Nursing Fees: *$30*

Circle 92 on reader card   See in-depth profile for more information

OWENSBORO COMMUNITY COLLEGE

Address: 4800 New Hartford Road, Owensboro, KY 42303
Phone: 270-686-4459
Fax: 270-686-4623
Contact: Freida Pagan, MSN, RN, Coordinator
Email: Freida.Pagan@kctcs.edu

GENERAL INFORMATION

Type of School: *2-Year College or University, Public* • Accreditation: *Southern Association of Colleges and Schools* • Total Enrollment: *2614*

PROGRAM INFORMATION

LPN/LVN Exit: *No* • NLNAC Accreditation: *No*

NURSING STUDENT PROFILE

Total Nursing Enrollment: *36* • Full-Time Enrollment: *10* • Part-Time Enrollment: *26* • Female Enrollment: *35* • Male Enrollment: *1* • Total New Admissions Who Enrolled for Fall: *40* • Total Graduates: *12*

FINANCES

Residential Annual Tuition: *$2,370* • Non-Residential Annual Tuition: *$7,110* • General Institution Fees: *$10* • Additional Nursing Fees: *$185*

PADUCAH COMMUNITY COLLEGE

Address: PO Box 7380, Paducah, KY 42002
Phone: 270-554-6265
Fax: .   270-554-6227
Contact: Tena Payne, EdD, RN, Nursing Coordinator
Email: tena.payne@kctcs.net

GENERAL INFORMATION

Type of School: *2-Year College or University, Public* • Accreditation: *Southern Association of Colleges and Schools* • Total Enrollment: *3257*

PROGRAM INFORMATION

LPN/LVN Exit: *No* • NLNAC Accreditation: *Yes*

NURSING STUDENT PROFILE

Total Nursing Enrollment: *115* • Full-Time Enrollment: *62* • Part-Time Enrollment: *53* • Female Enrollment: *105* • Male Enrollment: *10* • Total New Admissions Who Enrolled for Fall: *41* • Total Graduates: *52*

FINANCES

Residential Annual Tuition: *$1,230* • Non-Residential Annual Tuition: *$3,530* • General Institution Fees: *$40* • Additional Nursing Fees: *$12*

PIKEVILLE COLLEGE

Address: 147 Sycamore Street, Pikeville, KY 41501
Phone: 606-218-5750
Fax: 606-218-5768
Contact: Mary Rado Simpson, MSN, PhD, RN, Chair
Email: msimpson@pc.edu

GENERAL INFORMATION

Type of School: *4-Year College or University, Private (Independent)* • Accreditation: *Southern Association of Colleges and Schools* • Total Enrollment: *917*

PROGRAM INFORMATION

LPN/LVN Exit: *No* • NLNAC Accreditation: *No*

NURSING STUDENT PROFILE

Total Nursing Enrollment: *54* • Full-Time Enrollment: *54* • Part-Time Enrollment: *0* • Female Enrollment: *46* • Male Enrollment: *8* • Total New Admissions Who Enrolled for Fall: *27* • Total Graduates: *17*

FINANCES

Residential Annual Tuition: *$7,800* • Non-Residential Annual Tuition: *$7,800* • General Institution Fees: *$0* • Additional Nursing Fees: *$130*

PRESTONSBURG COMMUNITY COLLEGE

Address: One Bert Combs Drive, Prestonburg, KY 41653
Phone: 606-886-3863
Fax: 606-886-6200
Contact: Paula J. Gibson, MSN, RN, ADN Program Coordinator
Email: paula.gibson@kctcs.net

GENERAL INFORMATION

Type of School: *2-Year College or University, Public* • Accreditation: *Southern Association of Colleges and Schools* • Total Enrollment: *2100*

PROGRAM INFORMATION

LPN/LVN Exit: *No* • NLNAC Accreditation: *No*

NURSING STUDENT PROFILE

Total Nursing Enrollment: *43* • Full-Time Enrollment: *32* • Part-Time Enrollment: *11* • Female Enrollment: *41* • Male Enrollment: *2* • Total New Admissions Who Enrolled for Fall: *32* • Total Graduates: *11*

FINANCES

Residential Annual Tuition: *$1,450* • Non-Residential Annual Tuition: *$4,350* • General Institution Fees: *$172* • Additional Nursing Fees: *$12*

SOMERSET COMMUNITY COLLEGE

Address: 808 Monticello Street, Somerset, KY 42501
Phone: 606-679-8501
Fax: 606-676-9065
Contact: Linda Ballard, MSN, RN, Nursing Coordinator
Email: Linda.Ballard@kctcs.net

GENERAL INFORMATION

Type of School: *2-Year College or University, Public* •
Accreditation: *Southern Association of Colleges and Schools* •
Total Enrollment: *2400*

PROGRAM INFORMATION

LPN/LVN Exit: *No* • NLNAC Accreditation: *Yes*

NURSING STUDENT PROFILE

Total Nursing Enrollment: *70* • Full-Time Enrollment: *48* •
Part-Time Enrollment: *22* • Female Enrollment: *64* • Male
Enrollment: *6* • Total New Admissions Who Enrolled for
Fall: *45* • Total Graduates: *31*

FINANCES

Residential Annual Tuition: *$2,370* • Non-Residential
Annual Tuition: *$7,110* • General Institution Fees: *$40* •
Additional Nursing Fees: *$637*

SOUTHEAST COMMUNITY COLLEGE—PINEVILLE

Address: PO Box 187, Pineville, KY 40977
Phone: 606-589-2145
Fax: 606-589-5758
Contact: Milton Borntrager, MSN, RN, Program
Coordinator
Email: Milton.Borntrager@kctcs.edu

GENERAL INFORMATION

Type of School: *Vocational/Technical School, Public* •
Accreditation: *Southern Association of Colleges and Schools* •
Total Enrollment: *240*

PROGRAM INFORMATION

LPN/LVN Exit: *No* • NLNAC Accreditation: *Yes*

NURSING STUDENT PROFILE

Total Nursing Enrollment: *92* • Full-Time Enrollment: *68* •
Part-Time Enrollment: *24* • Female Enrollment: *78* • Male
Enrollment: *14* • Total New Admissions Who Enrolled for
Fall: *56* • Total Graduates: *29*

FINANCES

Residential Annual Tuition: *$725* • Non-Residential Annual
Tuition: *$2,175* • General Institution Fees: *$102* •
Additional Nursing Fees: *$12*

SPENCERIAN COLLEGE

Address: 4627 Dixie Highway, Louisville, KY 40216
Phone: 502-447-1000
Fax: 502-447-4574
Contact: Jane Younger, MSN, RN, Associate Degree
           Nursing Director
Email: jyounger@spencerian.edu

GENERAL INFORMATION

Type of School: *4-Year College or University, Private
(Independent)* • Accreditation: *Southern Association of Colleges
and Schools* • Total Enrollment: *5600*

PROGRAM INFORMATION

LPN/LVN Exit: *No* • NLNAC Accreditation: *No*

NURSING STUDENT PROFILE

Total Nursing Enrollment: *39* • Full-Time Enrollment: *Not
Reported* • Part-Time Enrollment: *Not Reported* • Female
Enrollment: *36* • Male Enrollment: *3* • Total New
Admissions Who Enrolled for Fall: *39* • Total Graduates: *Not
Reported*

FINANCES

Residential Annual Tuition: *$14,240* • Non-Residential
Annual Tuition: *$14,240* • General Institution Fees: *$685* •
Additional Nursing Fees: *$1,840*

ST. CATHARINE COLLEGE

Address: 2735 Bardstown Road, Saint Catharine, KY
           40061
Phone: 859-336-5082
Fax: 856-336-5031
Contact: Fannie Jean Spencer, MSN, RN, Chair of
           Nursing
Email: jspencer@sccky.edu

GENERAL INFORMATION

Type of School: *2-Year College or University, Private
(Independent)* • Accreditation: *Southern Association of Colleges
and Schools* • Total Enrollment: *525*

PROGRAM INFORMATION

LPN/LVN Exit: *No* • NLNAC Accreditation: *Not Reported*

NURSING STUDENT PROFILE

Total Nursing Enrollment: *20* • Full-Time Enrollment: *20* •
Part-Time Enrollment: *0* • Female Enrollment: *18* • Male
Enrollment: *2* • Total New Admissions Who Enrolled for
Fall: *14* • Total Graduates: *17*

FINANCES

Residential Annual Tuition: *$9,716* • Non-Residential
Annual Tuition: *$9,716* • General Institution Fees: *Not
Reported* • Additional Nursing Fees: *Not Reported*

WESTERN KENTUCKY UNIVERSITY

Address: 1 Big Red Way, Academic Complex WKU,
              Bowling Green, KY 42101
Phone: 270-780-2502
Fax: 270-780-2560
Contact: Martha Houchin, MSN, RN, Program Director
Email: martha.houchin@wku.edu

GENERAL INFORMATION

Type of School: *4-Year College or University, Public* •
Accreditation: *Southern Association of Colleges and Schools* •
Total Enrollment: *15516*

PROGRAM INFORMATION

LPN/LVN Exit: *No* • NLNAC Accreditation: *Yes*

NURSING STUDENT PROFILE

Total Nursing Enrollment: *152* • Full-Time Enrollment: *37* •
Part-Time Enrollment: *115* • Female Enrollment: *137* • Male
Enrollment: *15* • Total New Admissions Who Enrolled for
Fall: *44* • Total Graduates: *64*

FINANCES

Residential Annual Tuition: *$2,404* • Non-Residential
Annual Tuition: *$6,444* • General Institution Fees: *$50* •
Additional Nursing Fees: *$50*

DELGADO COMMUNITY COLLEGE

Address: 450 South Claiborne Avenue, New Orleans, LA
              70112
Phone: 504-568-6466
Fax: 504-568-5494
Contact: Patricia Egers, RN, MS, Interim Director
Email: pegers@dcc.edu

GENERAL INFORMATION

Type of School: *2-Year College or University, Public* •
Accreditation: *Southern Association of Colleges and Schools* •
Total Enrollment: *12500*

PROGRAM INFORMATION

LPN/LVN Exit: *No* • NLNAC Accreditation: *Yes*

NURSING STUDENT PROFILE

Total Nursing Enrollment: *432* • Full-Time Enrollment:
108 • Part-Time Enrollment: *324* • Female Enrollment:
354 • Male Enrollment: *78* • Total New Admissions Who
Enrolled for Fall: *103* • Total Graduates: *172*

FINANCES

Residential Annual Tuition: *$587* • Non-Residential Annual
Tuition: *$1,747* • General Institution Fees: *$0* • Additional
Nursing Fees: *$190*

LOUISIANA STATE UNIVERSITY

Address: 433 Bolivar Street, New Orleans, LA 70112
Phone: 504-568-4106
Fax: Not Reported
Contact: Elizabeth A. Humphrey, RN, EdD, Dean
Email: ehumph@lsumc.edu

LOUISIANA STATE UNIVERSITY—ALEXANDRIA

Address: 8100 Highway 71 South, Alexandria, LA 71302
Phone: 318-473-6459
Fax: 318-473-6567
Contact: Wanda J Guidry, MSN, RN, Division Head
            Nursing
Email: wguidry@pobox.lsua.edu

GENERAL INFORMATION

Type of School: *Other, Public* • Accreditation: *Southern Association of Colleges and Schools* • Total Enrollment: *2755*

GENERAL INFORMATION

Type of School: *2-Year College or University, Public* • Accreditation: *Southern Association of Colleges and Schools* • Total Enrollment: *2400*

PROGRAM INFORMATION

LPN/LVN Exit: *No* • NLNAC Accreditation: *Yes*

PROGRAM INFORMATION

LPN/LVN Exit: *No* • NLNAC Accreditation: *Yes*

NURSING STUDENT PROFILE

Total Nursing Enrollment: *34* • Full-Time Enrollment: *32* • Part-Time Enrollment: *2* • Female Enrollment: *30* • Male Enrollment: *4* • Total New Admissions Who Enrolled for Fall: *0* • Total Graduates: *33*

NURSING STUDENT PROFILE

Total Nursing Enrollment: *176* • Full-Time Enrollment: *27* • Part-Time Enrollment: *149* • Female Enrollment: *144* • Male Enrollment: *32* • Total New Admissions Who Enrolled for Fall: *51* • Total Graduates: *85*

FINANCES

Residential Annual Tuition: *$1,946* • Non-Residential Annual Tuition: *$3,546* • General Institution Fees: *Not Reported* • Additional Nursing Fees: *Not Reported*

FINANCES

Residential Annual Tuition: *$1,250* • Non-Residential Annual Tuition: *$3,900* • General Institution Fees: *$75* • Additional Nursing Fees: *$200*

LOUISIANA STATE UNIVERSITY—EUNICE

Address: P.O.Box 1129, Eunice, LA 70535
Phone: 337-550-1357
Fax: 337-550-1289
Contact: Theresa H. deBeche, MN, RN, Head, Division
            of Nursing and Allied Health
Email: tdebeche@lsue.edu

GENERAL INFORMATION

Type of School: *2-Year College or University, Public* •
Accreditation: *Southern Association of Colleges and Schools* •
Total Enrollment: *2742*

PROGRAM INFORMATION

LPN/LVN Exit: *No* • NLNAC Accreditation: *Yes*

NURSING STUDENT PROFILE

Total Nursing Enrollment: *121* • Full-Time Enrollment: *15* •
Part-Time Enrollment: *106* • Female Enrollment: *96* • Male
Enrollment: *25* • Total New Admissions Who Enrolled for
Fall: *61* • Total Graduates: *55*

FINANCES

Residential Annual Tuition: *$1,141* • Non-Residential
Annual Tuition: *$4,414* • General Institution Fees: *Not
Reported* • Additional Nursing Fees: *Not Reported*

LOUISIANA TECHNICAL UNIVERSITY—RUSTON CAMPUS

Address: PO Box 3152TS, Ruston, LA 71273
Phone: 318-257-3036
Fax: Not Reported
Contact: Virginia Pennington, PhD, RN, Chairperson
Email: Not Reported

GENERAL INFORMATION

Type of School: *Vocational/Technical School, Public* •
Accreditation: *None* • Total Enrollment: *188*

PROGRAM INFORMATION

LPN/LVN Exit: *No* • NLNAC Accreditation: *Yes*

NURSING STUDENT PROFILE

Total Nursing Enrollment: *148* • Full-Time Enrollment: *72* •
Part-Time Enrollment: *76* • Female Enrollment: *Not
Reported* • Male Enrollment: *Not Reported* • Total New
Admissions Who Enrolled for Fall: *85* • Total Graduates: *80*

FINANCES

Residential Annual Tuition: *Not Reported* • Non-Residential
Annual Tuition: *Not Reported* • General Institution Fees: *Not
Reported* • Additional Nursing Fees: *Not Reported*

MCNEESE STATE UNIVERSITY

Address: P.O. Box 90415, Lake Charles, LA 70609
Phone: 337-475-5998
Fax: 337-475-5996
Contact: Jeannine Babineaux, PhD, RN, Coordinator, Associate Degree Program
Email: jbabinea@mail.mcneese.edu

GENERAL INFORMATION

Type of School: *4-Year College or University, Public* •
Accreditation: *Southern Association of Colleges and Schools* •
Total Enrollment: *7780*

PROGRAM INFORMATION

LPN/LVN Exit: *No* • NLNAC Accreditation: *Not Reported*

NURSING STUDENT PROFILE

Total Nursing Enrollment: *94* • Full-Time Enrollment: *70* •
Part-Time Enrollment: *24* • Female Enrollment: *77* • Male
Enrollment: *17* • Total New Admissions Who Enrolled for
Fall: *26* • Total Graduates: *24*

FINANCES

Residential Annual Tuition: *$1,213* • Non-Residential
Annual Tuition: *$3,170* • General Institution Fees: *$598* •
Additional Nursing Fees: *$100*

NICHOLLS STATE UNIVERSITY

Address: P.O. Box 2143, Thibodaux, LA 70310
Phone: 985-448-4696
Fax: 985-448-4932
Contact: Cheryl P. Franklin, MN, RN, ASN Program Director and Associate Professor
Email: nurs-cpf@nich-nsunet.nich.edu

GENERAL INFORMATION

Type of School: *4-Year College or University, Public* •
Accreditation: *Southern Association of Colleges and Schools* •
Total Enrollment: *7400*

PROGRAM INFORMATION

LPN/LVN Exit: *No* • NLNAC Accreditation: *Yes*

NURSING STUDENT PROFILE

Total Nursing Enrollment: *37* • Full-Time Enrollment: *37* •
Part-Time Enrollment: *0* • Female Enrollment: *32* • Male
Enrollment: *5* • Total New Admissions Who Enrolled for
Fall: *13* • Total Graduates: *30*

FINANCES

Residential Annual Tuition: *$1,058* • Non-Residential
Annual Tuition: *$3,626* • General Institution Fees: *$300* •
Additional Nursing Fees: *$150*

NORTHWESTERN STATE UNIVERSITY OF LOUISIANA

Address: 1800 Line Avenue, Natchitoches, LA 71497
Phone: 318-677-3100
Fax: 318-677-3127
Contact: Shirley Cashio, MSN, RN, Director, Undergraduate Studies in Nursing
Email: cashios@nsula.edu

GENERAL INFORMATION

Type of School: *4-Year College or University, Public* • Accreditation: *Southern Association of Colleges and Schools* • Total Enrollment: *9415*

PROGRAM INFORMATION

LPN/LVN Exit: *No* • NLNAC Accreditation: *Yes*

NURSING STUDENT PROFILE

Total Nursing Enrollment: *769* • Full-Time Enrollment: *345* • Part-Time Enrollment: *424* • Female Enrollment: *661* • Male Enrollment: *108* • Total New Admissions Who Enrolled for Fall: *50* • Total Graduates: *86*

FINANCES

Residential Annual Tuition: *$2,250* • Non-Residential Annual Tuition: *$7,050* • General Institution Fees: *$128* • Additional Nursing Fees: *$250*

OUR LADY OF THE LAKE COLLEGE

Address: 7500 Hennesy Blvd, Baton Rouge, LA 70808
Phone: 225-768-1709
Fax: 225-768-1760
Contact: Louise Plaisan, DNS, RN, Acting Dean, Division of Nursing
Email: lplaisan@ololcollege.edu

GENERAL INFORMATION

Type of School: *4-Year College or University, Private (Religious)* • Accreditation: *Southern Association of Colleges and Schools* • Total Enrollment: *1200*

PROGRAM INFORMATION

LPN/LVN Exit: *No* • NLNAC Accreditation: *Yes*

NURSING STUDENT PROFILE

Total Nursing Enrollment: *207* • Full-Time Enrollment: *207* • Part-Time Enrollment: *0* • Female Enrollment: *192* • Male Enrollment: *15* • Total New Admissions Who Enrolled for Fall: *54* • Total Graduates: *119*

FINANCES

Residential Annual Tuition: *Not Reported* • Non-Residential Annual Tuition: *Not Reported* • General Institution Fees: *Not Reported* • Additional Nursing Fees: *Not Reported*

CENTRAL MAINE MEDICAL CENTER

Address:　70 Middle Street, Lewiston, ME 04240
Phone:　207-795-2841
Fax:　207-795-2849
Contact:　Sharon L. Kuhrt, RNC, MSN, Director
Email:　skuhrt@cmhc.org

GENERAL INFORMATION

Type of School: *Independent, Private (Independent)* •
Accreditation: *New England Association of Schools and
Colleges* • Total Enrollment: *98*

PROGRAM INFORMATION

LPN/LVN Exit: *No* • NLNAC Accreditation: *Yes*

NURSING STUDENT PROFILE

Total Nursing Enrollment: *98* • Full-Time Enrollment: *25* •
Part-Time Enrollment: *73* • Female Enrollment: *88* • Male
Enrollment: *10* • Total New Admissions Who Enrolled for
Fall: *51* • Total Graduates: *31*

FINANCES

Residential Annual Tuition: *$2,310* • Non-Residential
Annual Tuition: *$2,310* • General Institution Fees: *$935* •
Additional Nursing Fees: *Not Reported*

CENTRAL MAINE TECHNICAL COLLEGE

Address:　1250 Turner Street, Auburn, ME 04210
Phone:　207-755-5408
Fax:　207-755-5496
Contact:　Anne Schuettinger, RN, MS, CS, Chair of
　　　　　Nursing
Email:　aschuet@cmtc.net

GENERAL INFORMATION

Type of School: *2-Year College or University, Public* •
Accreditation: *New England Association of Schools and
Colleges* • Total Enrollment: *1435*

PROGRAM INFORMATION

LPN/LVN Exit: *Yes* • NLNAC Accreditation: *Yes*

NURSING STUDENT PROFILE

Total Nursing Enrollment: *47* • Full-Time Enrollment: *25* •
Part-Time Enrollment: *22* • Female Enrollment: *44* • Male
Enrollment: *3* • Total New Admissions Who Enrolled for
Fall: *22* • Total Graduates: *18*

FINANCES

Residential Annual Tuition: *$2,176* • Non-Residential
Annual Tuition: *$4,768* • General Institution Fees: *$90* •
Additional Nursing Fees: *$100*

EASTERN MAINE TECHNICAL COLLEGE

Address: 354 Hogan Road, Bangor, ME 04401
Phone: 207-941-4657
Fax: 207-941-4608
Contact: Marilyn A. Lavelle, MS, RN, Chairperson
Email: mlavelle@emtc.org

GENERAL INFORMATION

Type of School: *2-Year College or University, Public* •
Accreditation: *New England Association of Schools and Colleges* • Total Enrollment: *1250*

PROGRAM INFORMATION

LPN/LVN Exit: *Yes* • NLNAC Accreditation: *Yes*

NURSING STUDENT PROFILE

Total Nursing Enrollment: *48* • Full-Time Enrollment: *15* •
Part-Time Enrollment: *33* • Female Enrollment: *42* • Male
Enrollment: *6* • Total New Admissions Who Enrolled for
Fall: *31* • Total Graduates: *28*

FINANCES

Residential Annual Tuition: *$2,312* • Non-Residential
Annual Tuition: *$5,066* • General Institution Fees: *$518* •
Additional Nursing Fees: *$230*

KENNEBEC VALLEY TECHNICAL COLLEGE

Address: 92 Western Ave, Fairfield, ME 04937-1367
Phone: 207-453-5167
Fax: 207-453-5194
Contact: Marcia J. Parker, RN, MS, Nursing Department
   Chairperson
Email: mparker@kvtc.net

GENERAL INFORMATION

Type of School: *2-Year College or University, Public* •
Accreditation: *New England Association of Schools and Colleges* • Total Enrollment: *1135*

PROGRAM INFORMATION

LPN/LVN Exit: *Yes* • NLNAC Accreditation: *Yes*

NURSING STUDENT PROFILE

Total Nursing Enrollment: *83* • Full-Time Enrollment: *17* •
Part-Time Enrollment: *66* • Female Enrollment: *78* • Male
Enrollment: *5* • Total New Admissions Who Enrolled for
Fall: *48* • Total Graduates: *26*

FINANCES

Residential Annual Tuition: *$2,176* • Non-Residential
Annual Tuition: *$4,768* • General Institution Fees: *$600* •
Additional Nursing Fees: *$500*

NORTHERN MAINE TECHNICAL COLLEGE

Address: 33 Edgemont Drive, Presque Isle, ME 04769
Phone: 207-768-2749
Fax: 207-768-2831
Contact: Betty Kent-Conant, MSN, RN, Department Chair, Nursing
Email: nbconant@nmtc.net

GENERAL INFORMATION

Type of School: *Vocational/Technical School, Public* • Accreditation: *New England Association of Schools and Colleges* • Total Enrollment: *45*

PROGRAM INFORMATION

LPN/LVN Exit: *Yes* • NLNAC Accreditation: *Yes*

NURSING STUDENT PROFILE

Total Nursing Enrollment: *49* • Full-Time Enrollment: *49* • Part-Time Enrollment: *0* • Female Enrollment: *43* • Male Enrollment: *6* • Total New Admissions Who Enrolled for Fall: *34* • Total Graduates: *27*

FINANCES

Residential Annual Tuition: *$2,244* • Non-Residential Annual Tuition: *$4,917* • General Institution Fees: *$222* • Additional Nursing Fees: *$115*

SOUTHERN MAINE TECHNICAL COLLEGE

Address: 2 Fort Road, South Portland, ME 04106
Phone: 207-767-9588
Fax: 207-767-9690
Contact: Nancy E. Smith, MS, RN, Chairperson
Email: nsmith@smtc.net

GENERAL INFORMATION

Type of School: *Other, Private (Religious)* • Accreditation: *New England Association of Schools and Colleges* • Total Enrollment: *90*

PROGRAM INFORMATION

LPN/LVN Exit: *Yes* • NLNAC Accreditation: *Yes*

NURSING STUDENT PROFILE

Total Nursing Enrollment: *79* • Full-Time Enrollment: *60* • Part-Time Enrollment: *19* • Female Enrollment: *69* • Male Enrollment: *10* • Total New Admissions Who Enrolled for Fall: *Not Reported* • Total Graduates: *30*

FINANCES

Residential Annual Tuition: *$1,140* • Non-Residential Annual Tuition: *$2,020* • General Institution Fees: *$200* • Additional Nursing Fees: *$1,000*

UNIVERSITY OF MAINE— AUGUSTA

Address: 46 University Dr, Augusta, ME 04330-9488
Phone: 207-621-3469
Fax: 207-621-3293
Contact: Nancy J. Cooley, MSN, RN, CS-FNP, Coordinator
Email: ncooley@maine.edu

GENERAL INFORMATION

Type of School: *4-Year College or University, Public* • Accreditation: *New England Association of Schools and Colleges* • Total Enrollment: *5617*

PROGRAM INFORMATION

LPN/LVN Exit: *No* • NLNAC Accreditation: *Yes*

NURSING STUDENT PROFILE

Total Nursing Enrollment: *112* • Full-Time Enrollment: *Not Reported* • Part-Time Enrollment: *Not Reported* • Female Enrollment: *104* • Male Enrollment: *8* • Total New Admissions Who Enrolled for Fall: *71* • Total Graduates: *58*

FINANCES

Residential Annual Tuition: *$2,520* • Non-Residential Annual Tuition: *$6,168* • General Institution Fees: *$60* • Additional Nursing Fees: *$133*

UNIVERSITY OF NEW ENGLAND

Address: 716 Stevens Avenue, Portland, ME 04103
Phone: 207-797-7688
Fax: 207-878-4895
Contact: Jean Dyer, PhD(c), MSN, BSN, RN, Chair
Email: jdyer@une.edu

GENERAL INFORMATION

Type of School: *4-Year College or University, Private (Independent)* • Accreditation: *New England Association of Schools and Colleges* • Total Enrollment: *3887*

PROGRAM INFORMATION

LPN/LVN Exit: *No* • NLNAC Accreditation: *Yes*

NURSING STUDENT PROFILE

Total Nursing Enrollment: *102* • Full-Time Enrollment: *84* • Part-Time Enrollment: *18* • Female Enrollment: *95* • Male Enrollment: *7* • Total New Admissions Who Enrolled for Fall: *50* • Total Graduates: *22*

FINANCES

Residential Annual Tuition: *$15,740* • Non-Residential Annual Tuition: *$15,740* • General Institution Fees: *$210* • Additional Nursing Fees: *$125*

ALLEGANY COLLEGE OF MARYLAND

Address: 12401 Willowbrook Road, Cumberland, MD
             21502
Phone: 301-784-5567
Fax: 301-784-5016
Contact: Fran Leibfreid, MEd, BSN, RN, Director of
             Nursing Education
Email: fleibfreid@ac.cc.md.us

GENERAL INFORMATION

Type of School: *2-Year College or University, Public* •
Accreditation: *Middle States Association of Colleges and
Schools* • Total Enrollment: *Not Reported*

PROGRAM INFORMATION

LPN/LVN Exit: *Yes* • NLNAC Accreditation: *Yes*

NURSING STUDENT PROFILE

Total Nursing Enrollment: *128* • Full-Time Enrollment:
128 • Part-Time Enrollment: *0* • Female Enrollment: *115* •
Male Enrollment: *13* • Total New Admissions Who Enrolled
for Fall: *40* • Total Graduates: *42*

FINANCES

Residential Annual Tuition: *$2,040* • Non-Residential
Annual Tuition: *$4,008* • General Institution Fees: *$110* •
Additional Nursing Fees: *$490*

ANNE ARUNDEL COMMUNITY COLLEGE

Address: 101 College Parkway, Arnold, MD 21012
Phone: 410-315-7352
Fax: 410-315-7099
Contact: Linda J. Epstein, RN, MS, Chair, Department of
             Nursing
Email: ljepstein@mail.aacc.cc.md.us

GENERAL INFORMATION

Type of School: *2-Year College or University, Public* •
Accreditation: *Middle States Association of Colleges and
Schools* • Total Enrollment: *Not Reported*

PROGRAM INFORMATION

LPN/LVN Exit: *Yes* • NLNAC Accreditation: *Yes*

NURSING STUDENT PROFILE

Total Nursing Enrollment: *209* • Full-Time Enrollment:
209 • Part-Time Enrollment: *0* • Female Enrollment: *192* •
Male Enrollment: *17* • Total New Admissions Who Enrolled
for Fall: *106* • Total Graduates: *84*

FINANCES

Residential Annual Tuition: *Not Reported* • Non-Residential
Annual Tuition: *Not Reported* • General Institution Fees: *Not
Reported* • Additional Nursing Fees: *Not Reported*

BALTIMORE CITY COMMUNITY COLLEGE

Address: 2901 Liberty Hts Ave, Baltimore, MD 21215
Phone: 410-462-7786
Fax: Not Reported
Contact: Dorothy N. Holley, RN,MSN, Chairperson
Email: dholley@bccc.state.md.us

GENERAL INFORMATION

Type of School: *2-Year College or University, Public* •
Accreditation: *Middle States Association of Colleges and Schools* • Total Enrollment: *Not Reported*

PROGRAM INFORMATION

LPN/LVN Exit: *Not Reported* • NLNAC Accreditation: *No*

NURSING STUDENT PROFILE

Total Nursing Enrollment: *Not Reported* • Full-Time Enrollment: *Not Reported* • Part-Time Enrollment: *Not Reported* • Female Enrollment: *Not Reported* • Male Enrollment: *Not Reported* • Total New Admissions Who Enrolled for Fall: *Not Reported* • Total Graduates: *Not Reported*

FINANCES

Residential Annual Tuition: *Not Reported* • Non-Residential Annual Tuition: *Not Reported* • General Institution Fees: *Not Reported* • Additional Nursing Fees: *Not Reported*

CECIL COMMUNITY COLLEGE

Address: One Seahawk Dr, North East, MD 21901
Phone: 410-287-6060
Fax: 410-287-1040
Contact: Mary Way Bolt, RN, EdD, Director of Nursing Education
Email: mbolt@cecilcc.edu

GENERAL INFORMATION

Type of School: *2-Year College or University, Public* •
Accreditation: *Middle States Association of Colleges and Schools* • Total Enrollment: *Not Reported*

PROGRAM INFORMATION

LPN/LVN Exit: *Yes* • NLNAC Accreditation: *Yes*

NURSING STUDENT PROFILE

Total Nursing Enrollment: *76* • Full-Time Enrollment: *16* • Part-Time Enrollment: *60* • Female Enrollment: *70* • Male Enrollment: *6* • Total New Admissions Who Enrolled for Fall: *51* • Total Graduates: *24*

FINANCES

Residential Annual Tuition: *$780* • Non-Residential Annual Tuition: *$2,400* • General Institution Fees: *$100* • Additional Nursing Fees: *$100*

CHESAPEAKE COLLEGE

Address:　PO BOX 8, Wye Mills, MD 21676
Phone:　　410-639-2982
Fax:　　　Not Reported
Contact:　Judith E. Stetson, PhD, RN, Director, MGW
　　　　　Nursing
Email:　　jstetson@chesapeake.edu

GENERAL INFORMATION

Type of School: *2-Year College or University, Public* •
Accreditation: *Middle States Association of Colleges and
Schools* • Total Enrollment: *Not Reported*

PROGRAM INFORMATION

LPN/LVN Exit: *Yes* • NLNAC Accreditation: *No*

NURSING STUDENT PROFILE

Total Nursing Enrollment: *69* • Full-Time Enrollment: *69* •
Part-Time Enrollment: *0* • Female Enrollment: *65* • Male
Enrollment: *4* • Total New Admissions Who Enrolled for
Fall: *40* • Total Graduates: *0*

FINANCES

Residential Annual Tuition: *Not Reported* • Non-Residential
Annual Tuition: *Not Reported* • General Institution Fees: *Not
Reported* • Additional Nursing Fees: *Not Reported*

COLLEGE OF SOUTHERN MARYLAND

Address:　PO BOX 910, La Plata, MD 20646
Phone:　　301-934-7535
Fax:　　　301-934-7672
Contact:　Margaret DeStefanis, RN, BSN, MN, Chair,
　　　　　Nursing and Health Technology
Email:　　peggyd@csm.cc.md.us

GENERAL INFORMATION

Type of School: *2-Year College or University, Public* •
Accreditation: *Middle States Association of Colleges and
Schools* • Total Enrollment: *Not Reported*

PROGRAM INFORMATION

LPN/LVN Exit: *Not Reported* • NLNAC Accreditation: *Yes*

NURSING STUDENT PROFILE

Total Nursing Enrollment: *101* • Full-Time Enrollment: *23* •
Part-Time Enrollment: *78* • Female Enrollment: *94* • Male
Enrollment: *7* • Total New Admissions Who Enrolled for
Fall: *55* • Total Graduates: *51*

FINANCES

Residential Annual Tuition: *$1,752* • Non-Residential
Annual Tuition: *$4,560* • General Institution Fees: *$200* •
Additional Nursing Fees: *$155*

THE COMMUNITY COLLEGE OF BALTIMORE

Address: 800 South Rolling Road, Catonsville, MD
            21228
Phone: 410-455-4570
Fax: Not Reported
Contact: Ann E Miller, MS, BSN, RN, Chairperson
Email: amiller@ccbc.cc.md.us

GENERAL INFORMATION

Type of School: *Not Reported* • Accreditation: *Not Reported* •
Total Enrollment: *Not Reported*

PROGRAM INFORMATION

LPN/LVN Exit: *No* • NLNAC Accreditation: *Yes*

NURSING STUDENT PROFILE

Total Nursing Enrollment: *133* • Full-Time Enrollment:
133 • Part-Time Enrollment: *0* • Female Enrollment: *Not
Reported* • Male Enrollment: *Not Reported* • Total New
Admissions Who Enrolled for Fall: *52* • Total Graduates: *58*

FINANCES

Residential Annual Tuition: *Not Reported* • Non-Residential
Annual Tuition: *Not Reported* • General Institution Fees: *Not
Reported* • Additional Nursing Fees: *Not Reported*

THE COMMUNITY COLLEGE OF BALTIMORE COUNTY

Address: 7201 Rossville Blvd, Baltimore, MD 21237
Phone: 410-780-6360
Fax: 410-780-6405
Contact: Roberta Raymond, PhD, RN, Nursing Program
            Administrator
Email: rraymond@ccbc.cc.md.us

GENERAL INFORMATION

Type of School: *2-Year College or University, Public* •
Accreditation: *Middle States Association of Colleges and
Schools* • Total Enrollment: *Not Reported*

PROGRAM INFORMATION

LPN/LVN Exit: *No* • NLNAC Accreditation: *No*

NURSING STUDENT PROFILE

Total Nursing Enrollment: *335* • Full-Time Enrollment: *54* •
Part-Time Enrollment: *281* • Female Enrollment: *304* • Male
Enrollment: *31* • Total New Admissions Who Enrolled for
Fall: *133* • Total Graduates: *104*

FINANCES

Residential Annual Tuition: *$2,904* • Non-Residential
Annual Tuition: *$4,224* • General Institution Fees: *$60* •
Additional Nursing Fees: *$100*

FREDERICK COMMUNITY COLLEGE

Address: 7932 Opossumtown Pike, Frederick, MD 21702
Phone: 301-846-2525
Fax: 301-846-2498
Contact: Jane A. Garvin, MSN, RN, CS-P, Director of
          Nursing Education and Chair, Department of
          Allied Health and Wellness
Email: jgarvin@fcc.cc.md.us

GENERAL INFORMATION

Type of School: *2-Year College or University, Public* •
Accreditation: *Middle States Association of Colleges and
Schools* • Total Enrollment: *Not Reported*

PROGRAM INFORMATION

LPN/LVN Exit: *Yes* • NLNAC Accreditation: *No*

NURSING STUDENT PROFILE

Total Nursing Enrollment: *83* • Full-Time Enrollment: *0* •
Part-Time Enrollment: *83* • Female Enrollment: *78* • Male
Enrollment: *5* • Total New Admissions Who Enrolled for
Fall: *41* • Total Graduates: *34*

FINANCES

Residential Annual Tuition: *$2,298* • Non-Residential
Annual Tuition: *$5,754* • General Institution Fees: *Not
Reported* • Additional Nursing Fees: *$65*

HAGERSTOWN COMMUNITY COLLEGE

Address: 11400 Robinwood Dr, Hagerstown, MD 21742
Phone: 301-790-2800
Fax: 301-739-0737
Contact: Diana K. Foley, MSN, RN, EdD, Chair,
          Division of Health Sciences and Director of
          Nursing
Email: foleyd@hcc.cc.md.us

GENERAL INFORMATION

Type of School: *2-Year College or University, Public* •
Accreditation: *Middle States Association of Colleges and
Schools* • Total Enrollment: *Not Reported*

PROGRAM INFORMATION

LPN/LVN Exit: *Not Reported* • NLNAC Accreditation: *No*

NURSING STUDENT PROFILE

Total Nursing Enrollment: *75* • Full-Time Enrollment: *17* •
Part-Time Enrollment: *58* • Female Enrollment: *69* • Male
Enrollment: *6* • Total New Admissions Who Enrolled for
Fall: *42* • Total Graduates: *20*

FINANCES

Residential Annual Tuition: *$1,492* • Non-Residential
Annual Tuition: *$2,028* • General Institution Fees: *$60* •
Additional Nursing Fees: *$95*

HARFORD COMMUNITY COLLEGE

Address: 401 Thomas Run Rd, Bel Air, MD 21015
Phone: 410-836-4389
Fax: Not Reported
Contact: Joyce Jordan, MS, RNCS, Division Chair, Nursing, Allied Health and PE
Email: jjordan@harford.cc.md.us

GENERAL INFORMATION

Type of School: *Not Reported* • Accreditation: *Middle States Association of Colleges and Schools* • Total Enrollment: *Not Reported*

PROGRAM INFORMATION

LPN/LVN Exit: *Yes* • NLNAC Accreditation: *Yes*

NURSING STUDENT PROFILE

Total Nursing Enrollment: *Not Reported* • Full-Time Enrollment: *Not Reported* • Part-Time Enrollment: *Not Reported* • Female Enrollment: *Not Reported* • Male Enrollment: *Not Reported* • Total New Admissions Who Enrolled for Fall: *Not Reported* • Total Graduates: *Not Reported*

FINANCES

Residential Annual Tuition: *Not Reported* • Non-Residential Annual Tuition: *Not Reported* • General Institution Fees: *Not Reported* • Additional Nursing Fees: *Not Reported*

HOWARD COMMUNITY COLLEGE

Address: 19001 Little Patuxent Parkway, Columbia, MD 21044
Phone: 410-772-4888
Fax: 410-772-4494
Contact: Emily Slunt, PhD, RN, Health Sciences Division Chair and Director of Nursing
Email: eslunt@howardcc.edu

GENERAL INFORMATION

Type of School: *2-Year College or University, Public* • Accreditation: *Middle States Association of Colleges and Schools* • Total Enrollment: *Not Reported*

PROGRAM INFORMATION

LPN/LVN Exit: *Yes* • NLNAC Accreditation: *Yes*

NURSING STUDENT PROFILE

Total Nursing Enrollment: *137* • Full-Time Enrollment: *14* • Part-Time Enrollment: *123* • Female Enrollment: *126* • Male Enrollment: *11* • Total New Admissions Who Enrolled for Fall: *61* • Total Graduates: *34*

FINANCES

Residential Annual Tuition: *$1,944* • Non-Residential Annual Tuition: *$4,272* • General Institution Fees: *$100* • Additional Nursing Fees: *$100*

MONTGOMERY COLLEGE

Address: 900 Hungerford Dr, Rockville, MD 20850
Phone: 301-650-1355
Fax: 301-650-1346
Contact: Sharon L. Bernier, PhD, RN, CS-P, Director
Email: sbernier@mc.cc.md.us

GENERAL INFORMATION

Type of School: *2-Year College or University, Public* •
Accreditation: *Middle States Association of Colleges and
Schools* • Total Enrollment: *Not Reported*

PROGRAM INFORMATION

LPN/LVN Exit: *No* • NLNAC Accreditation: *Yes*

NURSING STUDENT PROFILE

Total Nursing Enrollment: *178* • Full-Time Enrollment:
178 • Part-Time Enrollment: *0* • Female Enrollment: *161* •
Male Enrollment: *17* • Total New Admissions Who Enrolled
for Fall: *61* • Total Graduates: *49*

FINANCES

Residential Annual Tuition: *$1,836* • Non-Residential
Annual Tuition: *$2,400* • General Institution Fees: *$450* •
Additional Nursing Fees: *$0*

PRINCE GEORGES COMMUNITY COLLEGE

Address: 301 Largo Rd, Largo, MD 20774-2144
Phone: 301-322-0734
Fax: 301-386-7528
Contact: Lois H. Neuman, PhD, RN, Dean
Email: lnz@pgstumail.pg.cc.md.us

GENERAL INFORMATION

Type of School: *2-Year College or University, Public* •
Accreditation: *Middle States Association of Colleges and
Schools* • Total Enrollment: *Not Reported*

PROGRAM INFORMATION

LPN/LVN Exit: *Yes* • NLNAC Accreditation: *Yes*

NURSING STUDENT PROFILE

Total Nursing Enrollment: *197* • Full-Time Enrollment: *Not
Reported* • Part-Time Enrollment: *Not Reported* • Female
Enrollment: *Not Reported* • Male Enrollment: *Not Reported* •
Total New Admissions Who Enrolled for Fall: *Not Reported* •
Total Graduates: *88*

FINANCES

Residential Annual Tuition: *$2,304* • Non-Residential
Annual Tuition: *$5,760* • General Institution Fees: *Not
Reported* • Additional Nursing Fees: *Not Reported*

WOR-WIC COMMUNITY COLLEGE

Address: 32000 Campus Dr, Salisbury, MD 21804
Phone: 410-572-8700
Fax: 410-572-8710
Contact: Denise Marshall, RN, MEd, Department Head
Email: dmarshall@mail.worwic.edu

GENERAL INFORMATION

Type of School: *2-Year College or University, Public* •
Accreditation: *Middle States Association of Colleges and
Schools* • Total Enrollment: *Not Reported*

PROGRAM INFORMATION

LPN/LVN Exit: *Yes* • NLNAC Accreditation: *No*

NURSING STUDENT PROFILE

Total Nursing Enrollment: *50* • Full-Time Enrollment: *15* •
Part-Time Enrollment: *35* • Female Enrollment: *49* • Male
Enrollment: *1* • Total New Admissions Who Enrolled for
Fall: *50* • Total Graduates: *25*

FINANCES

Residential Annual Tuition: *$1,711* • Non-Residential
Annual Tuition: *$3,633* • General Institution Fees: *$73* •
Additional Nursing Fees: *$124*

ATLANTIC UNION COLLEGE

Address: 338 Main Street, Box 1000, South Lancaster,
MA 01561
Phone: 978-368-2404
Fax: 978-368-2518
Contact: Ninon P. Amertil, PhD, FNP, RN, Chairperson
Email: namertil@atlanticus.edu

GENERAL INFORMATION

Type of School: *4-Year College or University, Private
(Religious)* • Accreditation: *New England Association of Schools
and Colleges* • Total Enrollment: *720*

PROGRAM INFORMATION

LPN/LVN Exit: *No* • NLNAC Accreditation: *Yes*

NURSING STUDENT PROFILE

Total Nursing Enrollment: *44* • Full-Time Enrollment: *44* •
Part-Time Enrollment: *0* • Female Enrollment: *39* • Male
Enrollment: *5* • Total New Admissions Who Enrolled for
Fall: *17* • Total Graduates: *14*

FINANCES

Residential Annual Tuition: *$12,624* • Non-Residential
Annual Tuition: *$12,624* • General Institution Fees: *$325* •
Additional Nursing Fees: *$360*

Circle 5 on reader card   See in-depth profile for more information

BECKER COLLEGE

Address: 61 Sever Street, Worcester, MA 01615
Phone: 508-791-8241
Fax: 508-849-5213
Contact: Valerie A. McCarthy, EdD, RN, C, Director of
            the Nursing Program
Email: vmccarthy@beckercollege.edu

GENERAL INFORMATION

Type of School: *4-Year College or University, Private
(Independent)* • Accreditation: *New England Association of
Schools and Colleges* • Total Enrollment: *965*

PROGRAM INFORMATION

LPN/LVN Exit: *No* • NLNAC Accreditation: *Yes*

NURSING STUDENT PROFILE

Total Nursing Enrollment: *47* • Full-Time Enrollment: *35* •
Part-Time Enrollment: *12* • Female Enrollment: *43* • Male
Enrollment: *4* • Total New Admissions Who Enrolled for
Fall: *23* • Total Graduates: *29*

FINANCES

Residential Annual Tuition: *$12,900* • Non-Residential
Annual Tuition: *$12,900* • General Institution Fees: *$110* •
Additional Nursing Fees: *$20*

BERKSHIRE COMMUNITY COLLEGE

Address: 1350 West Street, Pittsfield, MA 01201
Phone: 413-499-4660
Fax: 413-447-7840
Contact: Patricia E. Brien, MSN, RN, MEd, Department
            Chairperson
Email: pbrien@cc.berkshire.org

GENERAL INFORMATION

Type of School: *2-Year College or University, Public* •
Accreditation: *New England Association of Schools and
Colleges* • Total Enrollment: *2494*

PROGRAM INFORMATION

LPN/LVN Exit: *Not Reported* • NLNAC Accreditation: *Yes*

NURSING STUDENT PROFILE

Total Nursing Enrollment: *98* • Full-Time Enrollment: *30* •
Part-Time Enrollment: *68* • Female Enrollment: *90* • Male
Enrollment: *8* • Total New Admissions Who Enrolled for
Fall: *45* • Total Graduates: *34*

FINANCES

Residential Annual Tuition: *$614* • Non-Residential Annual
Tuition: *$936* • General Institution Fees: *$1,536* •
Additional Nursing Fees: *$1,000*

BRISTOL COMMUNITY COLLEGE

Address: 777 Elsbree St, Fall River, MA 02720-7307
Phone: 508-678-2318
Fax: 508-675-2318
Contact: Marie Marshall, EdD, RN, FN, PC, Chairperson
Email: mmarshal@bristol.mass.edu

GENERAL INFORMATION

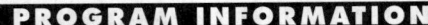

Type of School: *2-Year College or University, Private (Independent)* • Accreditation: *New England Association of Schools and Colleges* • Total Enrollment: *Not Reported*

PROGRAM INFORMATION

LPN/LVN Exit: *No* • NLNAC Accreditation: *Yes*

NURSING STUDENT PROFILE

Total Nursing Enrollment: *87* • Full-Time Enrollment: *83* • Part-Time Enrollment: *4* • Female Enrollment: *79* • Male Enrollment: *8* • Total New Admissions Who Enrolled for Fall: *57* • Total Graduates: *43*

FINANCES

Residential Annual Tuition: *Not Reported* • Non-Residential Annual Tuition: *Not Reported* • General Institution Fees: *Not Reported* • Additional Nursing Fees: *Not Reported*

BUNKER HILL COMMUNITY COLLEGE

Address: 250 New Rutherford Ave, Boston, MA 01950
Phone: 617-228-2443
Fax: 617-228-2052
Contact: Anne M. Zabriskie, MS, RN, Chairperson
Email: azabriskie@bhcc.mass.edu

GENERAL INFORMATION

Type of School: *Not Reported* • Accreditation: *New England Association of Schools and Colleges* • Total Enrollment: *Not Reported*

PROGRAM INFORMATION

LPN/LVN Exit: *No* • NLNAC Accreditation: *Yes*

NURSING STUDENT PROFILE

Total Nursing Enrollment: *86* • Full-Time Enrollment: *86* • Part-Time Enrollment: *0* • Female Enrollment: *69* • Male Enrollment: *17* • Total New Admissions Who Enrolled for Fall: *56* • Total Graduates: *35*

FINANCES

Residential Annual Tuition: *$3,200* • Non-Residential Annual Tuition: *$9,792* • General Institution Fees: *$50* • Additional Nursing Fees: *$15*

CAPE COD COMMUNITY COLLEGE

Address: 2240 Iyanough Road, West Barnstable, MA
             02668-1599
Phone: 508-362-2131
Fax: 508-375-4086
Contact: Luise Speakman, PhD, RN, Coordinator,
             Nursing Program
Email: lspeakman@capecod.mass.edu

GENERAL INFORMATION

Type of School: *2-Year College or University, Public* •
Accreditation: *New England Association of Schools and
Colleges* • Total Enrollment: *Not Reported*

PROGRAM INFORMATION

LPN/LVN Exit: *No* • NLNAC Accreditation: *Yes*

NURSING STUDENT PROFILE

Total Nursing Enrollment: *133* • Full-Time Enrollment:
133 • Part-Time Enrollment: *0* • Female Enrollment: *118* •
Male Enrollment: *15* • Total New Admissions Who Enrolled
for Fall: *76* • Total Graduates: *61*

FINANCES

Residential Annual Tuition: *Not Reported* • Non-Residential
Annual Tuition: *Not Reported* • General Institution Fees: *Not
Reported* • Additional Nursing Fees: *Not Reported*

GREENFIELD COMMUNITY COLLEGE

Address: 270 Main Street, Greenfield, MA 01301
Phone: 413-775-1631
Fax: 413-774-2285
Contact: Jean A. Simmons, MSN, RN, Program
             Coordinator
Email: simmons@gcc.mass.edu

GENERAL INFORMATION

Type of School: *2-Year College or University, Public* •
Accreditation: *New England Association of Schools and
Colleges* • Total Enrollment: *Not Reported*

PROGRAM INFORMATION

LPN/LVN Exit: *Not Reported* • NLNAC Accreditation: *Yes*

NURSING STUDENT PROFILE

Total Nursing Enrollment: *70* • Full-Time Enrollment: *68* •
Part-Time Enrollment: *2* • Female Enrollment: *59* • Male
Enrollment: *11* • Total New Admissions Who Enrolled for
Fall: *44* • Total Graduates: *34*

FINANCES

Residential Annual Tuition: *$832* • Non-Residential Annual
Tuition: *$8,992* • General Institution Fees: *$1,284* •
Additional Nursing Fees: *$65*

HOLYOKE COMMUNITY COLLEGE

Address: 303 Homestead Ave, Holyoke, MA 01040
Phone: 413-552-2458
Fax: 413-534-8975
Contact: Joan M. Culley, RN, CWOCN, MS, MPH, BSN, Director of Nursing
Email: jculley@hcc.mass.edu

GENERAL INFORMATION

Type of School: *2-Year College or University, Public* • Accreditation: *New England Association of Schools and Colleges* • Total Enrollment: *Not Reported*

PROGRAM INFORMATION

LPN/LVN Exit: *No* • NLNAC Accreditation: *Yes*

NURSING STUDENT PROFILE

Total Nursing Enrollment: *81* • Full-Time Enrollment: *81* • Part-Time Enrollment: *0* • Female Enrollment: *70* • Male Enrollment: *11* • Total New Admissions Who Enrolled for Fall: *43* • Total Graduates: *26*

FINANCES

Residential Annual Tuition: *$1,152* • Non-Residential Annual Tuition: *$5,520* • General Institution Fees: *$1,244* • Additional Nursing Fees: *$250*

LABOURE' COLLEGE

Address: 2120 Dorchester Avenue, Boston, MA 02124
Phone: 617-296-8300
Fax: 617-296-7947
Contact: Nancy Pedranti, MSN in Education, Chairperson, Nursing Division
Email: Not Reported

GENERAL INFORMATION

Type of School: *Not Reported, Private (Independent)* • Accreditation: *New England Association of Schools and Colleges* • Total Enrollment: *Not Reported*

PROGRAM INFORMATION

LPN/LVN Exit: *No* • NLNAC Accreditation: *Yes*

NURSING STUDENT PROFILE

Total Nursing Enrollment: *132* • Full-Time Enrollment: *44* • Part-Time Enrollment: *88* • Female Enrollment: *122* • Male Enrollment: *10* • Total New Admissions Who Enrolled for Fall: *26* • Total Graduates: *52*

FINANCES

Residential Annual Tuition: *$2,000* • Non-Residential Annual Tuition: *$5,000* • General Institution Fees: *Not Reported* • Additional Nursing Fees: *$490*

LAWRENCE MEMORIAL/ REGIS COLLEGE

Address: 170 Governors Avenue, Medford, MA 02155
Phone: 781-306-6600
Fax: 781-306-6655
Contact: Marie B. McCarthy, MSN, RN, Vice President
          for Education
Email: mmc2m@hhs.lmh.edu

GENERAL INFORMATION

Type of School: *Not Reported* • Accreditation: *None* • Total
Enrollment: *Not Reported*

PROGRAM INFORMATION

LPN/LVN Exit: *No* • NLNAC Accreditation: *Yes*

NURSING STUDENT PROFILE

Total Nursing Enrollment: *147* • Full-Time Enrollment:
108 • Part-Time Enrollment: *39* • Female Enrollment: *133* •
Male Enrollment: *14* • Total New Admissions Who Enrolled
for Fall: *50* • Total Graduates: *47*

FINANCES

Residential Annual Tuition: *Not Reported* • Non-Residential
Annual Tuition: *Not Reported* • General Institution Fees: *Not
Reported* • Additional Nursing Fees: *Not Reported*

MASSACHUSETTS BAY COMMUNITY COLLEGE

Address: 50 Oakland Street, Wellesley Hills, MA 02481
Phone: 781-239-2205
Fax: 781-239-2483
Contact: Susan M. Mullaney, MA, MS, RN, Department
          Chair, Evening ADN
Email: mullan01@mbcc.mass.edu

GENERAL INFORMATION

Type of School: *2-Year College or University, Public* •
Accreditation: *New England Association of Schools and
Colleges* • Total Enrollment: *Not Reported*

PROGRAM INFORMATION

LPN/LVN Exit: *No* • NLNAC Accreditation: *Yes*

NURSING STUDENT PROFILE

Total Nursing Enrollment: *260* • Full-Time Enrollment:
130 • Part-Time Enrollment: *130* • Female Enrollment:
234 • Male Enrollment: *26* • Total New Admissions Who
Enrolled for Fall: *78* • Total Graduates: *89*

FINANCES

Residential Annual Tuition: *Not Reported* • Non-Residential
Annual Tuition: *Not Reported* • General Institution Fees: *Not
Reported* • Additional Nursing Fees: *Not Reported*

MASSASOIT COMMUNITY COLLEGE

Address: 1 Massasoit Blvd., Brockton, MA 02302
Phone: 508-588-9100
Fax: 508-427-1250
Contact: Barbara Waible, MSN, RN, Chairperson, Nurse Education Department
Email: bwaible@massasoit.mass.edu

GENERAL INFORMATION

Type of School: *2-Year College or University, Public* • Accreditation: *New England Association of Schools and Colleges* • Total Enrollment: *Not Reported*

PROGRAM INFORMATION

LPN/LVN Exit: *No* • NLNAC Accreditation: *Yes*

NURSING STUDENT PROFILE

Total Nursing Enrollment: *106* • Full-Time Enrollment: *106* • Part-Time Enrollment: *0* • Female Enrollment: *96* • Male Enrollment: *10* • Total New Admissions Who Enrolled for Fall: *63* • Total Graduates: *57*

FINANCES

Residential Annual Tuition: *$768* • Non-Residential Annual Tuition: *$7,360* • General Institution Fees: *$1,290* • Additional Nursing Fees: *$340*

MIDDLESEX COMMUNITY COLLEGE

Address: 33 Kearney Square, Lowell, MA 01852
Phone: 978-656-3046
Fax: 978-656-3078
Contact: Ann M. Montminy, MS, RN, Assistant Division Dean for Nursing
Email: montminya@middlesex.cc.ma.us

GENERAL INFORMATION

Type of School: *2-Year College or University, Public* • Accreditation: *New England Association of Schools and Colleges* • Total Enrollment: *Not Reported*

PROGRAM INFORMATION

LPN/LVN Exit: *No* • NLNAC Accreditation: *Yes*

NURSING STUDENT PROFILE

Total Nursing Enrollment: *92* • Full-Time Enrollment: *92* • Part-Time Enrollment: *0* • Female Enrollment: *84* • Male Enrollment: *8* • Total New Admissions Who Enrolled for Fall: *39* • Total Graduates: *26*

FINANCES

Residential Annual Tuition: *$3,552* • Non-Residential Annual Tuition: *$10,144* • General Institution Fees: *$600* • Additional Nursing Fees: *$65*

Circle 76 on reader card   **See in-depth profile for more information**

MOUNT WACHUSETT COMMUNITY COLLEGE

Address: 444 Green Street, Gardner, MA 01440
Phone: 978-632-6600
Fax: 978-632-6155
Contact: Paula d'Entremont, MS, RN, Chairperson,
            Nursing Department
Email: p_dentremont@mwcc.mass.edu

GENERAL INFORMATION

Type of School: *2-Year College or University, Public* •
Accreditation: *New England Association of Schools and
Colleges* • Total Enrollment: *Not Reported*

PROGRAM INFORMATION

LPN/LVN Exit: *No* • NLNAC Accreditation: *Yes*

NURSING STUDENT PROFILE

Total Nursing Enrollment: *98* • Full-Time Enrollment: *8* •
Part-Time Enrollment: *90* • Female Enrollment: *94* • Male
Enrollment: *4* • Total New Admissions Who Enrolled for
Fall: *70* • Total Graduates: *36*

FINANCES

Residential Annual Tuition: *$1,992* • Non-Residential
Annual Tuition: *$6,912* • General Institution Fees: *$40* •
Additional Nursing Fees: *$0*

NORTH SHORE COMMUNITY COLLEGE

Address: 1 Ferncroft Road, Danvers, MA 01923
Phone: 978-762-4160
Fax: 978-762-4022
Contact: Susan Maciewicz, MSN, RN, Department
            Chairperson
Email: Smaciewi@nscc.mass.edu

GENERAL INFORMATION

Type of School: *2-Year College or University, Public* •
Accreditation: *New England Association of Schools and
Colleges* • Total Enrollment: *Not Reported*

PROGRAM INFORMATION

LPN/LVN Exit: *Not Reported* • NLNAC Accreditation: *Yes*

NURSING STUDENT PROFILE

Total Nursing Enrollment: *117* • Full-Time Enrollment:
117 • Part-Time Enrollment: *0* • Female Enrollment: *108* •
Male Enrollment: *9* • Total New Admissions Who Enrolled
for Fall: *52* • Total Graduates: *51*

FINANCES

Residential Annual Tuition: *Not Reported* • Non-Residential
Annual Tuition: *Not Reported* • General Institution Fees: *Not
Reported* • Additional Nursing Fees: *Not Reported*

NORTHERN ESSEX COMMUNITY COLLEGE

Address: 45 Franklin Street, Lawrence, MA 01841
Phone: 978-738-7447
Fax: 978-738-7450
Contact: Sylvia C. Hallsworth, RN, CD, EdD, Assistant Dean, Health Professions
Email: shallsworth@necc.mass.edu

GENERAL INFORMATION

Type of School: *2-Year College or University, Public* • Accreditation: *New England Association of Schools and Colleges* • Total Enrollment: *Not Reported*

PROGRAM INFORMATION

LPN/LVN Exit: *No* • NLNAC Accreditation: *Yes*

NURSING STUDENT PROFILE

Total Nursing Enrollment: *130* • Full-Time Enrollment: *1* • Part-Time Enrollment: *129* • Female Enrollment: *109* • Male Enrollment: *21* • Total New Admissions Who Enrolled for Fall: *79* • Total Graduates: *Not Reported*

FINANCES

Residential Annual Tuition: *Not Reported* • Non-Residential Annual Tuition: *Not Reported* • General Institution Fees: *Not Reported* • Additional Nursing Fees: *Not Reported*

QUINCY COLLEGE

Address: 34 Coddington St., Quincy, MA 02169
Phone: 617-984-1742
Fax: 617-984-1792
Contact: Kristin M Parks, MSN, RNC, Program Chair
Email: kparks@quincycollege.com

GENERAL INFORMATION

Type of School: *2-Year College or University, Other* • Accreditation: *New England Association of Schools and Colleges* • Total Enrollment: *Not Reported*

PROGRAM INFORMATION

LPN/LVN Exit: *No* • NLNAC Accreditation: *Yes*

NURSING STUDENT PROFILE

Total Nursing Enrollment: *262* • Full-Time Enrollment: *148* • Part-Time Enrollment: *114* • Female Enrollment: *245* • Male Enrollment: *17* • Total New Admissions Who Enrolled for Fall: *106* • Total Graduates: *130*

FINANCES

Residential Annual Tuition: *$3,300* • Non-Residential Annual Tuition: *$3,300* • General Institution Fees: *$100* • Additional Nursing Fees: *$100*

QUINSIGAMOND COMMUNITY COLLEGE

Address: 670 W. Boylston St, Worcester, MA 01606-2092
Phone: 508-854-4334
Fax: 508-854-2704
Contact: Allison Shields, RN, MS, Director, Nurse
          Education Program
Email: allisons@gcc.mass.edu

GENERAL INFORMATION

Type of School: *2-Year College or University, Public* •
Accreditation: *New England Association of Schools and
Colleges* • Total Enrollment: *Not Reported*

PROGRAM INFORMATION

LPN/LVN Exit: *No* • NLNAC Accreditation: *Yes*

NURSING STUDENT PROFILE

Total Nursing Enrollment: *152* • Full-Time Enrollment: *53* •
Part-Time Enrollment: *99* • Female Enrollment: *139* • Male
Enrollment: *13* • Total New Admissions Who Enrolled for
Fall: *48* • Total Graduates: *53*

FINANCES

Residential Annual Tuition: *$3,680* • Non-Residential
Annual Tuition: *$10,272* • General Institution Fees: *$468* •
Additional Nursing Fees: *Not Reported*

ROXBURY COMMUNITY COLLEGE

Address: 1234 Columbus Avenue, Roxbury Crossing, MA
          02120
Phone: 617-427-0060
Fax: 617-427-4689
Contact: Jo Ann Mulread, RN, MS, Program Coordinator
Email: jmulre@rcc.mass.edu

GENERAL INFORMATION

Type of School: *2-Year College or University, Public* •
Accreditation: *New England Association of Schools and
Colleges* • Total Enrollment: *Not Reported*

PROGRAM INFORMATION

LPN/LVN Exit: *No* • NLNAC Accreditation: *Yes*

NURSING STUDENT PROFILE

Total Nursing Enrollment: *65* • Full-Time Enrollment: *65* •
Part-Time Enrollment: *0* • Female Enrollment: *56* • Male
Enrollment: *9* • Total New Admissions Who Enrolled for
Fall: *36* • Total Graduates: *22*

FINANCES

Residential Annual Tuition: *Not Reported* • Non-Residential
Annual Tuition: *Not Reported* • General Institution Fees: *Not
Reported* • Additional Nursing Fees: *Not Reported*

SPRINGFIELD TECHNICAL COMMUNITY COLLEGE

Address: One Armory Square, Springfield, MA 01105
Phone: 413-755-4666
Fax: 413-733-0023
Contact: Eileen Neville, EdD, MS, CS, RN, Dean, School of Nursing
Email: eneville@stcc.edu

GENERAL INFORMATION

Type of School: *2-Year College or University, Public* • Accreditation: *New England Association of Schools and Colleges* • Total Enrollment: *Not Reported*

PROGRAM INFORMATION

LPN/LVN Exit: *No* • NLNAC Accreditation: *Yes*

NURSING STUDENT PROFILE

Total Nursing Enrollment: *102* • Full-Time Enrollment: *2* • Part-Time Enrollment: *100* • Female Enrollment: *86* • Male Enrollment: *16* • Total New Admissions Who Enrolled for Fall: *60* • Total Graduates: *47*

FINANCES

Residential Annual Tuition: *$3,072* • Non-Residential Annual Tuition: *$10,016* • General Institution Fees: *$44* • Additional Nursing Fees: *$45*

ALPENA COMMUNITY COLLEGE

Address: 666 Johnson, Alpena, MI 49707
Phone: 989-358-7226
Fax: 989-358-7559
Contact: Kathleen McGillis, RN, BSN, MS, Assistant Dean, Health Occupations
Email: mcgillik@alpena.cc.mi.us

GENERAL INFORMATION

Type of School: *2-Year College or University, Public* • Accreditation: *North Central Association of Colleges and Schools* • Total Enrollment: *Not Reported*

PROGRAM INFORMATION

LPN/LVN Exit: *Not Reported* • NLNAC Accreditation: *No*

NURSING STUDENT PROFILE

Total Nursing Enrollment: *16* • Full-Time Enrollment: *16* • Part-Time Enrollment: *0* • Female Enrollment: *14* • Male Enrollment: *2* • Total New Admissions Who Enrolled for Fall: *16* • Total Graduates: *15*

FINANCES

Residential Annual Tuition: *$2,112* • Non-Residential Annual Tuition: *$4,224* • General Institution Fees: *$13* • Additional Nursing Fees: *Not Reported*

BAY DE NOC COMMUNITY COLLEGE

Address: 2001 North Lincoln Road, Escabana, MI 49829
Phone: 906-786-5802
Fax: 906-789-6919
Contact: Patricia Valensky, MSN, RN, Dean of Allied
             Health and Wellness Programs
Email: valenskp@baydenoc.cc.mi.us

GENERAL INFORMATION

Type of School: *2-Year College or University, Public* •
Accreditation: *North Central Association of Colleges and
Schools* • Total Enrollment: *2084*

PROGRAM INFORMATION

LPN/LVN Exit: *Not Reported* • NLNAC Accreditation: *No*

NURSING STUDENT PROFILE

Total Nursing Enrollment: *65* • Full-Time Enrollment: *26* •
Part-Time Enrollment: *39* • Female Enrollment: *56* • Male
Enrollment: *9* • Total New Admissions Who Enrolled for
Fall: *50* • Total Graduates: *46*

FINANCES

Residential Annual Tuition: *$1,320* • Non-Residential
Annual Tuition: *$2,880* • General Institution Fees: *$101* •
Additional Nursing Fees: *$78*

DAVENPORT UNIVERSITY SYSTEM

Address: 3555 East Patrick Road, Midland, MI 48642
Phone: 517-835-4501
Fax: 517-835-8363
Contact: Barbara Carter, MSN, RN, Dean of Nursing
Email: mdbcarter@davenport.edu

GENERAL INFORMATION

Type of School: *Not Reported* • Accreditation: *North Central
Association of Colleges and Schools* • Total Enrollment: *15000*

PROGRAM INFORMATION

LPN/LVN Exit: *Yes* • NLNAC Accreditation: *No*

NURSING STUDENT PROFILE

Total Nursing Enrollment: *106* • Full-Time Enrollment: *69* •
Part-Time Enrollment: *37* • Female Enrollment: *98* • Male
Enrollment: *8* • Total New Admissions Who Enrolled for
Fall: *126* • Total Graduates: *63*

FINANCES

Residential Annual Tuition: *Not Reported* • Non-Residential
Annual Tuition: *Not Reported* • General Institution Fees: *Not
Reported* • Additional Nursing Fees: *Not Reported*

DELTA COLLEGE

Address: 1961 Delta Road, University Center, MI 48710
Phone: 517-686-9274
Fax: Not Reported
Contact: Louise K. Brentin, MSN, RN, Nursing Division
           Chairperson
Email: lkbrenti@alpha.delta.edu

GENERAL INFORMATION

Type of School: *2-Year College or University, Public* •
Accreditation: *North Central Association of Colleges and
Schools* • Total Enrollment: *9599*

PROGRAM INFORMATION

LPN/LVN Exit: *No* • NLNAC Accreditation: *Yes*

NURSING STUDENT PROFILE

Total Nursing Enrollment: *141* • Full-Time Enrollment:
141 • Part-Time Enrollment: *0* • Female Enrollment: *122* •
Male Enrollment: *19* • Total New Admissions Who Enrolled
for Fall: *Not Reported* • Total Graduates: *69*

FINANCES

Residential Annual Tuition: *$1,044* • Non-Residential
Annual Tuition: *$1,422* • General Institution Fees: *$69* •
Additional Nursing Fees: *$50*

FERRIS STATE UNIVERSITY

Address: 200 Ferris Drive, Big Rapids, MI 49307-2740
Phone: 231-591-2267
Fax: 231-591-2325
Contact: Sally K Johnson, EdD, RN, Department Head,
           Nursing and Dental Hygiene
Email: johnson@ferris.edu

GENERAL INFORMATION

Type of School: *4-Year College or University, Public* •
Accreditation: *North Central Association of Colleges and
Schools* • Total Enrollment: *9000*

PROGRAM INFORMATION

LPN/LVN Exit: *Not Reported* • NLNAC Accreditation: *No*

NURSING STUDENT PROFILE

Total Nursing Enrollment: *48* • Full-Time Enrollment: *37* •
Part-Time Enrollment: *11* • Female Enrollment: *46* • Male
Enrollment: *2* • Total New Admissions Who Enrolled for
Fall: *130* • Total Graduates: *33*

FINANCES

Residential Annual Tuition: *$4,300* • Non-Residential
Annual Tuition: *$9,050* • General Institution Fees: *$125* •
Additional Nursing Fees: *$0*

FINLANDIA UNIVERSITY

Address: 601 Quincy Street, Hancock, MI 49930
Phone: 906-487-7306
Fax: 906-487-7297
Contact: Elizabeth Reynolds, MSN, RN, Interim Chair
Email: finnsg@ccisd.k12.mi.us

GLEN OAKS COMMUNITY COLLEGE

Address: 62249 Shimmel Road, Centreville, MI 49032
Phone: 616-467-9945
Fax: Not Reported
Contact: Karen Ganger, MS, MEd, RN, CS, CARN, Director of Nursing and Allied Health
Email: kganger@glenoaks.cc.mi.us

GENERAL INFORMATION

Type of School: *4-Year College or University, Private (Independent)* • Accreditation: *North Central Association of Colleges and Schools* • Total Enrollment: *420*

GENERAL INFORMATION

Type of School: *2-Year College or University, Public* • Accreditation: *North Central Association of Colleges and Schools* • Total Enrollment: *1608*

PROGRAM INFORMATION

LPN/LVN Exit: *Not Reported* • NLNAC Accreditation: *No*

PROGRAM INFORMATION

LPN/LVN Exit: *No* • NLNAC Accreditation: *No*

NURSING STUDENT PROFILE

Total Nursing Enrollment: *35* • Full-Time Enrollment: *30* • Part-Time Enrollment: *5* • Female Enrollment: *32* • Male Enrollment: *3* • Total New Admissions Who Enrolled for Fall: *10* • Total Graduates: *13*

NURSING STUDENT PROFILE

Total Nursing Enrollment: *Not Reported* • Full-Time Enrollment: *Not Reported* • Part-Time Enrollment: *Not Reported* • Female Enrollment: *Not Reported* • Male Enrollment: *Not Reported* • Total New Admissions Who Enrolled for Fall: *Not Reported* • Total Graduates: *Not Reported*

FINANCES

Residential Annual Tuition: *Not Reported* • Non-Residential Annual Tuition: *Not Reported* • General Institution Fees: *Not Reported* • Additional Nursing Fees: *Not Reported*

FINANCES

Residential Annual Tuition: *Not Reported* • Non-Residential Annual Tuition: *Not Reported* • General Institution Fees: *Not Reported* • Additional Nursing Fees: *Not Reported*

GOGEBIC COMMUNITY COLLEGE

Address: East 4946 Jackson Road, Ironwood, MI 49938
Phone: 906-932-4231
Fax: 906-932-5541
Contact: Kathryn A. Encalada, MSN, RN, Director of Allied Health Programs
Email: encalada@gogebic.cc.mi.us

GENERAL INFORMATION

Type of School: *2-Year College or University, Public* • Accreditation: *North Central Association of Colleges and Schools* • Total Enrollment: *1121*

PROGRAM INFORMATION

LPN/LVN Exit: *Yes* • NLNAC Accreditation: *No*

NURSING STUDENT PROFILE

Total Nursing Enrollment: *28* • Full-Time Enrollment: *18* • Part-Time Enrollment: *10* • Female Enrollment: *26* • Male Enrollment: *2* • Total New Admissions Who Enrolled for Fall: *26* • Total Graduates: *8*

FINANCES

Residential Annual Tuition: *$1,440* • Non-Residential Annual Tuition: *$2,784* • General Institution Fees: *$90* • Additional Nursing Fees: *$300*

GRAND RAPIDS COMMUNITY COLLEGE

Address: 143 Bostwick Avenue North East, Grand Rapids, MI 49503
Phone: 616-234-4231
Fax: 616-234-4234
Contact: Marilyn Smidt, MSN, RN, Director of Nursing Program
Email: msmidt@grcc.edu

GENERAL INFORMATION

Type of School: *2-Year College or University, Public* • Accreditation: *North Central Association of Colleges and Schools* • Total Enrollment: *13000*

PROGRAM INFORMATION

LPN/LVN Exit: *No* • NLNAC Accreditation: *Yes*

NURSING STUDENT PROFILE

Total Nursing Enrollment: *182* • Full-Time Enrollment: *94* • Part-Time Enrollment: *88* • Female Enrollment: *172* • Male Enrollment: *10* • Total New Admissions Who Enrolled for Fall: *75* • Total Graduates: *70*

FINANCES

Residential Annual Tuition: *$7,072* • Non-Residential Annual Tuition: *$10,350* • General Institution Fees: *$155* • Additional Nursing Fees: *Not Reported*

HENRY FORD COMMUNITY COLLEGE

Address: 5101 Evergreen Road, Dearborn, MI 48128
Phone: 313-845-9661
Fax: 313-845-9845
Contact: Katherine M. Bradley, PhD, RN, Director of Nursing
Email: kbradley@hfcc.net

GENERAL INFORMATION

Type of School: *2-Year College or University, Public* • Accreditation: *North Central Association of Colleges and Schools* • Total Enrollment: *12000*

PROGRAM INFORMATION

LPN/LVN Exit: *No* • NLNAC Accreditation: *Yes*

NURSING STUDENT PROFILE

Total Nursing Enrollment: *337* • Full-Time Enrollment: *337* • Part-Time Enrollment: *0* • Female Enrollment: *304* • Male Enrollment: *33* • Total New Admissions Who Enrolled for Fall: *182* • Total Graduates: *136*

FINANCES

Residential Annual Tuition: *$2,136* • Non-Residential Annual Tuition: *$2,472* • General Institution Fees: *$66* • Additional Nursing Fees: *Not Reported*

JACKSON COMMUNITY COLLEGE

Address: 2111 Emmons Road, Jackson, MI 49203
Phone: 517-796-8515
Fax: Not Reported
Contact: Kathleen Kelley Walsh, MS, RN, Department Chair of Nursing
Email: kathy-walsh@joekson.cc.mi.us

GENERAL INFORMATION

Type of School: *Other* • Accreditation: *North Central Association of Colleges and Schools* • Total Enrollment: *Not Reported*

PROGRAM INFORMATION

LPN/LVN Exit: *Not Reported* • NLNAC Accreditation: *No*

NURSING STUDENT PROFILE

Total Nursing Enrollment: *Not Reported* • Full-Time Enrollment: *Not Reported* • Part-Time Enrollment: *Not Reported* • Female Enrollment: *Not Reported* • Male Enrollment: *Not Reported* • Total New Admissions Who Enrolled for Fall: *Not Reported* • Total Graduates: *Not Reported*

FINANCES

Residential Annual Tuition: *Not Reported* • Non-Residential Annual Tuition: *Not Reported* • General Institution Fees: *Not Reported* • Additional Nursing Fees: *Not Reported*

KALAMAZOO VALLEY COMMUNITY COLLEGE

Address: 6767 West O Avenue, P. O. Box 4070, Kalamazoo, MI 49003-4070
Phone: 616-372-5108
Fax: 616-372-5458
Contact: Dennis A Bertch, MSN, RN, Director of Nursing
Email: dbertch@kvcc.edu

GENERAL INFORMATION

Type of School: *2-Year College or University, Public* • Accreditation: *North Central Association of Colleges and Schools* • Total Enrollment: *19300*

PROGRAM INFORMATION

LPN/LVN Exit: *Yes* • NLNAC Accreditation: *No*

NURSING STUDENT PROFILE

Total Nursing Enrollment: *162* • Full-Time Enrollment: *130* • Part-Time Enrollment: *32* • Female Enrollment: *145* • Male Enrollment: *17* • Total New Admissions Who Enrolled for Fall: *43* • Total Graduates: *51*

FINANCES

Residential Annual Tuition: *$4,525* • Non-Residential Annual Tuition: *$11,425* • General Institution Fees: *$0* • Additional Nursing Fees: *$135*

KIRTLAND COMMUNITY COLLEGE

Address: 10775 North Street Helen Road, Roscommon, MI 48653
Phone: 989-275-5000
Fax: 989-275-6715
Contact: Karen Brown, RNC, BSN, MS, CNAA, Director of Health Careers
Email: brownk@kirtland.edu

GENERAL INFORMATION

Type of School: *2-Year College or University, Public* • Accreditation: *North Central Association of Colleges and Schools* • Total Enrollment: *1631*

PROGRAM INFORMATION

LPN/LVN Exit: *Yes* • NLNAC Accreditation: *No*

NURSING STUDENT PROFILE

Total Nursing Enrollment: *98* • Full-Time Enrollment: *Not Reported* • Part-Time Enrollment: *Not Reported* • Female Enrollment: *Not Reported* • Male Enrollment: *Not Reported* • Total New Admissions Who Enrolled for Fall: *Not Reported* • Total Graduates: *Not Reported*

FINANCES

Residential Annual Tuition: *Not Reported* • Non-Residential Annual Tuition: *Not Reported* • General Institution Fees: *Not Reported* • Additional Nursing Fees: *Not Reported*

LAKE MICHIGAN COLLEGE

Address:　2755 East Napier, Benton Harbor, MI 49022
Phone:　　616-927-8100
Fax:　　　616-927-8186
Contact:　Alice Rasmussen, RN, BSN, MSN, Nursing
　　　　　　Coordinator
Email:　　rasmuss@lmc.cc.mi.us

GENERAL INFORMATION

Type of School: *2-Year College or University, Public* •
Accreditation: *North Central Association of Colleges and
Schools* • Total Enrollment: *Not Reported*

PROGRAM INFORMATION

LPN/LVN Exit: *Yes* • NLNAC Accreditation: *Yes*

NURSING STUDENT PROFILE

Total Nursing Enrollment: *114* • Full-Time Enrollment: *40* •
Part-Time Enrollment: *74* • Female Enrollment: *96* • Male
Enrollment: *18* • Total New Admissions Who Enrolled for
Fall: *64* • Total Graduates: *39*

FINANCES

Residential Annual Tuition: *$2,080* • Non-Residential
Annual Tuition: *$3,136* • General Institution Fees: *$2,062* •
Additional Nursing Fees: *$0*

LANSING COMMUNITY COLLEGE

Address:　3400 Human Health and Public Service Career,
　　　　　　P. O. Box 40010, Lansing, MI 48901-7210
Phone:　　517-483-1461
Fax:　　　517-483-1508
Contact:　Margie Clark, MSN, RN, CS, GNP, CCRN,
　　　　　　Nursing Program Director
Email:　　mclark@lansing.cc.mi.us

GENERAL INFORMATION

Type of School: *2-Year College or University, Public* •
Accreditation: *North Central Association of Colleges and
Schools* • Total Enrollment: *Not Reported*

PROGRAM INFORMATION

LPN/LVN Exit: *Yes* • NLNAC Accreditation: *Yes*

NURSING STUDENT PROFILE

Total Nursing Enrollment: *167* • Full-Time Enrollment:
167 • Part-Time Enrollment: *0* • Female Enrollment: *149* •
Male Enrollment: *18* • Total New Admissions Who Enrolled
for Fall: *50* • Total Graduates: *77*

FINANCES

Residential Annual Tuition: *$1,872* • Non-Residential
Annual Tuition: *$2,568* • General Institution Fees: *$40* •
Additional Nursing Fees: *$200*

MACOMB COMMUNITY COLLEGE

Address: 44575 Garfield Road, Clinton Township, MI
48038-1139
Phone: 586-286-2074
Fax: 586-286-2098
Contact: Bernadette Pieczynski, MSN, RN, CS, Director
of Nursing
Email: pieczynskib@macomb.edu

GENERAL INFORMATION

Type of School: *2-Year College or University, Public* •
Accreditation: *North Central Association of Colleges and
Schools* • Total Enrollment: *21416*

PROGRAM INFORMATION

LPN/LVN Exit: *No* • NLNAC Accreditation: *Yes*

NURSING STUDENT PROFILE

Total Nursing Enrollment: *210* • Full-Time Enrollment:
210 • Part-Time Enrollment: *0* • Female Enrollment: *197* •
Male Enrollment: *13* • Total New Admissions Who Enrolled
for Fall: *120* • Total Graduates: *98*

FINANCES

Residential Annual Tuition: *Not Reported* • Non-Residential
Annual Tuition: *Not Reported* • General Institution Fees: *Not
Reported* • Additional Nursing Fees: *Not Reported*

MID-MICHIGAN COMMUNITY COLLEGE

Address: 1375 South Clare Avenue, Harrison, MI 48625
Phone: 989-386-6645
Fax: 989-386-6666
Contact: Beth L Sendre, MSN, RN, Dean of Nursing and
Academic Sciences
Email: bsendre@midmich.cc.mi.us

GENERAL INFORMATION

Type of School: *2-Year College or University, Public* •
Accreditation: *North Central Association of Colleges and
Schools* • Total Enrollment: *Not Reported*

PROGRAM INFORMATION

LPN/LVN Exit: *Not Reported* • NLNAC Accreditation: *No*

NURSING STUDENT PROFILE

Total Nursing Enrollment: *30* • Full-Time Enrollment: *20* •
Part-Time Enrollment: *10* • Female Enrollment: *29* • Male
Enrollment: *1* • Total New Admissions Who Enrolled for
Fall: *30* • Total Graduates: *Not Reported*

FINANCES

Residential Annual Tuition: *$1,736* • Non-Residential
Annual Tuition: *$2,816* • General Institution Fees: *$175* •
Additional Nursing Fees: *Not Reported*

MONROE COUNTY COMMUNITY

Address: 1555 South Raisinville Road, Monroe, MI 48161
Phone: 734-384-4101
Fax: 734-384-4187
Contact: Gail Odneal, MSN, RN, Dean of Health Sciences Division
Email: godneal@mail.monroe.cc.mi.us

GENERAL INFORMATION

Type of School: *2-Year College or University, Public* • Accreditation: *North Central Association of Colleges and Schools* • Total Enrollment: *3649*

PROGRAM INFORMATION

LPN/LVN Exit: *No* • NLNAC Accreditation: *Yes*

NURSING STUDENT PROFILE

Total Nursing Enrollment: *71* • Full-Time Enrollment: *25* • Part-Time Enrollment: *46* • Female Enrollment: *66* • Male Enrollment: *5* • Total New Admissions Who Enrolled for Fall: *41* • Total Graduates: *34*

FINANCES

Residential Annual Tuition: *$2,736* • Non-Residential Annual Tuition: *$4,704* • General Institution Fees: *$92* • Additional Nursing Fees: *$2,137*

MONTCALM COMMUNITY COLLEGE

Address: 2800 College Drive, Sidney, MI 48885
Phone: 989-328-1240
Fax: 989-328-2950
Contact: Susan Wambach, MSN, RN, Associate Dean of Health Occupations
Email: swambach@montcalm.cc.mi.us

GENERAL INFORMATION

Type of School: *2-Year College or University, Public* • Accreditation: *North Central Association of Colleges and Schools* • Total Enrollment: *1540*

PROGRAM INFORMATION

LPN/LVN Exit: *Yes* • NLNAC Accreditation: *Yes*

NURSING STUDENT PROFILE

Total Nursing Enrollment: *25* • Full-Time Enrollment: *25* • Part-Time Enrollment: *0* • Female Enrollment: *25* • Male Enrollment: *0* • Total New Admissions Who Enrolled for Fall: *25* • Total Graduates: *30*

FINANCES

Residential Annual Tuition: *$3,667* • Non-Residential Annual Tuition: *$5,626* • General Institution Fees: *$192* • Additional Nursing Fees: *$1,870*

MOTT COMMUNITY COLLEGE

Address: 1401 East Court Street, Flint, MI 48503
Phone: 810-232-3271
Fax: 810-762-5619
Contact: Patricia Markowicz, BSN, MSN, RN, Associate Dean, Division of Health Sciences
Email: pmarkowi@mcc.edu

GENERAL INFORMATION

Type of School: *2-Year College or University, Public* • Accreditation: *North Central Association of Colleges and Schools* • Total Enrollment: *9019*

PROGRAM INFORMATION

LPN/LVN Exit: *No* • NLNAC Accreditation: *Yes*

NURSING STUDENT PROFILE

Total Nursing Enrollment: *277* • Full-Time Enrollment: *277* • Part-Time Enrollment: *0* • Female Enrollment: *254* • Male Enrollment: *23* • Total New Admissions Who Enrolled for Fall: *100* • Total Graduates: *86*

FINANCES

Residential Annual Tuition: *$3,142* • Non-Residential Annual Tuition: *$6,050* • General Institution Fees: *$100* • Additional Nursing Fees: *$50*

MUSKEGON COMMUNITY COLLEGE

Address: 221 South Quarterline Road, Muskegon, MI 49442
Phone: 231-777-0281
Fax: 231-777-0435
Contact: Pam Brown, RNCS, MSN, Instructor
Email: Brownp@muskegon.cc.mi.us

GENERAL INFORMATION

Type of School: *2-Year College or University, Public* • Accreditation: *North Central Association of Colleges and Schools* • Total Enrollment: *Not Reported*

PROGRAM INFORMATION

LPN/LVN Exit: *No* • NLNAC Accreditation: *Not Reported*

NURSING STUDENT PROFILE

Total Nursing Enrollment: *140* • Full-Time Enrollment: *140* • Part-Time Enrollment: *0* • Female Enrollment: *137* • Male Enrollment: *3* • Total New Admissions Who Enrolled for Fall: *40* • Total Graduates: *47*

FINANCES

Residential Annual Tuition: *Not Reported* • Non-Residential Annual Tuition: *Not Reported* • General Institution Fees: *Not Reported* • Additional Nursing Fees: *Not Reported*

NORTH CENTRAL MICHIGAN COLLEGE

Address: 1515 Howard Street, Petoskey, MI 49770
Phone: 231-348-6681
Fax: 231-348-6628
Contact: Polly Flippo, MSN, RN, Director, Health and
          Human Services
Email: pflip@ncmc.cc.mi.us

GENERAL INFORMATION

Type of School: *2-Year College or University, Public* •
Accreditation: *North Central Association of Colleges and
Schools* • Total Enrollment: *2400*

PROGRAM INFORMATION

LPN/LVN Exit: *No* • NLNAC Accreditation: *Not Reported*

NURSING STUDENT PROFILE

Total Nursing Enrollment: *57* • Full-Time Enrollment: *57* •
Part-Time Enrollment: *0* • Female Enrollment: *50* • Male
Enrollment: *7* • Total New Admissions Who Enrolled for
Fall: *24* • Total Graduates: *31*

FINANCES

Residential Annual Tuition: *Not Reported* • Non-Residential
Annual Tuition: *Not Reported* • General Institution Fees:
$1,850 • Additional Nursing Fees: *$100*

NORTHWESTERN MICHIGAN COLLEGE

Address: 1701 East Front Street, Traverse City, MI 49686
Phone: 231-995-1245
Fax: 231-995-1950
Contact: Laura Schmidt, MSN, RN, Director, Nursing
          Programs
Email: lschmidt@nmc.edu

GENERAL INFORMATION

Type of School: *2-Year College or University, Public* •
Accreditation: *North Central Association of Colleges and
Schools* • Total Enrollment: *4173*

PROGRAM INFORMATION

LPN/LVN Exit: *Yes* • NLNAC Accreditation: *Not Reported*

NURSING STUDENT PROFILE

Total Nursing Enrollment: *48* • Full-Time Enrollment: *46* •
Part-Time Enrollment: *2* • Female Enrollment: *42* • Male
Enrollment: *6* • Total New Admissions Who Enrolled for
Fall: *23* • Total Graduates: *30*

FINANCES

Residential Annual Tuition: *$10,444* • Non-Residential
Annual Tuition: *$11,900* • General Institution Fees: *$200* •
Additional Nursing Fees: *$1,300*

OAKLAND COMMUNITY COLLEGE

Address: H. L. Campus 7350 Cooley Lake Road, Waterford, MI 48327
Phone: 248-942-3337
Fax: 248-942-3338
Contact: Nadia E. Boulos, PhD, RN, Dean, Nursing and Allied Health
Email: neboulos@occ.cc.mi.us

GENERAL INFORMATION

Type of School: *2-Year College or University, Public* • Accreditation: *North Central Association of Colleges and Schools* • Total Enrollment: *Not Reported*

PROGRAM INFORMATION

LPN/LVN Exit: *No* • NLNAC Accreditation: *Yes*

NURSING STUDENT PROFILE

Total Nursing Enrollment: *338* • Full-Time Enrollment: *0* • Part-Time Enrollment: *338* • Female Enrollment: *313* • Male Enrollment: *25* • Total New Admissions Who Enrolled for Fall: *233* • Total Graduates: *105*

FINANCES

Residential Annual Tuition: *$1,131* • Non-Residential Annual Tuition: *$2,688* • General Institution Fees: *$105* • Additional Nursing Fees: *$378*

SAINT CLAIR COUNTY COMMUNITY COLLEGE

Address: 323 Erie Street, P. O. Box 5015, Port Huron, MI 48061-5015
Phone: 810-989-5680
Fax: 810-989-5702
Contact: Susan Meeker, BSN, MSN, RN, Director of Nursing
Email: smeeker@stclair.cc.mi.us

GENERAL INFORMATION

Type of School: *2-Year College or University, Public* • Accreditation: *North Central Association of Colleges and Schools* • Total Enrollment: *5400*

PROGRAM INFORMATION

LPN/LVN Exit: *No* • NLNAC Accreditation: *Not Reported*

NURSING STUDENT PROFILE

Total Nursing Enrollment: *151* • Full-Time Enrollment: *151* • Part-Time Enrollment: *0* • Female Enrollment: *140* • Male Enrollment: *11* • Total New Admissions Who Enrolled for Fall: *78* • Total Graduates: *80*

FINANCES

Residential Annual Tuition: *$1,458* • Non-Residential Annual Tuition: *$2,136* • General Institution Fees: *$50* • Additional Nursing Fees: *Not Reported*

SCHOOLCRAFT COLLEGE

Address: 18600 Haggerty Road, Livonia, MI 48152
Phone: 734-462-4528
Fax: 734-462-4531
Contact: Midge Carleton, RN, MS, Associate Dean for
          Science and Director of Nursing
Email: mcarleto@schoolcraft.cc.mi.us

GENERAL INFORMATION

Type of School: *2-Year College or University, Public* •
Accreditation: *North Central Association of Colleges and
Schools* • Total Enrollment: *22036*

PROGRAM INFORMATION

LPN/LVN Exit: *Not Reported* • NLNAC Accreditation: *Not
Reported*

NURSING STUDENT PROFILE

Total Nursing Enrollment: *160* • Full-Time Enrollment:
160 • Part-Time Enrollment: *0* • Female Enrollment: *150* •
Male Enrollment: *10* • Total New Admissions Who Enrolled
for Fall: *93* • Total Graduates: *40*

FINANCES

Residential Annual Tuition: *$4,015* • Non-Residential
Annual Tuition: *$5,986* • General Institution Fees: *$1,571* •
Additional Nursing Fees: *$2,506*

SOUTHWESTERN MICHIGAN COLLEGE

Address: 58900 Cherry Grove Rd, Dowagiac, MI 49047
Phone: 616-782-1237
Fax: Not Reported
Contact: Elaine Foster, RNC, MSN, Chair, School of
          Nursing and Allied Health
Email: efoster@smc.cc.mi.us

GENERAL INFORMATION

Type of School: *2-Year College or University, Public* •
Accreditation: *North Central Association of Colleges and
Schools* • Total Enrollment: *1600*

PROGRAM INFORMATION

LPN/LVN Exit: *Not Reported* • NLNAC Accreditation: *Not
Reported*

NURSING STUDENT PROFILE

Total Nursing Enrollment: *Not Reported* • Full-Time
Enrollment: *Not Reported* • Part-Time Enrollment: *Not
Reported* • Female Enrollment: *Not Reported* • Male
Enrollment: *Not Reported* • Total New Admissions Who
Enrolled for Fall: *40* • Total Graduates: *Not Reported*

FINANCES

Residential Annual Tuition: *Not Reported* • Non-Residential
Annual Tuition: *Not Reported* • General Institution Fees:
$4,650 • Additional Nursing Fees: *$9*

WASHTENAW COMMUNITY COLLEGE

Address: 4800 East Huron River Drive, Ann Arbor, MI
            48106
Phone: 734-973-3474
Fax: 734-677-5078
Contact: Phyllis Grzegorczyk, BS, MS, SA, PhD, Dean,
            Health and Public Service
Email: phylg@wccnet.org

GENERAL INFORMATION

Type of School: *2-Year College or University, Public* •
Accreditation: *North Central Association of Colleges and
Schools* • Total Enrollment: *17500*

PROGRAM INFORMATION

LPN/LVN Exit: *No* • NLNAC Accreditation: *Yes*

NURSING STUDENT PROFILE

Total Nursing Enrollment: *239* • Full-Time Enrollment:
214 • Part-Time Enrollment: *25* • Female Enrollment: *212* •
Male Enrollment: *27* • Total New Admissions Who Enrolled
for Fall: *62* • Total Graduates: *68*

FINANCES

Residential Annual Tuition: *Not Reported* • Non-Residential
Annual Tuition: *Not Reported* • General Institution Fees: *Not
Reported* • Additional Nursing Fees: *Not Reported*

WAYNE COUNTY COMMUNITY COLLEGE

Address: 8551 Greenfield, Detroit, MI 48228-9987
Phone: 313-943-4490
Fax: Not Reported
Contact: Rosellen Burkart, RN, C, MSN, Associate Dean,
            Nursing
Email: nnurrb@admin.wccc.edu

GENERAL INFORMATION

Type of School: *Other* • Accreditation: *None* • Total
Enrollment: *Not Reported*

PROGRAM INFORMATION

LPN/LVN Exit: *No* • NLNAC Accreditation: *Yes*

NURSING STUDENT PROFILE

Total Nursing Enrollment: *314* • Full-Time Enrollment:
236 • Part-Time Enrollment: *78* • Female Enrollment: *Not
Reported* • Male Enrollment: *Not Reported* • Total New
Admissions Who Enrolled for Fall: *Not Reported* • Total
Graduates: *Not Reported*

FINANCES

Residential Annual Tuition: *Not Reported* • Non-Residential
Annual Tuition: *Not Reported* • General Institution Fees: *Not
Reported* • Additional Nursing Fees: *Not Reported*

WEST SHORE COMMUNITY COLLEGE

Address: PO Box 277, Scottville, MI 49545
Phone: 231-845-6511
Fax: 231-845-6511
Contact: Patricia Collins, MSN, RN, MSEd, Director of Nurse Education
Email: pcollins@westshore.cc.mi.us

GENERAL INFORMATION

Type of School: *2-Year College or University, Public* • Accreditation: *North Central Association of Colleges and Schools* • Total Enrollment: *1300*

PROGRAM INFORMATION

LPN/LVN Exit: *Yes* • NLNAC Accreditation: *No*

NURSING STUDENT PROFILE

Total Nursing Enrollment: *44* • Full-Time Enrollment: *40* • Part-Time Enrollment: *4* • Female Enrollment: *41* • Male Enrollment: *3* • Total New Admissions Who Enrolled for Fall: *39* • Total Graduates: *21*

FINANCES

Residential Annual Tuition: *$1,236* • Non-Residential Annual Tuition: *$2,400* • General Institution Fees: *$50* • Additional Nursing Fees: *Not Reported*

ANOKA-RAMSEY COMMUNITY COLLEGE

Address: 11200 Mississippi Blvd. NW, Coon Rapids, MN 55433-3470
Phone: 763-422-3440
Fax: 763-422-3341
Contact: Ann Holand, MA, RN, Dean of Educational Services
Email: aholland@an.cc.mn.us

GENERAL INFORMATION

Type of School: *Other, Public* • Accreditation: *North Central Association of Colleges and Schools* • Total Enrollment: *5954*

PROGRAM INFORMATION

LPN/LVN Exit: *No* • NLNAC Accreditation: *Yes*

NURSING STUDENT PROFILE

Total Nursing Enrollment: *233* • Full-Time Enrollment: *44* • Part-Time Enrollment: *189* • Female Enrollment: *220* • Male Enrollment: *13* • Total New Admissions Who Enrolled for Fall: *159* • Total Graduates: *89*

FINANCES

Residential Annual Tuition: *$3,381* • Non-Residential Annual Tuition: *$6,361* • General Institution Fees: *$380* • Additional Nursing Fees: *$100*

CENTRAL LAKES COLLEGE

Address: 501 West College Drive, Brainerd, MN 56401
Phone: 218-855-8192
Fax: 218-855-8259
Contact: Linda M Anderson, RN, MA, Nursing Director
Email: landers1@gwmail.clc.mnscu.edu

GENERAL INFORMATION

Type of School: *2-Year College or University, Public* •
Accreditation: *North Central Association of Colleges and
Schools* • Total Enrollment: *Not Reported*

PROGRAM INFORMATION

LPN/LVN Exit: *Yes* • NLNAC Accreditation: *No*

NURSING STUDENT PROFILE

Total Nursing Enrollment: *40* • Full-Time Enrollment: *40* •
Part-Time Enrollment: *0* • Female Enrollment: *37* • Male
Enrollment: *3* • Total New Admissions Who Enrolled for
Fall: *40* • Total Graduates: *35*

FINANCES

Residential Annual Tuition: *$7,815* • Non-Residential
Annual Tuition: *$15,630* • General Institution Fees: *$300* •
Additional Nursing Fees: *$42*

COLLEGE OF SAINT CATHERINE

Address: 2004 Randolph Ave, St. Paul, MN 55105
Phone: 651-690-7733
Fax: 651-690-7849
Contact: Kathleen Bell, RN, MS, Associate Nursing
            Program Director
Email: kmbell@stkate.edu

GENERAL INFORMATION

Type of School: *4-Year College or University, Private
(Religious)* • Accreditation: *North Central Association of
Colleges and Schools* • Total Enrollment: *Not Reported*

PROGRAM INFORMATION

LPN/LVN Exit: *No* • NLNAC Accreditation: *Yes*

NURSING STUDENT PROFILE

Total Nursing Enrollment: *400* • Full-Time Enrollment:
101 • Part-Time Enrollment: *299* • Female Enrollment:
372 • Male Enrollment: *28* • Total New Admissions Who
Enrolled for Fall: *200* • Total Graduates: *121*

FINANCES

Annual Tuition: *$19,520* • General Institution Fees: *$250* •
Additional Nursing Fees: *Not Reported*

HIBBING COMMUNITY COLLEGE

Address: 1515 East 25th Street, Hibbing, MN 55476
Phone: 218-262-6743
Fax: 218-262-6717
Contact: Susan Hyndman, RN, MN, Ed.D., Associate Vice President, Academic Affairs
Email: s.hyndman@ins.hcc.mnscu.edu

GENERAL INFORMATION

Type of School: *Other, Public* • Accreditation: *North Central Association of Colleges and Schools* • Total Enrollment: *Not Reported*

PROGRAM INFORMATION

LPN/LVN Exit: *No* • NLNAC Accreditation: *Not Reported*

NURSING STUDENT PROFILE

Total Nursing Enrollment: *106* • Full-Time Enrollment: *105* • Part-Time Enrollment: *1* • Female Enrollment: *93* • Male Enrollment: *13* • Total New Admissions Who Enrolled for Fall: *73* • Total Graduates: *33*

FINANCES

Residential Annual Tuition: *$7,660* • Non-Residential Annual Tuition: *$15,320* • General Institution Fees: *$1,325* • Additional Nursing Fees: *Not Reported*

INVER HILLS COMMUNITY COLLEGE

Address: 2500 80th Street East, Inver Grove Heights, MN 55076
Phone: 651-450-8372
Fax: Not Reported
Contact: LeeAnn Joy, MSN, RN, Dean of Allied Health Services and Director of Nursing
Email: ljoy@ih.cc.mn.us

GENERAL INFORMATION

Type of School: *2-Year College or University, Public* • Accreditation: *North Central Association of Colleges and Schools* • Total Enrollment: *Not Reported*

PROGRAM INFORMATION

LPN/LVN Exit: *No* • NLNAC Accreditation: *Yes*

NURSING STUDENT PROFILE

Total Nursing Enrollment: *274* • Full-Time Enrollment: *36* • Part-Time Enrollment: *238* • Female Enrollment: *251* • Male Enrollment: *23* • Total New Admissions Who Enrolled for Fall: *162* • Total Graduates: *160*

FINANCES

Residential Annual Tuition: *Not Reported* • Non-Residential Annual Tuition: *Not Reported* • General Institution Fees: *$1,002* • Additional Nursing Fees: *$12*

MINNEAPOLIS COMMUNITY AND TECHNICAL COLLEGE

Address: 1501 Hennepin Avenue, Minneapolis, MN
55403
Phone: 612-341-7063
Fax: 612-359-1367
Contact: Jane Foote, RN, BSN, MSN, Dean of Health
Sciences and Human Services
Email: footja@mctm.mnscu.edu

GENERAL INFORMATION

Type of School: *Other, Public* • Accreditation: *North Central Association of Colleges and Schools* • Total Enrollment: *Not Reported*

PROGRAM INFORMATION

LPN/LVN Exit: *Yes* • NLNAC Accreditation: *Yes*

NURSING STUDENT PROFILE

Total Nursing Enrollment: *210* • Full-Time Enrollment: *210* • Part-Time Enrollment: *0* • Female Enrollment: *175* • Male Enrollment: *35* • Total New Admissions Who Enrolled for Fall: *0* • Total Graduates: *76*

FINANCES

Residential Annual Tuition: *$8,275* • Non-Residential Annual Tuition: *$16,550* • General Institution Fees: *$10* • Additional Nursing Fees: *$65*

MINNESOTA WEST COMMUNITY & TECHNICAL COLLEGE

Address: 1450 Collegeway, Worthington, MN 56187
Phone: 507-372-3443
Fax: 507-372-5803
Contact: Kathi Haberman, RN, MS, Dean of Nursing
and Allied Health
Email: khaberman@wr.mnwest.mnscu.edu

GENERAL INFORMATION

Type of School: *Vocational/Technical School, Public* • Accreditation: *North Central Association of Colleges and Schools* • Total Enrollment: *Not Reported*

PROGRAM INFORMATION

LPN/LVN Exit: *No* • NLNAC Accreditation: *Yes*

NURSING STUDENT PROFILE

Total Nursing Enrollment: *21* • Full-Time Enrollment: *8* • Part-Time Enrollment: *13* • Female Enrollment: *20* • Male Enrollment: *1* • Total New Admissions Who Enrolled for Fall: *22* • Total Graduates: *18*

FINANCES

Residential Annual Tuition: *Not Reported* • Non-Residential Annual Tuition: *Not Reported* • General Institution Fees: *$725* • Additional Nursing Fees: *$40*

NORMANDALE COMMUNITY COLLEGE

Address: 9700 France Ave South, Minneapolis, MN 55431
Phone: 952-487-8158
Fax: 952-487-8101
Contact: Kathleen F Manahan, EdD, RN, Dean of Health Sciences
Email: k.manahan@nr.cc.mn.us

GENERAL INFORMATION

Type of School: *2-Year College or University, Public* • Accreditation: *North Central Association of Colleges and Schools* • Total Enrollment: *Not Reported*

PROGRAM INFORMATION

LPN/LVN Exit: *No* • NLNAC Accreditation: *Yes*

NURSING STUDENT PROFILE

Total Nursing Enrollment: *172* • Full-Time Enrollment: *52* • Part-Time Enrollment: *120* • Female Enrollment: *159* • Male Enrollment: *13* • Total New Admissions Who Enrolled for Fall: *80* • Total Graduates: *93*

FINANCES

Residential Annual Tuition: *Not Reported* • Non-Residential Annual Tuition: *Not Reported* • General Institution Fees: *$1,375* • Additional Nursing Fees: *$12*

NORTH HENNEPIN COMMUNITY COLLEGE

Address: 7411 85th Ave North, Brooklyn Park, MN 55445-2231
Phone: 763-424-0759
Fax: 763-493-0547
Contact: Mary Reuland, EdD, RN, Dean of Sciences and Health Careers
Email: mreuland@nh.cc.mn.us

GENERAL INFORMATION

Type of School: *Other, Public* • Accreditation: *North Central Association of Colleges and Schools* • Total Enrollment: *Not Reported*

PROGRAM INFORMATION

LPN/LVN Exit: *No* • NLNAC Accreditation: *Yes*

NURSING STUDENT PROFILE

Total Nursing Enrollment: *175* • Full-Time Enrollment: *175* • Part-Time Enrollment: *0* • Female Enrollment: *150* • Male Enrollment: *25* • Total New Admissions Who Enrolled for Fall: *93* • Total Graduates: *86*

FINANCES

Residential Annual Tuition: *Not Reported* • Non-Residential Annual Tuition: *Not Reported* • General Institution Fees: *$1,225* • Additional Nursing Fees: *$15*

NORTHLAND COMMUNITY AND TECHNICAL COLLEGE

Address: 1101 Hwy 1 East, Thief River Falls, MN 56701
Phone: 218-681-0841
Fax: 218-681-0774
Contact: Deb Filer, RN, MS, Dean of Nursing
Email: dfiler@nctc.mnscu.edu

GENERAL INFORMATION

Type of School: *2-Year College or University, Public* •
Accreditation: *North Central Association of Colleges and
Schools* • Total Enrollment: *Not Reported*

PROGRAM INFORMATION

LPN/LVN Exit: *Not Reported* • NLNAC Accreditation: *No*

NURSING STUDENT PROFILE

Total Nursing Enrollment: *58* • Full-Time Enrollment: *Not
Reported* • Part-Time Enrollment: *Not Reported* • Female
Enrollment: *56* • Male Enrollment: *2* • Total New
Admissions Who Enrolled for Fall: *71* • Total Graduates: *51*

FINANCES

Residential Annual Tuition: *Not Reported* • Non-Residential
Annual Tuition: *Not Reported* • General Institution Fees:
$1,155 • Additional Nursing Fees: *$25*

RIDGEWATER COLLEGE

Address: 2101 15th Ave NW Box 1097, Willmar, MN
            56201
Phone: 320-231-6034
Fax: Not Reported
Contact: Lynn Johnson, MSN, RN, Director of Nursing
Email: jojnsoly@ridgewater.mnscu.edu

GENERAL INFORMATION

Type of School: *Other, Public* • Accreditation: *North Central
Association of Colleges and Schools* • Total Enrollment: *Not
Reported*

PROGRAM INFORMATION

LPN/LVN Exit: *Not Reported* • NLNAC Accreditation: *Yes*

NURSING STUDENT PROFILE

Total Nursing Enrollment: *Not Reported* • Full-Time
Enrollment: *Not Reported* • Part-Time Enrollment: *Not
Reported* • Female Enrollment: *Not Reported* • Male
Enrollment: *Not Reported* • Total New Admissions Who
Enrolled for Fall: *Not Reported* • Total Graduates: *Not
Reported*

FINANCES

Residential Annual Tuition: *Not Reported* • Non-Residential
Annual Tuition: *Not Reported* • General Institution Fees: *Not
Reported* • Additional Nursing Fees: *Not Reported*

RIVERLAND COMMUNITY COLLEGE

Address: 1900 8th Ave NW, Austin, MN 55912-1470
Phone: 507-433-0826
Fax: Not Reported
Contact: Patricia A Parsons, MSN, RN, Director of Nursing Programs
Email: pparsons@river.cc.mn.us

GENERAL INFORMATION

Type of School: *Other, Public* • Accreditation: *North Central Association of Colleges and Schools* • Total Enrollment: *Not Reported*

PROGRAM INFORMATION

LPN/LVN Exit: *No* • NLNAC Accreditation: *Yes*

NURSING STUDENT PROFILE

Total Nursing Enrollment: *88* • Full-Time Enrollment: *Not Reported* • Part-Time Enrollment: *Not Reported* • Female Enrollment: *80* • Male Enrollment: *8* • Total New Admissions Who Enrolled for Fall: *49* • Total Graduates: *31*

FINANCES

Residential Annual Tuition: *Not Reported* • Non-Residential Annual Tuition: *Not Reported* • General Institution Fees: *$105* • Additional Nursing Fees: *$408*

ROCHESTER COMMUNITY & TECHNICAL COLLEGE

Address: 851 30th Ave SE, Rochester, MN 55904
Phone: 507-285-7143
Fax: 507-280-3166
Contact: Diane Nicholls, MSN, RN, Interim Director of Nursing
Email: diane.nicholls@roch.edu

GENERAL INFORMATION

Type of School: *2-Year College or University, Private (Religious)* • Accreditation: *North Central Association of Colleges and Schools* • Total Enrollment: *Not Reported*

PROGRAM INFORMATION

LPN/LVN Exit: *No* • NLNAC Accreditation: *Yes*

NURSING STUDENT PROFILE

Total Nursing Enrollment: *242* • Full-Time Enrollment: *233* • Part-Time Enrollment: *9* • Female Enrollment: *212* • Male Enrollment: *30* • Total New Admissions Who Enrolled for Fall: *74* • Total Graduates: *75*

FINANCES

Residential Annual Tuition: *$7,865* • Non-Residential Annual Tuition: *$15,730* • General Institution Fees: *$1,430* • Additional Nursing Fees: *$2,990*

ALCORN STATE UNIVERSITY

Address: 1000 ASU Drive, Alcorn State, MS 39096
Phone: 601-304-4315
Fax: 601-304-4398
Contact: Linda Godley, MSN, RN, Chairperson
Email: godley@lorman.alcorn.edu

GENERAL INFORMATION

Type of School: *4-Year College or University, Public •*
Accreditation: *Southern Association of Colleges and Schools •*
Total Enrollment: *3109*

PROGRAM INFORMATION

LPN/LVN Exit: *No* • NLNAC Accreditation: *Yes*

NURSING STUDENT PROFILE

Total Nursing Enrollment: *75* • Full-Time Enrollment: *53* •
Part-Time Enrollment: *22* • Female Enrollment: *72* • Male
Enrollment: *3* • Total New Admissions Who Enrolled for
Fall: *47* • Total Graduates: *16*

FINANCES

Residential Annual Tuition: *$1,601* • Non-Residential
Annual Tuition: *$3,687* • General Institution Fees: *$200* •
Additional Nursing Fees: *$30*

COPIAH-LINCOLN COMMUNITY COLLEGE

Address: PO Box 649, Wesson, MS 39191
Phone: 601-643-8413
Fax: 601-643-8212
Contact: Mary Ann Canterbury, MSN, RN, Director, Associate Degree Nursing
Email: maryann.catnerbury@colin.cc.ms.us

GENERAL INFORMATION

Type of School: *2-Year College or University, Public •*
Accreditation: *Southern Association of Colleges and Schools •*
Total Enrollment: *1800*

PROGRAM INFORMATION

LPN/LVN Exit: *No* • NLNAC Accreditation: *Yes*

NURSING STUDENT PROFILE

Total Nursing Enrollment: *69* • Full-Time Enrollment: *67* •
Part-Time Enrollment: *2* • Female Enrollment: *62* • Male
Enrollment: *7* • Total New Admissions Who Enrolled for
Fall: *39* • Total Graduates: *25*

FINANCES

Residential Annual Tuition: *$1,300* • Non-Residential
Annual Tuition: *$2,900* • General Institution Fees: *$50* •
Additional Nursing Fees: *$1,800*

EAST CENTRAL COMMUNITY COLLEGE

Address: 275 West Broad Street, Decatur, MS 39327
Phone: 601-635-2111
Fax: 601-635-5472
Contact: Melanie Gilmore, MSN, RN, Dean
Email: mgilmore@eccc.cc.ms.us

GENERAL INFORMATION

Type of School: *2-Year College or University, Public* •
Accreditation: *Southern Association of Colleges and Schools* •
Total Enrollment: *2361*

PROGRAM INFORMATION

LPN/LVN Exit: *No* • NLNAC Accreditation: *Yes*

NURSING STUDENT PROFILE

Total Nursing Enrollment: *84* • Full-Time Enrollment: *84* •
Part-Time Enrollment: *0* • Female Enrollment: *74* • Male
Enrollment: *10* • Total New Admissions Who Enrolled for
Fall: *50* • Total Graduates: *16*

FINANCES

Residential Annual Tuition: *$600* • Non-Residential Annual
Tuition: *$1,475* • General Institution Fees: *$50* • Additional
Nursing Fees: *$150*

HINDS COMMUNITY COLLEGE

Address: 1750 Chadwick Drive, Jackson, MS 39204
Phone: 601-371-3503
Fax: 604-371-3529
Contact: Gloria Coxwell, BSN, MN, Assistant Dean and
          Director, AD Nursing
Email: gjcoxwell@hinds.cc.ms.us

GENERAL INFORMATION

Type of School: *2-Year College or University, Public* •
Accreditation: *Southern Association of Colleges and Schools* •
Total Enrollment: *16074*

PROGRAM INFORMATION

LPN/LVN Exit: *No* • NLNAC Accreditation: *Yes*

NURSING STUDENT PROFILE

Total Nursing Enrollment: *328* • Full-Time Enrollment:
328 • Part-Time Enrollment: *0* • Female Enrollment: *286* •
Male Enrollment: *42* • Total New Admissions Who Enrolled
for Fall: *104* • Total Graduates: *112*

FINANCES

Residential Annual Tuition: *$1,120* • Non-Residential
Annual Tuition: *$3,326* • General Institution Fees: *$152* •
Additional Nursing Fees: *$66*

HOLMES COMMUNITY COLLEGE

Address: 1060 Avent Drive, Grenada, MS 38901
Phone: 662-227-2305
Fax: 662-227-2290
Contact: Joyce C. Vaughn, MSN, RN, Director
Email: jvaughn@holmes.cc.ms.us

GENERAL INFORMATION

Type of School: *2-Year College or University, Public* •
Accreditation: *Southern Association of Colleges and Schools* •
Total Enrollment: *Not Reported*

PROGRAM INFORMATION

LPN/LVN Exit: *No* • NLNAC Accreditation: *Yes*

NURSING STUDENT PROFILE

Total Nursing Enrollment: *108* • Full-Time Enrollment:
108 • Part-Time Enrollment: *0* • Female Enrollment: *103* •
Male Enrollment: *5* • Total New Admissions Who Enrolled
for Fall: *64* • Total Graduates: *32*

FINANCES

Residential Annual Tuition: *$950* • Non-Residential Annual
Tuition: *$1,700* • General Institution Fees: *$127* •
Additional Nursing Fees: *$75*

ITAWAMBA COMMUNITY COLLEGE

Address: 602 West Hill Street, Fulton, MS 38843
Phone: 662-862-8328
Fax: 662-862-8350
Contact: Melisa Lepard, RNC, MSN, Program Director
Email: mrlepard@icc.cc.ms.us

GENERAL INFORMATION

Type of School: *2-Year College or University, Public* •
Accreditation: *Southern Association of Colleges and Schools* •
Total Enrollment: *3834*

PROGRAM INFORMATION

LPN/LVN Exit: *No* • NLNAC Accreditation: *Yes*

NURSING STUDENT PROFILE

Total Nursing Enrollment: *175* • Full-Time Enrollment:
168 • Part-Time Enrollment: *7* • Female Enrollment: *160* •
Male Enrollment: *15* • Total New Admissions Who Enrolled
for Fall: *104* • Total Graduates: *72*

FINANCES

Residential Annual Tuition: *$1,000* • Non-Residential
Annual Tuition: *$2,750* • General Institution Fees: *$100* •
Additional Nursing Fees: *$170*

JONES COUNTY JUNIOR COLLEGE

Address: 900 South Court Street, Ellisville, MS 39437
Phone: 604-477-4019
Fax: 601-477-4099
Contact: Linda Suttle, RN, MS, Director, AD Nursing
Email: *linda.suttle@jcjc.cc.ms.us*

GENERAL INFORMATION

Type of School: *2-Year College or University, Public* •
Accreditation: *Southern Association of Colleges and Schools* •
Total Enrollment: *4879*

PROGRAM INFORMATION

LPN/LVN Exit: *No* • NLNAC Accreditation: *Yes*

NURSING STUDENT PROFILE

Total Nursing Enrollment: *110* • Full-Time Enrollment:
110 • Part-Time Enrollment: *0* • Female Enrollment: *90* •
Male Enrollment: *20* • Total New Admissions Who Enrolled
for Fall: *50* • Total Graduates: *44*

FINANCES

Residential Annual Tuition: *$1,200* • Non-Residential
Annual Tuition: *$1,200* • General Institution Fees: *$48* •
Additional Nursing Fees: *$40*

MERIDIAN COMMUNITY COLLEGE

Address: 910 Highway 19 North, Meridian, MS 39307
Phone: 601-484-8745
Fax: 601-482-3936
Contact: Betty W. Davis, MSN, RN, Assistant Dean,
           Nursing
Email: *bdavis@mcc.cc.ms.us*

GENERAL INFORMATION

Type of School: *2-Year College or University, Public* •
Accreditation: *Southern Association of Colleges and Schools* •
Total Enrollment: *2900*

PROGRAM INFORMATION

LPN/LVN Exit: *No* • NLNAC Accreditation: *Yes*

NURSING STUDENT PROFILE

Total Nursing Enrollment: *224* • Full-Time Enrollment:
224 • Part-Time Enrollment: *0* • Female Enrollment: *Not
Reported* • Male Enrollment: *Not Reported* • Total New
Admissions Who Enrolled for Fall: *75* • Total Graduates: *95*

FINANCES

Residential Annual Tuition: *$1,320* • Non-Residential
Annual Tuition: *$3,168* • General Institution Fees: *$65* •
Additional Nursing Fees: *$55*

MISSISSIPPI DELTA COMMUNITY COLLEGE

Address: PO Box 668, Moorhead, MS 38761
Phone: 662-246-6407
Fax: Not Reported
Contact: Martha Catlette, RN, DSN(c), Director
Email: mcatlette@mdcc.cc.ms.us

GENERAL INFORMATION

Type of School: *Other* • Accreditation: *Southern Association of Colleges and Schools* • Total Enrollment: *Not Reported*

PROGRAM INFORMATION

LPN/LVN Exit: *Not Reported* • NLNAC Accreditation: *Yes*

NURSING STUDENT PROFILE

Total Nursing Enrollment: *85* • Full-Time Enrollment: *Not Reported* • Part-Time Enrollment: *Not Reported* • Female Enrollment: *Not Reported* • Male Enrollment: *Not Reported* • Total New Admissions Who Enrolled for Fall: *80* • Total Graduates: *32*

FINANCES

Residential Annual Tuition: *Not Reported* • Non-Residential Annual Tuition: *Not Reported* • General Institution Fees: *Not Reported* • Additional Nursing Fees: *Not Reported*

MISSISSIPPI GULF COAST COMMUNITY COLLEGE

Address: 10298 Express Drive, Gulfport, MS 39503
Phone: 228-897-3702
Fax: 228-897-3918
Contact: Wanda Brignac, RN, MS, Chairperson ADN Department
Email: wanda.brignac@mgccc.edu

GENERAL INFORMATION

Type of School: *Not Reported* • Accreditation: *Southern Association of Colleges and Schools* • Total Enrollment: *Not Reported*

PROGRAM INFORMATION

LPN/LVN Exit: *No* • NLNAC Accreditation: *Yes*

NURSING STUDENT PROFILE

Total Nursing Enrollment: *130* • Full-Time Enrollment: *130* • Part-Time Enrollment: *0* • Female Enrollment: *115* • Male Enrollment: *15* • Total New Admissions Who Enrolled for Fall: *50* • Total Graduates: *59*

FINANCES

Residential Annual Tuition: *$1,090* • Non-Residential Annual Tuition: *$2,936* • General Institution Fees: *$112* • Additional Nursing Fees: *$132*

MISSISSIPPI GULF COAST COMMUNITY COLLEGE— JACKSON COUNTY CAMPUS

Address: P.O. Box 1000, Gulfport, MS 39503
Phone: 228-497-7660
Fax: 228-497-7676
Contact: Nica Cason, MS, RN, Chairperson
Email: nica.cason@mgccc.cc.ms.us

GENERAL INFORMATION

Type of School: *2-Year College or University, Public* •
Accreditation: *Southern Association of Colleges and Schools* •
Total Enrollment: *25000*

PROGRAM INFORMATION

LPN/LVN Exit: *No* • NLNAC Accreditation: *Yes*

NURSING STUDENT PROFILE

Total Nursing Enrollment: *180* • Full-Time Enrollment:
180 • Part-Time Enrollment: *0* • Female Enrollment: *156* •
Male Enrollment: *24* • Total New Admissions Who Enrolled
for Fall: *50* • Total Graduates: *54*

FINANCES

Residential Annual Tuition: *$1,090* • Non-Residential
Annual Tuition: *$2,936* • General Institution Fees: *$112* •
Additional Nursing Fees: *$132*

MISSISSIPPI UNIVERSITY FOR WOMEN

Address: Taylor Hall, P.O. Box W910, Columbus, MS
            39701
Phone: 662-329-7312
Fax: Not Reported
Contact: Jessica Alexander, MSN, RN, Interim Director of
            ASN Program
Email: jalexander@muw.edu

GENERAL INFORMATION

Type of School: *4-Year College or University, Public* •
Accreditation: *Southern Association of Colleges and Schools* •
Total Enrollment: *3000*

PROGRAM INFORMATION

LPN/LVN Exit: *No* • NLNAC Accreditation: *Yes*

NURSING STUDENT PROFILE

Total Nursing Enrollment: *75* • Full-Time Enrollment: *69* •
Part-Time Enrollment: *6* • Female Enrollment: *69* • Male
Enrollment: *6* • Total New Admissions Who Enrolled for
Fall: *32* • Total Graduates: *34*

FINANCES

Residential Annual Tuition: *$2,556* • Non-Residential
Annual Tuition: *$5,546* • General Institution Fees: *$0* •
Additional Nursing Fees: *$1,074*

NORTHEAST MISSISSIPPI COMMUNITY COLLEGE

Address: Cunningham Blvd., Booneville, MS 38829
Phone: 662-720-7215
Fax: 662-728-1165
Contact: Debbie G. Ricks, MSN, RN, Academic Head, Division of Nursing
Email: dricks@necc.cc.ms.us

GENERAL INFORMATION

Type of School: *2-Year College or University, Public* •
Accreditation: *Southern Association of Colleges and Schools* •
Total Enrollment: *2962*

PROGRAM INFORMATION

LPN/LVN Exit: *No* • NLNAC Accreditation: *Yes*

NURSING STUDENT PROFILE

Total Nursing Enrollment: *146* • Full-Time Enrollment: *140* • Part-Time Enrollment: *6* • Female Enrollment: *137* • Male Enrollment: *9* • Total New Admissions Who Enrolled for Fall: *108* • Total Graduates: *56*

FINANCES

Residential Annual Tuition: *$1,296* • Non-Residential Annual Tuition: *$3,016* • General Institution Fees: *$33* • Additional Nursing Fees: *$250*

PEARL RIVER COMMUNITY COLLEGE

Address: 101 Highway 11 North, Poplarville, MS 39470
Phone: 601-403-1017
Fax: 601-403-1275
Contact: Peggy Dease, RN, MS, Director, Associate Degree Nursing
Email: pdease@prcc.cc.ms.us

GENERAL INFORMATION

Type of School: *2-Year College or University, Public* •
Accreditation: *Southern Association of Colleges and Schools* •
Total Enrollment: *3154*

PROGRAM INFORMATION

LPN/LVN Exit: *Yes* • NLNAC Accreditation: *Yes*

NURSING STUDENT PROFILE

Total Nursing Enrollment: *158* • Full-Time Enrollment: *158* • Part-Time Enrollment: *0* • Female Enrollment: *135* • Male Enrollment: *23* • Total New Admissions Who Enrolled for Fall: *63* • Total Graduates: *65*

FINANCES

Residential Annual Tuition: *$1,250* • Non-Residential Annual Tuition: *$2,180* • General Institution Fees: *$20* • Additional Nursing Fees: *$257*

SOUTHWEST MISSISSIPPI COMMUNITY COLLEGE

Address: College Drive, Summit, MS 39666
Phone: 601-276-2008
Fax: 601-276-3824
Contact: Truda Jane McGrew, RN, MN, Director
Email: mcgrew@smcc.cc.ms.us

GENERAL INFORMATION

Type of School: *2-Year College or University, Public* •
Accreditation: *Southern Association of Colleges and Schools* •
Total Enrollment: *1651*

PROGRAM INFORMATION

LPN/LVN Exit: *No* • NLNAC Accreditation: *Yes*

NURSING STUDENT PROFILE

Total Nursing Enrollment: *197* • Full-Time Enrollment:
197 • Part-Time Enrollment: *0* • Female Enrollment: *176* •
Male Enrollment: *21* • Total New Admissions Who Enrolled
for Fall: *119* • Total Graduates: *67*

FINANCES

Residential Annual Tuition: *$575* • Non-Residential Annual
Tuition: *$1,475* • General Institution Fees: *$50* • Additional
Nursing Fees: *$500*

COLUMBIA COLLEGE

Address: 500 Strawn Road, Columbia, MO 65203
Phone: 787-743-4041
Fax: Not Reported
Contact: Carmen Lopez, MSN, RN, Associate Degree
Coordinator
Email: Not Reported

GENERAL INFORMATION

Type of School: *Independent, Private (Independent)* •
Accreditation: *North Central Association of Colleges and
Schools* • Total Enrollment: *2000*

PROGRAM INFORMATION

LPN/LVN Exit: *No* • NLNAC Accreditation: *Yes*

NURSING STUDENT PROFILE

Total Nursing Enrollment: *295* • Full-Time Enrollment:
295 • Part-Time Enrollment: *Not Reported* • Female
Enrollment: *Not Reported* • Male Enrollment: *Not Reported* •
Total New Admissions Who Enrolled for Fall: *103* • Total
Graduates: *128*

FINANCES

Residential Annual Tuition: *Not Reported* • Non-Residential
Annual Tuition: *Not Reported* • General Institution Fees: *Not
Reported* • Additional Nursing Fees: *Not Reported*

Circle 32 on reader card

CROWDER COLLEGE

Address: 601 Laclede, Neosho, MO 64850
Phone: 417-451-3223
Fax: Not Reported
Contact: Karen Vinyard, RN, MS, Director
Email: kvinyard@crowdercollege.net

GENERAL INFORMATION

Type of School: *Other* • Accreditation: *None* • Total Enrollment: *Not Reported*

PROGRAM INFORMATION

LPN/LVN Exit: *No* • NLNAC Accreditation: *No*

NURSING STUDENT PROFILE

Total Nursing Enrollment: *55* • Full-Time Enrollment: *Not Reported* • Part-Time Enrollment: *Not Reported* • Female Enrollment: *Not Reported* • Male Enrollment: *Not Reported* • Total New Admissions Who Enrolled for Fall: *35* • Total Graduates: *27*

FINANCES

Residential Annual Tuition: *Not Reported* • Non-Residential Annual Tuition: *Not Reported* • General Institution Fees: *Not Reported* • Additional Nursing Fees: *Not Reported*

DEACONESS COLLEGE OF NURSING

Address: 6150 Oakland Avenue, Saint Louis, MO 63139
Phone: 314-768-3042
Fax: 314-768-3843
Contact: Janet Barrett, PhD, MSN, BSN, Academic Dean
Email: janet.barrett(college)@tenethealth.com

GENERAL INFORMATION

Type of School: *4-Year College or University, Other* • Accreditation: *North Central Association of Colleges and Schools* • Total Enrollment: *220*

PROGRAM INFORMATION

LPN/LVN Exit: *No* • NLNAC Accreditation: *Yes*

NURSING STUDENT PROFILE

Total Nursing Enrollment: *34* • Full-Time Enrollment: *11* • Part-Time Enrollment: *23* • Female Enrollment: *32* • Male Enrollment: *2* • Total New Admissions Who Enrolled for Fall: *15* • Total Graduates: *14*

FINANCES

Residential Annual Tuition: *$8,900* • Non-Residential Annual Tuition: *$8,900* • General Institution Fees: *$150* • Additional Nursing Fees: *$100*

EAST CENTRAL COLLEGE

Address: 500 Forum, Rolla, MO 65401
Phone: 636-583-5193
Fax: 636-583-6637
Contact: Patrice O'Conner, PhD, RN, Director of
            Nursing and Allied Health
Email: oconnomp@ecmail.ecc.cc.mo.us

GENERAL INFORMATION

Type of School: *Other* • Accreditation: *None* • Total
Enrollment: *Not Reported*

PROGRAM INFORMATION

LPN/LVN Exit: *Not Reported* • NLNAC Accreditation: *No*

NURSING STUDENT PROFILE

Total Nursing Enrollment: *11* • Full-Time Enrollment: *11* •
Part-Time Enrollment: *0* • Female Enrollment: *11* • Male
Enrollment: *0* • Total New Admissions Who Enrolled for
Fall: *13* • Total Graduates: *10*

FINANCES

Residential Annual Tuition: *$3,000* • Non-Residential
Annual Tuition: *$3,000* • General Institution Fees: *Not
Reported* • Additional Nursing Fees: *$75*

EAST CENTRAL COLLEGE— UNION

Address: PO Box 529, Union, MO 63084-3720
Phone: 636-583-5193
Fax: 636-583-6637
Contact: Patricia O'Connor, PhD, RN, Director of
            Nursing and Allied Health
Email: oconnomp@ecmail.ecc.cc.mo.us

GENERAL INFORMATION

Type of School: *2-Year College or University, Public* •
Accreditation: *North Central Association of Colleges and
Schools* • Total Enrollment: *3000*

PROGRAM INFORMATION

LPN/LVN Exit: *No* • NLNAC Accreditation: *No*

NURSING STUDENT PROFILE

Total Nursing Enrollment: *30* • Full-Time Enrollment: *30* •
Part-Time Enrollment: *0* • Female Enrollment: *26* • Male
Enrollment: *4* • Total New Admissions Who Enrolled for
Fall: *14* • Total Graduates: *Not Reported*

FINANCES

Residential Annual Tuition: *$7,500* • Non-Residential
Annual Tuition: *$9,000* • General Institution Fees: *Not
Reported* • Additional Nursing Fees: *$42*

HANNIBAL LAGRANGE COLLEGE

Address: 2800 Palmyra Road, Hannibal, MO 63401
Phone: 573-221-3675
Fax: 573-248-1294
Contact: Senda Guertzgen, RN, MS, Director
Email: sguertzg@hlg.edu

GENERAL INFORMATION

Type of School: *4-Year College or University, Private (Religious)* • Accreditation: *North Central Association of Colleges and Schools* • Total Enrollment: *1152*

PROGRAM INFORMATION

LPN/LVN Exit: *No* • NLNAC Accreditation: *Yes*

NURSING STUDENT PROFILE

Total Nursing Enrollment: *15* • Full-Time Enrollment: *15* • Part-Time Enrollment: *0* • Female Enrollment: *14* • Male Enrollment: *1* • Total New Admissions Who Enrolled for Fall: *9* • Total Graduates: *10*

FINANCES

Residential Annual Tuition: *$6,840* • Non-Residential Annual Tuition: *$6,840* • General Institution Fees: *$260* • Additional Nursing Fees: *$1,158*

JEFFERSON COLLEGE

Address: 1000 Viking Drive, Hillsboro, MO 63050
Phone: 636-789-3000
Fax: 636-789-2047
Contact: Michele Soest, MSN, RN, BC, ANP, Director of Health Technologies
Email: msoest@jeffco.edu

GENERAL INFORMATION

Type of School: *2-Year College or University, Public* • Accreditation: *North Central Association of Colleges and Schools* • Total Enrollment: *Not Reported*

PROGRAM INFORMATION

LPN/LVN Exit: *Yes* • NLNAC Accreditation: *No*

NURSING STUDENT PROFILE

Total Nursing Enrollment: *30* • Full-Time Enrollment: *30* • Part-Time Enrollment: *0* • Female Enrollment: *29* • Male Enrollment: *1* • Total New Admissions Who Enrolled for Fall: *30* • Total Graduates: *22*

FINANCES

Residential Annual Tuition: *$1,976* • Non-Residential Annual Tuition: *$2,584* • General Institution Fees: *$25* • Additional Nursing Fees: *$327*

JEWISH HOSPITAL

Address: 306 South Kingshighway Boulevard, St. Louis, MO 63110
Phone: 314-454-8416
Fax: 314-454-5239
Contact: Elizabeth A. Buck, PhD, RN, Academic Dean, Nursing Division
Email: eab1458@bjc.org

GENERAL INFORMATION

Type of School: *Hospital, Private (Independent)* • Accreditation: *North Central Association of Colleges and Schools* • Total Enrollment: *Not Reported*

PROGRAM INFORMATION

LPN/LVN Exit: *Not Reported* • NLNAC Accreditation: *Yes*

NURSING STUDENT PROFILE

Total Nursing Enrollment: *217* • Full-Time Enrollment: *76* • Part-Time Enrollment: *141* • Female Enrollment: *199* • Male Enrollment: *18* • Total New Admissions Who Enrolled for Fall: *68* • Total Graduates: *74*

FINANCES

Residential Annual Tuition: *$9,240* • Non-Residential Annual Tuition: *Not Reported* • General Institution Fees: *$200* • Additional Nursing Fees: *$0*

LESTER L. COX COLLEGE

Address: 1423 North Jefferson, Springfield, MO 65802
Phone: 417-269-3067
Fax: 417-269-3581
Contact: Vickie L. Donnell, RN, MS, MED, Director, Associate Degree Program
Email: vdonnel@coxcollege.edu

GENERAL INFORMATION

Type of School: *Hospital, Private (Independent)* • Accreditation: *North Central Association of Colleges and Schools* • Total Enrollment: *294*

PROGRAM INFORMATION

LPN/LVN Exit: *No* • NLNAC Accreditation: *No*

NURSING STUDENT PROFILE

Total Nursing Enrollment: *275* • Full-Time Enrollment: *170* • Part-Time Enrollment: *105* • Female Enrollment: *257* • Male Enrollment: *18* • Total New Admissions Who Enrolled for Fall: *126* • Total Graduates: *69*

FINANCES

Residential Annual Tuition: *$6,288* • Non-Residential Annual Tuition: *$6,288* • General Institution Fees: *$260* • Additional Nursing Fees: *$380*

LINCOLN UNIVERSITY

Address: 820 Chestnut, Jefferson City, MO 65102
Phone: 573-681-5421
Fax: 573-681-5422
Contact: Connie Hamacher, PhD, RN, Department Head
Email: hamacher@lincolnu.edu

GENERAL INFORMATION

Type of School: *4-Year College or University, Public* •
Accreditation: *North Central Association of Colleges and Schools* • Total Enrollment: *3347*

PROGRAM INFORMATION

LPN/LVN Exit: *No* • NLNAC Accreditation: *Yes*

NURSING STUDENT PROFILE

Total Nursing Enrollment: *65* • Full-Time Enrollment: *32* •
Part-Time Enrollment: *33* • Female Enrollment: *59* • Male
Enrollment: *6* • Total New Admissions Who Enrolled for
Fall: *48* • Total Graduates: *29*

FINANCES

Residential Annual Tuition: *$2,424* • Non-Residential
Annual Tuition: *$4,848* • General Institution Fees: *$374* •
Additional Nursing Fees: *$50*

LINCOLN UNIVERSITY— FORT LEONARD WOOD

Address: Truman Education Center, Building 499, Fort
Leonard Wood, MO 65473
Phone: 573-681-5421
Fax: 573-681-5422
Contact: Connie Hamacher, PhD, RN, Chairperson,
Department of Nursing Science
Email: hamacher@lincolnu.edu

GENERAL INFORMATION

Type of School: *Not Reported* • Accreditation: *Not Reported* •
Total Enrollment: *Not Reported*

PROGRAM INFORMATION

LPN/LVN Exit: *No* • NLNAC Accreditation: *Yes*

NURSING STUDENT PROFILE

Total Nursing Enrollment: *54* • Full-Time Enrollment: *5* •
Part-Time Enrollment: *49* • Female Enrollment: *46* • Male
Enrollment: *8* • Total New Admissions Who Enrolled for
Fall: *34* • Total Graduates: *24*

FINANCES

Residential Annual Tuition: *Not Reported* • Non-Residential
Annual Tuition: *Not Reported* • General Institution Fees: *Not
Reported* • Additional Nursing Fees: *$50*

METROPOLITAN COMMUNITY COLLEGE

Address: 3201 Southwest Trafficway, Kansas City, MO
             64111
Phone: 402-457-2664
Fax: 402-457-2833
Contact: Nina Wardell, MSN, RN, Director of Nursing
             Programs
Email: nwardell@metropo.mccneb.edu

GENERAL INFORMATION

Type of School: *2-Year College or University, Public* •
Accreditation: *North Central Association of Colleges and
Schools* • Total Enrollment: *5000*

PROGRAM INFORMATION

LPN/LVN Exit: *No* • NLNAC Accreditation: *No*

NURSING STUDENT PROFILE

Total Nursing Enrollment: *71* • Full-Time Enrollment: *16* •
Part-Time Enrollment: *55* • Female Enrollment: *61* • Male
Enrollment: *10* • Total New Admissions Who Enrolled for
Fall: *37* • Total Graduates: *30*

FINANCES

Residential Annual Tuition: *$2,240* • Non-Residential
Annual Tuition: *$5,280* • General Institution Fees: *$98* •
Additional Nursing Fees: *$15*

MINERAL AREA COLLEGE

Address: PO Box 1000, 5270 Flat River Road, Park Hills,
             MO 63601
Phone: 573-518-2103
Fax: 573-518-2292
Contact: Teri Douglas, MSN, RN, Chairperson
Email: TDouglas@mail.mac.cc.mo.us

GENERAL INFORMATION

Type of School: *2-Year College or University, Public* •
Accreditation: *North Central Association of Colleges and
Schools* • Total Enrollment: *3200*

PROGRAM INFORMATION

LPN/LVN Exit: *No* • NLNAC Accreditation: *No*

NURSING STUDENT PROFILE

Total Nursing Enrollment: *72* • Full-Time Enrollment: *72* •
Part-Time Enrollment: *0* • Female Enrollment: *66* • Male
Enrollment: *6* • Total New Admissions Who Enrolled for
Fall: *37* • Total Graduates: *43*

FINANCES

Residential Annual Tuition: *Not Reported* • Non-Residential
Annual Tuition: *Not Reported* • General Institution Fees: *Not
Reported* • Additional Nursing Fees: *Not Reported*

MOBERLY AREA COMMUNITY COLLEGE

Address: 101 College Avenue, Moberly, MO 65270
Phone: 660-263-4110
Fax: Not Reported
Contact: Ruth J. Jones, MSN, RN, Director
Email: ruthj@hp9000.mapp.mo.us

GENERAL INFORMATION

Type of School: *2-Year College or University, Public* • Accreditation: *North Central Association of Colleges and Schools* • Total Enrollment: *Not Reported*

PROGRAM INFORMATION

LPN/LVN Exit: *Not Reported* • NLNAC Accreditation: *No*

NURSING STUDENT PROFILE

Total Nursing Enrollment: *72* • Full-Time Enrollment: *72* • Part-Time Enrollment: *0* • Female Enrollment: *Not Reported* • Male Enrollment: *Not Reported* • Total New Admissions Who Enrolled for Fall: *41* • Total Graduates: *28*

FINANCES

Residential Annual Tuition: *Not Reported* • Non-Residential Annual Tuition: *Not Reported* • General Institution Fees: *Not Reported* • Additional Nursing Fees: *Not Reported*

NORTH CENTRAL MISSOURI COLLEGE

Address: 1301 Main, Trenton, MO 64683
Phone: 800-880-6180
Fax: 660-359-2211
Contact: Patricia J. Dixon, MSN, RN, Associate Dean, Allied Health Sciences
Email: Pdixon@ncmc.cc.mo.us

GENERAL INFORMATION

Type of School: *Other* • Accreditation: *None* • Total Enrollment: *Not Reported*

PROGRAM INFORMATION

LPN/LVN Exit: *Yes* • NLNAC Accreditation: *No*

NURSING STUDENT PROFILE

Total Nursing Enrollment: *31* • Full-Time Enrollment: *31* • Part-Time Enrollment: *0* • Female Enrollment: *Not Reported* • Male Enrollment: *Not Reported* • Total New Admissions Who Enrolled for Fall: *32* • Total Graduates: *29*

FINANCES

Residential Annual Tuition: *$1,582* • Non-Residential Annual Tuition: *$1,782* • General Institution Fees: *$444* • Additional Nursing Fees: *Not Reported*

PARK UNIVERSITY

Web site: www.park.edu
Address: 8700 NW River Park Dr, Parkville, MO 64152
Phone: (816) 741-2000, Ext. 6256
Contact: Miss Margaret Monahan, Director

GENERAL INFORMATION

Type of School: *Private* • Campus Setting: *Urban* • Total Enrollment: *14,000*

PROGRAM INFORMATION

Programs Offered: *Associate Degree* • Options: *Evening Classes, Weekend Classes, Distance Learning, Other Alternative Schedules, Continuing Education* • Articulations: *LPN to ADN, ADN to BSN* • NLNAC Accredited

NURSING STUDENT PROFILE

First-Year Undergraduate Enrollment: *35* • Total Graduates: *33* • Total Enrollment: *32*

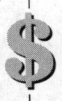

FINANCES

Resident Annual Tuition: *n/a* • Non-Resident Annual Tuition: *n/a* • Grants: *Institutionally-Sponsored Need-Based and Non-Need-Based Grants, Federal Pell Grants, Supplemental Educational Opportunity Grants, Missouri Grants* • Scholarships: *Institutionally-Sponsored Need-Based and Non-Need-Based Scholarships, Endowed* • Loans: *Institutionally-Sponsored Loans, Federal Perkins Loans, Federal PLUS Loans, Federal Stafford Loans* • Work Programs: *Fellowships, Federal Work-Study, Institutional* • % of Students Receiving Some Type of Aid: *25%* • Financial Aid Application Deadline: *April 1- MO Grant* • Financial Aid Office Phone: *(816) 741-2000 Ext. 6290*

PENN VALLEY COMMUNITY COLLEGE

Address: 3201 South West Trafficway, Kansas City, MO 64111
Phone: 816-759-4174
Fax: 816-759-4361
Contact: Karen S. Komoroski, EdS, MN, RN, Chairperson, Division of Nursing
Email: komok@pennvalley.cc.mo.us

GENERAL INFORMATION

Type of School: *Not Reported* • Accreditation: *Not Reported* • Total Enrollment: *Not Reported*

PROGRAM INFORMATION

LPN/LVN Exit: *No* • NLNAC Accreditation: *Yes*

NURSING STUDENT PROFILE

Total Nursing Enrollment: *167* • Full-Time Enrollment: *155* • Part-Time Enrollment: *12* • Female Enrollment: *151* • Male Enrollment: *16* • Total New Admissions Who Enrolled for Fall: *63* • Total Graduates: *90*

FINANCES

Residential Annual Tuition: *Not Reported* • Non-Residential Annual Tuition: *Not Reported* • General Institution Fees: *Not Reported* • Additional Nursing Fees: *$150*

SAINT LOUIS COMMUNITY COLLEGE—FOREST PARK

Address: 5600 Oakland, St. Louis, MO 63110-1393
Phone: 314-984-7750
Fax: 314-984-7114
Contact: Sharon Godwin, MSN, RN, Chairperson,
Department of Nursing Education
Email: sgodwin@stlcc.cc.mo.us

GENERAL INFORMATION

Type of School: *Not Reported* • Accreditation: *None* • Total Enrollment: *Not Reported*

PROGRAM INFORMATION

LPN/LVN Exit: *No* • NLNAC Accreditation: *Yes*

NURSING STUDENT PROFILE

Total Nursing Enrollment: *136* • Full-Time Enrollment: *136* • Part-Time Enrollment: *0* • Female Enrollment: *127* • Male Enrollment: *9* • Total New Admissions Who Enrolled for Fall: *38* • Total Graduates: *66*

FINANCES

Residential Annual Tuition: *$1,272* • Non-Residential Annual Tuition: *$1,608* • General Institution Fees: *$24* • Additional Nursing Fees: *$0*

SAINT LOUIS COMMUNITY COLLEGE—ST. LOUIS

Address: 3400 Pershall Road, Saint Louis, MO 63135
Phone: 314-595-2310
Fax: 314-595-2218
Contact: Karen Mayes, MSN, RN, Chairperson
Email: kmayes@stlcc.cc.mo.us

GENERAL INFORMATION

Type of School: *2-Year College or University, Public* • Accreditation: *North Central Association of Colleges and Schools* • Total Enrollment: *7000*

PROGRAM INFORMATION

LPN/LVN Exit: *No* • NLNAC Accreditation: *Yes*

NURSING STUDENT PROFILE

Total Nursing Enrollment: *81* • Full-Time Enrollment: *10* • Part-Time Enrollment: *71* • Female Enrollment: *78* • Male Enrollment: *3* • Total New Admissions Who Enrolled for Fall: *37* • Total Graduates: *22*

FINANCES

Residential Annual Tuition: *$1,008* • Non-Residential Annual Tuition: *$1,608* • General Institution Fees: *Not Reported* • Additional Nursing Fees: *$8*

SANFORD BROWN COLLEGE

Address: 1203 Smizer Mill Road, Fenton, MO 63026
Phone: 816-472-0275
Fax: 816-472-0688
Contact: Renee Stafford, MSN, RN, Nursing Department Chair
Email: renee.stafford@wix.net

GENERAL INFORMATION

Type of School: *Other* • Accreditation: *None* • Total Enrollment: *Not Reported*

PROGRAM INFORMATION

LPN/LVN Exit: *No* • NLNAC Accreditation: *No*

NURSING STUDENT PROFILE

Total Nursing Enrollment: *54* • Full-Time Enrollment: *54* • Part-Time Enrollment: *0* • Female Enrollment: *49* • Male Enrollment: *5* • Total New Admissions Who Enrolled for Fall: *34* • Total Graduates: *51*

FINANCES

Residential Annual Tuition: *Not Reported* • Non-Residential Annual Tuition: *Not Reported* • General Institution Fees: *$100* • Additional Nursing Fees: *$100*

SOUTHEAST MISSOURI HOSPITAL

Address: 1819 Broadway, Cape Girardeau, MO 63701
Phone: 573-334-6825
Fax: 573-339-7805
Contact: Tonya Buttry, RNC, MSN, President
Email: tbuttry@sehosp.org

GENERAL INFORMATION

Type of School: *Independent, Private (Independent)* • Accreditation: *North Central Association of Colleges and Schools* • Total Enrollment: *100*

PROGRAM INFORMATION

LPN/LVN Exit: *No* • NLNAC Accreditation: *No*

NURSING STUDENT PROFILE

Total Nursing Enrollment: *62* • Full-Time Enrollment: *19* • Part-Time Enrollment: *43* • Female Enrollment: *55* • Male Enrollment: *7* • Total New Admissions Who Enrolled for Fall: *34* • Total Graduates: *12*

FINANCES

Residential Annual Tuition: *$5,280* • Non-Residential Annual Tuition: *$5,280* • General Institution Fees: *$0* • Additional Nursing Fees: *$20*

SOUTHWEST BAPTIST UNIVERSITY

Address: 4431 South Freemont Street, Springfield, MO 65804
Phone: 417-885-2098
Fax: 417-887-4847
Contact: Virginia Mayeux, MSN, RN, Director
Email: vmayeux@sprg.smhs.com

GENERAL INFORMATION

Type of School: *4-Year College or University, Private (Religious)* • Accreditation: *North Central Association of Colleges and Schools* • Total Enrollment: *3593*

PROGRAM INFORMATION

LPN/LVN Exit: *No* • NLNAC Accreditation: *Yes*

NURSING STUDENT PROFILE

Total Nursing Enrollment: *169* • Full-Time Enrollment: *169* • Part-Time Enrollment: *0* • Female Enrollment: *160* • Male Enrollment: *9* • Total New Admissions Who Enrolled for Fall: *49* • Total Graduates: *57*

FINANCES

Annual Tuition: *$10,600* • General Institution Fees: *$466* • Additional Nursing Fees: *$415*

SOUTHWEST MISSOURI STATE UNIVERSITY— WEST PLAINS

Address: 128 Garfield Avenue, West Plains, MO 65775
Phone: 417-255-7247
Fax: 417-255-7241
Contact: Juanita J. Roth, EdD, RN, MS, Director
Email: NitaRoth@wp.smsu.edu

GENERAL INFORMATION

Type of School: *2-Year College or University, Public* • Accreditation: *North Central Association of Colleges and Schools* • Total Enrollment: *1653*

PROGRAM INFORMATION

LPN/LVN Exit: *No* • NLNAC Accreditation: *Yes*

NURSING STUDENT PROFILE

Total Nursing Enrollment: *64* • Full-Time Enrollment: *64* • Part-Time Enrollment: *0* • Female Enrollment: *54* • Male Enrollment: *10* • Total New Admissions Who Enrolled for Fall: *36* • Total Graduates: *22*

FINANCES

Residential Annual Tuition: *$4,416* • Non-Residential Annual Tuition: *$8,832* • General Institution Fees: *$190* • Additional Nursing Fees: *$365*

ST. CHARLES COUNTY COMMUNITY COLLEGE

Address: 4601 Mid River Mall Drive, Saint Peters, MO
             63376
Phone: 636-922-8280
Fax: 636-922-8478
Contact: Patricia Porterfield, MSN, RN, Dean, Health
             and Wellness
Email: pporterfield@stchas.edu

STATE FAIR COMMUNITY COLLEGE

Address: 3201 West 16th Street, Sedalia, MO 62901
Phone: 660-530-5800
Fax: 660-530-5827
Contact: Sandy Whitehead, RN, BSN, MSN, Director,
             ADN Programs
Email: whitehea@sfcc.cc.mo.us

GENERAL INFORMATION

Type of School: *2-Year College or University, Public* •
Accreditation: *North Central Association of Colleges and Schools* • Total Enrollment: *6000*

GENERAL INFORMATION

Type of School: *2-Year College or University, Public* •
Accreditation: *North Central Association of Colleges and Schools* • Total Enrollment: *3356*

PROGRAM INFORMATION

LPN/LVN Exit: *No* • NLNAC Accreditation: *Yes*

PROGRAM INFORMATION

LPN/LVN Exit: *No* • NLNAC Accreditation: *No*

NURSING STUDENT PROFILE

Total Nursing Enrollment: *105* • Full-Time Enrollment: *60* •
Part-Time Enrollment: *45* • Female Enrollment: *101* • Male
Enrollment: *4* • Total New Admissions Who Enrolled for
Fall: *56* • Total Graduates: *53*

NURSING STUDENT PROFILE

Total Nursing Enrollment: *27* • Full-Time Enrollment: *27* •
Part-Time Enrollment: *0* • Female Enrollment: *26* • Male
Enrollment: *1* • Total New Admissions Who Enrolled for
Fall: *36* • Total Graduates: *28*

FINANCES

Residential Annual Tuition: *Not Reported* • Non-Residential
Annual Tuition: *Not Reported* • General Institution Fees:
$1,500 • Additional Nursing Fees: *Not Reported*

FINANCES

Residential Annual Tuition: *$1,617* • Non-Residential
Annual Tuition: *$2,503* • General Institution Fees: *$257* •
Additional Nursing Fees: *$1,054*

THREE RIVERS COMMUNITY COLLEGE—POPLAR BLUFF

Address: 2080 Three Rivers Boulevard, Poplar Bluff, MO 63901
Phone: 573-840-9681
Fax: 573-840-9657
Contact: Catherine F. Wampler, RN, BSN, MN, Division Chair, Health and Human Services
Email: cwampler@trcc.cc.mo.us

GENERAL INFORMATION

Type of School: *2-Year College or University, Public* • Accreditation: *North Central Association of Colleges and Schools* • Total Enrollment: *2824*

PROGRAM INFORMATION

LPN/LVN Exit: *No* • NLNAC Accreditation: *Yes*

NURSING STUDENT PROFILE

Total Nursing Enrollment: *62* • Full-Time Enrollment: *25* • Part-Time Enrollment: *37* • Female Enrollment: *59* • Male Enrollment: *3* • Total New Admissions Who Enrolled for Fall: *44* • Total Graduates: *33*

FINANCES

Residential Annual Tuition: *$1,285* • Non-Residential Annual Tuition: *$2,627* • General Institution Fees: *$450* • Additional Nursing Fees: *$535*

MILES COMMUNITY COLLEGE

Address: 2715 Dickinson Street, Miles City, MT 59301
Phone: 406-234-3543
Fax: 406-234-6598
Contact: Kathleen K. Wankel, RN, MN, Director, Nursing Program
Email: wankelk@milescc.edu

GENERAL INFORMATION

Type of School: *2-Year College or University, Public* • Accreditation: *Northwestern Association of Schools and Colleges* • Total Enrollment: *493*

PROGRAM INFORMATION

LPN/LVN Exit: *No* • NLNAC Accreditation: *Yes*

NURSING STUDENT PROFILE

Total Nursing Enrollment: *35* • Full-Time Enrollment: *33* • Part-Time Enrollment: *2* • Female Enrollment: *33* • Male Enrollment: *2* • Total New Admissions Who Enrolled for Fall: *20* • Total Graduates: *14*

FINANCES

Residential Annual Tuition: *$1,800* • Non-Residential Annual Tuition: *$3,750* • General Institution Fees: *$840* • Additional Nursing Fees: *$400*

MONTANA TECHNOLOGY OF THE UNIVERSITY OF MONTANA

Address: 1300 West Park, Butte, MT 59701
Phone: 406-496-3722
Fax: 406-496-3710
Contact: Karen Pafhausen Vandaveer, MSN, RN, Director of Nursing
Email: KVandaveer@mtech.edu

SALISH KOOTENAI COLLEGE

Address: PO Box 117, Pablo, MT 58555-0117
Phone: 406-675-4800
Fax: Not Reported
Contact: Jacque Dolberry, RN, MS, Director of Nursing Department
Email: jacque_dolberry@skc.edu

GENERAL INFORMATION

Type of School: *4-Year College or University, Public* • Accreditation: *Northwestern Association of Schools and Colleges* • Total Enrollment: *2067*

GENERAL INFORMATION

Type of School: *Independent, Private (Independent)* • Accreditation: *Northwestern Association of Schools and Colleges* • Total Enrollment: *989*

PROGRAM INFORMATION

LPN/LVN Exit: *Not Reported* • NLNAC Accreditation: *No*

PROGRAM INFORMATION

LPN/LVN Exit: *Not Reported* • NLNAC Accreditation: *Yes*

NURSING STUDENT PROFILE

Total Nursing Enrollment: *Not Reported* • Full-Time Enrollment: *Not Reported* • Part-Time Enrollment: *Not Reported* • Female Enrollment: *Not Reported* • Male Enrollment: *Not Reported* • Total New Admissions Who Enrolled for Fall: *Not Reported* • Total Graduates: *Not Reported*

NURSING STUDENT PROFILE

Total Nursing Enrollment: *51* • Full-Time Enrollment: *51* • Part-Time Enrollment: *0* • Female Enrollment: *44* • Male Enrollment: *7* • Total New Admissions Who Enrolled for Fall: *28* • Total Graduates: *25*

FINANCES

Residential Annual Tuition: *Not Reported* • Non-Residential Annual Tuition: *Not Reported* • General Institution Fees: *Not Reported* • Additional Nursing Fees: *Not Reported*

FINANCES

Residential Annual Tuition: *$2,264* • Non-Residential Annual Tuition: *$1,560* • General Institution Fees: *$219* • Additional Nursing Fees: *$200*

CENTRAL COMMUNITY COLLEGE

Address: PO Box 4903, 3134 W Hwy 34, Grand Island, NE 68802
Phone: 308-398-7455
Fax: 308-385-6414
Contact: Linda K. Walline, RN, BS, BSN, MSN, Associate Dean of Instruction
Email: lwalline@cccneb.edu

GENERAL INFORMATION

Type of School: *2-Year College or University, Public* • Accreditation: *North Central Association of Colleges and Schools* • Total Enrollment: *2048*

PROGRAM INFORMATION

LPN/LVN Exit: *Yes* • NLNAC Accreditation: *Yes*

NURSING STUDENT PROFILE

Total Nursing Enrollment: *73* • Full-Time Enrollment: *73* • Part-Time Enrollment: *0* • Female Enrollment: *67* • Male Enrollment: *6* • Total New Admissions Who Enrolled for Fall: *39* • Total Graduates: *33*

FINANCES

Residential Annual Tuition: *$1,080* • Non-Residential Annual Tuition: *$1,620* • General Institution Fees: *$4* • Additional Nursing Fees: *$143*

COLLEGE OF SAINT MARY

Address: 1901 S. 72nd St., Omaha, NE 68124
Phone: 402-399-2636
Fax: Not Reported
Contact: Peggy L. Hawkins, MSN, RN, ASN Program Director and Associate Professor
Email: phawkins@csm.edu

GENERAL INFORMATION

Type of School: *4-Year College or University, Private (Religious)* • Accreditation: *North Central Association of Colleges and Schools* • Total Enrollment: *930*

PROGRAM INFORMATION

LPN/LVN Exit: *No* • NLNAC Accreditation: *Yes*

NURSING STUDENT PROFILE

Total Nursing Enrollment: *86* • Full-Time Enrollment: *62* • Part-Time Enrollment: *24* • Female Enrollment: *86* • Male Enrollment: *0* • Total New Admissions Who Enrolled for Fall: *47* • Total Graduates: *31*

FINANCES

Residential Annual Tuition: *$13,136* • Non-Residential Annual Tuition: *Not Reported* • General Institution Fees: *$408* • Additional Nursing Fees: *$300*

MID-PLAINS COMMUNITY COLLEGE AREA

Address: 1101 Halligan Drive, North Platte, NE 69101
Phone: 308-535-3623
Fax: Not Reported
Contact: Diane Hoffmann, MSN, RN, Health Division Chair
Email: hoffmannd@mpcca.cc.ne.us

GENERAL INFORMATION

Type of School: *2-Year College or University, Public* • Accreditation: *North Central Association of Colleges and Schools* • Total Enrollment: *650*

PROGRAM INFORMATION

LPN/LVN Exit: *No* • NLNAC Accreditation: *Yes*

NURSING STUDENT PROFILE

Total Nursing Enrollment: *40* • Full-Time Enrollment: *40* • Part-Time Enrollment: *0* • Female Enrollment: *40* • Male Enrollment: *0* • Total New Admissions Who Enrolled for Fall: *24* • Total Graduates: *23*

FINANCES

Residential Annual Tuition: *$1,152* • Non-Residential Annual Tuition: *Not Reported* • General Institution Fees: *Not Reported* • Additional Nursing Fees: *Not Reported*

NORTHEAST COMMUNITY COLLEGE

Address: 801 East Benjamin Ave, PO Box 469, Norfolk, NE 68701
Phone: 402-644-0612
Fax: Not Reported
Contact: Elaine Gardner, MSN, RN, ADN Program Director
Email: elaine@alpha.necc.ne.us

GENERAL INFORMATION

Type of School: *2-Year College or University, Public* • Accreditation: *North Central Association of Colleges and Schools* • Total Enrollment: *4520*

PROGRAM INFORMATION

LPN/LVN Exit: *No* • NLNAC Accreditation: *Yes*

NURSING STUDENT PROFILE

Total Nursing Enrollment: *195* • Full-Time Enrollment: *45* • Part-Time Enrollment: *150* • Female Enrollment: *180* • Male Enrollment: *15* • Total New Admissions Who Enrolled for Fall: *24* • Total Graduates: *24*

FINANCES

Residential Annual Tuition: *$1,008* • Non-Residential Annual Tuition: *$1,056* • General Institution Fees: *Not Reported* • Additional Nursing Fees: *Not Reported*

SOUTHEAST COMMUNITY COLLEGE—LINCOLN

Address: 8800 O Street, Lincoln, NE 68520
Phone: 402-437-2730
Fax: 402-437-2404
Contact: Virginia Hess, RN, MS in Nursing, Program Chair
Email: vhess@scc.cc.ne.us

GENERAL INFORMATION

Type of School: *Other, Public* • Accreditation: *North Central Association of Colleges and Schools* • Total Enrollment: *7396*

PROGRAM INFORMATION

LPN/LVN Exit: *Not Reported* • NLNAC Accreditation: *Yes*

NURSING STUDENT PROFILE

Total Nursing Enrollment: *85* • Full-Time Enrollment: *44* • Part-Time Enrollment: *41* • Female Enrollment: *82* • Male Enrollment: *3* • Total New Admissions Who Enrolled for Fall: *65* • Total Graduates: *34*

FINANCES

Residential Annual Tuition: *$1,072* • Non-Residential Annual Tuition: *$1,296* • General Institution Fees: *$48* • Additional Nursing Fees: *$200*

COMMUNITY COLLEGE OF SOUTHERN NEVADA

Address: 6375 W. Charleston Blvd., Las Vegas, NV 89146
Phone: 702-651-5676
Fax: 702-651-5641
Contact: Shirlee Snyder, EdD, RN, Nursing Program Director
Email: shirlee_snyder@ccsn.nevada.edu

GENERAL INFORMATION

Type of School: *2-Year College or University, Public* • Accreditation: *Northwestern Association of Schools and Colleges* • Total Enrollment: *33364*

PROGRAM INFORMATION

LPN/LVN Exit: *No* • NLNAC Accreditation: *Yes*

NURSING STUDENT PROFILE

Total Nursing Enrollment: *163* • Full-Time Enrollment: *163* • Part-Time Enrollment: *0* • Female Enrollment: *150* • Male Enrollment: *13* • Total New Admissions Who Enrolled for Fall: *62* • Total Graduates: *74*

FINANCES

Residential Annual Tuition: *$3,410* • Non-Residential Annual Tuition: *$11,400* • General Institution Fees: *$100* • Additional Nursing Fees: *$100*

GREAT BASIN COLLEGE

Address: 1500 College Parkway, Elko, NV 89801
Phone: 775-753-2216
Fax: Not Reported
Contact: Georgeanna Smith, MSN, RN, Nursing Program Director
Email: gsmith@gbcnv.edu

GENERAL INFORMATION

Type of School: *Other, Public* • Accreditation: *Northwestern Association of Schools and Colleges* • Total Enrollment: *1300*

PROGRAM INFORMATION

LPN/LVN Exit: *Yes* • NLNAC Accreditation: *Yes*

NURSING STUDENT PROFILE

Total Nursing Enrollment: *26* • Full-Time Enrollment: *8* • Part-Time Enrollment: *18* • Female Enrollment: *25* • Male Enrollment: *1* • Total New Admissions Who Enrolled for Fall: *12* • Total Graduates: *14*

FINANCES

Residential Annual Tuition: *$2,700* • Non-Residential Annual Tuition: *$4,700* • General Institution Fees: *$0* • Additional Nursing Fees: *$300*

WESTERN NEVADA COMMUNITY COLLEGE

Address: 2201 W. College Pkwy, Carson City, NV 89701
Phone: 775-445-3295
Fax: Not Reported
Contact: Mildred R. Wade, RN, MS, Director of Allied Health Programs
Email: wade@wncc.nevada.edu

GENERAL INFORMATION

Type of School: *2-Year College or University, Public* • Accreditation: *Northwestern Association of Schools and Colleges* • Total Enrollment: *5682*

PROGRAM INFORMATION

LPN/LVN Exit: *Yes* • NLNAC Accreditation: *Yes*

NURSING STUDENT PROFILE

Total Nursing Enrollment: *42* • Full-Time Enrollment: *34* • Part-Time Enrollment: *8* • Female Enrollment: *38* • Male Enrollment: *4* • Total New Admissions Who Enrolled for Fall: *28* • Total Graduates: *45*

FINANCES

Residential Annual Tuition: *$1,204* • Non-Residential Annual Tuition: *$3,199* • General Institution Fees: *$101* • Additional Nursing Fees: *$0*

NEW HAMPSHIRE COMMUNITY TECHNICAL COLLEGE—BERLIN

Address: 2020 Riverside Dr, Berlin, NH 3570
Phone: 603-752-1113
Fax: 603-752-6335
Contact: John D. Colbath, MSN, MBA, RNc, ARNP,
            Professor of Nursing and Program Director
Email: jcolbath@tec.nh.us

GENERAL INFORMATION

Type of School: *2-Year College or University, Public* •
Accreditation: *New England Association of Schools and Colleges* • Total Enrollment: *Not Reported*

PROGRAM INFORMATION

LPN/LVN Exit: *No* • NLNAC Accreditation: *Yes*

NURSING STUDENT PROFILE

Total Nursing Enrollment: *43* • Full-Time Enrollment: *24* • Part-Time Enrollment: *19* • Female Enrollment: *37* • Male Enrollment: *6* • Total New Admissions Who Enrolled for Fall: *32* • Total Graduates: *22*

FINANCES

Residential Annual Tuition: *Not Reported* • Non-Residential Annual Tuition: *Not Reported* • General Institution Fees: *Not Reported* • Additional Nursing Fees: *Not Reported*

NEW HAMPSHIRE COMMUNITY TECHNICAL COLLEGE— CLAREMONT/NASHUA

Address: One College Dr, Claremont, NH 03743-9707
Phone: 603-542-7744
Fax: 603-543-1844
Contact: Susan Jane Henderson, EdD, RN, Chairperson,
            Nursing
Email: shenderson@tec.nh.us

GENERAL INFORMATION

Type of School: *2-Year College or University, Public* •
Accreditation: *New England Association of Schools and Colleges* • Total Enrollment: *Not Reported*

PROGRAM INFORMATION

LPN/LVN Exit: *No* • NLNAC Accreditation: *Yes*

NURSING STUDENT PROFILE

Total Nursing Enrollment: *57* • Full-Time Enrollment: *30* • Part-Time Enrollment: *27* • Female Enrollment: *52* • Male Enrollment: *5* • Total New Admissions Who Enrolled for Fall: *29* • Total Graduates: *26*

FINANCES

Residential Annual Tuition: *$3,740* • Non-Residential Annual Tuition: *$8,602* • General Institution Fees: *$180* • Additional Nursing Fees: *$1,042*

NEW HAMPSHIRE COMMUNITY TECHNICAL COLLEGE—MANCHESTER

Address: 1066 Front St, Manchester, NH 3102
Phone: 603-668-6706
Fax: 603-668-5354
Contact: Lisa McCurley, MS, RN, CS-ANP, Director and
             Regional Chairperson
Email: lmccurley@tech.nh.us

GENERAL INFORMATION

Type of School: *2-Year College or University, Public* •
Accreditation: *New England Association of Schools and
Colleges* • Total Enrollment: *Not Reported*

PROGRAM INFORMATION

LPN/LVN Exit: *No* • NLNAC Accreditation: *Yes*

NURSING STUDENT PROFILE

Total Nursing Enrollment: *141* • Full-Time Enrollment: *64* •
Part-Time Enrollment: *77* • Female Enrollment: *129* • Male
Enrollment: *12* • Total New Admissions Who Enrolled for
Fall: *80* • Total Graduates: *49*

FINANCES

Residential Annual Tuition: *$2,000* • Non-Residential
Annual Tuition: *$4,692* • General Institution Fees: *$150* •
Additional Nursing Fees: *$400*

NEW HAMPSHIRE TECHNICAL INSTITUTE

Address: 11 Institute Dr, Concord, NH 03301-7400
Phone: 603-271-7177
Fax: 603-271-7148
Contact: Joyce P. Myles, RN, MA, Department Head
Email: jmyles@tec.nh.us

GENERAL INFORMATION

Type of School: *Governmental Agency, Public* • Accreditation:
New England Association of Schools and Colleges • Total
Enrollment: *Not Reported*

PROGRAM INFORMATION

LPN/LVN Exit: *Not Reported* • NLNAC Accreditation: *Yes*

NURSING STUDENT PROFILE

Total Nursing Enrollment: *172* • Full-Time Enrollment: *60* •
Part-Time Enrollment: *112* • Female Enrollment: *160* • Male
Enrollment: *12* • Total New Admissions Who Enrolled for
Fall: *97* • Total Graduates: *59*

FINANCES

Residential Annual Tuition: *$3,740* • Non-Residential
Annual Tuition: *$8,602* • General Institution Fees: *$374* •
Additional Nursing Fees: *$700*

RIVIER COLLEGE

Address: 420 Main St, Nashua, NH 3060
Phone: 603-897-8598
Fax: Not Reported
Contact: Susan Buchholz, RN, MS, Chair Associate
            Degree Program
Email: sbuchholz@river.edu

GENERAL INFORMATION

Type of School: *Other* • Accreditation: *None* • Total
Enrollment: *Not Reported*

PROGRAM INFORMATION

LPN/LVN Exit: *Not Reported* • NLNAC Accreditation: *Yes*

NURSING STUDENT PROFILE

Total Nursing Enrollment: *319* • Full-Time Enrollment:
124 • Part-Time Enrollment: *195* • Female Enrollment: *Not
Reported* • Male Enrollment: *Not Reported* • Total New
Admissions Who Enrolled for Fall: *83* • Total Graduates: *97*

FINANCES

Residential Annual Tuition: *Not Reported* • Non-Residential
Annual Tuition: *Not Reported* • General Institution Fees: *Not
Reported* • Additional Nursing Fees: *Not Reported*

ATLANTIC CAPE COMMUNITY COLLEGE

Address: 5100 Black Horse Pike, Mays Landing, NJ 8330
Phone: 609-343-5035
Fax: Not Reported
Contact: Barbara Warner, DNS, RNC, Chair, Allied
            Health
Email: bwarner@atlantic.edu

GENERAL INFORMATION

Type of School: *2-Year College or University, Public* •
Accreditation: *Middle States Association of Colleges and
Schools* • Total Enrollment: *7300*

PROGRAM INFORMATION

LPN/LVN Exit: *No* • NLNAC Accreditation: *Yes*

NURSING STUDENT PROFILE

Total Nursing Enrollment: *72* • Full-Time Enrollment: *72* •
Part-Time Enrollment: *0* • Female Enrollment: *63* • Male
Enrollment: *9* • Total New Admissions Who Enrolled for
Fall: *28* • Total Graduates: *34*

FINANCES

Residential Annual Tuition: *$2,100* • Non-Residential
Annual Tuition: *$2,310* • General Institution Fees: *Not
Reported* • Additional Nursing Fees: *$1,700*

BERGEN COMMUNITY COLLEGE

Address: 400 Paramus Road, Paramus, NJ 7652
Phone: 201-447-7181
Fax: 201-612-3876
Contact: Joan G. Murko, RN, MA, Director
Email: jmurko@bergen.edu

GENERAL INFORMATION

Type of School: *2-Year College or University, Public* •
Accreditation: *Middle States Association of Colleges and
Schools* • Total Enrollment: *12145*

PROGRAM INFORMATION

LPN/LVN Exit: *No* • NLNAC Accreditation: *Yes*

NURSING STUDENT PROFILE

Total Nursing Enrollment: *224* • Full-Time Enrollment: *31* •
Part-Time Enrollment: *193* • Female Enrollment: *203* • Male
Enrollment: *21* • Total New Admissions Who Enrolled for
Fall: *88* • Total Graduates: *76*

FINANCES

Residential Annual Tuition: *$2,285* • Non-Residential
Annual Tuition: *$5,056* • General Institution Fees: *Not
Reported* • Additional Nursing Fees: *$20*

BROOKDALE COMMUNITY COLLEGE

Address: 765 Newman Springs Road, Lincroft, NJ 7738
Phone: 732-224-2417
Fax: 732-224-2998
Contact: Maris A. Lown, RN, MS, Director, Health
           Sciences
Email: mlown@brookdalecc.edu

GENERAL INFORMATION

Type of School: *2-Year College or University, Public* •
Accreditation: *Middle States Association of Colleges and
Schools* • Total Enrollment: *12000*

PROGRAM INFORMATION

LPN/LVN Exit: *No* • NLNAC Accreditation: *Yes*

NURSING STUDENT PROFILE

Total Nursing Enrollment: *240* • Full-Time Enrollment: *62* •
Part-Time Enrollment: *178* • Female Enrollment: *218* • Male
Enrollment: *22* • Total New Admissions Who Enrolled for
Fall: *75* • Total Graduates: *101*

FINANCES

Residential Annual Tuition: *$1,256* • Non-Residential
Annual Tuition: *$3,375* • General Institution Fees: *$15* •
Additional Nursing Fees: *$30*

BURLINGTON COUNTY COLLEGE

Address: County Route 530, Pemberton, NJ 8068
Phone: 609-894-9311
Fax: 609-726-1781
Contact: Charlotte McCarrahor, MSN, RN, Director of Nursing and Allied Health
Email: cmccarra@bcc.edu

GENERAL INFORMATION

Type of School: *2-Year College or University, Public* • Accreditation: *Middle States Association of Colleges and Schools* • Total Enrollment: *6467*

PROGRAM INFORMATION

LPN/LVN Exit: *No* • NLNAC Accreditation: *Yes*

NURSING STUDENT PROFILE

Total Nursing Enrollment: *73* • Full-Time Enrollment: *2* • Part-Time Enrollment: *71* • Female Enrollment: *63* • Male Enrollment: *10* • Total New Admissions Who Enrolled for Fall: *30* • Total Graduates: *18*

FINANCES

Residential Annual Tuition: *$1,572* • Non-Residential Annual Tuition: *$3,360* • General Institution Fees: *$228* • Additional Nursing Fees: *$443*

COUNTY COLLEGE OF MORRIS

Address: 214 Center Grove Road, Randolph, NJ 7869
Phone: 973-328-5351
Fax: Not Reported
Contact: Joan M. Cunningham, RN, MA, Chairperson, Department of Nursing and Allied Health
Email: jcunningham@ccm.edu

GENERAL INFORMATION

Type of School: *2-Year College or University, Public* • Accreditation: *Middle States Association of Colleges and Schools* • Total Enrollment: *7798*

PROGRAM INFORMATION

LPN/LVN Exit: *No* • NLNAC Accreditation: *Yes*

NURSING STUDENT PROFILE

Total Nursing Enrollment: *337* • Full-Time Enrollment: *67* • Part-Time Enrollment: *270* • Female Enrollment: *312* • Male Enrollment: *25* • Total New Admissions Who Enrolled for Fall: *60* • Total Graduates: *94*

FINANCES

Residential Annual Tuition: *$2,618* • Non-Residential Annual Tuition: *$6,596* • General Institution Fees: *Not Reported* • Additional Nursing Fees: *$50*

CUMBERLAND COUNTY COLLEGE

Address: Box 517, Vineland, NJ 08362-0517
Phone: 856-691-8600
Fax: 856-691-9489
Contact: Marianne J. Hoy, MSN, Director of Nursing
Email: mhoy@cccnj.net

ESSEX COUNTY COLLEGE

Address: 303 University Avenue, Newark, NJ 7102
Phone: 973-877-1885
Fax: Not Reported
Contact: Marlene Dey, MSN, RN, CNS-C, NP-C,
            Associate Professor and Chairperson
Email: dey@essex.edu

GENERAL INFORMATION

Type of School: *2-Year College or University, Public* •
Accreditation: *Middle States Association of Colleges and
Schools* • Total Enrollment: *2739*

GENERAL INFORMATION

Type of School: *2-Year College or University, Public* •
Accreditation: *Middle States Association of Colleges and
Schools* • Total Enrollment: *8868*

PROGRAM INFORMATION

LPN/LVN Exit: *Yes* • NLNAC Accreditation: *Yes*

PROGRAM INFORMATION

LPN/LVN Exit: *No* • NLNAC Accreditation: *Yes*

NURSING STUDENT PROFILE

Total Nursing Enrollment: *89* • Full-Time Enrollment: *52* •
Part-Time Enrollment: *37* • Female Enrollment: *80* • Male
Enrollment: *9* • Total New Admissions Who Enrolled for
Fall: *59* • Total Graduates: *28*

NURSING STUDENT PROFILE

Total Nursing Enrollment: *75* • Full-Time Enrollment: *Not
Reported* • Part-Time Enrollment: *Not Reported* • Female
Enrollment: *67* • Male Enrollment: *8* • Total New
Admissions Who Enrolled for Fall: *36* • Total Graduates: *18*

FINANCES

Residential Annual Tuition: *$1,680* • Non-Residential
Annual Tuition: *$6,720* • General Institution Fees: *$336* •
Additional Nursing Fees: *$312*

FINANCES

Residential Annual Tuition: *$2,458* • Non-Residential
Annual Tuition: *$4,754* • General Institution Fees: *$100* •
Additional Nursing Fees: *$100*

Circle 46 on reader card   **See in-depth profile for more information**

FELICIAN COLLEGE

Address: 262 South Main Street, Lodi, NJ 07644-2117
Phone: 201-559-6030
Fax: 201-559-6188
Contact: Joann Frazier, RN, MA, Chair, Department of Associate Nursing
Email: frazierj@inet.felician.edu

GENERAL INFORMATION

Type of School: *4-Year College or University, Private (Religious)* • Accreditation: *Middle States Association of Colleges and Schools* • Total Enrollment: *1374*

PROGRAM INFORMATION

LPN/LVN Exit: *Yes* • NLNAC Accreditation: *Yes*

NURSING STUDENT PROFILE

Total Nursing Enrollment: *121* • Full-Time Enrollment: *73* • Part-Time Enrollment: *48* • Female Enrollment: *112* • Male Enrollment: *9* • Total New Admissions Who Enrolled for Fall: *Not Reported* • Total Graduates: *42*

FINANCES

Residential Annual Tuition: *$10,560* • Non-Residential Annual Tuition: *Not Reported* • General Institution Fees: *$250* • Additional Nursing Fees: *$150*

GLOUCESTER COUNTY COLLEGE

Address: 1400 Tanyard Road, Sewell, NJ 8080
Phone: 856-415-2178
Fax: 856-464-8463
Contact: Yvonne M. Burgess, MSN, APRN, BC, Chairperson Division of Nursing, Allied Health and Science
Email: yburgess@gccnj.edu

GENERAL INFORMATION

Type of School: *2-Year College or University, Public* • Accreditation: *Middle States Association of Colleges and Schools* • Total Enrollment: *4901*

PROGRAM INFORMATION

LPN/LVN Exit: *No* • NLNAC Accreditation: *Yes*

NURSING STUDENT PROFILE

Total Nursing Enrollment: *100* • Full-Time Enrollment: *40* • Part-Time Enrollment: *60* • Female Enrollment: *92* • Male Enrollment: *8* • Total New Admissions Who Enrolled for Fall: *63* • Total Graduates: *27*

FINANCES

Residential Annual Tuition: *$1,600* • Non-Residential Annual Tuition: *$1,650* • General Institution Fees: *$250* • Additional Nursing Fees: *$250*

Circle 49 on reader card   See in-depth profile for more information

MERCER COUNTY COMMUNITY COLLEGE

Address: 1200 Old Trenton Rd, Box B, Trenton, NJ 8690
Phone: 609-586-4800
Fax: Not Reported
Contact: Clara G. Lidz, MSN, RN, Director
Email: lidz@mccc.edu

GENERAL INFORMATION

Type of School: *2-Year College or University, Public* •
Accreditation: *Middle States Association of Colleges and Schools* • Total Enrollment: *292*

PROGRAM INFORMATION

LPN/LVN Exit: *No* • NLNAC Accreditation: *Yes*

NURSING STUDENT PROFILE

Total Nursing Enrollment: *106* • Full-Time Enrollment: *19* • Part-Time Enrollment: *87* • Female Enrollment: *95* • Male Enrollment: *11* • Total New Admissions Who Enrolled for Fall: *40* • Total Graduates: *31*

FINANCES

Residential Annual Tuition: *$2,328* • Non-Residential Annual Tuition: *$3,888* • General Institution Fees: *$17* • Additional Nursing Fees: *$100*

RARITAN VALLEY COMMUNITY COLLEGE

Address: PO Box 3300, Somerville, NJ 8876
Phone: 908-218-8877
Fax: 908-429-1125
Contact: Maureen S. Hreha, RN,MSN,PNP, Chairperson
           and Associate Professor
Email: mhreha@raritanval.edu

GENERAL INFORMATION

Type of School: *2-Year College or University, Public* •
Accreditation: *Middle States Association of Colleges and Schools* • Total Enrollment: *5751*

PROGRAM INFORMATION

LPN/LVN Exit: *Yes* • NLNAC Accreditation: *Yes*

NURSING STUDENT PROFILE

Total Nursing Enrollment: *262* • Full-Time Enrollment: *78* • Part-Time Enrollment: *184* • Female Enrollment: *237* • Male Enrollment: *25* • Total New Admissions Who Enrolled for Fall: *178* • Total Graduates: *64*

FINANCES

Residential Annual Tuition: *$2,555* • Non-Residential Annual Tuition: *$5,110* • General Institution Fees: *$13* • Additional Nursing Fees: *Not Reported*

UNIVERSITY OF MEDICAL DENTISTRY OF NEW JERSEY/NJIT JOINT BSN PROGRAM

Address: 65 Bergen Street, Rm. 1141, Newark, NJ 07107-3001
Phone: 732-906-4660
Fax: Not Reported
Contact: Ellen Ehrlich, EdD, RN, On-site Faculty Administrator
Email: ellen@nac.net

GENERAL INFORMATION

Type of School: *Other, Public* • Accreditation: *Middle States Association of Colleges and Schools* • Total Enrollment: *600*

PROGRAM INFORMATION

LPN/LVN Exit: *No* • NLNAC Accreditation: *Yes*

NURSING STUDENT PROFILE

Total Nursing Enrollment: *67* • Full-Time Enrollment: *19* • Part-Time Enrollment: *48* • Female Enrollment: *57* • Male Enrollment: *10* • Total New Admissions Who Enrolled for Fall: *40* • Total Graduates: *26*

FINANCES

Residential Annual Tuition: *$1,573* • Non-Residential Annual Tuition: *$3,146* • General Institution Fees: *$15* • Additional Nursing Fees: *$250*

ALBUQUERQUE TECHNICAL VOCATIONAL INSTITUTE

Address: 525 Buena Vista SE, Albuquerque, NM 87106
Phone: 505-224-4144
Fax: Not Reported
Contact: Patricia S Stephens, MSN, RN, MA, Director of Nursing Programs
Email: pats@tvi.cc.nm.us

GENERAL INFORMATION

Type of School: *2-Year College or University, Public* • Accreditation: *North Central Association of Colleges and Schools* • Total Enrollment: *18000*

PROGRAM INFORMATION

LPN/LVN Exit: *No* • NLNAC Accreditation: *Yes*

NURSING STUDENT PROFILE

Total Nursing Enrollment: *145* • Full-Time Enrollment: *29* • Part-Time Enrollment: *116* • Female Enrollment: *126* • Male Enrollment: *19* • Total New Admissions Who Enrolled for Fall: *52* • Total Graduates: *95*

FINANCES

Residential Annual Tuition: *$888* • Non-Residential Annual Tuition: *$3,802* • General Institution Fees: *$67* • Additional Nursing Fees: *Not Reported*

CLOVIS COMMUNITY COLLEGE

Address: 417 Shepps Boulevard, Clovis, NM 88101
Phone: 505-769-4954
Fax: 505-769-4190
Contact: Robin Jones, MSN, RN, Nursing Program
          Director and Chair, Allied Health and Human
          Services
Email: jonesr@clovis.cc.nm.us

GENERAL INFORMATION

Type of School: *2-Year College or University, Public* •
Accreditation: *North Central Association of Colleges and
Schools* • Total Enrollment: *3838*

PROGRAM INFORMATION

LPN/LVN Exit: *Yes* • NLNAC Accreditation: *Yes*

NURSING STUDENT PROFILE

Total Nursing Enrollment: *51* • Full-Time Enrollment: *51* •
Part-Time Enrollment: *0* • Female Enrollment: *46* • Male
Enrollment: *5* • Total New Admissions Who Enrolled for
Fall: *21* • Total Graduates: *50*

FINANCES

Residential Annual Tuition: *$888* • Non-Residential Annual
Tuition: *$1,320* • General Institution Fees: *$0* • Additional
Nursing Fees: *$185*

EASTERN NEW MEXICO UNIVERSITY-ROSWELL

Address: PO Box 6000, Roswell, NM 88202-6000
Phone: 505-624-7237
Fax: Not Reported
Contact: Tammy Bennett, MSN,BSN, Nursing Instructor
Email: BennettT@lib.enmuros.cc.nm.us

GENERAL INFORMATION

Type of School: *2-Year College or University, Public* •
Accreditation: *North Central Association of Colleges and
Schools* • Total Enrollment: *2666*

PROGRAM INFORMATION

LPN/LVN Exit: *Yes* • NLNAC Accreditation: *Yes*

NURSING STUDENT PROFILE

Total Nursing Enrollment: *47* • Full-Time Enrollment: *45* •
Part-Time Enrollment: *2* • Female Enrollment: *41* • Male
Enrollment: *6* • Total New Admissions Who Enrolled for
Fall: *29* • Total Graduates: *36*

FINANCES

Residential Annual Tuition: *$684* • Non-Residential Annual
Tuition: *$1,944* • General Institution Fees: *$54* • Additional
Nursing Fees: *$20*

LUNA COMMUNITY COLLEGE

Address: PO Box 1510, Las Vegas, NM 87701
Phone: 505-454-2524
Fax: 505-454-2588
Contact: Beatrice Hurtado, MSN, RN, Nursing Director
Email: bhurtado@luna.cc.nm.us

GENERAL INFORMATION

Type of School: *2-Year College or University, Public* • Accreditation: *North Central Association of Colleges and Schools* • Total Enrollment: *1920*

PROGRAM INFORMATION

LPN/LVN Exit: *Yes* • NLNAC Accreditation: *No*

NURSING STUDENT PROFILE

Total Nursing Enrollment: *49* • Full-Time Enrollment: *49* • Part-Time Enrollment: *0* • Female Enrollment: *42* • Male Enrollment: *7* • Total New Admissions Who Enrolled for Fall: *31* • Total Graduates: *8*

FINANCES

Residential Annual Tuition: *$444* • Non-Residential Annual Tuition: *$912* • General Institution Fees: *$44* • Additional Nursing Fees: *$88*

NEW MEXICO JUNIOR COLLEGE

Address: 5317 Lovington Highway, Hobbs, NM 88240
Phone: 505-392-5714
Fax: 505-392-0368
Contact: Karen Cummings, MSN, RN, Director of Health
Email: kcummings@nmjc.cc.nm.us

GENERAL INFORMATION

Type of School: *2-Year College or University, Public* • Accreditation: *North Central Association of Colleges and Schools* • Total Enrollment: *98*

PROGRAM INFORMATION

LPN/LVN Exit: *Yes* • NLNAC Accreditation: *Yes*

NURSING STUDENT PROFILE

Total Nursing Enrollment: *98* • Full-Time Enrollment: *98* • Part-Time Enrollment: *0* • Female Enrollment: *93* • Male Enrollment: *5* • Total New Admissions Who Enrolled for Fall: *60* • Total Graduates: *38*

FINANCES

Residential Annual Tuition: *$204* • Non-Residential Annual Tuition: *$468* • General Institution Fees: *$162* • Additional Nursing Fees: *$187*

NEW MEXICO STATE UNIVERSITY

Address: PO Box 30001, Las Cruces, NM 88003-8001
Phone: 505-527-7335
Fax: Not Reported
Contact: Leslie Robbins, RNCS, MSN, Program
Coordinator
Email: lerobbin@nmsu.edu

GENERAL INFORMATION

Type of School: *4-Year College or University, Public* •
Accreditation: *North Central Association of Colleges and
Schools* • Total Enrollment: *Not Reported*

PROGRAM INFORMATION

LPN/LVN Exit: *Not Reported* • NLNAC Accreditation: *Yes*

NURSING STUDENT PROFILE

Total Nursing Enrollment: *62* • Full-Time Enrollment: *60* •
Part-Time Enrollment: *2* • Female Enrollment: *62* • Male
Enrollment: *0* • Total New Admissions Who Enrolled for
Fall: *35* • Total Graduates: *15*

FINANCES

Residential Annual Tuition: *$816* • Non-Residential Annual
Tuition: *$2,112* • General Institution Fees: *$24* • Additional
Nursing Fees: *$35*

NEW MEXICO STATE UNIVERSITY—ALAMOGORDO

Address: 2400 North Scenic Drive, Alamogordo, NM
88317
Phone: 505-439-3662
Fax: 505-439-3684
Contact: Dennis L. Ellis, MSN, NCMC, CNAA, Nursing
Area Coordinator
Email: dellis@nmsua.nmsu.edu

GENERAL INFORMATION

Type of School: *4-Year College or University, Public* •
Accreditation: *North Central Association of Colleges and
Schools* • Total Enrollment: *Not Reported*

PROGRAM INFORMATION

LPN/LVN Exit: *No* • NLNAC Accreditation: *Yes*

NURSING STUDENT PROFILE

Total Nursing Enrollment: *56* • Full-Time Enrollment: *56* •
Part-Time Enrollment: *0* • Female Enrollment: *52* • Male
Enrollment: *4* • Total New Admissions Who Enrolled for
Fall: *22* • Total Graduates: *30*

FINANCES

Residential Annual Tuition: *$864* • Non-Residential Annual
Tuition: *$2,208* • General Institution Fees: *$15* • Additional
Nursing Fees: *$20*

NEW MEXICO STATE UNIVERSITY—CARLSBAD

Address: 1500 University Drive, Carlsbad, NM 88220
Phone: 505-234-9301
Fax: 505-885-4951
Contact: Sharon Souter, RN, BSN, MSN, Program Director
Email: ssouter@cavern.nmsu.edu

GENERAL INFORMATION

Type of School: *2-Year College or University, Public* •
Accreditation: *North Central Association of Colleges and Schools* • Total Enrollment: *1011*

PROGRAM INFORMATION

LPN/LVN Exit: *Yes* • NLNAC Accreditation: *Yes*

NURSING STUDENT PROFILE

Total Nursing Enrollment: *63* • Full-Time Enrollment: *63* • Part-Time Enrollment: *0* • Female Enrollment: *61* • Male Enrollment: *2* • Total New Admissions Who Enrolled for Fall: *33* • Total Graduates: *18*

FINANCES

Residential Annual Tuition: *$840* • Non-Residential Annual Tuition: *$2,208* • General Institution Fees: *Not Reported* • Additional Nursing Fees: *$45*

NORTHERN NEW MEXICO COMMUNITY COLLEGE

Address: 921 Paseo de Onate, Espanola, NM 87532
Phone: 505-747-2209
Fax: Not Reported
Contact: Ramona Gonzales, BSN, RN, Director of Nursing Education
Email: ramonag@nnm.cc.nm.us

GENERAL INFORMATION

Type of School: *2-Year College or University, Public* •
Accreditation: *North Central Association of Colleges and Schools* • Total Enrollment: *Not Reported*

PROGRAM INFORMATION

LPN/LVN Exit: *Yes* • NLNAC Accreditation: *No*

NURSING STUDENT PROFILE

Total Nursing Enrollment: *37* • Full-Time Enrollment: *37* • Part-Time Enrollment: *0* • Female Enrollment: *33* • Male Enrollment: *4* • Total New Admissions Who Enrolled for Fall: *37* • Total Graduates: *14*

FINANCES

Residential Annual Tuition: *$576* • Non-Residential Annual Tuition: *$1,392* • General Institution Fees: *$46* • Additional Nursing Fees: *$175*

SAN JUAN COLLEGE

Address:　4601 College Boulevard, Farmington, NM
　　　　　87402
Phone:　505-599-0224
Fax:　Not Reported
Contact:　Judy Lund-Green, RN, BSN, MSN, Director of
　　　　　the Nursing Program
Email:　Lund_Green@sjc.cc.nm.us

GENERAL INFORMATION

Type of School: *2-Year College or University, Public* •
Accreditation: *North Central Association of Colleges and
Schools* • Total Enrollment: *8300*

PROGRAM INFORMATION

LPN/LVN Exit: *No* • NLNAC Accreditation: *Yes*

NURSING STUDENT PROFILE

Total Nursing Enrollment: *71* • Full-Time Enrollment: *71* •
Part-Time Enrollment: *0* • Female Enrollment: *56* • Male
Enrollment: *15* • Total New Admissions Who Enrolled for
Fall: *32* • Total Graduates: *29*

FINANCES

Residential Annual Tuition: *$680* • Non-Residential Annual
Tuition: *$840* • General Institution Fees: *$0* • Additional
Nursing Fees: *$1,000*

SANTA FE COMMUNITY COLLEGE—SANTA FE

Address:　6401 Richards Avenue, Santa Fe, NM 87505
Phone:　505-428-1324
Fax:　Not Reported
Contact:　Sue MacMillan, MSN, RN, Director
Email:　smacmillan@santa-fe.cc.nm.us

GENERAL INFORMATION

Type of School: *2-Year College or University, Public* •
Accreditation: *North Central Association of Colleges and
Schools* • Total Enrollment: *5000*

PROGRAM INFORMATION

LPN/LVN Exit: *No* • NLNAC Accreditation: *Yes*

NURSING STUDENT PROFILE

Total Nursing Enrollment: *44* • Full-Time Enrollment: *30* •
Part-Time Enrollment: *14* • Female Enrollment: *36* • Male
Enrollment: *8* • Total New Admissions Who Enrolled for
Fall: *25* • Total Graduates: *15*

FINANCES

Residential Annual Tuition: *$504* • Non-Residential Annual
Tuition: *$810* • General Institution Fees: *$20* • Additional
Nursing Fees: *$80*

UNIVERSITY OF NEW MEXICO—GALLUP

Address: 200 College Rd, Gallup, NM 87131
Phone: 505-863-7516
Fax: Not Reported
Contact: Jane Bruker, RNCS, MSN, Coordinator
Email: JKBru@AOL.COM

GENERAL INFORMATION

Type of School: *4-Year College or University, Public* •
Accreditation: *North Central Association of Colleges and Schools* • Total Enrollment: *23659*

PROGRAM INFORMATION

LPN/LVN Exit: *No* • NLNAC Accreditation: *Yes*

NURSING STUDENT PROFILE

Total Nursing Enrollment: *75* • Full-Time Enrollment: *75* •
Part-Time Enrollment: *0* • Female Enrollment: *70* • Male
Enrollment: *5* • Total New Admissions Who Enrolled for
Fall: *16* • Total Graduates: *19*

FINANCES

Residential Annual Tuition: *$1,657* • Non-Residential
Annual Tuition: *$5,977* • General Institution Fees: *$0* •
Additional Nursing Fees: *$50*

WESTERN NEW MEXICO UNIVERSITY

Address: PO Box 680, Silver City, NM 88062
Phone: 505-574-5140
Fax: Not Reported
Contact: Patricia McIntire, MS, C-FNP, Chair, Nursing
Department
Email: mcintirep@silver.wnmu.edu

GENERAL INFORMATION

Type of School: *4-Year College or University, Public* •
Accreditation: *North Central Association of Colleges and Schools* • Total Enrollment: *2585*

PROGRAM INFORMATION

LPN/LVN Exit: *No* • NLNAC Accreditation: *Yes*

NURSING STUDENT PROFILE

Total Nursing Enrollment: *32* • Full-Time Enrollment: *30* •
Part-Time Enrollment: *2* • Female Enrollment: *26* • Male
Enrollment: *6* • Total New Admissions Who Enrolled for
Fall: *20* • Total Graduates: *17*

FINANCES

Residential Annual Tuition: *$1,768* • Non-Residential
Annual Tuition: *$6,156* • General Institution Fees: *$0* •
Additional Nursing Fees: *$80*

ADIRONDACK COMMUNITY COLLEGE

Address: 640 Bay Rd., Queensbury, NY 12804
Phone: 518-743-2300
Fax: 518-743-2288
Contact: Normadine Keller, MSN, RN, Program Director
Email: kellern@acc.sunyacc.edu

GENERAL INFORMATION

Type of School: *2-Year College or University, Private (Independent)* • Accreditation: *Middle States Association of Colleges and Schools* • Total Enrollment: *3000*

PROGRAM INFORMATION

LPN/LVN Exit: *No* • NLNAC Accreditation: *Yes*

NURSING STUDENT PROFILE

Total Nursing Enrollment: *101* • Full-Time Enrollment: *57* • Part-Time Enrollment: *44* • Female Enrollment: *89* • Male Enrollment: *12* • Total New Admissions Who Enrolled for Fall: *43* • Total Graduates: *36*

FINANCES

Residential Annual Tuition: *$2,300* • Non-Residential Annual Tuition: *$4,600* • General Institution Fees: *$1,150* • Additional Nursing Fees: *$83*

BOROUGH OF MANHATTAN COMMUNITY COLLEGE

Address: 199 Chambers St., New York, NY 10007
Phone: 212-220-8230
Fax: 212-346-8698
Contact: Barbara Tacinelli, MA, RN, Chairperson
Email: btacinelli@bmcc.cuny.edu

GENERAL INFORMATION

Type of School: *2-Year College or University, Public* • Accreditation: *Middle States Association of Colleges and Schools* • Total Enrollment: *15000*

PROGRAM INFORMATION

LPN/LVN Exit: *No* • NLNAC Accreditation: *Yes*

NURSING STUDENT PROFILE

Total Nursing Enrollment: *398* • Full-Time Enrollment: *259* • Part-Time Enrollment: *139* • Female Enrollment: *348* • Male Enrollment: *50* • Total New Admissions Who Enrolled for Fall: *112* • Total Graduates: *108*

FINANCES

Residential Annual Tuition: *$1,250* • Non-Residential Annual Tuition: *$1,538* • General Institution Fees: *$80* • Additional Nursing Fees: *$20*

BRONX COMMUNITY COLLEGE

Address: West 181 St. and University Ave., Bronx, NY
            10453
Phone: 718-289-5426
Fax: 718-289-6059
Contact: Lois Augustus, MA, RN, Associate Professor
Email: lois.augustus@bcc.cuny.edu

GENERAL INFORMATION

Type of School: *2-Year College or University, Public* •
Accreditation: *Middle States Association of Colleges and
Schools* • Total Enrollment: *7200*

PROGRAM INFORMATION

LPN/LVN Exit: *No* • NLNAC Accreditation: *Yes*

NURSING STUDENT PROFILE

Total Nursing Enrollment: *130* • Full-Time Enrollment: *Not
Reported* • Part-Time Enrollment: *Not Reported* • Female
Enrollment: *113* • Male Enrollment: *17* • Total New
Admissions Who Enrolled for Fall: *Not Reported* • Total
Graduates: *27*

FINANCES

Residential Annual Tuition: *$2,500* • Non-Residential
Annual Tuition: *$3,076* • General Institution Fees: *$190* •
Additional Nursing Fees: *$15*

BROOME COMMUNITY COLLEGE

Address: P.O. Box 1017, Binghamton, NY 13902
Phone: 607-778-5059
Fax: 607-778-5467
Contact: Claire Ligeikis-Clayton, RN, EdD, Chairperson
Email: ligeikis_c@sunybroome.edu

GENERAL INFORMATION

Type of School: *2-Year College or University, Private
(Independent)* • Accreditation: *Middle States Association of
Colleges and Schools* • Total Enrollment: *5472*

PROGRAM INFORMATION

LPN/LVN Exit: *No* • NLNAC Accreditation: *Yes*

NURSING STUDENT PROFILE

Total Nursing Enrollment: *157* • Full-Time Enrollment:
130 • Part-Time Enrollment: *27* • Female Enrollment: *142* •
Male Enrollment: *15* • Total New Admissions Who Enrolled
for Fall: *102* • Total Graduates: *51*

FINANCES

Residential Annual Tuition: *$2,438* • Non-Residential
Annual Tuition: *$4,876* • General Institution Fees: *$180* •
Additional Nursing Fees: *$400*

CAYUGA COMMUNITY COLLEGE

Address: 197 Franklin St., Auburn, NY 13021
Phone: 315-255-1743
Fax: 315-255-1996
Contact: Vicki Cook Condie, MSN, RN, CAS, Director
             of Nursing
Email: condiev@cayuga-cc.edu

GENERAL INFORMATION

Type of School: *2-Year College or University, Public* •
Accreditation: *Middle States Association of Colleges and
Schools* • Total Enrollment: *2498*

PROGRAM INFORMATION

LPN/LVN Exit: *No* • NLNAC Accreditation: *Yes*

NURSING STUDENT PROFILE

Total Nursing Enrollment: *81* • Full-Time Enrollment: *46* •
Part-Time Enrollment: *35* • Female Enrollment: *75* • Male
Enrollment: *6* • Total New Admissions Who Enrolled for
Fall: *44* • Total Graduates: *39*

FINANCES

Residential Annual Tuition: *$2,500* • Non-Residential
Annual Tuition: *$5,000* • General Institution Fees: *Not
Reported* • Additional Nursing Fees: *Not Reported*

CLINTON COMMUNITY COLLEGE

Address: 136 Clinton Point Dr., Plattsburg, NY 12901
Phone: 518-562-4162
Fax: 518-562-4158
Contact: Patricia L. Shinn, Masters Degree, Acting
             Associate Academic Dean and Director of
             Nursing
Email: shinpl@clinconcc.suny.edu

GENERAL INFORMATION

Type of School: *2-Year College or University, Public* •
Accreditation: *Middle States Association of Colleges and
Schools* • Total Enrollment: *1700*

PROGRAM INFORMATION

LPN/LVN Exit: *No* • NLNAC Accreditation: *Yes*

NURSING STUDENT PROFILE

Total Nursing Enrollment: *85* • Full-Time Enrollment: *55* •
Part-Time Enrollment: *30* • Female Enrollment: *77* • Male
Enrollment: *8* • Total New Admissions Who Enrolled for
Fall: *44* • Total Graduates: *30*

FINANCES

Residential Annual Tuition: *$2,320* • Non-Residential
Annual Tuition: *$4,350* • General Institution Fees: *$86* •
Additional Nursing Fees: *$50*

THE COLLEGE OF STATEN ISLAND

Address: 2800 Victory Boulvard, Marcus Hall, Staten Island, NY 10314
Phone: 718-982-3810
Fax: 718-982-3813
Contact: Linda E Reese, MA, RN, Chairperson, Dept. of Nursing
Email: reese@postbox.csi.cuny.edu

GENERAL INFORMATION

Type of School: *4-Year College or University, Public* • Accreditation: *Middle States Association of Colleges and Schools* • Total Enrollment: *11000*

PROGRAM INFORMATION

LPN/LVN Exit: *Not Reported* • NLNAC Accreditation: *Yes*

NURSING STUDENT PROFILE

Total Nursing Enrollment: *176* • Full-Time Enrollment: *60* • Part-Time Enrollment: *116* • Female Enrollment: *151* • Male Enrollment: *25* • Total New Admissions Who Enrolled for Fall: *40* • Total Graduates: *75*

FINANCES

Residential Annual Tuition: *$3,200* • Non-Residential Annual Tuition: *$6,800* • General Institution Fees: *$79* • Additional Nursing Fees: *$1,220*

CORNING COMMUNITY COLLEGE

Address: 1 Academic Dr., Corning, NY 14830
Phone: 607-962-9241
Fax: 607-962-9287
Contact: Gail Ropelewski-Ryan, MS, RN, Chairperson, Division of Nurse Education and Health
Email: ryan@corning-cc.edu

GENERAL INFORMATION

Type of School: *2-Year College or University, Public* • Accreditation: *Middle States Association of Colleges and Schools* • Total Enrollment: *Not Reported*

PROGRAM INFORMATION

LPN/LVN Exit: *No* • NLNAC Accreditation: *Yes*

NURSING STUDENT PROFILE

Total Nursing Enrollment: *138* • Full-Time Enrollment: *93* • Part-Time Enrollment: *45* • Female Enrollment: *125* • Male Enrollment: *13* • Total New Admissions Who Enrolled for Fall: *97* • Total Graduates: *31*

FINANCES

Residential Annual Tuition: *$1,287* • Non-Residential Annual Tuition: *$2,574* • General Institution Fees: *$365* • Additional Nursing Fees: *$127*

CROUSE HOSPITAL SCHOOL OF NURSING

Address: 736 Irving Ave., Syracuse, NY 13210
Phone: 315-470-7481
Fax: 315-470-7925
Contact: Sherry Pearsall, RN, BSN, MSN, CAS, Director
Email: sherrypearsall@crouse.org

GENERAL INFORMATION

Type of School: *Hospital, Private (Independent)* •
Accreditation: *None* • Total Enrollment: *180*

PROGRAM INFORMATION

LPN/LVN Exit: *No* • NLNAC Accreditation: *No*

NURSING STUDENT PROFILE

Total Nursing Enrollment: *180* • Full-Time Enrollment: *127* • Part-Time Enrollment: *53* • Female Enrollment: *172* • Male Enrollment: *8* • Total New Admissions Who Enrolled for Fall: *75* • Total Graduates: *65*

FINANCES

Residential Annual Tuition: *$6,129* • Non-Residential Annual Tuition: *$9,682* • General Institution Fees: *$250* • Additional Nursing Fees: *$99*

DUTCHESS COMMUNITY COLLEGE

Address: 53 Pendell Rd., Poughkeepsie, NY 12601
Phone: 845-431-8571
Fax: 845-431-8991
Contact: Toni Doherty, MSN, RN, Department Head
Email: doherty@sunydutchess.edu

GENERAL INFORMATION

Type of School: *2-Year College or University, Public* •
Accreditation: *Middle States Association of Colleges and Schools* • Total Enrollment: *6739*

PROGRAM INFORMATION

LPN/LVN Exit: *Not Reported* • NLNAC Accreditation: *Yes*

NURSING STUDENT PROFILE

Total Nursing Enrollment: *537* • Full-Time Enrollment: *Not Reported* • Part-Time Enrollment: *Not Reported* • Female Enrollment: *Not Reported* • Male Enrollment: *Not Reported* • Total New Admissions Who Enrolled for Fall: *98* • Total Graduates: *67*

FINANCES

Residential Annual Tuition: *$2,300* • Non-Residential Annual Tuition: *$4,600* • General Institution Fees: *$95* • Additional Nursing Fees: *$100*

ELLIS HOSPITAL

Address: 1101 Nott St., Schenectady, NY 12308
Phone: 518-243-4471
Fax: 518-243-4470
Contact: Mary Lee Pollard, RNCS, MS, Director
Email: pollardM@shine.org

GENERAL INFORMATION

Type of School: *Hospital, Private (Independent)* •
Accreditation: *None* • Total Enrollment: *69*

PROGRAM INFORMATION

LPN/LVN Exit: *No* • NLNAC Accreditation: *No*

NURSING STUDENT PROFILE

Total Nursing Enrollment: *69* • Full-Time Enrollment: *44* •
Part-Time Enrollment: *25* • Female Enrollment: *66* • Male
Enrollment: *3* • Total New Admissions Who Enrolled for
Fall: *49* • Total Graduates: *18*

FINANCES

Residential Annual Tuition: *$4,400* • Non-Residential
Annual Tuition: *$5,820* • General Institution Fees: *$0* •
Additional Nursing Fees: *$100*

ERIE COMMUNITY COLLEGE

Address: 6805 Main St., Williamsville, NY 14221
Phone: 716-851-1357
Fax: 716-851-1349
Contact: Theresa M. Ranne, RN, MEd, MS, EdD,
Professor and Department Head of Nursing
Email: ranne@ecc.edu

GENERAL INFORMATION

Type of School: *2-Year College or University, Public* •
Accreditation: *Middle States Association of Colleges and
Schools* • Total Enrollment: *Not Reported*

PROGRAM INFORMATION

LPN/LVN Exit: *No* • NLNAC Accreditation: *Yes*

NURSING STUDENT PROFILE

Total Nursing Enrollment: *215* • Full-Time Enrollment:
145 • Part-Time Enrollment: *70* • Female Enrollment: *189* •
Male Enrollment: *26* • Total New Admissions Who Enrolled
for Fall: *97* • Total Graduates: *116*

FINANCES

Residential Annual Tuition: *Not Reported* • Non-Residential
Annual Tuition: *Not Reported* • General Institution Fees: *Not
Reported* • Additional Nursing Fees: *Not Reported*

EXCELSIOR COLLEGE

Address:　7 Columbia Cr., Albany, NY 12203
Phone:　518-464-8776
Fax:　518-464-8777
Contact:　Marianne Lettus, EdD, RN, Associate Dean
Email:　mlettus@excelsior.edu

GENERAL INFORMATION

Type of School: *4-Year College or University, Private (Independent)* • Accreditation: *Middle States Association of Colleges and Schools* • Total Enrollment: *17250*

PROGRAM INFORMATION

LPN/LVN Exit: *Not Reported* • NLNAC Accreditation: *Yes*

NURSING STUDENT PROFILE

Total Nursing Enrollment: *7549* • Full-Time Enrollment: *0* • Part-Time Enrollment: *7549* • Female Enrollment: *6012* • Male Enrollment: *1537* • Total New Admissions Who Enrolled for Fall: *3598* • Total Graduates: *1607*

FINANCES

Residential Annual Tuition: *Not Reported* • Non-Residential Annual Tuition: *Not Reported* • General Institution Fees: *Not Reported* • Additional Nursing Fees: *Not Reported*

FINGER LAKES COMMUNITY COLLEGE

Address:　4355 Lakeshore Dr., Canandaigua, NY 14424
Phone:　716-394-3500
Fax:　716-394-5005
Contact:　Ann P Robinson, RN, MS, Professor and
　　　　　Chairperson
Email:　robinsap@flcc.edu

GENERAL INFORMATION

Type of School: *2-Year College or University, Public* • Accreditation: *Middle States Association of Colleges and Schools* • Total Enrollment: *4667*

PROGRAM INFORMATION

LPN/LVN Exit: *No* • NLNAC Accreditation: *Yes*

NURSING STUDENT PROFILE

Total Nursing Enrollment: *102* • Full-Time Enrollment: *46* • Part-Time Enrollment: *56* • Female Enrollment: *94* • Male Enrollment: *8* • Total New Admissions Who Enrolled for Fall: *73* • Total Graduates: *46*

FINANCES

Residential Annual Tuition: *$2,350* • Non-Residential Annual Tuition: *$4,700* • General Institution Fees: *$1,175* • Additional Nursing Fees: *$87*

FULTON-MONTGOMERY COMMUNITY COLLEGE

Address: 2805 St. Hwy. 67, Johnstown, NY 12095
Phone: 518-762-5651
Fax: 518-762-4035
Contact: Judy Munn, MS, RN, Director of Nursing
Email: jmunn@fmcc.suny.edu

GENERAL INFORMATION

Type of School: *2-Year College or University, Public* •
Accreditation: *Middle States Association of Colleges and Schools* • Total Enrollment: *1949*

PROGRAM INFORMATION

LPN/LVN Exit: *Not Reported* • NLNAC Accreditation: *No*

NURSING STUDENT PROFILE

Total Nursing Enrollment: *57* • Full-Time Enrollment: *29* • Part-Time Enrollment: *28* • Female Enrollment: *49* • Male Enrollment: *8* • Total New Admissions Who Enrolled for Fall: *32* • Total Graduates: *26*

FINANCES

Residential Annual Tuition: *$2,380* • Non-Residential Annual Tuition: *$4,760* • General Institution Fees: *$300* • Additional Nursing Fees: *$55*

HELENE FULD COLLEGE OF NURSING

Address: 26 East 120th Street, New York, NY 10035
Phone: 212-423-1000
Fax: Not Reported
Contact: Margaret Wines, PhD, RN, President
Email: drpwines@aol.com

GENERAL INFORMATION

Type of School: *2-Year College or University, Other* •
Accreditation: *None* • Total Enrollment: *Not Reported*

PROGRAM INFORMATION

LPN/LVN Exit: *No* • NLNAC Accreditation: *Yes*

NURSING STUDENT PROFILE

Total Nursing Enrollment: *188* • Full-Time Enrollment: *100* • Part-Time Enrollment: *88* • Female Enrollment: *170* • Male Enrollment: *18* • Total New Admissions Who Enrolled for Fall: *87* • Total Graduates: *129*

FINANCES

Residential Annual Tuition: *$10,472* • Non-Residential Annual Tuition: *$10,472* • General Institution Fees: *$64* • Additional Nursing Fees: *Not Reported*

HUDSON VALLEY COMMUNITY COLLEGE

Address: 80 Vandenburgh Ave., Troy, NY 12180
Phone: 518-629-7469
Fax: 518-629-8121
Contact: Dicey O'Malley, PhD, RN, Department
            Chairperson
Email: omalldic@hvcc.edu

GENERAL INFORMATION

Type of School: *2-Year College or University, Public* •
Accreditation: *Middle States Association of Colleges and
Schools* • Total Enrollment: *10000*

PROGRAM INFORMATION

LPN/LVN Exit: *No* • NLNAC Accreditation: *Yes*

NURSING STUDENT PROFILE

Total Nursing Enrollment: *242* • Full-Time Enrollment:
150 • Part-Time Enrollment: *92* • Female Enrollment: *215* •
Male Enrollment: *27* • Total New Admissions Who Enrolled
for Fall: *114* • Total Graduates: *53*

FINANCES

Residential Annual Tuition: *$2,350* • Non-Residential
Annual Tuition: *$6,125* • General Institution Fees: *$100* •
Additional Nursing Fees: *$70*

JAMESTOWN COMMUNITY COLLEGE

Address: 525 Falconer St., Jamestown, NY 14701
Phone: 716-665-5220
Fax: 716-665-3679
Contact: Dawn Columbare, RN, MS, Director, Nursing
            Education
Email: dawncolumbare@mail.sunyjcc.edu

GENERAL INFORMATION

Type of School: *2-Year College or University, Public* •
Accreditation: *Middle States Association of Colleges and
Schools* • Total Enrollment: *110*

PROGRAM INFORMATION

LPN/LVN Exit: *No* • NLNAC Accreditation: *Yes*

NURSING STUDENT PROFILE

Total Nursing Enrollment: *108* • Full-Time Enrollment: *43* •
Part-Time Enrollment: *65* • Female Enrollment: *99* • Male
Enrollment: *9* • Total New Admissions Who Enrolled for
Fall: *64* • Total Graduates: *46*

FINANCES

Residential Annual Tuition: *$1,250* • Non-Residential
Annual Tuition: *$2,600* • General Institution Fees: *$30* •
Additional Nursing Fees: *$100*

JEFFERSON COMMUNITY COLLEGE

Address: Outer Coffenn St., Watertown, NY 13601
Phone: 315-786-2340
Fax: 315-786-0716
Contact: Debra Marsala, MS, RN, ANP, Chair, Nursing Department
Email: debra_marsala@ccmgate.sunyjefferson.edu

GENERAL INFORMATION

Type of School: *2-Year College or University, Public* • Accreditation: *Middle States Association of Colleges and Schools* • Total Enrollment: *1623*

PROGRAM INFORMATION

LPN/LVN Exit: *No* • NLNAC Accreditation: *Yes*

NURSING STUDENT PROFILE

Total Nursing Enrollment: *66* • Full-Time Enrollment: *38* • Part-Time Enrollment: *28* • Female Enrollment: *58* • Male Enrollment: *8* • Total New Admissions Who Enrolled for Fall: *33* • Total Graduates: *28*

FINANCES

Residential Annual Tuition: *$2,320* • Non-Residential Annual Tuition: *$3,000* • General Institution Fees: *$181* • Additional Nursing Fees: *$5*

KINGSBOROUGH COMMUNITY COLLEGE—CUNY

Address: 2001 Oriental Blvd., Brooklyn, NY 11235
Phone: 718-368-5522
Fax: 718-368-4867
Contact: Dolores M. Shrimpton, RN, MA, Chairperson
Email: Not Reported

GENERAL INFORMATION

Type of School: *2-Year College or University, Public* • Accreditation: *Middle States Association of Colleges and Schools* • Total Enrollment: *10000*

PROGRAM INFORMATION

LPN/LVN Exit: *No* • NLNAC Accreditation: *Yes*

NURSING STUDENT PROFILE

Total Nursing Enrollment: *183* • Full-Time Enrollment: *82* • Part-Time Enrollment: *101* • Female Enrollment: *166* • Male Enrollment: *17* • Total New Admissions Who Enrolled for Fall: *55* • Total Graduates: *57*

FINANCES

Residential Annual Tuition: *$2,500* • Non-Residential Annual Tuition: *$3,096* • General Institution Fees: *$100* • Additional Nursing Fees: *$20*

LAGUARDIA COMMUNITY COLLEGE

Address: 31-10 Thompson Ave., Floral Park, NY 11001
Phone: 718-482-5772
Fax: 718-482-5599
Contact: Barbara Svitlik, RN, CS, MSN, PhD, Acting
             Director
Email: svitlikba@lagcc.cuny.edu

GENERAL INFORMATION

Type of School: *2-Year College or University, Public* •
Accreditation: *Middle States Association of Colleges and
Schools* • Total Enrollment: *11778*

PROGRAM INFORMATION

LPN/LVN Exit: *No* • NLNAC Accreditation: *Yes*

NURSING STUDENT PROFILE

Total Nursing Enrollment: *87* • Full-Time Enrollment: *67* •
Part-Time Enrollment: *20* • Female Enrollment: *78* • Male
Enrollment: *9* • Total New Admissions Who Enrolled for
Fall: *38* • Total Graduates: *38*

FINANCES

Residential Annual Tuition: *$2,500* • Non-Residential
Annual Tuition: *$3,100* • General Institution Fees: *$60* •
Additional Nursing Fees: *$80*

LONG ISLAND COLLEGE HOSPITAL

Address: 397 Hicks St., Brooklyn, NY 11201
Phone: 718-780-1998
Fax: 718-780-1936
Contact: Stephen Paul Hozemer, Phd, RN, Dean
Email: Not Reported

GENERAL INFORMATION

Type of School: *Hospital, Private (Independent)* •
Accreditation: *None* • Total Enrollment: *86*

PROGRAM INFORMATION

LPN/LVN Exit: *No* • NLNAC Accreditation: *Yes*

NURSING STUDENT PROFILE

Total Nursing Enrollment: *86* • Full-Time Enrollment: *15* •
Part-Time Enrollment: *71* • Female Enrollment: *83* • Male
Enrollment: *3* • Total New Admissions Who Enrolled for
Fall: *41* • Total Graduates: *Not Reported*

FINANCES

Residential Annual Tuition: *$8,470* • Non-Residential
Annual Tuition: *$8,470* • General Institution Fees: *$160* •
Additional Nursing Fees: *$250*

MARIA COLLEGE

Address: 700 New Scotland Ave., Albany, NY 12208
Phone: 518-489-7436
Fax: Not Reported
Contact: Esther K. McEvoy, MS, RN, Program Chair
Email: Not Reported

GENERAL INFORMATION

Type of School: *Other* • Accreditation: *None* • Total Enrollment: *Not Reported*

PROGRAM INFORMATION

LPN/LVN Exit: *No* • NLNAC Accreditation: *Yes*

NURSING STUDENT PROFILE

Total Nursing Enrollment: *183* • Full-Time Enrollment: *83* • Part-Time Enrollment: *100* • Female Enrollment: *161* • Male Enrollment: *22* • Total New Admissions Who Enrolled for Fall: *90* • Total Graduates: *78*

FINANCES

Residential Annual Tuition: *$5,750* • Non-Residential Annual Tuition: *$5,700* • General Institution Fees: *$200* • Additional Nursing Fees: *$150*

MEDGAR EVERS COLLEGE— CUNY

Address: 1150 Caroll Street, Brooklyn, NY 11225
Phone: 718-270-6222
Fax: 718-270-6296
Contact: Georgia McDuffie, PhD, RN, Director and Chairperson
Email: gmcduffie@mec.cuny.edu

GENERAL INFORMATION

Type of School: *Not Reported* • Accreditation: *None* • Total Enrollment: *Not Reported*

PROGRAM INFORMATION

LPN/LVN Exit: *Not Reported* • NLNAC Accreditation: *Yes*

NURSING STUDENT PROFILE

Total Nursing Enrollment: *480* • Full-Time Enrollment: *191* • Part-Time Enrollment: *289* • Female Enrollment: *440* • Male Enrollment: *40* • Total New Admissions Who Enrolled for Fall: *Not Reported* • Total Graduates: *50*

FINANCES

Residential Annual Tuition: *Not Reported* • Non-Residential Annual Tuition: *Not Reported* • General Institution Fees: *Not Reported* • Additional Nursing Fees: *Not Reported*

MOHAWK VALLEY COMMUNITY COLLEGE

Address: 1101 Sherman Dr., Utica, NY 13501
Phone: 315-792-5499
Fax: 315-731-5666
Contact: Nancy Caputo, MSN, RN, Department Head
Email: ncaputo@mvcc.edu

GENERAL INFORMATION

Type of School: *2-Year College or University, Public* •
Accreditation: *Middle States Association of Colleges and
Schools* • Total Enrollment: *4800*

PROGRAM INFORMATION

LPN/LVN Exit: *No* • NLNAC Accreditation: *Yes*

NURSING STUDENT PROFILE

Total Nursing Enrollment: *269* • Full-Time Enrollment:
150 • Part-Time Enrollment: *119* • Female Enrollment:
200 • Male Enrollment: *69* • Total New Admissions Who
Enrolled for Fall: *80* • Total Graduates: *56*

FINANCES

Residential Annual Tuition: *$2,500* • Non-Residential
Annual Tuition: *$3,750* • General Institution Fees: *$350* •
Additional Nursing Fees: *$500*

MONROE COMMUNITY COLLEGE

Address: 1000 E. Henrietta Rd., Rochester, NY 14623
Phone: 585-292-3866
Fax: 585-292-3866
Contact: Janice Volland, RN, MS, Professor and
            Chairman
Email: jvolland@monroecc.edu

GENERAL INFORMATION

Type of School: *2-Year College or University, Public* •
Accreditation: *Middle States Association of Colleges and
Schools* • Total Enrollment: *15315*

PROGRAM INFORMATION

LPN/LVN Exit: *No* • NLNAC Accreditation: *Yes*

NURSING STUDENT PROFILE

Total Nursing Enrollment: *259* • Full-Time Enrollment: *89* •
Part-Time Enrollment: *170* • Female Enrollment: *243* • Male
Enrollment: *16* • Total New Admissions Who Enrolled for
Fall: *77* • Total Graduates: *106*

FINANCES

Residential Annual Tuition: *$1,250* • Non-Residential
Annual Tuition: *$2,500* • General Institution Fees: *$250* •
Additional Nursing Fees: *$124*

MOUNT SAINT MARY COLLEGE

Address: 330 Powell Ave., Newburgh, NY 12550
Phone: 213-746-0450
Fax: 213-477-2519
Contact: Rebecca Otten, MSN, RN, Director, ADN Program
Email: Not Reported

GENERAL INFORMATION

Type of School: *Independent, Private (Independent)* • Accreditation: *Middle States Association of Colleges and Schools* • Total Enrollment: *2221*

PROGRAM INFORMATION

LPN/LVN Exit: *Not Reported* • NLNAC Accreditation: *No*

NURSING STUDENT PROFILE

Total Nursing Enrollment: *Not Reported* • Full-Time Enrollment: *Not Reported* • Part-Time Enrollment: *Not Reported* • Female Enrollment: *Not Reported* • Male Enrollment: *Not Reported* • Total New Admissions Who Enrolled for Fall: *Not Reported* • Total Graduates: *Not Reported*

FINANCES

Residential Annual Tuition: *Not Reported* • Non-Residential Annual Tuition: *Not Reported* • General Institution Fees: *Not Reported* • Additional Nursing Fees: *Not Reported*

THE MOUNT VERNON HOSPITAL

Address: 53 Valetine St., Mount Vernon, NY 10550
Phone: 914-664-8000
Fax: 914-665-7047
Contact: Beatrice Dunajski, RN, CS, PhD, Dean
Email: beatricetdunajsk@aol.com

GENERAL INFORMATION

Type of School: *Hospital, Private (Independent)* • Accreditation: *None* • Total Enrollment: *56*

PROGRAM INFORMATION

LPN/LVN Exit: *No* • NLNAC Accreditation: *No*

NURSING STUDENT PROFILE

Total Nursing Enrollment: *56* • Full-Time Enrollment: *18* • Part-Time Enrollment: *38* • Female Enrollment: *48* • Male Enrollment: *8* • Total New Admissions Who Enrolled for Fall: *22* • Total Graduates: *16*

FINANCES

Residential Annual Tuition: *$1,800* • Non-Residential Annual Tuition: *$0* • General Institution Fees: *$420* • Additional Nursing Fees: *$0*

NASSAU COMMUNITY COLLEGE

Address: 1 Education Dr., Garden City, NY 11530
Phone: 516-572-9630
Fax: 516-572-0697
Contact: Carol A. Mottola, PhD, RN, Chairperson
Email: mottolc@ncc.edu

GENERAL INFORMATION

Type of School: *2-Year College or University, Public* •
Accreditation: *Middle States Association of Colleges and
Schools* • Total Enrollment: *19049*

PROGRAM INFORMATION

LPN/LVN Exit: *No* • NLNAC Accreditation: *Yes*

NURSING STUDENT PROFILE

Total Nursing Enrollment: *358* • Full-Time Enrollment: *89* •
Part-Time Enrollment: *269* • Female Enrollment: *315* • Male
Enrollment: *43* • Total New Admissions Who Enrolled for
Fall: *170* • Total Graduates: *107*

FINANCES

Residential Annual Tuition: *$2,150* • Non-Residential
Annual Tuition: *$4,300* • General Institution Fees: *$200* •
Additional Nursing Fees: *$75*

NEW YORK CITY TECHNICAL COLLEGE

Address: 300 Jay St., Brooklyn, NY 11201
Phone: 718-260-5660
Fax: Not Reported
Contact: Kathryn P Richardson, RN, MS, Chairperson,
            Department of Nursing
Email: krichardson@nyctc.cuny.edu

GENERAL INFORMATION

Type of School: *Not Reported* • Accreditation: *Not Reported* •
Total Enrollment: *Not Reported*

PROGRAM INFORMATION

LPN/LVN Exit: *No* • NLNAC Accreditation: *Yes*

NURSING STUDENT PROFILE

Total Nursing Enrollment: *Not Reported* • Full-Time
Enrollment: *Not Reported* • Part-Time Enrollment: *Not
Reported* • Female Enrollment: *Not Reported* • Male
Enrollment: *Not Reported* • Total New Admissions Who
Enrolled for Fall: *Not Reported* • Total Graduates: *Not
Reported*

FINANCES

Residential Annual Tuition: *Not Reported* • Non-Residential
Annual Tuition: *Not Reported* • General Institution Fees: *Not
Reported* • Additional Nursing Fees: *Not Reported*

NIAGARA COUNTY COMMUNITY COLLEGE

Address: 3111 Saunders Settlement Rd., Sanborn, NY
           14132
Phone: 716-614-5940
Fax: 716-614-6827
Contact: Katherine B. Collard, MSN, RN, Professor and
           Interim Director
Email: collard@niagaracc.suny.edu

GENERAL INFORMATION

Type of School: *2-Year College or University, Public* •
Accreditation: *Middle States Association of Colleges and
Schools* • Total Enrollment: *4915*

PROGRAM INFORMATION

LPN/LVN Exit: *No* • NLNAC Accreditation: *Yes*

NURSING STUDENT PROFILE

Total Nursing Enrollment: *187* • Full-Time Enrollment:
121 • Part-Time Enrollment: *66* • Female Enrollment: *168* •
Male Enrollment: *19* • Total New Admissions Who Enrolled
for Fall: *70* • Total Graduates: *46*

FINANCES

Residential Annual Tuition: *$1,300* • Non-Residential
Annual Tuition: *$1,950* • General Institution Fees: *$248* •
Additional Nursing Fees: *$200*

ONONDAGA COMMUNITY COLLEGE

Address: 4941 Onondaga Rd., Syracuse, NY 13215
Phone: 315-498-2630
Fax: 315-498-2098
Contact: Pamela F. Ryan, MS, RNC, Chairperson
Email: raynp@sunyocc.edu

GENERAL INFORMATION

Type of School: *2-Year College or University, Public* •
Accreditation: *Middle States Association of Colleges and
Schools* • Total Enrollment: *8180*

PROGRAM INFORMATION

LPN/LVN Exit: *No* • NLNAC Accreditation: *Yes*

NURSING STUDENT PROFILE

Total Nursing Enrollment: *170* • Full-Time Enrollment: *92* •
Part-Time Enrollment: *78* • Female Enrollment: *147* • Male
Enrollment: *23* • Total New Admissions Who Enrolled for
Fall: *58* • Total Graduates: *30*

FINANCES

Residential Annual Tuition: *$2,500* • Non-Residential
Annual Tuition: *$7,500* • General Institution Fees: *$126* •
Additional Nursing Fees: *$84*

ORANGE COUNTY COMMUNITY COLLEGE

Address: 115 South Street, Middletown, NY 10940
Phone: 845-341-4108
Fax: 845-343-1228
Contact: Margaret E. Scribner, RN, MS, Chairperson
Email: mscribne@mail.sunyorange.edu

PHILLIPS BETH ISRAEL MEDICAL CENTER

Address: 3310 East 22nd St., New York, NY 10010
Phone: 212-614-6107
Fax: 212-614-6109
Contact: Janet Mackin, RN, EdD, Dean
Email: jmackin@slrhc.org

GENERAL INFORMATION

Type of School: *2-Year College or University, Public* •
Accreditation: *Middle States Association of Colleges and Schools* • Total Enrollment: *5532*

GENERAL INFORMATION

Type of School: *Hospital, Private (Independent)* •
Accreditation: *None* • Total Enrollment: *84*

PROGRAM INFORMATION

LPN/LVN Exit: *No* • NLNAC Accreditation: *Yes*

PROGRAM INFORMATION

LPN/LVN Exit: *No* • NLNAC Accreditation: *No*

NURSING STUDENT PROFILE

Total Nursing Enrollment: *181* • Full-Time Enrollment: *52* •
Part-Time Enrollment: *129* • Female Enrollment: *161* • Male
Enrollment: *20* • Total New Admissions Who Enrolled for
Fall: *100* • Total Graduates: *70*

NURSING STUDENT PROFILE

Total Nursing Enrollment: *84* • Full-Time Enrollment: *17* •
Part-Time Enrollment: *67* • Female Enrollment: *69* • Male
Enrollment: *15* • Total New Admissions Who Enrolled for
Fall: *40* • Total Graduates: *18*

FINANCES

Residential Annual Tuition: *$2,260* • Non-Residential
Annual Tuition: *$5,520* • General Institution Fees: *$100* •
Additional Nursing Fees: *$60*

FINANCES

Residential Annual Tuition: *$5,225* • Non-Residential
Annual Tuition: *$5,225* • General Institution Fees: *$210* •
Additional Nursing Fees: *$210*

QUEENSBOROUGH COMMUNITY COLLEGE— CUNY

Address: 222-05 56th Ave., Bayside, NY 11364
Phone: 718-631-6205
Fax: 718-631-6067
Contact: Maureen Wallace, EdD, RN, Chairperson
Email: mwallace@qcc.cuny.edu

RIVERSIDE HEALTH SYSTEM

Address: 967 North Broadway, Yonkers, NY 10701
Phone: 914-964-4282
Fax: 914-964-4266
Contact: Kathleen Dirschel, PhD, RN, VP of Education
           and Director
Email: kdirschel@riversidehealth.org

GENERAL INFORMATION

Type of School: *2-Year College or University, Public* •
Accreditation: *Middle States Association of Colleges and Schools* • Total Enrollment: *10*

GENERAL INFORMATION

Type of School: *Other* • Accreditation: *None* • Total Enrollment: *136*

PROGRAM INFORMATION

LPN/LVN Exit: *Not Reported* • NLNAC Accreditation: *Yes*

PROGRAM INFORMATION

LPN/LVN Exit: *No* • NLNAC Accreditation: *No*

NURSING STUDENT PROFILE

Total Nursing Enrollment: *861* • Full-Time Enrollment: *328* • Part-Time Enrollment: *533* • Female Enrollment: *773* • Male Enrollment: *88* • Total New Admissions Who Enrolled for Fall: *182* • Total Graduates: *74*

NURSING STUDENT PROFILE

Total Nursing Enrollment: *94* • Full-Time Enrollment: *63* • Part-Time Enrollment: *31* • Female Enrollment: *85* • Male Enrollment: *9* • Total New Admissions Who Enrolled for Fall: *46* • Total Graduates: *48*

FINANCES

Residential Annual Tuition: *$2,800* • Non-Residential Annual Tuition: *$6,080* • General Institution Fees: *$53* • Additional Nursing Fees: *$158*

FINANCES

Residential Annual Tuition: *$6,000* • Non-Residential Annual Tuition: *Not Reported* • General Institution Fees: *Not Reported* • Additional Nursing Fees: *$720*

SAINT ELIZABETH MEDICAL CENTER

Address: 2215 Genesee St., Utica, NY 13501
Phone: 315-798-8125
Fax: 315-798-8271
Contact: Sister Walter Marie, MS, RN, Dean
Email: condir@stemc.org

GENERAL INFORMATION

Type of School: *Hospital, Private (Religious)* • Accreditation: *None* • Total Enrollment: *Not Reported*

PROGRAM INFORMATION

LPN/LVN Exit: *No* • NLNAC Accreditation: *No*

NURSING STUDENT PROFILE

Total Nursing Enrollment: *160* • Full-Time Enrollment: *100* • Part-Time Enrollment: *60* • Female Enrollment: *141* • Male Enrollment: *19* • Total New Admissions Who Enrolled for Fall: *106* • Total Graduates: *Not Reported*

FINANCES

Residential Annual Tuition: *$6,094* • Non-Residential Annual Tuition: *$6,094* • General Institution Fees: *$200* • Additional Nursing Fees: *$650*

SAINT JOSEPH'S HOSPITAL HEALTH CENTER

Address: 206 Prospect Ave., Syracuse, NY 290413203
Phone: 315-448-5040
Fax: 315-448-5745
Contact: Marianne Markowitz, MS, RN, Director
Email: marianne.markiwitz@sjhsyr.org

GENERAL INFORMATION

Type of School: *Hospital, Private (Religious)* • Accreditation: *None* • Total Enrollment: *Not Reported*

PROGRAM INFORMATION

LPN/LVN Exit: *No* • NLNAC Accreditation: *No*

NURSING STUDENT PROFILE

Total Nursing Enrollment: *191* • Full-Time Enrollment: *132* • Part-Time Enrollment: *59* • Female Enrollment: *181* • Male Enrollment: *10* • Total New Admissions Who Enrolled for Fall: *85* • Total Graduates: *47*

FINANCES

Residential Annual Tuition: *$5,907* • Non-Residential Annual Tuition: *$9,142* • General Institution Fees: *$524* • Additional Nursing Fees: *$24*

SAINT VINCENT CATHOLIC MEDICAL CENTER OF NY

Address: 130 West 12th St., Ste 1G, New York, NY 10011
Phone: 718-357-0500
Fax: 718-357-4683
Contact: Genevieve M. Jensen, MS, RN, Administrative
            Director
Email: gjensen@cmcny.com

GENERAL INFORMATION

Type of School: *Hospital, Private (Religious)* • Accreditation:
None • Total Enrollment: *153*

PROGRAM INFORMATION

LPN/LVN Exit: *Not Reported* • NLNAC Accreditation: *No*

NURSING STUDENT PROFILE

Total Nursing Enrollment: *89* • Full-Time Enrollment: *40* •
Part-Time Enrollment: *49* • Female Enrollment: *78* • Male
Enrollment: *11* • Total New Admissions Who Enrolled for
Fall: *58* • Total Graduates: *34*

FINANCES

Residential Annual Tuition: *$5,397* • Non-Residential
Annual Tuition: *$5,397* • General Institution Fees: *$185* •
Additional Nursing Fees: *$900*

STATE UNIVERSITY OF NEW YORK COLLEGE OF TECHNOLOGY AT ALFRED

Address: Allied Health Building, SUNY Alfred, Alfred,
             NY 14802
Phone: 607-587-3680
Fax: 607-587-3684
Contact: Cynthie Luehman, MS, RN, Department Chair
Email: luehmacr@alfredstate.edu

GENERAL INFORMATION

Type of School: *Other, Public* • Accreditation: *Middle States
Association of Colleges and Schools* • Total Enrollment: *Not
Reported*

PROGRAM INFORMATION

LPN/LVN Exit: *No* • NLNAC Accreditation: *Yes*

NURSING STUDENT PROFILE

Total Nursing Enrollment: *101* • Full-Time Enrollment: *97* •
Part-Time Enrollment: *4* • Female Enrollment: *94* • Male
Enrollment: *7* • Total New Admissions Who Enrolled for
Fall: *55* • Total Graduates: *29*

FINANCES

Residential Annual Tuition: *$3,200* • Non-Residential
Annual Tuition: *$5,000* • General Institution Fees: *$740* •
Additional Nursing Fees: *$0*

STATE UNIVERSITY OF NEW YORK-FARMINGDALE

Address: Gleason Hall Rm. 304, Farmingdale, NY 11735
Phone: 631-420-2229
Fax: 631-420-2784
Contact: Marie Hayden Miles, PhD, RN, Chairperson
Email: haydenm@farmingdale.edu

GENERAL INFORMATION

Type of School: *Governmental Agency, Public* • Accreditation: *Middle States Association of Colleges and Schools* • Total Enrollment: *5000*

PROGRAM INFORMATION

LPN/LVN Exit: *No* • NLNAC Accreditation: *Yes*

NURSING STUDENT PROFILE

Total Nursing Enrollment: *178* • Full-Time Enrollment: *55* • Part-Time Enrollment: *123* • Female Enrollment: *159* • Male Enrollment: *19* • Total New Admissions Who Enrolled for Fall: *80* • Total Graduates: *Not Reported*

FINANCES

Residential Annual Tuition: *$3,200* • Non-Residential Annual Tuition: *$8,300* • General Institution Fees: *$675* • Additional Nursing Fees: *$55*

SUFFOLK COUNTY COMMUNITY COLLEGE

Address: 533 College Rd., Riverhead Bldg., RM 106, Selden, NY 11784
Phone: 631-451-4265
Fax: 631-451-4671
Contact: Susan Dewey-Hammer, MN, RN, CS, Academic Chair
Email: deweyhs@sunysuffolk.edu

GENERAL INFORMATION

Type of School: *2-Year College or University, Public* • Accreditation: *Middle States Association of Colleges and Schools* • Total Enrollment: *18264*

PROGRAM INFORMATION

LPN/LVN Exit: *No* • NLNAC Accreditation: *Yes*

NURSING STUDENT PROFILE

Total Nursing Enrollment: *303* • Full-Time Enrollment: *197* • Part-Time Enrollment: *106* • Female Enrollment: *265* • Male Enrollment: *38* • Total New Admissions Who Enrolled for Fall: *153* • Total Graduates: *130*

FINANCES

Residential Annual Tuition: *$2,330* • Non-Residential Annual Tuition: *$4,660* • General Institution Fees: *$99* • Additional Nursing Fees: *$55*

SULLIVAN COUNTY COMMUNITY COLLEGE

Address: 112 College Rd., Lochsheldrake, NY 12752
Phone: 845-434-5750
Fax: 845-434-4806
Contact: Anne Lavelle, MA, RN, Chairperson
Email: alavelle@sullivan.suny.edu

GENERAL INFORMATION

Type of School: *2-Year College or University, Public* •
Accreditation: *Middle States Association of Colleges and Schools* • Total Enrollment: 925

PROGRAM INFORMATION

LPN/LVN Exit: *No* • NLNAC Accreditation: *Yes*

NURSING STUDENT PROFILE

Total Nursing Enrollment: *61* • Full-Time Enrollment: *35* •
Part-Time Enrollment: *26* • Female Enrollment: *54* • Male
Enrollment: *7* • Total New Admissions Who Enrolled for
Fall: *27* • Total Graduates: *Not Reported*

FINANCES

Residential Annual Tuition: *$2,500* • Non-Residential
Annual Tuition: *$5,000* • General Institution Fees: *$156* •
Additional Nursing Fees: *$310*

SUNY ROCKLAND COMMUNITY COLLEGE

Address: 145 College Rd., Suffern, NY 10901
Phone: 845-574-4223
Fax: 845-574-4462
Contact: Frances D. Monahan, PhD, RN, Coordinator,
           Department of Nursing
Email: fmonahan@sunyrockland.edu

GENERAL INFORMATION

Type of School: *Other* • Accreditation: *None* • Total
Enrollment: *Not Reported*

PROGRAM INFORMATION

LPN/LVN Exit: *No* • NLNAC Accreditation: *Yes*

NURSING STUDENT PROFILE

Total Nursing Enrollment: *304* • Full-Time Enrollment:
188 • Part-Time Enrollment: *116* • Female Enrollment:
278 • Male Enrollment: *26* • Total New Admissions Who
Enrolled for Fall: *78* • Total Graduates: *63*

FINANCES

Residential Annual Tuition: *$2,325* • Non-Residential
Annual Tuition: *$4,650* • General Institution Fees: *$51* •
Additional Nursing Fees: *$50*

TOMPKINS CORTLAND

Address: 170 North St., Dryden, NY 13053
Phone: 607-844-8211
Fax: 607-844-9665
Contact: Catherine Milnor, RN, BSN, MSN, Professor
          and Chair
Email: milnorc@sunytccc.edu

GENERAL INFORMATION

Type of School: *2-Year College or University, Public* •
Accreditation: *Middle States Association of Colleges and
Schools* • Total Enrollment: *2674*

PROGRAM INFORMATION

LPN/LVN Exit: *No* • NLNAC Accreditation: *Yes*

NURSING STUDENT PROFILE

Total Nursing Enrollment: *88* • Full-Time Enrollment: *Not
Reported* • Part-Time Enrollment: *Not Reported* • Female
Enrollment: *83* • Male Enrollment: *5* • Total New
Admissions Who Enrolled for Fall: *58* • Total Graduates: *40*

FINANCES

Residential Annual Tuition: *$2,600* • Non-Residential
Annual Tuition: *$5,200* • General Institution Fees: *$84* •
Additional Nursing Fees: *$30*

TROCAIRE COLLEGE

Address: 360 Choate Ave., Buffalo, NY 14220
Phone: 716-827-2462
Fax: 716-828-6107
Contact: Carol A. Fanutti, EdD, RN, Director of Nursing
Email: fanuttic@trocaire.edu

GENERAL INFORMATION

Type of School: *Independent, Private (Independent)* •
Accreditation: *Middle States Association of Colleges and
Schools* • Total Enrollment: *709*

PROGRAM INFORMATION

LPN/LVN Exit: *No* • NLNAC Accreditation: *Yes*

NURSING STUDENT PROFILE

Total Nursing Enrollment: *124* • Full-Time Enrollment: *60* •
Part-Time Enrollment: *64* • Female Enrollment: *114* • Male
Enrollment: *10* • Total New Admissions Who Enrolled for
Fall: *54* • Total Graduates: *57*

FINANCES

Residential Annual Tuition: *$8,980* • Non-Residential
Annual Tuition: *$8,980* • General Institution Fees: *$200* •
Additional Nursing Fees: *$450*

ULSTER COUNTY COMMUNITY COLLEGE

Address: Cottekill Rd., Ulster County Community
College, Stone Ridge, NY 12484
Phone: 845-687-5235
Fax: 845-687-5083
Contact: Joan Gilbert, RN, MA, Chairperson
Email: gilbertj@sunnyulster.edu

GENERAL INFORMATION

Type of School: *2-Year College or University, Public* •
Accreditation: *Middle States Association of Colleges and
Schools* • Total Enrollment: *2525*

PROGRAM INFORMATION

LPN/LVN Exit: *No* • NLNAC Accreditation: *Yes*

NURSING STUDENT PROFILE

Total Nursing Enrollment: *67* • Full-Time Enrollment: *28* •
Part-Time Enrollment: *39* • Female Enrollment: *55* • Male
Enrollment: *12* • Total New Admissions Who Enrolled for
Fall: *44* • Total Graduates: *29*

FINANCES

Residential Annual Tuition: *$1,235* • Non-Residential
Annual Tuition: *$2,470* • General Institution Fees: *Not
Reported* • Additional Nursing Fees: *$20*

WESTCHESTER COMMUNITY COLLEGE

Address: 75 Grasslands Rd., Valhalla, NY 10595
Phone: 914-785-6891
Fax: 914-785-7832
Contact: Joanna Scalabrini, MSN, MHEd, RNC,
Department Chairperson
Email: joanna.scalabrini@sunywcc.com

GENERAL INFORMATION

Type of School: *2-Year College or University, Public* •
Accreditation: *Middle States Association of Colleges and
Schools* • Total Enrollment: *11000*

PROGRAM INFORMATION

LPN/LVN Exit: *No* • NLNAC Accreditation: *No*

NURSING STUDENT PROFILE

Total Nursing Enrollment: *86* • Full-Time Enrollment: *86* •
Part-Time Enrollment: *0* • Female Enrollment: *81* • Male
Enrollment: *5* • Total New Admissions Who Enrolled for
Fall: *58* • Total Graduates: *35*

FINANCES

Residential Annual Tuition: *$2,200* • Non-Residential
Annual Tuition: *$4,400* • General Institution Fees: *$85* •
Additional Nursing Fees: *$200*

ALAMANCE COMMUNITY COLLEGE

Address: PO Box 8000, Graham, NC 27253
Phone: 336-506-4162
Fax: 336-578-1987
Contact: Susan E. Holt, RN, MSN, Nursing Department Head and Director
Email: holts@alamance.cc.nc.us

GENERAL INFORMATION

Type of School: *2-Year College or University, Public* •
Accreditation: *Southern Association of Colleges and Schools* •
Total Enrollment: *3600*

PROGRAM INFORMATION

LPN/LVN Exit: *Not Reported* • NLNAC Accreditation: *No*

NURSING STUDENT PROFILE

Total Nursing Enrollment: *73* • Full-Time Enrollment: *73* •
Part-Time Enrollment: *0* • Female Enrollment: *69* • Male
Enrollment: *4* • Total New Admissions Who Enrolled for
Fall: *Not Reported* • Total Graduates: *30*

FINANCES

Residential Annual Tuition: *Not Reported* • Non-Residential
Annual Tuition: *Not Reported* • General Institution Fees: *Not
Reported* • Additional Nursing Fees: *Not Reported*

ASHEVILLE-BUNCOMBE TECHNICAL COMMUNITY COLLEGE

Address: 340 Victoria Road, Asheville, NC 28801
Phone: 828-254-1921
Fax: 828-251-6355
Contact: Brenda Causey, MSN, RN, Chairperson, Nursing Programs
Email: bcausey@asheville.cc.nc.us

GENERAL INFORMATION

Type of School: *2-Year College or University, Public* •
Accreditation: *Southern Association of Colleges and Schools* •
Total Enrollment: *4937*

PROGRAM INFORMATION

LPN/LVN Exit: *No* • NLNAC Accreditation: *No*

NURSING STUDENT PROFILE

Total Nursing Enrollment: *120* • Full-Time Enrollment: *Not
Reported* • Part-Time Enrollment: *Not Reported* • Female
Enrollment: *101* • Male Enrollment: *19* • Total New
Admissions Who Enrolled for Fall: *62* • Total Graduates: *44*

FINANCES

Residential Annual Tuition: *$1,182* • Non-Residential
Annual Tuition: *$7,299* • General Institution Fees: *Not
Reported* • Additional Nursing Fees: *$34*

BEAUFORT COUNTY COMMUNITY COLLEGE

Address: PO Box 1069, Washington, NC 27889
Phone: 252-946-6194
Fax: Not Reported
Contact: Sandra Edwards, MSN, RN, Chairperson Allied Health
Email: sandrae@email.beaufort.cc.nc.us

GENERAL INFORMATION

Type of School: *2-Year College or University, Public* •
Accreditation: *Southern Association of Colleges and Schools* •
Total Enrollment: *Not Reported*

PROGRAM INFORMATION

LPN/LVN Exit: *Not Reported* • NLNAC Accreditation: *No*

NURSING STUDENT PROFILE

Total Nursing Enrollment: *68* • Full-Time Enrollment: *68* •
Part-Time Enrollment: *0* • Female Enrollment: *61* • Male
Enrollment: *7* • Total New Admissions Who Enrolled for
Fall: *43* • Total Graduates: *21*

FINANCES

Residential Annual Tuition: *$1,457* • Non-Residential
Annual Tuition: *$8,143* • General Institution Fees: *$42* •
Additional Nursing Fees: *$0*

BLUE RIDGE COMMUNITY COLLEGE—NORTH CAROLINA

Address: College Drive, Flat Rock, NC 28731
Phone: 828-692-3572
Fax: 828-692-2441
Contact: Rita D. Conner, MSN, RN, Director, Allied Health Programs
Email: ritac@blueridge.cc.nc.us

GENERAL INFORMATION

Type of School: *2-Year College or University, Public* •
Accreditation: *Southern Association of Colleges and Schools* •
Total Enrollment: *1887*

PROGRAM INFORMATION

LPN/LVN Exit: *No* • NLNAC Accreditation: *No*

NURSING STUDENT PROFILE

Total Nursing Enrollment: *56* • Full-Time Enrollment: *29* •
Part-Time Enrollment: *27* • Female Enrollment: *51* • Male
Enrollment: *5* • Total New Admissions Who Enrolled for
Fall: *30* • Total Graduates: *24*

FINANCES

Residential Annual Tuition: *Not Reported* • Non-Residential
Annual Tuition: *Not Reported* • General Institution Fees: *$8* •
Additional Nursing Fees: *$15*

CABARRUS COLLEGE OF HEALTH SCIENCES

Address: 431 Copperfield Blvd NE, Concord, NC 28025
Phone: 704-783-1629
Fax: 704-783-1764
Contact: Elizabeth Baucom, MSN, RN, ADN Program
            Chairman
Email: ebaucom@northeastmedical.org

GENERAL INFORMATION

Type of School: *4-Year College or University, Private
(Independent)* • Accreditation: *Southern Association of Colleges
and Schools* • Total Enrollment: *250*

PROGRAM INFORMATION

LPN/LVN Exit: *No* • NLNAC Accreditation: *Yes*

NURSING STUDENT PROFILE

Total Nursing Enrollment: *129* • Full-Time Enrollment: *91* •
Part-Time Enrollment: *38* • Female Enrollment: *120* • Male
Enrollment: *9* • Total New Admissions Who Enrolled for
Fall: *77* • Total Graduates: *54*

FINANCES

Residential Annual Tuition: *$5,760* • Non-Residential
Annual Tuition: *$5,760* • General Institution Fees: *$450* •
Additional Nursing Fees: *Not Reported*

CALDWELL COMMUNITY COLLEGE & TECHNICAL INSTITUTE

Address: 2855 Hickory Blvd, Hudson, NC 28638
Phone: 828-726-2353
Fax: 828-726-2489
Contact: Fredel T. Reighard, MSN, MA, RN, Director,
            Nursing Programs
Email: freighard@caldwell.cc.nc.us

GENERAL INFORMATION

Type of School: *2-Year College or University, Public* •
Accreditation: *Southern Association of Colleges and Schools* •
Total Enrollment: *Not Reported*

PROGRAM INFORMATION

LPN/LVN Exit: *No* • NLNAC Accreditation: *No*

NURSING STUDENT PROFILE

Total Nursing Enrollment: *78* • Full-Time Enrollment: *78* •
Part-Time Enrollment: *0* • Female Enrollment: *67* • Male
Enrollment: *11* • Total New Admissions Who Enrolled for
Fall: *53* • Total Graduates: *29*

FINANCES

Residential Annual Tuition: *$1,108* • Non-Residential
Annual Tuition: *$9,506* • General Institution Fees: *$32* •
Additional Nursing Fees: *$429*

CAPE FEAR COMMUNITY COLLEGE

Address: 411 N. Front Street, Wilmington, NC 28401
Phone: 910-251-5182
Fax: 910-251-5187
Contact: Susan Vinson-Greene, MSN, RN, Director, Nursing and Allied Health
Email: svgreene@capefear.cc.nc.us

GENERAL INFORMATION

Type of School: *2-Year College or University, Public* • Accreditation: *Southern Association of Colleges and Schools* • Total Enrollment: *5550*

PROGRAM INFORMATION

LPN/LVN Exit: *No* • NLNAC Accreditation: *Yes*

NURSING STUDENT PROFILE

Total Nursing Enrollment: *58* • Full-Time Enrollment: *58* • Part-Time Enrollment: *0* • Female Enrollment: *Not Reported* • Male Enrollment: *Not Reported* • Total New Admissions Who Enrolled for Fall: *40* • Total Graduates: *24*

FINANCES

Residential Annual Tuition: *$660* • Non-Residential Annual Tuition: *$4,074* • General Institution Fees: *$34* • Additional Nursing Fees: *$15*

CAROLINAS COLLEGE OF HEALTH SCIENCES

Address: 1200 Blythe Blvd, Charlotte, NC 28232
Phone: 704-355-5970
Fax: 704-355-5967
Contact: Claire B. Corbin, RN, MS, Dean
Email: ccorbin@carolinas.org

GENERAL INFORMATION

Type of School: *Hospital, Public* • Accreditation: *Southern Association of Colleges and Schools* • Total Enrollment: *3000*

PROGRAM INFORMATION

LPN/LVN Exit: *No* • NLNAC Accreditation: *Yes*

NURSING STUDENT PROFILE

Total Nursing Enrollment: *173* • Full-Time Enrollment: *52* • Part-Time Enrollment: *121* • Female Enrollment: *163* • Male Enrollment: *10* • Total New Admissions Who Enrolled for Fall: *97* • Total Graduates: *74*

FINANCES

Residential Annual Tuition: *$3,500* • Non-Residential Annual Tuition: *$3,500* • General Institution Fees: *$130* • Additional Nursing Fees: *$150*

CATAWBA VALLEY COMMUNITY COLLEGE

Address: 2550 Highway, 70 SE, Hickory, NC 28602
Phone: 828-327-7000
Fax: 828-327-7276
Contact: Jackie Lawrence, MSN, RN, Department Head
Email: jlawrenc@cvcc.cc.nc.us

GENERAL INFORMATION

Type of School: *2-Year College or University, Public* •
Accreditation: *Southern Association of Colleges and Schools* •
Total Enrollment: *3500*

PROGRAM INFORMATION

LPN/LVN Exit: *No* • NLNAC Accreditation: *Yes*

NURSING STUDENT PROFILE

Total Nursing Enrollment: *105* • Full-Time Enrollment:
105 • Part-Time Enrollment: *0* • Female Enrollment: *96* •
Male Enrollment: *9* • Total New Admissions Who Enrolled
for Fall: *81* • Total Graduates: *30*

FINANCES

Residential Annual Tuition: *$642* • Non-Residential Annual
Tuition: *$4,074* • General Institution Fees: *$24* • Additional
Nursing Fees: *$28*

CENTRAL CAROLINA COMMUNITY COLLEGE

Address: Route 1, Box 447-C, Lillington, NC 27546
Phone: 919-775-5401
Fax: Not Reported
Contact: Rhonda Evans, MSN, RN, Department Chair,
            Nursing and Allied Health
Email: revans@gw.ccarolina.cc.nc.us

GENERAL INFORMATION

Type of School: *2-Year College or University, Public* •
Accreditation: *Southern Association of Colleges and Schools* •
Total Enrollment: *3000*

PROGRAM INFORMATION

LPN/LVN Exit: *Yes* • NLNAC Accreditation: *No*

NURSING STUDENT PROFILE

Total Nursing Enrollment: *65* • Full-Time Enrollment: *27* •
Part-Time Enrollment: *38* • Female Enrollment: *60* • Male
Enrollment: *5* • Total New Admissions Who Enrolled for
Fall: *61* • Total Graduates: *37*

FINANCES

Residential Annual Tuition: *$642* • Non-Residential Annual
Tuition: *$4,074* • General Institution Fees: *$36* • Additional
Nursing Fees: *$20*

CENTRAL PIEDMONT COMMUNITY COLLEGE

Address: PO Box 35009, Charlotte, NC 28235
Phone: 704-330-6379
Fax: 704-330-6677
Contact: Patti McCahan, RN, MS, Program Chair
Email: patricia_mccahan@cpcc.cc.nc.us

GENERAL INFORMATION

Type of School: *2-Year College or University, Public* •
Accreditation: *Southern Association of Colleges and Schools* •
Total Enrollment: *70000*

PROGRAM INFORMATION

LPN/LVN Exit: *Not Reported* • NLNAC Accreditation: *No*

NURSING STUDENT PROFILE

Total Nursing Enrollment: *95* • Full-Time Enrollment: *95* •
Part-Time Enrollment: *0* • Female Enrollment: *87* • Male
Enrollment: *8* • Total New Admissions Who Enrolled for
Fall: *60* • Total Graduates: *41*

FINANCES

Residential Annual Tuition: *$992* • Non-Residential Annual
Tuition: *$5,544* • General Institution Fees: *$40* • Additional
Nursing Fees: *$100*

COASTAL CAROLINA COMMUNITY COLLEGE

Address: 444 Western Boulevard, Jacksonville, NC 28546
Phone: 910-938-6273
Fax: 910-455-7027
Contact: Paula V. Gribble, RN,BSN,MSAS, Chair,
Nursing and Allied Health
Email: gribblep@coastal.cc.nc.us

GENERAL INFORMATION

Type of School: *2-Year College or University, Public* •
Accreditation: *Southern Association of Colleges and Schools* •
Total Enrollment: *4039*

PROGRAM INFORMATION

LPN/LVN Exit: *No* • NLNAC Accreditation: *No*

NURSING STUDENT PROFILE

Total Nursing Enrollment: *54* • Full-Time Enrollment: *54* •
Part-Time Enrollment: *0* • Female Enrollment: *51* • Male
Enrollment: *3* • Total New Admissions Who Enrolled for
Fall: *30* • Total Graduates: *25*

FINANCES

Residential Annual Tuition: *$1,085* • Non-Residential
Annual Tuition: *$6,064* • General Institution Fees: *$15* •
Additional Nursing Fees: *$15*

COLLEGE OF THE ALBEMARLE

Address:　PO Box 2327, Elizabeth City, NC 27906
Phone:　252-335-0821
Fax:　252-337-6797
Contact:　Mary Pat Omer, RN, MS, Program Coordinator
Email:　momer@albermarle.cc.nc.us

GENERAL INFORMATION

Type of School: *2-Year College or University, Public* •
Accreditation: *Southern Association of Colleges and Schools* •
Total Enrollment: *2309*

PROGRAM INFORMATION

LPN/LVN Exit: *No* • NLNAC Accreditation: *Yes*

NURSING STUDENT PROFILE

Total Nursing Enrollment: *56* • Full-Time Enrollment: *17* •
Part-Time Enrollment: *39* • Female Enrollment: *54* • Male
Enrollment: *2* • Total New Admissions Who Enrolled for
Fall: *30* • Total Graduates: *21*

FINANCES

Residential Annual Tuition: *$880* • Non-Residential Annual
Tuition: *$5,432* • General Institution Fees: *$28* • Additional
Nursing Fees: *$35*

CRAVEN COMMUNITY COLLEGE

Address:　800 College Court, New Bern, NC 28562
Phone:　252-638-7342
Fax:　252-638-4232
Contact:　Carolyn S. Jones, RN, MAEd, MSN, Director of
　　　　　Health Care Programs
Email:　jonesc@admin.craven.cc.nc.us

GENERAL INFORMATION

Type of School: *2-Year College or University, Public* •
Accreditation: *Southern Association of Colleges and Schools* •
Total Enrollment: *2865*

PROGRAM INFORMATION

LPN/LVN Exit: *No* • NLNAC Accreditation: *No*

NURSING STUDENT PROFILE

Total Nursing Enrollment: *76* • Full-Time Enrollment: *76* •
Part-Time Enrollment: *0* • Female Enrollment: *73* • Male
Enrollment: *3* • Total New Admissions Who Enrolled for
Fall: *46* • Total Graduates: *30*

FINANCES

Residential Annual Tuition: *$1,488* • Non-Residential
Annual Tuition: *$8,316* • General Institution Fees: *$28* •
Additional Nursing Fees: *$23*

DAVIDSON COUNTY COMMUNITY COLLEGE

Address: PO Box 1287, Lexington, NC 27293
Phone: 336-249-8186
Fax: 336-249-9060
Contact: Jeannine Woody, RN, MSN, Chair, Health Technology
Email: jwoody@davidson.cc.nc.us

GENERAL INFORMATION

Type of School: *Governmental Agency, Public* • Accreditation: *Southern Association of Colleges and Schools* • Total Enrollment: *2800*

PROGRAM INFORMATION

LPN/LVN Exit: *Yes* • NLNAC Accreditation: *Yes*

NURSING STUDENT PROFILE

Total Nursing Enrollment: *79* • Full-Time Enrollment: *75* • Part-Time Enrollment: *4* • Female Enrollment: *72* • Male Enrollment: *7* • Total New Admissions Who Enrolled for Fall: *48* • Total Graduates: *35*

FINANCES

Residential Annual Tuition: *$568* • Non-Residential Annual Tuition: *$3,312* • General Institution Fees: *$31* • Additional Nursing Fees: *$0*

DUN TECHNICAL COMMUNITY COLLEGE

Address: 1637 Lawson Street, Durham, NC 27703
Phone: 919-686-3689
Fax: Not Reported
Contact: Margaret Skulnik, RN, MS, CDE, Program Director
Email: skulnikm@gwmail.dtcc.cc.nc.us

GENERAL INFORMATION

Type of School: *Other, Public* • Accreditation: *Southern Association of Colleges and Schools* • Total Enrollment: *5000*

PROGRAM INFORMATION

LPN/LVN Exit: *Not Reported* • NLNAC Accreditation: *No*

NURSING STUDENT PROFILE

Total Nursing Enrollment: *64* • Full-Time Enrollment: *10* • Part-Time Enrollment: *54* • Female Enrollment: *Not Reported* • Male Enrollment: *Not Reported* • Total New Admissions Who Enrolled for Fall: *37* • Total Graduates: *21*

FINANCES

Residential Annual Tuition: *Not Reported* • Non-Residential Annual Tuition: *Not Reported* • General Institution Fees: *Not Reported* • Additional Nursing Fees: *Not Reported*

EDGECOMBE COMMUNITY COLLEGE

Address: 225 Tarboro Street, Rocky Mount, NC 27801
Phone: 252-446-0436
Fax: Not Reported
Contact: Katherine Williford, MSN, Director of Nursing
Email: willifordk@edgecombe.ncus

GENERAL INFORMATION

Type of School: *Not Reported* • Accreditation: *Southern Association of Colleges and Schools* • Total Enrollment: *Not Reported*

PROGRAM INFORMATION

LPN/LVN Exit: *Not Reported* • NLNAC Accreditation: *No*

NURSING STUDENT PROFILE

Total Nursing Enrollment: *Not Reported* • Full-Time Enrollment: *Not Reported* • Part-Time Enrollment: *Not Reported* • Female Enrollment: *Not Reported* • Male Enrollment: *Not Reported* • Total New Admissions Who Enrolled for Fall: *Not Reported* • Total Graduates: *Not Reported*

FINANCES

Residential Annual Tuition: *Not Reported* • Non-Residential Annual Tuition: *Not Reported* • General Institution Fees: *Not Reported* • Additional Nursing Fees: *Not Reported*

FAYETTEVILLE TECHNICAL COMMUNITY COLLEGE

Address: PO Box 35236, Fayetteville, NC 28303
Phone: 910-678-8482
Fax: 910-678-8500
Contact: Kathy T. Weeks, RN, MSN, Chair, Nursing Department
Email: weeksk@ftccmail.faytech.cc.nc.us

GENERAL INFORMATION

Type of School: *Not Reported* • Accreditation: *Southern Association of Colleges and Schools* • Total Enrollment: *Not Reported*

PROGRAM INFORMATION

LPN/LVN Exit: *No* • NLNAC Accreditation: *Yes*

NURSING STUDENT PROFILE

Total Nursing Enrollment: *134* • Full-Time Enrollment: *80* • Part-Time Enrollment: *54* • Female Enrollment: *122* • Male Enrollment: *12* • Total New Admissions Who Enrolled for Fall: *85* • Total Graduates: *47*

FINANCES

Residential Annual Tuition: *$1,073* • Non-Residential Annual Tuition: *$6,620* • General Institution Fees: *$9* • Additional Nursing Fees: *$18*

FOOTHILLS NURSING CONSORTIUM

Address: PO Box 804, Spindale, NC 28160
Phone: 828-286-3636
Fax: 828-286-4014
Contact: Jeanette M. Cheshire, RN, MPH, Director, Foothills Nursing Consortium
Email: jcheshir@isothermal.cc.nc.us

GENERAL INFORMATION

Type of School: *2-Year College or University, Public* • Accreditation: *Southern Association of Colleges and Schools* • Total Enrollment: *1800*

PROGRAM INFORMATION

LPN/LVN Exit: *No* • NLNAC Accreditation: *No*

NURSING STUDENT PROFILE

Total Nursing Enrollment: *65* • Full-Time Enrollment: *51* • Part-Time Enrollment: *14* • Female Enrollment: *58* • Male Enrollment: *7* • Total New Admissions Who Enrolled for Fall: *33* • Total Graduates: *26*

FINANCES

Residential Annual Tuition: *$744* • Non-Residential Annual Tuition: *$4,158* • General Institution Fees: *$28* • Additional Nursing Fees: *$0*

FORSYTH TECHNICAL COMMUNITY COLLEGE

Address: 2100 Silas Creek Parkway, Winston-Salem, NC 27103
Phone: 336-734-7428
Fax: 336-761-2399
Contact: Phyllis D. Bonds, MS, BSN, Assistant Dean, ADN Program
Email: psample@forsyth.cc.nc.us

GENERAL INFORMATION

Type of School: *Other, Public* • Accreditation: *Southern Association of Colleges and Schools* • Total Enrollment: *4000*

PROGRAM INFORMATION

LPN/LVN Exit: *No* • NLNAC Accreditation: *No*

NURSING STUDENT PROFILE

Total Nursing Enrollment: *136* • Full-Time Enrollment: *136* • Part-Time Enrollment: *0* • Female Enrollment: *126* • Male Enrollment: *10* • Total New Admissions Who Enrolled for Fall: *53* • Total Graduates: *63*

FINANCES

Residential Annual Tuition: *$660* • Non-Residential Annual Tuition: *$4,070* • General Institution Fees: *Not Reported* • Additional Nursing Fees: *$40*

GARDNER-WEBB UNIVERSITY

Address: Box 7268, Boiling Springs, NC 28017
Phone: 704-406-4359
Fax: 704-406-3919
Contact: Tracy T. Caldwell, RN, MN, Chair, Associate Degree Nursing Program
Email: tcaldwell@gardner-webb.edu

GENERAL INFORMATION

Type of School: *4-Year College or University, Private (Religious)* • Accreditation: *Southern Association of Colleges and Schools* • Total Enrollment: *3400*

PROGRAM INFORMATION

LPN/LVN Exit: *No* • NLNAC Accreditation: *Yes*

NURSING STUDENT PROFILE

Total Nursing Enrollment: *120* • Full-Time Enrollment: *120* • Part-Time Enrollment: *0* • Female Enrollment: *114* • Male Enrollment: *6* • Total New Admissions Who Enrolled for Fall: *70* • Total Graduates: *44*

FINANCES

Residential Annual Tuition: *$12,520* • Non-Residential Annual Tuition: *$12,520* • General Institution Fees: *Not Reported* • Additional Nursing Fees: *$14*

GASTON COLLEGE

Address: 201 Highway, 321 South, Dallas, NC 28034
Phone: 704-922-6367
Fax: 704-922-6468
Contact: Lois B. Bradley, RN, BSN, MEd, Chairperson of Nursing
Email: bradley.lois@gaston.cc.nc.us

GENERAL INFORMATION

Type of School: *2-Year College or University, Public* • Accreditation: *Southern Association of Colleges and Schools* • Total Enrollment: *4000*

PROGRAM INFORMATION

LPN/LVN Exit: *No* • NLNAC Accreditation: *No*

NURSING STUDENT PROFILE

Total Nursing Enrollment: *109* • Full-Time Enrollment: *109* • Part-Time Enrollment: *0* • Female Enrollment: *106* • Male Enrollment: *3* • Total New Admissions Who Enrolled for Fall: *72* • Total Graduates: *28*

FINANCES

Residential Annual Tuition: *$1,320* • Non-Residential Annual Tuition: *$8,148* • General Institution Fees: *$32* • Additional Nursing Fees: *$50*

GUILFORD TECHNICAL COMMUNITY COLLEGE

Address: PO Box 309, Jamestown, NC 27282
Phone: 336-334-4822
Fax: Not Reported
Contact: Cecelia G. Ray, RN, MEd, Department Chair
Email: rayc@gtec.cc.nc.us

GENERAL INFORMATION

Type of School: *Not Reported* • Accreditation: *None* • Total Enrollment: *Not Reported*

PROGRAM INFORMATION

LPN/LVN Exit: *Yes* • NLNAC Accreditation: *No*

NURSING STUDENT PROFILE

Total Nursing Enrollment: *135* • Full-Time Enrollment: *126* • Part-Time Enrollment: *9* • Female Enrollment: *118* • Male Enrollment: *17* • Total New Admissions Who Enrolled for Fall: *107* • Total Graduates: *62*

FINANCES

Residential Annual Tuition: *$480* • Non-Residential Annual Tuition: *$3,912* • General Institution Fees: *$56* • Additional Nursing Fees: *$8*

JAMES SPRUNT COMMUNITY COLLEGE

Address: PO Box 398, Kenansville, NC 28349
Phone: 910-296-2450
Fax: 910-296-6032
Contact: Rhonda B. Ferrell, RN, BSN, MSN, Department Chair Health Education
Email: rferrell@fscc.cc.nc.us

GENERAL INFORMATION

Type of School: *2-Year College or University, Other* • Accreditation: *Southern Association of Colleges and Schools* • Total Enrollment: *1200*

PROGRAM INFORMATION

LPN/LVN Exit: *No* • NLNAC Accreditation: *No*

NURSING STUDENT PROFILE

Total Nursing Enrollment: *77* • Full-Time Enrollment: *77* • Part-Time Enrollment: *0* • Female Enrollment: *74* • Male Enrollment: *3* • Total New Admissions Who Enrolled for Fall: *40* • Total Graduates: *32*

FINANCES

Residential Annual Tuition: *$496* • Non-Residential Annual Tuition: *$2,772* • General Institution Fees: *$38* • Additional Nursing Fees: *$71*

LENOIR COMMUNITY COLLEGE

Address: PO Box 188, Kinston, NC 28502
Phone: 252-527-6223
Fax: 252-527-2712
Contact: Alexis B. Welch, RN, BSN, MAEd, Dean of
           Allied Health and Director of Nursing Programs
Email: abw801@email.lenoir.cc.nc.us

GENERAL INFORMATION

Type of School: *2-Year College or University, Public* •
Accreditation: *Southern Association of Colleges and Schools* •
Total Enrollment: *1990*

PROGRAM INFORMATION

LPN/LVN Exit: *No* • NLNAC Accreditation: *No*

NURSING STUDENT PROFILE

Total Nursing Enrollment: *49* • Full-Time Enrollment: *39* •
Part-Time Enrollment: *10* • Female Enrollment: *2* • Male
Enrollment: *47* • Total New Admissions Who Enrolled for
Fall: *29* • Total Graduates: *19*

FINANCES

Residential Annual Tuition: *$660* • Non-Residential Annual
Tuition: *$4,074* • General Institution Fees: *$38* • Additional
Nursing Fees: *$16*

MAYLAND COMMUNITY COLLEGE

Address: PO Box 547, Spruce Pine, NC 28777
Phone: 828-765-7351
Fax: 828-765-2327
Contact: Fredel Reighard, RN, MA, MSN, Dean, Nursing
           Programs
Email: freighard@mayland.cc.nc.us

GENERAL INFORMATION

Type of School: *2-Year College or University, Public* •
Accreditation: *Southern Association of Colleges and Schools* •
Total Enrollment: *1342*

PROGRAM INFORMATION

LPN/LVN Exit: *No* • NLNAC Accreditation: *No*

NURSING STUDENT PROFILE

Total Nursing Enrollment: *40* • Full-Time Enrollment: *40* •
Part-Time Enrollment: *0* • Female Enrollment: *35* • Male
Enrollment: *5* • Total New Admissions Who Enrolled for
Fall: *24* • Total Graduates: *24*

FINANCES

Residential Annual Tuition: *$1,650* • Non-Residential
Annual Tuition: *Not Reported* • General Institution Fees:
$56 • Additional Nursing Fees: *$1,621*

MITCHELL COMMUNITY COLLEGE

Address: 500 West Broad Street, Statesville, NC 28677
Phone: 704-878-4261
Fax: 704-878-3282
Contact: Kaye Miller, RNC, MSN, Director, Allied
           Health and Public Service Technologies
Email: kmiller@mitchell.cc.nc.us

GENERAL INFORMATION

Type of School: *2-Year College or University, Public* •
Accreditation: *Southern Association of Colleges and Schools* •
Total Enrollment: *1958*

PROGRAM INFORMATION

LPN/LVN Exit: *No* • NLNAC Accreditation: *No*

NURSING STUDENT PROFILE

Total Nursing Enrollment: *87* • Full-Time Enrollment: *87* •
Part-Time Enrollment: *0* • Female Enrollment: *80* • Male
Enrollment: *7* • Total New Admissions Who Enrolled for
Fall: *47* • Total Graduates: *38*

FINANCES

Residential Annual Tuition: *$28* • Non-Residential Annual
Tuition: *$170* • General Institution Fees: *$1* • Additional
Nursing Fees: *$118*

PIEDMONT COMMUNITY COLLEGE

Address: PO Box 1197, Roxboro, NC 27573
Phone: 336-599-1181
Fax: 336-598-0453
Contact: James W. Bevill, MSN, RN, Director, ADN
           Education
Email: bevillb@piedmont.cc.nc.us

GENERAL INFORMATION

Type of School: *2-Year College or University, Public* •
Accreditation: *Southern Association of Colleges and Schools* •
Total Enrollment: *1934*

PROGRAM INFORMATION

LPN/LVN Exit: *Yes* • NLNAC Accreditation: *No*

NURSING STUDENT PROFILE

Total Nursing Enrollment: *31* • Full-Time Enrollment: *31* •
Part-Time Enrollment: *0* • Female Enrollment: *28* • Male
Enrollment: *3* • Total New Admissions Who Enrolled for
Fall: *17* • Total Graduates: *13*

FINANCES

Residential Annual Tuition: *$913* • Non-Residential Annual
Tuition: *$5,465* • General Institution Fees: *$33* • Additional
Nursing Fees: *$16*

PITT COMMUNITY COLLEGE

Address: Highway 11 South, PO Drawer 7007, Greenville, NC 27835
Phone: 919-321-4337
Fax: 919-321-4451
Contact: Carla Lewis, MSN, RN, Chair
Email: clewis@pcc.pitt.nc.us

GENERAL INFORMATION

Type of School: *Not Reported* • Accreditation: *None* • Total Enrollment: *Not Reported*

PROGRAM INFORMATION

LPN/LVN Exit: *Yes* • NLNAC Accreditation: *No*

NURSING STUDENT PROFILE

Total Nursing Enrollment: *117* • Full-Time Enrollment: *117* • Part-Time Enrollment: *0* • Female Enrollment: *Not Reported* • Male Enrollment: *Not Reported* • Total New Admissions Who Enrolled for Fall: *75* • Total Graduates: *36*

FINANCES

Residential Annual Tuition: *$480* • Non-Residential Annual Tuition: *$1,512* • General Institution Fees: *$27* • Additional Nursing Fees: *Not Reported*

RANDOLPH COMMUNITY COLLEGE

Address: PO Box 1009, Asheboro, NC 27204
Phone: 336-633-0264
Fax: 336-629-4695
Contact: Bonnie W. Baker, MSN, RN, OCN, Department Chair, Health Occupations
Email: bwbaker@randolph.cc.nc.us

GENERAL INFORMATION

Type of School: *2-Year College or University, Public* • Accreditation: *Southern Association of Colleges and Schools* • Total Enrollment: *1949*

PROGRAM INFORMATION

LPN/LVN Exit: *No* • NLNAC Accreditation: *Yes*

NURSING STUDENT PROFILE

Total Nursing Enrollment: *66* • Full-Time Enrollment: *53* • Part-Time Enrollment: *13* • Female Enrollment: *62* • Male Enrollment: *4* • Total New Admissions Who Enrolled for Fall: *40* • Total Graduates: *28*

FINANCES

Residential Annual Tuition: *$1,127* • Non-Residential Annual Tuition: *$6,959* • General Institution Fees: *Not Reported* • Additional Nursing Fees: *$30*

RICHMOND COMMUNITY COLLEGE

Address: P.O. Box 1169, Hamlet, NC 28345
Phone: 910-582-7061
Fax: Not Reported
Contact: Fran Irby, MEd, BSN, RN, Division
           Chairperson, Health Sciences
Email: Fran@richmond.cc.nc.us

GENERAL INFORMATION

Type of School: *Not Reported* • Accreditation: *Not Reported* • Total Enrollment: *Not Reported*

PROGRAM INFORMATION

LPN/LVN Exit: *Not Reported* • NLNAC Accreditation: *No*

NURSING STUDENT PROFILE

Total Nursing Enrollment: *80* • Full-Time Enrollment: *80* • Part-Time Enrollment: *0* • Female Enrollment: *Not Reported* • Male Enrollment: *Not Reported* • Total New Admissions Who Enrolled for Fall: *40* • Total Graduates: *37*

FINANCES

Residential Annual Tuition: *Not Reported* • Non-Residential Annual Tuition: *Not Reported* • General Institution Fees: *Not Reported* • Additional Nursing Fees: *Not Reported*

ROANOKE-CHOWAN COMMUNITY COLLEGE

Address: 109 Community College Road, Ahoskie, NC
           27910
Phone: 252-862-1286
Fax: 252-862-1358
Contact: Jean Matthews, RN, MSN, ADN Director
Email: jeanm@roanoke.cc.nc.us

GENERAL INFORMATION

Type of School: *2-Year College or University, Public* • Accreditation: *Southern Association of Colleges and Schools* • Total Enrollment: *1000*

PROGRAM INFORMATION

LPN/LVN Exit: *No* • NLNAC Accreditation: *No*

NURSING STUDENT PROFILE

Total Nursing Enrollment: *50* • Full-Time Enrollment: *50* • Part-Time Enrollment: *0* • Female Enrollment: *49* • Male Enrollment: *1* • Total New Admissions Who Enrolled for Fall: *31* • Total Graduates: *19*

FINANCES

Residential Annual Tuition: *$660* • Non-Residential Annual Tuition: *$4,074* • General Institution Fees: *$30* • Additional Nursing Fees: *$19*

ROBESON COMMUNITY COLLEGE

Address: P.O. Box 1420, Lamberton, NC 28359
Phone: 910-618-5680
Fax: 910-618-5685
Contact: Barbara N. Brown, BSN, MHEd, Director of
             ADN Program
Email: bbrown@robeson.cc.nc.us

GENERAL INFORMATION

Type of School: *2-Year College or University, Public* •
Accreditation: *Southern Association of Colleges and Schools* •
Total Enrollment: *2125*

PROGRAM INFORMATION

LPN/LVN Exit: *Yes* • NLNAC Accreditation: *Yes*

NURSING STUDENT PROFILE

Total Nursing Enrollment: *72* • Full-Time Enrollment: *72* •
Part-Time Enrollment: *0* • Female Enrollment: *66* • Male
Enrollment: *6* • Total New Admissions Who Enrolled for
Fall: *50* • Total Graduates: *30*

FINANCES

Residential Annual Tuition: *$960* • Non-Residential Annual
Tuition: *$4,374* • General Institution Fees: *$40* • Additional
Nursing Fees: *$15*

ROCKINGHAM COMMUNITY COLLEGE

Address: PO Box 38, Wentworth, NC 27375
Phone: 336-342-4261
Fax: Not Reported
Contact: Cindy Yount, MSN, RN, Nursing Program
             Director
Email: yountc@rcc.cc.nc.us

GENERAL INFORMATION

Type of School: *2-Year College or University, Public* •
Accreditation: *Southern Association of Colleges and Schools* •
Total Enrollment: *2000*

PROGRAM INFORMATION

LPN/LVN Exit: *Not Reported* • NLNAC Accreditation: *No*

NURSING STUDENT PROFILE

Total Nursing Enrollment: *42* • Full-Time Enrollment: *42* •
Part-Time Enrollment: *0* • Female Enrollment: *37* • Male
Enrollment: *5* • Total New Admissions Who Enrolled for
Fall: *32* • Total Graduates: *19*

FINANCES

Residential Annual Tuition: *$1,512* • Non-Residential
Annual Tuition: *$4,926* • General Institution Fees: *$70* •
Additional Nursing Fees: *$1,250*

ROWAN-CABARRUS COMMUNITY COLLEGE

Address: PO Box 1595, Salisbury, NC 28145
Phone: 704-637-0760
Fax: 704-642-0750
Contact: Cathy Norris, MSN, RN, Director of Nursing Education
Email: norrisc@rccc.cc.nc.us

GENERAL INFORMATION

Type of School: *Other, Public* • Accreditation: *Southern Association of Colleges and Schools* • Total Enrollment: *4724*

PROGRAM INFORMATION

LPN/LVN Exit: *No* • NLNAC Accreditation: *Yes*

NURSING STUDENT PROFILE

Total Nursing Enrollment: *106* • Full-Time Enrollment: *53* • Part-Time Enrollment: *53* • Female Enrollment: *96* • Male Enrollment: *10* • Total New Admissions Who Enrolled for Fall: *60* • Total Graduates: *56*

FINANCES

Residential Annual Tuition: *$568* • Non-Residential Annual Tuition: *$3,152* • General Institution Fees: *$69* • Additional Nursing Fees: *$52*

SAMPSON COMMUNITY COLLEGE

Address: PO Box 318, Clinton, NC 28329
Phone: 910-592-8081
Fax: 910-592-8048
Contact: Mary B. Brown, RN, MS, BSN, Division Chair of Health Programs
Email: mbrown@sampson.cc.nc.us

GENERAL INFORMATION

Type of School: *2-Year College or University, Public* • Accreditation: *Southern Association of Colleges and Schools* • Total Enrollment: *1400*

PROGRAM INFORMATION

LPN/LVN Exit: *No* • NLNAC Accreditation: *No*

NURSING STUDENT PROFILE

Total Nursing Enrollment: *75* • Full-Time Enrollment: *75* • Part-Time Enrollment: *0* • Female Enrollment: *69* • Male Enrollment: *6* • Total New Admissions Who Enrolled for Fall: *40* • Total Graduates: *29*

FINANCES

Residential Annual Tuition: *$440* • Non-Residential Annual Tuition: *$2,716* • General Institution Fees: *Not Reported* • Additional Nursing Fees: *$750*

SANDHILL COMMUNITY COLLEGE

Address: 2200 Airport Road, Pinehurst, NC 28374
Phone: 910-692-6185
Fax: 610-692-6918
Contact: Star Mitchell, MSN, RN, Director
Email: Not Reported

GENERAL INFORMATION

Type of School: *Not Reported* • Accreditation: *Not Reported* • Total Enrollment: *Not Reported*

PROGRAM INFORMATION

LPN/LVN Exit: *Not Reported* • NLNAC Accreditation: *No*

NURSING STUDENT PROFILE

Total Nursing Enrollment: *115* • Full-Time Enrollment: *Not Reported* • Part-Time Enrollment: *Not Reported* • Female Enrollment: *Not Reported* • Male Enrollment: *Not Reported* • Total New Admissions Who Enrolled for Fall: *Not Reported* • Total Graduates: *60*

FINANCES

Residential Annual Tuition: *Not Reported* • Non-Residential Annual Tuition: *Not Reported* • General Institution Fees: *Not Reported* • Additional Nursing Fees: *Not Reported*

SOUTHEASTERN COMMUNITY COLLEGE

Address: 4564 Chadbourn Highway, PO Box 151, Whiteville, NC 28472
Phone: Not Reported
Fax: Not Reported
Contact: Pamela Bradley, MSN, RN, Director
Email: Not Reported

GENERAL INFORMATION

Type of School: *2-Year College or University, Public* • Accreditation: *Southern Association of Colleges and Schools* • Total Enrollment: *1900*

PROGRAM INFORMATION

LPN/LVN Exit: *Not Reported* • NLNAC Accreditation: *No*

NURSING STUDENT PROFILE

Total Nursing Enrollment: *87* • Full-Time Enrollment: *87* • Part-Time Enrollment: *0* • Female Enrollment: *81* • Male Enrollment: *6* • Total New Admissions Who Enrolled for Fall: *54* • Total Graduates: *32*

FINANCES

Residential Annual Tuition: *$1,216* • Non-Residential Annual Tuition: *$6,304* • General Institution Fees: *$47* • Additional Nursing Fees: *$18*

STANLY COMMUNITY COLLEGE

Address: 141 College Drive, Albermarle, NC 28001
Phone: 704-991-0276
Fax: 704-982-0819
Contact: Joan D. Eudy, PhD, RN, CS, Associate Dean for Allied Health/Nursing
Email: eudyjc@stanly.cc.nc.us

GENERAL INFORMATION

Type of School: *2-Year College or University, Public* •
Accreditation: *Southern Association of Colleges and Schools* •
Total Enrollment: *1500*

PROGRAM INFORMATION

LPN/LVN Exit: *Yes* • NLNAC Accreditation: *No*

NURSING STUDENT PROFILE

Total Nursing Enrollment: *80* • Full-Time Enrollment: *Not Reported* • Part-Time Enrollment: *Not Reported* • Female Enrollment: *73* • Male Enrollment: *7* • Total New Admissions Who Enrolled for Fall: *52* • Total Graduates: *21*

FINANCES

Residential Annual Tuition: *$800* • Non-Residential Annual Tuition: *$4,800* • General Institution Fees: *$38* • Additional Nursing Fees: *$8*

SURRY COMMUNITY COLLEGE—ALLIED HEALTH DIVISION

Address: PO Box 304, Dobson, NC 27017
Phone: 336-386-8121
Fax: 336-386-4723
Contact: Sharon Kallam, RN, BSN, MSN, Chairperson, Allied Health Division
Email: kallams@surry.cc.nc.us

GENERAL INFORMATION

Type of School: *2-Year College or University, Public* •
Accreditation: *Southern Association of Colleges and Schools* •
Total Enrollment: *3390*

PROGRAM INFORMATION

LPN/LVN Exit: *Not Reported* • NLNAC Accreditation: *No*

NURSING STUDENT PROFILE

Total Nursing Enrollment: *119* • Full-Time Enrollment: *99* • Part-Time Enrollment: *20* • Female Enrollment: *116* • Male Enrollment: *3* • Total New Admissions Who Enrolled for Fall: *191* • Total Graduates: *36*

FINANCES

Residential Annual Tuition: *$512* • Non-Residential Annual Tuition: *$2,788* • General Institution Fees: *$43* • Additional Nursing Fees: *$14*

VANCE GRANVILLE COMMUNITY COLLEGE

Address: PO Box 917, Henderson, NC 27536
Phone: 252-492-2061
Fax: 252-492-2019
Contact: Beth C. Phillips, MSN, RN, Program Director
Email: phillips@admin.vgcc.cc.nc.us

GENERAL INFORMATION

Type of School: *Not Reported* • Accreditation: *Southern Association of Colleges and Schools* • Total Enrollment: *Not Reported*

PROGRAM INFORMATION

LPN/LVN Exit: *No* • NLNAC Accreditation: *No*

NURSING STUDENT PROFILE

Total Nursing Enrollment: *71* • Full-Time Enrollment: *71* • Part-Time Enrollment: *0* • Female Enrollment: *67* • Male Enrollment: *4* • Total New Admissions Who Enrolled for Fall: *42* • Total Graduates: *26*

FINANCES

Residential Annual Tuition: *$660* • Non-Residential Annual Tuition: *$5,433* • General Institution Fees: *$0* • Additional Nursing Fees: *$0*

WAYNE COMMUNITY COLLEGE

Address: PO Box 8002, Goldsboro, NC 27533
Phone: 919-735-5151
Fax: 919-736-1707
Contact: Rachel B. Hall, RN, MSN, BSN, Department Head, Nursing
Email: rabh@wcc.wayne.cc.nc.us

GENERAL INFORMATION

Type of School: *2-Year College or University, Public* • Accreditation: *Southern Association of Colleges and Schools* • Total Enrollment: *3162*

PROGRAM INFORMATION

LPN/LVN Exit: *No* • NLNAC Accreditation: *No*

NURSING STUDENT PROFILE

Total Nursing Enrollment: *66* • Full-Time Enrollment: *66* • Part-Time Enrollment: *0* • Female Enrollment: *65* • Male Enrollment: *1* • Total New Admissions Who Enrolled for Fall: *40* • Total Graduates: *27*

FINANCES

Residential Annual Tuition: *$1,320* • Non-Residential Annual Tuition: *$8,148* • General Institution Fees: *$48* • Additional Nursing Fees: *$0*

WESTERN PIEDMONT COMMUNITY COLLEGE

Address: 1001 Burkemont Avenue, Morganton, NC 28655
Phone: 828-438-6122
Fax: 828-430-7183
Contact: Betty L. Miller, PhD, RN, BSN, MSN, ADN Program Coordinator
Email: bmiller@wp.cc.nc.us

GENERAL INFORMATION

Type of School: *2-Year College or University, Public* • Accreditation: *Southern Association of Colleges and Schools* • Total Enrollment: *Not Reported*

PROGRAM INFORMATION

LPN/LVN Exit: *No* • NLNAC Accreditation: *Yes*

NURSING STUDENT PROFILE

Total Nursing Enrollment: *97* • Full-Time Enrollment: *97* • Part-Time Enrollment: *0* • Female Enrollment: *86* • Male Enrollment: *11* • Total New Admissions Who Enrolled for Fall: *61* • Total Graduates: *38*

FINANCES

Residential Annual Tuition: *$936* • Non-Residential Annual Tuition: *$5,941* • General Institution Fees: *$17* • Additional Nursing Fees: *$50*

WILKES COMMUNITY COLLEGE

Address: PO Drawer 120, Wilkesboro, NC 28697
Phone: 336-838-6257
Fax: 338-838-6255
Contact: Kathryn Tinsdale, MSN, RN, Chairperson
Email: Not Reported

GENERAL INFORMATION

Type of School: *Not Reported* • Accreditation: *Not Reported* • Total Enrollment: *Not Reported*

PROGRAM INFORMATION

LPN/LVN Exit: *Not Reported* • NLNAC Accreditation: *No*

NURSING STUDENT PROFILE

Total Nursing Enrollment: *Not Reported* • Full-Time Enrollment: *Not Reported* • Part-Time Enrollment: *Not Reported* • Female Enrollment: *Not Reported* • Male Enrollment: *Not Reported* • Total New Admissions Who Enrolled for Fall: *Not Reported* • Total Graduates: *Not Reported*

FINANCES

Residential Annual Tuition: *Not Reported* • Non-Residential Annual Tuition: *Not Reported* • General Institution Fees: *Not Reported* • Additional Nursing Fees: *Not Reported*

JAMESTOWN COLLEGE

Address: 6000 College Lane, Jamestown, ND 58405
Phone: 716-665-5220
Fax: 716-665-3679
Contact: Dawn T. Columbare, RN, MS, Director, Nursing Education
Email: dawncolumbare@mail.sunyjcc.edu

BELMONT TECHNICAL COLLEGE

Address: 120 Fox - Shannon Place, St. Craisville, OH 43950
Phone: 740-695-9500
Fax: 740-695-2247
Contact: Rebecca J. Kurtz, MSN, RN, Dean of Program Coordination and Nursing
Email: bkurtz@belmont.cc.oh.us

GENERAL INFORMATION

Type of School: *4-Year College or University, Private (Religious)* • Accreditation: *North Central Association of Colleges and Schools* • Total Enrollment: *Not Reported*

GENERAL INFORMATION

Type of School: *2-Year College or University, Public* • Accreditation: *North Central Association of Colleges and Schools* • Total Enrollment: *1800*

PROGRAM INFORMATION

LPN/LVN Exit: *No* • NLNAC Accreditation: *Yes*

PROGRAM INFORMATION

LPN/LVN Exit: *No* • NLNAC Accreditation: *No*

NURSING STUDENT PROFILE

Total Nursing Enrollment: *108* • Full-Time Enrollment: *43* • Part-Time Enrollment: *65* • Female Enrollment: *99* • Male Enrollment: *9* • Total New Admissions Who Enrolled for Fall: *64* • Total Graduates: *46*

NURSING STUDENT PROFILE

Total Nursing Enrollment: *65* • Full-Time Enrollment: *65* • Part-Time Enrollment: *0* • Female Enrollment: *60* • Male Enrollment: *5* • Total New Admissions Who Enrolled for Fall: *48* • Total Graduates: *25*

FINANCES

Residential Annual Tuition: *$1,250* • Non-Residential Annual Tuition: *$2,600* • General Institution Fees: *Not Reported* • Additional Nursing Fees: *$100*

FINANCES

Residential Annual Tuition: *$2,272* • Non-Residential Annual Tuition: *$4,000* • General Institution Fees: *$140* • Additional Nursing Fees: *$160*

CENTRAL OHIO TECHNICAL COLLEGE

Address: 1179 University Drive, Newark, OH 43055
Phone: 740-366-9288
Fax: 740-366-9478
Contact: Tamar J. Gilson, MS, RN, Nursing Programs Administrator
Email: tgilson@cotc.tec.oh.us

GENERAL INFORMATION

Type of School: *2-Year College or University, Public* • Accreditation: *North Central Association of Colleges and Schools* • Total Enrollment: *1973*

PROGRAM INFORMATION

LPN/LVN Exit: *No* • NLNAC Accreditation: *Yes*

NURSING STUDENT PROFILE

Total Nursing Enrollment: *141* • Full-Time Enrollment: *57* • Part-Time Enrollment: *84* • Female Enrollment: *126* • Male Enrollment: *15* • Total New Admissions Who Enrolled for Fall: *109* • Total Graduates: *48*

FINANCES

Residential Annual Tuition: *$3,672* • Non-Residential Annual Tuition: *$5,664* • General Institution Fees: *Not Reported* • Additional Nursing Fees: *$100*

CINCINNATI STATE TECHNICAL & COMMUNITY COLLEGE

Address: 3520 Central Parkway, Cincinnati, OH 45223
Phone: 513-569-1476
Fax: 513-569-1659
Contact: Alice Palmer, RN, MS, ANP-C, Program Chair and Director
Email: palmera@cinstate.cc.oh.us

GENERAL INFORMATION

Type of School: *2-Year College or University, Public* • Accreditation: *North Central Association of Colleges and Schools* • Total Enrollment: *7184*

PROGRAM INFORMATION

LPN/LVN Exit: *No* • NLNAC Accreditation: *Yes*

NURSING STUDENT PROFILE

Total Nursing Enrollment: *162* • Full-Time Enrollment: *32* • Part-Time Enrollment: *130* • Female Enrollment: *154* • Male Enrollment: *8* • Total New Admissions Who Enrolled for Fall: *70* • Total Graduates: *85*

FINANCES

Residential Annual Tuition: *$1,500* • Non-Residential Annual Tuition: *$3,000* • General Institution Fees: *$24* • Additional Nursing Fees: *$200*

CLARK STATE COMMUNITY COLLEGE

Address: 570 East Leffel Lane, Springfield, OH 45505
Phone: 937-328-6060
Fax: 937-328-6138
Contact: Barbara Burcham, BSN, MS, Dean of Health Technologies
Email: burchamb@clarkstate.edu

GENERAL INFORMATION

Type of School: *2-Year College or University, Public* • Accreditation: *North Central Association of Colleges and Schools* • Total Enrollment: *2985*

PROGRAM INFORMATION

LPN/LVN Exit: *No* • NLNAC Accreditation: *Yes*

NURSING STUDENT PROFILE

Total Nursing Enrollment: *127* • Full-Time Enrollment: *Not Reported* • Part-Time Enrollment: *Not Reported* • Female Enrollment: *117* • Male Enrollment: *10* • Total New Admissions Who Enrolled for Fall: *85* • Total Graduates: *44*

FINANCES

Residential Annual Tuition: *$2,300* • Non-Residential Annual Tuition: *$5,000* • General Institution Fees: *$420* • Additional Nursing Fees: *$180*

COLUMBUS STATE COMMUNITY COLLEGE— COLUMBUS

Address: 550 East Spring Street, Columbus, OH 43216-1609
Phone: 614-287-2507
Fax: 614-287-3854
Contact: Polly Owens, PhD, RN, Chairpersons, Nursing and Related Services
Email: psowen@cscc.edu

GENERAL INFORMATION

Type of School: *2-Year College or University, Public* • Accreditation: *North Central Association of Colleges and Schools* • Total Enrollment: *19642*

PROGRAM INFORMATION

LPN/LVN Exit: *No* • NLNAC Accreditation: *Yes*

NURSING STUDENT PROFILE

Total Nursing Enrollment: *266* • Full-Time Enrollment: *39* • Part-Time Enrollment: *227* • Female Enrollment: *251* • Male Enrollment: *15* • Total New Admissions Who Enrolled for Fall: *108* • Total Graduates: *68*

FINANCES

Residential Annual Tuition: *$3,660* • Non-Residential Annual Tuition: *$9,720* • General Institution Fees: *Not Reported* • Additional Nursing Fees: *$218*

CUYAHOGA COMMUNITY COLLEGE

Address: 2900 Community College Avenue, Cleveland, OH 44115
Phone: 216-987-4106
Fax: 216-987-4287
Contact: Barbara A. Pennell, PhD, RN, Assistant Dean and Director
Email: Barbara.pennell@tri-c.cc.oh.us

GENERAL INFORMATION

Type of School: *2-Year College or University, Public* • Accreditation: *North Central Association of Colleges and Schools* • Total Enrollment: *20321*

PROGRAM INFORMATION

LPN/LVN Exit: *No* • NLNAC Accreditation: *Yes*

NURSING STUDENT PROFILE

Total Nursing Enrollment: *205* • Full-Time Enrollment: *205* • Part-Time Enrollment: *0* • Female Enrollment: *181* • Male Enrollment: *24* • Total New Admissions Who Enrolled for Fall: *70* • Total Graduates: *68*

FINANCES

Residential Annual Tuition: *$1,864* • Non-Residential Annual Tuition: *$3,806* • General Institution Fees: *$5* • Additional Nursing Fees: *$1,705*

EDISON COMMUNITY COLLEGE—PIQUA

Address: 1973 Edison Drive, Piqua, OH 45356
Phone: 937-778-8600
Fax: 937-778-1920
Contact: Sharon Brown, MSN, BSN, RN, Dean of Health and Human Systems
Email: brown@edison.cc.oh.us

GENERAL INFORMATION

Type of School: *2-Year College or University, Public* • Accreditation: *North Central Association of Colleges and Schools* • Total Enrollment: *2700*

PROGRAM INFORMATION

LPN/LVN Exit: *No* • NLNAC Accreditation: *Yes*

NURSING STUDENT PROFILE

Total Nursing Enrollment: *77* • Full-Time Enrollment: *55* • Part-Time Enrollment: *22* • Female Enrollment: *69* • Male Enrollment: *8* • Total New Admissions Who Enrolled for Fall: *38* • Total Graduates: *39*

FINANCES

Residential Annual Tuition: *$1,584* • Non-Residential Annual Tuition: *$3,264* • General Institution Fees: *$792* • Additional Nursing Fees: *$309*

GOOD SAMARITAN HOSPITAL

Address: 375 Dixmyth Avenue, Cincinnati, OH 45220-2489
Phone: 513-872-3736
Fax: 513-872-3572
Contact: Pat McMahon, MSN, RN, NP-C, Dean of Academic Affairs
Email: Pat_McMahon@trihealth.com

GENERAL INFORMATION

Type of School: *Independent, Private (Religious)* • Accreditation: *None* • Total Enrollment: *263*

PROGRAM INFORMATION

LPN/LVN Exit: *No* • NLNAC Accreditation: *No*

NURSING STUDENT PROFILE

Total Nursing Enrollment: *263* • Full-Time Enrollment: *151* • Part-Time Enrollment: *112* • Female Enrollment: *253* • Male Enrollment: *10* • Total New Admissions Who Enrolled for Fall: *79* • Total Graduates: *68*

FINANCES

Residential Annual Tuition: *$7,630* • Non-Residential Annual Tuition: *$7,630* • General Institution Fees: *$276* • Additional Nursing Fees: *$220*

HOCKING TECHNICAL COLLEGE

Address: 3301 Hocking Parkway, Nelsonville, OH 45764
Phone: 740-753-3591
Fax: 740-753-5105
Contact: Mary B. Weiland, PhD, MSN, RN, Dean, School of Health and Nursing
Email: weiland_m@hocking.edu

GENERAL INFORMATION

Type of School: *Other, Public* • Accreditation: *North Central Association of Colleges and Schools* • Total Enrollment: *5316*

PROGRAM INFORMATION

LPN/LVN Exit: *Yes* • NLNAC Accreditation: *Yes*

NURSING STUDENT PROFILE

Total Nursing Enrollment: *358* • Full-Time Enrollment: *Not Reported* • Part-Time Enrollment: *Not Reported* • Female Enrollment: *327* • Male Enrollment: *31* • Total New Admissions Who Enrolled for Fall: *110* • Total Graduates: *313*

FINANCES

Residential Annual Tuition: *$2,448* • Non-Residential Annual Tuition: *$4,896* • General Institution Fees: *$912* • Additional Nursing Fees: *$1,053*

KENT STATE UNIVERSITY

Address: 113 Henderson Hall PO Box 5190, Kent, OH
            44242
Phone: 330-672-3777
Fax: Not Reported
Contact: Davina Gosnell, PhD, RN, FAAN, Dean,
            College of Nursing
Email: dgosnell@kent.edu

GENERAL INFORMATION

Type of School: *Not Reported* • Accreditation: *Not Reported* •
Total Enrollment: *Not Reported*

PROGRAM INFORMATION

LPN/LVN Exit: *No* • NLNAC Accreditation: *Yes*

NURSING STUDENT PROFILE

Total Nursing Enrollment: *221* • Full-Time Enrollment: *73* •
Part-Time Enrollment: *148* • Female Enrollment: *205* • Male
Enrollment: *16* • Total New Admissions Who Enrolled for
Fall: *97* • Total Graduates: *112*

FINANCES

Residential Annual Tuition: *$3,164* • Non-Residential
Annual Tuition: *$7,824* • General Institution Fees: *$0* •
Additional Nursing Fees: *$96*

KETTERING COLLEGE OF MEDICAL ARTS

Address: 3737 Southern Boulevard, Kettering, OH 45429
Phone: 937-296-7219
Fax: 937-296-7810
Contact: Brenda Stevenson, PhD, RN, Director
Email: brenda.stevenson@kmcnetwork.org

GENERAL INFORMATION

Type of School: *4-Year College or University, Private
(Religious)* • Accreditation: *North Central Association of
Colleges and Schools* • Total Enrollment: *505*

PROGRAM INFORMATION

LPN/LVN Exit: *No* • NLNAC Accreditation: *Yes*

NURSING STUDENT PROFILE

Total Nursing Enrollment: *112* • Full-Time Enrollment:
112 • Part-Time Enrollment: *0* • Female Enrollment: *102* •
Male Enrollment: *10* • Total New Admissions Who Enrolled
for Fall: *30* • Total Graduates: *34*

FINANCES

Residential Annual Tuition: *$6,150* • Non-Residential
Annual Tuition: *$6,150* • General Institution Fees: *$144* •
Additional Nursing Fees: *$360*

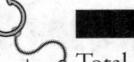

Circle 159 on reader card

LAKELAND COMMUNITY COLLEGE

Address: 7700 Clocktower Drive, Kirtland, OH 44094-5198
Phone: 440-953-7172
Fax: 440-975-4733
Contact: Judith C. Greig, MSN, RN, Nursing Program Director
Email: jgreig@lakeland.cc.oh.us

GENERAL INFORMATION

Type of School: *Not Reported* • Accreditation: *Not Reported* • Total Enrollment: *Not Reported*

PROGRAM INFORMATION

LPN/LVN Exit: *No* • NLNAC Accreditation: *Yes*

NURSING STUDENT PROFILE

Total Nursing Enrollment: *164* • Full-Time Enrollment: *56* • Part-Time Enrollment: *108* • Female Enrollment: *153* • Male Enrollment: *11* • Total New Admissions Who Enrolled for Fall: *52* • Total Graduates: *58*

FINANCES

Residential Annual Tuition: *$2,283* • Non-Residential Annual Tuition: *$5,979* • General Institution Fees: *$29* • Additional Nursing Fees: *$220*

LIMA TECHNICAL COLLEGE

Address: 4240 Campus Drive, Lima, OH 45804-3597
Phone: 419-995-8218
Fax: 419-995-8818
Contact: Lois Deleryyelle, PhD, RN, Chairperson
Email: deleruyl@ltc.tcc.oh.uu

GENERAL INFORMATION

Type of School: *2-Year College or University, Public* • Accreditation: *North Central Association of Colleges and Schools* • Total Enrollment: *2521*

PROGRAM INFORMATION

LPN/LVN Exit: *Not Reported* • NLNAC Accreditation: *No*

NURSING STUDENT PROFILE

Total Nursing Enrollment: *Not Reported* • Full-Time Enrollment: *Not Reported* • Part-Time Enrollment: *Not Reported* • Female Enrollment: *Not Reported* • Male Enrollment: *Not Reported* • Total New Admissions Who Enrolled for Fall: *Not Reported* • Total Graduates: *Not Reported*

FINANCES

Residential Annual Tuition: *Not Reported* • Non-Residential Annual Tuition: *Not Reported* • General Institution Fees: *Not Reported* • Additional Nursing Fees: *Not Reported*

LORAIN COUNTY COMMUNITY COLLEGE

Address: 1005 North Abbe Road, Elyria, OH 44035
Phone: 440-366-7186
Fax: 440-366-4116
Contact: Hope M. Moon, MSN, RN, CNS, Program Director
Email: hmoon@lorainccc.edu

GENERAL INFORMATION

Type of School: *2-Year College or University, Public* • Accreditation: *North Central Association of Colleges and Schools* • Total Enrollment: *421*

PROGRAM INFORMATION

LPN/LVN Exit: *No* • NLNAC Accreditation: *Yes*

NURSING STUDENT PROFILE

Total Nursing Enrollment: *421* • Full-Time Enrollment: *Not Reported* • Part-Time Enrollment: *Not Reported* • Female Enrollment: *335* • Male Enrollment: *86* • Total New Admissions Who Enrolled for Fall: *158* • Total Graduates: *53*

FINANCES

Residential Annual Tuition: *$2,750* • Non-Residential Annual Tuition: *$6,750* • General Institution Fees: *$0* • Additional Nursing Fees: *$155*

MARION TECHNICAL COLLEGE

Address: 1467 Mount Vernon Avenue, Marion, OH 43302-5628
Phone: 740-389-4636
Fax: 740-725-4018
Contact: Carol Hoffman, RN, MS, Director of Nursing
Email: hoffmanc@mtc.tec.oh.us

GENERAL INFORMATION

Type of School: *Technical/Specialized Institution, Public* • Accreditation: *North Central Association of Colleges and Schools* • Total Enrollment: *1595*

PROGRAM INFORMATION

LPN/LVN Exit: *No* • NLNAC Accreditation: *Yes*

NURSING STUDENT PROFILE

Total Nursing Enrollment: *1665* • Full-Time Enrollment: *596* • Part-Time Enrollment: *1069* • Female Enrollment: *1025* • Male Enrollment: *640* • Total New Admissions Who Enrolled for Fall: *52* • Total Graduates: *40*

FINANCES

Residential Annual Tuition: *$2,484* • Non-Residential Annual Tuition: *$4,248* • General Institution Fees: *$0* • Additional Nursing Fees: *$600*

MERCY COLLEGE OF NORTHWEST OHIO

Address: 2221 Madison Avenue, Toledo, OH 43624-1132
Phone: 419-251-1583
Fax: 419-251-1570
Contact: Maria E. Nowicki, PhD, RN, Director of Nursing
Email: Maria.Nowicki@mercycollege.edu

GENERAL INFORMATION

Type of School: *4-Year College or University, Private (Religious)* • Accreditation: *North Central Association of Colleges and Schools* • Total Enrollment: *222*

PROGRAM INFORMATION

LPN/LVN Exit: *Not Reported* • NLNAC Accreditation: *Not Reported*

NURSING STUDENT PROFILE

Total Nursing Enrollment: *105* • Full-Time Enrollment: *30* • Part-Time Enrollment: *75* • Female Enrollment: *103* • Male Enrollment: *2* • Total New Admissions Who Enrolled for Fall: *19* • Total Graduates: *33*

FINANCES

Residential Annual Tuition: *$4,000* • Non-Residential Annual Tuition: *$4,000* • General Institution Fees: *$65* • Additional Nursing Fees: *$250*

MIAMI UNIVERSITY

Address: 501 East High Street, Oxford, OH 45056
Phone: 513-785-3280
Fax: 513-785-3284
Contact: Eugenia M. Mills, PhD, RN, Chair and Director
Email: millsem@muohio.edu

GENERAL INFORMATION

Type of School: *4-Year College or University, Public* • Accreditation: *North Central Association of Colleges and Schools* • Total Enrollment: *19600*

PROGRAM INFORMATION

LPN/LVN Exit: *No* • NLNAC Accreditation: *Yes*

NURSING STUDENT PROFILE

Total Nursing Enrollment: *140* • Full-Time Enrollment: *128* • Part-Time Enrollment: *12* • Female Enrollment: *131* • Male Enrollment: *9* • Total New Admissions Who Enrolled for Fall: *89* • Total Graduates: *65*

FINANCES

Residential Annual Tuition: *$2,813* • Non-Residential Annual Tuition: *$10,486* • General Institution Fees: *$299* • Additional Nursing Fees: *$550*

NORTH CENTRAL STATE COLLEGE

Address: 2441 Kenwood Circle, Box 698, Mansfield, OH
            44901-0698
Phone: 419-755-4823
Fax: 419-755-5630
Contact: Janet Boeckman, MSN, RN, CPNP, Director of
            Nursing Programs
Email: jboeckma@nstate.tec.oh.us

GENERAL INFORMATION

Type of School: *Vocational/Technical School, Public* •
Accreditation: *North Central Association of Colleges and
Schools* • Total Enrollment: *2813*

PROGRAM INFORMATION

LPN/LVN Exit: *Yes* • NLNAC Accreditation: *Yes*

NURSING STUDENT PROFILE

Total Nursing Enrollment: *142* • Full-Time Enrollment:
142 • Part-Time Enrollment: *0* • Female Enrollment: *131* •
Male Enrollment: *11* • Total New Admissions Who Enrolled
for Fall: *72* • Total Graduates: *48*

FINANCES

Residential Annual Tuition: *$2,324* • Non-Residential
Annual Tuition: *$4,372* • General Institution Fees: *$369* •
Additional Nursing Fees: *$300*

NORTHWEST STATE COMMUNITY COLLEGE

Address: 22600 State Route 34, Archbold, OH 43502-
            9542
Phone: 419-267-5511
Fax: 419-267-3688
Contact: Cindy A. Krueger, MSN, RN, Dean, Allied
            Health and Public Service
Email: cindykru@nscc.cc.oh.us

GENERAL INFORMATION

Type of School: *2-Year College or University, Public* •
Accreditation: *North Central Association of Colleges and
Schools* • Total Enrollment: *2942*

PROGRAM INFORMATION

LPN/LVN Exit: *No* • NLNAC Accreditation: *Yes*

NURSING STUDENT PROFILE

Total Nursing Enrollment: *84* • Full-Time Enrollment: *55* •
Part-Time Enrollment: *29* • Female Enrollment: *76* • Male
Enrollment: *8* • Total New Admissions Who Enrolled for
Fall: *30* • Total Graduates: *31*

FINANCES

Residential Annual Tuition: *$3,600* • Non-Residential
Annual Tuition: *$6,804* • General Institution Fees: *$35* •
Additional Nursing Fees: *$244*

OHIO UNIVERSITY

Address: Grover Center E 365, Athens, OH 45701
Phone: 740-774-7282
Fax: 740-774-7711
Contact: Barbara Montgomery, PhD, RN, Associate
           Director
Email: montgob1@ohio.edu

GENERAL INFORMATION

Type of School: *4-Year College or University, Public* •
Accreditation: *North Central Association of Colleges and
Schools* • Total Enrollment: *17000*

PROGRAM INFORMATION

LPN/LVN Exit: *No* • NLNAC Accreditation: *Yes*

NURSING STUDENT PROFILE

Total Nursing Enrollment: *76* • Full-Time Enrollment: *45* •
Part-Time Enrollment: *31* • Female Enrollment: *62* • Male
Enrollment: *14* • Total New Admissions Who Enrolled for
Fall: *39* • Total Graduates: *27*

FINANCES

Residential Annual Tuition: *$3,383* • Non-Residential
Annual Tuition: *$8,328* • General Institution Fees: *Not
Reported* • Additional Nursing Fees: *$15*

OHIO UNIVERSITY— ZANESVILLE

Address: 1425 Newark Road, Zanesville, OH 43701
Phone: 740-453-0762
Fax: 740-588-1527
Contact: Sally F. Fusner, MS, RN, Interim Associate
           Director
Email: fusner@ohio.edu

GENERAL INFORMATION

Type of School: *4-Year College or University, Public* •
Accreditation: *North Central Association of Colleges and
Schools* • Total Enrollment: *1200*

PROGRAM INFORMATION

LPN/LVN Exit: *No* • NLNAC Accreditation: *Yes*

NURSING STUDENT PROFILE

Total Nursing Enrollment: *150* • Full-Time Enrollment: *Not
Reported* • Part-Time Enrollment: *Not Reported* • Female
Enrollment: *140* • Male Enrollment: *10* • Total New
Admissions Who Enrolled for Fall: *57* • Total Graduates: *75*

FINANCES

Residential Annual Tuition: *$3,261* • Non-Residential
Annual Tuition: *$7,782* • General Institution Fees: *$2,874* •
Additional Nursing Fees: *$190*

OWENS STATE COMMUNITY COLLEGE

Address: 10000 Oregon Road, Toledo, OH 43699-1947
Phone: 419-661-7338
Fax: Not Reported
Contact: Dawn E. Wetmore, MSN, RN, Chairman, Nursing and Surgical Technologies
Email: dwetmore@owens.cc.oh.us

GENERAL INFORMATION

Type of School: *2-Year College or University, Public* • Accreditation: *North Central Association of Colleges and Schools* • Total Enrollment: *16688*

PROGRAM INFORMATION

LPN/LVN Exit: *No* • NLNAC Accreditation: *Yes*

NURSING STUDENT PROFILE

Total Nursing Enrollment: *401* • Full-Time Enrollment: *112* • Part-Time Enrollment: *289* • Female Enrollment: *357* • Male Enrollment: *44* • Total New Admissions Who Enrolled for Fall: *114* • Total Graduates: *184*

FINANCES

Residential Annual Tuition: *$1,656* • Non-Residential Annual Tuition: *$3,312* • General Institution Fees: *$240* • Additional Nursing Fees: *$296*

SHAWNEE STATE UNIVERSITY

Address: 940 Second Street, Portsmouth, OH 45662
Phone: 740-355-2382
Fax: Not Reported
Contact: Gayle Massie, MSN, RN, Associate Professor; Acting Co-Chair
Email: gmassie@shawnee.edu

GENERAL INFORMATION

Type of School: *4-Year College or University, Public* • Accreditation: *North Central Association of Colleges and Schools* • Total Enrollment: *3613*

PROGRAM INFORMATION

LPN/LVN Exit: *No* • NLNAC Accreditation: *No*

NURSING STUDENT PROFILE

Total Nursing Enrollment: *198* • Full-Time Enrollment: *156* • Part-Time Enrollment: *42* • Female Enrollment: *172* • Male Enrollment: *26* • Total New Admissions Who Enrolled for Fall: *44* • Total Graduates: *37*

FINANCES

Residential Annual Tuition: *$2,745* • Non-Residential Annual Tuition: *$5,148* • General Institution Fees: *$732* • Additional Nursing Fees: *$0*

SINCLAIR COMMUNITY COLLEGE

Address: 444 West Third Street, Dyton, OH 45402
Phone: 937-512-2424
Fax: 937-512-3331
Contact: Gloria Goldman, PhD, RN, Chair, Nursing Department
Email: gloria.goldman@sinclair.edu

GENERAL INFORMATION

Type of School: *2-Year College or University, Public* • Accreditation: *North Central Association of Colleges and Schools* • Total Enrollment: *23000*

PROGRAM INFORMATION

LPN/LVN Exit: *No* • NLNAC Accreditation: *Yes*

NURSING STUDENT PROFILE

Total Nursing Enrollment: *304* • Full-Time Enrollment: *74* • Part-Time Enrollment: *230* • Female Enrollment: *279* • Male Enrollment: *25* • Total New Admissions Who Enrolled for Fall: *47* • Total Graduates: *86*

FINANCES

Residential Annual Tuition: *$1,179* • Non-Residential Annual Tuition: *$3,179* • General Institution Fees: *$10* • Additional Nursing Fees: *$30*

SOUTHERN STATE COMMUNITY COLLEGE

Address: 100 Hobert Drive, Hillsboro, OH 45133
Phone: 937-393-3431
Fax: 937-393-9831
Contact: Marsha R. Snyder, RN, MS, CCM, Dean of Health Sciences
Email: msnyder@soucc.southern.cc.oh.us

GENERAL INFORMATION

Type of School: *2-Year College or University, Public* • Accreditation: *North Central Association of Colleges and Schools* • Total Enrollment: *1847*

PROGRAM INFORMATION

LPN/LVN Exit: *No* • NLNAC Accreditation: *Yes*

NURSING STUDENT PROFILE

Total Nursing Enrollment: *74* • Full-Time Enrollment: *74* • Part-Time Enrollment: *0* • Female Enrollment: *72* • Male Enrollment: *2* • Total New Admissions Who Enrolled for Fall: *41* • Total Graduates: *20*

FINANCES

Residential Annual Tuition: *$1,680* • Non-Residential Annual Tuition: *Not Reported* • General Institution Fees: *Not Reported* • Additional Nursing Fees: *$300*

STARK STATE COLLEGE OF TECHNOLOGY

Address: 218 Frank Avenue NorthWest C, Canton, OH 44720
Phone: 330-949-6170
Fax: Not Reported
Contact: Gloria Kline, MSN, RN, Department Head
Email: Not Reported

GENERAL INFORMATION

Type of School: *Not Reported* • Accreditation: *Not Reported* • Total Enrollment: *Not Reported*

PROGRAM INFORMATION

LPN/LVN Exit: *Not Reported* • NLNAC Accreditation: *Yes*

NURSING STUDENT PROFILE

Total Nursing Enrollment: *Not Reported* • Full-Time Enrollment: *Not Reported* • Part-Time Enrollment: *Not Reported* • Female Enrollment: *Not Reported* • Male Enrollment: *Not Reported* • Total New Admissions Who Enrolled for Fall: *Not Reported* • Total Graduates: *Not Reported*

FINANCES

Residential Annual Tuition: *Not Reported* • Non-Residential Annual Tuition: *Not Reported* • General Institution Fees: *Not Reported* • Additional Nursing Fees: *Not Reported*

UNIVERSITY OF CINCINNATI—RAYMOND WALTERS COLLEGE

Address: 9555 Plainfield Road, Cincinnati, OH 45236
Phone: 513-745-5665
Fax: 513-558-8736
Contact: Joan E Purdon, MSN, RN, CS, Chairperson
Email: joan-purdon@uc.edu

GENERAL INFORMATION

Type of School: *2-Year College or University, Public* • Accreditation: *North Central Association of Colleges and Schools* • Total Enrollment: *3500*

PROGRAM INFORMATION

LPN/LVN Exit: *Not Reported* • NLNAC Accreditation: *Yes*

NURSING STUDENT PROFILE

Total Nursing Enrollment: *136* • Full-Time Enrollment: *65* • Part-Time Enrollment: *71* • Female Enrollment: *124* • Male Enrollment: *12* • Total New Admissions Who Enrolled for Fall: *102* • Total Graduates: *44*

FINANCES

Residential Annual Tuition: *$3,393* • Non-Residential Annual Tuition: *$8,994* • General Institution Fees: *$114* • Additional Nursing Fees: *Not Reported*

UNIVERSITY OF RIO GRANDE HOLZER

Address: 218 North College Avenue, Rio Grande, OH
45674
Phone: 740-245-7308
Fax: Not Reported
Contact: Donna Mitchell, PhD, RN, CS, Chairperson and
Associate Professor
Email: mitchell@urgrgcc.edu

GENERAL INFORMATION

Type of School: *Not Reported* • Accreditation: *Not Reported* •
Total Enrollment: *Not Reported*

PROGRAM INFORMATION

LPN/LVN Exit: *Not Reported* • NLNAC Accreditation: *Yes*

NURSING STUDENT PROFILE

Total Nursing Enrollment: *Not Reported* • Full-Time
Enrollment: *Not Reported* • Part-Time Enrollment: *Not
Reported* • Female Enrollment: *Not Reported* • Male
Enrollment: *Not Reported* • Total New Admissions Who
Enrolled for Fall: *Not Reported* • Total Graduates: *Not
Reported*

FINANCES

Residential Annual Tuition: *Not Reported* • Non-Residential
Annual Tuition: *Not Reported* • General Institution Fees: *Not
Reported* • Additional Nursing Fees: *Not Reported*

UNIVERSITY OF TOLEDO

Address: 2801 Bancroft, Toledo, OH 43606-3390
Phone: 419-530-3374
Fax: 419-530-3096
Contact: Celeste Baldwin, PhD, RN, CNS, Director of
Nursing
Email: cbaldwi@utnet.utoledo.edu

GENERAL INFORMATION

Type of School: *4-Year College or University, Public* •
Accreditation: *North Central Association of Colleges and
Schools* • Total Enrollment: *Not Reported*

PROGRAM INFORMATION

LPN/LVN Exit: *No* • NLNAC Accreditation: *Yes*

NURSING STUDENT PROFILE

Total Nursing Enrollment: *98* • Full-Time Enrollment: *90* •
Part-Time Enrollment: *8* • Female Enrollment: *88* • Male
Enrollment: *10* • Total New Admissions Who Enrolled for
Fall: *16* • Total Graduates: *50*

FINANCES

Residential Annual Tuition: *Not Reported* • Non-Residential
Annual Tuition: *Not Reported* • General Institution Fees: *Not
Reported* • Additional Nursing Fees: *$80*

WALSH UNIVERSITY

Address: 2020 Easton Street NW, North Canton, OH
                44720-3396
Phone: 330-490-7250
Fax: 330-490-7206
Contact: Mary E. Meeker, RN, DNSc, CNS, Chair,
                Nursing Division
Email: mmeeker@walsh.edu

GENERAL INFORMATION

Type of School: *4-Year College or University, Private (Religious)* • Accreditation: *North Central Association of Colleges and Schools* • Total Enrollment: *4500*

PROGRAM INFORMATION

LPN/LVN Exit: *Not Reported* • NLNAC Accreditation: *Yes*

NURSING STUDENT PROFILE

Total Nursing Enrollment: *8* • Full-Time Enrollment: *5* • Part-Time Enrollment: *3* • Female Enrollment: *7* • Male Enrollment: *1* • Total New Admissions Who Enrolled for Fall: *0* • Total Graduates: *18*

FINANCES

Residential Annual Tuition: *$12,050* • Non-Residential Annual Tuition: *$12,050* • General Institution Fees: *$288* • Additional Nursing Fees: *Not Reported*

BACONE COLLEGE

Address: 2299 Old Bacone Road, Muskogee, OK 74403
Phone: 918-781-7325
Fax: 918-781-7310
Contact: Nancy Diede, MS, APRN, BC, Dean, School of
                Health Sciences and Director, Nursing
Email: dieden@bacone.edu

GENERAL INFORMATION

Type of School: *4-Year College or University, Private (Religious)* • Accreditation: *North Central Association of Colleges and Schools* • Total Enrollment: *800*

PROGRAM INFORMATION

LPN/LVN Exit: *No* • NLNAC Accreditation: *Yes*

NURSING STUDENT PROFILE

Total Nursing Enrollment: *41* • Full-Time Enrollment: *30* • Part-Time Enrollment: *11* • Female Enrollment: *34* • Male Enrollment: *7* • Total New Admissions Who Enrolled for Fall: *24* • Total Graduates: *24*

FINANCES

Residential Annual Tuition: *$7,900* • Non-Residential Annual Tuition: *$7,900* • General Institution Fees: *$200* • Additional Nursing Fees: *$150*

BARTLESVILLE WESLEYAN COLLEGE

Address:　2201 Silver Lake Rd, Bartesville, OK 74006-6233
Phone:　918-335-6218
Fax:　918-335-6204
Contact:　Elizabeth A. VonBuchwald, MS, BSN, RN, Chairperson, Nursing Division
Email:　elbethanne@bwc.edu

GENERAL INFORMATION

Type of School: *4-Year College or University, Private (Religious)* • Accreditation: *North Central Association of Colleges and Schools* • Total Enrollment: *23*

PROGRAM INFORMATION

LPN/LVN Exit: *Not Reported* • NLNAC Accreditation: *Yes*

NURSING STUDENT PROFILE

Total Nursing Enrollment: *14* • Full-Time Enrollment: *7* • Part-Time Enrollment: *7* • Female Enrollment: *13* • Male Enrollment: *1* • Total New Admissions Who Enrolled for Fall: *5* • Total Graduates: *6*

FINANCES

Residential Annual Tuition: *$9,200* • Non-Residential Annual Tuition: *$9,200* • General Institution Fees: *$290* • Additional Nursing Fees: *$13*

CARL ALBERT STATE COLLEGE

Address:　1507 S McKenna, Poteau, OK 74953
Phone:　918-647-1350
Fax:　Not Reported
Contact:　Abbie R. Bailey, MSN, RN, Health Sciences Chairperson and Director, Nursing Education
Email:　abailey@casc.cc.ok.us

GENERAL INFORMATION

Type of School: *2-Year College or University, Public* • Accreditation: *North Central Association of Colleges and Schools* • Total Enrollment: *1999*

PROGRAM INFORMATION

LPN/LVN Exit: *No* • NLNAC Accreditation: *Yes*

NURSING STUDENT PROFILE

Total Nursing Enrollment: *72* • Full-Time Enrollment: *38* • Part-Time Enrollment: *34* • Female Enrollment: *63* • Male Enrollment: *9* • Total New Admissions Who Enrolled for Fall: *45* • Total Graduates: *27*

FINANCES

Residential Annual Tuition: *$1,056* • Non-Residential Annual Tuition: *$2,772* • General Institution Fees: *$0* • Additional Nursing Fees: *$25*

CONNORS STATE COLLEGE

Address: Rt 1 Box 1000, Warner, OK 74469-1000
Phone: 918-463-2931
Fax: 918-463-4272
Contact: Glenda Shockley, RN, MS, Director of Nursing
Email: gshockl@connors.cc.ok.us

GENERAL INFORMATION

Type of School: *2-Year College or University, Public* • Accreditation: *North Central Association of Colleges and Schools* • Total Enrollment: *1985*

PROGRAM INFORMATION

LPN/LVN Exit: *Yes* • NLNAC Accreditation: *Yes*

NURSING STUDENT PROFILE

Total Nursing Enrollment: *104* • Full-Time Enrollment: *Not Reported* • Part-Time Enrollment: *Not Reported* • Female Enrollment: *95* • Male Enrollment: *9* • Total New Admissions Who Enrolled for Fall: *26* • Total Graduates: *34*

FINANCES

Residential Annual Tuition: *$1,026* • Non-Residential Annual Tuition: *$2,610* • General Institution Fees: *$70* • Additional Nursing Fees: *$103*

EASTERN OKLAHOMA STATE COLLEGE

Address: 1301 W Main St, Wilburton, OK 74578-4901
Phone: 918-465-2361
Fax: 918-465-4465
Contact: Marsha Green, RN, MS, BS, Director of Nursing Education
Email: mgreen@eosc.cc.ok.us

GENERAL INFORMATION

Type of School: *2-Year College or University, Public* • Accreditation: *North Central Association of Colleges and Schools* • Total Enrollment: *Not Reported*

PROGRAM INFORMATION

LPN/LVN Exit: *No* • NLNAC Accreditation: *Yes*

NURSING STUDENT PROFILE

Total Nursing Enrollment: *66* • Full-Time Enrollment: *16* • Part-Time Enrollment: *50* • Female Enrollment: *61* • Male Enrollment: *5* • Total New Admissions Who Enrolled for Fall: *55* • Total Graduates: *47*

FINANCES

Residential Annual Tuition: *$1,152* • Non-Residential Annual Tuition: *$2,772* • General Institution Fees: *$25* • Additional Nursing Fees: *$100*

MURRAY STATE COLLEGE

Address: One Murray Campus Suite N/AH 105,
            Tishomingo, OK 73460
Phone: 580-371-2371
Fax: 580-371-2297
Contact: Joni Jeter, RN, MS, Nursing Program Director
Email: jojeter@mscok.edu

GENERAL INFORMATION

Type of School: *2-Year College or University, Public* •
Accreditation: *North Central Association of Colleges and
Schools* • Total Enrollment: *1909*

PROGRAM INFORMATION

LPN/LVN Exit: *No* • NLNAC Accreditation: *Yes*

NURSING STUDENT PROFILE

Total Nursing Enrollment: *76* • Full-Time Enrollment: *21* •
Part-Time Enrollment: *55* • Female Enrollment: *68* • Male
Enrollment: *8* • Total New Admissions Who Enrolled for
Fall: *42* • Total Graduates: *41*

FINANCES

Residential Annual Tuition: *$808* • Non-Residential Annual
Tuition: *$2,574* • General Institution Fees: *$391* •
Additional Nursing Fees: *$313*

NORTHEASTERN OKLAHOMA A&M COLLEGE

Address: 200 1st Ave NE, Miami, OK 74354-6306
Phone: 918-504-6312
Fax: 918-540-6471
Contact: Patricia L. Hempsmyer, MSN, RN, Interim
            Director and Department Chair
Email: phempsmyer@neoam.cc.ok.us

GENERAL INFORMATION

Type of School: *2-Year College or University, Public* •
Accreditation: *North Central Association of Colleges and
Schools* • Total Enrollment: *1918*

PROGRAM INFORMATION

LPN/LVN Exit: *No* • NLNAC Accreditation: *Yes*

NURSING STUDENT PROFILE

Total Nursing Enrollment: *103* • Full-Time Enrollment:
103 • Part-Time Enrollment: *0* • Female Enrollment: *96* •
Male Enrollment: *7* • Total New Admissions Who Enrolled
for Fall: *58* • Total Graduates: *33*

FINANCES

Residential Annual Tuition: *$1,092* • Non-Residential
Annual Tuition: *$2,712* • General Institution Fees: *$0* •
Additional Nursing Fees: *$100*

NORTHERN OKLAHOMA COLLEGE

Address: 1220 E Grand Ave # 310, Tonkawa, OK 74653-
            4022
Phone: 580-628-6649
Fax: 580-628-6674
Contact: Kim Webb, RN,MN, Nursing Chair
Email: kimwebb@nocaxp.north-ok.edu

GENERAL INFORMATION

Type of School: *2-Year College or University, Public* •
Accreditation: *North Central Association of Colleges and
Schools* • Total Enrollment: *2000*

PROGRAM INFORMATION

LPN/LVN Exit: *No* • NLNAC Accreditation: *Yes*

NURSING STUDENT PROFILE

Total Nursing Enrollment: *88* • Full-Time Enrollment: *67* •
Part-Time Enrollment: *21* • Female Enrollment: *76* • Male
Enrollment: *12* • Total New Admissions Who Enrolled for
Fall: *45* • Total Graduates: *51*

FINANCES

Residential Annual Tuition: *$1,008* • Non-Residential
Annual Tuition: *$2,628* • General Institution Fees: *$20* •
Additional Nursing Fees: *$80*

OKLAHOMA BAPTIST UNIVERSITY

Address: 500 W. University, Shawnee, OK 74804
Phone: 405-878-2081
Fax: 405-878-2083
Contact: Lana Bolhouse, PhD, RN, Dean, School of
            Nursing
Email: lana_lolhouse@mail.okbu.edu

GENERAL INFORMATION

Type of School: *4-Year College or University, Private
(Independent)* • Accreditation: *North Central Association of
Colleges and Schools* • Total Enrollment: *1933*

PROGRAM INFORMATION

LPN/LVN Exit: *No* • NLNAC Accreditation: *No*

NURSING STUDENT PROFILE

Total Nursing Enrollment: *112* • Full-Time Enrollment:
111 • Part-Time Enrollment: *1* • Female Enrollment: *111* •
Male Enrollment: *1* • Total New Admissions Who Enrolled
for Fall: *16* • Total Graduates: *26*

FINANCES

Residential Annual Tuition: *$4,750* • Non-Residential
Annual Tuition: *$4,750* • General Institution Fees: *$369* •
Additional Nursing Fees: *$560*

OKLAHOMA CITY COMMUNITY COLLEGE

Address: 7777 S. May Ave., Oklahoma City, OK 73159
Phone: 405-682-1611
Fax: 405-682-7826
Contact: Lea Ann Loftis, MSN, RN, Program Director
Email: lloftis@okc.cc.ok.us

GENERAL INFORMATION

Type of School: *2-Year College or University, Public* •
Accreditation: *North Central Association of Colleges and Schools* • Total Enrollment: *10667*

PROGRAM INFORMATION

LPN/LVN Exit: *No* • NLNAC Accreditation: *Yes*

NURSING STUDENT PROFILE

Total Nursing Enrollment: *200* • Full-Time Enrollment: *48* • Part-Time Enrollment: *152* • Female Enrollment: *181* • Male Enrollment: *19* • Total New Admissions Who Enrolled for Fall: *75* • Total Graduates: *88*

FINANCES

Residential Annual Tuition: *$1,842* • Non-Residential Annual Tuition: *$4,816* • General Institution Fees: *$14* • Additional Nursing Fees: *$125*

OKLAHOMA STATE UNIVERSITY-OKLAHOMA CITY

Address: 900 N Portland Ave, Oklahoma City, OK
            73107-6120
Phone: 405-945-3295
Fax: 405-945-8613
Contact: Lois L. Salmeron, EdD, RNC, MSN, Division
            Head, Health Services
Email: loiss@suokc.edu

GENERAL INFORMATION

Type of School: *2-Year College or University, Public* •
Accreditation: *North Central Association of Colleges and Schools* • Total Enrollment: *22000*

PROGRAM INFORMATION

LPN/LVN Exit: *No* • NLNAC Accreditation: *Yes*

NURSING STUDENT PROFILE

Total Nursing Enrollment: *202* • Full-Time Enrollment: *202* • Part-Time Enrollment: *0* • Female Enrollment: *176* • Male Enrollment: *26* • Total New Admissions Who Enrolled for Fall: *51* • Total Graduates: *106*

FINANCES

Residential Annual Tuition: *$1,056* • Non-Residential Annual Tuition: *$1,800* • General Institution Fees: *$27* • Additional Nursing Fees: *$50*

REDLANDS COMMUNITY COLLEGE

Address: 1300 South Country Club Road, El Reno, OK
            73036-5304
Phone: 405-422-1126
Fax: 405-422-1215
Contact: Rose Marie Bolton, RN, MS, Division Director
            and Nursing Director
Email: boltonr@redlandscc.net

GENERAL INFORMATION

Type of School: *2-Year College or University, Public* •
Accreditation: *North Central Association of Colleges and
Schools* • Total Enrollment: *2178*

PROGRAM INFORMATION

LPN/LVN Exit: *No* • NLNAC Accreditation: *Yes*

NURSING STUDENT PROFILE

Total Nursing Enrollment: *87* • Full-Time Enrollment: *49* •
Part-Time Enrollment: *38* • Female Enrollment: *81* • Male
Enrollment: *6* • Total New Admissions Who Enrolled for
Fall: *48* • Total Graduates: *44*

FINANCES

Residential Annual Tuition: *$756* • Non-Residential Annual
Tuition: *$1,620* • General Institution Fees: *$414* •
Additional Nursing Fees: *$200*

ROGERS STATE UNIVERSITY

Address: 1701 West Will Rogers Boulevard, Claremore,
            OK 74017
Phone: 918-343-7635
Fax: 918-343-7628
Contact: Linda D. Andrews, RN, MS, Department Head,
            Health Sciences and Assistant Professor
Email: landrews@rsu.edu

GENERAL INFORMATION

Type of School: *4-Year College or University, Public* •
Accreditation: *North Central Association of Colleges and
Schools* • Total Enrollment: *27925*

PROGRAM INFORMATION

LPN/LVN Exit: *No* • NLNAC Accreditation: *Yes*

NURSING STUDENT PROFILE

Total Nursing Enrollment: *82* • Full-Time Enrollment: *41* •
Part-Time Enrollment: *41* • Female Enrollment: *78* • Male
Enrollment: *4* • Total New Admissions Who Enrolled for
Fall: *46* • Total Graduates: *40*

FINANCES

Residential Annual Tuition: *$2,110* • Non-Residential
Annual Tuition: *$4,860* • General Institution Fees: *$40* •
Additional Nursing Fees: *$215*

ROSE STATE COLLEGE

Address: 6420 S.E. 15th Street, Midwest City, OK 73110
Phone: 405-733-7546
Fax: 405-736-0338
Contact: Lynn Korvick, RN, MS, Director, Nursing Science Program
Email: lkorvick@rose.edu

GENERAL INFORMATION

Type of School: *2-Year College or University, Public* • Accreditation: *North Central Association of Colleges and Schools* • Total Enrollment: *7500*

PROGRAM INFORMATION

LPN/LVN Exit: *Not Reported* • NLNAC Accreditation: *Yes*

NURSING STUDENT PROFILE

Total Nursing Enrollment: *144* • Full-Time Enrollment: *144* • Part-Time Enrollment: *0* • Female Enrollment: *127* • Male Enrollment: *17* • Total New Admissions Who Enrolled for Fall: *61* • Total Graduates: *80*

FINANCES

Residential Annual Tuition: *$1,269* • Non-Residential Annual Tuition: *$4,090* • General Institution Fees: *$500* • Additional Nursing Fees: *$300*

SEMINOLE STATE COLLEGE

Address: 2701 Boren Blvd - PO Box 351, Seminole, OK 74868-1901
Phone: 405-382-9269
Fax: 405-382-9586
Contact: Jorge Neuhaus, PhD, RN, Nursing and Health Sciences Division Chair
Email: neuhaus_j@ssc.cc.ok.us

GENERAL INFORMATION

Type of School: *2-Year College or University, Public* • Accreditation: *North Central Association of Colleges and Schools* • Total Enrollment: *1935*

PROGRAM INFORMATION

LPN/LVN Exit: *Yes* • NLNAC Accreditation: *Yes*

NURSING STUDENT PROFILE

Total Nursing Enrollment: *38* • Full-Time Enrollment: *38* • Part-Time Enrollment: *0* • Female Enrollment: *34* • Male Enrollment: *4* • Total New Admissions Who Enrolled for Fall: *25* • Total Graduates: *24*

FINANCES

Residential Annual Tuition: *$1,169* • Non-Residential Annual Tuition: *$2,789* • General Institution Fees: *$20* • Additional Nursing Fees: *$15*

TULSA COMMUNITY COLLEGE

Address: 909 S. Boston, Tulsa, OK 74119
Phone: 918-595-7188
Fax: 918-595-7198
Contact: Ann Strong Anthony, MSN, RN, Associate
            Dean, Nursing
Email: aanthony@tulsa.cc.ok.us

GENERAL INFORMATION

Type of School: *2-Year College or University, Public* •
Accreditation: *North Central Association of Colleges and
Schools* • Total Enrollment: *20000*

PROGRAM INFORMATION

LPN/LVN Exit: *No* • NLNAC Accreditation: *Yes*

NURSING STUDENT PROFILE

Total Nursing Enrollment: *224* • Full-Time Enrollment:
171 • Part-Time Enrollment: *53* • Female Enrollment: *202* •
Male Enrollment: *22* • Total New Admissions Who Enrolled
for Fall: *73* • Total Graduates: *84*

FINANCES

Residential Annual Tuition: *$1,024* • Non-Residential
Annual Tuition: *$3,232* • General Institution Fees: *$718* •
Additional Nursing Fees: *$297*

WESTERN OKLAHOMA STATE COLLEGE

Address: 2801 N Main St, Altus, OK 73521-1310
Phone: 580-477-7832
Fax: 580-477-7862
Contact: Margaret Thomas, RN, MEd, MSN, Director
Email: mathomas@western.cc.ok.us

GENERAL INFORMATION

Type of School: *2-Year College or University, Public* •
Accreditation: *North Central Association of Colleges and
Schools* • Total Enrollment: *1750*

PROGRAM INFORMATION

LPN/LVN Exit: *No* • NLNAC Accreditation: *Yes*

NURSING STUDENT PROFILE

Total Nursing Enrollment: *44* • Full-Time Enrollment: *0* •
Part-Time Enrollment: *44* • Female Enrollment: *39* • Male
Enrollment: *5* • Total New Admissions Who Enrolled for
Fall: *31* • Total Graduates: *17*

FINANCES

Residential Annual Tuition: *$1,465* • Non-Residential
Annual Tuition: *$3,726* • General Institution Fees: *$120* •
Additional Nursing Fees: *$1,000*

BLUE MOUNTAIN COMMUNITY COLLEGE

Address: P.O.Box 100, Pendleton, OR 97801
Phone: 541-278-5877
Fax: Not Reported
Contact: Elizabeth S. Sullivan, RN, MS, Program Coordinator
Email: lsullivan@bmcc.cc.or.us

GENERAL INFORMATION

Type of School: *2-Year College or University, Private (Independent)* • Accreditation: *Northwestern Association of Schools and Colleges* • Total Enrollment: *1816*

PROGRAM INFORMATION

LPN/LVN Exit: *Yes* • NLNAC Accreditation: *No*

NURSING STUDENT PROFILE

Total Nursing Enrollment: *45* • Full-Time Enrollment: *45* • Part-Time Enrollment: *0* • Female Enrollment: *40* • Male Enrollment: *5* • Total New Admissions Who Enrolled for Fall: *18* • Total Graduates: *14*

FINANCES

Residential Annual Tuition: *$1,332* • Non-Residential Annual Tuition: *$3,996* • General Institution Fees: *$80* • Additional Nursing Fees: *$160*

CENTRAL OREGON COMMUNITY COLLEGE

Address: 2600 North West College Way, Bend, OR 97001
Phone: 541-383-7543
Fax: 541-317-3064
Contact: Kiri Simning, RN, MS, Chair
Email: Ksimning@cocc.edu

GENERAL INFORMATION

Type of School: *2-Year College or University, Public* • Accreditation: *Northwestern Association of Schools and Colleges* • Total Enrollment: *1457*

PROGRAM INFORMATION

LPN/LVN Exit: *Yes* • NLNAC Accreditation: *No*

NURSING STUDENT PROFILE

Total Nursing Enrollment: *59* • Full-Time Enrollment: *Not Reported* • Part-Time Enrollment: *Not Reported* • Female Enrollment: *50* • Male Enrollment: *9* • Total New Admissions Who Enrolled for Fall: *28* • Total Graduates: *40*

FINANCES

Residential Annual Tuition: *$1,728* • Non-Residential Annual Tuition: *4,928* • General Institution Fees: *$1,032* • Additional Nursing Fees: *$6*

CHEMEKETA COMMUNITY COLLEGE

Address: 4000Lancaster Drive North East, PO Box 14007, Salem, OR 97309-7070
Phone: 503-399-5058
Fax: 503-399-5496
Contact: Kay Carnegie, RN, MS, Nursing Program Coordinator
Email: cark@chemeketa.edu

GENERAL INFORMATION

Type of School: *2-Year College or University, Public* • Accreditation: *Northwestern Association of Schools and Colleges* • Total Enrollment: *50000*

PROGRAM INFORMATION

LPN/LVN Exit: *Yes* • NLNAC Accreditation: *Yes*

NURSING STUDENT PROFILE

Total Nursing Enrollment: *126* • Full-Time Enrollment: *126* • Part-Time Enrollment: *0* • Female Enrollment: *107* • Male Enrollment: *19* • Total New Admissions Who Enrolled for Fall: *70* • Total Graduates: *35*

FINANCES

Residential Annual Tuition: *$1,677* • Non-Residential Annual Tuition: *$0* • General Institution Fees: *$0* • Additional Nursing Fees: *$67*

CLACKAMAS COMMUNITY COLLEGE

Address: 19600 South Molalla Avenue, Oregon City, OR 97045
Phone: 503-657-6958
Fax: 503-655-5153
Contact: Arlene Jurgens, RN, MN, Chairperson
Email: arlenej@clackamas.cc.or.us

GENERAL INFORMATION

Type of School: *2-Year College or University, Public* • Accreditation: *Northwestern Association of Schools and Colleges* • Total Enrollment: *8438*

PROGRAM INFORMATION

LPN/LVN Exit: *No* • NLNAC Accreditation: *Yes*

NURSING STUDENT PROFILE

Total Nursing Enrollment: *72* • Full-Time Enrollment: *72* • Part-Time Enrollment: *0* • Female Enrollment: *63* • Male Enrollment: *9* • Total New Admissions Who Enrolled for Fall: *40* • Total Graduates: *31*

FINANCES

Residential Annual Tuition: *$1,665* • Non-Residential Annual Tuition: *$5,895* • General Institution Fees: *$0* • Additional Nursing Fees: *$300*

CLATSOP COMMUNITY COLLEGE

Address: 1653 Jerome Avenue, Astoria, OR 97103
Phone: 503-338-2496
Fax: 503-325-5738
Contact: Karen Burke, RN, MS, Director of Health Occupations
Email: kburke@clatsop.cc.or.us

GENERAL INFORMATION

Type of School: *2-Year College or University, Public* • Accreditation: *North Central Association of Colleges and Schools* • Total Enrollment: *Not Reported*

PROGRAM INFORMATION

LPN/LVN Exit: *Yes* • NLNAC Accreditation: *No*

NURSING STUDENT PROFILE

Total Nursing Enrollment: *40* • Full-Time Enrollment: *35* • Part-Time Enrollment: *5* • Female Enrollment: *34* • Male Enrollment: *6* • Total New Admissions Who Enrolled for Fall: *18* • Total Graduates: *12*

FINANCES

Residential Annual Tuition: *$2,340* • Non-Residential Annual Tuition: *$6,000* • General Institution Fees: *$120* • Additional Nursing Fees: *$160*

LANE COMMUNITY COLLEGE

Address: 4000 East 30th Avenue, Eugene, OR 97405
Phone: 541-747-4501
Fax: 541-744-4151
Contact: Joyce H. Godels, MSN, RN, Family Health Careers Division Chair and Nursing Program Coordinator
Email: godelsj@lanecc.edu

GENERAL INFORMATION

Type of School: *2-Year College or University, Public* • Accreditation: *Northwestern Association of Schools and Colleges* • Total Enrollment: *10626*

PROGRAM INFORMATION

LPN/LVN Exit: *Yes* • NLNAC Accreditation: *Yes*

NURSING STUDENT PROFILE

Total Nursing Enrollment: *110* • Full-Time Enrollment: *110* • Part-Time Enrollment: *0* • Female Enrollment: *85* • Male Enrollment: *25* • Total New Admissions Who Enrolled for Fall: *56* • Total Graduates: *104*

FINANCES

Residential Annual Tuition: *$864* • Non-Residential Annual Tuition: *Not Reported* • General Institution Fees: *$152* • Additional Nursing Fees: *$200*

LINN–BENTON COMMUNITY COLLEGE

Address: 6500 Pacific Boulevard South West, Albany, OR 97321
Phone: 541-917-4514
Fax: 541-917-4527
Contact: Faye Melius, RN, MS, Nursing Program Chair
Email: meliusf@gw.lbcc.cc.or.us

GENERAL INFORMATION

Type of School: *2-Year College or University, Public* • Accreditation: *Northwestern Association of Schools and Colleges* • Total Enrollment: *25000*

PROGRAM INFORMATION

LPN/LVN Exit: *Yes* • NLNAC Accreditation: *Yes*

NURSING STUDENT PROFILE

Total Nursing Enrollment: *84* • Full-Time Enrollment: *84* • Part-Time Enrollment: *0* • Female Enrollment: *74* • Male Enrollment: *10* • Total New Admissions Who Enrolled for Fall: *48* • Total Graduates: *24*

FINANCES

Residential Annual Tuition: *$1,600* • Non-Residential Annual Tuition: *$4,832* • General Institution Fees: *$7* • Additional Nursing Fees: *$600*

MT. HOOD COMMUNITY COLLEGE

Address: 2600 SouthEast Stark, Gresham, OR 97030
Phone: 503-491-7446
Fax: Not Reported
Contact: Paula Gubrud, MSN, RN, Program Director
Email: gubrudp@mhcc.edu

GENERAL INFORMATION

Type of School: *Not Reported* • Accreditation: *Not Reported* • Total Enrollment: *Not Reported*

PROGRAM INFORMATION

LPN/LVN Exit: *Not Reported* • NLNAC Accreditation: *Yes*

NURSING STUDENT PROFILE

Total Nursing Enrollment: *88* • Full-Time Enrollment: *88* • Part-Time Enrollment: *0* • Female Enrollment: *Not Reported* • Male Enrollment: *Not Reported* • Total New Admissions Who Enrolled for Fall: *47* • Total Graduates: *38*

FINANCES

Residential Annual Tuition: *$1,088* • Non-Residential Annual Tuition: *$3,744* • General Institution Fees: *Not Reported* • Additional Nursing Fees: *Not Reported*

PORTLAND COMMUNITY COLLEGE

Address: 12000 South West 49th Avenue, Portland, OR 97219
Phone: 503-977-4205
Fax: 503-977-8860
Contact: Shelly Quint, RN, MS, Program Director
Email: squint@pcc.edu

GENERAL INFORMATION

Type of School: *2-Year College or University, Private (Independent)* • Accreditation: *Northwestern Association of Schools and Colleges* • Total Enrollment: *88000*

PROGRAM INFORMATION

LPN/LVN Exit: *Yes* • NLNAC Accreditation: *Yes*

NURSING STUDENT PROFILE

Total Nursing Enrollment: *170* • Full-Time Enrollment: *170* • Part-Time Enrollment: *0* • Female Enrollment: *140* • Male Enrollment: *30* • Total New Admissions Who Enrolled for Fall: *85* • Total Graduates: *67*

FINANCES

Residential Annual Tuition: *$2,067* • Non-Residential Annual Tuition: *$7,685* • General Institution Fees: *$250* • Additional Nursing Fees: *$300*

ROGUE COMMUNITY COLLEGE

Address: 3345 Redwood Highway, Grants Pass, OR 97527
Phone: 541-956-7308
Fax: 541-471-3566
Contact: Linda Wagner, RN, MN, Allied Health Department Head and Director of Nursing Programs
Email: lwagner@roguecc.edu

GENERAL INFORMATION

Type of School: *2-Year College or University, Public* • Accreditation: *Northwestern Association of Schools and Colleges* • Total Enrollment: *Not Reported*

PROGRAM INFORMATION

LPN/LVN Exit: *Yes* • NLNAC Accreditation: *Yes*

NURSING STUDENT PROFILE

Total Nursing Enrollment: *52* • Full-Time Enrollment: *52* • Part-Time Enrollment: *0* • Female Enrollment: *45* • Male Enrollment: *7* • Total New Admissions Who Enrolled for Fall: *32* • Total Graduates: *19*

FINANCES

Residential Annual Tuition: *$1,888* • Non-Residential Annual Tuition: *$2,272* • General Institution Fees: *$228* • Additional Nursing Fees: *Not Reported*

SOUTHWESTERN OREGON COMMUNITY COLLEGE

Address: 1988 Newmark, Coos Bay, OR 97420
Phone: 541-888-7340
Fax: 541-888-7285
Contact: Barbara A. Davey, MS, RN, Coordinator
Email: D.DAVEY@SOUTHWESTERN.CC.OR.US

GENERAL INFORMATION

Type of School: *2-Year College or University, Public* •
Accreditation: *Northwestern Association of Schools and
Colleges* • Total Enrollment: *3500*

PROGRAM INFORMATION

LPN/LVN Exit: *Not Reported* • NLNAC Accreditation: *No*

NURSING STUDENT PROFILE

Total Nursing Enrollment: *Not Reported* • Full-Time
Enrollment: *Not Reported* • Part-Time Enrollment: *Not
Reported* • Female Enrollment: *Not Reported* • Male
Enrollment: *Not Reported* • Total New Admissions Who
Enrolled for Fall: *Not Reported* • Total Graduates: *Not
Reported*

FINANCES

Residential Annual Tuition: *Not Reported* • Non-Residential
Annual Tuition: *Not Reported* • General Institution Fees: *Not
Reported* • Additional Nursing Fees: *Not Reported*

TREASURE VALLEY COMMUNITY COLLEGE

Address: 650 College Boulevard, Ontario, OR 97914
Phone: 541-881-8822
Fax: 541-881-2768
Contact: Maureen McDonough, RN, MS, Nursing
             Program Director
Email: mmcdonou@tvcc.cc

GENERAL INFORMATION

Type of School: *2-Year College or University, Public* •
Accreditation: *Northwestern Association of Schools and
Colleges* • Total Enrollment: *1300*

PROGRAM INFORMATION

LPN/LVN Exit: *Yes* • NLNAC Accreditation: *No*

NURSING STUDENT PROFILE

Total Nursing Enrollment: *19* • Full-Time Enrollment: *19* •
Part-Time Enrollment: *0* • Female Enrollment: *19* • Male
Enrollment: *0* • Total New Admissions Who Enrolled for
Fall: *19* • Total Graduates: *17*

FINANCES

Residential Annual Tuition: *$2,052* • Non-Residential
Annual Tuition: *$2,916* • General Institution Fees: *$345* •
Additional Nursing Fees: *$1,000*

UMPQUA COMMUNITY COLLEGE

Address: P.O. Box 967, Roseburg, OR 97470
Phone: 541-440-4613
Fax: 541-440-3298
Contact: Sandra Henny, MSN, RN, Director of Health
          Occupations
Email: hendys@umpqua.cc.or.us

GENERAL INFORMATION

Type of School: *2-Year College or University, Public* •
Accreditation: *Northwestern Association of Schools and
Colleges* • Total Enrollment: *4388*

PROGRAM INFORMATION

LPN/LVN Exit: *Not Reported* • NLNAC Accreditation: *Yes*

NURSING STUDENT PROFILE

Total Nursing Enrollment: *Not Reported* • Full-Time
Enrollment: *Not Reported* • Part-Time Enrollment: *Not
Reported* • Female Enrollment: *Not Reported* • Male
Enrollment: *Not Reported* • Total New Admissions Who
Enrolled for Fall: *Not Reported* • Total Graduates: *Not
Reported*

FINANCES

Residential Annual Tuition: *Not Reported* • Non-Residential
Annual Tuition: *Not Reported* • General Institution Fees: *Not
Reported* • Additional Nursing Fees: *Not Reported*

ALVERNIA COLLEGE

Address: 400 St. Bernadine Street, Reading, PA 19607
Phone: 610-796-8306
Fax: 610-796-8464
Contact: Karen S. Thacker, MSN, RN, CS, Assistant
          Professor and Nursing Department Chair
Email: karen.thacker@alvernia.edu

GENERAL INFORMATION

Type of School: *4-Year College or University, Private
(Religious)* • Accreditation: *Middle States Association of
Colleges and Schools* • Total Enrollment: *1400*

PROGRAM INFORMATION

LPN/LVN Exit: *No* • NLNAC Accreditation: *Yes*

NURSING STUDENT PROFILE

Total Nursing Enrollment: *33* • Full-Time Enrollment: *18* •
Part-Time Enrollment: *15* • Female Enrollment: *33* • Male
Enrollment: *0* • Total New Admissions Who Enrolled for
Fall: *10* • Total Graduates: *20*

FINANCES

Residential Annual Tuition: *$1,400* • Non-Residential
Annual Tuition: *$1,400* • General Institution Fees: *$500* •
Additional Nursing Fees: *$400*

BUCKS COUNTY COMMUNITY COLLEGE

Address: 275 Swamp Road, Newtown, PA 18940
Phone: 215-968-8319
Fax: 215-968-8330
Contact: Martha F. Pollick, EdD, RN, CNAA, Director of Nursing
Email: pollickm@bucks.edu

GENERAL INFORMATION

Type of School: *2-Year College or University, Public* • Accreditation: *Middle States Association of Colleges and Schools* • Total Enrollment: *8831*

PROGRAM INFORMATION

LPN/LVN Exit: *No* • NLNAC Accreditation: *Yes*

NURSING STUDENT PROFILE

Total Nursing Enrollment: *332* • Full-Time Enrollment: *53* • Part-Time Enrollment: *279* • Female Enrollment: *246* • Male Enrollment: *86* • Total New Admissions Who Enrolled for Fall: *77* • Total Graduates: *82*

FINANCES

Residential Annual Tuition: *$3,552* • Non-Residential Annual Tuition: *$5,328* • General Institution Fees: *$100* • Additional Nursing Fees: *$350*

BUTLER COUNTY COMMUNITY COLLEGE

Address: PO Box 1203, College Drive, Oak Hills, Butler, PA 67042
Phone: 316-322-3140
Fax: 316-733-3158
Contact: Patricia Bayles, MN, MS, RN, Dean
Email: THUTCHIN@BUTLERCC.EDU

GENERAL INFORMATION

Type of School: *2-Year College or University, Public* • Accreditation: *Middle States Association of Colleges and Schools* • Total Enrollment: *3078*

PROGRAM INFORMATION

LPN/LVN Exit: *Yes* • NLNAC Accreditation: *Yes*

NURSING STUDENT PROFILE

Total Nursing Enrollment: *176* • Full-Time Enrollment: *176* • Part-Time Enrollment: *0* • Female Enrollment: *163* • Male Enrollment: *13* • Total New Admissions Who Enrolled for Fall: *40* • Total Graduates: *88*

FINANCES

Residential Annual Tuition: *$4,650* • Non-Residential Annual Tuition: *Not Reported* • General Institution Fees: *Not Reported* • Additional Nursing Fees: *$33*

CLARION UNIVERSITY

Address: 1801 West 1st Street, Oil City, PA 16301
Phone: 814-676-6591
Fax: 814-676-0251
Contact: T. Audean Duespohl, PhD, RN, Dean, School of
             Nursing
Email: ADuespohl@clarion.edu

GENERAL INFORMATION

Type of School: *4-Year College or University, Public* •
Accreditation: *Middle States Association of Colleges and
Schools* • Total Enrollment: *6192*

PROGRAM INFORMATION

LPN/LVN Exit: *No* • NLNAC Accreditation: *Yes*

NURSING STUDENT PROFILE

Total Nursing Enrollment: *58* • Full-Time Enrollment: *40* •
Part-Time Enrollment: *18* • Female Enrollment: *51* • Male
Enrollment: *7* • Total New Admissions Who Enrolled for
Fall: *38* • Total Graduates: *10*

FINANCES

Residential Annual Tuition: *$7,584* • Non-Residential
Annual Tuition: *$11,376* • General Institution Fees: *$1,399* •
Additional Nursing Fees: *$35*

COMMUNITY COLLEGE OF BEAVER COUNTY

Address: 1 Campus Drive, Monaca, PA 15061
Phone: 724-775-8561
Fax: 724-775-3003
Contact: Linda M. Gallagher, MSN, RN, Director, Allied
             Health
Email: linda.gallagher@ccbc.cc.pa.us

GENERAL INFORMATION

Type of School: *2-Year College or University, Public* •
Accreditation: *Middle States Association of Colleges and
Schools* • Total Enrollment: *2322*

PROGRAM INFORMATION

LPN/LVN Exit: *Yes* • NLNAC Accreditation: *Yes*

NURSING STUDENT PROFILE

Total Nursing Enrollment: *87* • Full-Time Enrollment: *80* •
Part-Time Enrollment: *7* • Female Enrollment: *80* • Male
Enrollment: *7* • Total New Admissions Who Enrolled for
Fall: *65* • Total Graduates: *28*

FINANCES

Residential Annual Tuition: *$2,555* • Non-Residential
Annual Tuition: *$8,365* • General Institution Fees: *$280* •
Additional Nursing Fees: *$500*

COMMUNITY COLLEGE OF PHILADELPHIA

Address: 1700 Spring Garden Street, Philadelphia, PA 19130
Phone: 215-751-8853
Fax: 215-751-8937
Contact: Andrea Mengel, PhD, RN, Head, Department of Nursing
Email: amengel@ccp.cc.pa.us

GENERAL INFORMATION

Type of School: *2-Year College or University, Public* • Accreditation: *Middle States Association of Colleges and Schools* • Total Enrollment: *18000*

PROGRAM INFORMATION

LPN/LVN Exit: *No* • NLNAC Accreditation: *Yes*

NURSING STUDENT PROFILE

Total Nursing Enrollment: *173* • Full-Time Enrollment: *173* • Part-Time Enrollment: *0* • Female Enrollment: *146* • Male Enrollment: *27* • Total New Admissions Who Enrolled for Fall: *Not Reported* • Total Graduates: *87*

FINANCES

Residential Annual Tuition: *$2,528* • Non-Residential Annual Tuition: *Not Reported* • General Institution Fees: *$293* • Additional Nursing Fees: *$1,000*

DELAWARE COUNTY COMMUNITY COLLEGE

Address: 901 S Media Line Road, Media, PA 19063
Phone: 610-359-5285
Fax: 610-359-7350
Contact: Carol Lillis, MSN, RN, Dean, Allied Health and Nursing
Email: clillis@dcccnet.dccc.edu

GENERAL INFORMATION

Type of School: *2-Year College or University, Public* • Accreditation: *Middle States Association of Colleges and Schools* • Total Enrollment: *23000*

PROGRAM INFORMATION

LPN/LVN Exit: *No* • NLNAC Accreditation: *Yes*

NURSING STUDENT PROFILE

Total Nursing Enrollment: *230* • Full-Time Enrollment: *48* • Part-Time Enrollment: *182* • Female Enrollment: *198* • Male Enrollment: *32* • Total New Admissions Who Enrolled for Fall: *145* • Total Graduates: *56*

FINANCES

Residential Annual Tuition: *$1,560* • Non-Residential Annual Tuition: *$4,728* • General Institution Fees: *$30* • Additional Nursing Fees: *$25*

GWYNEDD-MERCY COLLEGE

Address: Sunnytown Pike Box 901, Gwynedd Valley, PA
            19437
Phone: 215-751-8853
Fax: 215-751-8937
Contact: Andrea Mengel, PhD, RN, Department Head
Email: amengel@ccp.cc.ga.us

GENERAL INFORMATION

Type of School: *Independent, Private (Religious)* •
Accreditation: *Middle States Association of Colleges and
Schools* • Total Enrollment: *1750*

PROGRAM INFORMATION

LPN/LVN Exit: *Not Reported* • NLNAC Accreditation: *Yes*

NURSING STUDENT PROFILE

Total Nursing Enrollment: *Not Reported* • Full-Time
Enrollment: *Not Reported* • Part-Time Enrollment: *Not
Reported* • Female Enrollment: *Not Reported* • Male
Enrollment: *Not Reported* • Total New Admissions Who
Enrolled for Fall: *Not Reported* • Total Graduates: *Not
Reported*

FINANCES

Residential Annual Tuition: *Not Reported* • Non-Residential
Annual Tuition: *Not Reported* • General Institution Fees: *Not
Reported* • Additional Nursing Fees: *Not Reported*

HARRISBURG AREA COMMUNITY COLLEGE

Address: 1 Hacc Drive, Harrisburg, PA 17110
Phone: 717-780-2316
Fax: 717-780-2551
Contact: Diana Wells, MSN, RN, Director
Email: dkwells@hacc.edu

GENERAL INFORMATION

Type of School: *2-Year College or University, Public* •
Accreditation: *Middle States Association of Colleges and
Schools* • Total Enrollment: *10991*

PROGRAM INFORMATION

LPN/LVN Exit: *No* • NLNAC Accreditation: *Yes*

NURSING STUDENT PROFILE

Total Nursing Enrollment: *179* • Full-Time Enrollment: *59* •
Part-Time Enrollment: *120* • Female Enrollment: *160* • Male
Enrollment: *19* • Total New Admissions Who Enrolled for
Fall: *105* • Total Graduates: *69*

FINANCES

Residential Annual Tuition: *$3,360* • Non-Residential
Annual Tuition: *$5,100* • General Institution Fees: *$500* •
Additional Nursing Fees: *$90*

LEHIGH CARBON COMMUNITY COLLEGE

Address: 4525 Education Park Dr., Schnecksville, PA 18078
Phone: 610-799-1550
Fax: 610-799-1527
Contact: Nancy Becker, RN, MS, Dean of Allied Health and Director of Nursing
Email: nbecker@lccc.edu

GENERAL INFORMATION

Type of School: *2-Year College or University, Public* • Accreditation: *Middle States Association of Colleges and Schools* • Total Enrollment: *3768*

PROGRAM INFORMATION

LPN/LVN Exit: *No* • NLNAC Accreditation: *Yes*

NURSING STUDENT PROFILE

Total Nursing Enrollment: *67* • Full-Time Enrollment: *0* • Part-Time Enrollment: *67* • Female Enrollment: *59* • Male Enrollment: *8* • Total New Admissions Who Enrolled for Fall: *47* • Total Graduates: *30*

FINANCES

Residential Annual Tuition: *$3,216* • Non-Residential Annual Tuition: *$4,824* • General Institution Fees: *$216* • Additional Nursing Fees: *$55*

LOCK HAVEN UNIVERSITY OF PENNSYLVANIA

Address: 119 Byers St., Clearfield, PA 16830
Phone: 814-765-0619
Fax: 814-765-0611
Contact: Therese M. Sayers, RN, MS, Chairperson, Nursing Department
Email: tsayers@lhup.edu

GENERAL INFORMATION

Type of School: *4-Year College or University, Public* • Accreditation: *Middle States Association of Colleges and Schools* • Total Enrollment: *3650*

PROGRAM INFORMATION

LPN/LVN Exit: *No* • NLNAC Accreditation: *Yes*

NURSING STUDENT PROFILE

Total Nursing Enrollment: *55* • Full-Time Enrollment: *55* • Part-Time Enrollment: *0* • Female Enrollment: *51* • Male Enrollment: *4* • Total New Admissions Who Enrolled for Fall: *30* • Total Graduates: *22*

FINANCES

Residential Annual Tuition: *$4,280* • Non-Residential Annual Tuition: *$7,480* • General Institution Fees: *$244* • Additional Nursing Fees: *$33*

LUZERNE COUNTY COMMUNITY COLLEGE

Address: 1333 South Prospect St., Nanticoke, PA 18634
Phone: 570-740-0463
Fax: Not Reported
Contact: Jane E. Brown, PhD, RN, Associate Dean of
            Nursing
Email: jbrown@luzerne.edu

GENERAL INFORMATION

Type of School: *2-Year College or University, Public* •
Accreditation: *Middle States Association of Colleges and
Schools* • Total Enrollment: *5800*

PROGRAM INFORMATION

LPN/LVN Exit: *Not Reported* • NLNAC Accreditation: *Yes*

NURSING STUDENT PROFILE

Total Nursing Enrollment: *Not Reported* • Full-Time
Enrollment: *Not Reported* • Part-Time Enrollment: *Not
Reported* • Female Enrollment: *Not Reported* • Male
Enrollment: *Not Reported* • Total New Admissions Who
Enrolled for Fall: *Not Reported* • Total Graduates: *Not
Reported*

FINANCES

Residential Annual Tuition: *Not Reported* • Non-Residential
Annual Tuition: *Not Reported* • General Institution Fees: *Not
Reported* • Additional Nursing Fees: *Not Reported*

MERCYHURST COLLEGE— NORTH EAST

Address: 16 W Division, North East, PA 16428
Phone: 814-725-6139
Fax: 814-725-6133
Contact: Susan A. Vitron, MSN, RN, Director of Nursing
Email: svitron@mercyhurst.edu

GENERAL INFORMATION

Type of School: *4-Year College or University, Private
(Religious)* • Accreditation: *Middle States Association of
Colleges and Schools* • Total Enrollment: *Not Reported*

PROGRAM INFORMATION

LPN/LVN Exit: *No* • NLNAC Accreditation: *No*

NURSING STUDENT PROFILE

Total Nursing Enrollment: *78* • Full-Time Enrollment: *78* •
Part-Time Enrollment: *0* • Female Enrollment: *71* • Male
Enrollment: *7* • Total New Admissions Who Enrolled for
Fall: *54* • Total Graduates: *20*

FINANCES

Residential Annual Tuition: *$8,070* • Non-Residential
Annual Tuition: *Not Reported* • General Institution Fees:
$750 • Additional Nursing Fees: *$900*

MONTGOMERY COUNTY COMMUNITY COLLEGE

Address: PO Box 400, 340 DeKalb Pike, Blue Bell, PA 19422-0796
Phone: 215-641-6471
Fax: 215-619-7180
Contact: Beverly L. Welhan, RN, DNSc, Director and Professor, Nursing Program
Email: bwelhan@admin.mc3.edu

GENERAL INFORMATION

Type of School: *2-Year College or University, Private (Religious)* • Accreditation: *Middle States Association of Colleges and Schools* • Total Enrollment: *9592*

PROGRAM INFORMATION

LPN/LVN Exit: *No* • NLNAC Accreditation: *Yes*

NURSING STUDENT PROFILE

Total Nursing Enrollment: *142* • Full-Time Enrollment: *22* • Part-Time Enrollment: *120* • Female Enrollment: *125* • Male Enrollment: *17* • Total New Admissions Who Enrolled for Fall: *37* • Total Graduates: *43*

FINANCES

Residential Annual Tuition: *$3,600* • Non-Residential Annual Tuition: *$5,400* • General Institution Fees: *$168* • Additional Nursing Fees: *$160*

MOUNT ALOYSIUS COLLEGE

Address: 7373 Admiral Peary Highway, Cresson, PA 16630
Phone: 814-886-6401
Fax: 814-886-4906
Contact: Cheryl A. Webb, PhD, RN, CS, Chairperson
Email: cwebb@mtaloy.edu

GENERAL INFORMATION

Type of School: *4-Year College or University, Private (Religious)* • Accreditation: *Middle States Association of Colleges and Schools* • Total Enrollment: *900*

PROGRAM INFORMATION

LPN/LVN Exit: *No* • NLNAC Accreditation: *Yes*

NURSING STUDENT PROFILE

Total Nursing Enrollment: *116* • Full-Time Enrollment: *115* • Part-Time Enrollment: *1* • Female Enrollment: *100* • Male Enrollment: *16* • Total New Admissions Who Enrolled for Fall: *59* • Total Graduates: *21*

FINANCES

Residential Annual Tuition: *$12,430* • Non-Residential Annual Tuition: *$12,430* • General Institution Fees: *$100* • Additional Nursing Fees: *$55*

NORTHAMPTON COMMUNITY COLLEGE

Address:　3835 Green Pond Road, Bethlehem, PA 18020
Phone:　　610-861-5376
Fax:　　　610-861-4132
Contact:　Carolyn Kern, MSN, RN, Director of Nursing
　　　　　　Programs
Email:　　ckern@northampton.edu

GENERAL INFORMATION

Type of School: *2-Year College or University, Public* •
Accreditation: *Middle States Association of Colleges and
Schools* • Total Enrollment: *5666*

PROGRAM INFORMATION

LPN/LVN Exit: *No* • NLNAC Accreditation: *Yes*

NURSING STUDENT PROFILE

Total Nursing Enrollment: *90* • Full-Time Enrollment: *19* •
Part-Time Enrollment: *71* • Female Enrollment: *82* • Male
Enrollment: *8* • Total New Admissions Who Enrolled for
Fall: *41* • Total Graduates: *58*

FINANCES

Residential Annual Tuition: *$1,560* • Non-Residential
Annual Tuition: *$4,680* • General Institution Fees: *$384* •
Additional Nursing Fees: *$384*

PENNSYLVANIA COLLEGE OF TECHNOLOGY

Address:　One College Avenue, Williamsport, PA 17701
Phone:　　570-327-4525
Fax:　　　570-321-5556
Contact:　Pamela L. Starcher, PhD, RN, MN, Director of
　　　　　　Nursing
Email:　　pstarche@pct.edu

GENERAL INFORMATION

Type of School: *4-Year College or University, Public* •
Accreditation: *Middle States Association of Colleges and
Schools* • Total Enrollment: *5320*

PROGRAM INFORMATION

LPN/LVN Exit: *No* • NLNAC Accreditation: *Yes*

NURSING STUDENT PROFILE

Total Nursing Enrollment: *77* • Full-Time Enrollment: *68* •
Part-Time Enrollment: *9* • Female Enrollment: *70* • Male
Enrollment: *7* • Total New Admissions Who Enrolled for
Fall: *10* • Total Graduates: *43*

FINANCES

Residential Annual Tuition: *$8,940* • Non-Residential
Annual Tuition: *$11,250* • General Institution Fees: *$0* •
Additional Nursing Fees: *$1,208*

PENNSYLVANIA STATE UNIVERSITY

Address: 201 Health and Human Dev East, University Park, PA 16802-6508
Phone: 814-863-0245
Fax: 814-865-3779
Contact: Sarah Hall Gueldner, DSN, RN, FAAN, Director
Email: shg9@psu.edu

GENERAL INFORMATION

Type of School: *4-Year College or University, Public* • Accreditation: *Middle States Association of Colleges and Schools* • Total Enrollment: *15582*

PROGRAM INFORMATION

LPN/LVN Exit: *Not Reported* • NLNAC Accreditation: *Yes*

NURSING STUDENT PROFILE

Total Nursing Enrollment: *279* • Full-Time Enrollment: *194* • Part-Time Enrollment: *85* • Female Enrollment: *258* • Male Enrollment: *21* • Total New Admissions Who Enrolled for Fall: *166* • Total Graduates: *122*

FINANCES

Residential Annual Tuition: *$6,546* • Non-Residential Annual Tuition: *$14,088* • General Institution Fees: *$286* • Additional Nursing Fees: *$44*

PITTSBURGH MERCY HEALTH SYSTEM

Address: 1401 Bulevard of the Allies, Pittsburgh, PA 15219
Phone: 412-232-7964
Fax: 412-232-7951
Contact: Joanne Sperry, MN, BSN, RN, Director
Email: jsperry#@mercy.pmhs.org

GENERAL INFORMATION

Type of School: *Hospital, Private (Religious)* • Accreditation: *None* • Total Enrollment: *Not Reported*

PROGRAM INFORMATION

LPN/LVN Exit: *No* • NLNAC Accreditation: *No*

NURSING STUDENT PROFILE

Total Nursing Enrollment: *42* • Full-Time Enrollment: *42* • Part-Time Enrollment: *0* • Female Enrollment: *37* • Male Enrollment: *5* • Total New Admissions Who Enrolled for Fall: *23* • Total Graduates: *24*

FINANCES

Residential Annual Tuition: *$7,685* • Non-Residential Annual Tuition: *$7,685* • General Institution Fees: *Not Reported* • Additional Nursing Fees: *$65*

READING AREA COMMUNITY COLLEGE

Address: 10 S Second St. PO Box 1706, Reading, PA 19603
Phone: 610-372-4721
Fax: Not Reported
Contact: Elissa Sauer, MSN, RN, Assistant Dean, Health Services
Email: es1568@email.racc.cc.pa.us

GENERAL INFORMATION

Type of School: *2-Year College or University, Public* • Accreditation: *Middle States Association of Colleges and Schools* • Total Enrollment: *2900*

PROGRAM INFORMATION

LPN/LVN Exit: *Not Reported* • NLNAC Accreditation: *Yes*

NURSING STUDENT PROFILE

Total Nursing Enrollment: *Not Reported* • Full-Time Enrollment: *Not Reported* • Part-Time Enrollment: *Not Reported* • Female Enrollment: *Not Reported* • Male Enrollment: *Not Reported* • Total New Admissions Who Enrolled for Fall: *Not Reported* • Total Graduates: *Not Reported*

FINANCES

Residential Annual Tuition: *Not Reported* • Non-Residential Annual Tuition: *Not Reported* • General Institution Fees: *Not Reported* • Additional Nursing Fees: *Not Reported*

READING HOSPITAL SCHOOL OF NURSING

Web site: www.chc.hcwp.org/rndread.htm
Address: 6th & Spruce Sts, West Reading, PA 19612
Phone: (610) 378-6331
Contact: Miss Lorna Ramsay, Director

GENERAL INFORMATION

Type of School: *Public* • Campus Setting: *n/a* • Total Enrollment: *141*

PROGRAM INFORMATION

Programs Offered: *Diploma* • Options: *Evening Classes, Weekend Classes, Distance Learning, Other Alternative Schedules, Continuing Education* • Articulations: *Diploma to BSN* • NLNAC Accredited

NURSING STUDENT PROFILE

First-Year Undergraduate Enrollment: *62* • Total Graduates: *35* • Total Enrollment: *141*

FINANCES

Resident Annual Tuition: *n/a* • Non-Resident Annual Tuition: *n/a* • Grants: *Federal Pell Grants* • Scholarships: *Institutionally-Sponsored Need-Based Scholarships* • Loans: *Federal PLUS Loans, Federal Stafford Loans* • % of Students Receiving Some Type of Aid: *94%* • Financial Aid Application Deadline: *None* • Financial Aid Office Phone: *(610) 378-6958*

UNIVERSITY OF PITTSBURGH AT BRADFORD

Address: 300 Campus Drive, Bradford, PA 16701
Phone: 814-362-7640
Fax: 814-362-0919
Contact: Lisa M. Fiorentino, PhD, RN, Director,
           Department of Nursing
Email: lmfl+@pitt.edu

GENERAL INFORMATION

Type of School: *4-Year College or University, Other* •
Accreditation: *Middle States Association of Colleges and
Schools* • Total Enrollment: *1024*

PROGRAM INFORMATION

LPN/LVN Exit: *No* • NLNAC Accreditation: *Yes*

NURSING STUDENT PROFILE

Total Nursing Enrollment: *29* • Full-Time Enrollment: *26* •
Part-Time Enrollment: *3* • Female Enrollment: *25* • Male
Enrollment: *4* • Total New Admissions Who Enrolled for
Fall: *16* • Total Graduates: *14*

FINANCES

Residential Annual Tuition: *$8,264* • Non-Residential
Annual Tuition: *$18,026* • General Institution Fees: *$544* •
Additional Nursing Fees: *$11*

WESTMORELAND COUNTY COMMUNITY COLLEGE

Address: 400 Armbrust Road, Youngwood, PA 15697
Phone: 724-925-4028
Fax: 724-925-4293
Contact: Patricia E. Mihalcin, PhD, RN, Division Chair,
           Social Science and Health Professionals
Email: mihalcpe@wccc.westmoreland.cc.pa.us

GENERAL INFORMATION

Type of School: *Not Reported* • Accreditation: *Middle States
Association of Colleges and Schools* • Total Enrollment: *Not
Reported*

PROGRAM INFORMATION

LPN/LVN Exit: *Yes* • NLNAC Accreditation: *No*

NURSING STUDENT PROFILE

Total Nursing Enrollment: *91* • Full-Time Enrollment: *69* •
Part-Time Enrollment: *22* • Female Enrollment: *82* • Male
Enrollment: *9* • Total New Admissions Who Enrolled for
Fall: *44* • Total Graduates: *55*

FINANCES

Residential Annual Tuition: *$1,200* • Non-Residential
Annual Tuition: *$3,600* • General Institution Fees: *Not
Reported* • Additional Nursing Fees: *Not Reported*

ANTILLEAN ADVENTIST UNIVERSITY

Address: PO Box 118, Mayaguez, PR 00681
Phone: 787-834-9595
Fax: 787-834-9597
Contact: Maria L Cruz, MSN RN, Director of Nursing Department
Email: *Not Reported*

GENERAL INFORMATION

Type of School: *4-Year College or University, Private (Religious)* • Accreditation: *Middle States Association of Colleges and Schools* • Total Enrollment: *719*

PROGRAM INFORMATION

LPN/LVN Exit: *No* • NLNAC Accreditation: *No*

NURSING STUDENT PROFILE

Total Nursing Enrollment: *194* • Full-Time Enrollment: *182* • Part-Time Enrollment: *12* • Female Enrollment: *162* • Male Enrollment: *32* • Total New Admissions Who Enrolled for Fall: *19* • Total Graduates: *46*

FINANCES

Residential Annual Tuition: *$4,070* • Non-Residential Annual Tuition: *$4,070* • General Institution Fees: *$770* • Additional Nursing Fees: *$380*

BAYAMON CENTRAL UNIVERSITY

Address: Box 1725, Bayamon, PR 00960-1725
Phone: 787-786-3030
Fax: 787-740-2200
Contact: Norma I Moctezuma Rodriguez, EdD, RN, Coordinator
Email: nmoctezuma@ucb.edu.pr.com

GENERAL INFORMATION

Type of School: *4-Year College or University, Private (Religious)* • Accreditation: *Middle States Association of Colleges and Schools* • Total Enrollment: *Not Reported*

PROGRAM INFORMATION

LPN/LVN Exit: *No* • NLNAC Accreditation: *No*

NURSING STUDENT PROFILE

Total Nursing Enrollment: *155* • Full-Time Enrollment: *123* • Part-Time Enrollment: *32* • Female Enrollment: *133* • Male Enrollment: *22* • Total New Admissions Who Enrolled for Fall: *31* • Total Graduates: *13*

FINANCES

Residential Annual Tuition: *Not Reported* • Non-Residential Annual Tuition: *Not Reported* • General Institution Fees: *Not Reported* • Additional Nursing Fees: *Not Reported*

ELECTRONIC DATA PROCESSING COLLEGE

Address: PO Box 1674, San Sebastian, PR 00685
Phone: 787-765-3560
Fax: Not Reported
Contact: Gladys Nieves, MSN, RN, Chairperson
Email: *Not Reported*

GENERAL INFORMATION

Type of School: *Not Reported* • Accreditation: *Not Reported* • Total Enrollment: *Not Reported*

PROGRAM INFORMATION

LPN/LVN Exit: *Not Reported* • NLNAC Accreditation: *No*

NURSING STUDENT PROFILE

Total Nursing Enrollment: *Not Reported* • Full-Time Enrollment: *Not Reported* • Part-Time Enrollment: *Not Reported* • Female Enrollment: *Not Reported* • Male Enrollment: *Not Reported* • Total New Admissions Who Enrolled for Fall: *Not Reported* • Total Graduates: *Not Reported*

FINANCES

Residential Annual Tuition: *Not Reported* • Non-Residential Annual Tuition: *Not Reported* • General Institution Fees: *Not Reported* • Additional Nursing Fees: *Not Reported*

INTERAMERICAN UNIVERSITY

Address: PO Box 5700, San German, PR 00683
Phone: 787-264-1912
Fax: 787-751-3375
Contact: Leida Madera-Cruz, MSN, RN, Director
Email: lmadera@sg.inter.edu

GENERAL INFORMATION

Type of School: *Not Reported* • Accreditation: *None* • Total Enrollment: *Not Reported*

PROGRAM INFORMATION

LPN/LVN Exit: *Not Reported* • NLNAC Accreditation: *Not Reported*

NURSING STUDENT PROFILE

Total Nursing Enrollment: *16* • Full-Time Enrollment: *16* • Part-Time Enrollment: *0* • Female Enrollment: *14* • Male Enrollment: *2* • Total New Admissions Who Enrolled for Fall: *7* • Total Graduates: *10*

FINANCES

Residential Annual Tuition: *Not Reported* • Non-Residential Annual Tuition: *Not Reported* • General Institution Fees: *Not Reported* • Additional Nursing Fees: *Not Reported*

INTERAMERICAN UNIVERSITY—AGUADILLA

Address: Apartado 20000, Aguadilla, PR 00605
Phone: 787-891-0925
Fax: 787-882-3020
Contact: Rosa M Mercado, Master in Public Health, Nursing Program Coordinator
Email: *Not Reported*

GENERAL INFORMATION

Type of School: *Not Reported* • Accreditation: *Not Reported* • Total Enrollment: *Not Reported*

PROGRAM INFORMATION

LPN/LVN Exit: *No* • NLNAC Accreditation: *Not Reported*

NURSING STUDENT PROFILE

Total Nursing Enrollment: *24* • Full-Time Enrollment: *24* • Part-Time Enrollment: *Not Reported* • Female Enrollment: *20* • Male Enrollment: *4* • Total New Admissions Who Enrolled for Fall: *20* • Total Graduates: *38*

FINANCES

Residential Annual Tuition: *$3,960* • Non-Residential Annual Tuition: *$3,960* • General Institution Fees: *$338* • Additional Nursing Fees: *$1,170*

INTERAMERICAN UNIVERSITY—SAN GERMAN

Address: PO Box 5106, San German, PR 00683
Phone: 787-264-1912
Fax: 787-751-3375
Contact: Leida Madera Cruz, MN, RN, Director of Program
Email: lmadera@sg.inter.edu

GENERAL INFORMATION

Type of School: *Not Reported* • Accreditation: *Not Reported* • Total Enrollment: *Not Reported*

PROGRAM INFORMATION

LPN/LVN Exit: *Not Reported* • NLNAC Accreditation: *Not Reported*

NURSING STUDENT PROFILE

Total Nursing Enrollment: *16* • Full-Time Enrollment: *16* • Part-Time Enrollment: *0* • Female Enrollment: *14* • Male Enrollment: *2* • Total New Admissions Who Enrolled for Fall: *7* • Total Graduates: *10*

FINANCES

Residential Annual Tuition: *Not Reported* • Non-Residential Annual Tuition: *Not Reported* • General Institution Fees: *Not Reported* • Additional Nursing Fees: *Not Reported*

INTERAMERICAN UNIVERSITY—SAN JUAN

Address: P.O. Box 191293, San Juan, PR 00919
Phone: 787-763-3066
Fax: 787-250-1242
Contact: Gloria E Ortiz, EdD, RN, Director
Email: glortiz@inter.edu

INTERAMERICAN UNIVERSITY OF PUERTO RICO

Address: Metropolitan Campus, PO Box 191293, San Juan, PR 00919-1293
Phone: 787-864-2222
Fax: 787-866-4986
Contact: Carlos Cobeo, MSN, RN, CSN, Director of the Nursing Program
Email: ccobeo@ns.inter.edu

GENERAL INFORMATION

Type of School: *Not Reported* • Accreditation: *Not Reported* • Total Enrollment: *Not Reported*

GENERAL INFORMATION

Type of School: *4-Year College or University, Private (Independent)* • Accreditation: *Middle States Association of Colleges and Schools* • Total Enrollment: *40000*

PROGRAM INFORMATION

LPN/LVN Exit: *No* • NLNAC Accreditation: *Not Reported*

PROGRAM INFORMATION

LPN/LVN Exit: *Not Reported* • NLNAC Accreditation: *Not Reported*

NURSING STUDENT PROFILE

Total Nursing Enrollment: *130* • Full-Time Enrollment: *130* • Part-Time Enrollment: *0* • Female Enrollment: *109* • Male Enrollment: *21* • Total New Admissions Who Enrolled for Fall: *130* • Total Graduates: *52*

NURSING STUDENT PROFILE

Total Nursing Enrollment: *150* • Full-Time Enrollment: *150* • Part-Time Enrollment: *Not Reported* • Female Enrollment: *140* • Male Enrollment: *10* • Total New Admissions Who Enrolled for Fall: *59* • Total Graduates: *43*

FINANCES

Residential Annual Tuition: *$4,838* • Non-Residential Annual Tuition: *Not Reported* • General Institution Fees: *$440* • Additional Nursing Fees: *$880*

FINANCES

Residential Annual Tuition: *$2,640* • Non-Residential Annual Tuition: *Not Reported* • General Institution Fees: *$580* • Additional Nursing Fees: *$580*

INTERAMERICAN UNIVERSITY OF PUERTO RICO—GUAYAMA

Address: PO Box 10004, Guayama, PR 00785
Phone: 787-864-2222
Fax: 787-866-4986
Contact: Carlos Cobeo, MSN, RN, CNS, Director of the Nursing Program
Email: ccobeo@ns.inter.edu

GENERAL INFORMATION

Type of School: *Not Reported* • Accreditation: *Not Reported* • Total Enrollment: *Not Reported*

PROGRAM INFORMATION

LPN/LVN Exit: *Not Reported* • NLNAC Accreditation: *Not Reported*

NURSING STUDENT PROFILE

Total Nursing Enrollment: *150* • Full-Time Enrollment: *150* • Part-Time Enrollment: *0* • Female Enrollment: *140* • Male Enrollment: *10* • Total New Admissions Who Enrolled for Fall: *59* • Total Graduates: *43*

FINANCES

Residential Annual Tuition: *$2,640* • Non-Residential Annual Tuition: *$2,640* • General Institution Fees: *$580* • Additional Nursing Fees: *$580*

TECHNOLOGICAL COLLEGE OF SAN JUAN

Address: Box 70179, San Juan, PR 00936
Phone: 787-250-7111
Fax: Not Reported
Contact: Sinthia Fernnandez, Director
Email: ctmsj2@prtc.net

GENERAL INFORMATION

Type of School: *2-Year College or University, Public* • Accreditation: *Middle States Association of Colleges and Schools* • Total Enrollment: *881*

PROGRAM INFORMATION

LPN/LVN Exit: *No* • NLNAC Accreditation: *Yes*

NURSING STUDENT PROFILE

Total Nursing Enrollment: *881* • Full-Time Enrollment: *736* • Part-Time Enrollment: *145* • Female Enrollment: *421* • Male Enrollment: *460* • Total New Admissions Who Enrolled for Fall: *53* • Total Graduates: *92*

FINANCES

Residential Annual Tuition: *$2,240* • Non-Residential Annual Tuition: *Not Reported* • General Institution Fees: *$85* • Additional Nursing Fees: *$80*

UNIVERSIDAD DEL SAGRADO CORAZÓN

Address: PO Box 12383, Loiza Street, Santurce, PR 00914
Phone: 787-728-1515
Fax: 787-727-1250
Contact: Amelia E Yordan
Email: *Not Reported*

GENERAL INFORMATION

Type of School: *4-Year College or University, Private (Independent)* • Accreditation: *Middle States Association of Colleges and Schools* • Total Enrollment: *5500*

PROGRAM INFORMATION

LPN/LVN Exit: *Not Reported* • NLNAC Accreditation: *No*

NURSING STUDENT PROFILE

Total Nursing Enrollment: *121* • Full-Time Enrollment: *92* • Part-Time Enrollment: *29* • Female Enrollment: *Not Reported* • Male Enrollment: *Not Reported* • Total New Admissions Who Enrolled for Fall: *50* • Total Graduates: *22*

FINANCES

Residential Annual Tuition: *Not Reported* • Non-Residential Annual Tuition: *Not Reported* • General Institution Fees: *$350* • Additional Nursing Fees: *Not Reported*

UNIVERSIDAD INTERAMERICANA DE PUERTO RICO

Address: Universidad Interamericana De Puerto Rico, Apartado 20000, Aguadilla, PR 00605
Phone: 787-891-0925
Fax: *Not Reported*
Contact: Rosa M. Mercado, MPH, RN, Nursing Program Director
Email: *Not Reported*

GENERAL INFORMATION

Type of School: *4-Year College or University, Private (Independent)* • Accreditation: *Middle States Association of Colleges and Schools* • Total Enrollment: *3564*

PROGRAM INFORMATION

LPN/LVN Exit: *No* • NLNAC Accreditation: *Not Reported*

NURSING STUDENT PROFILE

Total Nursing Enrollment: *58* • Full-Time Enrollment: *58* • Part-Time Enrollment: *0* • Female Enrollment: *Not Reported* • Male Enrollment: *Not Reported* • Total New Admissions Who Enrolled for Fall: *64* • Total Graduates: *24*

FINANCES

Residential Annual Tuition: *Not Reported* • Non-Residential Annual Tuition: *Not Reported* • General Institution Fees: *Not Reported* • Additional Nursing Fees: *Not Reported*

UNIVERSIDAD METROPOLITANA

Address: PO Box 21150, San Juan, PR 00928-1150
Phone: *Not Reported*
Fax: *Not Reported*
Contact: *Not Reported*
Email: *Not Reported*

GENERAL INFORMATION

Type of School: *4-Year College or University, Private (Independent)* • Accreditation: *Middle States Association of Colleges and Schools* • Total Enrollment: *6501*

PROGRAM INFORMATION

LPN/LVN Exit: *Not Reported* • NLNAC Accreditation: *Yes*

NURSING STUDENT PROFILE

Total Nursing Enrollment: *Not Reported* • Full-Time Enrollment: *Not Reported* • Part-Time Enrollment: *Not Reported* • Female Enrollment: *Not Reported* • Male Enrollment: *Not Reported* • Total New Admissions Who Enrolled for Fall: *Not Reported* • Total Graduates: *Not Reported*

FINANCES

Residential Annual Tuition: *Not Reported* • Non-Residential Annual Tuition: *Not Reported* • General Institution Fees: *Not Reported* • Additional Nursing Fees: *Not Reported*

UNIVERSITY OF PUERTO RICO

Address: GPO Box 365067, San Juan, PR 00936-5067
Phone: 787-850-9346
Fax: 787-850-9411
Contact: Francisca Rodriguez-Trinidad, EdD, MSN, RN, Director of Nursing Department
Email: f_rodriguez@cuhac.upr.clu.edu

GENERAL INFORMATION

Type of School: *Independent, Public* • Accreditation: *Middle States Association of Colleges and Schools* • Total Enrollment: *3154*

PROGRAM INFORMATION

LPN/LVN Exit: *Not Reported* • NLNAC Accreditation: *Yes*

NURSING STUDENT PROFILE

Total Nursing Enrollment: *50* • Full-Time Enrollment: *48* • Part-Time Enrollment: *2* • Female Enrollment: *40* • Male Enrollment: *10* • Total New Admissions Who Enrolled for Fall: *50* • Total Graduates: *16*

FINANCES

Residential Annual Tuition: *$1,245* • Non-Residential Annual Tuition: *Not Reported* • General Institution Fees: *$75* • Additional Nursing Fees: *$150*

UNIVERSITY OF PUERTO RICO—HUMACAO

Address: CUH Station 100 Road 1908, Humacao, PR
00791-4300
Phone: 787-850-9346
Fax: 787-850-9411
Contact: Francisca Rodriguez-Trinidad, Ed.D., MSN, RN,
Director of Nursing Department
Email: f_rodriguez@cuhac.upr.clu.edu

GENERAL INFORMATION

Type of School: *4-Year College or University, Public* •
Accreditation: *Middle States Association of Colleges and
Schools* • Total Enrollment: *4592*

PROGRAM INFORMATION

LPN/LVN Exit: *No* • NLNAC Accreditation: *Yes*

NURSING STUDENT PROFILE

Total Nursing Enrollment: *50* • Full-Time Enrollment: *48* •
Part-Time Enrollment: *2* • Female Enrollment: *40* • Male
Enrollment: *10* • Total New Admissions Who Enrolled for
Fall: *50* • Total Graduates: *16*

FINANCES

Residential Annual Tuition: *$1,245* • Non-Residential
Annual Tuition: *Not Reported* • General Institution Fees:
$623 • Additional Nursing Fees: *$30*

COMMUNITY COLLEGE OF RHODE ISLAND

Address: 1762 Louisquisett Pike, Lincoln, RI 2865
Phone: 401-825-2162
Fax: 401-825-1102
Contact: Elizabeth Murphy, MSN, RN, Department
Chairperson
Email: Emurphy@ccri.cc.ri.us

GENERAL INFORMATION

Type of School: *2-Year College or University, Public* •
Accreditation: *New England Association of Schools and
Colleges* • Total Enrollment: *15000*

PROGRAM INFORMATION

LPN/LVN Exit: *Not Reported* • NLNAC Accreditation: *Yes*

NURSING STUDENT PROFILE

Total Nursing Enrollment: *454* • Full-Time Enrollment: *15* •
Part-Time Enrollment: *439* • Female Enrollment: *401* • Male
Enrollment: *53* • Total New Admissions Who Enrolled for
Fall: *195* • Total Graduates: *182*

FINANCES

Residential Annual Tuition: *$1,616* • Non-Residential
Annual Tuition: *$4,742* • General Institution Fees: *$120* •
Additional Nursing Fees: *$20*

CENTRAL CAROLINA TECHNICAL COLLEGE

Address: 506 North Guignard Dr, Sumter, SC 29150
Phone: 803-778-7822
Fax: 803-778-7868
Contact: Beverly H Gulledge, MN, RN, ADN/PN
             Department Chair
Email: gulledgebh@cctc6.sum.tec.sc.us

GENERAL INFORMATION

Type of School: *2-Year College or University, Public* •
Accreditation: *Southern Association of Colleges and Schools* •
Total Enrollment: *Not Reported*

PROGRAM INFORMATION

LPN/LVN Exit: *No* • NLNAC Accreditation: *Yes*

NURSING STUDENT PROFILE

Total Nursing Enrollment: *70* • Full-Time Enrollment: *Not
Reported* • Part-Time Enrollment: *70* • Female Enrollment:
66 • Male Enrollment: *4* • Total New Admissions Who
Enrolled for Fall: *46* • Total Graduates: *43*

FINANCES

Residential Annual Tuition: *$850* • Non-Residential Annual
Tuition: *$1,922* • General Institution Fees: *$0* • Additional
Nursing Fees: *$0*

FLORENCE DARLINGTON TECHNICAL COLLEGE

Address: 2715 W. Lucas Street, Florence, SC 29501-0548
Phone: 803-661-8180
Fax: 803-661-8116
Contact: Anne-Marie Goff, , Department Head for
             Nursing
Email: goff@flo.tec.sc.us

GENERAL INFORMATION

Type of School: *Not Reported* • Accreditation: *None* • Total
Enrollment: *Not Reported*

PROGRAM INFORMATION

LPN/LVN Exit: *No* • NLNAC Accreditation: *Yes*

NURSING STUDENT PROFILE

Total Nursing Enrollment: *145* • Full-Time Enrollment: *79* •
Part-Time Enrollment: *66* • Female Enrollment: *128* • Male
Enrollment: *17* • Total New Admissions Who Enrolled for
Fall: *112* • Total Graduates: *46*

FINANCES

Residential Annual Tuition: *$1,100* • Non-Residential
Annual Tuition: *$1,476* • General Institution Fees: *$4* •
Additional Nursing Fees: *Not Reported*

GREENVILLE TECHNICAL COLLEGE

Address: PO Box 5616, Greenville, SC 29606
Phone: 864-250-8240
Fax: 864-250-8549
Contact: Alethia Walker, MSN, Co-Department Head
Email: walkerarw@gvltec.edu

GENERAL INFORMATION

Type of School: *Vocational/Technical School, Public* •
Accreditation: *Southern Association of Colleges and Schools* •
Total Enrollment: *Not Reported*

PROGRAM INFORMATION

LPN/LVN Exit: *No* • NLNAC Accreditation: *Yes*

NURSING STUDENT PROFILE

Total Nursing Enrollment: *324* • Full-Time Enrollment: *139* • Part-Time Enrollment: *185* • Female Enrollment: *305* • Male Enrollment: *19* • Total New Admissions Who Enrolled for Fall: *90* • Total Graduates: *85*

FINANCES

Residential Annual Tuition: *$1,450* • Non-Residential Annual Tuition: *$3,450* • General Institution Fees: *$50* • Additional Nursing Fees: *$90*

MIDLANDS TECHNICAL COLLEGE

Address: PO Box 2408, Columbia, SC 29202
Phone: 803-822-3402
Fax: 803-822-3343
Contact: Janet H Lee, MSN, RN, Department Chair, Nursing
Email: leej@midlandstech.com

GENERAL INFORMATION

Type of School: *2-Year College or University, Public* •
Accreditation: *Southern Association of Colleges and Schools* •
Total Enrollment: *Not Reported*

PROGRAM INFORMATION

LPN/LVN Exit: *No* • NLNAC Accreditation: *Yes*

NURSING STUDENT PROFILE

Total Nursing Enrollment: *306* • Full-Time Enrollment: *40* • Part-Time Enrollment: *266* • Female Enrollment: *266* • Male Enrollment: *40* • Total New Admissions Who Enrolled for Fall: *104* • Total Graduates: *142*

FINANCES

Residential Annual Tuition: *$1,700* • Non-Residential Annual Tuition: *$3,100* • General Institution Fees: *$26* • Additional Nursing Fees: *Not Reported*

ORANGEBURG CALHOUN TECHNICAL COLLEGE

Address: 3250 Saint Mathews Road, Orangeburg, SC 29118
Phone: 803-535-1354
Fax: 803-535-1388
Contact: Delura R Knight, MSN, Nursing Group Director
Email: knightd@org.tec.sc.us

GENERAL INFORMATION

Type of School: *2-Year College or University, Public* •
Accreditation: *Southern Association of Colleges and Schools* •
Total Enrollment: *Not Reported*

PROGRAM INFORMATION

LPN/LVN Exit: *No* • NLNAC Accreditation: *Yes*

NURSING STUDENT PROFILE

Total Nursing Enrollment: *118* • Full-Time Enrollment: *44* •
Part-Time Enrollment: *74* • Female Enrollment: *112* • Male
Enrollment: *6* • Total New Admissions Who Enrolled for
Fall: *70* • Total Graduates: *43*

FINANCES

Residential Annual Tuition: *$1,700* • Non-Residential
Annual Tuition: *$3,624* • General Institution Fees: *Not
Reported* • Additional Nursing Fees: *$250*

PIEDMONT TECHNICAL COLLEGE

Address: Emerald Road Drawer 1467, Greenwood, SC 29648
Phone: 864-941-8536
Fax: 864-941-8684
Contact: Lena W Warren, MSN, BSN, Dean of Health Science
Email: warren_l@peidmont.tec.sc.us

GENERAL INFORMATION

Type of School: *2-Year College or University, Public* •
Accreditation: *Southern Association of Colleges and Schools* •
Total Enrollment: *Not Reported*

PROGRAM INFORMATION

LPN/LVN Exit: *No* • NLNAC Accreditation: *Yes*

NURSING STUDENT PROFILE

Total Nursing Enrollment: *83* • Full-Time Enrollment: *76* •
Part-Time Enrollment: *7* • Female Enrollment: *82* • Male
Enrollment: *1* • Total New Admissions Who Enrolled for
Fall: *30* • Total Graduates: *30*

FINANCES

Residential Annual Tuition: *$1,872* • Non-Residential
Annual Tuition: *$3,060* • General Institution Fees: *$15* •
Additional Nursing Fees: *$216*

TECHNICAL COLLEGE OF THE LOWCOUNTRY

Address: PO Box 1288, Beaufort, SC 29901
Phone: 843-525-8267
Fax: 843-525-8268
Contact: Patricia A Slachta, PhD, RN, CWOCN
Email: pslachta@tcl.edu

GENERAL INFORMATION

Type of School: *2-Year College or University, Public •*
Accreditation: *Southern Association of Colleges and Schools •*
Total Enrollment: *Not Reported*

PROGRAM INFORMATION

LPN/LVN Exit: *Not Reported* • NLNAC Accreditation: *Yes*

NURSING STUDENT PROFILE

Total Nursing Enrollment: *61* • Full-Time Enrollment: *0* •
Part-Time Enrollment: *61* • Female Enrollment: *58* • Male
Enrollment: *3* • Total New Admissions Who Enrolled for
Fall: *70* • Total Graduates: *24*

FINANCES

Residential Annual Tuition: *$1,700* • Non-Residential
Annual Tuition: *$3,710* • General Institution Fees: *$50* •
Additional Nursing Fees: *$112*

TRI- COUNTY TECHNICAL COLLEGE

Address: PO Box 587, Pendleton, SC 29670
Phone: 864-646-8361
Fax: Not Reported
Contact: Polly D Fehler, MSN, BSN, AS, RN,
            Department Head
Email: pfehler@tricty.tricounty.tec.sc.us

GENERAL INFORMATION

Type of School: *Vocational/Technical School, Other •*
Accreditation: *Southern Association of Colleges and Schools •*
Total Enrollment: *Not Reported*

PROGRAM INFORMATION

LPN/LVN Exit: *No* • NLNAC Accreditation: *Yes*

NURSING STUDENT PROFILE

Total Nursing Enrollment: *106* • Full-Time Enrollment: *9* •
Part-Time Enrollment: *97* • Female Enrollment: *98* • Male
Enrollment: *8* • Total New Admissions Who Enrolled for
Fall: *60* • Total Graduates: *34*

FINANCES

Residential Annual Tuition: *$1,650* • Non-Residential
Annual Tuition: *$2,688* • General Institution Fees: *Not
Reported* • Additional Nursing Fees: *$15*

TRIDENT TECHNICAL COLLEGE

Address: PO Box 118067, Charleston, SC 29423
Phone: 843-572-6138
Fax: 843-574-6585
Contact: Muriel Horton, MSN, RN, Dean
Email: zphortonm@trident.tec.sc.us

GENERAL INFORMATION

Type of School: *2-Year College or University, Public* •
Accreditation: *Southern Association of Colleges and Schools* •
Total Enrollment: *Not Reported*

PROGRAM INFORMATION

LPN/LVN Exit: *No* • NLNAC Accreditation: *Yes*

NURSING STUDENT PROFILE

Total Nursing Enrollment: *265* • Full-Time Enrollment: *34* •
Part-Time Enrollment: *231* • Female Enrollment: *235* • Male
Enrollment: *30* • Total New Admissions Who Enrolled for
Fall: *104* • Total Graduates: *87*

FINANCES

Residential Annual Tuition: *$1,256* • Non-Residential
Annual Tuition: *$3,628* • General Institution Fees: *$44* •
Additional Nursing Fees: *$2*

UNIVERSITY OF SOUTH CAROLINA—AIKEN

Address: 471 University Parkway, Aiken, SC 29801
Phone: 803-641-3333
Fax: 803-641-3725
Contact: Iris Walliser, MSN, RN, Coordinator, ADN
Program
Email: irisw@usca.edu

GENERAL INFORMATION

Type of School: *4-Year College or University, Public* •
Accreditation: *Southern Association of Colleges and Schools* •
Total Enrollment: *Not Reported*

PROGRAM INFORMATION

LPN/LVN Exit: *No* • NLNAC Accreditation: *Yes*

NURSING STUDENT PROFILE

Total Nursing Enrollment: *149* • Full-Time Enrollment:
119 • Part-Time Enrollment: *30* • Female Enrollment: *143* •
Male Enrollment: *6* • Total New Admissions Who Enrolled
for Fall: *37* • Total Graduates: *60*

FINANCES

Residential Annual Tuition: *$3,638* • Non-Residential
Annual Tuition: *$8,164* • General Institution Fees: *$140* •
Additional Nursing Fees: *$300*

UNIVERSITY OF SOUTH CAROLINA—SPARTANBURG

Address: 800 University Way, Spartanburg, SC 29303
Phone: 864-503-5455
Fax: 864-503-5411
Contact: Mary Jo Tone, MSN, RN, Associate Professor and Division Chair
Email: mjtone@gw.uscs.edu

GENERAL INFORMATION

Type of School: *4-Year College or University, Public* •
Accreditation: *Southern Association of Colleges and Schools* •
Total Enrollment: *Not Reported*

PROGRAM INFORMATION

LPN/LVN Exit: *No* • NLNAC Accreditation: *Yes*

NURSING STUDENT PROFILE

Total Nursing Enrollment: *116* • Full-Time Enrollment: *52* •
Part-Time Enrollment: *64* • Female Enrollment: *111* • Male
Enrollment: *5* • Total New Admissions Who Enrolled for
Fall: *30* • Total Graduates: *43*

FINANCES

Residential Annual Tuition: *$3,844* • Non-Residential
Annual Tuition: *$8,736* • General Institution Fees: *$220* •
Additional Nursing Fees: *$114*

YORK TECHNICAL COLLEGE

Address: 452 South Anderson Road, Rock Hill, SC 29730
Phone: 803-981-7067
Fax: 803-327-8059
Contact: Mary Anne Laney, MSN, RN, Program Director
Email: MLaney@york.tec.sc.us

GENERAL INFORMATION

Type of School: *2-Year College or University, Public* •
Accreditation: *Southern Association of Colleges and Schools* •
Total Enrollment: *Not Reported*

PROGRAM INFORMATION

LPN/LVN Exit: *No* • NLNAC Accreditation: *Yes*

NURSING STUDENT PROFILE

Total Nursing Enrollment: *111* • Full-Time Enrollment: *15* •
Part-Time Enrollment: *96* • Female Enrollment: *107* • Male
Enrollment: *4* • Total New Admissions Who Enrolled for
Fall: *64* • Total Graduates: *28*

FINANCES

Residential Annual Tuition: *$1,224* • Non-Residential
Annual Tuition: *$5,016* • General Institution Fees: *Not
Reported* • Additional Nursing Fees: *Not Reported*

DAKOTA WESLEYAN UNIVERSITY

Address: 1200 West University Avenue, Mitchell, SD
           57301
Phone: 605-995-2889
Fax: 605-995-2701
Contact: Gloria Thompson, MS, RN, Administrative
           Chair
Email: glthomps@dwu.edu

GENERAL INFORMATION

Type of School: *4-Year College or University, Private (Religious)* • Accreditation: *North Central Association of Colleges and Schools* • Total Enrollment: *700*

PROGRAM INFORMATION

LPN/LVN Exit: *No* • NLNAC Accreditation: *Yes*

NURSING STUDENT PROFILE

Total Nursing Enrollment: *79* • Full-Time Enrollment: *62* • Part-Time Enrollment: *17* • Female Enrollment: *75* • Male Enrollment: *4* • Total New Admissions Who Enrolled for Fall: *46* • Total Graduates: *33*

FINANCES

Residential Annual Tuition: *$11,354* • Non-Residential Annual Tuition: *$11,354* • General Institution Fees: *$300* • Additional Nursing Fees: *Not Reported*

HURON UNIVERSITY

Address: 333 9th Street South West, Huron, SD 57350
Phone: 600-535-2874
Fax: 605-352-7421
Contact: Ella M Brooks, PhD, RN, Dean
Email: ebrooks@huron.edu

GENERAL INFORMATION

Type of School: *4-Year College or University, Private (Independent)* • Accreditation: *North Central Association of Colleges and Schools* • Total Enrollment: *598*

PROGRAM INFORMATION

LPN/LVN Exit: *No* • NLNAC Accreditation: *Yes*

NURSING STUDENT PROFILE

Total Nursing Enrollment: *22* • Full-Time Enrollment: *16* • Part-Time Enrollment: *6* • Female Enrollment: *21* • Male Enrollment: *1* • Total New Admissions Who Enrolled for Fall: *9* • Total Graduates: *12*

FINANCES

Residential Annual Tuition: *Not Reported* • Non-Residential Annual Tuition: *Not Reported* • General Institution Fees: *$400* • Additional Nursing Fees: *Not Reported*

OGLALA LAKOTA COLLEGE

Address:　Box 861, Pine Ridge, SD 57770
Phone:　605-867-5856
Fax:　Not Reported
Contact:　Margaret Hart, MSN, RN, Chair
Email:　mhart@old.edu

GENERAL INFORMATION

Type of School: *4-Year College or University, Other* •
Accreditation: *North Central Association of Colleges and
Schools* • Total Enrollment: *45*

PROGRAM INFORMATION

LPN/LVN Exit: *No* • NLNAC Accreditation: *No*

NURSING STUDENT PROFILE

Total Nursing Enrollment: *18* • Full-Time Enrollment: *18* •
Part-Time Enrollment: *Not Reported* • Female Enrollment:
18 • Male Enrollment: *Not Reported* • Total New Admissions
Who Enrolled for Fall: *9* • Total Graduates: *7*

FINANCES

Residential Annual Tuition: *Not Reported* • Non-Residential
Annual Tuition: *Not Reported* • General Institution Fees: *Not
Reported* • Additional Nursing Fees: *$18*

PRESENTATION COLLEGE

Address:　1500 North Main, Aberdeen, SD 57401
Phone:　605-229-8473
Fax:　605-229-8489
Contact:　Janice S Williams, ND, MSN, RN, CDE, Chair
　　　　and Associate Professor
Email:　janicesw@presentation.edu

GENERAL INFORMATION

Type of School: *4-Year College or University, Private
(Religious)* • Accreditation: *North Central Association of
Colleges and Schools* • Total Enrollment: *615*

PROGRAM INFORMATION

LPN/LVN Exit: *No* • NLNAC Accreditation: *Yes*

NURSING STUDENT PROFILE

Total Nursing Enrollment: *58* • Full-Time Enrollment: *34* •
Part-Time Enrollment: *24* • Female Enrollment: *57* • Male
Enrollment: *1* • Total New Admissions Who Enrolled for
Fall: *54* • Total Graduates: *5*

FINANCES

Residential Annual Tuition: *$8,500* • Non-Residential
Annual Tuition: *$8,500* • General Institution Fees: *$150* •
Additional Nursing Fees: *$600*

UNIVERSITY OF SOUTH DAKOTA

Address: 414 East Clark, Julian Hall 212, Vermillion, SD 57069
Phone: 605-677-5251
Fax: 605-677-5886
Contact: June Larson, MS, RN, Chair
Email: jclarson@usd.edu

AQUINAS COLLEGE

Address: 4210 Harding Road, Nashville, TN 37205
Phone: 615-297-2008
Fax: 615-297-7970
Contact: Peggy Daniel, MSN, BSN, ASN Program Director
Email: daniel@aquinad-tn.edu

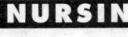

GENERAL INFORMATION

Type of School: *4-Year College or University, Public* • Accreditation: *North Central Association of Colleges and Schools* • Total Enrollment: *7349*

GENERAL INFORMATION

Type of School: *4-Year College or University, Private (Religious)* • Accreditation: *Southern Association of Colleges and Schools* • Total Enrollment: *Not Reported*

PROGRAM INFORMATION

LPN/LVN Exit: *No* • NLNAC Accreditation: *Yes*

PROGRAM INFORMATION

LPN/LVN Exit: *No* • NLNAC Accreditation: *Yes*

NURSING STUDENT PROFILE

Total Nursing Enrollment: *253* • Full-Time Enrollment: *253* • Part-Time Enrollment: *Not Reported* • Female Enrollment: *231* • Male Enrollment: *22* • Total New Admissions Who Enrolled for Fall: *133* • Total Graduates: *117*

NURSING STUDENT PROFILE

Total Nursing Enrollment: *137* • Full-Time Enrollment: *80* • Part-Time Enrollment: *57* • Female Enrollment: *125* • Male Enrollment: *12* • Total New Admissions Who Enrolled for Fall: *78* • Total Graduates: *44*

FINANCES

Residential Annual Tuition: *$2,685* • Non-Residential Annual Tuition: *$5,849* • General Institution Fees: *$54* • Additional Nursing Fees: *$326*

FINANCES

Residential Annual Tuition: *Not Reported* • Non-Residential Annual Tuition: *Not Reported* • General Institution Fees: *Not Reported* • Additional Nursing Fees: *Not Reported*

CHATTANOOGA STATE TECHNICAL COMMUNITY COLLEGE

Address: 4501 Amnicola Highway, Chattanooga, TN
             37406
Phone: 423-778-8080
Fax: 423-267-4624
Contact: Cynthia Swafford, EdD, RN, Director
Email: swaffard@cstcc.cc.tn.us

GENERAL INFORMATION

Type of School: *2-Year College or University, Public* •
Accreditation: *Southern Association of Colleges and Schools* •
Total Enrollment: *4800*

PROGRAM INFORMATION

LPN/LVN Exit: *No* • NLNAC Accreditation: *Yes*

NURSING STUDENT PROFILE

Total Nursing Enrollment: *182* • Full-Time Enrollment:
182 • Part-Time Enrollment: *Not Reported* • Female
Enrollment: *154* • Male Enrollment: *28* • Total New
Admissions Who Enrolled for Fall: *111* • Total Graduates: *82*

FINANCES

Residential Annual Tuition: *$1,294* • Non-Residential
Annual Tuition: *$3,876* • General Institution Fees: *$161* •
Additional Nursing Fees: *$112*

CLEVELAND STATE COMMUNITY COLLEGE

Address: PO Box 3570, Cleveland, TN 37320
Phone: 423-478-6227
Fax: 423-614-8722
Contact: Mary Purnell, EdS, MSN,RN, Chair of Health
             Sciences and Director of Nursing
Email: mpurnell@clscc.cc.tn.us

GENERAL INFORMATION

Type of School: *Other, Public* • Accreditation: *Southern
Association of Colleges and Schools* • Total Enrollment: *3006*

PROGRAM INFORMATION

LPN/LVN Exit: *No* • NLNAC Accreditation: *Yes*

NURSING STUDENT PROFILE

Total Nursing Enrollment: *121* • Full-Time Enrollment:
121 • Part-Time Enrollment: *Not Reported* • Female
Enrollment: *115* • Male Enrollment: *6* • Total New
Admissions Who Enrolled for Fall: *66* • Total Graduates: *33*

FINANCES

Residential Annual Tuition: *$1,294* • Non-Residential
Annual Tuition: *$3,170* • General Institution Fees: *Not
Reported* • Additional Nursing Fees: *$55*

COLUMBIA STATE COMMUNITY COLLEGE

Address: PO Box 1315, Columbia, TN 38402
Phone: 931-540-2600
Fax: 931-540-2794
Contact: Lois L. Ewen, PhD, MSN, RN, Chair Health
           Sciences and Director of Nursing
Email: ewen@coscc.cc.tn.us

GENERAL INFORMATION

Type of School: *Not Reported* • Accreditation: *Southern Association of Colleges and Schools* • Total Enrollment: *Not Reported*

PROGRAM INFORMATION

LPN/LVN Exit: *Yes* • NLNAC Accreditation: *Yes*

NURSING STUDENT PROFILE

Total Nursing Enrollment: *273* • Full-Time Enrollment: *273* • Part-Time Enrollment: *0* • Female Enrollment: *251* • Male Enrollment: *22* • Total New Admissions Who Enrolled for Fall: *84* • Total Graduates: *98*

FINANCES

Residential Annual Tuition: *$1,640* • Non-Residential Annual Tuition: *$5,940* • General Institution Fees: *$50* • Additional Nursing Fees: *$15*

COLUMBUS STATE COMMUNITY COLLEGE

Address: PO Box 1315, Columbia, TN 38402-1315
Phone: 931-540-2600
Fax: 931-540-2794
Contact: Lois L Ewen, PhD, MSN, RN, Chair Health
           Sciences and Director of Nursing
Email: ewen@cocss.cc.tn.us

GENERAL INFORMATION

Type of School: *2-Year College or University, Public* • Accreditation: *Southern Association of Colleges and Schools* • Total Enrollment: *4500*

PROGRAM INFORMATION

LPN/LVN Exit: *Yes* • NLNAC Accreditation: *No*

NURSING STUDENT PROFILE

Total Nursing Enrollment: *273* • Full-Time Enrollment: *273* • Part-Time Enrollment: *Not Reported* • Female Enrollment: *251* • Male Enrollment: *22* • Total New Admissions Who Enrolled for Fall: *84* • Total Graduates: *98*

FINANCES

Residential Annual Tuition: *$1,640* • Non-Residential Annual Tuition: *$5,940* • General Institution Fees: *$50* • Additional Nursing Fees: *$15*

DYERSBURG STATE COMMUNITY COLLEGE

Address: 1510 Lake Road, Dyesburg, TN 38024
Phone: 731-286-3398
Fax: 731-288-7744
Contact: Faye Sigman, MSN, RN, Dean of Nursing and Allied Health
Email: sigman@dscc.edu

GENERAL INFORMATION

Type of School: *2-Year College or University, Public* •
Accreditation: *Southern Association of Colleges and Schools* •
Total Enrollment: *2284*

PROGRAM INFORMATION

LPN/LVN Exit: *No* • NLNAC Accreditation: *Yes*

NURSING STUDENT PROFILE

Total Nursing Enrollment: *62* • Full-Time Enrollment: *25* •
Part-Time Enrollment: *37* • Female Enrollment: *61* • Male
Enrollment: *1* • Total New Admissions Who Enrolled for
Fall: *26* • Total Graduates: *34*

FINANCES

Residential Annual Tuition: *$744* • Non-Residential Annual
Tuition: *$2,973* • General Institution Fees: *$151* •
Additional Nursing Fees: *$75*

EAST TENNESSEE STATE UNIVERSITY

Address: 807 University Parkway, Johnson City, TN 37614
Phone: Not Reported
Fax: Not Reported
Contact: Not Reported
Email: Not Reported

GENERAL INFORMATION

Type of School: *4-Year College or University, Public* •
Accreditation: *Southern Association of Colleges and Schools* •
Total Enrollment: *11000*

PROGRAM INFORMATION

LPN/LVN Exit: *Not Reported* • NLNAC Accreditation: *No*

NURSING STUDENT PROFILE

Total Nursing Enrollment: *Not Reported* • Full-Time
Enrollment: *Not Reported* • Part-Time Enrollment: *Not
Reported* • Female Enrollment: *Not Reported* • Male
Enrollment: *Not Reported* • Total New Admissions Who
Enrolled for Fall: *Not Reported* • Total Graduates: *Not
Reported*

FINANCES

Residential Annual Tuition: *Not Reported* • Non-Residential
Annual Tuition: *Not Reported* • General Institution Fees: *Not
Reported* • Additional Nursing Fees: *Not Reported*

JACKSON STATE COMMUNITY COLLEGE

Address: 2046 North Parkway East, Jackson, TN 38301-3797
Phone: 901-425-2662
Fax: Not Reported
Contact: Leslie West Sands, DSN, RN, CS, Program Director and Department Chair
Email: lsands@jscc.cc.tn.us

GENERAL INFORMATION

Type of School: *2-Year College or University, Public* • Accreditation: *Southern Association of Colleges and Schools* • Total Enrollment: *4000*

PROGRAM INFORMATION

LPN/LVN Exit: *No* • NLNAC Accreditation: *Yes*

NURSING STUDENT PROFILE

Total Nursing Enrollment: *104* • Full-Time Enrollment: *100* • Part-Time Enrollment: *4* • Female Enrollment: *96* • Male Enrollment: *8* • Total New Admissions Who Enrolled for Fall: *54* • Total Graduates: *41*

FINANCES

Residential Annual Tuition: *$1,198* • Non-Residential Annual Tuition: *$4,786* • General Institution Fees: *$12* • Additional Nursing Fees: *$9*

LINCOLN MEMORIAL UNIVERSITY

Address: Cumberland Gap Parkway, Harrogate, TN 37752
Phone: 423-869-6319
Fax: 423-869-6244
Contact: Mary Anne Modrcin Talbott, PhD, RN, Chair Department of Nursing
Email: Drtalbott@aol.com

GENERAL INFORMATION

Type of School: *4-Year College or University, Private (Independent)* • Accreditation: *Southern Association of Colleges and Schools* • Total Enrollment: *1753*

PROGRAM INFORMATION

LPN/LVN Exit: *No* • NLNAC Accreditation: *Yes*

NURSING STUDENT PROFILE

Total Nursing Enrollment: *163* • Full-Time Enrollment: *87* • Part-Time Enrollment: *76* • Female Enrollment: *146* • Male Enrollment: *17* • Total New Admissions Who Enrolled for Fall: *103* • Total Graduates: *54*

FINANCES

Residential Annual Tuition: *$5,400* • Non-Residential Annual Tuition: *$5,400* • General Institution Fees: *$30* • Additional Nursing Fees: *Not Reported*

MOTLOW STATE COMMUNITY COLLEGE

Address: PO Box 8500, Lynchburg, TN 37352
Phone: 931-393-1631
Fax: 931-393-1656
Contact: Susan T Sanders, MSN, RN, CNAA, Director of
           Nursing Education
Email: ssanders@mscc.cc.tn.us

GENERAL INFORMATION

Type of School: *2-Year College or University, Public* •
Accreditation: *Southern Association of Colleges and Schools* •
Total Enrollment: *3300*

PROGRAM INFORMATION

LPN/LVN Exit: *No* • NLNAC Accreditation: *Yes*

NURSING STUDENT PROFILE

Total Nursing Enrollment: *99* • Full-Time Enrollment: *74* •
Part-Time Enrollment: *25* • Female Enrollment: *90* • Male
Enrollment: *9* • Total New Admissions Who Enrolled for
Fall: *52* • Total Graduates: *39*

FINANCES

Residential Annual Tuition: *$767* • Non-Residential Annual
Tuition: *$1,534* • General Institution Fees: *$1,534* •
Additional Nursing Fees: *$200*

ROANE STATE COMMUNITY COLLEGE

Address: 276 Patton Lane, Harriman, TN 37748
Phone: 865-882-4594
Fax: 865-882-4549
Contact: Sharon J Tanner, MSN RN, Dean of Nursing
           and Health Sciences
Email: tanner_sj@rscc.cc.tn.us

GENERAL INFORMATION

Type of School: *2-Year College or University, Public* •
Accreditation: *Southern Association of Colleges and Schools* •
Total Enrollment: *5099*

PROGRAM INFORMATION

LPN/LVN Exit: *No* • NLNAC Accreditation: *Yes*

NURSING STUDENT PROFILE

Total Nursing Enrollment: *182* • Full-Time Enrollment:
130 • Part-Time Enrollment: *52* • Female Enrollment: *170* •
Male Enrollment: *12* • Total New Admissions Who Enrolled
for Fall: *106* • Total Graduates: *56*

FINANCES

Residential Annual Tuition: *$1,419* • Non-Residential
Annual Tuition: *$5,295* • General Institution Fees: *Not
Reported* • Additional Nursing Fees: *$325*

SOUTHERN ADVENTIST UNIVERSITY

Address: PO Box 370, Collegedale, TN 37315
Phone: 423-238-2942
Fax: 423-238-3004
Contact: L Phil Hunt, EdD, MEd, RN, Dean and Professor
Email: phunt@southern.edu

GENERAL INFORMATION

Type of School: *4-Year College or University, Private (Religious)* • Accreditation: *Southern Association of Colleges and Schools* • Total Enrollment: *1900*

PROGRAM INFORMATION

LPN/LVN Exit: *No* • NLNAC Accreditation: *Yes*

NURSING STUDENT PROFILE

Total Nursing Enrollment: *122* • Full-Time Enrollment: *110* • Part-Time Enrollment: *12* • Female Enrollment: *100* • Male Enrollment: *22* • Total New Admissions Who Enrolled for Fall: *61* • Total Graduates: *33*

FINANCES

Residential Annual Tuition: *$11,250* • Non-Residential Annual Tuition: *$11,250* • General Institution Fees: *$360* • Additional Nursing Fees: *$720*

SOUTHWEST TENNESSEE COMMUNITY COLLEGE

Address: 301 Walnut Street, Memphis, TN 38126
Phone: 901-333-5425
Fax: Not Reported
Contact: Carolyn Brown, MSN, RN, Interim Department Head
Email: cbrown@sscc.cc.tn.us

GENERAL INFORMATION

Type of School: *Not Reported* • Accreditation: *Southern Association of Colleges and Schools* • Total Enrollment: *Not Reported*

PROGRAM INFORMATION

LPN/LVN Exit: *No* • NLNAC Accreditation: *Yes*

NURSING STUDENT PROFILE

Total Nursing Enrollment: *206* • Full-Time Enrollment: *35* • Part-Time Enrollment: *171* • Female Enrollment: *184* • Male Enrollment: *22* • Total New Admissions Who Enrolled for Fall: *109* • Total Graduates: *82*

FINANCES

Residential Annual Tuition: *$1,198* • Non-Residential Annual Tuition: *$4,786* • General Institution Fees: *$80* • Additional Nursing Fees: *$170*

TENNESSEE STATE UNIVERSITY

Address: 3500 John A. Merritt Boulevard, Box 9596, Nashville, TN 37209
Phone: 615-693-5254
Fax: 615-963-5059
Contact: Marion G Anema, PhD, RN, Dean
Email: menema@tnstate.edu

WALTERS STATE COMMUNITY COLLEGE

Address: 2073 Ridgewood Drive, Jefferson City, TN 37760
Phone: 423-585-6993
Fax: 423-585-6955
Contact: Martel K Rucker, MSN, RNC, Director of Nursing
Email: Marty.Rucker@wscc.cc.tn.us

GENERAL INFORMATION

Type of School: *4-Year College or University, Public* •
Accreditation: *Southern Association of Colleges and Schools* •
Total Enrollment: *10000*

GENERAL INFORMATION

Type of School: *2-Year College or University, Public* •
Accreditation: *Southern Association of Colleges and Schools* •
Total Enrollment: *6000*

PROGRAM INFORMATION

LPN/LVN Exit: *Yes* • NLNAC Accreditation: *Yes*

PROGRAM INFORMATION

LPN/LVN Exit: *No* • NLNAC Accreditation: *Yes*

NURSING STUDENT PROFILE

Total Nursing Enrollment: *190* • Full-Time Enrollment: *160* • Part-Time Enrollment: *30* • Female Enrollment: *160* • Male Enrollment: *30* • Total New Admissions Who Enrolled for Fall: *80* • Total Graduates: *86*

NURSING STUDENT PROFILE

Total Nursing Enrollment: *232* • Full-Time Enrollment: *159* • Part-Time Enrollment: *73* • Female Enrollment: *210* • Male Enrollment: *22* • Total New Admissions Who Enrolled for Fall: *132* • Total Graduates: *99*

FINANCES

Residential Annual Tuition: *$3,000* • Non-Residential Annual Tuition: *$6,000* • General Institution Fees: *Not Reported* • Additional Nursing Fees: *$200*

FINANCES

Residential Annual Tuition: *$1,198* • Non-Residential Annual Tuition: *$3,588* • General Institution Fees: *$13* • Additional Nursing Fees: *$20*

ALVIN COMMUNITY COLLEGE

Address: 3110 Mustang Rd, Alvin, TX 77511-4898
Phone: 281-756-3634
Fax: 281-756-3860
Contact: Sally J Durand, MSN, RN, Director Associate Degree Nursing
Email: sdurand@alvin.cc.tx.us

GENERAL INFORMATION

Type of School: *2-Year College or University, Public* •
Accreditation: *Southern Association of Colleges and Schools* •
Total Enrollment: *3690*

PROGRAM INFORMATION

LPN/LVN Exit: *No* • NLNAC Accreditation: *Yes*

NURSING STUDENT PROFILE

Total Nursing Enrollment: *98* • Full-Time Enrollment: *61* •
Part-Time Enrollment: *37* • Female Enrollment: *93* • Male
Enrollment: *5* • Total New Admissions Who Enrolled for
Fall: *58* • Total Graduates: *43*

FINANCES

Residential Annual Tuition: *$832* • Non-Residential Annual
Tuition: *$2,144* • General Institution Fees: *$272* •
Additional Nursing Fees: *$45*

AMARILLO COLLEGE

Address: PO Box 447, Amarillo, TX 79178
Phone: 806-354-6010
Fax: 806-354-6096
Contact: Sue McGee, MSN, RN, Chairman, Nursing Division
Email: mcgee-sk@actx.edu

GENERAL INFORMATION

Type of School: *2-Year College or University, Public* •
Accreditation: *Southern Association of Colleges and Schools* •
Total Enrollment: *Not Reported*

PROGRAM INFORMATION

LPN/LVN Exit: *Yes* • NLNAC Accreditation: *Yes*

NURSING STUDENT PROFILE

Total Nursing Enrollment: *374* • Full-Time Enrollment: *Not
Reported* • Part-Time Enrollment: *Not Reported* • Female
Enrollment: *298* • Male Enrollment: *76* • Total New
Admissions Who Enrolled for Fall: *67* • Total Graduates: *90*

FINANCES

Residential Annual Tuition: *$950* • Non-Residential Annual
Tuition: *$2,150* • General Institution Fees: *$10* • Additional
Nursing Fees: *$72*

ANGELINA COLLEGE

Address: PO Box 1768, Lufkin, TX 75901
Phone: 936-633-5445
Fax: 936-633-5241
Contact: Sharon Buffalo, MSN, RN, Nursing Program
            Coordinator
Email: sbuffalo@angelina.cc.tx.us

GENERAL INFORMATION

Type of School: *2-Year College or University, Public* •
Accreditation: *Southern Association of Colleges and Schools* •
Total Enrollment: *4000*

PROGRAM INFORMATION

LPN/LVN Exit: *Yes* • NLNAC Accreditation: *No*

NURSING STUDENT PROFILE

Total Nursing Enrollment: *101* • Full-Time Enrollment:
101 • Part-Time Enrollment: *0* • Female Enrollment: *Not
Reported* • Male Enrollment: *Not Reported* • Total New
Admissions Who Enrolled for Fall: *77* • Total Graduates: *32*

FINANCES

Residential Annual Tuition: *$1,248* • Non-Residential
Annual Tuition: *Not Reported* • General Institution Fees:
$80 • Additional Nursing Fees: *$285*

ANGELO STATE UNIVERSITY

Address: 2601 W. Ave. N, San Angelo, TX 76909
Phone: 915-942-2224
Fax: 915-942-2236
Contact: Sherry Halfmann, PhD, CNS, RN, Program
            Director, AASN
Email: sherry.halfmann@angelo.edu

GENERAL INFORMATION

Type of School: *4-Year College or University, Public* •
Accreditation: *Southern Association of Colleges and Schools* •
Total Enrollment: *6000*

PROGRAM INFORMATION

LPN/LVN Exit: *No* • NLNAC Accreditation: *Yes*

NURSING STUDENT PROFILE

Total Nursing Enrollment: *115* • Full-Time Enrollment: *80* •
Part-Time Enrollment: *35* • Female Enrollment: *96* • Male
Enrollment: *19* • Total New Admissions Who Enrolled for
Fall: *65* • Total Graduates: *45*

FINANCES

Residential Annual Tuition: *$1,043* • Non-Residential
Annual Tuition: *$3,623* • General Institution Fees: *$563* •
Additional Nursing Fees: *$30*

AUSTIN COMMUNITY COLLEGE

Address: 5930 Middle Fiskville Rd., Austin, TX 78752
Phone: 512-223-6109
Fax: 512-223-6750
Contact: Jere Hammer, MSN, RN, Program Coordinator
Email: jhammer@austin.cc.tx.us

BLINN COLLEGE

Address: PO Box 6030, Bryan, TX 77805
Phone: 979-821-0204
Fax: Not Reported
Contact: Thena E Parrott, PhD, RN, Director, ADN
Program and Division Chair, Allied Health
Email: tparrott@acmail.blinncol.edu

GENERAL INFORMATION

Type of School: *2-Year College or University, Public* •
Accreditation: *Southern Association of Colleges and Schools* •
Total Enrollment: *27577*

GENERAL INFORMATION

Type of School: *2-Year College or University, Public* •
Accreditation: *Southern Association of Colleges and Schools* •
Total Enrollment: *11352*

PROGRAM INFORMATION

LPN/LVN Exit: *No* • NLNAC Accreditation: *Yes*

PROGRAM INFORMATION

LPN/LVN Exit: *No* • NLNAC Accreditation: *Yes*

NURSING STUDENT PROFILE

Total Nursing Enrollment: *161* • Full-Time Enrollment: *92* •
Part-Time Enrollment: *69* • Female Enrollment: *143* • Male
Enrollment: *18* • Total New Admissions Who Enrolled for
Fall: *70* • Total Graduates: *140*

NURSING STUDENT PROFILE

Total Nursing Enrollment: *82* • Full-Time Enrollment: *82* •
Part-Time Enrollment: *Not Reported* • Female Enrollment:
69 • Male Enrollment: *13* • Total New Admissions Who
Enrolled for Fall: *40* • Total Graduates: *40*

FINANCES

Residential Annual Tuition: *$1,038* • Non-Residential
Annual Tuition: *$2,214* • General Institution Fees: *$135* •
Additional Nursing Fees: *$27*

FINANCES

Residential Annual Tuition: *Not Reported* • Non-Residential
Annual Tuition: *Not Reported* • General Institution Fees: *Not
Reported* • Additional Nursing Fees: *Not Reported*

Circle 7 on reader card   See in-depth profile for more information

CENTRAL TEXAS COLLEGE

Address: PO Box 1800, Killeen, TX 76540-1800
Phone: 254-526-1300
Fax: 254-526-1765
Contact: Shirley R Robertson, PhD, RN, Department Chair, Nursing
Email: sroberts@ctcd.cc.tx.us

GENERAL INFORMATION

Type of School: *2-Year College or University, Public* •
Accreditation: *Southern Association of Colleges and Schools* •
Total Enrollment: *1480*

PROGRAM INFORMATION

LPN/LVN Exit: *No* • NLNAC Accreditation: *Yes*

NURSING STUDENT PROFILE

Total Nursing Enrollment: *204* • Full-Time Enrollment: *183* • Part-Time Enrollment: *21* • Female Enrollment: *191* • Male Enrollment: *13* • Total New Admissions Who Enrolled for Fall: *67* • Total Graduates: *52*

FINANCES

Residential Annual Tuition: *$704* • Non-Residential Annual Tuition: *$3,250* • General Institution Fees: *$8* • Additional Nursing Fees: *$146*

CISCO JUNIOR COLLEGE

Address: Rt. 3, Box 3, Cisco, TX 76437
Phone: 915-673-4567
Fax: 915-673-4575
Contact: Jackolyn Morgan, MSN, RN, Director of Nursing Programs
Email: jmorgan@cisco.cc.tx.us

GENERAL INFORMATION

Type of School: *2-Year College or University, Public* •
Accreditation: *Southern Association of Colleges and Schools* •
Total Enrollment: *663*

PROGRAM INFORMATION

LPN/LVN Exit: *No* • NLNAC Accreditation: *No*

NURSING STUDENT PROFILE

Total Nursing Enrollment: *28* • Full-Time Enrollment: *28* • Part-Time Enrollment: *0* • Female Enrollment: *26* • Male Enrollment: *2* • Total New Admissions Who Enrolled for Fall: *30* • Total Graduates: *28*

FINANCES

Residential Annual Tuition: *$1,796* • Non-Residential Annual Tuition: *$2,294* • General Institution Fees: *Not Reported* • Additional Nursing Fees: *$315*

COLLEGE OF THE MAINLAND

Address: 1200 Amburn Road, Texas City, TX 77591
Phone: 409-938-1211
Fax: 409-933-4369
Contact: Gay Reeves, EdD, MSN, RN, Interim Director
Email: greeves@mail.mainland.cc.tx.us

GENERAL INFORMATION

Type of School: *2-Year College or University, Public* •
Accreditation: *Southern Association of Colleges and Schools* •
Total Enrollment: *3175*

PROGRAM INFORMATION

LPN/LVN Exit: *Yes* • NLNAC Accreditation: *Yes*

NURSING STUDENT PROFILE

Total Nursing Enrollment: *9* • Full-Time Enrollment: *Not Reported* • Part-Time Enrollment: *9* • Female Enrollment: *8* • Male Enrollment: *1* • Total New Admissions Who Enrolled for Fall: *9* • Total Graduates: *17*

FINANCES

Residential Annual Tuition: *$672* • Non-Residential Annual Tuition: *$1,856* • General Institution Fees: *$50* • Additional Nursing Fees: *$105*

COLLIN COUNTY COMMUNITY COLLEGE

Address: 220 W. University Dr., Mc Kinney, TX 75070
Phone: 972-548-6883
Fax: 972-548-6722
Contact: Vivian C Lilly, PhD, MBA, RN, Associate Dean
           Health Services
Email: vlillu@ccccd.edu

GENERAL INFORMATION

Type of School: *2-Year College or University, Public* •
Accreditation: *Southern Association of Colleges and Schools* •
Total Enrollment: *11000*

PROGRAM INFORMATION

LPN/LVN Exit: *No* • NLNAC Accreditation: *Yes*

NURSING STUDENT PROFILE

Total Nursing Enrollment: *73* • Full-Time Enrollment: *73* • Part-Time Enrollment: *Not Reported* • Female Enrollment: *69* • Male Enrollment: *4* • Total New Admissions Who Enrolled for Fall: *37* • Total Graduates: *18*

FINANCES

Residential Annual Tuition: *Not Reported* • Non-Residential Annual Tuition: *Not Reported* • General Institution Fees: *$20* • Additional Nursing Fees: *$48*

DEL MAR COLLEGE

Address: 101 Baldwin, Corpus Christi, TX 78404
Phone: 361-698-1320
Fax: 361-698-1173
Contact: Blanca Rosa Garcia, PhD, RN, Chairperson
Email: rgarcia@delmar.edu

GENERAL INFORMATION

Type of School: *2-Year College or University, Public* •
Accreditation: *Southern Association of Colleges and Schools* •
Total Enrollment: *9900*

PROGRAM INFORMATION

LPN/LVN Exit: *No* • NLNAC Accreditation: *Yes*

NURSING STUDENT PROFILE

Total Nursing Enrollment: *278* • Full-Time Enrollment:
276 • Part-Time Enrollment: *2* • Female Enrollment: *227* •
Male Enrollment: *51* • Total New Admissions Who Enrolled
for Fall: *75* • Total Graduates: *130*

FINANCES

Residential Annual Tuition: *Not Reported* • Non-Residential
Annual Tuition: *Not Reported* • General Institution Fees:
$200 • Additional Nursing Fees: *$78*

EL CENTRO COLLEGE

Address: Main and Lamar Sts, Dallas, TX 75202
Phone: 214-860-2141
Fax: Not Reported
Contact: Sondra Flemmings, MS, RN, Executive Dean
Email: sgf5540@dcccd.edu

GENERAL INFORMATION

Type of School: *2-Year College or University, Public* •
Accreditation: *Southern Association of Colleges and Schools* •
Total Enrollment: *4187*

PROGRAM INFORMATION

LPN/LVN Exit: *No* • NLNAC Accreditation: *Yes*

NURSING STUDENT PROFILE

Total Nursing Enrollment: *417* • Full-Time Enrollment:
417 • Part-Time Enrollment: *Not Reported* • Female
Enrollment: *361* • Male Enrollment: *56* • Total New
Admissions Who Enrolled for Fall: *150* • Total Graduates:
165

FINANCES

Residential Annual Tuition: *$960* • Non-Residential Annual
Tuition: *$2,560* • General Institution Fees: *Not Reported* •
Additional Nursing Fees: *Not Reported*

EL PASO COMMUNITY COLLEGE

Address: PO Box 20500, El Paso, TX 79778
Phone: 915-831-4030
Fax: Not Reported
Contact: Paula R Mitchell, EdD, RNC, Dean, Health Occupations
Email: pauam@epcc.edu

GENERAL INFORMATION

Type of School: *2-Year College or University, Public* •
Accreditation: *Southern Association of Colleges and Schools* •
Total Enrollment: *28974*

PROGRAM INFORMATION

LPN/LVN Exit: *Not Reported* • NLNAC Accreditation: *Yes*

NURSING STUDENT PROFILE

Total Nursing Enrollment: *197* • Full-Time Enrollment: *Not Reported* • Part-Time Enrollment: *197* • Female Enrollment: *152* • Male Enrollment: *45* • Total New Admissions Who Enrolled for Fall: *Not Reported* • Total Graduates: *Not Reported*

FINANCES

Residential Annual Tuition: *Not Reported* • Non-Residential Annual Tuition: *Not Reported* • General Institution Fees: *Not Reported* • Additional Nursing Fees: *Not Reported*

GALVESTON COLLEGE

Address: 4015 Avenue Q, Galveston, TX 77550-7447
Phone: 409-763-6551
Fax: 809-762-9367
Contact: Elizabeth K Michel, MSN, RN, C, Dean, Health Occupations
Email: bmichel@gc.edu

GENERAL INFORMATION

Type of School: *2-Year College or University, Public* •
Accreditation: *Southern Association of Colleges and Schools* •
Total Enrollment: *2600*

PROGRAM INFORMATION

LPN/LVN Exit: *No* • NLNAC Accreditation: *Yes*

NURSING STUDENT PROFILE

Total Nursing Enrollment: *147* • Full-Time Enrollment: *147* • Part-Time Enrollment: *Not Reported* • Female Enrollment: *122* • Male Enrollment: *25* • Total New Admissions Who Enrolled for Fall: *70* • Total Graduates: *34*

FINANCES

Residential Annual Tuition: *$960* • Non-Residential Annual Tuition: *$1,920* • General Institution Fees: *$454* • Additional Nursing Fees: *$200*

GRAYSON COUNTY COLLEGE

Address: 6101 Grayson Drive, Denison, TX 75020
Phone: 903-463-8643
Fax: 903-463-8779
Contact: Jeanie Hardin, MS, RN, Assistant Dean and Director, Health Sciences
Email: hardinj@grayson.edu

GENERAL INFORMATION

Type of School: *2-Year College or University, Public* • Accreditation: *Southern Association of Colleges and Schools* • Total Enrollment: *3500*

PROGRAM INFORMATION

LPN/LVN Exit: *No* • NLNAC Accreditation: *Yes*

NURSING STUDENT PROFILE

Total Nursing Enrollment: *210* • Full-Time Enrollment: *210* • Part-Time Enrollment: *0* • Female Enrollment: *186* • Male Enrollment: *24* • Total New Admissions Who Enrolled for Fall: *100* • Total Graduates: *81*

FINANCES

Residential Annual Tuition: *$1,048* • Non-Residential Annual Tuition: *$2,408* • General Institution Fees: *$50* • Additional Nursing Fees: *$100*

HOUSTON BAPTIST UNIVERSITY

Address: 7502 Fondren, Houston, TX 77074
Phone: 281-649-3300
Fax: 281-649-3340
Contact: Nancy Yuill, PhD, RN, Dean
Email: nyuill@hbu.edu

GENERAL INFORMATION

Type of School: *4-Year College or University, Private (Independent)* • Accreditation: *Southern Association of Colleges and Schools* • Total Enrollment: *2300*

PROGRAM INFORMATION

LPN/LVN Exit: *No* • NLNAC Accreditation: *Yes*

NURSING STUDENT PROFILE

Total Nursing Enrollment: *36* • Full-Time Enrollment: *36* • Part-Time Enrollment: *Not Reported* • Female Enrollment: *35* • Male Enrollment: *1* • Total New Admissions Who Enrolled for Fall: *10* • Total Graduates: *14*

FINANCES

Residential Annual Tuition: *$10,048* • Non-Residential Annual Tuition: *$10,148* • General Institution Fees: *$1,040* • Additional Nursing Fees: *$100*

HOWARD COLLEGE— BIG SPRING

Address: 1001 N. Birdwell Lane, Big Spring, TX 79720
Phone: 915-264-5070
Fax: 915-264-5142
Contact: Cindy Stokes, MSN, RN, CNM, Dean of Nursing and Director of Allied Health
Email: cstokes@hc.cc.tx.us

GENERAL INFORMATION

Type of School: *2-Year College or University, Public* •
Accreditation: *Southern Association of Colleges and Schools* •
Total Enrollment: *1100*

PROGRAM INFORMATION

LPN/LVN Exit: *Yes* • NLNAC Accreditation: *Yes*

NURSING STUDENT PROFILE

Total Nursing Enrollment: *28* • Full-Time Enrollment: *28* •
Part-Time Enrollment: *0* • Female Enrollment: *25* • Male
Enrollment: *3* • Total New Admissions Who Enrolled for
Fall: *16* • Total Graduates: *5*

FINANCES

Residential Annual Tuition: *$1,198* • Non-Residential
Annual Tuition: *$2,020* • General Institution Fees: *$171* •
Additional Nursing Fees: *$364*

KILGORE COLLEGE

Address: 1100 Broadway Boulevard, Kilgore, TX 75662
Phone: 903-983-8168
Fax: Not Reported
Contact: Genie Bartlett, MSN, RN, Director
Email: genie@texramp.net

GENERAL INFORMATION

Type of School: *2-Year College or University, Public* •
Accreditation: *Southern Association of Colleges and Schools* •
Total Enrollment: *3600*

PROGRAM INFORMATION

LPN/LVN Exit: *No* • NLNAC Accreditation: *Not Reported*

NURSING STUDENT PROFILE

Total Nursing Enrollment: *90* • Full-Time Enrollment: *90* •
Part-Time Enrollment: *Not Reported* • Female Enrollment:
Not Reported • Male Enrollment: *Not Reported* • Total New
Admissions Who Enrolled for Fall: *30* • Total Graduates: *46*

FINANCES

Residential Annual Tuition: *Not Reported* • Non-Residential
Annual Tuition: *Not Reported* • General Institution Fees: *Not
Reported* • Additional Nursing Fees: *Not Reported*

LAMAR STATE COLLEGE— ORANGE

Address: 410 Front St, Orange, TX 77630
Phone: 409-882-3307
Fax: Not Reported
Contact: Nancy McAfee, MSN, RN, Program Director
Email: mfafent@lub002.lamar.edu

GENERAL INFORMATION

Type of School: *2-Year College or University, Public* •
Accreditation: *Southern Association of Colleges and Schools* •
Total Enrollment: *1500*

PROGRAM INFORMATION

LPN/LVN Exit: *No* • NLNAC Accreditation: *No*

NURSING STUDENT PROFILE

Total Nursing Enrollment: *70* • Full-Time Enrollment: *70* •
Part-Time Enrollment: *Not Reported* • Female Enrollment:
56 • Male Enrollment: *14* • Total New Admissions Who
Enrolled for Fall: *0* • Total Graduates: *61*

FINANCES

Residential Annual Tuition: *$2,760* • Non-Residential
Annual Tuition: *$10,536* • General Institution Fees: *$128* •
Additional Nursing Fees: *$848*

LAMAR STATE COLLEGE— PORT ARTHUR

Address: Box 310, Port Arthur, TX 77641
Phone: 409-984-6356
Fax: Not Reported
Contact: Janet R Hamilton, MSN, RN, Allied Health
Department Chair
Email: janet.hamilton@lamarpa.edu

GENERAL INFORMATION

Type of School: *2-Year College or University, Public* •
Accreditation: *Southern Association of Colleges and Schools* •
Total Enrollment: *2600*

PROGRAM INFORMATION

LPN/LVN Exit: *No* • NLNAC Accreditation: *No*

NURSING STUDENT PROFILE

Total Nursing Enrollment: *31* • Full-Time Enrollment: *Not
Reported* • Part-Time Enrollment: *31* • Female Enrollment:
Not Reported • Male Enrollment: *Not Reported* • Total New
Admissions Who Enrolled for Fall: *30* • Total Graduates: *27*

FINANCES

Residential Annual Tuition: *Not Reported* • Non-Residential
Annual Tuition: *Not Reported* • General Institution Fees: *Not
Reported* • Additional Nursing Fees: *Not Reported*

LAMAR UNIVERSITY

Address: PO Box 10081, Beaumont, TX 77710
Phone: 409-880-8832
Fax: Not Reported
Contact: Iva L Hall, MSN, RN, Undergraduate Program
            Coordinator
Email: hallil@hal.lamar.edu

GENERAL INFORMATION

Type of School: *4-Year College or University, Public* •
Accreditation: *Southern Association of Colleges and Schools* •
Total Enrollment: *8149*

PROGRAM INFORMATION

LPN/LVN Exit: *No* • NLNAC Accreditation: *Yes*

NURSING STUDENT PROFILE

Total Nursing Enrollment: *74* • Full-Time Enrollment: *74* •
Part-Time Enrollment: *Not Reported* • Female Enrollment:
Not Reported • Male Enrollment: *Not Reported* • Total New
Admissions Who Enrolled for Fall: *47* • Total Graduates: *73*

FINANCES

Residential Annual Tuition: *Not Reported* • Non-Residential
Annual Tuition: *Not Reported* • General Institution Fees: *Not
Reported* • Additional Nursing Fees: *Not Reported*

LAREDO COMMUNITY COLLEGE

Address: W. End Washington Street, Laredo, TX 78040
Phone: 956-721-5252
Fax: 956-764-5930
Contact: Dianna Miller, MSN, RN, ADN Department
            Chair
Email: dmiller@laredo.cc.tx.us

GENERAL INFORMATION

Type of School: *2-Year College or University, Public* •
Accreditation: *Southern Association of Colleges and Schools* •
Total Enrollment: *7493*

PROGRAM INFORMATION

LPN/LVN Exit: *No* • NLNAC Accreditation: *Yes*

NURSING STUDENT PROFILE

Total Nursing Enrollment: *108* • Full-Time Enrollment:
104 • Part-Time Enrollment: *4* • Female Enrollment: *89* •
Male Enrollment: *19* • Total New Admissions Who Enrolled
for Fall: *24* • Total Graduates: *39*

FINANCES

Residential Annual Tuition: *$1,096* • Non-Residential
Annual Tuition: *$1,096* • General Institution Fees: *$312* •
Additional Nursing Fees: *$54*

LEE COLLEGE

Address: 511 S Whiting, Baytown, TX 77522
Phone: 281-425-6449
Fax: 281-425-6520
Contact: Lorena Maher, EdD, RN, Chairperson, Allied
Health Division
Email: rmaher@lee.edu

GENERAL INFORMATION

Type of School: *2-Year College or University, Public* •
Accreditation: *Southern Association of Colleges and Schools* •
Total Enrollment: *6225*

PROGRAM INFORMATION

LPN/LVN Exit: *No* • NLNAC Accreditation: *Yes*

NURSING STUDENT PROFILE

Total Nursing Enrollment: *110* • Full-Time Enrollment:
110 • Part-Time Enrollment: *0* • Female Enrollment: *97* •
Male Enrollment: *13* • Total New Admissions Who Enrolled
for Fall: *70* • Total Graduates: *32*

FINANCES

Residential Annual Tuition: *Not Reported* • Non-Residential
Annual Tuition: *Not Reported* • General Institution Fees: *Not
Reported* • Additional Nursing Fees: *$56*

MCLENNAN COMMUNITY COLLEGE

Address: 1400 College Drive, Waco, TX 76708
Phone: 254-299-8349
Fax: 254-299-8435
Contact: Alice Myers, MSN, RN, Program Director
Email: afm@mcc.cc.tx.us

GENERAL INFORMATION

Type of School: *2-Year College or University, Public* •
Accreditation: *Southern Association of Colleges and Schools* •
Total Enrollment: *Not Reported*

PROGRAM INFORMATION

LPN/LVN Exit: *Yes* • NLNAC Accreditation: *Yes*

NURSING STUDENT PROFILE

Total Nursing Enrollment: *218* • Full-Time Enrollment:
218 • Part-Time Enrollment: *Not Reported* • Female
Enrollment: *202* • Male Enrollment: *16* • Total New
Admissions Who Enrolled for Fall: *54* • Total Graduates: *96*

FINANCES

Residential Annual Tuition: *$832* • Non-Residential Annual
Tuition: *$1,792* • General Institution Fees: *$306* •
Additional Nursing Fees: *$41*

MIDLAND COLLEGE

Address: 3600 North Garfield, Midland, TX 79705
Phone: 915-658-4590
Fax: 915-685-4752
Contact: Dorothy Joy, MSN, RN, Program Director
Email: djoy@midland.edu

GENERAL INFORMATION

Type of School: *2-Year College or University, Public* •
Accreditation: *Southern Association of Colleges and Schools* •
Total Enrollment: *5065*

PROGRAM INFORMATION

LPN/LVN Exit: *No* • NLNAC Accreditation: *Yes*

NURSING STUDENT PROFILE

Total Nursing Enrollment: *77* • Full-Time Enrollment: *24* •
Part-Time Enrollment: *53* • Female Enrollment: *65* • Male
Enrollment: *12* • Total New Admissions Who Enrolled for
Fall: *24* • Total Graduates: *31*

FINANCES

Residential Annual Tuition: *$1,400* • Non-Residential
Annual Tuition: *$2,568* • General Institution Fees: *$5* •
Additional Nursing Fees: *$65*

NAVARRO COLLEGE

Address: 3200 W 7th Avenue, Corsicana, TX 75110
Phone: 903-875-7585
Fax: 903-875-7577
Contact: Judy W Howden, PhD, RN, Assistant Dean for
            Health Professions
Email: jhowd@nav.cc.tx.us

GENERAL INFORMATION

Type of School: *2-Year College or University, Public* •
Accreditation: *Southern Association of Colleges and Schools* •
Total Enrollment: *3800*

PROGRAM INFORMATION

LPN/LVN Exit: *No* • NLNAC Accreditation: *Yes*

NURSING STUDENT PROFILE

Total Nursing Enrollment: *66* • Full-Time Enrollment: *66* •
Part-Time Enrollment: *Not Reported* • Female Enrollment:
58 • Male Enrollment: *8* • Total New Admissions Who
Enrolled for Fall: *30* • Total Graduates: *31*

FINANCES

Residential Annual Tuition: *$2,134* • Non-Residential
Annual Tuition: *$2,926* • General Institution Fees: *Not
Reported* • Additional Nursing Fees: *$50*

NORTH CENTRAL TEXAS COLLEGE

Address: 1525 W California, Gainesville, TX 76240
Phone: 940-668-426
Fax: 940-668-6049
Contact: Patrick J Lilley, MBA, MS, RN, Chair,
       Department of Nursing
Email: plilley@nctc.cc.tx.us

GENERAL INFORMATION

Type of School: *2-Year College or University, Public* •
Accreditation: *Southern Association of Colleges and Schools* •
Total Enrollment: *4800*

PROGRAM INFORMATION

LPN/LVN Exit: *No* • NLNAC Accreditation: *Yes*

NURSING STUDENT PROFILE

Total Nursing Enrollment: *123* • Full-Time Enrollment:
122 • Part-Time Enrollment: *1* • Female Enrollment: *100* •
Male Enrollment: *23* • Total New Admissions Who Enrolled
for Fall: *48* • Total Graduates: *56*

FINANCES

Residential Annual Tuition: *Not Reported* • Non-Residential
Annual Tuition: *Not Reported* • General Institution Fees: *Not
Reported* • Additional Nursing Fees: *$126*

NORTH HARRIS MONTGOMERY COMMUNITY COLLEGE DISTRICT

Address: 30555 Tomball Pkwr, Tomball, TX 77375
Phone: 281-618-5751
Fax: 218-618-5756
Contact: Patricia S. Crotwell, MSN, RN, Interim Director
Email: patricia.s.crotwell@nh.mccd.edu

GENERAL INFORMATION

Type of School: *2-Year College or University, Public* •
Accreditation: *Southern Association of Colleges and Schools* •
Total Enrollment: *17615*

PROGRAM INFORMATION

LPN/LVN Exit: *Not Reported* • NLNAC Accreditation: *Yes*

NURSING STUDENT PROFILE

Total Nursing Enrollment: *Not Reported* • Full-Time
Enrollment: *Not Reported* • Part-Time Enrollment: *Not
Reported* • Female Enrollment: *Not Reported* • Male
Enrollment: *Not Reported* • Total New Admissions Who
Enrolled for Fall: *Not Reported* • Total Graduates: *Not
Reported*

FINANCES

Residential Annual Tuition: *Not Reported* • Non-Residential
Annual Tuition: *Not Reported* • General Institution Fees: *Not
Reported* • Additional Nursing Fees: *Not Reported*

NORTHEAST TEXAS COMMUNITY COLLEGE

Address: PO Box 1307, Mt. Pleasant, TX 75455
Phone: 903-572-1911
Fax: 903-572-6712
Contact: Cynthia Amerson, MS, BSN, RN, Director, Nursing
Email: camerson@ntcc.cc.tx.us

GENERAL INFORMATION

Type of School: *2-Year College or University, Public* •
Accreditation: *Southern Association of Colleges and Schools* •
Total Enrollment: *1950*

PROGRAM INFORMATION

LPN/LVN Exit: *Not Reported* • NLNAC Accreditation: *No*

NURSING STUDENT PROFILE

Total Nursing Enrollment: *39* • Full-Time Enrollment: *39* •
Part-Time Enrollment: *Not Reported* • Female Enrollment:
36 • Male Enrollment: *3* • Total New Admissions Who
Enrolled for Fall: *26* • Total Graduates: *19*

FINANCES

Residential Annual Tuition: *$1,124* • Non-Residential
Annual Tuition: *$1,924* • General Institution Fees: *$336* •
Additional Nursing Fees: *$70*

ODESSA COLLEGE

Address: 201 W University, Odessa, TX 79764
Phone: 915-335-6463
Fax: 915-355-6846
Contact: Becky Hammack, MSN, RN, Director of Nursing Program
Email: bhammack@odessa.edu

GENERAL INFORMATION

Type of School: *2-Year College or University, Public* •
Accreditation: *Southern Association of Colleges and Schools* •
Total Enrollment: *5000*

PROGRAM INFORMATION

LPN/LVN Exit: *Yes* • NLNAC Accreditation: *Yes*

NURSING STUDENT PROFILE

Total Nursing Enrollment: *107* • Full-Time Enrollment:
107 • Part-Time Enrollment: *Not Reported* • Female
Enrollment: *85* • Male Enrollment: *22* • Total New
Admissions Who Enrolled for Fall: *48* • Total Graduates: *54*

FINANCES

Residential Annual Tuition: *$656* • Non-Residential Annual
Tuition: *$966* • General Institution Fees: *$424* • Additional
Nursing Fees: *$50*

PANOLA COLLEGE

Address: 1109 W Panola, Curthage, TX 15633
Phone: 903-694-4003
Fax: 903-694-4010
Contact: Barbara Cordull, PhD, RN, HNC, Director, ADN program
Email: bcordell@panola.cc.tx.us

GENERAL INFORMATION

Type of School: *2-Year College or University, Public* •
Accreditation: *Southern Association of Colleges and Schools* •
Total Enrollment: *1424*

PROGRAM INFORMATION

LPN/LVN Exit: *No* • NLNAC Accreditation: *No*

NURSING STUDENT PROFILE

Total Nursing Enrollment: *50* • Full-Time Enrollment: *50* •
Part-Time Enrollment: *Not Reported* • Female Enrollment: *41* • Male Enrollment: *9* • Total New Admissions Who Enrolled for Fall: *25* • Total Graduates: *25*

FINANCES

Residential Annual Tuition: *Not Reported* • Non-Residential Annual Tuition: *Not Reported* • General Institution Fees: *$390* • Additional Nursing Fees: *$688*

PARIS JUNIOR COLLEGE

Address: 2400 Clarksville, Paris, TX 75460
Phone: 903-782-0734
Fax: Not Reported
Contact: Virginia Holmes, MSN, RN, Director, Health Occupations
Email: vholmes@paris.cc.tx.us

GENERAL INFORMATION

Type of School: *2-Year College or University, Public* •
Accreditation: *Southern Association of Colleges and Schools* •
Total Enrollment: *2942*

PROGRAM INFORMATION

LPN/LVN Exit: *Not Reported* • NLNAC Accreditation: *Yes*

NURSING STUDENT PROFILE

Total Nursing Enrollment: *47* • Full-Time Enrollment: *47* •
Part-Time Enrollment: *Not Reported* • Female Enrollment: *43* • Male Enrollment: *4* • Total New Admissions Who Enrolled for Fall: *47* • Total Graduates: *35*

FINANCES

Residential Annual Tuition: *$1,236* • Non-Residential Annual Tuition: *$2,740* • General Institution Fees: *$80* • Additional Nursing Fees: *$50*

SAINT PHILLIP'S COLLEGE

Address: 1801 M.L. King Dr., San Antonio, TX 78203
Phone: 210-531-3415
Fax: Not Reported
Contact: Frannie Rettig, , Program Director
Email: frettig@accd.edu

GENERAL INFORMATION

Type of School: *Other* • Accreditation: *None* • Total Enrollment: *Not Reported*

PROGRAM INFORMATION

LPN/LVN Exit: *Not Reported* • NLNAC Accreditation: *No*

NURSING STUDENT PROFILE

Total Nursing Enrollment: *18* • Full-Time Enrollment: *18* • Part-Time Enrollment: *Not Reported* • Female Enrollment: *Not Reported* • Male Enrollment: *Not Reported* • Total New Admissions Who Enrolled for Fall: *20* • Total Graduates: *15*

FINANCES

Residential Annual Tuition: *Not Reported* • Non-Residential Annual Tuition: *Not Reported* • General Institution Fees: *Not Reported* • Additional Nursing Fees: *Not Reported*

SAN ANTONIO COLLEGE

Address: 1300 San Pedro Avenue, San Antonio, TX
           78212-4299
Phone: 210-733-2367
Fax: 210-733-2323
Contact: Lula Westrup Pelayo, PhD, RN, Chairperson
Email: LPelayo@accd.edu

GENERAL INFORMATION

Type of School: *2-Year College or University, Public* • Accreditation: *Southern Association of Colleges and Schools* • Total Enrollment: *448*

PROGRAM INFORMATION

LPN/LVN Exit: *Not Reported* • NLNAC Accreditation: *Yes*

NURSING STUDENT PROFILE

Total Nursing Enrollment: *448* • Full-Time Enrollment: *448* • Part-Time Enrollment: *0* • Female Enrollment: *359* • Male Enrollment: *89* • Total New Admissions Who Enrolled for Fall: *157* • Total Graduates: *173*

FINANCES

Residential Annual Tuition: *$560* • Non-Residential Annual Tuition: *$2,240* • General Institution Fees: *$109* • Additional Nursing Fees: *$75*

SAN JACINTO COLLEGE

Address: 8060 Spencer Hwy, Pasadena, TX 77501
Phone: 281-476-1842
Fax: 281-478-2754
Contact: Edna Robinson, MS, RN, Department
Chairperson
Email: erobin@sjcd.cc.tx.us

GENERAL INFORMATION

Type of School: *2-Year College or University, Public* •
Accreditation: *Southern Association of Colleges and Schools* •
Total Enrollment: *20603*

PROGRAM INFORMATION

LPN/LVN Exit: *No* • NLNAC Accreditation: *Yes*

NURSING STUDENT PROFILE

Total Nursing Enrollment: *300* • Full-Time Enrollment:
300 • Part-Time Enrollment: *0* • Female Enrollment: *260* •
Male Enrollment: *40* • Total New Admissions Who Enrolled
for Fall: *105* • Total Graduates: *102*

FINANCES

Residential Annual Tuition: *$1,324* • Non-Residential
Annual Tuition: *$2,732* • General Institution Fees: *$812* •
Additional Nursing Fees: *Not Reported*

SAN JACINTO COLLEGE— SOUTH

Address: 13735 Beamer Road, Houston, TX 77089
Phone: 281-922-3466
Fax: 281-922-3487
Contact: Joyce M. Adams, PhD, RN, Dean
Email: jadams@sice.cc.tx.us

GENERAL INFORMATION

Type of School: *Not Reported* • Accreditation: *Not Reported* •
Total Enrollment: *Not Reported*

PROGRAM INFORMATION

LPN/LVN Exit: *Yes* • NLNAC Accreditation: *Yes*

NURSING STUDENT PROFILE

Total Nursing Enrollment: *63* • Full-Time Enrollment: *0* •
Part-Time Enrollment: *63* • Female Enrollment: *61* • Male
Enrollment: *2* • Total New Admissions Who Enrolled for
Fall: *30* • Total Graduates: *30*

FINANCES

Residential Annual Tuition: *Not Reported* • Non-Residential
Annual Tuition: *Not Reported* • General Institution Fees:
$70 • Additional Nursing Fees: *$27*

SOUTH PLAINS COLLEGE

Address: 1401 College Avenue, Levelland, TX 79336
Phone: 806-894-9611
Fax: 806-894-1608
Contact: Sue Ann Lopez, MSN, RN, Chair, Department
            of Nursing and Director, ADNP
Email: salopez@spc.cc.tx.us

GENERAL INFORMATION

Type of School: *2-Year College or University, Public* •
Accreditation: *Southern Association of Colleges and Schools* •
Total Enrollment: *7481*

PROGRAM INFORMATION

LPN/LVN Exit: *Not Reported* • NLNAC Accreditation: *Yes*

NURSING STUDENT PROFILE

Total Nursing Enrollment: *102* • Full-Time Enrollment:
102 • Part-Time Enrollment: *0* • Female Enrollment: *86* •
Male Enrollment: *16* • Total New Admissions Who Enrolled
for Fall: *42* • Total Graduates: *39*

FINANCES

Residential Annual Tuition: *$1,082* • Non-Residential
Annual Tuition: *$1,466* • General Institution Fees: *$94* •
Additional Nursing Fees: *$170*

SOUTH TEXAS COMMUNITY COLLEGE

Address: 3201 W. Pecan Blvd, McAllen, TX 78501
Phone: 956-683-3124
Fax: 956-683-3115
Contact: Paula A Olesen, MSN, RN, Program Director
Email: polesen@stcc.cc.tx.us

GENERAL INFORMATION

Type of School: *2-Year College or University, Public* •
Accreditation: *Southern Association of Colleges and Schools* •
Total Enrollment: *11500*

PROGRAM INFORMATION

LPN/LVN Exit: *Not Reported* • NLNAC Accreditation: *No*

NURSING STUDENT PROFILE

Total Nursing Enrollment: *117* • Full-Time Enrollment:
116 • Part-Time Enrollment: *1* • Female Enrollment: *83* •
Male Enrollment: *34* • Total New Admissions Who Enrolled
for Fall: *86* • Total Graduates: *40*

FINANCES

Residential Annual Tuition: *$1,637* • Non-Residential
Annual Tuition: *$3,650* • General Institution Fees: *$0* •
Additional Nursing Fees: *$40*

SOUTHWESTERN ADVENTIST UNIVERSITY

Address: PO Box 58, Keene, TX 76059
Phone: 817-645-3921
Fax: 817-556-4713
Contact: Bonnie Gnadt, MSN, RN, Chair
Email: gnadtb@swau.edu

GENERAL INFORMATION

Type of School: *4-Year College or University, Private (Religious)* • Accreditation: *Southern Association of Colleges and Schools* • Total Enrollment: *1200*

PROGRAM INFORMATION

LPN/LVN Exit: *No* • NLNAC Accreditation: *Yes*

NURSING STUDENT PROFILE

Total Nursing Enrollment: *84* • Full-Time Enrollment: *84* • Part-Time Enrollment: *Not Reported* • Female Enrollment: *73* • Male Enrollment: *11* • Total New Admissions Who Enrolled for Fall: *44* • Total Graduates: *41*

FINANCES

Residential Annual Tuition: *$9,400* • Non-Residential Annual Tuition: *$9,400* • General Institution Fees: *$50* • Additional Nursing Fees: *$250*

TARRANT COUNTY COLLEGE

Address: May Owen Center - 1500 Houston Street, Fort Worth, TX 76102
Phone: 817-515-6052
Fax: 817-515-5730
Contact: Eva Williams, MS, RN, Interim Director
Email: Eva.Williams@tccd.net

GENERAL INFORMATION

Type of School: *2-Year College or University, Public* • Accreditation: *Southern Association of Colleges and Schools* • Total Enrollment: *26907*

PROGRAM INFORMATION

LPN/LVN Exit: *No* • NLNAC Accreditation: *Yes*

NURSING STUDENT PROFILE

Total Nursing Enrollment: *310* • Full-Time Enrollment: *310* • Part-Time Enrollment: *0* • Female Enrollment: *265* • Male Enrollment: *45* • Total New Admissions Who Enrolled for Fall: *77* • Total Graduates: *141*

FINANCES

Residential Annual Tuition: *$992* • Non-Residential Annual Tuition: *$4,480* • General Institution Fees: *$56* • Additional Nursing Fees: *$585*

TEMPLE COLLEGE

Address: 2600 S 1st, Temple, TX 76504
Phone: 254-298-8666
Fax: 254-771-3726
Contact: Virginia N Leak, MS, RN, Division Director, Nursing
Email: virginia.leak@templejc.edu

GENERAL INFORMATION

Type of School: *2-Year College or University, Public* •
Accreditation: *Southern Association of Colleges and Schools* •
Total Enrollment: *3405*

PROGRAM INFORMATION

LPN/LVN Exit: *No* • NLNAC Accreditation: *Yes*

NURSING STUDENT PROFILE

Total Nursing Enrollment: *68* • Full-Time Enrollment: *68* •
Part-Time Enrollment: *0* • Female Enrollment: *62* • Male
Enrollment: *6* • Total New Admissions Who Enrolled for
Fall: *28* • Total Graduates: *31*

FINANCES

Residential Annual Tuition: *$2,340* • Non-Residential
Annual Tuition: *$8,576* • General Institution Fees: *Not
Reported* • Additional Nursing Fees: *Not Reported*

TEXARKANA COLLEGE

Address: 2500 North Robison Rd, Texarkana, TX 75599
Phone: 903-832-5565
Fax: 903-831-1037
Contact: Carol Hodgsom, PhD, RN, Division Chair, Health Occupations Director of ADN Program
Email: chodgson@tc.cc.tx.us

GENERAL INFORMATION

Type of School: *2-Year College or University, Public* •
Accreditation: *Southern Association of Colleges and Schools* •
Total Enrollment: *3735*

PROGRAM INFORMATION

LPN/LVN Exit: *No* • NLNAC Accreditation: *Yes*

NURSING STUDENT PROFILE

Total Nursing Enrollment: *176* • Full-Time Enrollment:
175 • Part-Time Enrollment: *1* • Female Enrollment: *153* •
Male Enrollment: *23* • Total New Admissions Who Enrolled
for Fall: *69* • Total Graduates: *73*

FINANCES

Residential Annual Tuition: *$932* • Non-Residential Annual
Tuition: *$2,000* • General Institution Fees: *$100* •
Additional Nursing Fees: *$110*

TRINITY VALLEY COMMUNITY COLLEGE

Address: 100 Cardinal Drive, Athens, TX 75751
Phone: 972-932-4309
Fax: 972-932-5010
Contact: Helen Reid, EdD, MSN, RN, Dean of Health Occupations
Email: reid@tvcc.edu

GENERAL INFORMATION

Type of School: *2-Year College or University, Public* •
Accreditation: *Southern Association of Colleges and Schools* •
Total Enrollment: *5094*

PROGRAM INFORMATION

LPN/LVN Exit: *No* • NLNAC Accreditation: *Yes*

NURSING STUDENT PROFILE

Total Nursing Enrollment: *184* • Full-Time Enrollment: *184* • Part-Time Enrollment: *Not Reported* • Female Enrollment: *169* • Male Enrollment: *15* • Total New Admissions Who Enrolled for Fall: *100* • Total Graduates: *71*

FINANCES

Residential Annual Tuition: *$764* • Non-Residential Annual Tuition: *$2,056* • General Institution Fees: *$240* • Additional Nursing Fees: *$70*

TYLER JUNIOR COLLEGE

Address: P.O. Box 9020, Tyler, TX 75711
Phone: 903-510-2864
Fax: 903-510-2542
Contact: Lylith Nicholson, MSN, RN, Instructor and Director
Email: inic@tj.tyler.cc.tx.us

GENERAL INFORMATION

Type of School: *Not Reported* • Accreditation: *Not Reported* • Total Enrollment: *Not Reported*

PROGRAM INFORMATION

LPN/LVN Exit: *Not Reported* • NLNAC Accreditation: *No*

NURSING STUDENT PROFILE

Total Nursing Enrollment: *115* • Full-Time Enrollment: *115* • Part-Time Enrollment: *0* • Female Enrollment: *91* • Male Enrollment: *24* • Total New Admissions Who Enrolled for Fall: *39* • Total Graduates: *56*

FINANCES

Residential Annual Tuition: *$716* • Non-Residential Annual Tuition: *$1,292* • General Institution Fees: *$24* • Additional Nursing Fees: *$120*

THE UNIVERSITY OF TEXAS— BROWNSVILLE AND TEXAS SOUTHMOST COLLEGE

Address: 80 Fort Brown, Brownsville, TX 78520
Phone: 956-544-8924
Fax: Not Reported
Contact: Edna Iris Garza-Escobedo, PhD, RN, Program Director ADN/Nursing Department
Email: eige@utbl.utb.edu

GENERAL INFORMATION

Type of School: *Not Reported* • Accreditation: *Not Reported* • Total Enrollment: *Not Reported*

PROGRAM INFORMATION

LPN/LVN Exit: *No* • NLNAC Accreditation: *Yes*

NURSING STUDENT PROFILE

Total Nursing Enrollment: *93* • Full-Time Enrollment: *93* • Part-Time Enrollment: *Not Reported* • Female Enrollment: *Not Reported* • Male Enrollment: *Not Reported* • Total New Admissions Who Enrolled for Fall: *40* • Total Graduates: *68*

FINANCES

Residential Annual Tuition: *Not Reported* • Non-Residential Annual Tuition: *Not Reported* • General Institution Fees: *Not Reported* • Additional Nursing Fees: *Not Reported*

UNIVERSITY OF TEXAS— PAN AMERICAN

Address: 1201 W. University Drive, Edinburg, TX 78539
Phone: Not Reported
Fax: Not Reported
Contact: Not Reported
Email: Not Reported

GENERAL INFORMATION

Type of School: *4-Year College or University, Public* • Accreditation: *Southern Association of Colleges and Schools* • Total Enrollment: *12500*

PROGRAM INFORMATION

LPN/LVN Exit: *Not Reported* • NLNAC Accreditation: *No*

NURSING STUDENT PROFILE

Total Nursing Enrollment: *Not Reported* • Full-Time Enrollment: *Not Reported* • Part-Time Enrollment: *Not Reported* • Female Enrollment: *Not Reported* • Male Enrollment: *Not Reported* • Total New Admissions Who Enrolled for Fall: *Not Reported* • Total Graduates: *Not Reported*

FINANCES

Residential Annual Tuition: *Not Reported* • Non-Residential Annual Tuition: *Not Reported* • General Institution Fees: *Not Reported* • Additional Nursing Fees: *Not Reported*

VERNON REGIONAL JR COLLEGE

Address: 4105 Maplewood Ave, Wichita Falls, TX 76308
Phone: 940-552-6291
Fax: 940-553-3902
Contact: Cathy Bolton, Director of Health Sciences
Email: cbolton@vrjc.cc.tx.us

VICTORIA COLLEGE

Address: 2200 E. Red River, Victoria, TX 77901
Phone: 361-582-2425
Fax: 361-572-6441
Contact: Kathie Aduddell, EdD, RN, CNABC, Associate Degree Nursing Program Director
Email: kadduddel@vc.cc.tx.us

GENERAL INFORMATION

Type of School: *Independent, Public* • Accreditation: *Southern Association of Colleges and Schools* • Total Enrollment: *933*

GENERAL INFORMATION

Type of School: *2-Year College or University, Public* • Accreditation: *Southern Association of Colleges and Schools* • Total Enrollment: *4022*

PROGRAM INFORMATION

LPN/LVN Exit: *Not Reported* • NLNAC Accreditation: *No*

PROGRAM INFORMATION

LPN/LVN Exit: *Yes* • NLNAC Accreditation: *Yes*

NURSING STUDENT PROFILE

Total Nursing Enrollment: *80* • Full-Time Enrollment: *Not Reported* • Part-Time Enrollment: *Not Reported* • Female Enrollment: *Not Reported* • Male Enrollment: *Not Reported* • Total New Admissions Who Enrolled for Fall: *50* • Total Graduates: *41*

NURSING STUDENT PROFILE

Total Nursing Enrollment: *157* • Full-Time Enrollment: *157* • Part-Time Enrollment: *Not Reported* • Female Enrollment: *144* • Male Enrollment: *13* • Total New Admissions Who Enrolled for Fall: *49* • Total Graduates: *50*

FINANCES

Residential Annual Tuition: *Not Reported* • Non-Residential Annual Tuition: *Not Reported* • General Institution Fees: *Not Reported* • Additional Nursing Fees: *Not Reported*

FINANCES

Residential Annual Tuition: *Not Reported* • Non-Residential Annual Tuition: *Not Reported* • General Institution Fees: *Not Reported* • Additional Nursing Fees: *Not Reported*

WHARTON COUNTY JUNIOR COLLEGE

Address: 911 Boling Highway, Wharton, TX 77488
Phone: 979-532-6404
Fax: 979-532-6489
Contact: Sarah Clark, MS, RN, Director
Email: sarahc@wcjc.cc.tx.us

GENERAL INFORMATION

Type of School: *2-Year College or University, Public* •
Accreditation: *Southern Association of Colleges and Schools* •
Total Enrollment: *5100*

PROGRAM INFORMATION

LPN/LVN Exit: *No* • NLNAC Accreditation: *No*

NURSING STUDENT PROFILE

Total Nursing Enrollment: *68* • Full-Time Enrollment: *68* •
Part-Time Enrollment: *0* • Female Enrollment: *60* • Male
Enrollment: *8* • Total New Admissions Who Enrolled for
Fall: *38* • Total Graduates: *27*

FINANCES

Residential Annual Tuition: *$870* • Non-Residential Annual
Tuition: *$1,830* • General Institution Fees: *$100* •
Additional Nursing Fees: *$80*

COLLEGE OF EASTERN UTAH

Address: 451 East 400 North, Price, UT 84501
Phone: 435-613-5347
Fax: 435-613-5801
Contact: Frances Swasey, MN, RN, Department of
            Nursing Chair
Email: fswasey@ceu.edu

GENERAL INFORMATION

Type of School: *2-Year College or University, Public* •
Accreditation: *Northwestern Association of Schools and
Colleges* • Total Enrollment: *2704*

PROGRAM INFORMATION

LPN/LVN Exit: *No* • NLNAC Accreditation: *Yes*

NURSING STUDENT PROFILE

Total Nursing Enrollment: *19* • Full-Time Enrollment: *19* •
Part-Time Enrollment: *Not Reported* • Female Enrollment:
15 • Male Enrollment: *4* • Total New Admissions Who
Enrolled for Fall: *24* • Total Graduates: *11*

FINANCES

Residential Annual Tuition: *$1,365* • Non-Residential
Annual Tuition: *$4,648* • General Institution Fees: *$361* •
Additional Nursing Fees: *$97*

Circle 28 on reader card   See in-depth profile for more information

DIXIE STATE COLLEGE

Address: 225 S. 700 E., St. George, UT 84770
Phone: 435-652-7863
Fax: 435-656-4025
Contact: Kevin Tipton, MSN, RN, Director
Email: tipton@dixie.edu

GENERAL INFORMATION

Type of School: *2-Year College or University, Public* •
Accreditation: *Northwestern Association of Schools and Colleges* • Total Enrollment: *6100*

PROGRAM INFORMATION

LPN/LVN Exit: *Not Reported* • NLNAC Accreditation: *No*

NURSING STUDENT PROFILE

Total Nursing Enrollment: *Not Reported* • Full-Time Enrollment: *Not Reported* • Part-Time Enrollment: *Not Reported* • Female Enrollment: *Not Reported* • Male Enrollment: *Not Reported* • Total New Admissions Who Enrolled for Fall: *Not Reported* • Total Graduates: *Not Reported*

FINANCES

Residential Annual Tuition: *Not Reported* • Non-Residential Annual Tuition: *Not Reported* • General Institution Fees: *Not Reported* • Additional Nursing Fees: *Not Reported*

SALT LAKE COMMUNITY COLLEGE

Address: PO Box 31808, Salt Lake City, UT 84131
Phone: 801-957-5704
Fax: Not Reported
Contact: Marilyn Little, MSN, APRN, Coordinator
Email: littlema@slcc.edu

GENERAL INFORMATION

Type of School: *Not Reported* • Accreditation: *Not Reported* • Total Enrollment: *Not Reported*

PROGRAM INFORMATION

LPN/LVN Exit: *Yes* • NLNAC Accreditation: *Yes*

NURSING STUDENT PROFILE

Total Nursing Enrollment: *219* • Full-Time Enrollment: *219* • Part-Time Enrollment: *Not Reported* • Female Enrollment: *185* • Male Enrollment: *34* • Total New Admissions Who Enrolled for Fall: *219* • Total Graduates: *196*

FINANCES

Residential Annual Tuition: *Not Reported* • Non-Residential Annual Tuition: *Not Reported* • General Institution Fees: *$100* • Additional Nursing Fees: *$51*

UTAH VALLEY STATE COLLEGE

Address: 800 West University Parkway, Orem, UT 84058
Phone: 801-222-8979
Fax: 801-226-5207
Contact: Alene Harrison, EdD, RN, Director,
            Department of Nursing
Email: harrisal@uvsc.edu

GENERAL INFORMATION

Type of School: *Governmental Agency, Public* • Accreditation: *Northwestern Association of Schools and Colleges* • Total Enrollment: *21000*

PROGRAM INFORMATION

LPN/LVN Exit: *Yes* • NLNAC Accreditation: *Yes*

NURSING STUDENT PROFILE

Total Nursing Enrollment: *74* • Full-Time Enrollment: *74* • Part-Time Enrollment: *Not Reported* • Female Enrollment: *59* • Male Enrollment: *15* • Total New Admissions Who Enrolled for Fall: *40* • Total Graduates: *77*

FINANCES

Residential Annual Tuition: *$1,682* • Non-Residential Annual Tuition: *$5,262* • General Institution Fees: *$320* • Additional Nursing Fees: *$62*

WEBER STATE UNIVERSITY

Address: 3903 University Circle, Ogden, UT 84408
Phone: 801-626-6161
Fax: 801-626-6397
Contact: Pamela Rice, MS, RN, PN/AD Coordinator
Email: price@weber.edu

GENERAL INFORMATION

Type of School: *4-Year College or University, Public* • Accreditation: *Northwestern Association of Schools and Colleges* • Total Enrollment: *Not Reported*

PROGRAM INFORMATION

LPN/LVN Exit: *Yes* • NLNAC Accreditation: *Yes*

NURSING STUDENT PROFILE

Total Nursing Enrollment: *346* • Full-Time Enrollment: *346* • Part-Time Enrollment: *Not Reported* • Female Enrollment: *313* • Male Enrollment: *33* • Total New Admissions Who Enrolled for Fall: *221* • Total Graduates: *253*

FINANCES

Residential Annual Tuition: *$2,118* • Non-Residential Annual Tuition: *$6,294* • General Institution Fees: *Not Reported* • Additional Nursing Fees: *Not Reported*

CASTLETON STATE COLLEGE

Address: 251 South Street, Castleton, VT 05735
Phone: 802-468-1236
Fax: Not Reported
Contact: Susan O Farrell, MS, RN, Chairperson
Email: susan.farrell@castleton.edu

GENERAL INFORMATION

Type of School: *4-Year College or University, Public* •
Accreditation: *New England Association of Schools and Colleges* • Total Enrollment: *Not Reported*

PROGRAM INFORMATION

LPN/LVN Exit: *No* • NLNAC Accreditation: *Yes*

NURSING STUDENT PROFILE

Total Nursing Enrollment: *56* • Full-Time Enrollment: *42* •
Part-Time Enrollment: *14* • Female Enrollment: *52* • Male
Enrollment: *4* • Total New Admissions Who Enrolled for
Fall: *24* • Total Graduates: *18*

FINANCES

Residential Annual Tuition: *$3,924* • Non-Residential
Annual Tuition: *$9,192* • General Institution Fees: *$752* •
Additional Nursing Fees: *$110*

NORWICH UNIVERSITY

Address: 158 Harmon Drive, Northfield, VT 05663
Phone: 802-485-2609
Fax: 802-485-2607
Contact: Marilyn Rinker, MSN, BS, RN, APN, Interim
Program Chair
Email: mrinker@norwich.edu

GENERAL INFORMATION

Type of School: *Not Reported* • Accreditation: *New England Association of Schools and Colleges* • Total Enrollment: *Not Reported*

PROGRAM INFORMATION

LPN/LVN Exit: *No* • NLNAC Accreditation: *Yes*

NURSING STUDENT PROFILE

Total Nursing Enrollment: *15* • Full-Time Enrollment: *0* •
Part-Time Enrollment: *15* • Female Enrollment: *13* • Male
Enrollment: *2* • Total New Admissions Who Enrolled for
Fall: *Not Reported* • Total Graduates: *12*

FINANCES

Residential Annual Tuition: *$15,550* • Non-Residential
Annual Tuition: *$15,550* • General Institution Fees: *$0* •
Additional Nursing Fees: *$0*

SOUTHERN VERMONT COLLEGE

Address: 982 Mansion Dr., Bennington, VT 05201
Phone: 802-447-4656
Fax: Not Reported
Contact: Holly Evans Madison, MS, RN, Chair, Nursing
             Division
Email: hmadison@svc.edu

GENERAL INFORMATION

Type of School: *4-Year College or University, Private (Independent)* • Accreditation: *New England Association of Schools and Colleges* • Total Enrollment: *Not Reported*

PROGRAM INFORMATION

LPN/LVN Exit: *No* • NLNAC Accreditation: *Yes*

NURSING STUDENT PROFILE

Total Nursing Enrollment: *33* • Full-Time Enrollment: *33* • Part-Time Enrollment: *Not Reported* • Female Enrollment: *Not Reported* • Male Enrollment: *Not Reported* • Total New Admissions Who Enrolled for Fall: *15* • Total Graduates: *24*

FINANCES

Residential Annual Tuition: *Not Reported* • Non-Residential Annual Tuition: *Not Reported* • General Institution Fees: *Not Reported* • Additional Nursing Fees: *Not Reported*

VERMONT TECHNICAL COLLEGE

Address: PO Box 500, Randolph Center, VT 05061
Phone: 802-447-5419
Fax: 802-477-5218
Contact: Patricia Menchini, MS, RN, Director
Email: pmenchini@yahoo.com

GENERAL INFORMATION

Type of School: *Other, Public* • Accreditation: *New England Association of Schools and Colleges* • Total Enrollment: *Not Reported*

PROGRAM INFORMATION

LPN/LVN Exit: *No* • NLNAC Accreditation: *Yes*

NURSING STUDENT PROFILE

Total Nursing Enrollment: *35* • Full-Time Enrollment: *19* • Part-Time Enrollment: *16* • Female Enrollment: *33* • Male Enrollment: *2* • Total New Admissions Who Enrolled for Fall: *35* • Total Graduates: *29*

FINANCES

Residential Annual Tuition: *$6,264* • Non-Residential Annual Tuition: *$11,712* • General Institution Fees: *$869* • Additional Nursing Fees: *Not Reported*

UNIVERSITY OF THE VIRGIN ISLANDS

Address: #2 John Brewers Bay, Saint Thomas, VI 00802
Phone: 340-692-4011
Fax: 340-692-4015
Contact: Kathy Sheats, MSN, RN, Chairperson, Nursing
          Education
Email: ksheats@uni.edu

GENERAL INFORMATION

Type of School: *4-Year College or University, Public* •
Accreditation: *Middle States Association of Colleges and
Schools* • Total Enrollment: *Not Reported*

PROGRAM INFORMATION

LPN/LVN Exit: *Not Reported* • NLNAC Accreditation: *Yes*

NURSING STUDENT PROFILE

Total Nursing Enrollment: *15* • Full-Time Enrollment: *15* •
Part-Time Enrollment: *0* • Female Enrollment: *15* • Male
Enrollment: *0* • Total New Admissions Who Enrolled for
Fall: *8* • Total Graduates: *3*

FINANCES

Residential Annual Tuition: *$1,365* • Non-Residential
Annual Tuition: *$4,095* • General Institution Fees: *$128* •
Additional Nursing Fees: *$30*

BLUE RIDGE COMMUNITY COLLEGE—VIRGINIA

Address: PO Box 80, College Lane, Weyers Cave, VA
          24486
Phone: 540-453-2321
Fax: 540-234-9066
Contact: Loretta Wack, MSN, PNP, FNP, RN, Nursing
          Program Coordinator
Email: brwackl@br.cc.va.us

GENERAL INFORMATION

Type of School: *2-Year College or University, Public* •
Accreditation: *Southern Association of Colleges and Schools* •
Total Enrollment: *2033*

PROGRAM INFORMATION

LPN/LVN Exit: *No* • NLNAC Accreditation: *Yes*

NURSING STUDENT PROFILE

Total Nursing Enrollment: *70* • Full-Time Enrollment: *70* •
Part-Time Enrollment: *Not Reported* • Female Enrollment:
68 • Male Enrollment: *2* • Total New Admissions Who
Enrolled for Fall: *34* • Total Graduates: *34*

FINANCES

Residential Annual Tuition: *Not Reported* • Non-Residential
Annual Tuition: *Not Reported* • General Institution Fees: *Not
Reported* • Additional Nursing Fees: *$32*

COLLEGE OF HEALTH SCIENCES

Address:	PO Box 13186, Roanoke, VA 24031
Phone:	540-985-8531
Fax:	Not Reported
Contact:	Linda R Rickabaugh, MSN, RN, Director, Associate Degree Nursing
Email:	linda@health.chs.edu

GENERAL INFORMATION

Type of School: *Not Reported* • Accreditation: *Not Reported* • Total Enrollment: *Not Reported*

PROGRAM INFORMATION

LPN/LVN Exit: *No* • NLNAC Accreditation: *Yes*

NURSING STUDENT PROFILE

Total Nursing Enrollment: *85* • Full-Time Enrollment: *80* • Part-Time Enrollment: *5* • Female Enrollment: *78* • Male Enrollment: *7* • Total New Admissions Who Enrolled for Fall: *35* • Total Graduates: *19*

FINANCES

Residential Annual Tuition: *Not Reported* • Non-Residential Annual Tuition: *Not Reported* • General Institution Fees: *Not Reported* • Additional Nursing Fees: *$200*

DABNEYS LANCASTER

Address:	PO Box 1000, Clifton Forge, VA 24422
Phone:	540-863-2843
Fax:	540-863-2915
Contact:	Joan B Hawse, MS, RN, Program Head
Email:	dlhawsj@dl.cc.va.us

GENERAL INFORMATION

Type of School: *2-Year College or University, Public* • Accreditation: *Southern Association of Colleges and Schools* • Total Enrollment: *690*

PROGRAM INFORMATION

LPN/LVN Exit: *Yes* • NLNAC Accreditation: *Yes*

NURSING STUDENT PROFILE

Total Nursing Enrollment: *40* • Full-Time Enrollment: *Not Reported* • Part-Time Enrollment: *Not Reported* • Female Enrollment: *Not Reported* • Male Enrollment: *Not Reported* • Total New Admissions Who Enrolled for Fall: *18* • Total Graduates: *16*

FINANCES

Residential Annual Tuition: *Not Reported* • Non-Residential Annual Tuition: *Not Reported* • General Institution Fees: *Not Reported* • Additional Nursing Fees: *Not Reported*

GERMANNA COMMUNITY COLLEGE

Address: 2130 Germanna Highway, Locust Grove, VA
22508
Phone: 540-727-3071
Fax: 540-727-3207
Contact: Jane R. Ingalls, Director
Email: gcingaj@gc.cc.va.us

GENERAL INFORMATION

Type of School: *2-Year College or University, Public* •
Accreditation: *Southern Association of Colleges and Schools* •
Total Enrollment: *7300*

PROGRAM INFORMATION

LPN/LVN Exit: *No* • NLNAC Accreditation: *Yes*

NURSING STUDENT PROFILE

Total Nursing Enrollment: *62* • Full-Time Enrollment: *62* •
Part-Time Enrollment: *0* • Female Enrollment: *62* • Male
Enrollment: *0* • Total New Admissions Who Enrolled for
Fall: *36* • Total Graduates: *36*

FINANCES

Residential Annual Tuition: *$1,147* • Non-Residential
Annual Tuition: *$3,792* • General Institution Fees: *Not
Reported* • Additional Nursing Fees: *Not Reported*

J. SARGEANT REYNOLDS COMMUNITY COLLEGE

Address: 700 East Jackson St., Richmond, VA 23219
Phone: 804-786-1379
Fax: Not Reported
Contact: Fran Stanley, MN, RN, Coordinator, Nursing
Email: fstanley@jsr.cc.va.us

GENERAL INFORMATION

Type of School: *Other* • Accreditation: *None* • Total
Enrollment: *Not Reported*

PROGRAM INFORMATION

LPN/LVN Exit: *No* • NLNAC Accreditation: *Yes*

NURSING STUDENT PROFILE

Total Nursing Enrollment: *287* • Full-Time Enrollment:
287 • Part-Time Enrollment: *0* • Female Enrollment: *Not
Reported* • Male Enrollment: *Not Reported* • Total New
Admissions Who Enrolled for Fall: *119* • Total Graduates:
119

FINANCES

Residential Annual Tuition: *Not Reported* • Non-Residential
Annual Tuition: *Not Reported* • General Institution Fees: *Not
Reported* • Additional Nursing Fees: *Not Reported*

JOHN TYLER COMMUNITY COLLEGE

Address: 13101 Jefferson Davis Highway, Chester, VA 23831
Phone: 804-796-4076
Fax: 804-796-4359
Contact: Shelley F Conroy, EdD, MS, RN, Nursing Program Director
Email: sconroy@jt.cc.va.us

GENERAL INFORMATION

Type of School: *2-Year College or University, Public* •
Accreditation: *Southern Association of Colleges and Schools* •
Total Enrollment: *8400*

PROGRAM INFORMATION

LPN/LVN Exit: *No* • NLNAC Accreditation: *Yes*

NURSING STUDENT PROFILE

Total Nursing Enrollment: *162* • Full-Time Enrollment: *27* •
Part-Time Enrollment: *135* • Female Enrollment: *157* • Male
Enrollment: *5* • Total New Admissions Who Enrolled for
Fall: *54* • Total Graduates: *44*

FINANCES

Residential Annual Tuition: *Not Reported* • Non-Residential
Annual Tuition: *Not Reported* • General Institution Fees: *Not
Reported* • Additional Nursing Fees: *$100*

LORD FAIRFAX COMMUNITY COLLEGE

Address: 173 Skirmisher Lane, Middletown, VA 22645
Phone: 540-868-7000
Fax: 540-868-7100
Contact: Betty J Ward, MS, BSN, ADN Program Director
Email: lfwardb@lf.cc.va.us

GENERAL INFORMATION

Type of School: *2-Year College or University, Public* •
Accreditation: *Southern Association of Colleges and Schools* •
Total Enrollment: *Not Reported*

PROGRAM INFORMATION

LPN/LVN Exit: *No* • NLNAC Accreditation: *No*

NURSING STUDENT PROFILE

Total Nursing Enrollment: *48* • Full-Time Enrollment: *27* •
Part-Time Enrollment: *21* • Female Enrollment: *45* • Male
Enrollment: *3* • Total New Admissions Who Enrolled for
Fall: *48* • Total Graduates: *Not Reported*

FINANCES

Residential Annual Tuition: *Not Reported* • Non-Residential
Annual Tuition: *Not Reported* • General Institution Fees:
$60 • Additional Nursing Fees: *$200*

MARYMOUNT UNIVERSITY

Address: 2807 N. Glebe Road, Arlington, VA 22207-4299
Phone: 703-284-1580
Fax: 703-284-3819
Contact: Leslie Neal, PhD, RN, Co-Chair, AAS Program
Email: leslie.neal@marymount.edu

GENERAL INFORMATION

Type of School: *4-Year College or University, Private (Religious)* • Accreditation: *Southern Association of Colleges and Schools* • Total Enrollment: *3600*

PROGRAM INFORMATION

LPN/LVN Exit: *No* • NLNAC Accreditation: *Yes*

NURSING STUDENT PROFILE

Total Nursing Enrollment: *175* • Full-Time Enrollment: *91* • Part-Time Enrollment: *84* • Female Enrollment: *150* • Male Enrollment: *25* • Total New Admissions Who Enrolled for Fall: *78* • Total Graduates: *77*

FINANCES

Annual Tuition: *$16,300* • General Institution Fees: *$138* • Additional Nursing Fees: *$115*

NORFOLK STATE UNIVERSITY

Address: 700 Park Avenue, Norfolk, VA 23504
Phone: 757-823-9013
Fax: Not Reported
Contact: Willar F White-Parson, PhD, RN, CS, FAAN, Department Head
Email: wfwhiteparson@nsu.edu

GENERAL INFORMATION

Type of School: *4-Year College or University, Public* • Accreditation: *Southern Association of Colleges and Schools* • Total Enrollment: *6000*

PROGRAM INFORMATION

LPN/LVN Exit: *No* • NLNAC Accreditation: *Yes*

NURSING STUDENT PROFILE

Total Nursing Enrollment: *255* • Full-Time Enrollment: *201* • Part-Time Enrollment: *54* • Female Enrollment: *231* • Male Enrollment: *24* • Total New Admissions Who Enrolled for Fall: *137* • Total Graduates: *78*

FINANCES

Residential Annual Tuition: *$2,856* • Non-Residential Annual Tuition: *$8,056* • General Institution Fees: *$0* • Additional Nursing Fees: *$90*

NORTHERN VIRGINIA COMMUNITY COLLEGE

Address: 8333 Little River Turnpike, Annandale, VA 22003
Phone: 703-323-3405
Fax: 703-323-4576
Contact: Diane C Wilson, MSN, CS, RN, Acting Division Chair and Program Head, Nursing and Surgical Technology
Email: diwilson@nvcc.vccs.edu

GENERAL INFORMATION

Type of School: *2-Year College or University, Public* •
Accreditation: *Southern Association of Colleges and Schools* •
Total Enrollment: *60000*

PROGRAM INFORMATION

LPN/LVN Exit: *No* • NLNAC Accreditation: *Yes*

NURSING STUDENT PROFILE

Total Nursing Enrollment: *199* • Full-Time Enrollment: *199* • Part-Time Enrollment: *Not Reported* • Female Enrollment: *183* • Male Enrollment: *16* • Total New Admissions Who Enrolled for Fall: *106* • Total Graduates: *82*

FINANCES

Residential Annual Tuition: *$2,035* • Non-Residential Annual Tuition: *$6,753* • General Institution Fees: *$0* • Additional Nursing Fees: *$48*

PATRICK HENRY COMMUNITY COLLEGE

Address: PO Box 5311, Martinsville, VA 24115
Phone: 540-656-0248
Fax: 540-656-0261
Contact: Mildred Owings, MSN, RN, CS, Program Head of Nursing
Email: mowings@ph.cc.va.us

GENERAL INFORMATION

Type of School: *2-Year College or University, Public* •
Accreditation: *Southern Association of Colleges and Schools* •
Total Enrollment: *2400*

PROGRAM INFORMATION

LPN/LVN Exit: *No* • NLNAC Accreditation: *Yes*

NURSING STUDENT PROFILE

Total Nursing Enrollment: *54* • Full-Time Enrollment: *54* • Part-Time Enrollment: *Not Reported* • Female Enrollment: *52* • Male Enrollment: *2* • Total New Admissions Who Enrolled for Fall: *25* • Total Graduates: *19*

FINANCES

Residential Annual Tuition: *Not Reported* • Non-Residential Annual Tuition: *Not Reported* • General Institution Fees: *$5* • Additional Nursing Fees: *$64*

PIEDMONT VIRGINIA COMMUNITY COLLEGE

Address: 501 College Drive, Charlottesville, VA 22902
Phone: 434-961-5446
Fax: 434-971-8232
Contact: Kathleen Hudson, PhD,RN, Division Chair,
           Math, Science, and Human Services
Email: khudson@pvcc.vccs.edu

GENERAL INFORMATION

Type of School: *Governmental Agency, Public* • Accreditation:
Southern Association of Colleges and Schools • Total
Enrollment: *4470*

PROGRAM INFORMATION

LPN/LVN Exit: *No* • NLNAC Accreditation: *Yes*

NURSING STUDENT PROFILE

Total Nursing Enrollment: *110* • Full-Time Enrollment: *28* •
Part-Time Enrollment: *82* • Female Enrollment: *98* • Male
Enrollment: *12* • Total New Admissions Who Enrolled for
Fall: *68* • Total Graduates: *45*

FINANCES

Residential Annual Tuition: *$1,907* • Non-Residential
Annual Tuition: *$6,578* • General Institution Fees: *$142* •
Additional Nursing Fees: *$0*

RIVERSIDE SCHOOL OF PROFESSIONAL NURSING

Address: 500 J Clyde Morris Blvd, Newport News,
           VA 23601
Phone: (757) 594-2714
Contact: Ms. Mary A. Ford, Director

GENERAL INFORMATION

Type of School: *Private* • Campus Setting: *Suburban* • Total
Enrollment: *165*

PROGRAM INFORMATION

Programs Offered: *Diploma* • Options: *Evening Classes,
Weekend Classes, Distance Learning, Other Alternative
Schedules, Continuing Education* • NLNAC Accredited

NURSING STUDENT PROFILE

First-Year Undergraduate Enrollment: *54* • Total Graduates:
54 • Total Enrollment: *154*

FINANCES

Resident Annual Tuition: *Not Reported* • Non-Resident
Annual Tuition: *Not Reported* • Grants: *Institutionally-
Sponsored Non-Need-Based Grants, Federal Pell Grants* •
Scholarships: *Institutionally-Sponsored Need-Based
Scholarships* • Loans: *Federal Nursing Student Loans, Federal
PLUS Loans, Federal Stafford Loans* • % of Students Receiving
Some Type of Aid: *Not Reported* • Financial Aid Application
Deadline: *Not Reported* • Financial Aid Office Phone:
(757) 594-2700*

Circle 101 on reader card   See in-depth profile for more information

SHENANDOAH UNIVERSITY

Address: 1460 University Drive, Winchester, VA 22601
Phone: 540-678-4381
Fax: 540-665-5519
Contact: Sheila M Sparks, DNSc, RN, CS, Interim
            Director
Email: ssparks@su.edu

GENERAL INFORMATION

Type of School: *4-Year College or University, Private
(Independent)* • Accreditation: *Southern Association of Colleges
and Schools* • Total Enrollment: *2428*

PROGRAM INFORMATION

LPN/LVN Exit: *No* • NLNAC Accreditation: *Yes*

NURSING STUDENT PROFILE

Total Nursing Enrollment: *Not Reported* • Full-Time
Enrollment: *Not Reported* • Part-Time Enrollment: *Not
Reported* • Female Enrollment: *Not Reported* • Male
Enrollment: *Not Reported* • Total New Admissions Who
Enrolled for Fall: *Not Reported* • Total Graduates: *Not
Reported*

FINANCES

Residential Annual Tuition: *Not Reported* • Non-Residential
Annual Tuition: *Not Reported* • General Institution Fees: *Not
Reported* • Additional Nursing Fees: *Not Reported*

THOMAS NELSON COMMUNITY COLLEGE

Address: 99 Thomas Nelson Drive, PO Box 9407,
            Hampton, VA 23670
Phone: 757-825-2762
Fax: 757-825-3620
Contact: Catherine Curtis, MS, RN, Co-Program Head of
            Nursing
Email: curtisc@tncc.cc.va.us

GENERAL INFORMATION

Type of School: *2-Year College or University, Public* •
Accreditation: *Southern Association of Colleges and Schools* •
Total Enrollment: *7379*

PROGRAM INFORMATION

LPN/LVN Exit: *No* • NLNAC Accreditation: *Yes*

NURSING STUDENT PROFILE

Total Nursing Enrollment: *87* • Full-Time Enrollment: *47* •
Part-Time Enrollment: *40* • Female Enrollment: *82* • Male
Enrollment: *5* • Total New Admissions Who Enrolled for
Fall: *40* • Total Graduates: *43*

FINANCES

Residential Annual Tuition: *Not Reported* • Non-Residential
Annual Tuition: *Not Reported* • General Institution Fees:
$21 • Additional Nursing Fees: *$85*

TIDEWATER COMMUNITY COLLEGE

Address: 7000 College Drive, Portsmouth, VA 23703
Phone: 757-822-2308
Fax: 757-822-2310
Contact: Denise Bell, MSN, RN, Nursing Program Head
Email: tcbelld@tc.cc.va.us

VIRGINIA HIGHLANDS COMMUNITY COLLEGE / VIRGINIA APPALACHIAN TRICOLLEGE

Address: P.O. Box 828, Abingdon, VA 24212
Phone: 276-739-2439
Fax: 276-739-2594
Contact: Lois S. Caldwell, MSN, RN, Director
Email: lcaldwell@vh.ccs.edu

GENERAL INFORMATION

Type of School: *2-Year College or University, Public* •
Accreditation: *Southern Association of Colleges and Schools* •
Total Enrollment: *20184*

GENERAL INFORMATION

Type of School: *2-Year College or University, Public* •
Accreditation: *Southern Association of Colleges and Schools* •
Total Enrollment: *2383*

PROGRAM INFORMATION

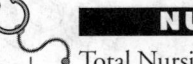

LPN/LVN Exit: *No* • NLNAC Accreditation: *Yes*

PROGRAM INFORMATION

LPN/LVN Exit: *No* • NLNAC Accreditation: *Yes*

NURSING STUDENT PROFILE

Total Nursing Enrollment: *152* • Full-Time Enrollment: *Not Reported* • Part-Time Enrollment: *Not Reported* • Female Enrollment: *139* • Male Enrollment: *13* • Total New Admissions Who Enrolled for Fall: *87* • Total Graduates: *68*

NURSING STUDENT PROFILE

Total Nursing Enrollment: *238* • Full-Time Enrollment: *238* • Part-Time Enrollment: *0* • Female Enrollment: *225* • Male Enrollment: *13* • Total New Admissions Who Enrolled for Fall: *150* • Total Graduates: *85*

FINANCES

Residential Annual Tuition: *Not Reported* • Non-Residential Annual Tuition: *Not Reported* • General Institution Fees: *$7* • Additional Nursing Fees: *$502*

FINANCES

Residential Annual Tuition: *$2,032* • Non-Residential Annual Tuition: *$6,750* • General Institution Fees: *$64* • Additional Nursing Fees: *$106*

VIRGINIA WESTERN COMMUNITY COLLEGE

Address: 3097 Colonial Avenue, SW, PO Box 14007,
            Roanoke, VA 24038
Phone: 540-857-6283
Fax: 540-857-7544
Contact: Martha S Barnas, MSN, MSEd, RN, Program
            Head of Nursing
Email: mbarnas@vw.vccs.edu

GENERAL INFORMATION

Type of School: *Governmental Agency, Public* • Accreditation:
Middle States Association of Colleges and Schools • Total
Enrollment: *8300*

PROGRAM INFORMATION

LPN/LVN Exit: *No* • NLNAC Accreditation: *Yes*

NURSING STUDENT PROFILE

Total Nursing Enrollment: *83* • Full-Time Enrollment: *83* •
Part-Time Enrollment: *Not Reported* • Female Enrollment:
77 • Male Enrollment: *6* • Total New Admissions Who
Enrolled for Fall: *49* • Total Graduates: *42*

FINANCES

Residential Annual Tuition: *$1,320* • Non-Residential
Annual Tuition: *$5,700* • General Institution Fees: *$8* •
Additional Nursing Fees: *$0*

WYTHEVILLE COMMUNITY COLLEGE

Address: 1000 East Main Street, Wytheville, VA 24382
Phone: 540-223-4845
Fax: 540-223-4778
Contact: Sue G Thacker, PhD, RN, C, Professor and
            Interim Program Head
Email: wcthacs@wc.cc.va.us

GENERAL INFORMATION

Type of School: *2-Year College or University, Public* •
Accreditation: *Southern Association of Colleges and Schools* •
Total Enrollment: *2396*

PROGRAM INFORMATION

LPN/LVN Exit: *No* • NLNAC Accreditation: *Yes*

NURSING STUDENT PROFILE

Total Nursing Enrollment: *199* • Full-Time Enrollment: *94* •
Part-Time Enrollment: *105* • Female Enrollment: *193* • Male
Enrollment: *6* • Total New Admissions Who Enrolled for
Fall: *102* • Total Graduates: *80*

FINANCES

Residential Annual Tuition: *Not Reported* • Non-Residential
Annual Tuition: *Not Reported* • General Institution Fees: *Not
Reported* • Additional Nursing Fees: *$15*

BELLEVUE COMMUNITY COLLEGE

Address: 3000 Landerholm Circle SE MSB134, Bellevue, WA 98007
Phone: 425-564-2554
Fax: 425-564-4135
Contact: Cheryl L Becker, MN, RN, Program Chair
Email: cbecker@bcc.ctc.edu

GENERAL INFORMATION

Type of School: *2-Year College or University, Public* • Accreditation: *Northwestern Association of Schools and Colleges* • Total Enrollment: *20000*

PROGRAM INFORMATION

LPN/LVN Exit: *No* • NLNAC Accreditation: *Yes*

NURSING STUDENT PROFILE

Total Nursing Enrollment: *89* • Full-Time Enrollment: *89* • Part-Time Enrollment: *Not Reported* • Female Enrollment: *75* • Male Enrollment: *14* • Total New Admissions Who Enrolled for Fall: *51* • Total Graduates: *37*

FINANCES

Residential Annual Tuition: *$1,671* • Non-Residential Annual Tuition: *$6,489* • General Institution Fees: *$105* • Additional Nursing Fees: *$75*

CLARK COLLEGE

Address: 1800 E McLoughlin Bulevard, Vancouver, WA 98663
Phone: 360-992-2192
Fax: 360-992-2880
Contact: Shelly Quint, MS, RN, Director of Nursing
Email: squint@clark.edu

GENERAL INFORMATION

Type of School: *2-Year College or University, Public* • Accreditation: *Northwestern Association of Schools and Colleges* • Total Enrollment: *12300*

PROGRAM INFORMATION

LPN/LVN Exit: *No* • NLNAC Accreditation: *Yes*

NURSING STUDENT PROFILE

Total Nursing Enrollment: *143* • Full-Time Enrollment: *142* • Part-Time Enrollment: *1* • Female Enrollment: *132* • Male Enrollment: *11* • Total New Admissions Who Enrolled for Fall: *9* • Total Graduates: *76*

FINANCES

Residential Annual Tuition: *$2,171* • General Institution Fees: *$200* • Additional Nursing Fees: *$125*

COLUMBIA BASIN COLLEGE

Address: 2600 N 20th, Pasco, WA 99301
Phone: 509-547-0511
Fax: Not Reported
Contact: Donna Campbell, MSN, RN, Dean
Email: dcambell@cbc2.org

COMMUNITY COLLEGES OF SPOKANE

Address: N. 2000 Greene St., Spokane, WA 99217
Phone: 509-533-8128
Fax: 509-533-8621
Contact: Claudia Kroll, EdD, MSN, RNC, Department
           Chairperson and Program Director
Email: ckroll@scc.spokane.cc.wa.us

GENERAL INFORMATION

Type of School: *Other* • Accreditation: *None* • Total Enrollment: *Not Reported*

GENERAL INFORMATION

Type of School: *Other* • Accreditation: *None* • Total Enrollment: *Not Reported*

PROGRAM INFORMATION

LPN/LVN Exit: *Yes* • NLNAC Accreditation: *No*

PROGRAM INFORMATION

LPN/LVN Exit: *Yes* • NLNAC Accreditation: *Yes*

NURSING STUDENT PROFILE

Total Nursing Enrollment: *50* • Full-Time Enrollment: *Not Reported* • Part-Time Enrollment: *Not Reported* • Female Enrollment: *Not Reported* • Male Enrollment: *Not Reported* • Total New Admissions Who Enrolled for Fall: *50* • Total Graduates: *38*

NURSING STUDENT PROFILE

Total Nursing Enrollment: *196* • Full-Time Enrollment: *132* • Part-Time Enrollment: *64* • Female Enrollment: *169* • Male Enrollment: *27* • Total New Admissions Who Enrolled for Fall: *65* • Total Graduates: *68*

FINANCES

Residential Annual Tuition: *Not Reported* • Non-Residential Annual Tuition: *Not Reported* • General Institution Fees: *Not Reported* • Additional Nursing Fees: *Not Reported*

FINANCES

Residential Annual Tuition: *$1,444* • Non-Residential Annual Tuition: *$2,154* • General Institution Fees: *$50* • Additional Nursing Fees: *$100*

EVERETT COMMUNITY COLLEGE

Address: 2000 Tower Street, Everett, WA 98201
Phone: 425-388-9471
Fax: 425-388-9135
Contact: Karen Heys, MN, RN, Nursing Department Chair
Email: kheys@evcc.ctc.edu

GENERAL INFORMATION

Type of School: *2-Year College or University, Public* • Accreditation: *Northwestern Association of Schools and Colleges* • Total Enrollment: *3360*

PROGRAM INFORMATION

LPN/LVN Exit: *No* • NLNAC Accreditation: *Yes*

NURSING STUDENT PROFILE

Total Nursing Enrollment: *117* • Full-Time Enrollment: *117* • Part-Time Enrollment: *0* • Female Enrollment: *107* • Male Enrollment: *10* • Total New Admissions Who Enrolled for Fall: *32* • Total Graduates: *50*

FINANCES

Residential Annual Tuition: *$1,738* • Non-Residential Annual Tuition: *$6,856* • General Institution Fees: *Not Reported* • Additional Nursing Fees: *$100*

GRAYS HARBOR COLLEGE

Address: 1620 Edward P. Smith Drive, Aberdeen, WA 98520
Phone: 360-538-4148
Fax: 360-538-4299
Contact: Penelope J Woodruff, MS, RN, Director, Nursing Programs and Chair, Health Science Division
Email: pwoodruf@ghc.ctc.edu

GENERAL INFORMATION

Type of School: *2-Year College or University, Public* • Accreditation: *Northwestern Association of Schools and Colleges* • Total Enrollment: *3200*

PROGRAM INFORMATION

LPN/LVN Exit: *No* • NLNAC Accreditation: *Yes*

NURSING STUDENT PROFILE

Total Nursing Enrollment: *33* • Full-Time Enrollment: *33* • Part-Time Enrollment: *Not Reported* • Female Enrollment: *31* • Male Enrollment: *2* • Total New Admissions Who Enrolled for Fall: *16* • Total Graduates: *9*

FINANCES

Residential Annual Tuition: *$1,449* • Non-Residential Annual Tuition: *$1,713* • General Institution Fees: *$12* • Additional Nursing Fees: *$83*

HIGHLINE COMMUNITY COLLEGE

Address: 2400 South 240th Street, PO Box 98000 MS 9-
            6, Des Moines, WA 98198
Phone: 206-878-3710
Fax: Not Reported
Contact: Mary Newell, MSN, RN, Nursing Program
            Director
Email: mnewell@hcc.ctc.edu

GENERAL INFORMATION

Type of School: *Other* • Accreditation: *None* • Total
Enrollment: *Not Reported*

PROGRAM INFORMATION

LPN/LVN Exit: *No* • NLNAC Accreditation: *Yes*

NURSING STUDENT PROFILE

Total Nursing Enrollment: *108* • Full-Time Enrollment:
108 • Part-Time Enrollment: *Not Reported* • Female
Enrollment: *Not Reported* • Male Enrollment: *Not Reported* •
Total New Admissions Who Enrolled for Fall: *45* • Total
Graduates: *68*

FINANCES

Residential Annual Tuition: *Not Reported* • Non-Residential
Annual Tuition: *Not Reported* • General Institution Fees: *Not
Reported* • Additional Nursing Fees: *Not Reported*

LOWER COLUMBIA COLLEGE

Address: 1600 Maple Street, Longview, WA 98632
Phone: 360-577-3446
Fax: 306-636-6759
Contact: Helen Kuebel, MSN, RN, Nursing Program
            Director
Email: hkuebel@lcc.ctc.edu

GENERAL INFORMATION

Type of School: *2-Year College or University, Public* •
Accreditation: *Northwestern Association of Schools and
Colleges* • Total Enrollment: *4200*

PROGRAM INFORMATION

LPN/LVN Exit: *Yes* • NLNAC Accreditation: *Yes*

NURSING STUDENT PROFILE

Total Nursing Enrollment: *122* • Full-Time Enrollment:
122 • Part-Time Enrollment: *Not Reported* • Female
Enrollment: *113* • Male Enrollment: *9* • Total New
Admissions Who Enrolled for Fall: *20* • Total Graduates: *36*

FINANCES

Residential Annual Tuition: *Not Reported* • Non-Residential
Annual Tuition: *Not Reported* • General Institution Fees: *Not
Reported* • Additional Nursing Fees: *$60*

NORTHWEST COLLEGE

Address: 231 West 6th Street, Powell, WA 82435
Phone: 307-754-6479
Fax: 307-754-6721
Contact: Marlys Ohman, MN, RN, Director of Nursing
Email: mfohman@nwc.cc.wy.us

OLYMPIC COLLEGE

Address: 1600 Chester Avenue, Bremeton, WA 98310
Phone: 360-475-7751
Fax: 360-475-7508
Contact: Marge Herzog, MN, RN, Assistant Dean for RN, PN, and Nursing Assistant Programs
Email: mherzog@oc.ctc.edu

GENERAL INFORMATION

Type of School: *2-Year College or University, Public* • Accreditation: *North Central Association of Colleges and Schools* • Total Enrollment: *1900*

GENERAL INFORMATION

Type of School: *2-Year College or University, Public* • Accreditation: *Northwestern Association of Schools and Colleges* • Total Enrollment: *12103*

PROGRAM INFORMATION

LPN/LVN Exit: *Yes* • NLNAC Accreditation: *No*

PROGRAM INFORMATION

LPN/LVN Exit: *No* • NLNAC Accreditation: *Yes*

NURSING STUDENT PROFILE

Total Nursing Enrollment: *43* • Full-Time Enrollment: *20* • Part-Time Enrollment: *23* • Female Enrollment: *37* • Male Enrollment: *6* • Total New Admissions Who Enrolled for Fall: *20* • Total Graduates: *16*

NURSING STUDENT PROFILE

Total Nursing Enrollment: *85* • Full-Time Enrollment: *85* • Part-Time Enrollment: *Not Reported* • Female Enrollment: *74* • Male Enrollment: *11* • Total New Admissions Who Enrolled for Fall: *47* • Total Graduates: *27*

FINANCES

Residential Annual Tuition: *$1,128* • Non-Residential Annual Tuition: *$3,384* • General Institution Fees: *$198* • Additional Nursing Fees: *$116*

FINANCES

Residential Annual Tuition: *$1,671* • Non-Residential Annual Tuition: *$6,489* • General Institution Fees: *Not Reported* • Additional Nursing Fees: *Not Reported*

PENINSULA COLLEGE

Address: 1502 E Lauridsen, Port Angeles, WA 98362
Phone: 360-452-9277
Fax: 360-457-8100
Contact: Marcia Davies, MSN, RN, Coordinator
Email: Not Reported

GENERAL INFORMATION

Type of School: *Not Reported* • Accreditation: *Not Reported* •
Total Enrollment: *Not Reported*

PROGRAM INFORMATION

LPN/LVN Exit: *Not Reported* • NLNAC Accreditation: *No*

NURSING STUDENT PROFILE

Total Nursing Enrollment: *Not Reported* • Full-Time
Enrollment: *Not Reported* • Part-Time Enrollment: *Not
Reported* • Female Enrollment: *Not Reported* • Male
Enrollment: *Not Reported* • Total New Admissions Who
Enrolled for Fall: *Not Reported* • Total Graduates: *Not
Reported*

FINANCES

Residential Annual Tuition: *Not Reported* • Non-Residential
Annual Tuition: *Not Reported* • General Institution Fees: *Not
Reported* • Additional Nursing Fees: *Not Reported*

SEATTLE CENTRAL COMMUNITY COLLEGE

Address: 1701 Broadway 2BE3210, Seattle, WA 98122
Phone: 206-344-4326
Fax: 206-344-4390
Contact: Maria Azpitarte, , Director
Email: Not Reported

GENERAL INFORMATION

Type of School: *Not Reported* • Accreditation: *Not Reported* •
Total Enrollment: *Not Reported*

PROGRAM INFORMATION

LPN/LVN Exit: *No* • NLNAC Accreditation: *Yes*

NURSING STUDENT PROFILE

Total Nursing Enrollment: *24* • Full-Time Enrollment: *24* •
Part-Time Enrollment: *Not Reported* • Female Enrollment:
15 • Male Enrollment: *9* • Total New Admissions Who
Enrolled for Fall: *18* • Total Graduates: *16*

FINANCES

Residential Annual Tuition: *$2,012* • Non-Residential
Annual Tuition: *$7,940* • General Institution Fees: *$108* •
Additional Nursing Fees: *Not Reported*

SHORELINE COMMUNITY COLLEGE

Address: 16101 Greenwood Ave N, Seattle, WA 98133
Phone: 206-546-4756
Fax: 206-533-5103
Contact: Janice R Ellis, PhD, RN, Director
Email: jellis@ctc.edu

GENERAL INFORMATION

Type of School: *2-Year College or University, Private (Independent)* • Accreditation: *Northwestern Association of Schools and Colleges* • Total Enrollment: *4500*

PROGRAM INFORMATION

LPN/LVN Exit: *No* • NLNAC Accreditation: *Yes*

NURSING STUDENT PROFILE

Total Nursing Enrollment: *171* • Full-Time Enrollment: *171* • Part-Time Enrollment: *Not Reported* • Female Enrollment: *141* • Male Enrollment: *30* • Total New Admissions Who Enrolled for Fall: *35* • Total Graduates: *72*

FINANCES

Residential Annual Tuition: *$1,632* • Non-Residential Annual Tuition: *$6,450* • General Institution Fees: *$165* • Additional Nursing Fees: *$107*

SKAGIT VALLEY COLLEGE

Address: 2405 East College Way, Mount Vernon, WA 98273
Phone: 360-416-7631
Fax: 360-416-6596
Contact: Flora Adams, MSN, RNC, Co-chair SVC Nursing
Email: adams@skagit.ctc.edu

GENERAL INFORMATION

Type of School: *2-Year College or University, Public* • Accreditation: *Northwestern Association of Schools and Colleges* • Total Enrollment: *6700*

PROGRAM INFORMATION

LPN/LVN Exit: *Yes* • NLNAC Accreditation: *Yes*

NURSING STUDENT PROFILE

Total Nursing Enrollment: *122* • Full-Time Enrollment: *101* • Part-Time Enrollment: *21* • Female Enrollment: *108* • Male Enrollment: *14* • Total New Admissions Who Enrolled for Fall: *93* • Total Graduates: *49*

FINANCES

Residential Annual Tuition: *$1,362* • Non-Residential Annual Tuition: *$5,808* • General Institution Fees: *$153* • Additional Nursing Fees: *$16*

SOUTH PUGET SOUND

Address: 2011 Mottman Road Southwest, Olympia, WA 98512
Phone: 360-754-7711
Fax: 360-664-0780
Contact: Marilyn Adair, MSN, RN, Director of Nursing
Email: madair@spscc.ctc.edu

TACOMA COMMUNITY COLLEGE

Address: 6501 South 19th Street, Tacoma, WA 98466
Phone: 253-566-5225
Fax: 253-566-5273
Contact: Susan Ford, MN, RN, Nursing Program Chair
Email: sford@rcc.tacoma.ctc.edu

GENERAL INFORMATION

Type of School: *2-Year College or University, Public* • Accreditation: *Northwestern Association of Schools and Colleges* • Total Enrollment: *5678*

GENERAL INFORMATION

Type of School: *2-Year College or University, Public* • Accreditation: *Northwestern Association of Schools and Colleges* • Total Enrollment: *8350*

PROGRAM INFORMATION

LPN/LVN Exit: *No* • NLNAC Accreditation: *Yes*

PROGRAM INFORMATION

LPN/LVN Exit: *No* • NLNAC Accreditation: *Yes*

NURSING STUDENT PROFILE

Total Nursing Enrollment: *57* • Full-Time Enrollment: *38* • Part-Time Enrollment: *19* • Female Enrollment: *49* • Male Enrollment: *8* • Total New Admissions Who Enrolled for Fall: *57* • Total Graduates: *27*

NURSING STUDENT PROFILE

Total Nursing Enrollment: *91* • Full-Time Enrollment: *91* • Part-Time Enrollment: *Not Reported* • Female Enrollment: *83* • Male Enrollment: *8* • Total New Admissions Who Enrolled for Fall: *36* • Total Graduates: *40*

FINANCES

Residential Annual Tuition: *$1,743* • Non-Residential Annual Tuition: *Not Reported* • General Institution Fees: *$170* • Additional Nursing Fees: *$155*

FINANCES

Residential Annual Tuition: *$1,749* • Non-Residential Annual Tuition: *$2,121* • General Institution Fees: *Not Reported* • Additional Nursing Fees: *$54*

WALLA WALLA COMMUNITY COLLEGE

Address: 500 Tausick Way, Walla Walla, WA 99362
Phone: 509-527-4240
Fax: 509-527-4226
Contact: Marilyn D Galusha, MS, RN, Director of Nursing
Email: marilyn.galusha@po.ww.cc.wa.us

GENERAL INFORMATION

Type of School: *Other* • Accreditation: *None* • Total Enrollment: *Not Reported*

PROGRAM INFORMATION

LPN/LVN Exit: *Yes* • NLNAC Accreditation: *Yes*

NURSING STUDENT PROFILE

Total Nursing Enrollment: *188* • Full-Time Enrollment: *188* • Part-Time Enrollment: *Not Reported* • Female Enrollment: *162* • Male Enrollment: *26* • Total New Admissions Who Enrolled for Fall: *101* • Total Graduates: *116*

FINANCES

Residential Annual Tuition: *Not Reported* • Non-Residential Annual Tuition: *Not Reported* • General Institution Fees: *$40* • Additional Nursing Fees: *Not Reported*

WENATCHEE VALLEY COLLEGE

Address: 1300 Fifth Street, Wenatchee, WA 98801
Phone: 509-665-2605
Fax: 509-664-2509
Contact: Connie Barnes, MSN, RN, Director of Allied Health and Safety
Email: cbarnes@wvcmail.ctc.edu

GENERAL INFORMATION

Type of School: *2-Year College or University, Public* • Accreditation: *Northwestern Association of Schools and Colleges* • Total Enrollment: *81*

PROGRAM INFORMATION

LPN/LVN Exit: *Yes* • NLNAC Accreditation: *Yes*

NURSING STUDENT PROFILE

Total Nursing Enrollment: *81* • Full-Time Enrollment: *81* • Part-Time Enrollment: *Not Reported* • Female Enrollment: *75* • Male Enrollment: *6* • Total New Admissions Who Enrolled for Fall: *49* • Total Graduates: *32*

FINANCES

Residential Annual Tuition: *$2,188* • Non-Residential Annual Tuition: *$2,684* • General Institution Fees: *Not Reported* • Additional Nursing Fees: *$200*

YAKIMA VALLLEY COMMUNITY COLLEGE

Address: PO Box 22520, Yakima, WA 98907
Phone: 509-574-4909
Fax: 509-574-4669
Contact: Rhonda Taylor, MSN, ARNP, Program
            Coordinator
Email: rtaylor@yvcc.cc.wa.us

BLUEFIELD STATE COLLEGE

Address: 219 Rock Street, Bluefield, WV 24701
Phone: 304-327-4144
Fax: 304-327-4219
Contact: Carol Cofer, MSN, MEd, RN, CS, Director
Email: ccofer@bluefield.wvnet.edu

GENERAL INFORMATION

Type of School: *2-Year College or University, Public* •
Accreditation: *Northwestern Association of Schools and
Colleges* • Total Enrollment: *10277*

GENERAL INFORMATION

Type of School: *4-Year College or University, Public* •
Accreditation: *North Central Association of Colleges and
Schools* • Total Enrollment: *2648*

PROGRAM INFORMATION

LPN/LVN Exit: *Yes* • NLNAC Accreditation: *Yes*

PROGRAM INFORMATION

LPN/LVN Exit: *No* • NLNAC Accreditation: *Yes*

NURSING STUDENT PROFILE

Total Nursing Enrollment: *87* • Full-Time Enrollment: *87* •
Part-Time Enrollment: *Not Reported* • Female Enrollment:
76 • Male Enrollment: *11* • Total New Admissions Who
Enrolled for Fall: *24* • Total Graduates: *37*

NURSING STUDENT PROFILE

Total Nursing Enrollment: *105* • Full-Time Enrollment: *82* •
Part-Time Enrollment: *23* • Female Enrollment: *91* • Male
Enrollment: *14* • Total New Admissions Who Enrolled for
Fall: *61* • Total Graduates: *48*

FINANCES

Residential Annual Tuition: *$2,288* • Non-Residential
Annual Tuition: *$8,712* • General Institution Fees: *$75* •
Additional Nursing Fees: *$108*

FINANCES

Residential Annual Tuition: *$2,288* • Non-Residential
Annual Tuition: *$5,554* • General Institution Fees: *Not
Reported* • Additional Nursing Fees: *$230*

DAVIS & ELKINS COLLEGE

Address: 100 Campus Drive, Elkins, WV 26241
Phone: 304-637-1314
Fax: 304-637-1413
Contact: R Carol Cochran, DNSc, RN, Director and Chair, Department of Nursing
Email: ccochran@dne.edu

GENERAL INFORMATION

Type of School: *4-Year College or University, Private (Religious)* • Accreditation: *North Central Association of Colleges and Schools* • Total Enrollment: *600*

PROGRAM INFORMATION

LPN/LVN Exit: *No* • NLNAC Accreditation: *Yes*

NURSING STUDENT PROFILE

Total Nursing Enrollment: *64* • Full-Time Enrollment: *60* • Part-Time Enrollment: *4* • Female Enrollment: *59* • Male Enrollment: *5* • Total New Admissions Who Enrolled for Fall: *30* • Total Graduates: *17*

FINANCES

Residential Annual Tuition: *$12,624* • Non-Residential Annual Tuition: *$12,624* • General Institution Fees: *$400* • Additional Nursing Fees: *Not Reported*

FAIRMONT STATE COLLEGE

Address: 1201 Locust Avenue, Fairmont, WV 26554
Phone: 304-367-4767
Fax: 304-367-4268
Contact: Deborah M Kisner, EdD, RN, Chairperson and Director
Email: dkisner@mail.fscww.edu

GENERAL INFORMATION

Type of School: *4-Year College or University, Public* • Accreditation: *North Central Association of Colleges and Schools* • Total Enrollment: *6600*

PROGRAM INFORMATION

LPN/LVN Exit: *No* • NLNAC Accreditation: *Yes*

NURSING STUDENT PROFILE

Total Nursing Enrollment: *125* • Full-Time Enrollment: *81* • Part-Time Enrollment: *44* • Female Enrollment: *116* • Male Enrollment: *9* • Total New Admissions Who Enrolled for Fall: *80* • Total Graduates: *48*

FINANCES

Residential Annual Tuition: *$2,408* • Non-Residential Annual Tuition: *$5,672* • General Institution Fees: *$200* • Additional Nursing Fees: *$160*

SHEPHERD COLLEGE

Address:　PO Box 3210, Shepherdstown, WV 25443
Phone:　304-876-5341
Fax:　304-876-5169
Contact:　Lynn E Hanson, MSN, RN, Chair, Department
　　　　　of Nursing Education
Email:　lhanson@shepherd.edu

GENERAL INFORMATION

Type of School: *4-Year College or University, Public* •
Accreditation: *North Central Association of Colleges and
Schools* • Total Enrollment: *4600*

PROGRAM INFORMATION

LPN/LVN Exit: *Not Reported* • NLNAC Accreditation: *Yes*

NURSING STUDENT PROFILE

Total Nursing Enrollment: *43* • Full-Time Enrollment: *43* •
Part-Time Enrollment: *Not Reported* • Female Enrollment:
41 • Male Enrollment: *2* • Total New Admissions Who
Enrolled for Fall: *20* • Total Graduates: *18*

FINANCES

Residential Annual Tuition: *$2,608* • Non-Residential
Annual Tuition: *$6,294* • General Institution Fees: *$40* •
Additional Nursing Fees: *$140*

SOUTHERN WEST VIRGINIA COMMUNITY AND TECHNICAL COLLEGE

Address:　PO Box 2900, Mount Gay, WV 25637
Phone:　304-792-7098
Fax:　304-792-7053
Contact:　Barbara Donahue, MSN, RN, Nursing
　　　　　Coordinator
Email:　pollyd@southern.wvnet.edu

GENERAL INFORMATION

Type of School: *2-Year College or University, Public* •
Accreditation: *North Central Association of Colleges and
Schools* • Total Enrollment: *2357*

PROGRAM INFORMATION

LPN/LVN Exit: *No* • NLNAC Accreditation: *Yes*

NURSING STUDENT PROFILE

Total Nursing Enrollment: *101* • Full-Time Enrollment:
101 • Part-Time Enrollment: *0* • Female Enrollment: *79* •
Male Enrollment: *22* • Total New Admissions Who Enrolled
for Fall: *60* • Total Graduates: *26*

FINANCES

Residential Annual Tuition: *$1,440* • Non-Residential
Annual Tuition: *$5,564* • General Institution Fees: *Not
Reported* • Additional Nursing Fees: *Not Reported*

ST. MARY'S HOSPITAL AND MARSHALL UNIVERSITY

Address: 2900 First Avenue, Huntington, WV 25702
Phone: 304-526-1416
Fax: 304-526-1517
Contact: Barbara Stevens, EdD, MSN, RN, Director
Email: Bstevens@st-marys.org

GENERAL INFORMATION

Type of School: *4-Year College or University, Public* •
Accreditation: *North Central Association of Colleges and Schools* • Total Enrollment: *16000*

PROGRAM INFORMATION

LPN/LVN Exit: *No* • NLNAC Accreditation: *Yes*

NURSING STUDENT PROFILE

Total Nursing Enrollment: *121* • Full-Time Enrollment: *121* • Part-Time Enrollment: *Not Reported* • Female Enrollment: *104* • Male Enrollment: *17* • Total New Admissions Who Enrolled for Fall: *68* • Total Graduates: *46*

FINANCES

Residential Annual Tuition: *$3,174* • Non-Residential Annual Tuition: *$5,927* • General Institution Fees: *$270* • Additional Nursing Fees: *$180*

UNIVERSITY OF CHARLESTON

Address: 2300 McCorkle Avenue, SE, Charleston, WV 25304
Phone: 304-357-4836
Fax: 304-357-4965
Contact: Rosemary N Valentine, MSN, RN, ADN Program Coordinator
Email: rvalentine@ucwv.edu

GENERAL INFORMATION

Type of School: *4-Year College or University, Private (Independent)* • Accreditation: *North Central Association of Colleges and Schools* • Total Enrollment: *955*

PROGRAM INFORMATION

LPN/LVN Exit: *No* • NLNAC Accreditation: *Yes*

NURSING STUDENT PROFILE

Total Nursing Enrollment: *79* • Full-Time Enrollment: *53* • Part-Time Enrollment: *26* • Female Enrollment: *67* • Male Enrollment: *12* • Total New Admissions Who Enrolled for Fall: *42* • Total Graduates: *59*

FINANCES

Residential Annual Tuition: *$13,200* • Non-Residential Annual Tuition: *$13,200* • General Institution Fees: *Not Reported* • Additional Nursing Fees: *$85*

| Circle 122 on reader card | See in-depth profile for more information |

WEST VIRGINIA NORTHERN COMMUNITY COLLEGE

Address: 1704 Market Street, Wheeling, WV 26003
Phone: 304-233-5900
Fax: 304-233-5837
Contact: M Regina Jenette, MSN, EdD, RN, Professor
           and Director of Nursing
Email: rjennette@northern.wvnet.edu

WEST VIRGINIA UNIVERSITY

Address: PO Box 9600, Morgantown, WV 26506
Phone: 304-442-3221
Fax: 304-442-3479
Contact: Jean M Hoff, MPH, RN, Interim Chair
Email: Not Reported

GENERAL INFORMATION

Type of School: *2-Year College or University, Public* •
Accreditation: *North Central Association of Colleges and
Schools* • Total Enrollment: *2464*

GENERAL INFORMATION

Type of School: *4-Year College or University, Public* •
Accreditation: *North Central Association of Colleges and
Schools* • Total Enrollment: *22150*

PROGRAM INFORMATION

LPN/LVN Exit: *No* • NLNAC Accreditation: *Yes*

PROGRAM INFORMATION

LPN/LVN Exit: *No* • NLNAC Accreditation: *Yes*

NURSING STUDENT PROFILE

Total Nursing Enrollment: *157* • Full-Time Enrollment:
140 • Part-Time Enrollment: *17* • Female Enrollment: *143* •
Male Enrollment: *14* • Total New Admissions Who Enrolled
for Fall: *75* • Total Graduates: *64*

NURSING STUDENT PROFILE

Total Nursing Enrollment: *81* • Full-Time Enrollment: *81* •
Part-Time Enrollment: *Not Reported* • Female Enrollment:
68 • Male Enrollment: *13* • Total New Admissions Who
Enrolled for Fall: *48* • Total Graduates: *53*

FINANCES

Residential Annual Tuition: *Not Reported* • Non-Residential
Annual Tuition: *Not Reported* • General Institution Fees:
$10 • Additional Nursing Fees: *$54*

FINANCES

Residential Annual Tuition: *$2,370* • Non-Residential
Annual Tuition: *$5,946* • General Institution Fees: *$100* •
Additional Nursing Fees: *Not Reported*

WEST VIRGINIA UNIVERSITY OF PARKERSBURG

Address: 300 Campus Drive, Parkersburg, WV 26101
Phone: 304-424-8300
Fax: 304-424-8315
Contact: Alita K Sellers, PhD, RN, Chairperson, Health Sciences Division
Email: asellers@wvu.edu

GENERAL INFORMATION

Type of School: *2-Year College or University, Public* • Accreditation: *North Central Association of Colleges and Schools* • Total Enrollment: *3200*

PROGRAM INFORMATION

LPN/LVN Exit: *No* • NLNAC Accreditation: *Yes*

NURSING STUDENT PROFILE

Total Nursing Enrollment: *86* • Full-Time Enrollment: *86* • Part-Time Enrollment: *0* • Female Enrollment: *78* • Male Enrollment: *8* • Total New Admissions Who Enrolled for Fall: *48* • Total Graduates: *43*

FINANCES

Residential Annual Tuition: *$1,436* • Non-Residential Annual Tuition: *$4,410* • General Institution Fees: *$200* • Additional Nursing Fees: *$200*

BLACKHAWK TECHNICAL COLLEGE

Address: PO Box 5009, Janesville, WI 53547
Phone: 608-757-7678
Fax: 608-743-4407
Contact: Thomas Neumann, MSN, RN, Nursing Coordinator
Email: tneumann@blackhawk.tec.wi.us

GENERAL INFORMATION

Type of School: *Vocational/Technical School, Public* • Accreditation: *North Central Association of Colleges and Schools* • Total Enrollment: *13817*

PROGRAM INFORMATION

LPN/LVN Exit: *Yes* • NLNAC Accreditation: *Yes*

NURSING STUDENT PROFILE

Total Nursing Enrollment: *163* • Full-Time Enrollment: *18* • Part-Time Enrollment: *145* • Female Enrollment: *157* • Male Enrollment: *6* • Total New Admissions Who Enrolled for Fall: *60* • Total Graduates: *32*

FINANCES

Residential Annual Tuition: *$2,600* • Non-Residential Annual Tuition: *Not Reported* • General Institution Fees: *$150* • Additional Nursing Fees: *$100*

CARDINAL STRITCH UNIVERSITY

Address: 6801 North Yates Road, Milwaukee, WI 53217
Phone: 414-410-4390
Fax: 414-410-4385
Contact: Nancy Cervenansky, PhD, RN, NCC, Dean
Email: ncerven@stritch.edu

GENERAL INFORMATION

Type of School: *4-Year College or University, Private (Religious)* • Accreditation: *North Central Association of Colleges and Schools* • Total Enrollment: *5700*

PROGRAM INFORMATION

LPN/LVN Exit: *No* • NLNAC Accreditation: *Yes*

NURSING STUDENT PROFILE

Total Nursing Enrollment: *165* • Full-Time Enrollment: *87* • Part-Time Enrollment: *78* • Female Enrollment: *149* • Male Enrollment: *16* • Total New Admissions Who Enrolled for Fall: *71* • Total Graduates: *47*

FINANCES

Residential Annual Tuition: *$12,480* • Non-Residential Annual Tuition: *Not Reported* • General Institution Fees: *$300* • Additional Nursing Fees: *$0*

CHIPPEWA VALLEY TECHNICAL COLLEGE

Address: 620 West Clairmont Avenue, Eau Claire, WI 54701
Phone: 715-833-6419
Fax: 715-833-6470
Contact: Margaret Dickens, MSN, RN, Campus Administrator
Email: mdickens@chippewa.tec.wi.us

GENERAL INFORMATION

Type of School: *Vocational/Technical School, Public* • Accreditation: *North Central Association of Colleges and Schools* • Total Enrollment: *5060*

PROGRAM INFORMATION

LPN/LVN Exit: *No* • NLNAC Accreditation: *Yes*

NURSING STUDENT PROFILE

Total Nursing Enrollment: *151* • Full-Time Enrollment: *41* • Part-Time Enrollment: *110* • Female Enrollment: *144* • Male Enrollment: *7* • Total New Admissions Who Enrolled for Fall: *54* • Total Graduates: *42*

FINANCES

Residential Annual Tuition: *$2,176* • Non-Residential Annual Tuition: *$16,986* • General Institution Fees: *$39* • Additional Nursing Fees: *$28*

COLUMBIA COLLEGE OF NURSING

Address: 2121 East Newport Avenue, Milwaukee, WI 53211
Phone: 573-886-2276
Fax: 573-886-2080
Contact: Sharon K. Taylor, MSN, RN, Director
Email: staylor@columbia.k-12.mo.us

GENERAL INFORMATION

Type of School: *4-Year College or University, Private (Independent)* • Accreditation: *North Central Association of Colleges and Schools* • Total Enrollment: *194*

PROGRAM INFORMATION

LPN/LVN Exit: *Not Reported* • NLNAC Accreditation: *No*

NURSING STUDENT PROFILE

Total Nursing Enrollment: *18* • Full-Time Enrollment: *18* • Part-Time Enrollment: *0* • Female Enrollment: *16* • Male Enrollment: *2* • Total New Admissions Who Enrolled for Fall: *20* • Total Graduates: *15*

FINANCES

Residential Annual Tuition: *$5,400* • Non-Residential Annual Tuition: *Not Reported* • General Institution Fees: *$3,120* • Additional Nursing Fees: *$350*

FOX VALLEY TECHNICAL COLLEGE

Address: 1825 North Bluemound Drive, Appleton, WI 54912-2277
Phone: 920-735-5664
Fax: 920-735-2582
Contact: Ardythe Korpela, MSN, RN, Department Chair, Nursing
Email: korpela@foxvalleytech.com

GENERAL INFORMATION

Type of School: *Vocational/Technical School, Public* • Accreditation: *North Central Association of Colleges and Schools* • Total Enrollment: *6100*

PROGRAM INFORMATION

LPN/LVN Exit: *No* • NLNAC Accreditation: *Yes*

NURSING STUDENT PROFILE

Total Nursing Enrollment: *106* • Full-Time Enrollment: *35* • Part-Time Enrollment: *71* • Female Enrollment: *100* • Male Enrollment: *6* • Total New Admissions Who Enrolled for Fall: *31* • Total Graduates: *56*

FINANCES

Residential Annual Tuition: *$2,608* • Non-Residential Annual Tuition: *$15,672* • General Institution Fees: *$425* • Additional Nursing Fees: *$39*

GATEWAY TECHNICAL COLLEGE

Address: 3520 30th Ave, Kenosha, WI 53144
Phone: 262-564-3074
Fax: 262-564-2007
Contact: Kathleen L. Russ, MSN, RN, Dean of Student
            Support and Health Careers
Email: russk@gateway.tcc.wi.us

GENERAL INFORMATION

Type of School: *Not Reported* • Accreditation: *Not Reported* •
Total Enrollment: *Not Reported*

PROGRAM INFORMATION

LPN/LVN Exit: *No* • NLNAC Accreditation: *Yes*

NURSING STUDENT PROFILE

Total Nursing Enrollment: *204* • Full-Time Enrollment: *14* •
Part-Time Enrollment: *190* • Female Enrollment: *192* • Male
Enrollment: *12* • Total New Admissions Who Enrolled for
Fall: *60* • Total Graduates: *88*

FINANCES

Residential Annual Tuition: *$4,416* • Non-Residential
Annual Tuition: *Not Reported* • General Institution Fees: *Not
Reported* • Additional Nursing Fees: *Not Reported*

LAKESHORE TECHNICAL COLLEGE

Address: 1290 North Avenue, Cleveland, WI 53015
Phone: 920-693-1661
Fax: 920-693-8955
Contact: Marilyn Kaufmann, PhD, RN, Chair, Associate
            Degree Nursing Program
Email: maka@ltc.tec.wi.us

GENERAL INFORMATION

Type of School: *Vocational/Technical School, Public* •
Accreditation: *North Central Association of Colleges and
Schools* • Total Enrollment: *2886*

PROGRAM INFORMATION

LPN/LVN Exit: *Yes* • NLNAC Accreditation: *Yes*

NURSING STUDENT PROFILE

Total Nursing Enrollment: *107* • Full-Time Enrollment: *40* •
Part-Time Enrollment: *67* • Female Enrollment: *101* • Male
Enrollment: *6* • Total New Admissions Who Enrolled for
Fall: *47* • Total Graduates: *32*

FINANCES

Residential Annual Tuition: *Not Reported* • Non-Residential
Annual Tuition: *Not Reported* • General Institution Fees: *$0* •
Additional Nursing Fees: *$272*

MADISON AREA TECHNICAL COLLEGE

Address: 3550 Anderson Street, Madison, WI 53704-2599
Phone: 608-246-6674
Fax: 308-246-6013
Contact: Marilyn Rinehart, MSN, Associate Dean, Nursing
Email: mrinehart@madison.tec.wi.us

GENERAL INFORMATION

Type of School: *2-Year College or University, Public* • Accreditation: *North Central Association of Colleges and Schools* • Total Enrollment: *13921*

PROGRAM INFORMATION

LPN/LVN Exit: *Not Reported* • NLNAC Accreditation: *Yes*

NURSING STUDENT PROFILE

Total Nursing Enrollment: *269* • Full-Time Enrollment: *160* • Part-Time Enrollment: *109* • Female Enrollment: *246* • Male Enrollment: *23* • Total New Admissions Who Enrolled for Fall: *58* • Total Graduates: *100*

FINANCES

Residential Annual Tuition: *Not Reported* • Non-Residential Annual Tuition: *Not Reported* • General Institution Fees: *Not Reported* • Additional Nursing Fees: *Not Reported*

MID STATE TECHNICAL COLLEGE

Address: 500 32nd Street North, Wisconsin Rapids, WI 54494
Phone: 715-422-5510
Fax: 715-422-5313
Contact: Mary Moss, MSN, EdD, RN, Associate Dean, Health
Email: mmoss@midstate.tech.wi.us

GENERAL INFORMATION

Type of School: *2-Year College or University, Public* • Accreditation: *North Central Association of Colleges and Schools* • Total Enrollment: *500*

PROGRAM INFORMATION

LPN/LVN Exit: *No* • NLNAC Accreditation: *Yes*

NURSING STUDENT PROFILE

Total Nursing Enrollment: *96* • Full-Time Enrollment: *50* • Part-Time Enrollment: *46* • Female Enrollment: *89* • Male Enrollment: *7* • Total New Admissions Who Enrolled for Fall: *49* • Total Graduates: *26*

FINANCES

Residential Annual Tuition: *Not Reported* • Non-Residential Annual Tuition: *Not Reported* • General Institution Fees: *$15* • Additional Nursing Fees: *$60*

MILWAUKEE AREA TECHNICAL COLLEGE

Address: 700 West State Street, Milwaukee, WI 53233
Phone: 414-297-6241
Fax: 414-297-6851
Contact: Nancy J Vrabec, PhD, RNC, Associate Dean, Nursing
Email: Vrabecn@matc.edu

GENERAL INFORMATION

Type of School: *Vocational/Technical School, Public* •
Accreditation: *North Central Association of Colleges and Schools* • Total Enrollment: *60000*

PROGRAM INFORMATION

LPN/LVN Exit: *No* • NLNAC Accreditation: *Yes*

NURSING STUDENT PROFILE

Total Nursing Enrollment: *307* • Full-Time Enrollment: *307* • Part-Time Enrollment: *Not Reported* • Female Enrollment: *270* • Male Enrollment: *37* • Total New Admissions Who Enrolled for Fall: *90* • Total Graduates: *110*

FINANCES

Residential Annual Tuition: *$4,020* • Non-Residential Annual Tuition: *Not Reported* • General Institution Fees: *$30* • Additional Nursing Fees: *$35*

MORAINE PARK TECHNICAL COLLEGE

Address: 2151 North Main Street, West Bend, WI 53090
Phone: 262-335-5782
Fax: 262-335-5708
Contact: Anne Kersbergen, PhD, RN, Nursing Program Director
Email: akersbergen@moraine.tec.wi.us

GENERAL INFORMATION

Type of School: *2-Year College or University, Public* •
Accreditation: *North Central Association of Colleges and Schools* • Total Enrollment: *1200*

PROGRAM INFORMATION

LPN/LVN Exit: *No* • NLNAC Accreditation: *Yes*

NURSING STUDENT PROFILE

Total Nursing Enrollment: *116* • Full-Time Enrollment: *108* • Part-Time Enrollment: *8* • Female Enrollment: *114* • Male Enrollment: *2* • Total New Admissions Who Enrolled for Fall: *41* • Total Graduates: *31*

FINANCES

Residential Annual Tuition: *Not Reported* • Non-Residential Annual Tuition: *Not Reported* • General Institution Fees: *Not Reported* • Additional Nursing Fees: *Not Reported*

NICOLET AREA TECHNICAL COLLEGE

Address: PO Box 518, Rhinelander, WI 54501
Phone: 715-365-4638
Fax: 715-365-4603
Contact: Rena K Hemlock, MSN, RN, Program Director
Email: rhemlock@nicolet.tec.wi.us

GENERAL INFORMATION

Type of School: *Vocational/Technical School, Public* •
Accreditation: *North Central Association of Colleges and Schools* • Total Enrollment: *1458*

PROGRAM INFORMATION

LPN/LVN Exit: *No* • NLNAC Accreditation: *Yes*

NURSING STUDENT PROFILE

Total Nursing Enrollment: *53* • Full-Time Enrollment: *53* •
Part-Time Enrollment: *0* • Female Enrollment: *48* • Male
Enrollment: *5* • Total New Admissions Who Enrolled for
Fall: *27* • Total Graduates: *19*

FINANCES

Residential Annual Tuition: *$3,170* • Non-Residential
Annual Tuition: *Not Reported* • General Institution Fees: *Not Reported* • Additional Nursing Fees: *$350*

NORTHCENTRAL TECHNICAL COLLEGE

Address: 1000 West Campus Drive, Wausau, WI 54401
Phone: 715-675-3331
Fax: 715-675-9776
Contact: Jean Flood, MSN, RN, Team Leader, Nursing
Email: flood@ntc.edu

GENERAL INFORMATION

Type of School: *Vocational/Technical School, Public* •
Accreditation: *North Central Association of Colleges and Schools* • Total Enrollment: *3821*

PROGRAM INFORMATION

LPN/LVN Exit: *No* • NLNAC Accreditation: *Yes*

NURSING STUDENT PROFILE

Total Nursing Enrollment: *127* • Full-Time Enrollment: *27* •
Part-Time Enrollment: *100* • Female Enrollment: *118* • Male
Enrollment: *9* • Total New Admissions Who Enrolled for
Fall: *39* • Total Graduates: *39*

FINANCES

Residential Annual Tuition: *Not Reported* • Non-Residential
Annual Tuition: *Not Reported* • General Institution Fees: *$7* •
Additional Nursing Fees: *$0*

NORTHEAST WISCONSIN TECHNICAL COLLEGE

Address: 2740 West Mason Street, Green Bay, WI 54303
Phone: 920-498-5482
Fax: 920-498-5673
Contact: Kathleen Resch, MSN, RN, Liaison Coordinator
Email: kresch@nwtc.tec.wi.us

SOUTHWEST WISCONSIN TECHNICAL COLLEGE

Address: 1800 Bronson Boulevard, Fennimore, WI 53809
Phone: 608-822-3262
Fax: 608-822-6019
Contact: Sharon Sellech-Lehman, MSN, MSEd, RN,
           Dean of Health Occupations
Email: slehman@southwest.tec.wi.us

GENERAL INFORMATION

Type of School: *Vocational/Technical School, Public* • Accreditation: *North Central Association of Colleges and Schools* • Total Enrollment: *440*

GENERAL INFORMATION

Type of School: *Vocational/Technical School, Public* • Accreditation: *North Central Association of Colleges and Schools* • Total Enrollment: *1540*

PROGRAM INFORMATION

LPN/LVN Exit: *No* • NLNAC Accreditation: *Yes*

PROGRAM INFORMATION

LPN/LVN Exit: *No* • NLNAC Accreditation: *Yes*

NURSING STUDENT PROFILE

Total Nursing Enrollment: *125* • Full-Time Enrollment: *62* • Part-Time Enrollment: *63* • Female Enrollment: *119* • Male Enrollment: *6* • Total New Admissions Who Enrolled for Fall: *81* • Total Graduates: *45*

NURSING STUDENT PROFILE

Total Nursing Enrollment: *88* • Full-Time Enrollment: *44* • Part-Time Enrollment: *44* • Female Enrollment: *81* • Male Enrollment: *7* • Total New Admissions Who Enrolled for Fall: *17* • Total Graduates: *26*

FINANCES

Residential Annual Tuition: *Not Reported* • Non-Residential Annual Tuition: *Not Reported* • General Institution Fees: *$30* • Additional Nursing Fees: *$2,364*

FINANCES

Residential Annual Tuition: *$2,248* • Non-Residential Annual Tuition: *$17,399* • General Institution Fees: *Not Reported* • Additional Nursing Fees: *Not Reported*

WAUKESHA COUNTY TECHNICAL COLLEGE

Address: 800 Main Street, Pewaukee, WI 53072
Phone: 262-691-5368
Fax: 262-691-7835
Contact: Kitty Gotham, EdD, RN, Associate Dean, Nursing
Email: Kgotham@waukesha.tec.wi.us

GENERAL INFORMATION

Type of School: *Vocational/Technical School, Public* •
Accreditation: *North Central Association of Colleges and Schools* • Total Enrollment: *22715*

PROGRAM INFORMATION

LPN/LVN Exit: *No* • NLNAC Accreditation: *Yes*

NURSING STUDENT PROFILE

Total Nursing Enrollment: *123* • Full-Time Enrollment: *123* • Part-Time Enrollment: *Not Reported* • Female Enrollment: *120* • Male Enrollment: *3* • Total New Admissions Who Enrolled for Fall: *65* • Total Graduates: *43*

FINANCES

Residential Annual Tuition: *Not Reported* • Non-Residential Annual Tuition: *Not Reported* • General Institution Fees: *Not Reported* • Additional Nursing Fees: *$90*

WESTERN WISCONSIN TECHNICAL COLLEGE

Address: 304 North 6th Street, La Crosse, WI 54602
Phone: 608-785-9196
Fax: 608-785-9194
Contact: Donna Destree, MS, RN, Head of AD Nursing Program
Email: destreed@western.tec.wi.us

GENERAL INFORMATION

Type of School: *Technical/Specialized Institution, Public* •
Accreditation: *North Central Association of Colleges and Schools* • Total Enrollment: *4300*

PROGRAM INFORMATION

LPN/LVN Exit: *No* • NLNAC Accreditation: *Yes*

NURSING STUDENT PROFILE

Total Nursing Enrollment: *128* • Full-Time Enrollment: *43* • Part-Time Enrollment: *85* • Female Enrollment: *115* • Male Enrollment: *13* • Total New Admissions Who Enrolled for Fall: *48* • Total Graduates: *45*

FINANCES

Residential Annual Tuition: *$2,214* • Non-Residential Annual Tuition: *$12,328* • General Institution Fees: *$182* • Additional Nursing Fees: *$54*

WISCONSIN INDIANHEAD TECHNICAL COLLEGE

Address: 505 Pine Ridge Drive, Shell Lake, WI 54871
Phone: 715-468-2815
Fax: 715-468-2819
Contact: Piper Larson, MSN, Dean
Email: plarson@witc.tec.wi.us

GENERAL INFORMATION

Type of School: *Vocational/Technical School, Public* •
Accreditation: *North Central Association of Colleges and Schools* • Total Enrollment: *25000*

PROGRAM INFORMATION

LPN/LVN Exit: *No* • NLNAC Accreditation: *Yes*

NURSING STUDENT PROFILE

Total Nursing Enrollment: *133* • Full-Time Enrollment: *14* •
Part-Time Enrollment: *119* • Female Enrollment: *11* • Male
Enrollment: *122* • Total New Admissions Who Enrolled for
Fall: *121* • Total Graduates: *50*

FINANCES

Residential Annual Tuition: *Not Reported* • Non-Residential
Annual Tuition: *Not Reported* • General Institution Fees: *Not
Reported* • Additional Nursing Fees: *$300*

CASPER COLLEGE

Address: HS 202A, 125 College Drive, Casper, WY 82601
Phone: 307-268-2717
Fax: 307-268-2087
Contact: Jolene Knaus, MS, RN, Director
Email: jknaus@acad.cc.whecn.edu

GENERAL INFORMATION

Type of School: *2-Year College or University, Public* •
Accreditation: *North Central Association of Colleges and Schools* • Total Enrollment: *3853*

PROGRAM INFORMATION

LPN/LVN Exit: *No* • NLNAC Accreditation: *Yes*

NURSING STUDENT PROFILE

Total Nursing Enrollment: *105* • Full-Time Enrollment: *62* •
Part-Time Enrollment: *43* • Female Enrollment: *97* • Male
Enrollment: *8* • Total New Admissions Who Enrolled for
Fall: *56* • Total Graduates: *38*

FINANCES

Residential Annual Tuition: *$1,320* • Non-Residential
Annual Tuition: *$3,672* • General Institution Fees: *Not
Reported* • Additional Nursing Fees: *$160*

CENTRAL WYOMING COLLEGE

Address: 2660 Peck Avenue, Riverton, WY 82501
Phone: 307-855-2226
Fax: Not Reported
Contact: Manuelita A Burns, MS, RN, Director of Nursing
Email: lburns@cwc.cc.wy.us

GENERAL INFORMATION

Type of School: *2-Year College or University, Public* • Accreditation: *North Central Association of Colleges and Schools* • Total Enrollment: *1500*

PROGRAM INFORMATION

LPN/LVN Exit: *No* • NLNAC Accreditation: *Yes*

NURSING STUDENT PROFILE

Total Nursing Enrollment: *34* • Full-Time Enrollment: *34* • Part-Time Enrollment: *Not Reported* • Female Enrollment: *30* • Male Enrollment: *4* • Total New Admissions Who Enrolled for Fall: *17* • Total Graduates: *13*

FINANCES

Residential Annual Tuition: *$1,052* • Non-Residential Annual Tuition: *$3,156* • General Institution Fees: *$198* • Additional Nursing Fees: *$50*

LARAMIE COUNTY COMMUNITY COLLEGE

Address: 1400 East College Drive, Cheyenne, WY 82007
Phone: 307-778-1133
Fax: 307-778-4386
Contact: Carrie Deselms, MSN, RN, Nursing Coordinator
Email: cdeselms@lcc.cc.wy.us

GENERAL INFORMATION

Type of School: *2-Year College or University, Public* • Accreditation: *North Central Association of Colleges and Schools* • Total Enrollment: *3394*

PROGRAM INFORMATION

LPN/LVN Exit: *Yes* • NLNAC Accreditation: *Yes*

NURSING STUDENT PROFILE

Total Nursing Enrollment: *80* • Full-Time Enrollment: *Not Reported* • Part-Time Enrollment: *Not Reported* • Female Enrollment: *74* • Male Enrollment: *6* • Total New Admissions Who Enrolled for Fall: *52* • Total Graduates: *22*

FINANCES

Residential Annual Tuition: *Not Reported* • Non-Residential Annual Tuition: *Not Reported* • General Institution Fees: *$1,428* • Additional Nursing Fees: *$100*

NORTHERN WYOMING COMMUNITY COLLEGE DISTRICT—GILLETTE

Address: 3059 Coffeen Avenue, PO Box 1500, Sheridan, WY 82801
Phone: 307-686-1358
Fax: 307-686-0339
Contact: Nancy Larmer, MSN, RN, Assistant Dean
Email: nlarmer@mickey.gc.whecn.edu

GENERAL INFORMATION

Type of School: *2-Year College or University, Public* • Accreditation: *North Central Association of Colleges and Schools* • Total Enrollment: *2670*

PROGRAM INFORMATION

LPN/LVN Exit: *No* • NLNAC Accreditation: *Yes*

NURSING STUDENT PROFILE

Total Nursing Enrollment: *Not Reported* • Full-Time Enrollment: *Not Reported* • Part-Time Enrollment: *Not Reported* • Female Enrollment: *Not Reported* • Male Enrollment: *Not Reported* • Total New Admissions Who Enrolled for Fall: *Not Reported* • Total Graduates: *11*

FINANCES

Residential Annual Tuition: *$1,128* • Non-Residential Annual Tuition: *$3,384* • General Institution Fees: *$144* • Additional Nursing Fees: *$35*

NORTHERN WYOMING COMMUNITY COLLEGE DISTRICT—SHERIDAN COLLEGE

Address: 3059 Coffeen Ave., PO Box 1500, Sheridan, WY 828019133
Phone: 307-674-6446
Fax: 307-673-1641
Contact: Trudy R. Munsick, BSN, RN, Director
Email: tmunsick@sc.cc.wy.us

GENERAL INFORMATION

Type of School: *Not Reported* • Accreditation: *North Central Association of Colleges and Schools* • Total Enrollment: *Not Reported*

PROGRAM INFORMATION

LPN/LVN Exit: *No* • NLNAC Accreditation: *Yes*

NURSING STUDENT PROFILE

Total Nursing Enrollment: *24* • Full-Time Enrollment: *17* • Part-Time Enrollment: *7* • Female Enrollment: *19* • Male Enrollment: *5* • Total New Admissions Who Enrolled for Fall: *16* • Total Graduates: *13*

FINANCES

Residential Annual Tuition: *Not Reported* • Non-Residential Annual Tuition: *Not Reported* • General Institution Fees: *Not Reported* • Additional Nursing Fees: *$12*

WESTERN WYOMING COMMUNITY COLLEGE

Address:	2500 College Drive, Rock Springs, WY 82901
Phone:	307-382-1801
Fax:	307-382-7665
Contact:	Marlene Ethier, MS, RN, Director of Nursing Program
Email:	methier@wwcc.cc.wy.us

GENERAL INFORMATION

Type of School: *2-Year College or University, Public* • Accreditation: *North Central Association of Colleges and Schools* • Total Enrollment: *2612*

PROGRAM INFORMATION

LPN/LVN Exit: *Yes* • NLNAC Accreditation: *Yes*

NURSING STUDENT PROFILE

Total Nursing Enrollment: *43* • Full-Time Enrollment: *34* • Part-Time Enrollment: *9* • Female Enrollment: *43* • Male Enrollment: *0* • Total New Admissions Who Enrolled for Fall: *24* • Total Graduates: *13*

FINANCES

Residential Annual Tuition: *$1,400* • Non-Residential Annual Tuition: *$3,742* • General Institution Fees: *$222* • Additional Nursing Fees: *$75*

BACCALAUREATE DEGREE PROGRAMS

AUBURN UNIVERSITY

Address: 107 Samford Hall, Auburn University, AL 36849
Phone: 334-844-5662
Fax: 334-844-4177
Contact: Barbara S. Witt, EdD, RN, Dean
Email: wittbar@auburn.edu

AUBURN UNIVERSITY— MONTGOMERY

Address: P.O. Box 244023, Montgomery, AL 36124-4023
Phone: 334-244-3658
Fax: *Not Reported*
Contact: Barbara Witt, EdD, RN, Dean
Email: witt@micket.aum.edu

GENERAL INFORMATION

Type of School: *4-Year College or University, Public* •
Accreditation: *Southern Association of Colleges and Schools* •
Total Enrollment: *22000*

GENERAL INFORMATION

Type of School: *Not Reported* • Accreditation: *Not Reported* •
Total Enrollment: *Not Reported*

PROGRAM INFORMATION

Two Year Exit Option: *No* • NLNAC Accreditation: *Yes* •
CCNE Accreditation:

PROGRAM INFORMATION

Two Year Exit Option: *Not Reported* • NLNAC
Accreditation: *Not Reported* • CCNE Accreditation:

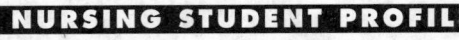

NURSING STUDENT PROFILE

Total Nursing Enrollment: *395* • Total Basic Student
Enrollment, Full Time: *391* • Total Basic Student
Enrollment, Part Time: *0* • Female Basic Student
Enrollment: *351* • Male Basic Student Enrollment: *40* • Total
RN Enrollment: *4* • Total New Fall Enrollments: *78* • Total
Graduates: *66* • Basic Student Graduates: *60* • RN Student
Graduates: *6*

NURSING STUDENT PROFILE

Total Nursing Enrollment: *Not Reported* • Total Basic Student
Enrollment, Full Time: *Not Reported* • Total Basic Student
Enrollment, Part Time: *Not Reported* • Female Basic Student
Enrollment: *Not Reported* • Male Basic Student Enrollment:
Not Reported • Total RN Enrollment: *Not Reported* • Total
New Fall Enrollments: *Not Reported* • Total Graduates: *Not
Reported* • Basic Student Graduates: *Not Reported* • RN
Student Graduates: *Not Reported*

FINANCES

Residential Annual Tuition: *$3,050* • Non-Residential
Annual Tuition: *$9,150* • General Institutional Fees: *$248* •
Additional Nursing Fees: *$147*

FINANCES

Residential Annual Tuition: *Not Reported* • Non-Residential
Annual Tuition: *Not Reported* • General Institutional Fees:
Not Reported • Additional Nursing Fees: *Not Reported*

IDA V. MOFFETT SCHOOL— SAMFORD UNIVERSITY

Address: 800 Lake Shore Drive, Birmingham, AL 35229
Phone: 205-726-2092
Fax: 205-726-4179
Contact: Joy Whatley, DSN, RN, Assistant Dean
Email: jhwhatle@samford.edu

GENERAL INFORMATION

Type of School: *4-Year College or University, Private (Religious)* • Accreditation: *Southern Association of Colleges and Schools* • Total Enrollment: *4500*

PROGRAM INFORMATION

Two Year Exit Option: *No* • NLNAC Accreditation: *Not Reported* • CCNE Accreditation: *Yes*

NURSING STUDENT PROFILE

Total Nursing Enrollment: *176* • Total Basic Student Enrollment, Full Time: *165* • Total Basic Student Enrollment, Part Time: *3* • Female Basic Student Enrollment: *163* • Male Basic Student Enrollment: *5* • Total RN Enrollment: *8* • Total New Fall Enrollments: *48* • Total Graduates: *52* • Basic Student Graduates: *40* • RN Student Graduates: *12*

FINANCES

Residential Annual Tuition: *$5,745* • Non-Residential Annual Tuition: *$5,745* • General Institutional Fees: *Not Reported* • Additional Nursing Fees: *Not Reported*

JACKSONVILLE STATE UNIVERSITY

Address: 700 Pelham Road North, Jacksonville, AL 36265-1602
Phone: 256-782-5428
Fax: 256-782-5406
Contact: Martha G. Lavender, DSN, RN, Dean and Professor
Email: lavender@jsucc.jsu.edu

GENERAL INFORMATION

Type of School: *4-Year College or University, Public* • Accreditation: *Southern Association of Colleges and Schools* • Total Enrollment: *8478*

PROGRAM INFORMATION

Two Year Exit Option: *No* • NLNAC Accreditation: *Not Reported* • CCNE Accreditation: *Yes*

NURSING STUDENT PROFILE

Total Nursing Enrollment: *181* • Total Basic Student Enrollment, Full Time: *174* • Total Basic Student Enrollment, Part Time: *0* • Female Basic Student Enrollment: *160* • Male Basic Student Enrollment: *14* • Total RN Enrollment: *7* • Total New Fall Enrollments: *48* • Total Graduates: *60* • Basic Student Graduates: *48* • RN Student Graduates: *12*

FINANCES

Residential Annual Tuition: *$2,940* • Non-Residential Annual Tuition: *$5,880* • General Institutional Fees: *$0* • Additional Nursing Fees: *$15*

SPRING HILL COLLEGE

Address: 4000 Dauphin Street, Mobile, AL 36608
Phone: 251-380-4490
Fax: 251-380-4495
Contact: Carol Harrison, PhD, RN, Chairperson
Email: charrison@shc.edu

TROY STATE UNIVERSITY

Address: 400 Pell Avenue, Troy, AL 36082
Phone: 334-670-3428
Fax: 334-670-3744
Contact: Brenda Riley, DSN, RN, Director, School of
          Nursing
Email: jriley@trojan.troyst.edu

GENERAL INFORMATION

Type of School: *Not Reported* • Accreditation: *Not Reported* •
Total Enrollment: *Not Reported*

GENERAL INFORMATION

Type of School: *4-Year College or University, Public* •
Accreditation: *Southern Association of Colleges and Schools* •
Total Enrollment: *6777*

PROGRAM INFORMATION

Two Year Exit Option: *Not Reported* • NLNAC
Accreditation: *Not Reported* • CCNE Accreditation:

PROGRAM INFORMATION

Two Year Exit Option: *No* • NLNAC Accreditation: *Yes* •
CCNE Accreditation:

NURSING STUDENT PROFILE

Total Nursing Enrollment: *Not Reported* • Total Basic Student
Enrollment, Full Time: *Not Reported* • Total Basic Student
Enrollment, Part Time: *Not Reported* • Female Basic Student
Enrollment: *Not Reported* • Male Basic Student Enrollment:
Not Reported • Total RN Enrollment: *Not Reported* • Total
New Fall Enrollments: *Not Reported* • Total Graduates: *Not
Reported* • Basic Student Graduates: *Not Reported* • RN
Student Graduates: *Not Reported*

NURSING STUDENT PROFILE

Total Nursing Enrollment: *260* • Total Basic Student
Enrollment, Full Time: *197* • Total Basic Student
Enrollment, Part Time: *63* • Female Basic Student
Enrollment: *233* • Male Basic Student Enrollment: *27* • Total
RN Enrollment: *0* • Total New Fall Enrollments: *27* • Total
Graduates: *34* • Basic Student Graduates: *34* • RN Student
Graduates: *0*

FINANCES

Residential Annual Tuition: *Not Reported* • Non-Residential
Annual Tuition: *Not Reported* • General Institutional Fees:
Not Reported • Additional Nursing Fees: *Not Reported*

FINANCES

Residential Annual Tuition: *$1,510* • Non-Residential
Annual Tuition: *$3,020* • General Institutional Fees: *$276* •
Additional Nursing Fees: *$325*

TUSKEGEE UNIVERSITY

Address: 209 Basil O'Connor Hall, Tuskegee, AL 36088
Phone: 334-727-8382
Fax: 334-727-5461
Contact: Doris S. Holeman, PhD, RN, Associate Dean and Director
Email: dholeman@acd.tusk.edu

GENERAL INFORMATION

Type of School: *4-Year College or University, Private (Independent)* • Accreditation: *Southern Association of Colleges and Schools* • Total Enrollment: *5000*

PROGRAM INFORMATION

Two Year Exit Option: *No* • NLNAC Accreditation: *Yes* • CCNE Accreditation:

NURSING STUDENT PROFILE

Total Nursing Enrollment: *71* • Total Basic Student Enrollment, Full Time: *70* • Total Basic Student Enrollment, Part Time: *1* • Female Basic Student Enrollment: *67* • Male Basic Student Enrollment: *4* • Total RN Enrollment: *0* • Total New Fall Enrollments: *35* • Total Graduates: *10* • Basic Student Graduates: *10* • RN Student Graduates: *0*

FINANCES

Residential Annual Tuition: *$10,326* • Non-Residential Annual Tuition: *$10,326* • General Institutional Fees: *$800* • Additional Nursing Fees: *$350*

THE UNIVERSITY OF ALABAMA

Address: 504 University Blvd., Box 870358, Tuscaloosa, AL 35487-0358
Phone: 205-348-1044
Fax: 205-348-1044
Contact: Donna R. Packa, DSN, RN, Associate Dean for Academic Affairs
Email: dpacka@bama.ua.edu

GENERAL INFORMATION

Type of School: *4-Year College or University, Public* • Accreditation: *Southern Association of Colleges and Schools* • Total Enrollment: *19171*

PROGRAM INFORMATION

Two Year Exit Option: *No* • NLNAC Accreditation: *Not Reported* • CCNE Accreditation: *Yes*

NURSING STUDENT PROFILE

Total Nursing Enrollment: *452* • Total Basic Student Enrollment, Full Time: *430* • Total Basic Student Enrollment, Part Time: *4* • Female Basic Student Enrollment: *389* • Male Basic Student Enrollment: *45* • Total RN Enrollment: *18* • Total New Fall Enrollments: *44* • Total Graduates: *67* • Basic Student Graduates: *56* • RN Student Graduates: *11*

FINANCES

Residential Annual Tuition: *$1,646* • Non-Residential Annual Tuition: *$4,456* • General Institutional Fees: *$374* • Additional Nursing Fees: *$20*

UNIVERSITY OF ALABAMA

Address: 1701 University Blvd, Birmingham, AL 35294-1210
Phone: 205-934-5360
Fax: *Not Reported*
Contact: Rachel Z. Booth, PhD, RN, Dean and Professor
Email: rzbooth@uab.edu

GENERAL INFORMATION

Type of School: *Other, Public* • Accreditation: *Southern Association of Colleges and Schools* • Total Enrollment: *10420*

PROGRAM INFORMATION

Two Year Exit Option: *No* • NLNAC Accreditation: *Yes* • CCNE Accreditation: *Yes*

NURSING STUDENT PROFILE

Total Nursing Enrollment: *220* • Total Basic Student Enrollment, Full Time: *162* • Total Basic Student Enrollment, Part Time: *28* • Female Basic Student Enrollment: *166* • Male Basic Student Enrollment: *24* • Total RN Enrollment: *30* • Total New Fall Enrollments: *41* • Total Graduates: *122* • Basic Student Graduates: *103* • RN Student Graduates: *19*

FINANCES

Residential Annual Tuition: *$3,978* • Non-Residential Annual Tuition: *$7,956* • General Institutional Fees: *$100* • Additional Nursing Fees: *$110*

UNIVERSITY OF ALABAMA—HUNTSVILLE

Address: 301 Sparkman Drive, Huntsville, AL 35899-0001
Phone: 256-824-6345
Fax: 256-824-6026
Contact: C Fay Raines, PhD, RN, Dean and Associate Provost
Email: rainesc@email.uah.edu

GENERAL INFORMATION

Type of School: *4-Year College or University, Public* • Accreditation: *Southern Association of Colleges and Schools* • Total Enrollment: *6500*

PROGRAM INFORMATION

Two Year Exit Option: *Not Reported* • NLNAC Accreditation: *Yes* • CCNE Accreditation: *Yes*

NURSING STUDENT PROFILE

Total Nursing Enrollment: *396* • Total Basic Student Enrollment, Full Time: *240* • Total Basic Student Enrollment, Part Time: *90* • Female Basic Student Enrollment: *309* • Male Basic Student Enrollment: *21* • Total RN Enrollment: *66* • Total New Fall Enrollments: *96* • Total Graduates: *114* • Basic Student Graduates: *77* • RN Student Graduates: *37*

FINANCES

Residential Annual Tuition: *$4,300* • Non-Residential Annual Tuition: *$9,000* • General Institutional Fees: *$600* • Additional Nursing Fees: *$450*

Circle 121 on reader card   See in-depth profile for more information

UNIVERSITY OF MOBILE

Address: Mobile, AL 36663
Phone: 334-675-5990
Fax: 334-442-2520
Contact: Rosemarie Adams, EdD, RN, Chairperson
Email: *Not Reported*

GENERAL INFORMATION

Type of School: *Not Reported* • Accreditation: *Not Reported* •
Total Enrollment: *Not Reported*

PROGRAM INFORMATION

Two Year Exit Option: *Not Reported* • NLNAC
Accreditation: *Yes* • CCNE Accreditation:

NURSING STUDENT PROFILE

Total Nursing Enrollment: *299* • Total Basic Student
Enrollment, Full Time: *220* • Total Basic Student
Enrollment, Part Time: *53* • Female Basic Student
Enrollment: *Not Reported* • Male Basic Student Enrollment:
Not Reported • Total RN Enrollment: *26* • Total New Fall
Enrollments: *Not Reported* • Total Graduates: *Not Reported* •
Basic Student Graduates: *Not Reported* • RN Student
Graduates: *Not Reported*

FINANCES

Residential Annual Tuition: *Not Reported* • Non-Residential
Annual Tuition: *Not Reported* • General Institutional Fees:
Not Reported • Additional Nursing Fees: *Not Reported*

UNIVERSITY OF NORTH ALABAMA

Address: P. O. Box 5054, Florence, AL 35632
Phone: 256-765-4984
Fax: 256-765-4935
Contact: Birdie Irene Bailey, PhD, RN, Dean and Professor
Email: bibailey@una.edu

GENERAL INFORMATION

Type of School: *4-Year College or University, Public* •
Accreditation: *Southern Association of Colleges and Schools* •
Total Enrollment: *5601*

PROGRAM INFORMATION

Two Year Exit Option: *No* • NLNAC Accreditation: *Yes* •
CCNE Accreditation:

NURSING STUDENT PROFILE

Total Nursing Enrollment: *218* • Total Basic Student
Enrollment, Full Time: *126* • Total Basic Student
Enrollment, Part Time: *8* • Female Basic Student
Enrollment: *120* • Male Basic Student Enrollment: *14* • Total
RN Enrollment: *84* • Total New Fall Enrollments: *48* • Total
Graduates: *81* • Basic Student Graduates: *63* • RN Student
Graduates: *18*

FINANCES

Residential Annual Tuition: *$1,272* • Non-Residential
Annual Tuition: *$2,544* • General Institutional Fees: *$150* •
Additional Nursing Fees: *$188*

UNIVERSITY OF SOUTH ALABAMA

Address: USA Springhill Avenue, Mobile, AL 36688
Phone: 334-434-3425
Fax: 334-434-3413
Contact: Rosemary S. Rhodes, DNS, RN, Associate Dean for Academic Affairs
Email: rrhodes@usamail.usouthal.edu

GENERAL INFORMATION

Type of School: *4-Year College or University, Public* • Accreditation: *Southern Association of Colleges and Schools* • Total Enrollment: *11792*

PROGRAM INFORMATION

Two Year Exit Option: *Not Reported* • NLNAC Accreditation: *Yes* • CCNE Accreditation: *Yes*

NURSING STUDENT PROFILE

Total Nursing Enrollment: *291* • Total Basic Student Enrollment, Full Time: *118* • Total Basic Student Enrollment, Part Time: *72* • Female Basic Student Enrollment: *160* • Male Basic Student Enrollment: *30* • Total RN Enrollment: *101* • Total New Fall Enrollments: *59* • Total Graduates: *162* • Basic Student Graduates: *107* • RN Student Graduates: *55*

FINANCES

Residential Annual Tuition: *$3,560* • Non-Residential Annual Tuition: *$7,120* • General Institutional Fees: *$291* • Additional Nursing Fees: *$120*

UNIVERSITY OF ALASKA-ANCHORAGE

Address: 3211 Providence Drive, Anchorage, AK 99508-8030
Phone: 907-786-4571
Fax: 907-786-4558
Contact: Tina D. DeLapp, EdD, RN, Director
Email: AFTDD@uaa.alaska.edu

GENERAL INFORMATION

Type of School: *4-Year College or University, Public* • Accreditation: *Northwestern Association of Schools and Colleges* • Total Enrollment: *17000*

PROGRAM INFORMATION

Two Year Exit Option: *No* • NLNAC Accreditation: *Yes* • CCNE Accreditation:

NURSING STUDENT PROFILE

Total Nursing Enrollment: *203* • Total Basic Student Enrollment, Full Time: *129* • Total Basic Student Enrollment, Part Time: *52* • Female Basic Student Enrollment: *148* • Male Basic Student Enrollment: *33* • Total RN Enrollment: *31* • Total New Fall Enrollments: *31* • Total Graduates: *54* • Basic Student Graduates: *51* • RN Student Graduates: *3*

FINANCES

Residential Annual Tuition: *Not Reported* • Non-Residential Annual Tuition: *Not Reported* • General Institutional Fees: *$9,450* • Additional Nursing Fees: *Not Reported*

| GRAND CANYON UNIVERSITY | NORTHERN ARIZONA UNIVERSITY |

GRAND CANYON UNIVERSITY

Address: 3300 West Camelback Road, Phoenix, AZ 85017
Phone: 602-589-2431
Fax: 602-589-2098
Contact: Cynthia A. Russell, DNSc, RN, CS, Dean and Professor
Email: crussell@grand-canyon.edu

NORTHERN ARIZONA UNIVERSITY

Address: PO BOX 15035, Flagstaff, AZ 86011-5015
Phone: 520-523-6712
Fax: 520-523-7171
Contact: Judith Sellers, PhD, RN, Interim Chair
Email: judith.sellers@nau.edu

GENERAL INFORMATION

Type of School: *4-Year College or University, Private (Religious)* • Accreditation: *North Central Association of Colleges and Schools* • Total Enrollment: *2000*

GENERAL INFORMATION

Type of School: *Not Reported* • Accreditation: *Not Reported* • Total Enrollment: *Not Reported*

PROGRAM INFORMATION

Two Year Exit Option: *No* • NLNAC Accreditation: *Yes* • CCNE Accreditation:

PROGRAM INFORMATION

Two Year Exit Option: *Not Reported* • NLNAC Accreditation: *Not Reported* • CCNE Accreditation:

NURSING STUDENT PROFILE

Total Nursing Enrollment: *147* • Total Basic Student Enrollment, Full Time: *Not Reported* • Total Basic Student Enrollment, Part Time: *Not Reported* • Female Basic Student Enrollment: *85* • Male Basic Student Enrollment: *6* • Total RN Enrollment: *56* • Total New Fall Enrollments: *21* • Total Graduates: *62* • Basic Student Graduates: *44* • RN Student Graduates: *18*

NURSING STUDENT PROFILE

Total Nursing Enrollment: *179* • Total Basic Student Enrollment, Full Time: *111* • Total Basic Student Enrollment, Part Time: *0* • Female Basic Student Enrollment: *Not Reported* • Male Basic Student Enrollment: *Not Reported* • Total RN Enrollment: *68* • Total New Fall Enrollments: *Not Reported* • Total Graduates: *Not Reported* • Basic Student Graduates: *Not Reported* • RN Student Graduates: *Not Reported*

FINANCES

Residential Annual Tuition: *Not Reported* • Non-Residential Annual Tuition: *Not Reported* • General Institutional Fees: *$4,452* • Additional Nursing Fees: *$377*

FINANCES

Residential Annual Tuition: *Not Reported* • Non-Residential Annual Tuition: *Not Reported* • General Institutional Fees: *Not Reported* • Additional Nursing Fees: *Not Reported*

UNIVERSITY OF ARIZONA

Address: 1305 North Martin, P.O. Box 210203, Tucson,
            AZ 85721-0203
Phone: 520-626-6152
Fax: 520-626-2669
Contact: Suzanne Van Ort, PhD, RN, FAAN, Dean and
            Professor
Email: svanort@nursing.arizona.edu

GENERAL INFORMATION

Type of School: *4-Year College or University, Public* •
Accreditation: *North Central Association of Colleges and
Schools* • Total Enrollment: *34300*

PROGRAM INFORMATION

Two Year Exit Option: *No* • NLNAC Accreditation: *Yes* •
CCNE Accreditation:

NURSING STUDENT PROFILE

Total Nursing Enrollment: *241* • Total Basic Student
Enrollment, Full Time: *179* • Total Basic Student
Enrollment, Part Time: *50* • Female Basic Student
Enrollment: *210* • Male Basic Student Enrollment: *19* • Total
RN Enrollment: *12* • Total New Fall Enrollments: *48* • Total
Graduates: *89* • Basic Student Graduates: *87* • RN Student
Graduates: *2*

FINANCES

Residential Annual Tuition: *$2,272* • Non-Residential
Annual Tuition: *$7,290* • General Institutional Fees:
$1,136 • Additional Nursing Fees: *$126*

ARKANSAS STATE UNIVERSITY

Address: P.O.Box 910, State University, AR 72467
Phone: 870-972-3074
Fax: 870-972-2954
Contact: Annette Stacy, MSN, RN, CS, AOCN, Program
            Director
Email: astacy@crow.astate.edu

GENERAL INFORMATION

Type of School: *4-Year College or University, Public* •
Accreditation: *North Central Association of Colleges and
Schools* • Total Enrollment: *10000*

PROGRAM INFORMATION

Two Year Exit Option: *No* • NLNAC Accreditation: *Yes* •
CCNE Accreditation:

NURSING STUDENT PROFILE

Total Nursing Enrollment: *176* • Total Basic Student
Enrollment, Full Time: *176* • Total Basic Student
Enrollment, Part Time: *0* • Female Basic Student
Enrollment: *159* • Male Basic Student Enrollment: *17* • Total
RN Enrollment: *0* • Total New Fall Enrollments: *65* • Total
Graduates: *58* • Basic Student Graduates: *45* • RN Student
Graduates: *13*

FINANCES

Residential Annual Tuition: *$2,520* • Non-Residential
Annual Tuition: *$6,456* • General Institutional Fees:
$1,260 • Additional Nursing Fees: *Not Reported*

ARKANSAS TECH UNIVERSITY

Address: 402 West O Street, Russellville, AR 72801-2222
Phone: 479-968-0383
Fax: 479-968-0219
Contact: Rebeca Burris, PhD, RN, Associate Professor and Department Head
Email: rebeca.buuris@mail.atu.edu

GENERAL INFORMATION

Type of School: *4-Year College or University, Public* • Accreditation: *North Central Association of Colleges and Schools* • Total Enrollment: *5600*

PROGRAM INFORMATION

Two Year Exit Option: *No* • NLNAC Accreditation: *Yes* • CCNE Accreditation:

NURSING STUDENT PROFILE

Total Nursing Enrollment: *69* • Total Basic Student Enrollment, Full Time: *57* • Total Basic Student Enrollment, Part Time: *4* • Female Basic Student Enrollment: *54* • Male Basic Student Enrollment: *7* • Total RN Enrollment: *8* • Total New Fall Enrollments: *38* • Total Graduates: *18* • Basic Student Graduates: *12* • RN Student Graduates: *6*

FINANCES

Residential Annual Tuition: *$2,796* • Non-Residential Annual Tuition: *$5,920* • General Institutional Fees: *$90* • Additional Nursing Fees: *$0*

HARDING UNIVERSITY

Address: 900 East Center, Searcy, AR 72149-0001
Phone: 501-279-4476
Fax: 501-279-4669
Contact: Cathleen M. Shultz, PhD, RN, FAAN, Professor and Dean
Email: shultz@harding.edu

GENERAL INFORMATION

Type of School: *4-Year College or University, Private (Religious)* • Accreditation: *North Central Association of Colleges and Schools* • Total Enrollment: *5050*

PROGRAM INFORMATION

Two Year Exit Option: *No* • NLNAC Accreditation: *Yes* • CCNE Accreditation:

NURSING STUDENT PROFILE

Total Nursing Enrollment: *266* • Total Basic Student Enrollment, Full Time: *196* • Total Basic Student Enrollment, Part Time: *0* • Female Basic Student Enrollment: *186* • Male Basic Student Enrollment: *10* • Total RN Enrollment: *70* • Total New Fall Enrollments: *22* • Total Graduates: *23* • Basic Student Graduates: *13* • RN Student Graduates: *10*

FINANCES

Residential Annual Tuition: *$8,730* • Non-Residential Annual Tuition: *$8,730* • General Institutional Fees: *$300* • Additional Nursing Fees: *$250*

HENDERSON STATE UNIVERSITY

Address: 100 Henderson Street, HSU Box 7803, Arkadelphia, AR 71999-0001
Phone: 870-230-5015
Fax: 870-230-5390
Contact: Laura Meeks, EdD, APRN-BC, Professor and Chair
Email: festal@hsu.edu

GENERAL INFORMATION

Type of School: *4-Year College or University, Public* • Accreditation: *North Central Association of Colleges and Schools* • Total Enrollment: *3300*

PROGRAM INFORMATION

Two Year Exit Option: *Not Reported* • NLNAC Accreditation: *Yes* • CCNE Accreditation:

NURSING STUDENT PROFILE

Total Nursing Enrollment: *221* • Total Basic Student Enrollment, Full Time: *79* • Total Basic Student Enrollment, Part Time: *8* • Female Basic Student Enrollment: *79* • Male Basic Student Enrollment: *8* • Total RN Enrollment: *134* • Total New Fall Enrollments: *31* • Total Graduates: *21* • Basic Student Graduates: *17* • RN Student Graduates: *4*

FINANCES

Residential Annual Tuition: *Not Reported* • Non-Residential Annual Tuition: *Not Reported* • General Institutional Fees: *Not Reported* • Additional Nursing Fees: *Not Reported*

UNIVERSITY OF ARKANSAS— FAYETTEVILLE

Address: 217 Ozark Hall, 1 University of Arkansas, Fayetteville, AR 72701
Phone: 479-575-3907
Fax: 479-575-3218
Contact: Barbara Conrad, PhD, RN, Director and Associate Professor
Email: bsconrad@uark.edu

GENERAL INFORMATION

Type of School: *4-Year College or University, Public* • Accreditation: *North Central Association of Colleges and Schools* • Total Enrollment: *14600*

PROGRAM INFORMATION

Two Year Exit Option: *No* • NLNAC Accreditation: *Yes* • CCNE Accreditation: *Yes*

NURSING STUDENT PROFILE

Total Nursing Enrollment: *59* • Total Basic Student Enrollment, Full Time: *55* • Total Basic Student Enrollment, Part Time: *0* • Female Basic Student Enrollment: *48* • Male Basic Student Enrollment: *7* • Total RN Enrollment: *4* • Total New Fall Enrollments: *0* • Total Graduates: *31* • Basic Student Graduates: *28* • RN Student Graduates: *3*

FINANCES

Residential Annual Tuition: *$3,573* • Non-Residential Annual Tuition: *$9,945* • General Institutional Fees: *$883* • Additional Nursing Fees: *$30*

UNIVERSITY OF ARKANSAS FOR MEDICAL SCIENCES

Address:　4301 West Markham, Slot 529, Little Rock, AR 72205
Phone:　501-686-7986
Fax:　501-686-8350
Contact:　Patricia E. Thompson, EdD, RN, Associate Dean for Baccalaureate Education
Email:　thompsonpatriciae@uams.edu

GENERAL INFORMATION

Type of School: *4-Year College or University, Public* • Accreditation: *North Central Association of Colleges and Schools* • Total Enrollment: *5000*

PROGRAM INFORMATION

Two Year Exit Option: *No* • NLNAC Accreditation: *Yes* • CCNE Accreditation: *Yes*

NURSING STUDENT PROFILE

Total Nursing Enrollment: *Not Reported* • Total Basic Student Enrollment, Full Time: *Not Reported* • Total Basic Student Enrollment, Part Time: *Not Reported* • Female Basic Student Enrollment: *Not Reported* • Male Basic Student Enrollment: *Not Reported* • Total RN Enrollment: *Not Reported* • Total New Fall Enrollments: *165* • Total Graduates: *92* • Basic Student Graduates: *72* • RN Student Graduates: *20*

FINANCES

Residential Annual Tuition: *$2,760* • Non-Residential Annual Tuition: *$6,888* • General Institutional Fees: *Not Reported* • Additional Nursing Fees: *Not Reported*

UNIVERSITY OF ARKANSAS— MONTICELLO

Address:　P.O.Box 3606, Monticello, AR 71656
Phone:　870-460-1069
Fax:　870-460-1969
Contact:　Brenda J. Mitchell, DSN, RN, Chair
Email:　mitchellbr@uamont.edu

GENERAL INFORMATION

Type of School: *4-Year College or University, Public* • Accreditation: *North Central Association of Colleges and Schools* • Total Enrollment: *1600*

PROGRAM INFORMATION

Two Year Exit Option: *No* • NLNAC Accreditation: *Yes* • CCNE Accreditation:

NURSING STUDENT PROFILE

Total Nursing Enrollment: *36* • Total Basic Student Enrollment, Full Time: *36* • Total Basic Student Enrollment, Part Time: *0* • Female Basic Student Enrollment: *34* • Male Basic Student Enrollment: *2* • Total RN Enrollment: *0* • Total New Fall Enrollments: *0* • Total Graduates: *14* • Basic Student Graduates: *14* • RN Student Graduates: *0*

FINANCES

Residential Annual Tuition: *Not Reported* • Non-Residential Annual Tuition: *Not Reported* • General Institutional Fees: *$980* • Additional Nursing Fees: *$70*

UNIVERSITY OF ARKANSAS— PINE BLUFF

Address: 1200 University Drive, Pine Bluff, AR 71601
Phone: 870-575-8220
Fax: 870-543-8229
Contact: Irene T. Henderson, EdD, RN, Chairperson
Email: henderson_i@uapb.edu

GENERAL INFORMATION

Type of School: *4-Year College or University, Public* •
Accreditation: *North Central Association of Colleges and
Schools* • Total Enrollment: *3030*

PROGRAM INFORMATION

Two Year Exit Option: *No* • NLNAC Accreditation: *Yes* •
CCNE Accreditation:

NURSING STUDENT PROFILE

Total Nursing Enrollment: *33* • Total Basic Student
Enrollment, Full Time: *32* • Total Basic Student Enrollment,
Part Time: *0* • Female Basic Student Enrollment: *31* • Male
Basic Student Enrollment: *1* • Total RN Enrollment: *1* •
Total New Fall Enrollments: *13* • Total Graduates: *12* • Basic
Student Graduates: *8* • RN Student Graduates: *4*

FINANCES

Residential Annual Tuition: *$2,400* • Non-Residential
Annual Tuition: *$5,550* • General Institutional Fees: *$258* •
Additional Nursing Fees: *$1*

UNIVERSITY OF CENTRAL ARKANSAS

Address: 201 Donaghey Avenue, Conway, AR 72035-
            0001
Phone: 501-450-3119
Fax: 501-450-5560
Contact: Barbara G. Williams, PhD, RN, Professor and
            Chair
Email: barbaraw@mail.uca.edu

GENERAL INFORMATION

Type of School: *4-Year College or University, Public* •
Accreditation: *North Central Association of Colleges and
Schools* • Total Enrollment: *8486*

PROGRAM INFORMATION

Two Year Exit Option: *No* • NLNAC Accreditation: *Yes* •
CCNE Accreditation:

NURSING STUDENT PROFILE

Total Nursing Enrollment: *146* • Total Basic Student
Enrollment, Full Time: *123* • Total Basic Student
Enrollment, Part Time: *22* • Female Basic Student
Enrollment: *117* • Male Basic Student Enrollment: *28* • Total
RN Enrollment: *1* • Total New Fall Enrollments: *50* • Total
Graduates: *43* • Basic Student Graduates: *43* • RN Student
Graduates: *0*

FINANCES

Residential Annual Tuition: *$1,530* • Non-Residential
Annual Tuition: *$3,060* • General Institutional Fees: *$340* •
Additional Nursing Fees: *$11*

AZUSA PACIFIC UNIVERSITY

Address: 901 East Alosta Avenue, Azusa, CA 91702-7000
Phone: 626-815-5386
Fax: 626-815-5414
Contact: Shila Wiebe, MSN, RN, Chair, Undergraduate
            Nursing
Email: swiebe@apu.edu

GENERAL INFORMATION

Type of School: *4-Year College or University, Private
(Religious)* • Accreditation: *Western Association of Schools and
Colleges* • Total Enrollment: *7000*

PROGRAM INFORMATION

Two Year Exit Option: *No* • NLNAC Accreditation: *Yes* •
CCNE Accreditation:

NURSING STUDENT PROFILE

Total Nursing Enrollment: *207* • Total Basic Student
Enrollment, Full Time: *149* • Total Basic Student
Enrollment, Part Time: *39* • Female Basic Student
Enrollment: *172* • Male Basic Student Enrollment: *16* • Total
RN Enrollment: *19* • Total New Fall Enrollments: *44* • Total
Graduates: *49* • Basic Student Graduates: *48* • RN Student
Graduates: *1*

FINANCES

Residential Annual Tuition: *$15,950* • Non-Residential
Annual Tuition: *$15,950* • General Institutional Fees: *$484* •
Additional Nursing Fees: *$270*

CALIFORNIA STATE UNIVERSITY—BAKERSFIELD

Address: 9001 Stockdale Highway, Bakersfield, CA
            93311-1099
Phone: 661-664-2093
Fax: 661-665-6903
Contact: Candace J. Meares, PhD, RN, CNAA, Chair
Email: cmeares@csub.edu

GENERAL INFORMATION

Type of School: *4-Year College or University, Public* •
Accreditation: *Western Association of Schools and Colleges* •
Total Enrollment: *6000*

PROGRAM INFORMATION

Two Year Exit Option: *No* • NLNAC Accreditation: *Yes* •
CCNE Accreditation:

NURSING STUDENT PROFILE

Total Nursing Enrollment: *128* • Total Basic Student
Enrollment, Full Time: *118* • Total Basic Student
Enrollment, Part Time: *0* • Female Basic Student
Enrollment: *107* • Male Basic Student Enrollment: *11* • Total
RN Enrollment: *10* • Total New Fall Enrollments: *56* • Total
Graduates: *35* • Basic Student Graduates: *31* • RN Student
Graduates: *4*

FINANCES

Residential Annual Tuition: *$1,364* • Non-Residential
Annual Tuition: *$7,380* • General Institutional Fees: *$254* •
Additional Nursing Fees: *Not Reported*

CALIFORNIA STATE UNIVERSITY—CHICO

Address: 1st and Orange Street, Holt Hall Rm 369, Chico, CA 95929
Phone: 530-898-5891
Fax: 530-898-4363
Contact: Sherry D. Fox, PhD, RN, Director
Email: sdfox@csuchico.edu

GENERAL INFORMATION

Type of School: *4-Year College or University, Public* • Accreditation: *Western Association of Schools and Colleges* • Total Enrollment: *14000*

PROGRAM INFORMATION

Two Year Exit Option: *No* • NLNAC Accreditation: *Yes* • CCNE Accreditation:

NURSING STUDENT PROFILE

Total Nursing Enrollment: *239* • Total Basic Student Enrollment, Full Time: *168* • Total Basic Student Enrollment, Part Time: *2* • Female Basic Student Enrollment: *152* • Male Basic Student Enrollment: *18* • Total RN Enrollment: *69* • Total New Fall Enrollments: *39* • Total Graduates: *67* • Basic Student Graduates: *55* • RN Student Graduates: *12*

FINANCES

Residential Annual Tuition: *$1,015* • Non-Residential Annual Tuition: *$3,967* • General Institutional Fees: *Not Reported* • Additional Nursing Fees: *$35*

CALIFORNIA STATE UNIVERSITY—FRESNO

Address: 2345 East San Ramon M/s MH25, Fresno, CA 93727
Phone: 559-278-2041
Fax: 559-278-6360
Contact: Mariama K. Mathai, EdD, RN, Chair, Department of Nursing
Email: mariamma_mathai@csufresno.edu

GENERAL INFORMATION

Type of School: *4-Year College or University, Public* • Accreditation: *Western Association of Schools and Colleges* • Total Enrollment: *19000*

PROGRAM INFORMATION

Two Year Exit Option: *No* • NLNAC Accreditation: *Yes* • CCNE Accreditation:

NURSING STUDENT PROFILE

Total Nursing Enrollment: *221* • Total Basic Student Enrollment, Full Time: *Not Reported* • Total Basic Student Enrollment, Part Time: *Not Reported* • Female Basic Student Enrollment: *163* • Male Basic Student Enrollment: *38* • Total RN Enrollment: *20* • Total New Fall Enrollments: *50* • Total Graduates: *65* • Basic Student Graduates: *63* • RN Student Graduates: *2*

FINANCES

Residential Annual Tuition: *$1,746* • Non-Residential Annual Tuition: *Not Reported* • General Institutional Fees: *$873* • Additional Nursing Fees: *$246*

CALIFORNIA STATE UNIVERSITY—HAYWARD

Address: 25800 Carlos Bee Boulevard, Hay ward, CA 94542
Phone: 510-885-2925
Fax: 510-885-2156
Contact: Brenda Bailey, DNSc, RN, Department Chair
Email: bbailey@csuhayward.edu

GENERAL INFORMATION

Type of School: *4-Year College or University, Public* •
Accreditation: *Western Association of Schools and Colleges* •
Total Enrollment: *13000*

PROGRAM INFORMATION

Two Year Exit Option: *No* • NLNAC Accreditation: *Yes* •
CCNE Accreditation:

NURSING STUDENT PROFILE

Total Nursing Enrollment: *183* • Total Basic Student
Enrollment, Full Time: *Not Reported* • Total Basic Student
Enrollment, Part Time: *Not Reported* • Female Basic Student
Enrollment: *144* • Male Basic Student Enrollment: *16* •
Total RN Enrollment: *23* • Total New Fall Enrollments: *58* •
Total Graduates: *57* • Basic Student Graduates: *48* • RN
Student Graduates: *9*

FINANCES

Residential Annual Tuition: *Not Reported* • Non-Residential
Annual Tuition: *Not Reported* • General Institutional Fees:
$576 • Additional Nursing Fees: *Not Reported*

CALIFORNIA STATE UNIVERSITY—LOS ANGELES

Address: 5151 State University Drive, Los Angeles, CA 90032
Phone: 323-343-4700
Fax: 323-343-6454
Contact: Judith L. Papenhausen, PhD, RN, Chairperson
Email: jpapenh@cslanet.calstatela.edu

GENERAL INFORMATION

Type of School: *Not Reported* • Accreditation: *Not Reported* •
Total Enrollment: *Not Reported*

PROGRAM INFORMATION

Two Year Exit Option: *No* • NLNAC Accreditation: *Yes* •
CCNE Accreditation:

NURSING STUDENT PROFILE

Total Nursing Enrollment: *268* • Total Basic Student
Enrollment, Full Time: *155* • Total Basic Student
Enrollment, Part Time: *0* • Female Basic Student
Enrollment: *130* • Male Basic Student Enrollment: *25* • Total
RN Enrollment: *113* • Total New Fall Enrollments: *70* •
Total Graduates: *93* • Basic Student Graduates: *43* • RN
Student Graduates: *50*

FINANCES

Residential Annual Tuition: *$1,428* • Non-Residential
Annual Tuition: *$1,428* • General Institutional Fees: *$476* •
Additional Nursing Fees: *$164*

CALIFORNIA STATE UNIVERSITY—SACRAMENTO

Address: 6000 J. Street, Sacramento, CA 95819-6096
Phone: 916-278-7543
Fax: 916-278-6311
Contact: Robyn Nelson, DNSc, RN, Chairperson and Professor
Email: nelsonrm@csus.edu

GENERAL INFORMATION

Type of School: *4-Year College or University, Public* •
Accreditation: *Western Association of Schools and Colleges* •
Total Enrollment: *26923*

PROGRAM INFORMATION

Two Year Exit Option: *No* • NLNAC Accreditation: *Not Reported* • CCNE Accreditation: *Yes*

NURSING STUDENT PROFILE

Total Nursing Enrollment: *278* • Total Basic Student Enrollment, Full Time: *245* • Total Basic Student Enrollment, Part Time: *7* • Female Basic Student Enrollment: *221* • Male Basic Student Enrollment: *31* • Total RN Enrollment: *26* • Total New Fall Enrollments: *54* • Total Graduates: *97* • Basic Student Graduates: *85* • RN Student Graduates: *12*

FINANCES

Residential Annual Tuition: *$1,572* • Non-Residential Annual Tuition: *$10,596* • General Institutional Fees: *$463* • Additional Nursing Fees: *$0*

CALIFORNIA STATE UNIVERSITY—SAN BERNARDINO

Address: 5500 University Parkway, San Bernardino, CA 92407
Phone: 909-880-5385
Fax: 909-880-7089
Contact: Marcia L. Raines, PhD, RN, CS, Department Chair
Email: mraines@csub.edu

GENERAL INFORMATION

Type of School: *4-Year College or University, Public* •
Accreditation: *Western Association of Schools and Colleges* •
Total Enrollment: *15000*

PROGRAM INFORMATION

Two Year Exit Option: *No* • NLNAC Accreditation: *Yes* •
CCNE Accreditation:

NURSING STUDENT PROFILE

Total Nursing Enrollment: *203* • Total Basic Student Enrollment, Full Time: *200* • Total Basic Student Enrollment, Part Time: *0* • Female Basic Student Enrollment: *178* • Male Basic Student Enrollment: *22* • Total RN Enrollment: *3* • Total New Fall Enrollments: *55* • Total Graduates: *72* • Basic Student Graduates: *69* • RN Student Graduates: *3*

FINANCES

Residential Annual Tuition: *$1,733* • Non-Residential Annual Tuition: *$7,749* • General Institutional Fees: *Not Reported* • Additional Nursing Fees: *$60*

DOMINICAN UNIVERSITY OF CALIFORNIA

Address: 50 Acacia Avenue, San Rafael, CA 94901
Phone: 415-257-1310
Fax: 415-257-0120
Contact: Martha A. Nelson, PhD, RN, Dean, School of Health Sciences
Email: nelson@dominican.edu

GENERAL INFORMATION

Type of School: *4-Year College or University, Private (Independent)* • Accreditation: *Western Association of Schools and Colleges* • Total Enrollment: *1478*

PROGRAM INFORMATION

Two Year Exit Option: *No* • NLNAC Accreditation: *Yes* • CCNE Accreditation:

NURSING STUDENT PROFILE

Total Nursing Enrollment: *193* • Total Basic Student Enrollment, Full Time: *139* • Total Basic Student Enrollment, Part Time: *36* • Female Basic Student Enrollment: *158* • Male Basic Student Enrollment: *17* • Total RN Enrollment: *18* • Total New Fall Enrollments: *20* • Total Graduates: *30* • Basic Student Graduates: *27* • RN Student Graduates: *3*

FINANCES

Residential Annual Tuition: *$17,256* • Non-Residential Annual Tuition: *$17,256* • General Institutional Fees: *$8,628* • Additional Nursing Fees: *$719*

HOLY NAMES COLLEGE

Address: 3500 Mountain Blvd, Oakwood, CA 94619
Phone: 510-436-1024
Fax: 510-436-1376
Contact: Fay L. Bower, DNSc, RN, FAAN, Chair
Email: bower@hnu.edu

GENERAL INFORMATION

Type of School: *4-Year College or University, Private (Religious)* • Accreditation: *Western Association of Schools and Colleges* • Total Enrollment: *832*

PROGRAM INFORMATION

Two Year Exit Option: *No* • NLNAC Accreditation: *Yes* • CCNE Accreditation:

NURSING STUDENT PROFILE

Total Nursing Enrollment: *175* • Total Basic Student Enrollment, Full Time: *0* • Total Basic Student Enrollment, Part Time: *0* • Female Basic Student Enrollment: *0* • Male Basic Student Enrollment: *0* • Total RN Enrollment: *175* • Total New Fall Enrollments: *10* • Total Graduates: *22* • Basic Student Graduates: *0* • RN Student Graduates: *22*

FINANCES

Residential Annual Tuition: *Not Reported* • Non-Residential Annual Tuition: *Not Reported* • General Institutional Fees: *Not Reported* • Additional Nursing Fees: *$495*

HUMBOLDT STATE UNIVERSITY

Address: 1 Harpst Street, Arcata, CA 95521
Phone: 707-826-5131
Fax: 707-826-5141
Contact: betty Jensen, PhD, RN, Director
Email: bjj2@axe.humboldt.edu

GENERAL INFORMATION

Type of School: *4-Year College or University, Public* •
Accreditation: *Western Association of Schools and Colleges* •
Total Enrollment: *7500*

PROGRAM INFORMATION

Two Year Exit Option: *Not Reported* • NLNAC
Accreditation: *Not Reported* • CCNE Accreditation: *Yes*

NURSING STUDENT PROFILE

Total Nursing Enrollment: *40* • Total Basic Student
Enrollment, Full Time: *Not Reported* • Total Basic Student
Enrollment, Part Time: *Not Reported* • Female Basic Student
Enrollment: *Not Reported* • Male Basic Student Enrollment:
Not Reported • Total RN Enrollment: *0* • Total New Fall
Enrollments: *Not Reported* • Total Graduates: *Not Reported* •
Basic Student Graduates: *Not Reported* • RN Student
Graduates: *Not Reported*

FINANCES

Residential Annual Tuition: *Not Reported* • Non-Residential
Annual Tuition: *Not Reported* • General Institutional Fees:
Not Reported • Additional Nursing Fees: *Not Reported*

LOMA LINDA UNIVERSITY

Address: 11262 Campus Street, Loma Linda, CA 92350
Phone: 909-558-8060
Fax: 909-558-0643
Contact: Marilyn Herrmann, PhD, RN, Associate Dean,
Undergraduate Program
Email: mherrmann@sn.llu.edu

GENERAL INFORMATION

Type of School: *4-Year College or University, Private
(Religious)* • Accreditation: *Western Association of Schools and
Colleges* • Total Enrollment: *3338*

PROGRAM INFORMATION

Two Year Exit Option: *No* • NLNAC Accreditation: *Yes* •
CCNE Accreditation:

NURSING STUDENT PROFILE

Total Nursing Enrollment: *293* • Total Basic Student
Enrollment, Full Time: *242* • Total Basic Student
Enrollment, Part Time: *33* • Female Basic Student
Enrollment: *216* • Male Basic Student Enrollment: *59* • Total
RN Enrollment: *18* • Total New Fall Enrollments: *54* • Total
Graduates: *55* • Basic Student Graduates: *49* • RN Student
Graduates: *6*

FINANCES

Residential Annual Tuition: *$17,640* • Non-Residential
Annual Tuition: *$17,640* • General Institutional Fees: *$0* •
Additional Nursing Fees: *$30*

MOUNT ST. MARY'S COLLEGE

Address: 10 Chester Place, Los Angeles, CA 90007-2518
Phone: 310-954-4231
Fax: *Not Reported*
Contact: Colette R. York, DNSc, RN, Chair, Department of Nursing
Email: cynk@msmc.la.edu

POINT LOMA NAZARENE UNIVERSITY

Address: 3900 Lomaland Drive, San Diego, CA 92106-2899
Phone: 619-849-2236
Fax: 619-849-2672
Contact: Dorothy E. Crummy, PhD, RN, Chair, Department of Nursing
Email: dcrummy@ptloma.edu

GENERAL INFORMATION

Type of School: *Not Reported* • Accreditation: *Not Reported* • Total Enrollment: *Not Reported*

GENERAL INFORMATION

Type of School: *4-Year College or University, Private (Religious)* • Accreditation: *Western Association of Schools and Colleges* • Total Enrollment: *2300*

PROGRAM INFORMATION

Two Year Exit Option: *No* • NLNAC Accreditation: *Yes* • CCNE Accreditation:

PROGRAM INFORMATION

Two Year Exit Option: *No* • NLNAC Accreditation: *Yes* • CCNE Accreditation: *Yes*

NURSING STUDENT PROFILE

Total Nursing Enrollment: *246* • Total Basic Student Enrollment, Full Time: *242* • Total Basic Student Enrollment, Part Time: *2* • Female Basic Student Enrollment: *232* • Male Basic Student Enrollment: *12* • Total RN Enrollment: *2* • Total New Fall Enrollments: *91* • Total Graduates: *63* • Basic Student Graduates: *63* • RN Student Graduates: *0*

NURSING STUDENT PROFILE

Total Nursing Enrollment: *136* • Total Basic Student Enrollment, Full Time: *122* • Total Basic Student Enrollment, Part Time: *13* • Female Basic Student Enrollment: *111* • Male Basic Student Enrollment: *24* • Total RN Enrollment: *1* • Total New Fall Enrollments: *45* • Total Graduates: *38* • Basic Student Graduates: *36* • RN Student Graduates: *2*

FINANCES

Residential Annual Tuition: *$15,452* • Non-Residential Annual Tuition: *Not Reported* • General Institutional Fees: *$7,726* • Additional Nursing Fees: *$588*

FINANCES

Residential Annual Tuition: *$18,000* • Non-Residential Annual Tuition: *$18,000* • General Institutional Fees: *$500* • Additional Nursing Fees: *$0*

SAINT FRANCIS CAREER COLLEGE

Address: 3630 East Imperial Highway, Lynwood, CA 90262
Phone: 814-472-3027
Fax: 814-472-3849
Contact: Jean M. Samii, PhD, RN, Chair and Professor
Email: Jsamii@francis.edu

GENERAL INFORMATION

Type of School: *Not Reported* • Accreditation: *Not Reported* • Total Enrollment: *Not Reported*

PROGRAM INFORMATION

Two Year Exit Option: *Not Reported* • NLNAC Accreditation: *Yes* • CCNE Accreditation:

NURSING STUDENT PROFILE

Total Nursing Enrollment: *Not Reported* • Total Basic Student Enrollment, Full Time: *Not Reported* • Total Basic Student Enrollment, Part Time: *Not Reported* • Female Basic Student Enrollment: *Not Reported* • Male Basic Student Enrollment: *Not Reported* • Total RN Enrollment: *Not Reported* • Total New Fall Enrollments: *14* • Total Graduates: *7* • Basic Student Graduates: *7* • RN Student Graduates: *0*

FINANCES

Residential Annual Tuition: *$16,796* • Non-Residential Annual Tuition: *$16,796* • General Institutional Fees: *Not Reported* • Additional Nursing Fees: *Not Reported*

SAMUEL MERRITT COLLEGE—SAINT MARY COLLEGE

Address: 370 Hawthorne Ave, Oakland, CA 94609
Phone: 510-869-6129
Fax: *Not Reported*
Contact: Sarah B. Keating, EdD, RN, FAAN, Dean
Email: skeating@samuelmerritt.edu

GENERAL INFORMATION

Type of School: *4-Year College or University, Private (Independent)* • Accreditation: *Western Association of Schools and Colleges* • Total Enrollment: *700*

PROGRAM INFORMATION

Two Year Exit Option: *No* • NLNAC Accreditation: *Not Reported* • CCNE Accreditation:

NURSING STUDENT PROFILE

Total Nursing Enrollment: *270* • Total Basic Student Enrollment, Full Time: *Not Reported* • Total Basic Student Enrollment, Part Time: *Not Reported* • Female Basic Student Enrollment: *Not Reported* • Male Basic Student Enrollment: *Not Reported* • Total RN Enrollment: *15* • Total New Fall Enrollments: *57* • Total Graduates: *95* • Basic Student Graduates: *85* • RN Student Graduates: *10*

FINANCES

Residential Annual Tuition: *Not Reported* • Non-Residential Annual Tuition: *Not Reported* • General Institutional Fees: *Not Reported* • Additional Nursing Fees: *Not Reported*

SAN DIEGO STATE UNIVERSITY

Address: 5300 Campantle Drive, San Diego, CA 92182-
             4158
Phone: 619-594-6384
Fax: *Not Reported*
Contact: Patricia R. Wahlfrd, PhD, RN, FAAN, Director
Email: pwrhl@mail.sdsu.edu

GENERAL INFORMATION

Type of School: *4-Year College or University, Public* •
Accreditation: *Western Association of Schools and Colleges* •
Total Enrollment: *28000*

PROGRAM INFORMATION

Two Year Exit Option: *No* • NLNAC Accreditation: *Yes* •
CCNE Accreditation:

NURSING STUDENT PROFILE

Total Nursing Enrollment: *288* • Total Basic Student
Enrollment, Full Time: *201* • Total Basic Student
Enrollment, Part Time: *79* • Female Basic Student
Enrollment: *243* • Male Basic Student Enrollment: *37* • Total
RN Enrollment: *8* • Total New Fall Enrollments: *102* • Total
Graduates: *73* • Basic Student Graduates: *65* • RN Student
Graduates: *8*

FINANCES

Residential Annual Tuition: *Not Reported* • Non-Residential
Annual Tuition: *Not Reported* • General Institutional Fees:
Not Reported • Additional Nursing Fees: *Not Reported*

SAN FRANCISCO STATE UNIVERSITY

Address: 1600 Holloway Avenue, San Francisco, CA
             94132-4161
Phone: 415-338-1801
Fax: *Not Reported*
Contact: Patricia Hess, PhD, RN, Associate Director of
             BSN Program
Email: phess@sfsu.edu

GENERAL INFORMATION

Type of School: *4-Year College or University, Public* •
Accreditation: *Western Association of Schools and Colleges* •
Total Enrollment: *29000*

PROGRAM INFORMATION

Two Year Exit Option: *No* • NLNAC Accreditation: *Yes* •
CCNE Accreditation: *Yes*

NURSING STUDENT PROFILE

Total Nursing Enrollment: *249* • Total Basic Student
Enrollment, Full Time: *214* • Total Basic Student
Enrollment, Part Time: *0* • Female Basic Student
Enrollment: *187* • Male Basic Student Enrollment: *27* • Total
RN Enrollment: *35* • Total New Fall Enrollments: *72* • Total
Graduates: *50* • Basic Student Graduates: *45* • RN Student
Graduates: *5*

FINANCES

Residential Annual Tuition: *Not Reported* • Non-Residential
Annual Tuition: *Not Reported* • General Institutional Fees:
$913 • Additional Nursing Fees: *Not Reported*

SAN JOSE STATE UNIVERSITY

Address: One Washington Square, San Jose, CA 95192-
            0057
Phone: 408-924-3132
Fax: 408-924-3135
Contact: Bobbye Gorenberg, DNSc, RN, Director
Email: bobbyedg@email.sjsu.edu

GENERAL INFORMATION

Type of School: *4-Year College or University, Public* •
Accreditation: *Western Association of Schools and Colleges* •
Total Enrollment: *25668*

PROGRAM INFORMATION

Two Year Exit Option: *No* • NLNAC Accreditation: *Yes* •
CCNE Accreditation:

NURSING STUDENT PROFILE

Total Nursing Enrollment: *447* • Total Basic Student
Enrollment, Full Time: *267* • Total Basic Student
Enrollment, Part Time: *69* • Female Basic Student
Enrollment: *Not Reported* • Male Basic Student Enrollment:
Not Reported • Total RN Enrollment: *111* • Total New Fall
Enrollments: *93* • Total Graduates: *113* • Basic Student
Graduates: *81* • RN Student Graduates: *32*

FINANCES

Residential Annual Tuition: *Not Reported* • Non-Residential
Annual Tuition: *Not Reported* • General Institutional Fees:
Not Reported • Additional Nursing Fees: *Not Reported*

SONOMA STATE UNIVERSITY

Address: 1801 East Cotati Avenue, Rohnert Park, CA
            94928
Phone: 707-664-2654
Fax: 707-664-2653
Contact: Liz Close, PhD, RN, Chair
Email: liz.close@sonoma.edu

GENERAL INFORMATION

Type of School: *Not Reported* • Accreditation: *Western
Association of Schools and Colleges* • Total Enrollment: *7000*

PROGRAM INFORMATION

Two Year Exit Option: *No* • NLNAC Accreditation: *Yes* •
CCNE Accreditation:

NURSING STUDENT PROFILE

Total Nursing Enrollment: *138* • Total Basic Student
Enrollment, Full Time: *85* • Total Basic Student Enrollment,
Part Time: *0* • Female Basic Student Enrollment: *80* • Male
Basic Student Enrollment: *5* • Total RN Enrollment: *53* •
Total New Fall Enrollments: *30* • Total Graduates: *60* • Basic
Student Graduates: *38* • RN Student Graduates: *22*

FINANCES

Residential Annual Tuition: *Not Reported* • Non-Residential
Annual Tuition: *Not Reported* • General Institutional Fees:
$1,001 • Additional Nursing Fees: *Not Reported*

SOUTHWESTERN COLLEGE

Address: 900 Otay Lakes Road, Chula Vista, CA 91910-7299
Phone: 316-229-6325
Fax: *Not Reported*
Contact: Martha R. Butler, PhD, RN, Nursing Program Director
Email: mbutler@sc

GENERAL INFORMATION

Type of School: *2-Year College or University, Public* •
Accreditation: *Western Association of Schools and Colleges* •
Total Enrollment: *19538*

PROGRAM INFORMATION

Two Year Exit Option: *Not Reported* • NLNAC
Accreditation: *Not Reported* • CCNE Accreditation:

NURSING STUDENT PROFILE

Total Nursing Enrollment: *Not Reported* • Total Basic Student Enrollment, Full Time: *Not Reported* • Total Basic Student Enrollment, Part Time: *Not Reported* • Female Basic Student Enrollment: *Not Reported* • Male Basic Student Enrollment: *Not Reported* • Total RN Enrollment: *Not Reported* • Total New Fall Enrollments: *Not Reported* • Total Graduates: *Not Reported* • Basic Student Graduates: *Not Reported* • RN Student Graduates: *Not Reported*

FINANCES

Residential Annual Tuition: *Not Reported* • Non-Residential Annual Tuition: *Not Reported* • General Institutional Fees: *Not Reported* • Additional Nursing Fees: *Not Reported*

UNIVERSITY OF CALIFORNIA, SAN FRANCISCO

Address: 500 Parnassus Avenue, San Francisco, CA 94143
Phone: 416-476-9710
Fax: 415-476-9707
Contact: Marilyn Flood, PhD, RN, Associate Dean
Email: marilyn.flood@nursing.ucf.edu

GENERAL INFORMATION

Type of School: *4-Year College or University, Public* •
Accreditation: *Western Association of Schools and Colleges* •
Total Enrollment: *2500*

PROGRAM INFORMATION

Two Year Exit Option: *Not Reported* • NLNAC
Accreditation: *Not Reported* • CCNE Accreditation:

NURSING STUDENT PROFILE

Total Nursing Enrollment: *Not Reported* • Total Basic Student Enrollment, Full Time: *Not Reported* • Total Basic Student Enrollment, Part Time: *Not Reported* • Female Basic Student Enrollment: *Not Reported* • Male Basic Student Enrollment: *Not Reported* • Total RN Enrollment: *Not Reported* • Total New Fall Enrollments: *Not Reported* • Total Graduates: *Not Reported* • Basic Student Graduates: *Not Reported* • RN Student Graduates: *Not Reported*

FINANCES

Residential Annual Tuition: *Not Reported* • Non-Residential Annual Tuition: *Not Reported* • General Institutional Fees: *Not Reported* • Additional Nursing Fees: *Not Reported*

UNIVERSITY OF SAN FRANCISCO

Address: 2130 Fulton Street, San Francisco, CA 94117-1080
Phone: 415-422-2959
Fax: 415-422-6877
Contact: John M. Lantz, PhD, RN, Dean
Email: lantzj@usfca.edu

GENERAL INFORMATION

Type of School: *4-Year College or University, Private (Independent)* • Accreditation: *Western Association of Schools and Colleges* • Total Enrollment: *7366*

PROGRAM INFORMATION

Two Year Exit Option: *No* • NLNAC Accreditation: *Yes* • CCNE Accreditation:

NURSING STUDENT PROFILE

Total Nursing Enrollment: *4,614* • Total Basic Student Enrollment, Full Time: *Not Reported* • Total Basic Student Enrollment, Part Time: *Not Reported* • Female Basic Student Enrollment: *Not Reported* • Male Basic Student Enrollment: *Not Reported* • Total RN Enrollment: *356* • Total New Fall Enrollments: *82* • Total Graduates: *67* • Basic Student Graduates: *59* • RN Student Graduates: *8*

FINANCES

Residential Annual Tuition: *$18,860* • Non-Residential Annual Tuition: *$18,860* • General Institutional Fees: *Not Reported* • Additional Nursing Fees: *Not Reported*

UNIVERSITY OF SOUTHERN CALIFORNIA

Address: 1540 Alcazar Street, CHP 222, Los Angeles, CA 90033
Phone: 323-442-2058
Fax: 323-442-2090
Contact: Wynne R. Waugaman, PhD, CRNA, FAAN, Interim Chair
Email: waugaman@usc.edu

GENERAL INFORMATION

Type of School: *4-Year College or University, Private (Independent)* • Accreditation: *Southern Association of Colleges and Schools* • Total Enrollment: *28766*

PROGRAM INFORMATION

Two Year Exit Option: *No* • NLNAC Accreditation: *Yes* • CCNE Accreditation:

NURSING STUDENT PROFILE

Total Nursing Enrollment: *226* • Total Basic Student Enrollment, Full Time: *210* • Total Basic Student Enrollment, Part Time: *16* • Female Basic Student Enrollment: *199* • Male Basic Student Enrollment: *27* • Total RN Enrollment: *0* • Total New Fall Enrollments: *88* • Total Graduates: *121* • Basic Student Graduates: *117* • RN Student Graduates: *4*

FINANCES

Residential Annual Tuition: *$23,664* • Non-Residential Annual Tuition: *$23,664* • General Institutional Fees: *Not Reported* • Additional Nursing Fees: *$797*

MESA STATE COLLEGE

Address: P.O.Box 2647, Grand Junction, CO 81502
Phone: 970-248-1774
Fax: 970-248-1133
Contact: Judy Goodhart, MSN, RN, Program Director
Email: goodhart@mesastate.edu

GENERAL INFORMATION

Type of School: *4-Year College or University, Public* •
Accreditation: *North Central Association of Colleges and
Schools* • Total Enrollment: *5210*

PROGRAM INFORMATION

Two Year Exit Option: *No* • NLNAC Accreditation: *Not
Reported* • CCNE Accreditation: *Yes*

NURSING STUDENT PROFILE

Total Nursing Enrollment: *91* • Total Basic Student
Enrollment, Full Time: *81* • Total Basic Student Enrollment,
Part Time: *9* • Female Basic Student Enrollment: *78* • Male
Basic Student Enrollment: *12* • Total RN Enrollment: *1* •
Total New Fall Enrollments: *20* • Total Graduates: *14* • Basic
Student Graduates: *13* • RN Student Graduates: *1*

FINANCES

Residential Annual Tuition: *$2,182* • Non-Residential
Annual Tuition: *$6,793* • General Institutional Fees:
$1,091 • Additional Nursing Fees: *$112*

REGIS UNIVERSITY

Address: 3333 Regis Boulevard, Mail Code:g-8, Denver,
           CO 80221-1099
Phone: 303-458-4181
Fax: 303-964-5533
Contact: Candace Berardinelli, PhD, ANP, Acting
           Director
Email: cberardi@regis.edu

GENERAL INFORMATION

Type of School: *4-Year College or University, Private
(Religious)* • Accreditation: *North Central Association of
Colleges and Schools* • Total Enrollment: *12000*

PROGRAM INFORMATION

Two Year Exit Option: *No* • NLNAC Accreditation: *Yes* •
CCNE Accreditation: *Yes*

NURSING STUDENT PROFILE

Total Nursing Enrollment: *161* • Total Basic Student
Enrollment, Full Time: *123* • Total Basic Student
Enrollment, Part Time: *0* • Female Basic Student
Enrollment: *116* • Male Basic Student Enrollment: *7* • Total
RN Enrollment: *38* • Total New Fall Enrollments: *61* • Total
Graduates: *122* • Basic Student Graduates: *79* • RN Student
Graduates: *43*

FINANCES

Residential Annual Tuition: *$20,235* • Non-Residential
Annual Tuition: *Not Reported* • General Institutional Fees:
$8,700 • Additional Nursing Fees: *$224*

Circle 100 on reader card   See in-depth profile for more information

UNIVERSITY OF COLORADO—COLORADO SPRINGS–BETH-EL COLLEGE OF NURSING

Address: 1420 Austin Bluffs Parkway, P. O. Box 7150, Colorado Springs, CO 80933-7150
Phone: 719-262-4429
Fax: 719-262-4416
Contact: Cindy Roach, DSN, RN, Chair, Undergraduate Nursing
Email: croach@mil.uccs.edu

GENERAL INFORMATION

Type of School: *4-Year College or University, Public* • Accreditation: *North Central Association of Colleges and Schools* • Total Enrollment: *Not Reported*

PROGRAM INFORMATION

Two Year Exit Option: *No* • NLNAC Accreditation: *Yes* • CCNE Accreditation:

NURSING STUDENT PROFILE

Total Nursing Enrollment: *316* • Total Basic Student Enrollment, Full Time: *279* • Total Basic Student Enrollment, Part Time: *20* • Female Basic Student Enrollment: *276* • Male Basic Student Enrollment: *23* • Total RN Enrollment: *17* • Total New Fall Enrollments: *Not Reported* • Total Graduates: *62* • Basic Student Graduates: *54* • RN Student Graduates: *8*

FINANCES

Residential Annual Tuition: *Not Reported* • Non-Residential Annual Tuition: *Not Reported* • General Institutional Fees: *Not Reported* • Additional Nursing Fees: *$155*

UNIVERSITY OF COLORADO HEALTH SCIENCES CENTER

Address: 4200 East 9th Avenue, Denver, CO 80262
Phone: 303-315-4824
Fax: 303-315-8660
Contact: Gayle Preheim, EdD, RN, CNAA, BS Program Director
Email: gayle.preheim@uchsc.edu

GENERAL INFORMATION

Type of School: *4-Year College or University, Public* • Accreditation: *North Central Association of Colleges and Schools* • Total Enrollment: *2400*

PROGRAM INFORMATION

Two Year Exit Option: *No* • NLNAC Accreditation: *Yes* • CCNE Accreditation:

NURSING STUDENT PROFILE

Total Nursing Enrollment: *216* • Total Basic Student Enrollment, Full Time: *186* • Total Basic Student Enrollment, Part Time: *22* • Female Basic Student Enrollment: *192* • Male Basic Student Enrollment: *16* • Total RN Enrollment: *8* • Total New Fall Enrollments: *121* • Total Graduates: *73* • Basic Student Graduates: *73* • RN Student Graduates: *0*

FINANCES

Residential Annual Tuition: *$5,222* • Non-Residential Annual Tuition: *$18,180* • General Institutional Fees: *$150* • Additional Nursing Fees: *$225*

UNIVERSITY OF NORTHERN COLORADO

Address: Campus Box 125, Gunte Hall 3080, Greeley, CO 80639
Phone: 970-351-1689
Fax: 970-351-1701
Contact: Sandra C. Baird, EdD, RN, Director
Email: sbaird@unco.edu

GENERAL INFORMATION

Type of School: *4-Year College or University, Public* • Accreditation: *North Central Association of Colleges and Schools* • Total Enrollment: *10500*

PROGRAM INFORMATION

Two Year Exit Option: *No* • NLNAC Accreditation: *Yes* • CCNE Accreditation:

NURSING STUDENT PROFILE

Total Nursing Enrollment: *169* • Total Basic Student Enrollment, Full Time: *140* • Total Basic Student Enrollment, Part Time: *0* • Female Basic Student Enrollment: *131* • Male Basic Student Enrollment: *9* • Total RN Enrollment: *29* • Total New Fall Enrollments: *72* • Total Graduates: *86* • Basic Student Graduates: *66* • RN Student Graduates: *20*

FINANCES

Residential Annual Tuition: *$2,014* • Non-Residential Annual Tuition: *$8,896* • General Institutional Fees: *$1,007* • Additional Nursing Fees: *$112*

UNIVERSITY OF SOUTHERN COLORADO

Address: 2200 Bonforte Boulevard, Pueblo, CO 81001
Phone: 719-549-2477
Fax: 719-549-2519
Contact: Melva Steen, PhD, RN, Department Chair
Email: thomas@uscolo.edu

GENERAL INFORMATION

Type of School: *4-Year College or University, Public* • Accreditation: *North Central Association of Colleges and Schools* • Total Enrollment: *4000*

PROGRAM INFORMATION

Two Year Exit Option: *No* • NLNAC Accreditation: *Yes* • CCNE Accreditation:

NURSING STUDENT PROFILE

Total Nursing Enrollment: *64* • Total Basic Student Enrollment, Full Time: *58* • Total Basic Student Enrollment, Part Time: *0* • Female Basic Student Enrollment: *50* • Male Basic Student Enrollment: *8* • Total RN Enrollment: *6* • Total New Fall Enrollments: *0* • Total Graduates: *32* • Basic Student Graduates: *26* • RN Student Graduates: *6*

FINANCES

Residential Annual Tuition: *$2,289* • Non-Residential Annual Tuition: *$17,861* • General Institutional Fees: *$651* • Additional Nursing Fees: *$120*

FAIRFIELD UNIVERSITY

Address: 1073 North Benson Boulevard, Fairfield, CT
06430
Phone: 203-254-4000
Fax: 203-254-4126
Contact: Jeanne M. Novotny, PhD, RN, Dean and
Professor
Email: jnovotny@mail.fairfield.edu

GENERAL INFORMATION

Type of School: *4-Year College or University, Private (Religious)* • Accreditation: *New England Association of Schools and Colleges* • Total Enrollment: *5188*

PROGRAM INFORMATION

Two Year Exit Option: *No* • NLNAC Accreditation: *Yes* • CCNE Accreditation:

NURSING STUDENT PROFILE

Total Nursing Enrollment: *204* • Total Basic Student Enrollment, Full Time: *Not Reported* • Total Basic Student Enrollment, Part Time: *Not Reported* • Female Basic Student Enrollment: *176* • Male Basic Student Enrollment: *6* • Total RN Enrollment: *22* • Total New Fall Enrollments: *45* • Total Graduates: *50* • Basic Student Graduates: *47* • RN Student Graduates: *3*

FINANCES

Residential Annual Tuition: *$22,000* • Non-Residential Annual Tuition: *$22,000* • General Institutional Fees: *$455* • Additional Nursing Fees: *$100*

QUINNIPIAC UNIVERSITY

Address: 275 Mount Carmel Avenue, Hamden, CT
06518-1961
Phone: 203-281-8678
Fax: 203-281-8706
Contact: Rita Hammer, EdD, RN, Chairperson
Email: hammer@quinnipiac.edu

GENERAL INFORMATION

Type of School: *4-Year College or University, Private (Independent)* • Accreditation: *New England Association of Schools and Colleges* • Total Enrollment: *Not Reported*

PROGRAM INFORMATION

Two Year Exit Option: *Not Reported* • NLNAC Accreditation: *Not Reported* • CCNE Accreditation:

NURSING STUDENT PROFILE

Total Nursing Enrollment: *146* • Total Basic Student Enrollment, Full Time: *131* • Total Basic Student Enrollment, Part Time: *7* • Female Basic Student Enrollment: *Not Reported* • Male Basic Student Enrollment: *Not Reported* • Total RN Enrollment: *8* • Total New Fall Enrollments: *0* • Total Graduates: *0* • Basic Student Graduates: *0* • RN Student Graduates: *0*

FINANCES

Residential Annual Tuition: *$21,120* • Non-Residential Annual Tuition: *$21,120* • General Institutional Fees: *Not Reported* • Additional Nursing Fees: *Not Reported*

SAINT JOSEPH COLLEGE— WEST HARTFORD

Address: 1678 Asylum Ave., West Hartford, CT 06117
Phone: 860-231-5258
Fax: 860-231-8396
Contact: Virginia Knowlden, EdD, RN, Professor and
           Chairperson
Email: vknowlden@sjc.edu

GENERAL INFORMATION

Type of School: *Not Reported* • Accreditation: *Not Reported* •
Total Enrollment: *Not Reported*

PROGRAM INFORMATION

Two Year Exit Option: *No* • NLNAC Accreditation: *Yes* •
CCNE Accreditation:

NURSING STUDENT PROFILE

Total Nursing Enrollment: *90* • Total Basic Student
Enrollment, Full Time: *45* • Total Basic Student Enrollment,
Part Time: *27* • Female Basic Student Enrollment: *72* • Male
Basic Student Enrollment: *0* • Total RN Enrollment: *18* •
Total New Fall Enrollments: *37* • Total Graduates: *31* • Basic
Student Graduates: *26* • RN Student Graduates: *5*

FINANCES

Residential Annual Tuition: *$20,350* • Non-Residential
Annual Tuition: *$20,350* • General Institutional Fees: *$550* •
Additional Nursing Fees: *$430*

SOUTHERN CONNECTICUT STATE UNIVERSITY

Address: 501 Crescent Street, New Haven, CT 06515
Phone: 203-392-6487
Fax: 203-392-6493
Contact: Cesarina Thompson, PhD, RN, Chairperson
Email: thompson_c@southernct.edu

GENERAL INFORMATION

Type of School: *4-Year College or University, Public* •
Accreditation: *New England Association of Schools and
Colleges* • Total Enrollment: *12000*

PROGRAM INFORMATION

Two Year Exit Option: *No* • NLNAC Accreditation: *Yes* •
CCNE Accreditation:

NURSING STUDENT PROFILE

Total Nursing Enrollment: *130* • Total Basic Student
Enrollment, Full Time: *113* • Total Basic Student
Enrollment, Part Time: *12* • Female Basic Student
Enrollment: *117* • Male Basic Student Enrollment: *8* • Total
RN Enrollment: *5* • Total New Fall Enrollments: *70* • Total
Graduates: *40* • Basic Student Graduates: *33* • RN Student
Graduates: *7*

FINANCES

Residential Annual Tuition: *$2,142* • Non-Residential
Annual Tuition: *$6,934* • General Institutional Fees:
$1,071 • Additional Nursing Fees: *$211*

UNIVERSITY OF CONNECTICUT

Address: 231 Glenbrook Road, Storrs Mansfield, CT 06269
Phone: 860-486-0537
Fax: 860-486-0001
Contact: Laura Cox Dzurec, PhD, RN, Dean
Email: laura.dzurec@uconn.edu

GENERAL INFORMATION

Type of School: *4-Year College or University, Public* • Accreditation: *New England Association of Schools and Colleges* • Total Enrollment: *16696*

PROGRAM INFORMATION

Two Year Exit Option: *Not Reported* • NLNAC Accreditation: *Yes* • CCNE Accreditation: *Yes*

NURSING STUDENT PROFILE

Total Nursing Enrollment: *341* • Total Basic Student Enrollment, Full Time: *316* • Total Basic Student Enrollment, Part Time: *17* • Female Basic Student Enrollment: *28* • Male Basic Student Enrollment: *28* • Total RN Enrollment: *8* • Total New Fall Enrollments: *93* • Total Graduates: *66* • Basic Student Graduates: *66* • RN Student Graduates: *0*

FINANCES

Residential Annual Tuition: *$4,282* • Non-Residential Annual Tuition: *$13,056* • General Institutional Fees: *$2,141* • Additional Nursing Fees: *Not Reported*

WESTERN CONNECTICUT STATE UNIVERSITY

Address: 181 White Street-WH Building, Room 107, Danbury, CT 06810
Phone: 203-837-8557
Fax: 202-383-7825
Contact: Barbara Piscopo, EdD, RN, Chair
Email: piscopob@wcsu.edu

GENERAL INFORMATION

Type of School: *4-Year College or University, Public* • Accreditation: *New England Association of Schools and Colleges* • Total Enrollment: *5806*

PROGRAM INFORMATION

Two Year Exit Option: *No* • NLNAC Accreditation: *Yes* • CCNE Accreditation:

NURSING STUDENT PROFILE

Total Nursing Enrollment: *241* • Total Basic Student Enrollment, Full Time: *123* • Total Basic Student Enrollment, Part Time: *80* • Female Basic Student Enrollment: *187* • Male Basic Student Enrollment: *16* • Total RN Enrollment: *38* • Total New Fall Enrollments: *0* • Total Graduates: *32* • Basic Student Graduates: *31* • RN Student Graduates: *1*

FINANCES

Residential Annual Tuition: *$2,142* • Non-Residential Annual Tuition: *$6,934* • General Institutional Fees: *$1,071* • Additional Nursing Fees: *$154*

DELAWARE STATE UNIVERSITY

Address: 1200 North DuPont Highway, Dover, DE 19901
Phone: 302-857-6750
Fax: 302-857-6755
Contact: Mary P. Watkins, PhD, RN, Department
            Chairperson
Email: mwatkins@dsc.edu

GENERAL INFORMATION

Type of School: *4-Year College or University, Public* •
Accreditation: *Middle States Association of Colleges and
Schools* • Total Enrollment: *3500*

PROGRAM INFORMATION

Two Year Exit Option: *No* • NLNAC Accreditation: *Yes* •
CCNE Accreditation:

NURSING STUDENT PROFILE

Total Nursing Enrollment: *175* • Total Basic Student
Enrollment, Full Time: *140* • Total Basic Student
Enrollment, Part Time: *25* • Female Basic Student
Enrollment: *150* • Male Basic Student Enrollment: *15* • Total
RN Enrollment: *10* • Total New Fall Enrollments: *65* • Total
Graduates: *21* • Basic Student Graduates: *20* • RN Student
Graduates: *1*

FINANCES

Residential Annual Tuition: *$2,814* • Non-Residential
Annual Tuition: *$6,562* • General Institutional Fees:
$1,407 • Additional Nursing Fees: *$117*

UNIVERSITY OF DELAWARE

Address: McDowell Hall, Newark, DE 19716
Phone: 302-831-2193
Fax: 302-831-2382
Contact: Janice Selekman, DNSc, RN, Chair
Email: selekman@udel.edu

GENERAL INFORMATION

Type of School: *4-Year College or University, Private
(Independent)* • Accreditation: *Middle States Association of
Colleges and Schools* • Total Enrollment: *20888*

PROGRAM INFORMATION

Two Year Exit Option: *No* • NLNAC Accreditation: *Yes* •
CCNE Accreditation:

NURSING STUDENT PROFILE

Total Nursing Enrollment: *698* • Total Basic Student
Enrollment, Full Time: *384* • Total Basic Student
Enrollment, Part Time: *43* • Female Basic Student
Enrollment: *398* • Male Basic Student Enrollment: *29* • Total
RN Enrollment: *271* • Total New Fall Enrollments: *95* •
Total Graduates: *155* • Basic Student Graduates: *107* • RN
Student Graduates: *48*

FINANCES

Residential Annual Tuition: *$4,510* • Non-Residential
Annual Tuition: *$13,260* • General Institutional Fees:
$2,255 • Additional Nursing Fees: *$188*

THE CATHOLIC UNIVERSITY OF AMERICA

Address: 620 Michigan Avenue, North East, Washington
             DC 20064
Phone: 202-319-6458
Fax: 203-319-6485
Contact: Shirley Jarecki, PhD, RN, Director
Email: jarecki@cua.edu

GENERAL INFORMATION

Type of School: *4-Year College or University, Private (Independent)* • Accreditation: *Middle States Association of Colleges and Schools* • Total Enrollment: *5500*

PROGRAM INFORMATION

Two Year Exit Option: *No* • NLNAC Accreditation: *Yes* • CCNE Accreditation:

NURSING STUDENT PROFILE

Total Nursing Enrollment: *129* • Total Basic Student Enrollment, Full Time: *120* • Total Basic Student Enrollment, Part Time: *3* • Female Basic Student Enrollment: *123* • Male Basic Student Enrollment: *0* • Total RN Enrollment: *6* • Total New Fall Enrollments: *23* • Total Graduates: *65* • Basic Student Graduates: *65* • RN Student Graduates: *0*

FINANCES

Residential Annual Tuition: *$10,025* • Non-Residential Annual Tuition: *$10,025* • General Institutional Fees: *Not Reported* • Additional Nursing Fees: *$500*

GEORGETOWN UNIVERSITY

Address: 3700 Reservoir Road North West, Washington
             DC 20007
Phone: 202-687-8415
Fax: 202-687-5553
Contact: Dorrie Fontaine, DNSc, RN, Associate Dean for
             Undergraduate Studies
Email: fontained@georgetown.edu

GENERAL INFORMATION

Type of School: *4-Year College or University, Private (Religious)* • Accreditation: *Middle States Association of Colleges and Schools* • Total Enrollment: *3174*

PROGRAM INFORMATION

Two Year Exit Option: *No* • NLNAC Accreditation: *Yes* • CCNE Accreditation:

NURSING STUDENT PROFILE

Total Nursing Enrollment: *316* • Total Basic Student Enrollment, Full Time: *307* • Total Basic Student Enrollment, Part Time: *2* • Female Basic Student Enrollment: *289* • Male Basic Student Enrollment: *20* • Total RN Enrollment: *7* • Total New Fall Enrollments: *100* • Total Graduates: *64* • Basic Student Graduates: *61* • RN Student Graduates: *3*

FINANCES

Residential Annual Tuition: *$22,260* • Non-Residential Annual Tuition: *Not Reported* • General Institutional Fees: *$11,130* • Additional Nursing Fees: *$92,750*

HOWARD UNIVERSITY

Address: 501 Bryant Street North West, Washington, DC
20059
Phone: 202-806-7460
Fax: 202-806-5958
Contact: Jacquelyn D. Jordan, PhD, RN, Assistant Dean
Email: jjordan@howard.edu

GENERAL INFORMATION

Type of School: *4-Year College or University, Private
(Independent)* • Accreditation: *Middle States Association of
Colleges and Schools* • Total Enrollment: *10000*

PROGRAM INFORMATION

Two Year Exit Option: *No* • NLNAC Accreditation: *Yes* •
CCNE Accreditation:

NURSING STUDENT PROFILE

Total Nursing Enrollment: *207* • Total Basic Student
Enrollment, Full Time: *Not Reported* • Total Basic Student
Enrollment, Part Time: *Not Reported* • Female Basic Student
Enrollment: *181* • Male Basic Student Enrollment: *15* • Total
RN Enrollment: *11* • Total New Fall Enrollments: *38* • Total
Graduates: *57* • Basic Student Graduates: *54* • RN Student
Graduates: *3*

FINANCES

Residential Annual Tuition: *$9,190* • Non-Residential
Annual Tuition: *Not Reported* • General Institutional Fees:
$4,595 • Additional Nursing Fees: *$383*

BARRY UNIVERSITY

Address: 11300 North East Second Avenue, Miami
Shores, FL 33161-6695
Phone: 305-899-3800
Fax: 305-899-3831
Contact: Linda K. Perkel, PhD, RN, Associate Dean of
Undergraduate Program
Email: lperkel@mail.barry.edu

GENERAL INFORMATION

Type of School: *4-Year College or University, Private
(Religious)* • Accreditation: *Southern Association of Colleges
and Schools* • Total Enrollment: *8700*

PROGRAM INFORMATION

Two Year Exit Option: *No* • NLNAC Accreditation: *Not
Reported* • CCNE Accreditation: *Yes*

NURSING STUDENT PROFILE

Total Nursing Enrollment: *273* • Total Basic Student
Enrollment, Full Time: *209* • Total Basic Student
Enrollment, Part Time: *26* • Female Basic Student
Enrollment: *198* • Male Basic Student Enrollment: *37* • Total
RN Enrollment: *38* • Total New Fall Enrollments: *62* • Total
Graduates: *86* • Basic Student Graduates: *65* • RN Student
Graduates: *21*

FINANCES

Residential Annual Tuition: *$16,600* • Non-Residential
Annual Tuition: *Not Reported* • General Institutional Fees:
Not Reported • Additional Nursing Fees: *$200*

BETHUNE–COOKMAN COLLEGE

Address: 640 Dr. Mary McLeod Bethune Boulevard, Daytona Beach, FL 32114
Phone: 386-481-2100
Fax: 386-481-2102
Contact: Alma Dixon, EdD, MPH, RN, Chair
Email: dixonal@cookman.edu

FLORIDA A&M UNIVERSITY

Address: P.O. Box 136, Tallahassee, FL 32307
Phone: 850-599-3017
Fax: 850-599-3847
Contact: Margaret W. Lewis, PhD, RN, Dean
Email: margaret.lewis@famu.edu

GENERAL INFORMATION

Type of School: *4-Year College or University, Private (Religious)* • Accreditation: *Southern Association of Colleges and Schools* • Total Enrollment: *2558*

GENERAL INFORMATION

Type of School: *4-Year College or University, Public* • Accreditation: *Southern Association of Colleges and Schools* • Total Enrollment: *12000*

PROGRAM INFORMATION

Two Year Exit Option: *No* • NLNAC Accreditation: *Yes* • CCNE Accreditation:

PROGRAM INFORMATION

Two Year Exit Option: *No* • NLNAC Accreditation: *Yes* • CCNE Accreditation:

NURSING STUDENT PROFILE

Total Nursing Enrollment: *185* • Total Basic Student Enrollment, Full Time: *182* • Total Basic Student Enrollment, Part Time: *0* • Female Basic Student Enrollment: *170* • Male Basic Student Enrollment: *12* • Total RN Enrollment: *3* • Total New Fall Enrollments: *36* • Total Graduates: *7* • Basic Student Graduates: *7* • RN Student Graduates: *0*

NURSING STUDENT PROFILE

Total Nursing Enrollment: *334* • Total Basic Student Enrollment, Full Time: *334* • Total Basic Student Enrollment, Part Time: *0* • Female Basic Student Enrollment: *318* • Male Basic Student Enrollment: *16* • Total RN Enrollment: *0* • Total New Fall Enrollments: *30* • Total Graduates: *50* • Basic Student Graduates: *50* • RN Student Graduates: *0*

FINANCES

Residential Annual Tuition: *$12,992* • Non-Residential Annual Tuition: *Not Reported* • General Institutional Fees: *$7,659* • Additional Nursing Fees: *$0*

FINANCES

Residential Annual Tuition: *$2,883* • Non-Residential Annual Tuition: *$13,928* • General Institutional Fees: *$108* • Additional Nursing Fees: *$7,688*

FLORIDA ATLANTIC UNIVERSITY

Address:　777 Glades Road, Boca Raton, FL 33431
Phone:　561-297-3206
Fax:　561-297-3687
Contact:　Anne Boykin, PhD, RN, Dean and Professor
Email:　boykina@fau.edu

GENERAL INFORMATION

Type of School: *4-Year College or University, Public* •
Accreditation: *Southern Association of Colleges and Schools* •
Total Enrollment: *25000*

PROGRAM INFORMATION

Two Year Exit Option: *No* • NLNAC Accreditation: *Yes* •
CCNE Accreditation:

NURSING STUDENT PROFILE

Total Nursing Enrollment: *431* • Total Basic Student
Enrollment, Full Time: *90* • Total Basic Student Enrollment,
Part Time: *23* • Female Basic Student Enrollment: *101* •
Male Basic Student Enrollment: *12* • Total RN Enrollment:
318 • Total New Fall Enrollments: *60* • Total Graduates:
163 • Basic Student Graduates: *66* • RN Student Graduates:
97

FINANCES

Residential Annual Tuition: *$2,845* • Non-Residential
Annual Tuition: *$11,160* • General Institutional Fees: *$948* •
Additional Nursing Fees: *$79*

FLORIDA GULF COAST UNIVERSITY

Address:　10501 FGCU Boulevard South, Fort Myers, FL
　　　　　33965-6565
Phone:　941-590-7505
Fax:　941-590-7474
Contact:　Carol E. Davis, PhD, RN, Director
Email:　cdavis@fgcu.edu

GENERAL INFORMATION

Type of School: *4-Year College or University, Public* •
Accreditation: *Southern Association of Colleges and Schools* •
Total Enrollment: *7500*

PROGRAM INFORMATION

Two Year Exit Option: *No* • NLNAC Accreditation: *Yes* •
CCNE Accreditation:

NURSING STUDENT PROFILE

Total Nursing Enrollment: *158* • Total Basic Student
Enrollment, Full Time: *95* • Total Basic Student Enrollment,
Part Time: *30* • Female Basic Student Enrollment: *112* •
Male Basic Student Enrollment: *13* • Total RN Enrollment:
33 • Total New Fall Enrollments: *70* • Total Graduates: *29* •
Basic Student Graduates: *20* • RN Student Graduates: *9*

FINANCES

Residential Annual Tuition: *$3,026* • Non-Residential
Annual Tuition: *$14,071* • General Institutional Fees: *$71* •
Additional Nursing Fees: *$200*

Circle 51 on reader card　　　　**See in-depth profile for more information**

FLORIDA INTERNATIONAL UNIVERSITY

Address: 3000 North East 151st Street, Building AC 2, Room 230, Miami, FL 33181-3605
Phone: 305-919-5000
Fax: 305-919-5001
Contact: Kathleen Blais, EdD, ARNP, Associate Dean
Email: blisk@fiu.edu

GENERAL INFORMATION

Type of School: *Not Reported* • Accreditation: *Southern Association of Colleges and Schools* • Total Enrollment: *31000*

PROGRAM INFORMATION

Two Year Exit Option: *Not Reported* • NLNAC Accreditation: *Yes* • CCNE Accreditation:

NURSING STUDENT PROFILE

Total Nursing Enrollment: *334* • Total Basic Student Enrollment, Full Time: *136* • Total Basic Student Enrollment, Part Time: *8* • Female Basic Student Enrollment: *112* • Male Basic Student Enrollment: *32* • Total RN Enrollment: *190* • Total New Fall Enrollments: *50* • Total Graduates: *150* • Basic Student Graduates: *80* • RN Student Graduates: *70*

FINANCES

Residential Annual Tuition: *$2,846* • Non-Residential Annual Tuition: *$14,609* • General Institutional Fees: *$231* • Additional Nursing Fees: *$7,472*

FLORIDA STATE UNIVERSITY

Address: 102 Vivian M. Duxbury Hall, Tallahassee, FL 32306-4310
Phone: 850-644-3299
Fax: 850-644-7660
Contact: Evelyn T. Singer, PhD, RN, Dean and Professor
Email: esinger@mailer.fsu.edu

GENERAL INFORMATION

Type of School: *4-Year College or University, Public* • Accreditation: *Southern Association of Colleges and Schools* • Total Enrollment: *33327*

PROGRAM INFORMATION

Two Year Exit Option: *No* • NLNAC Accreditation: *Yes* • CCNE Accreditation:

NURSING STUDENT PROFILE

Total Nursing Enrollment: *957* • Total Basic Student Enrollment, Full Time: *800* • Total Basic Student Enrollment, Part Time: *0* • Female Basic Student Enrollment: *745* • Male Basic Student Enrollment: *55* • Total RN Enrollment: *157* • Total New Fall Enrollments: *72* • Total Graduates: *159* • Basic Student Graduates: *121* • RN Student Graduates: *38*

FINANCES

Residential Annual Tuition: *$2,674* • Non-Residential Annual Tuition: *$11,235* • General Institutional Fees: *$993* • Additional Nursing Fees: *$7,642*

JACKSONVILLE UNIVERSITY

Address: 2800 University Boulevard North, Jacksonville, FL 32211
Phone: 904-745-7280
Fax: 904-745-7287
Contact: Linda Miller, EdD, RN, Director
Email: lmiller@ju.edu

GENERAL INFORMATION

Type of School: *4-Year College or University, Private (Independent)* • Accreditation: *Southern Association of Colleges and Schools* • Total Enrollment: *Not Reported*

PROGRAM INFORMATION

Two Year Exit Option: *No* • NLNAC Accreditation: *Yes* • CCNE Accreditation:

NURSING STUDENT PROFILE

Total Nursing Enrollment: *153* • Total Basic Student Enrollment, Full Time: *89* • Total Basic Student Enrollment, Part Time: *34* • Female Basic Student Enrollment: *102* • Male Basic Student Enrollment: *21* • Total RN Enrollment: *30* • Total New Fall Enrollments: *36* • Total Graduates: *38* • Basic Student Graduates: *28* • RN Student Graduates: *10*

FINANCES

Residential Annual Tuition: *$17,700* • Non-Residential Annual Tuition: *$17,700* • General Institutional Fees: *$240* • Additional Nursing Fees: *$509*

PENSACOLA CHRISTIAN COLLEGE

Address: 250 Brent Lane, Pensacola, FL 32503
Phone: 850-478-8496
Fax: *Not Reported*
Contact: Teresa Haughton, MSN, RN, Dean
Email: *Not Reported*

GENERAL INFORMATION

Type of School: *Not Reported* • Accreditation: *Not Reported* • Total Enrollment: *Not Reported*

PROGRAM INFORMATION

Two Year Exit Option: *No* • NLNAC Accreditation: *Not Reported* • CCNE Accreditation:

NURSING STUDENT PROFILE

Total Nursing Enrollment: *150* • Total Basic Student Enrollment, Full Time: *150* • Total Basic Student Enrollment, Part Time: *0* • Female Basic Student Enrollment: *Not Reported* • Male Basic Student Enrollment: *Not Reported* • Total RN Enrollment: *0* • Total New Fall Enrollments: *Not Reported* • Total Graduates: *50* • Basic Student Graduates: *50* • RN Student Graduates: *0*

FINANCES

Residential Annual Tuition: *Not Reported* • Non-Residential Annual Tuition: *Not Reported* • General Institutional Fees: *Not Reported* • Additional Nursing Fees: *Not Reported*

SOUTH COLLEGE

Address: 1760 North Congress Avenue, West Palm Beach, FL 33409
Phone: 561-697-9200
Fax: 561-697-9944
Contact: Rita A. Dekker, MSN, ARNP-C, Director
Email: t.dekker@southcollege.edu

GENERAL INFORMATION

Type of School: *4-Year College or University, Private (Independent)* • Accreditation: *Southern Association of Colleges and Schools* • Total Enrollment: *Not Reported*

PROGRAM INFORMATION

Two Year Exit Option: *Yes* • NLNAC Accreditation: *Not Reported* • CCNE Accreditation:

NURSING STUDENT PROFILE

Total Nursing Enrollment: 25 • Total Basic Student Enrollment, Full Time: 25 • Total Basic Student Enrollment, Part Time: 0 • Female Basic Student Enrollment: 21 • Male Basic Student Enrollment: 4 • Total RN Enrollment: 0 • Total New Fall Enrollments: 25 • Total Graduates: 0 • Basic Student Graduates: 0 • RN Student Graduates: 0

FINANCES

Residential Annual Tuition: *Not Reported* • Non-Residential Annual Tuition: *Not Reported* • General Institutional Fees: *Not Reported* • Additional Nursing Fees: *Not Reported*

ST. PETERSBURG COLLEGE

Address: P.O. Box 13489, Saint Petersburg, FL 33733
Phone: 727-345-7752
Fax: 727-341-3646
Contact: Verine J. Parks-Doyle, MSN, EdD, BSN, RN, Director of Nursing
Email: parksj@spjc.edu
Web: www.spjc.edu

GENERAL INFORMATION

Type of School: *4-Year College or University, Public* • Accreditation: *Southern Association of Colleges and Schools* • Total Enrollment: *58,000*

PROGRAM INFORMATION

LPN/LVN Exit: *No* • NLNAC Accreditation: *Yes*

NURSING STUDENT PROFILE

Total Nursing Enrollment: 362 • Full-Time Enrollment: 362 • Part-Time Enrollment: 0 • Female Enrollment: 335 • Male Enrollment: 27 • Total New Admissions Who Enrolled for Fall: 105 • Total Graduates: 233

FINANCES

Residential Annual Tuition: *$1,511* • Non-Residential Annual Tuition: *$5,580* • General Institution Fees: *Not Reported* • Additional Nursing Fees: *$267*

UNIVERSITY OF CENTRAL FLORIDA

Address: 4000 Central Florida Boulevard, Orlando, FL 32816
Phone: 407-823-2744
Fax: 407-823-5675
Contact: Patricia Leli, MSN, RN, Undergraduate Coordinator/ Instructor
Email: pleli@mail.ucf.edu

GENERAL INFORMATION

Type of School: *4-Year College or University, Public* •
Accreditation: *Southern Association of Colleges and Schools* •
Total Enrollment: *36000*

PROGRAM INFORMATION

Two Year Exit Option: *No* • NLNAC Accreditation: *Yes* •
CCNE Accreditation:

NURSING STUDENT PROFILE

Total Nursing Enrollment: *194* • Total Basic Student Enrollment, Full Time: *189* • Total Basic Student Enrollment, Part Time: *5* • Female Basic Student Enrollment: *179* • Male Basic Student Enrollment: *15* • Total RN Enrollment: *0* • Total New Fall Enrollments: *90* • Total Graduates: *70* • Basic Student Graduates: *70* • RN Student Graduates: *0*

FINANCES

Residential Annual Tuition: *$3,021* • Non-Residential Annual Tuition: *$14,785* • General Institutional Fees: *$180* • Additional Nursing Fees: *$50*

UNIVERSITY OF FLORIDA J. HILLIS MILLER HEALTH CENTER

Address: P.O. Box 100197, Gainesville, FL 32610
Phone: 352-273-6011
Fax: *Not Reported*
Contact: Kathleen Long, PhD, RN, Dean
Email: longka@nursing.ufl.edu

GENERAL INFORMATION

Type of School: *4-Year College or University, Public* •
Accreditation: *Southern Association of Colleges and Schools* •
Total Enrollment: *43000*

PROGRAM INFORMATION

Two Year Exit Option: *Not Reported* • NLNAC Accreditation: *Yes* • CCNE Accreditation:

NURSING STUDENT PROFILE

Total Nursing Enrollment: *315* • Total Basic Student Enrollment, Full Time: *282* • Total Basic Student Enrollment, Part Time: *2* • Female Basic Student Enrollment: *262* • Male Basic Student Enrollment: *22* • Total RN Enrollment: *31* • Total New Fall Enrollments: *140* • Total Graduates: *144* • Basic Student Graduates: *134* • RN Student Graduates: *10*

FINANCES

Residential Annual Tuition: *Not Reported* • Non-Residential Annual Tuition: *Not Reported* • General Institutional Fees: *Not Reported* • Additional Nursing Fees: *Not Reported*

UNIVERSITY OF MIAMI

Address: 58010 Red Road, Miami, FL 33143
Phone: 305-284-3666
Fax: 305-284-4370
Contact: Sharon Pontious, PhD, RN, Coordinator
Email: spontious@miami.edu

GENERAL INFORMATION

Type of School: *Independent, Private (Independent)* •
Accreditation: *Southern Association of Colleges and Schools* •
Total Enrollment: *13963*

PROGRAM INFORMATION

Two Year Exit Option: *No* • NLNAC Accreditation: *Yes* •
CCNE Accreditation:

NURSING STUDENT PROFILE

Total Nursing Enrollment: *246* • Total Basic Student
Enrollment, Full Time: *163* • Total Basic Student
Enrollment, Part Time: *28* • Female Basic Student
Enrollment: *165* • Male Basic Student Enrollment: *26* • Total
RN Enrollment: *55* • Total New Fall Enrollments: *70* • Total
Graduates: *93* • Basic Student Graduates: *62* • RN Student
Graduates: *31*

FINANCES

Residential Annual Tuition: *$25,838* • Non-Residential
Annual Tuition: *$25,838* • General Institutional Fees: *$442* •
Additional Nursing Fees: *$899*

UNIVERSITY OF NORTH FLORIDA

Address: 4567 Saint Johns Bluff Road South, Jacksonville,
             FL 32224-2673
Phone: 904-620-2684
Fax: 904-620-2848
Contact: Lucy B. Trice, PhD, ARNP, FNP, CS, Chair
Email: ltrice@unf.edu

GENERAL INFORMATION

Type of School: *4-Year College or University, Public* •
Accreditation: *Southern Association of Colleges and Schools* •
Total Enrollment: *12687*

PROGRAM INFORMATION

Two Year Exit Option: *Not Reported* • NLNAC
Accreditation: *Yes* • CCNE Accreditation:

NURSING STUDENT PROFILE

Total Nursing Enrollment: *191* • Total Basic Student
Enrollment, Full Time: *97* • Total Basic Student Enrollment,
Part Time: *39* • Female Basic Student Enrollment: *124* •
Male Basic Student Enrollment: *12* • Total RN Enrollment:
55 • Total New Fall Enrollments: *36* • Total Graduates: *103* •
Basic Student Graduates: *64* • RN Student Graduates: *39*

FINANCES

Residential Annual Tuition: *$2,913* • Non-Residential
Annual Tuition: *$13,268* • General Institutional Fees: *Not
Reported* • Additional Nursing Fees: *Not Reported*

UNIVERSITY OF SOUTH FLORIDA

Address: 12901 Bruce B. Downs Boulevard, MDC Box 22, Tampa, FL 33620
Phone: 813-974-5418
Fax: 813-974-5418
Contact: Patricia A. Burns, PhD, RN, FAAN, Dean and Professor
Email: pburns@hsc.usf.edu

GENERAL INFORMATION

Type of School: *4-Year College or University, Public* •
Accreditation: *Southern Association of Colleges and Schools* •
Total Enrollment: *37814*

PROGRAM INFORMATION

Two Year Exit Option: *No* • NLNAC Accreditation: *Yes* •
CCNE Accreditation: *Yes*

NURSING STUDENT PROFILE

Total Nursing Enrollment: *463* • Total Basic Student
Enrollment, Full Time: *157* • Total Basic Student
Enrollment, Part Time: *0* • Female Basic Student
Enrollment: *150* • Male Basic Student Enrollment: *7* • Total
RN Enrollment: *306* • Total New Fall Enrollments: *66* •
Total Graduates: *205* • Basic Student Graduates: *135* • RN
Student Graduates: *70*

FINANCES

Residential Annual Tuition: *$2,700* • Non-Residential
Annual Tuition: *$12,240* • General Institutional Fees: *$17* •
Additional Nursing Fees: *$89*

ALBANY STATE UNIVERSITY

Address: 504 College Drive, Albany, GA 31705
Phone: 229-430-4724
Fax: 229-430-3937
Contact: Lucille B. Wilson, EdD, RN, Dean
Email: lwilson@asurams.edu

GENERAL INFORMATION

Type of School: *4-Year College or University, Public* •
Accreditation: *Southern Association of Colleges and Schools* •
Total Enrollment: *3456*

PROGRAM INFORMATION

Two Year Exit Option: *No* • NLNAC Accreditation: *Yes* •
CCNE Accreditation:

NURSING STUDENT PROFILE

Total Nursing Enrollment: *209* • Total Basic Student
Enrollment, Full Time: *133* • Total Basic Student
Enrollment, Part Time: *44* • Female Basic Student
Enrollment: *164* • Male Basic Student Enrollment: *13* • Total
RN Enrollment: *32* • Total New Fall Enrollments: *14* • Total
Graduates: *15* • Basic Student Graduates: *7* • RN Student
Graduates: *8*

FINANCES

Residential Annual Tuition: *$1,238* • Non-Residential
Annual Tuition: *$3,864* • General Institutional Fees: *$272* •
Additional Nursing Fees: *$225*

ARMSTRONG ATLANTIC STATE UNIVERSITY

Address: 11935 Abercorn Street, Savannah, GA 31419
Phone: 912-927-5311
Fax: *Not Reported*
Contact: Sue W. Young, PhD, RN, Department Head
Email: youngsue@mail.armstrong.edu

GENERAL INFORMATION

Type of School: *4-Year College or University, Public* •
Accreditation: *Southern Association of Colleges and Schools* •
Total Enrollment: *5700*

PROGRAM INFORMATION

Two Year Exit Option: *No* • NLNAC Accreditation: *Yes* •
CCNE Accreditation:

NURSING STUDENT PROFILE

Total Nursing Enrollment: *126* • Total Basic Student
Enrollment, Full Time: *100* • Total Basic Student
Enrollment, Part Time: *8* • Female Basic Student
Enrollment: *104* • Male Basic Student Enrollment: *4* • Total
RN Enrollment: *18* • Total New Fall Enrollments: *55* • Total
Graduates: *71* • Basic Student Graduates: *43* • RN Student
Graduates: *28*

FINANCES

Residential Annual Tuition: *$2,098* • Non-Residential
Annual Tuition: *$7,522* • General Institutional Fees:
$1,049 • Additional Nursing Fees: *$221*

BRENAU UNIVERSITY

Address: One Centenial Circle, Gainesville, GA 39501
Phone: 770-534-6283
Fax: 770-538-4666
Contact: Cathy Dyches, PhD, RN, Chair
Email: cdyches@libibrenau.edu

GENERAL INFORMATION

Type of School: *4-Year College or University, Private
(Independent)* • Accreditation: *Southern Association of Colleges
and Schools* • Total Enrollment: *22139*

PROGRAM INFORMATION

Two Year Exit Option: *No* • NLNAC Accreditation: *Yes* •
CCNE Accreditation:

NURSING STUDENT PROFILE

Total Nursing Enrollment: *94* • Total Basic Student
Enrollment, Full Time: *76* • Total Basic Student Enrollment,
Part Time: *0* • Female Basic Student Enrollment: *73* • Male
Basic Student Enrollment: *3* • Total RN Enrollment: *18* •
Total New Fall Enrollments: *38* • Total Graduates: *125* •
Basic Student Graduates: *75* • RN Student Graduates: *50*

FINANCES

Residential Annual Tuition: *$19,350* • Non-Residential
Annual Tuition: *Not Reported* • General Institutional Fees:
$0 • Additional Nursing Fees: *$391*

CLAYTON COLLEGE AND STATE UNIVERSITY

Address: PO Box 285, Morrow, GA 30260
Phone: 770-961-3484
Fax: *Not Reported*
Contact: Linda F. Samson, PhD, RN, Dean
Email: lindasamson@mail.clayton.edu

GENERAL INFORMATION

Type of School: *4-Year College or University, Public* •
Accreditation: *Southern Association of Colleges and Schools* •
Total Enrollment: *4500*

PROGRAM INFORMATION

Two Year Exit Option: *No* • NLNAC Accreditation: *Yes* •
CCNE Accreditation: *Yes*

NURSING STUDENT PROFILE

Total Nursing Enrollment: *242* • Total Basic Student
Enrollment, Full Time: *100* • Total Basic Student
Enrollment, Part Time: *42* • Female Basic Student
Enrollment: *122* • Male Basic Student Enrollment: *20* • Total
RN Enrollment: *100* • Total New Fall Enrollments: *Not
Reported* • Total Graduates: *121* • Basic Student Graduates:
62 • RN Student Graduates: *59*

FINANCES

Residential Annual Tuition: *Not Reported* • Non-Residential
Annual Tuition: *Not Reported* • General Institutional Fees:
$904 • Additional Nursing Fees: *Not Reported*

COLUMBUS STATE UNIVERSITY

Address: 4225 University Avenue, Columbus, GA 31907
Phone: 706-568-2243
Fax: 706-569-3101
Contact: June Goyne, EdD, RN, BSN Program Director
Email: goyne_june@colstate.edu

GENERAL INFORMATION

Type of School: *4-Year College or University, Public* •
Accreditation: *Southern Association of Colleges and Schools* •
Total Enrollment: *5522*

PROGRAM INFORMATION

Two Year Exit Option: *No* • NLNAC Accreditation: *Yes* •
CCNE Accreditation:

NURSING STUDENT PROFILE

Total Nursing Enrollment: *72* • Total Basic Student
Enrollment, Full Time: *67* • Total Basic Student Enrollment,
Part Time: *0* • Female Basic Student Enrollment: *60* • Male
Basic Student Enrollment: *7* • Total RN Enrollment: *5* •
Total New Fall Enrollments: *34* • Total Graduates: *29* • Basic
Student Graduates: *29* • RN Student Graduates: *0*

FINANCES

Residential Annual Tuition: *$2,212* • Non-Residential
Annual Tuition: *$8,848* • General Institutional Fees: *$464* •
Additional Nursing Fees: *$0*

EMORY UNIVERSITY—NELL HODGSON WOODRUFF

Address: 1520 Clifton Rd. NE, Ste. 402, Atlanta, GA 30322
Phone: 404-727-7967
Fax: 404-727-8514
Contact: Helen O`Shea, PhD, RN, Chair, Adult and Elder Health, Baccalaureate Program
Email: hoshea@emory.edu

GENERAL INFORMATION

Type of School: *4-Year College or University, Private (Religious)* • Accreditation: *Southern Association of Colleges and Schools* • Total Enrollment: *11400*

PROGRAM INFORMATION

Two Year Exit Option: *No* • NLNAC Accreditation: *Not Reported* • CCNE Accreditation: *Yes*

NURSING STUDENT PROFILE

Total Nursing Enrollment: *130* • Total Basic Student Enrollment, Full Time: *126* • Total Basic Student Enrollment, Part Time: *1* • Female Basic Student Enrollment: *118* • Male Basic Student Enrollment: *9* • Total RN Enrollment: *3* • Total New Fall Enrollments: *60* • Total Graduates: *61* • Basic Student Graduates: *61* • RN Student Graduates: *0*

FINANCES

Residential Annual Tuition: *$24,240* • Non-Residential Annual Tuition: *$24,240* • General Institutional Fees: *$312* • Additional Nursing Fees: *$35*

GEORGIA BAPTIST COLLEGE OF NURSING

Address: 274 Boulevard NE, Atlanta, GA 30341-4115
Phone: 678-547-6798
Fax: 678-547-6796
Contact: Susan S. Gunby, PhD, RN, President
Email: gunby-ss@mercer.edu

GENERAL INFORMATION

Type of School: *Not Reported* • Accreditation: *Not Reported* • Total Enrollment: *Not Reported*

PROGRAM INFORMATION

Two Year Exit Option: *No* • NLNAC Accreditation: *Yes* • CCNE Accreditation:

NURSING STUDENT PROFILE

Total Nursing Enrollment: *311* • Total Basic Student Enrollment, Full Time: *248* • Total Basic Student Enrollment, Part Time: *52* • Female Basic Student Enrollment: *293* • Male Basic Student Enrollment: *7* • Total RN Enrollment: *11* • Total New Fall Enrollments: *80* • Total Graduates: *103* • Basic Student Graduates: *97* • RN Student Graduates: *6*

FINANCES

Residential Annual Tuition: *Not Reported* • Non-Residential Annual Tuition: *Not Reported* • General Institutional Fees: *Not Reported* • Additional Nursing Fees: *$335*

GEORGIA COLLEGE AND STATE UNIVERSITY

Address: 231 West Hancock St, PO 64, Milledgeville, GA 31062
Phone: 478-445-4004
Fax: 478-445-1913
Contact: Pamela C. Levi, EdD, RN, Dean, School of Health Sciences
Email: plevi@mail.gcsu.edu

GENERAL INFORMATION

Type of School: *4-Year College or University, Public* •
Accreditation: *Southern Association of Colleges and Schools* •
Total Enrollment: *5400*

PROGRAM INFORMATION

Two Year Exit Option: *No* • NLNAC Accreditation: *Yes* •
CCNE Accreditation:

NURSING STUDENT PROFILE

Total Nursing Enrollment: *144* • Total Basic Student
Enrollment, Full Time: *Not Reported* • Total Basic Student
Enrollment, Part Time: *Not Reported* • Female Basic Student
Enrollment: *104* • Male Basic Student Enrollment: *6* • Total
RN Enrollment: *34* • Total New Fall Enrollments: *45* • Total
Graduates: *82* • Basic Student Graduates: *59* • RN Student
Graduates: *23*

FINANCES

Residential Annual Tuition: *$1,876* • Non-Residential
Annual Tuition: *$7,506* • General Institutional Fees: *$938* •
Additional Nursing Fees: *$78*

GEORGIA SOUTHERN UNIVERSITY

Address: Box 8158, Statesboro, GA 30460-8158
Phone: 912-681-5454
Fax: 912-871-2115
Contact: Kathleen Koon, PhD, RN, CS, Director, BSN Program
Email: kkoon@gasou.edu

GENERAL INFORMATION

Type of School: *4-Year College or University, Public* •
Accreditation: *Southern Association of Colleges and Schools* •
Total Enrollment: *15000*

PROGRAM INFORMATION

Two Year Exit Option: *No* • NLNAC Accreditation: *Yes* •
CCNE Accreditation: *Yes*

NURSING STUDENT PROFILE

Total Nursing Enrollment: *183* • Total Basic Student
Enrollment, Full Time: *149* • Total Basic Student
Enrollment, Part Time: *0* • Female Basic Student
Enrollment: *136* • Male Basic Student Enrollment: *13* • Total
RN Enrollment: *34* • Total New Fall Enrollments: *34* • Total
Graduates: *50* • Basic Student Graduates: *43* • RN Student
Graduates: *7*

FINANCES

Residential Annual Tuition: *$1,876* • Non-Residential
Annual Tuition: *$9,380* • General Institutional Fees: *$938* •
Additional Nursing Fees: *$78*

GEORGIA SOUTHWESTERN STATE UNIVERSITY

Address: 800 Wheatley Street, Americus, GA 31709
Phone: 229-931-2662
Fax: 229-931-2288
Contact: Judith M. Malachowiski, PhD, RN, Chairperson
Email: jmm@canes.gsw.edu

GEORGIA STATE UNIVERSITY

Address: University Plaza, Atlanta, GA 30303
Phone: 404-651-2050
Fax: 404-651-4969
Contact: Judith L. Wold, PhD, RN, Director
Email: jwold@gsu.edu

GENERAL INFORMATION

Type of School: *4-Year College or University, Public* •
Accreditation: *Southern Association of Colleges and Schools* •
Total Enrollment: *2622*

GENERAL INFORMATION

Type of School: *4-Year College or University, Public* •
Accreditation: *Southern Association of Colleges and Schools* •
Total Enrollment: *24000*

PROGRAM INFORMATION

Two Year Exit Option: *Not Reported* • NLNAC
Accreditation: *Yes* • CCNE Accreditation: *Yes*

PROGRAM INFORMATION

Two Year Exit Option: *No* • NLNAC Accreditation: *Yes* •
CCNE Accreditation:

NURSING STUDENT PROFILE

Total Nursing Enrollment: *Not Reported* • Total Basic Student
Enrollment, Full Time: *Not Reported* • Total Basic Student
Enrollment, Part Time: *Not Reported* • Female Basic Student
Enrollment: *Not Reported* • Male Basic Student Enrollment:
Not Reported • Total RN Enrollment: *Not Reported* • Total
New Fall Enrollments: *Not Reported* • Total Graduates: *Not
Reported* • Basic Student Graduates: *Not Reported* • RN
Student Graduates: *Not Reported*

NURSING STUDENT PROFILE

Total Nursing Enrollment: *183* • Total Basic Student
Enrollment, Full Time: *133* • Total Basic Student
Enrollment, Part Time: *37* • Female Basic Student
Enrollment: *158* • Male Basic Student Enrollment: *12* • Total
RN Enrollment: *13* • Total New Fall Enrollments: *66* • Total
Graduates: *33* • Basic Student Graduates: *31* • RN Student
Graduates: *2*

FINANCES

Residential Annual Tuition: *Not Reported* • Non-Residential
Annual Tuition: *Not Reported* • General Institutional Fees:
Not Reported • Additional Nursing Fees: *Not Reported*

FINANCES

Residential Annual Tuition: *$2,506* • Non-Residential
Annual Tuition: *$10,024* • General Institutional Fees:
$1,253 • Additional Nursing Fees: *$104*

KENNESAW STATE UNIVERSITY

Address: 1000 Chastain Rd. Building 16, Kennesaw, GA
            30066
Phone: 770-423-6173
Fax: 770-423-6870
Contact: David N. Bennett, PhD, RN, Chair
Email: dbennett@kennesaw.edu

LA GRANGE COLLEGE

Address: 601 Broad Street, La Grange, GA 30240-2999
Phone: 706-880-8201
Fax: 706-880-8029
Contact: Maranah A. Sauter, PhD, RN, Professor and
            Chair
Email: msauter@lgc.edu

GENERAL INFORMATION

Type of School: *4-Year College or University, Public* •
Accreditation: *Southern Association of Colleges and Schools* •
Total Enrollment: *14000*

GENERAL INFORMATION

Type of School: *4-Year College or University, Private
(Religious)* • Accreditation: *Southern Association of Colleges
and Schools* • Total Enrollment: *918*

PROGRAM INFORMATION

Two Year Exit Option: *No* • NLNAC Accreditation: *Yes* •
CCNE Accreditation:

PROGRAM INFORMATION

Two Year Exit Option: *No* • NLNAC Accreditation: *Yes* •
CCNE Accreditation:

NURSING STUDENT PROFILE

Total Nursing Enrollment: *249* • Total Basic Student
Enrollment, Full Time: *83* • Total Basic Student Enrollment,
Part Time: *151* • Female Basic Student Enrollment: *213* •
Male Basic Student Enrollment: *21* • Total RN Enrollment:
15 • Total New Fall Enrollments: *61* • Total Graduates: *88* •
Basic Student Graduates: *69* • RN Student Graduates: *19*

NURSING STUDENT PROFILE

Total Nursing Enrollment: *35* • Total Basic Student
Enrollment, Full Time: *25* • Total Basic Student Enrollment,
Part Time: *5* • Female Basic Student Enrollment: *29* • Male
Basic Student Enrollment: *1* • Total RN Enrollment: *5* •
Total New Fall Enrollments: *15* • Total Graduates: *13* • Basic
Student Graduates: *11* • RN Student Graduates: *2*

FINANCES

Residential Annual Tuition: *$966* • Non-Residential Annual
Tuition: *$3,864* • General Institutional Fees: *$248* •
Additional Nursing Fees: *$115*

FINANCES

Residential Annual Tuition: *$12,000* • Non-Residential
Annual Tuition: *Not Reported* • General Institutional Fees:
$6,000 • Additional Nursing Fees: *$475*

MEDICAL COLLEGE OF GEORGIA

Address: 997 St. Sebastian Way, Augusta, GA 30912
Phone: 706-721-2787
Fax: 706-721-7390
Contact: Katherine E. Nugent, PhD, RN, Professor and
            Associate Dean, Academic Programs
Email: knugent@mail.mcg.edu

GENERAL INFORMATION

Type of School: *4-Year College or University, Public* •
Accreditation: *Southern Association of Colleges and Schools* •
Total Enrollment: *1939*

PROGRAM INFORMATION

Two Year Exit Option: *No* • NLNAC Accreditation: *Yes* •
CCNE Accreditation:

NURSING STUDENT PROFILE

Total Nursing Enrollment: *327* • Total Basic Student
Enrollment, Full Time: *281* • Total Basic Student
Enrollment, Part Time: *4* • Female Basic Student
Enrollment: *270* • Male Basic Student Enrollment: *15* • Total
RN Enrollment: *42* • Total New Fall Enrollments: *142* •
Total Graduates: *133* • Basic Student Graduates: *111* • RN
Student Graduates: *22*

FINANCES

Residential Annual Tuition: *$1,316* • Non-Residential
Annual Tuition: *$5,264* • General Institutional Fees: *$218* •
Additional Nursing Fees: *$15*

MERCER UNIVERSITY

Address: 1400 Coleman Avenue, Macon, GA 31207
Phone: 678-547-6798
Fax: 678-547-6796
Contact: Susan S. Gunby, PhD, RN, Dean
Email: gunby_ss@mercer.edu

GENERAL INFORMATION

Type of School: *4-Year College or University, Private
(Religious)* • Accreditation: *Southern Association of Colleges
and Schools* • Total Enrollment: *7000*

PROGRAM INFORMATION

Two Year Exit Option: *No* • NLNAC Accreditation: *Yes* •
CCNE Accreditation: *Yes*

NURSING STUDENT PROFILE

Total Nursing Enrollment: *313* • Total Basic Student
Enrollment, Full Time: *242* • Total Basic Student
Enrollment, Part Time: *62* • Female Basic Student
Enrollment: *296* • Male Basic Student Enrollment: *8* • Total
RN Enrollment: *9* • Total New Fall Enrollments: *97* • Total
Graduates: *84* • Basic Student Graduates: *77* • RN Student
Graduates: *7*

FINANCES

Residential Annual Tuition: *$11,200* • Non-Residential
Annual Tuition: *$11,200* • General Institutional Fees: *$500* •
Additional Nursing Fees: *$405*

PIEDMONT COLLEGE

Address: PO Box 10, Demorest, GA 30535
Phone: 706-776-0365
Fax: 706-776-0542
Contact: Frances W. Brown, PhD, RN, Dean
Email: fbrown@piedmont.edu

STATE UNIVERSITY OF WEST GEORGIA

Address: 1601 Maple St, Carrollton, GA 30118-4500
Phone: 770-836-4485
Fax: 770-836-4409
Contact: Jeanette Bernhardt, MSN, RN, Chairperson
Email: *Not Reported*

GENERAL INFORMATION

Type of School: *4-Year College or University, Private (Independent)* • Accreditation: *Southern Association of Colleges and Schools* • Total Enrollment: *2200*

GENERAL INFORMATION

Type of School: *4-Year College or University, Public* • Accreditation: *Southern Association of Colleges and Schools* • Total Enrollment: *8978*

PROGRAM INFORMATION

Two Year Exit Option: *Not Reported* • NLNAC Accreditation: *Not Reported* • CCNE Accreditation:

PROGRAM INFORMATION

Two Year Exit Option: *Not Reported* • NLNAC Accreditation: *Not Reported* • CCNE Accreditation:

NURSING STUDENT PROFILE

Total Nursing Enrollment: *33* • Total Basic Student Enrollment, Full Time: *33* • Total Basic Student Enrollment, Part Time: *0* • Female Basic Student Enrollment: *33* • Male Basic Student Enrollment: *0* • Total RN Enrollment: *0* • Total New Fall Enrollments: *19* • Total Graduates: *9* • Basic Student Graduates: *7* • RN Student Graduates: *2*

NURSING STUDENT PROFILE

Total Nursing Enrollment: *Not Reported* • Total Basic Student Enrollment, Full Time: *Not Reported* • Total Basic Student Enrollment, Part Time: *Not Reported* • Female Basic Student Enrollment: *Not Reported* • Male Basic Student Enrollment: *Not Reported* • Total RN Enrollment: *Not Reported* • Total New Fall Enrollments: *Not Reported* • Total Graduates: *Not Reported* • Basic Student Graduates: *Not Reported* • RN Student Graduates: *Not Reported*

FINANCES

Residential Annual Tuition: *$10,500* • Non-Residential Annual Tuition: *$10,500* • General Institutional Fees: *$0* • Additional Nursing Fees: *$300*

FINANCES

Residential Annual Tuition: *Not Reported* • Non-Residential Annual Tuition: *Not Reported* • General Institutional Fees: *Not Reported* • Additional Nursing Fees: *Not Reported*

VALDOSTA STATE UNIVERSITY

Address: 1300 N Patterson Street, Valdosta, GA 31698-0130
Phone: 229-333-5959
Fax: 229-333-7300
Contact: Maryann B. Reichenbach, PhD, RN, Dean
Email: mreichenbach@valdosta.edu

GENERAL INFORMATION

Type of School: *4-Year College or University, Public* •
Accreditation: *Southern Association of Colleges and Schools* •
Total Enrollment: *9700*

PROGRAM INFORMATION

Two Year Exit Option: *No* • NLNAC Accreditation: *Yes* •
CCNE Accreditation:

NURSING STUDENT PROFILE

Total Nursing Enrollment: *335* • Total Basic Student
Enrollment, Full Time: *290* • Total Basic Student
Enrollment, Part Time: *15* • Female Basic Student
Enrollment: *271* • Male Basic Student Enrollment: *34* • Total
RN Enrollment: *30* • Total New Fall Enrollments: *30* • Total
Graduates: *46* • Basic Student Graduates: *39* • RN Student
Graduates: *7*

FINANCES

Residential Annual Tuition: *$2,290* • Non-Residential
Annual Tuition: *$7,714* • General Institutional Fees:
$1,145 • Additional Nursing Fees: *$76*

UNIVERSITY OF GUAM

Address: Health Science Bldg. Rm 100, Mangilao, GM 96923
Phone: 671-735-2650
Fax: 671-734-1203
Contact: Maureen M. Fochtman, EdD, RN, Dean/Director
Email: fochtman@uog9.uog.edu

GENERAL INFORMATION

Type of School: *Not Reported* • Accreditation: *Not Reported* •
Total Enrollment: *Not Reported*

PROGRAM INFORMATION

Two Year Exit Option: *No* • NLNAC Accreditation: *Yes* •
CCNE Accreditation:

NURSING STUDENT PROFILE

Total Nursing Enrollment: *85* • Total Basic Student
Enrollment, Full Time: *80* • Total Basic Student Enrollment,
Part Time: *0* • Female Basic Student Enrollment: *70* • Male
Basic Student Enrollment: *10* • Total RN Enrollment: *5* •
Total New Fall Enrollments: *21* • Total Graduates: *32* • Basic
Student Graduates: *32* • RN Student Graduates: *0*

FINANCES

Residential Annual Tuition: *$3,424* • Non-Residential
Annual Tuition: *$10,208* • General Institutional Fees: *$420* •
Additional Nursing Fees: *$160*

HAWAII PACIFIC UNIVERSITY

Address: 45-045 Kamehameha Highway, Kaneohe, HI 96744
Phone: 808-236-5811
Fax: 808-236-5818
Contact: Carol E. Winters-Moorhead, PhD, RN, Dean and Academic Administrator
Email: cwinters@hpu.edu

GENERAL INFORMATION

Type of School: *4-Year College or University, Private (Independent)* • Accreditation: *Western Association of Schools and Colleges* • Total Enrollment: *768*

PROGRAM INFORMATION

Two Year Exit Option: *No* • NLNAC Accreditation: *Yes* • CCNE Accreditation:

NURSING STUDENT PROFILE

Total Nursing Enrollment: *722* • Total Basic Student Enrollment, Full Time: *492* • Total Basic Student Enrollment, Part Time: *210* • Female Basic Student Enrollment: *611* • Male Basic Student Enrollment: *91* • Total RN Enrollment: *20* • Total New Fall Enrollments: *0* • Total Graduates: *110* • Basic Student Graduates: *107* • RN Student Graduates: *3*

FINANCES

Residential Annual Tuition: *$4,230* • Non-Residential Annual Tuition: *$6,180* • General Institutional Fees: *$155* • Additional Nursing Fees: *$353*

UNIVERSITY OF HAWAII— HILO

Address: 200 W. Kawili Street, Hilo, HI 96720
Phone: 808-974-7761
Fax: *Not Reported*
Contact: Cecilia P. S. Wong Mukai, PhD, RN, FNP, Director
Email: cmukai@hawaii.edu

GENERAL INFORMATION

Type of School: *4-Year College or University, Public* • Accreditation: *Western Association of Schools and Colleges* • Total Enrollment: *2874*

PROGRAM INFORMATION

Two Year Exit Option: *No* • NLNAC Accreditation: *Yes* • CCNE Accreditation:

NURSING STUDENT PROFILE

Total Nursing Enrollment: *35* • Total Basic Student Enrollment, Full Time: *33* • Total Basic Student Enrollment, Part Time: *0* • Female Basic Student Enrollment: *27* • Male Basic Student Enrollment: *6* • Total RN Enrollment: *2* • Total New Fall Enrollments: *19* • Total Graduates: *19* • Basic Student Graduates: *18* • RN Student Graduates: *1*

FINANCES

Residential Annual Tuition: *Not Reported* • Non-Residential Annual Tuition: *Not Reported* • General Institutional Fees: *$50* • Additional Nursing Fees: *$108*

UNIVERSITY OF HAWAII— MANOA

Address: 2528 McCarthy Mall, Webster 330, Honolulu,
             HI 96822
Phone: 808-956-8522
Fax: *Not Reported*
Contact: Rosanne Harrigan, EdD, APRN, FAAN, Dean
Email: harrigan@hawaii.edu

BOISE STATE UNIVERSITY

Address: 1910 University Drive, Bosie, ID 83725-1840
Phone: 208-426-3783
Fax: 208-426-1370
Contact: Pat Taylor, MS, RN, Director
Email: ptaylor@boisestate.edu

GENERAL INFORMATION

Type of School: *4-Year College or University, Public* •
Accreditation: *Western Association of Schools and Colleges* •
Total Enrollment: *17498*

GENERAL INFORMATION

Type of School: *4-Year College or University, Public* •
Accreditation: *Northwestern Association of Schools and
Colleges* • Total Enrollment: *16300*

PROGRAM INFORMATION

Two Year Exit Option: *No* • NLNAC Accreditation: *Yes* •
CCNE Accreditation:

PROGRAM INFORMATION

Two Year Exit Option: *No* • NLNAC Accreditation: *Yes* •
CCNE Accreditation:

NURSING STUDENT PROFILE

Total Nursing Enrollment: *181* • Total Basic Student
Enrollment, Full Time: *143* • Total Basic Student
Enrollment, Part Time: *25* • Female Basic Student
Enrollment: *135* • Male Basic Student Enrollment: *33* • Total
RN Enrollment: *13* • Total New Fall Enrollments: *44* • Total
Graduates: *47* • Basic Student Graduates: *36* • RN Student
Graduates: *11*

NURSING STUDENT PROFILE

Total Nursing Enrollment: *147* • Total Basic Student
Enrollment, Full Time: *121* • Total Basic Student
Enrollment, Part Time: *0* • Female Basic Student
Enrollment: *107* • Male Basic Student Enrollment: *14* • Total
RN Enrollment: *26* • Total New Fall Enrollments: *44* • Total
Graduates: *72* • Basic Student Graduates: *43* • RN Student
Graduates: *29*

FINANCES

Residential Annual Tuition: *$3,024* • Non-Residential
Annual Tuition: *$9,304* • General Institutional Fees:
$1,512 • Additional Nursing Fees: *$126*

FINANCES

Residential Annual Tuition: *$0* • Non-Residential Annual
Tuition: *$6,000* • General Institutional Fees: *$1,722* •
Additional Nursing Fees: *$125*

IDAHO STATE UNIVERSITY

Address: 650 Memorial Drive, Builing 66, Campus Box
            8101, Pocatello, ID 83209-8101
Phone: 208-282-2185
Fax: 208-282-4476
Contact: Pamela N. Clarke, PhD, MPH, RN, Professor
            and Chair
Email: clarpame@isu.edu

GENERAL INFORMATION

Type of School: *4-Year College or University, Public* •
Accreditation: *Northwestern Association of Schools and
Colleges* • Total Enrollment: *12659*

PROGRAM INFORMATION

Two Year Exit Option: *No* • NLNAC Accreditation: *Yes* •
CCNE Accreditation:

NURSING STUDENT PROFILE

Total Nursing Enrollment: *154* • Total Basic Student
Enrollment, Full Time: *92* • Total Basic Student Enrollment,
Part Time: *0* • Female Basic Student Enrollment: *71* • Male
Basic Student Enrollment: *21* • Total RN Enrollment: *62* •
Total New Fall Enrollments: *50* • Total Graduates: *49* • Basic
Student Graduates: *36* • RN Student Graduates: *13*

FINANCES

Residential Annual Tuition: *$2,800* • Non-Residential
Annual Tuition: *$9,040* • General Institutional Fees:
$1,400 • Additional Nursing Fees: *$140*

LEWIS-CLARK STATE COLLEGE

Address: 500 8th Avenue, Lewiston, ID 83501
Phone: 208-792-2402
Fax: 208-792-2062
Contact: Donna Brandmeyer, EdD, RN, Division Chair
            and Professor
Email: dbrandmeyer@lcsc.edu

GENERAL INFORMATION

Type of School: *4-Year College or University, Public* •
Accreditation: *Northwestern Association of Schools and
Colleges* • Total Enrollment: *2702*

PROGRAM INFORMATION

Two Year Exit Option: *No* • NLNAC Accreditation: *Yes* •
CCNE Accreditation:

NURSING STUDENT PROFILE

Total Nursing Enrollment: *138* • Total Basic Student
Enrollment, Full Time: *89* • Total Basic Student Enrollment,
Part Time: *0* • Female Basic Student Enrollment: *78* • Male
Basic Student Enrollment: *11* • Total RN Enrollment: *49* •
Total New Fall Enrollments: *30* • Total Graduates: *45* • Basic
Student Graduates: *25* • RN Student Graduates: *20*

FINANCES

Residential Annual Tuition: *$3,126* • Non-Residential
Annual Tuition: *$9,124* • General Institutional Fees: *$348* •
Additional Nursing Fees: *$110*

NORTHWEST NAZARENE UNIVERSITY

Address: 623 Holly Street, Nampa, ID 83686
Phone: 208-467-8652
Fax: *Not Reported*
Contact: Judith P. Stocks, PhD, RN, Chair
Email: jpstocks@nnu.edu

GENERAL INFORMATION

Type of School: *4-Year College or University, Private (Independent)* • Accreditation: *Northwestern Association of Schools and Colleges* • Total Enrollment: *Not Reported*

PROGRAM INFORMATION

Two Year Exit Option: *Not Reported* • NLNAC Accreditation: *Not Reported* • CCNE Accreditation:

NURSING STUDENT PROFILE

Total Nursing Enrollment: *Not Reported* • Total Basic Student Enrollment, Full Time: *Not Reported* • Total Basic Student Enrollment, Part Time: *Not Reported* • Female Basic Student Enrollment: *Not Reported* • Male Basic Student Enrollment: *Not Reported* • Total RN Enrollment: *Not Reported* • Total New Fall Enrollments: *Not Reported* • Total Graduates: *Not Reported* • Basic Student Graduates: *Not Reported* • RN Student Graduates: *Not Reported*

FINANCES

Residential Annual Tuition: *Not Reported* • Non-Residential Annual Tuition: *Not Reported* • General Institutional Fees: *Not Reported* • Additional Nursing Fees: *Not Reported*

AURORA UNIVERSITY

Address: 347 South Gladstone, Aurora, IL 605064892
Phone: 630-844-5130
Fax: 630-844-7822
Contact: Marry A. Miller, PhD, RN, Dean and Professor
Email: mmiller@aurora.edu

GENERAL INFORMATION

Type of School: *4-Year College or University, Private (Independent)* • Accreditation: *North Central Association of Colleges and Schools* • Total Enrollment: *2371*

PROGRAM INFORMATION

Two Year Exit Option: *No* • NLNAC Accreditation: *Yes* • CCNE Accreditation: *Yes*

NURSING STUDENT PROFILE

Total Nursing Enrollment: *111* • Total Basic Student Enrollment, Full Time: *46* • Total Basic Student Enrollment, Part Time: *14* • Female Basic Student Enrollment: *57* • Male Basic Student Enrollment: *3* • Total RN Enrollment: *51* • Total New Fall Enrollments: *21* • Total Graduates: *36* • Basic Student Graduates: *30* • RN Student Graduates: *6*

FINANCES

Residential Annual Tuition: *$4,306* • Non-Residential Annual Tuition: *$4,306* • General Institutional Fees: *$442* • Additional Nursing Fees: *$344*

BLESSING-RIEMAN COLLEGE

Address: 33809 Broadway at 11th, Box 7005, Quinay, IL
Phone: 217-228-5520
Fax: 217-223-4661
Contact: Pamela Brown, MS, RN, President/CEO
Email: pbrown@blessinghospital.com

GENERAL INFORMATION

Type of School: *Not Reported* • Accreditation: *Not Reported* •
Total Enrollment: *Not Reported*

PROGRAM INFORMATION

Two Year Exit Option: *Not Reported* • NLNAC
Accreditation: *Yes* • CCNE Accreditation: *Yes*

NURSING STUDENT PROFILE

Total Nursing Enrollment: *124* • Total Basic Student
Enrollment, Full Time: *109* • Total Basic Student
Enrollment, Part Time: *7* • Female Basic Student
Enrollment: *109* • Male Basic Student Enrollment: *7* • Total
RN Enrollment: *8* • Total New Fall Enrollments: *38* • Total
Graduates: *21* • Basic Student Graduates: *16* • RN Student
Graduates: *5*

FINANCES

Residential Annual Tuition: *$10,650* • Non-Residential
Annual Tuition: *$14,300* • General Institutional Fees:
$5,325 • Additional Nursing Fees: *$300*

BRADLEY UNIVERSITY

Address: 1501 West Bradley Avenue, Burgess Hall, Peoria,
           IL 61625
Phone: 309-677-2528
Fax: 309-677-2527
Contact: Francesca A. Armmer, PhD, RN, Chairperson
Email: faa@bradley.edu

GENERAL INFORMATION

Type of School: *4-Year College or University, Private
(Independent)* • Accreditation: *North Central Association of
Colleges and Schools* • Total Enrollment: *5951*

PROGRAM INFORMATION

Two Year Exit Option: *No* • NLNAC Accreditation: *Yes* •
CCNE Accreditation:

NURSING STUDENT PROFILE

Total Nursing Enrollment: *134* • Total Basic Student
Enrollment, Full Time: *121* • Total Basic Student
Enrollment, Part Time: *3* • Female Basic Student
Enrollment: *118* • Male Basic Student Enrollment: *6* • Total
RN Enrollment: *10* • Total New Fall Enrollments: *44* • Total
Graduates: *40* • Basic Student Graduates: *35* • RN Student
Graduates: *5*

FINANCES

Residential Annual Tuition: *$7,250* • Non-Residential
Annual Tuition: *$7,250* • General Institutional Fees:
$14,500 • Additional Nursing Fees: *$489*

CHICAGO STATE UNIVERSITY

Address: 9501 South King Drive, Chicago, IL 60628
Phone: 773-995-3992
Fax: 773-821-2438
Contact: Meryl K. Price, PhD, RN, Chairperson
Email: mh-price@csu.edu

GENERAL INFORMATION

Type of School: *4-Year College or University, Public* • Accreditation: *North Central Association of Colleges and Schools* • Total Enrollment: *Not Reported*

PROGRAM INFORMATION

Two Year Exit Option: *No* • NLNAC Accreditation: *Yes* • CCNE Accreditation:

NURSING STUDENT PROFILE

Total Nursing Enrollment: *5060* • Total Basic Student Enrollment, Full Time: *3000* • Total Basic Student Enrollment, Part Time: *1683* • Female Basic Student Enrollment: *3560* • Male Basic Student Enrollment: *1123* • Total RN Enrollment: *377* • Total New Fall Enrollments: *383* • Total Graduates: *844* • Basic Student Graduates: *795* • RN Student Graduates: *49*

FINANCES

Residential Annual Tuition: *$4,382* • Non-Residential Annual Tuition: *$10,766* • General Institutional Fees: *Not Reported* • Additional Nursing Fees: *Not Reported*

CONCORDIA UNIVERSITY AND WEST SUBURBAN

Address: 3 Erie Court, Oak Park, IL 60302
Phone: 218-299-3883
Fax: 218-299-4308
Contact: Lois F. Nelson, EdD, RN, CNS, Chair and Professor
Email: lnelson@cord.edu

GENERAL INFORMATION

Type of School: *4-Year College or University, Private (Independent)* • Accreditation: *North Central Association of Colleges and Schools* • Total Enrollment: *119*

PROGRAM INFORMATION

Two Year Exit Option: *Not Reported* • NLNAC Accreditation: *Yes* • CCNE Accreditation: *Yes*

NURSING STUDENT PROFILE

Total Nursing Enrollment: *102* • Total Basic Student Enrollment, Full Time: *100* • Total Basic Student Enrollment, Part Time: *2* • Female Basic Student Enrollment: *92* • Male Basic Student Enrollment: *10* • Total RN Enrollment: *0* • Total New Fall Enrollments: *57* • Total Graduates: *49* • Basic Student Graduates: *49* • RN Student Graduates: *0*

FINANCES

Residential Annual Tuition: *$3,010* • Non-Residential Annual Tuition: *$7,359* • General Institutional Fees: *Not Reported* • Additional Nursing Fees: *Not Reported*

ELMHURST COLLEGE

Address: 190 Prospect Ave., Elmhurst, IL 60126
Phone: 630-617-3344
Fax: 630-617-3237
Contact: Linda K. Niedringhaus, PhD, RN, Director
Email: linda@elmhurst.edu

GENERAL INFORMATION

Type of School: *4-Year College or University, Private (Religious)* • Accreditation: *North Central Association of Colleges and Schools* • Total Enrollment: *3000*

PROGRAM INFORMATION

Two Year Exit Option: *Not Reported* • NLNAC Accreditation: *Not Reported* • CCNE Accreditation: *Yes*

NURSING STUDENT PROFILE

Total Nursing Enrollment: *130* • Total Basic Student Enrollment, Full Time: *115* • Total Basic Student Enrollment, Part Time: *10* • Female Basic Student Enrollment: *120* • Male Basic Student Enrollment: *5* • Total RN Enrollment: *5* • Total New Fall Enrollments: *30* • Total Graduates: *34* • Basic Student Graduates: *33* • RN Student Graduates: *1*

FINANCES

Residential Annual Tuition: *Not Reported* • Non-Residential Annual Tuition: *Not Reported* • General Institutional Fees: *Not Reported* • Additional Nursing Fees: *Not Reported*

ILLINOIS STATE UNIVERSITY

Address: Campus Box 5810, Normal, IL 61790
Phone: 309-438-2308
Fax: 309-438-2620
Contact: Pam Lindsey, MS, RN, CS, Interim
          Undergraduate Program Director
Email: pllindsey@ilstu.edu

GENERAL INFORMATION

Type of School: *4-Year College or University, Public* • Accreditation: *North Central Association of Colleges and Schools* • Total Enrollment: *20000*

PROGRAM INFORMATION

Two Year Exit Option: *Not Reported* • NLNAC Accreditation: *Yes* • CCNE Accreditation:

NURSING STUDENT PROFILE

Total Nursing Enrollment: *164* • Total Basic Student Enrollment, Full Time: *135* • Total Basic Student Enrollment, Part Time: *14* • Female Basic Student Enrollment: *142* • Male Basic Student Enrollment: *7* • Total RN Enrollment: *15* • Total New Fall Enrollments: *71* • Total Graduates: *67* • Basic Student Graduates: *60* • RN Student Graduates: *7*

FINANCES

Residential Annual Tuition: *$2,277* • Non-Residential Annual Tuition: *$5,710* • General Institutional Fees: *$1,430* • Additional Nursing Fees: *$60*

ILLINOIS WESLEYAN UNIVERSITY

Address: PO Box 2900, Bloomington, IL 61702
Phone: 309-556-3051
Fax: 309-556-3043
Contact: Donna L. Hartweg, PhD, RN, Director
Email: dhartweg@titan.iwu.edu

GENERAL INFORMATION

Type of School: *4-Year College or University, Private (Independent)* • Accreditation: *North Central Association of Colleges and Schools* • Total Enrollment: *2077*

PROGRAM INFORMATION

Two Year Exit Option: *No* • NLNAC Accreditation: *Not Reported* • CCNE Accreditation: *Yes*

NURSING STUDENT PROFILE

Total Nursing Enrollment: *77* • Total Basic Student Enrollment, Full Time: *77* • Total Basic Student Enrollment, Part Time: *0* • Female Basic Student Enrollment: *76* • Male Basic Student Enrollment: *1* • Total RN Enrollment: *0* • Total New Fall Enrollments: *22* • Total Graduates: *30* • Basic Student Graduates: *30* • RN Student Graduates: *0*

FINANCES

Residential Annual Tuition: *$24,390* • Non-Residential Annual Tuition: *$24,390* • General Institutional Fees: *$150* • Additional Nursing Fees: *$2,535*

LAKEVIEW COLLEGE

Address: 903 North Logan Ave., Danville, IL 61832
Phone: 217-477-2747
Fax: 217-477-2760
Contact: Jo-Ann Marrs, EdD, RN, FNP, President/ Dean
Email: jmarras@lakeviewcol.edu

GENERAL INFORMATION

Type of School: *Technical/Specialized Institution, Private (Independent)* • Accreditation: *North Central Association of Colleges and Schools* • Total Enrollment: *56*

PROGRAM INFORMATION

Two Year Exit Option: *Not Reported* • NLNAC Accreditation: *Yes* • CCNE Accreditation:

NURSING STUDENT PROFILE

Total Nursing Enrollment: *56* • Total Basic Student Enrollment, Full Time: *24* • Total Basic Student Enrollment, Part Time: *25* • Female Basic Student Enrollment: *48* • Male Basic Student Enrollment: *1* • Total RN Enrollment: *7* • Total New Fall Enrollments: *9* • Total Graduates: *24* • Basic Student Graduates: *12* • RN Student Graduates: *12*

FINANCES

Residential Annual Tuition: *Not Reported* • Non-Residential Annual Tuition: *Not Reported* • General Institutional Fees: *Not Reported* • Additional Nursing Fees: *$250*

LEWIS UNIVERSITY

Address: 500 S. Independence Blvd., Romeoville, IL 60446
Phone: 815-836-5878
Fax: 815-838-8306
Contact: Nan Yancey, MSN, RN, Undergraduate Director
Email: yanceyna@lewisu.edu

GENERAL INFORMATION

Type of School: *4-Year College or University, Private (Religious)* • Accreditation: *North Central Association of Colleges and Schools* • Total Enrollment: *4289*

PROGRAM INFORMATION

Two Year Exit Option: *No* • NLNAC Accreditation: *Yes* • CCNE Accreditation:

NURSING STUDENT PROFILE

Total Nursing Enrollment: *769* • Total Basic Student Enrollment, Full Time: *192* • Total Basic Student Enrollment, Part Time: *14* • Female Basic Student Enrollment: *193* • Male Basic Student Enrollment: *13* • Total RN Enrollment: *563* • Total New Fall Enrollments: *29* • Total Graduates: *159* • Basic Student Graduates: *66* • RN Student Graduates: *93*

FINANCES

Residential Annual Tuition: *Not Reported* • Non-Residential Annual Tuition: *Not Reported* • General Institutional Fees: *Not Reported* • Additional Nursing Fees: *$444*

LOYOLA UNIVERSITY— CHICAGO

Address: 6525 North Sheridan Rd., Chicago, IL 60625
Phone: 773-508-3255
Fax: 773-508-3241
Contact: Sheila A. Haas, PhD, RN, Dean and Professor
Email: shaas@luc.edu

GENERAL INFORMATION

Type of School: *4-Year College or University, Private (Religious)* • Accreditation: *North Central Association of Colleges and Schools* • Total Enrollment: *13358*

PROGRAM INFORMATION

Two Year Exit Option: *No* • NLNAC Accreditation: *Yes* • CCNE Accreditation:

NURSING STUDENT PROFILE

Total Nursing Enrollment: *335* • Total Basic Student Enrollment, Full Time: *278* • Total Basic Student Enrollment, Part Time: *40* • Female Basic Student Enrollment: *294* • Male Basic Student Enrollment: *24* • Total RN Enrollment: *17* • Total New Fall Enrollments: *88* • Total Graduates: *118* • Basic Student Graduates: *111* • RN Student Graduates: *7*

FINANCES

Residential Annual Tuition: *$18,266* • Non-Residential Annual Tuition: *$18,266* • General Institutional Fees: *$9,133* • Additional Nursing Fees: *$360*

MACMURRAY COLLEGE

Address: 447 East College Ave., Jacksonville, IL 62650
Phone: 217-479-7083
Fax: 217-479-7078
Contact: JoEllen Brannan, PhD(c), RN, Director and
           Associate Professor
Email: joellenb@mac.edu

GENERAL INFORMATION

Type of School: *4-Year College or University, Private (Religious)* • Accreditation: *North Central Association of Colleges and Schools* • Total Enrollment: *700*

PROGRAM INFORMATION

Two Year Exit Option: *No* • NLNAC Accreditation: *Not Reported* • CCNE Accreditation: *Yes*

NURSING STUDENT PROFILE

Total Nursing Enrollment: *46* • Total Basic Student Enrollment, Full Time: *44* • Total Basic Student Enrollment, Part Time: *1* • Female Basic Student Enrollment: *41* • Male Basic Student Enrollment: *4* • Total RN Enrollment: *1* • Total New Fall Enrollments: *23* • Total Graduates: *19* • Basic Student Graduates: *18* • RN Student Graduates: *1*

FINANCES

Residential Annual Tuition: *$13,140* • Non-Residential Annual Tuition: *$13,140* • General Institutional Fees: *Not Reported* • Additional Nursing Fees: *$325*

MILLIKIN UNIVERSITY

Address: 1184 W. Main St., Decatur, IL 62522
Phone: 217-424-6348
Fax: 217-424-3993
Contact: Nancy Creason, PhD, RN, Dean
Email: ncreason@mail.millikin.edu

GENERAL INFORMATION

Type of School: *4-Year College or University, Private (Independent)* • Accreditation: *North Central Association of Colleges and Schools* • Total Enrollment: *2307*

PROGRAM INFORMATION

Two Year Exit Option: *Not Reported* • NLNAC Accreditation: *Yes* • CCNE Accreditation:

NURSING STUDENT PROFILE

Total Nursing Enrollment: *102* • Total Basic Student Enrollment, Full Time: *99* • Total Basic Student Enrollment, Part Time: *2* • Female Basic Student Enrollment: *93* • Male Basic Student Enrollment: *8* • Total RN Enrollment: *1* • Total New Fall Enrollments: *18* • Total Graduates: *23* • Basic Student Graduates: *21* • RN Student Graduates: *2*

FINANCES

Residential Annual Tuition: *$16,192* • Non-Residential Annual Tuition: *$16,192* • General Institutional Fees: *$8,096* • Additional Nursing Fees: *$475*

NORTH PARK UNIVERSITY

Address: 3225 W. Foster Ave., Chcago, IL 60625
Phone: 773-244-5693
Fax: *Not Reported*
Contact: Elizabeth Ritt, EdD, RN, Interim Director
Email: eritt@northpark.edu

GENERAL INFORMATION

Type of School: *4-Year College or University, Private (Religious)* • Accreditation: *North Central Association of Colleges and Schools* • Total Enrollment: *2377*

PROGRAM INFORMATION

Two Year Exit Option: *Not Reported* • NLNAC Accreditation: *Not Reported* • CCNE Accreditation:

NURSING STUDENT PROFILE

Total Nursing Enrollment: *Not Reported* • Total Basic Student Enrollment, Full Time: *Not Reported* • Total Basic Student Enrollment, Part Time: *Not Reported* • Female Basic Student Enrollment: *Not Reported* • Male Basic Student Enrollment: *Not Reported* • Total RN Enrollment: *Not Reported* • Total New Fall Enrollments: *Not Reported* • Total Graduates: *Not Reported* • Basic Student Graduates: *Not Reported* • RN Student Graduates: *Not Reported*

FINANCES

Residential Annual Tuition: *Not Reported* • Non-Residential Annual Tuition: *Not Reported* • General Institutional Fees: *Not Reported* • Additional Nursing Fees: *Not Reported*

NORTHERN ILLINOIS UNIVERSITY

Address: 1240 Normal Road, De Kalb, IL 60115
Phone: 815-753-6390
Fax: 815-753-0814
Contact: Marilyn Stromborg, EdD, JD, FAAN, Professor and Chair
Email: cancer@niu.edu

GENERAL INFORMATION

Type of School: *Not Reported* • Accreditation: *Not Reported* • Total Enrollment: *Not Reported*

PROGRAM INFORMATION

Two Year Exit Option: *Not Reported* • NLNAC Accreditation: *Yes* • CCNE Accreditation:

NURSING STUDENT PROFILE

Total Nursing Enrollment: *390* • Total Basic Student Enrollment, Full Time: *254* • Total Basic Student Enrollment, Part Time: *50* • Female Basic Student Enrollment: *292* • Male Basic Student Enrollment: *12* • Total RN Enrollment: *86* • Total New Fall Enrollments: *92* • Total Graduates: *133* • Basic Student Graduates: *104* • RN Student Graduates: *29*

FINANCES

Residential Annual Tuition: *$2,736* • Non-Residential Annual Tuition: *$5,472* • General Institutional Fees: *$1,368* • Additional Nursing Fees: *$114*

OLIVET NAZARENE UNIVERSITY

Address: 1 University Ave., Bourbonnais, IL 60914
Phone: 815-939-5345
Fax: 815-939-5383
Contact: Norma R. Wood, PhD, RN, Chair
Email: nwood@olivet.edu

GENERAL INFORMATION

Type of School: *4-Year College or University, Private (Religious)* • Accreditation: *North Central Association of Colleges and Schools* • Total Enrollment: *2514*

PROGRAM INFORMATION

Two Year Exit Option: *Not Reported* • NLNAC Accreditation: *Yes* • CCNE Accreditation:

NURSING STUDENT PROFILE

Total Nursing Enrollment: *158* • Total Basic Student Enrollment, Full Time: *92* • Total Basic Student Enrollment, Part Time: *2* • Female Basic Student Enrollment: *91* • Male Basic Student Enrollment: *3* • Total RN Enrollment: *64* • Total New Fall Enrollments: *32* • Total Graduates: *63* • Basic Student Graduates: *19* • RN Student Graduates: *44*

FINANCES

Residential Annual Tuition: *$11,928* • Non-Residential Annual Tuition: *$11,928* • General Institutional Fees: *$5,964* • Additional Nursing Fees: *$497*

ROCKFORD COLLEGE

Address: 5050 E. State St., Rockford, IL 61108
Phone: 815-226-4196
Fax: 815-394-5166
Contact: Debra Gurney, EdDc, MSN, RN, Chair and
            Assistant Professor
Email: debra_gurney@rockford.edu

GENERAL INFORMATION

Type of School: *4-Year College or University, Private (Independent)* • Accreditation: *North Central Association of Colleges and Schools* • Total Enrollment: *1615*

PROGRAM INFORMATION

Two Year Exit Option: *No* • NLNAC Accreditation: *Yes* • CCNE Accreditation:

NURSING STUDENT PROFILE

Total Nursing Enrollment: *85* • Total Basic Student Enrollment, Full Time: *56* • Total Basic Student Enrollment, Part Time: *17* • Female Basic Student Enrollment: *70* • Male Basic Student Enrollment: *3* • Total RN Enrollment: *12* • Total New Fall Enrollments: *0* • Total Graduates: *23* • Basic Student Graduates: *23* • RN Student Graduates: *0*

FINANCES

Residential Annual Tuition: *$17,450* • Non-Residential Annual Tuition: *$17,450* • General Institutional Fees: *$100* • Additional Nursing Fees: *$0*

RUSH UNIVERSITY

Address: 600 S. Paulina, Chicago, IL 60612
Phone: 312-942-7117
Fax: 312-942-3043
Contact: Kathleen G. Andreoli, DSN, RN, FAAN, Dean
Email: kathleen_a_andreoli@rush.edu

GENERAL INFORMATION

Type of School: *Hospital, Private (Independent)* •
Accreditation: *North Central Association of Colleges and
Schools* • Total Enrollment: *1299*

PROGRAM INFORMATION

Two Year Exit Option: *No* • NLNAC Accreditation: *Not
Reported* • CCNE Accreditation: *Yes*

NURSING STUDENT PROFILE

Total Nursing Enrollment: *118* • Total Basic Student
Enrollment, Full Time: *110* • Total Basic Student
Enrollment, Part Time: *0* • Female Basic Student
Enrollment: *107* • Male Basic Student Enrollment: *3* • Total
RN Enrollment: *8* • Total New Fall Enrollments: *57* • Total
Graduates: *57* • Basic Student Graduates: *52* • RN Student
Graduates: *5*

FINANCES

Residential Annual Tuition: *$16,590* • Non-Residential
Annual Tuition: *Not Reported* • General Institutional Fees:
$0 • Additional Nursing Fees: *$0*

SAINT ANTHONY COLLEGE OF NURSING

Address: 5658 E. State St., Rockford, IL 61108
Phone: 815-395-5090
Fax: 815-395-2275
Contact: Terese Ann Burch, PhD, RN, Dean/ CEO
Email: terriburch@asn.edu

GENERAL INFORMATION

Type of School: *Other, Private (Religious)* • Accreditation:
North Central Association of Colleges and Schools • Total
Enrollment: *66*

PROGRAM INFORMATION

Two Year Exit Option: *No* • NLNAC Accreditation: *Yes* •
CCNE Accreditation: *Yes*

NURSING STUDENT PROFILE

Total Nursing Enrollment: *66* • Total Basic Student
Enrollment, Full Time: *53* • Total Basic Student Enrollment,
Part Time: *11* • Female Basic Student Enrollment: *61* • Male
Basic Student Enrollment: *3* • Total RN Enrollment: *2* •
Total New Fall Enrollments: *23* • Total Graduates: *29* • Basic
Student Graduates: *29* • RN Student Graduates: *0*

FINANCES

Residential Annual Tuition: *$12,000* • Non-Residential
Annual Tuition: *$12,000* • General Institutional Fees: *$100* •
Additional Nursing Fees: *$13*

SAINT FRANCIS MEDICAL CENTER

Address: 511 NE Greenleaf St., Peoria, IL 61603
Phone: 309-655-2086
Fax: 309-624-8973
Contact: Mary Ludgera Pieperbeck, PhD, RN, Dean
Email: sister.ludgera@osfhealthcare.org

GENERAL INFORMATION

Type of School: *Independent, Private (Religious)* •
Accreditation: *North Central Association of Colleges and Schools* • Total Enrollment: *134*

PROGRAM INFORMATION

Two Year Exit Option: *Not Reported* • NLNAC
Accreditation: *Yes* • CCNE Accreditation: *Yes*

NURSING STUDENT PROFILE

Total Nursing Enrollment: *134* • Total Basic Student
Enrollment, Full Time: *101* • Total Basic Student
Enrollment, Part Time: *15* • Female Basic Student
Enrollment: *108* • Male Basic Student Enrollment: *8* • Total
RN Enrollment: *18* • Total New Fall Enrollments: *34* • Total
Graduates: *54* • Basic Student Graduates: *48* • RN Student
Graduates: *6*

FINANCES

Residential Annual Tuition: *$9,048* • Non-Residential
Annual Tuition: *$9,048* • General Institutional Fees:
$4,524 • Additional Nursing Fees: *$377*

SAINT XAVIER UNIVERSITY

Address: 3700 W. 103 St., Chicago, IL 60655
Phone: 773-298-3700
Fax: 773-298-3704
Contact: Mary M. Lebold, EdD, RN, Dean
Email: lebold@sxu.edu

GENERAL INFORMATION

Type of School: *4-Year College or University, Private
(Religious)* • Accreditation: *North Central Association of
Colleges and Schools* • Total Enrollment: *4867*

PROGRAM INFORMATION

Two Year Exit Option: *No* • NLNAC Accreditation: *Yes* •
CCNE Accreditation:

NURSING STUDENT PROFILE

Total Nursing Enrollment: *438* • Total Basic Student
Enrollment, Full Time: *287* • Total Basic Student
Enrollment, Part Time: *52* • Female Basic Student
Enrollment: *325* • Male Basic Student Enrollment: *14* • Total
RN Enrollment: *99* • Total New Fall Enrollments: *83* • Total
Graduates: *95* • Basic Student Graduates: *88* • RN Student
Graduates: *7*

FINANCES

Residential Annual Tuition: *$15,000* • Non-Residential
Annual Tuition: *$15,000* • General Institutional Fees: *$130* •
Additional Nursing Fees: *$90*

SOUTHERN ILLINOIS UNIVERSITY— EDWARDSVILLE

Address: Alumni Hall Rm 2333, Edwardsville, IL 62026
Phone: 618-650-3972
Fax: 618-650-3854
Contact: Wendy M. Nehring, PhD, RN, FAAN, Acting Associate Dean for Educational Services
Email: wnehrin@siue.edu

GENERAL INFORMATION

Type of School: *Not Reported* • Accreditation: *Not Reported* • Total Enrollment: *Not Reported*

PROGRAM INFORMATION

Two Year Exit Option: *No* • NLNAC Accreditation: *Yes* • CCNE Accreditation: *Yes*

NURSING STUDENT PROFILE

Total Nursing Enrollment: *336* • Total Basic Student Enrollment, Full Time: *248* • Total Basic Student Enrollment, Part Time: *7* • Female Basic Student Enrollment: *224* • Male Basic Student Enrollment: *31* • Total RN Enrollment: *81* • Total New Fall Enrollments: *51* • Total Graduates: *140* • Basic Student Graduates: *111* • RN Student Graduates: *29*

FINANCES

Residential Annual Tuition: *$4,420* • Non-Residential Annual Tuition: *$8,004* • General Institutional Fees: *$7,540* • Additional Nursing Fees: *$180*

ST. JOHN'S COLLEGE

Address: 421 N. 9th St., Springfield, IL 62702
Phone: 217-525-5628
Fax: 217-757-6870
Contact: Kathleen Kay O'Neil, PhD, RN, Dean of Academic Affairs
Email: koneil@st-johns.org

GENERAL INFORMATION

Type of School: *4-Year College or University, Private (Religious)* • Accreditation: *North Central Association of Colleges and Schools* • Total Enrollment: *59*

PROGRAM INFORMATION

Two Year Exit Option: *Not Reported* • NLNAC Accreditation: *Yes* • CCNE Accreditation:

NURSING STUDENT PROFILE

Total Nursing Enrollment: *59* • Total Basic Student Enrollment, Full Time: *57* • Total Basic Student Enrollment, Part Time: *2* • Female Basic Student Enrollment: *56* • Male Basic Student Enrollment: *3* • Total RN Enrollment: *0* • Total New Fall Enrollments: *32* • Total Graduates: *47* • Basic Student Graduates: *47* • RN Student Graduates: *0*

FINANCES

Residential Annual Tuition: *$7,740* • Non-Residential Annual Tuition: *$7,740* • General Institutional Fees: *$3,870* • Additional Nursing Fees: *$254*

TRINITY CHRISTIAN COLLEGE

Address: 6601 W. College Dr., Palos Heights, IL 60463
Phone: 708-239-4723
Fax: 708-385-5665
Contact: Cynthia N. Sander, PhD, RN, Chairperson and Professor
Email: cynthia.sander@trnty.edu

GENERAL INFORMATION

Type of School: *4-Year College or University, Private (Religious)* • Accreditation: *North Central Association of Colleges and Schools* • Total Enrollment: *800*

PROGRAM INFORMATION

Two Year Exit Option: *No* • NLNAC Accreditation: *Yes* • CCNE Accreditation:

NURSING STUDENT PROFILE

Total Nursing Enrollment: *31* • Total Basic Student Enrollment, Full Time: *26* • Total Basic Student Enrollment, Part Time: *1* • Female Basic Student Enrollment: *26* • Male Basic Student Enrollment: *1* • Total RN Enrollment: *4* • Total New Fall Enrollments: *11* • Total Graduates: *12* • Basic Student Graduates: *12* • RN Student Graduates: *0*

FINANCES

Residential Annual Tuition: *$13,970* • Non-Residential Annual Tuition: *$13,970* • General Institutional Fees: *$0* • Additional Nursing Fees: *$85*

TRINITY COLLEGE OF NURSING

Address: 555 6th St., Ste 300, Moline, IL 61265
Phone: 309-757-2630
Fax: *Not Reported*
Contact: Sandra Bellinger, PhD, RN, Academic Dean
Email: bellinger@trinityqa.com

GENERAL INFORMATION

Type of School: *Hospital, Private (Independent)* • Accreditation: *North Central Association of Colleges and Schools* • Total Enrollment: *75*

PROGRAM INFORMATION

Two Year Exit Option: *No* • NLNAC Accreditation: *Not Reported* • CCNE Accreditation:

NURSING STUDENT PROFILE

Total Nursing Enrollment: *26* • Total Basic Student Enrollment, Full Time: *16* • Total Basic Student Enrollment, Part Time: *10* • Female Basic Student Enrollment: *26* • Male Basic Student Enrollment: *0* • Total RN Enrollment: *0* • Total New Fall Enrollments: *3* • Total Graduates: *12* • Basic Student Graduates: *0* • RN Student Graduates: *12*

FINANCES

Residential Annual Tuition: *$3,998* • Non-Residential Annual Tuition: *Not Reported* • General Institutional Fees: *$1,887* • Additional Nursing Fees: *$187*

UNIVERSITY OF ILLINOIS—CHICAGO

Address: 601 S. Morgan, Chicago, IL 60607
Phone: 312-996-1749
Fax: 312-413-4399
Contact: Joan Shaver, PhD, RN, FAAN, Dean
Email: jshaver@uic.edu

UNIVERSITY OF ST. FRANCIS—JOLIET

Address: 290 N. Springfield Ave., Joliet, IL 60435
Phone: 815-741-7130
Fax: 815-741-7131
Contact: JoAnn Glotfelty, MS, RN, Interim Dean
Email: jglotfelty@stfrancis.edu

GENERAL INFORMATION

Type of School: *4-Year College or University, Public* • Accreditation: *North Central Association of Colleges and Schools* • Total Enrollment: *25000*

GENERAL INFORMATION

Type of School: *4-Year College or University, Private (Religious)* • Accreditation: *North Central Association of Colleges and Schools* • Total Enrollment: *3974*

PROGRAM INFORMATION

Two Year Exit Option: *No* • NLNAC Accreditation: *Not Reported* • CCNE Accreditation: *Yes*

PROGRAM INFORMATION

Two Year Exit Option: *No* • NLNAC Accreditation: *Yes* • CCNE Accreditation: *Yes*

NURSING STUDENT PROFILE

Total Nursing Enrollment: *420* • Total Basic Student Enrollment, Full Time: *365* • Total Basic Student Enrollment, Part Time: *24* • Female Basic Student Enrollment: *357* • Male Basic Student Enrollment: *32* • Total RN Enrollment: *31* • Total New Fall Enrollments: *88* • Total Graduates: *125* • Basic Student Graduates: *107* • RN Student Graduates: *18*

NURSING STUDENT PROFILE

Total Nursing Enrollment: *112* • Total Basic Student Enrollment, Full Time: *88* • Total Basic Student Enrollment, Part Time: *7* • Female Basic Student Enrollment: *90* • Male Basic Student Enrollment: *5* • Total RN Enrollment: *17* • Total New Fall Enrollments: *46* • Total Graduates: *26* • Basic Student Graduates: *16* • RN Student Graduates: *10*

FINANCES

Residential Annual Tuition: *$1,915* • Non-Residential Annual Tuition: *$4,995* • General Institutional Fees: *$820* • Additional Nursing Fees: *$0*

FINANCES

Residential Annual Tuition: *$16,480* • Non-Residential Annual Tuition: *$16,480* • General Institutional Fees: *$340* • Additional Nursing Fees: *$200*

Circle 124 on reader card	See in-depth profile for more information

Circle 135 on reader card	See in-depth profile for more information

ANDERSON UNIVERSITY

Address: 1100 E. 5th Street, Anderson, IN 46012
Phone: 765-641-4383
Fax: 765-641-3095
Contact: Andrea W. Koepke, DNS, RN, Director
Email: awkoepke@anderson.edu

GENERAL INFORMATION

Type of School: *4-Year College or University, Private (Religious)* • Accreditation: *North Central Association of Colleges and Schools* • Total Enrollment: *1945*

PROGRAM INFORMATION

Two Year Exit Option: *No* • NLNAC Accreditation: *Yes* • CCNE Accreditation: *Yes*

NURSING STUDENT PROFILE

Total Nursing Enrollment: *112* • Total Basic Student Enrollment, Full Time: *80* • Total Basic Student Enrollment, Part Time: *32* • Female Basic Student Enrollment: *107* • Male Basic Student Enrollment: *5* • Total RN Enrollment: *0* • Total New Fall Enrollments: *44* • Total Graduates: *23* • Basic Student Graduates: *23* • RN Student Graduates: *0*

FINANCES

Residential Annual Tuition: *$14,680* • Non-Residential Annual Tuition: *$14,680* • General Institutional Fees: *$100* • Additional Nursing Fees: *$40*

BALL STATE UNIVERSITY

Address: 2000 University Ave., Muncie, IN 47306
Phone: 765-285-5589
Fax: 765-285-2169
Contact: Nancy L. Dillard, DNS, RN, CS, ANP, SANE, Associate Director, Baccalaureate Nursing Program
Email: ndillard@bsu.edu

GENERAL INFORMATION

Type of School: *4-Year College or University, Public* • Accreditation: *North Central Association of Colleges and Schools* • Total Enrollment: *18000*

PROGRAM INFORMATION

Two Year Exit Option: *No* • NLNAC Accreditation: *Yes* • CCNE Accreditation:

NURSING STUDENT PROFILE

Total Nursing Enrollment: *141* • Total Basic Student Enrollment, Full Time: *139* • Total Basic Student Enrollment, Part Time: *2* • Female Basic Student Enrollment: *135* • Male Basic Student Enrollment: *6* • Total RN Enrollment: *0* • Total New Fall Enrollments: *42* • Total Graduates: *48* • Basic Student Graduates: *48* • RN Student Graduates: *0*

FINANCES

Residential Annual Tuition: *$3,924* • Non-Residential Annual Tuition: *$10,800* • General Institutional Fees: *$110* • Additional Nursing Fees: *$120*

GOSHEN COLLEGE

Address: 1700 S. Main Street, Goshen, IN 46526
Phone: 574-535-7376
Fax: 574-535-7609
Contact: Vicky S. Kirkton, MA, RN, Director
Email: vickysk@goshen.edu

GENERAL INFORMATION

Type of School: *4-Year College or University, Private (Religious)* • Accreditation: *North Central Association of Colleges and Schools* • Total Enrollment: *970*

PROGRAM INFORMATION

Two Year Exit Option: *No* • NLNAC Accreditation: *Yes* • CCNE Accreditation:

NURSING STUDENT PROFILE

Total Nursing Enrollment: *62* • Total Basic Student Enrollment, Full Time: *52* • Total Basic Student Enrollment, Part Time: *0* • Female Basic Student Enrollment: *49* • Male Basic Student Enrollment: *3* • Total RN Enrollment: *10* • Total New Fall Enrollments: *25* • Total Graduates: *19* • Basic Student Graduates: *12* • RN Student Graduates: *7*

FINANCES

Residential Annual Tuition: *$13,600* • Non-Residential Annual Tuition: *$13,600* • General Institutional Fees: *$500* • Additional Nursing Fees: *$0*

INDIANA STATE UNIVERSITY

Address: 210 N. 7th Street, Terre Haute, IN 47809
Phone: 812-237-3688
Fax: 812-237-4300
Contact: Suzy Fletcher, DNS, RN, Interim Chair
Baccalaureate and Higher Degree Program
Email: s-fletcher@indstate.edu

GENERAL INFORMATION

Type of School: *4-Year College or University, Public* • Accreditation: *North Central Association of Colleges and Schools* • Total Enrollment: *11321*

PROGRAM INFORMATION

Two Year Exit Option: *No* • NLNAC Accreditation: *Yes* • CCNE Accreditation:

NURSING STUDENT PROFILE

Total Nursing Enrollment: *202* • Total Basic Student Enrollment, Full Time: *124* • Total Basic Student Enrollment, Part Time: *0* • Female Basic Student Enrollment: *122* • Male Basic Student Enrollment: *2* • Total RN Enrollment: *78* • Total New Fall Enrollments: *68* • Total Graduates: *23* • Basic Student Graduates: *23* • RN Student Graduates: *0*

FINANCES

Residential Annual Tuition: *$5,322* • Non-Residential Annual Tuition: *$11,790* • General Institutional Fees: *Not Reported* • Additional Nursing Fees: *$766*

INDIANA UNIVERSITY EAST

Address: 2325 Chester Boulevard, Richmond, IN 47374
Phone: 765-973-8257
Fax: 765-973-8220
Contact: Joanne Rains, DNS, RN, Dean
Email: jrains@indiana.edu

GENERAL INFORMATION

Type of School: *4-Year College or University, Public* •
Accreditation: *North Central Association of Colleges and
Schools* • Total Enrollment: *2600*

PROGRAM INFORMATION

Two Year Exit Option: *No* • NLNAC Accreditation: *Yes* •
CCNE Accreditation:

NURSING STUDENT PROFILE

Total Nursing Enrollment: *145* • Total Basic Student
Enrollment, Full Time: *86* • Total Basic Student Enrollment,
Part Time: *55* • Female Basic Student Enrollment: *132* •
Male Basic Student Enrollment: *9* • Total RN Enrollment:
4 • Total New Fall Enrollments: *41* • Total Graduates: *31* •
Basic Student Graduates: *27* • RN Student Graduates: *4*

FINANCES

Residential Annual Tuition: *$3,710* • Non-Residential
Annual Tuition: *$9,814* • General Institutional Fees: *$112* •
Additional Nursing Fees: *$464*

INDIANA UNIVERSITY— KOKOMO

Address: 2300 S. Washington Street, P.O. Box 9003,
           Bloomington, IN 46904-9003
Phone: 765-455-9334
Fax: 765-455-9421
Contact: Nancy Schlapman, PhD, RN, Coordinator,
           Baccalaureate and Higher Degree Programs
Email: nschlapm@iuk.edu

GENERAL INFORMATION

Type of School: *4-Year College or University, Public* •
Accreditation: *North Central Association of Colleges and
Schools* • Total Enrollment: *37963*

PROGRAM INFORMATION

Two Year Exit Option: *Not Reported* • CCNE Accreditation:
Yes

NURSING STUDENT PROFILE

Total Nursing Enrollment: *74* • Total Basic Student
Enrollment, Full Time: *31* • Total Basic Student Enrollment,
Part Time: *12* • Female Basic Student Enrollment: *42* • Male
Basic Student Enrollment: *1* • Total RN Enrollment: *31* •
Total New Fall Enrollments: *23* • Total Graduates: *34* • Basic
Student Graduates: *16* • RN Student Graduates: *18*

FINANCES

Residential Annual Tuition: *$3,710* • Non-Residential
Annual Tuition: *$9,814* • General Institutional Fees: *Not
Reported* • Additional Nursing Fees: *Not Reported*

INDIANA UNIVERSITY— NORTHWEST

Address:　3400 Broadway, Gary, IN 46408
Phone:　219-980-6604
Fax:　219-980-6578
Contact:　Linda A. Rooda, PhD, RN, Professor and Dean
Email:　lrooda@iun.edu

INDIANA UNIVERSITY— PURDUE UNIVERSITY

Address:　1111 Middle Drive, Indianapolis, IN 46202-2896
Phone:　317-274-8010
Fax:　317-274-2996
Contact:　Donna L. Boland, PhD, RN, Associate Dean for Undergraduate Programs
Email:　dboland@iupui.edu

GENERAL INFORMATION

Type of School: *4-Year College or University, Public* • Accreditation: *North Central Association of Colleges and Schools* • Total Enrollment: *4649*

GENERAL INFORMATION

Type of School: *4-Year College or University, Public* • Accreditation: *North Central Association of Colleges and Schools* • Total Enrollment: *27500*

PROGRAM INFORMATION

Two Year Exit Option: *Not Reported* • NLNAC Accreditation: *Yes* • CCNE Accreditation:

PROGRAM INFORMATION

Two Year Exit Option: *No* • NLNAC Accreditation: *Yes* • CCNE Accreditation: *Yes*

NURSING STUDENT PROFILE

Total Nursing Enrollment: *92* • Total Basic Student Enrollment, Full Time: *76* • Total Basic Student Enrollment, Part Time: *0* • Female Basic Student Enrollment: *70* • Male Basic Student Enrollment: *6* • Total RN Enrollment: *16* • Total New Fall Enrollments: *31* • Total Graduates: *73* • Basic Student Graduates: *26* • RN Student Graduates: *47*

NURSING STUDENT PROFILE

Total Nursing Enrollment: *736* • Total Basic Student Enrollment, Full Time: *629* • Total Basic Student Enrollment, Part Time: *51* • Female Basic Student Enrollment: *637* • Male Basic Student Enrollment: *43* • Total RN Enrollment: *56* • Total New Fall Enrollments: *156* • Total Graduates: *186* • Basic Student Graduates: *171* • RN Student Graduates: *15*

FINANCES

Residential Annual Tuition: *$3,859* • Non-Residential Annual Tuition: *$10,206* • General Institutional Fees: *Not Reported* • Additional Nursing Fees: *Not Reported*

FINANCES

Residential Annual Tuition: *$5,314* • Non-Residential Annual Tuition: *$15,926* • General Institutional Fees: *$350* • Additional Nursing Fees: *$450*

INDIANA UNIVERSITY— SOUTHEAST

Address: 4201 Grant Line Road, LF-102, New Albany, IN 47150
Phone: 812-941-2340
Fax: 812-941-2687
Contact: Lillian Yeager, EdD, RN, Interim Dean
Email: lyeager@ius.edu

GENERAL INFORMATION

Type of School: *4-Year College or University, Public* • Accreditation: *North Central Association of Colleges and Schools* • Total Enrollment: *Not Reported*

PROGRAM INFORMATION

Two Year Exit Option: *Not Reported* • NLNAC Accreditation: *Not Reported* • CCNE Accreditation: *Yes*

NURSING STUDENT PROFILE

Total Nursing Enrollment: *98* • Total Basic Student Enrollment, Full Time: *91* • Total Basic Student Enrollment, Part Time: *2* • Female Basic Student Enrollment: *92* • Male Basic Student Enrollment: *1* • Total RN Enrollment: *5* • Total New Fall Enrollments: *33* • Total Graduates: *57* • Basic Student Graduates: *35* • RN Student Graduates: *22*

FINANCES

Residential Annual Tuition: *$6,518* • Non-Residential Annual Tuition: *$17,552* • General Institutional Fees: *Not Reported* • Additional Nursing Fees: *Not Reported*

INDIANA WESLEYAN UNIVERSITY

Address: 4201 S. Washington Street, Marion, IN 46953
Phone: 765-677-2266
Fax: 765-677-2284
Contact: Susan D. Stranahan, PhD, RN, Chair
Email: sstranah@indwes.edu

GENERAL INFORMATION

Type of School: *4-Year College or University, Private (Religious)* • Accreditation: *North Central Association of Colleges and Schools* • Total Enrollment: *2135*

PROGRAM INFORMATION

Two Year Exit Option: *Not Reported* • CCNE Accreditation: *Yes*

NURSING STUDENT PROFILE

Total Nursing Enrollment: *432* • Total Basic Student Enrollment, Full Time: *135* • Total Basic Student Enrollment, Part Time: *19* • Female Basic Student Enrollment: *150* • Male Basic Student Enrollment: *4* • Total RN Enrollment: *278* • Total New Fall Enrollments: *34* • Total Graduates: *204* • Basic Student Graduates: *37* • RN Student Graduates: *167*

FINANCES

Residential Annual Tuition: *$12,250* • Non-Residential Annual Tuition: *$12,250* • General Institutional Fees: *$6,125* • Additional Nursing Fees: *$260*

MARIAN COLLEGE

Address: 3200 Cold Spring Rd, Indianapolis, IN 46222
Phone: 317-955-6155
Fax: 317-955-6135
Contact: Marian Pettengill, PhD, RN, Professor and Chair
Email: mpettengill@marian.edu

GENERAL INFORMATION

Type of School: *4-Year College or University, Private (Religious)* • Accreditation: *North Central Association of Colleges and Schools* • Total Enrollment: *1260*

PROGRAM INFORMATION

Two Year Exit Option: *No* • NLNAC Accreditation: *Yes* • CCNE Accreditation:

NURSING STUDENT PROFILE

Total Nursing Enrollment: *73* • Total Basic Student Enrollment, Full Time: *59* • Total Basic Student Enrollment, Part Time: *5* • Female Basic Student Enrollment: *62* • Male Basic Student Enrollment: *2* • Total RN Enrollment: *9* • Total New Fall Enrollments: *21* • Total Graduates: *25* • Basic Student Graduates: *25* • RN Student Graduates: *0*

FINANCES

Residential Annual Tuition: *$14,499* • Non-Residential Annual Tuition: *$14,499* • General Institutional Fees: *$100* • Additional Nursing Fees: *$950*

PURDUE UNIVERSITY

Address: 1337 Helen R. Johnson Hall, West Lafayette, IN 47907-1337
Phone: 765-494-2849
Fax: 765-496-1800
Contact: Linda A. Simunek, PhD, JD, RN, Head
Email: simunek@nursing.purdue.edu

GENERAL INFORMATION

Type of School: *Governmental Agency, Public* • Accreditation: *North Central Association of Colleges and Schools* • Total Enrollment: *37762*

PROGRAM INFORMATION

Two Year Exit Option: *Not Reported* • NLNAC Accreditation: *Yes* • CCNE Accreditation:

NURSING STUDENT PROFILE

Total Nursing Enrollment: *500* • Total Basic Student Enrollment, Full Time: *480* • Total Basic Student Enrollment, Part Time: *5* • Female Basic Student Enrollment: *465* • Male Basic Student Enrollment: *20* • Total RN Enrollment: *15* • Total New Fall Enrollments: *114* • Total Graduates: *96* • Basic Student Graduates: *92* • RN Student Graduates: *4*

FINANCES

Residential Annual Tuition: *Not Reported* • Non-Residential Annual Tuition: *Not Reported* • General Institutional Fees: *$1,936* • Additional Nursing Fees: *$139*

SAINT JOSEPH'S COLLEGE

Address: PO Box 849 Highway 231, Rensselaer, IN
            47978-0849
Phone: 207-893-7970
Fax: 207-893-7520
Contact: Margaret Hourigan, PhD, RN, CHE, Interim
            Chairperson
Email: mhouriga@sjcme.edu

GENERAL INFORMATION

Type of School: *Other* • Accreditation: *Not Reported* • Total
Enrollment: *Not Reported*

PROGRAM INFORMATION

Two Year Exit Option: *No* • NLNAC Accreditation: *Yes* •
CCNE Accreditation:

NURSING STUDENT PROFILE

Total Nursing Enrollment: *603* • Total Basic Student
Enrollment, Full Time: *99* • Total Basic Student Enrollment,
Part Time: *4* • Female Basic Student Enrollment: *98* • Male
Basic Student Enrollment: *5* • Total RN Enrollment: *500* •
Total New Fall Enrollments: *41* • Total Graduates: *38* • Basic
Student Graduates: *14* • RN Student Graduates: *24*

FINANCES

Residential Annual Tuition: *$13,920* • Non-Residential
Annual Tuition: *$13,920* • General Institutional Fees: *$155* •
Additional Nursing Fees: *$200*

SAINT MARY'S COLLEGE

Address: Havican Hall #6, Notre Dame, IN 46556-5032
Phone: 219-284-4680
Fax: 219-284-4716
Contact: Mary Jo Regan-Kubinski, PhD, RN, Chair
Email: regankub@saintmarys.edu

GENERAL INFORMATION

Type of School: *4-Year College or University, Private
(Religious)* • Accreditation: *North Central Association of
Colleges and Schools* • Total Enrollment: *1565*

PROGRAM INFORMATION

Two Year Exit Option: *Not Reported* • NLNAC
Accreditation: *Yes* • CCNE Accreditation:

NURSING STUDENT PROFILE

Total Nursing Enrollment: *82* • Total Basic Student
Enrollment, Full Time: *82* • Total Basic Student Enrollment,
Part Time: *0* • Female Basic Student Enrollment: *82* • Male
Basic Student Enrollment: *0* • Total RN Enrollment: *0* •
Total New Fall Enrollments: *32* • Total Graduates: *20* • Basic
Student Graduates: *10* • RN Student Graduates: *10*

FINANCES

Residential Annual Tuition: *$16,994* • Non-Residential
Annual Tuition: *$16,994* • General Institutional Fees: *Not
Reported* • Additional Nursing Fees: *Not Reported*

UNIVERSITY OF EVANSVILLE

Address: 1800 Lincoln Avenue, Evansville, IN 47722
Phone: 812-479-2717
Fax: 812-479-2717
Contact: Jane Allen, MSN, RN, Chair
Email: ja2@evansville.edu

GENERAL INFORMATION

Type of School: *Independent, Private (Religious)* •
Accreditation: *North Central Association of Colleges and Schools* • Total Enrollment: *2478*

PROGRAM INFORMATION

Two Year Exit Option: *No* • NLNAC Accreditation: *Yes* •
CCNE Accreditation:

NURSING STUDENT PROFILE

Total Nursing Enrollment: *49* • Total Basic Student
Enrollment, Full Time: *49* • Total Basic Student Enrollment,
Part Time: *0* • Female Basic Student Enrollment: *49* • Male
Basic Student Enrollment: *0* • Total RN Enrollment: *0* •
Total New Fall Enrollments: *15* • Total Graduates: *23* • Basic
Student Graduates: *23* • RN Student Graduates: *0*

FINANCES

Residential Annual Tuition: *$17,050* • Non-Residential
Annual Tuition: *$17,050* • General Institutional Fees:
$5,100 • Additional Nursing Fees: *$730*

UNIVERSITY OF INDIANAPOLIS

Address: 1400 E Hanna Ave, Indianapolis, IN 46227-3630
Phone: 317-788-3324
Fax: 317-788-3542
Contact: Karla Backer, PhD, RN, BSN Program Director
Email: backer@uindy.edu

GENERAL INFORMATION

Type of School: *4-Year College or University, Private
(Religious)* • Accreditation: *North Central Association of
Colleges and Schools* • Total Enrollment: *2839*

PROGRAM INFORMATION

Two Year Exit Option: *Not Reported* • NLNAC
Accreditation: *Yes* • CCNE Accreditation:

NURSING STUDENT PROFILE

Total Nursing Enrollment: *150* • Total Basic Student
Enrollment, Full Time: *63* • Total Basic Student Enrollment,
Part Time: *12* • Female Basic Student Enrollment: *73* • Male
Basic Student Enrollment: *2* • Total RN Enrollment: *75* •
Total New Fall Enrollments: *31* • Total Graduates: *20* • Basic
Student Graduates: *20* • RN Student Graduates: *0*

FINANCES

Residential Annual Tuition: *$14,630* • Non-Residential
Annual Tuition: *$14,630* • General Institutional Fees:
$7,315 • Additional Nursing Fees: *$610*

UNIVERSITY OF SAINT FRANCIS—FORT WAYNE

Address: 2701 Spring Street, Fort Wayne, IN 46808
Phone: 260-434-3284
Fax: 260-434-7404
Contact: Stephanie Oefting, MS, RN, BSN Program Director
Email: soefting@sf.edu

GENERAL INFORMATION

Type of School: *Not Reported* • Accreditation: *Not Reported* • Total Enrollment: *Not Reported*

PROGRAM INFORMATION

Two Year Exit Option: *No* • NLNAC Accreditation: *Not Reported* • CCNE Accreditation: *Yes*

NURSING STUDENT PROFILE

Total Nursing Enrollment: *Not Reported* • Total Basic Student Enrollment, Full Time: *Not Reported* • Total Basic Student Enrollment, Part Time: *Not Reported* • Female Basic Student Enrollment: *Not Reported* • Male Basic Student Enrollment: *Not Reported* • Total RN Enrollment: *Not Reported* • Total New Fall Enrollments: *Not Reported* • Total Graduates: *Not Reported* • Basic Student Graduates: *Not Reported* • RN Student Graduates: *Not Reported*

FINANCES

Residential Annual Tuition: *Not Reported* • Non-Residential Annual Tuition: *Not Reported* • General Institutional Fees: *Not Reported* • Additional Nursing Fees: *Not Reported*

UNIVERSITY OF SOUTHERN INDIANA

Address: 8600 University Blvd., Evansville, IN 47712
Phone: 812-465-1173
Fax: 812-465-7092
Contact: Ann White, PhD, MBA, RN, Undergraduate Program Director
Email: awhite@usi.edu

GENERAL INFORMATION

Type of School: *4-Year College or University, Public* • Accreditation: *North Central Association of Colleges and Schools* • Total Enrollment: *9600*

PROGRAM INFORMATION

Two Year Exit Option: *Not Reported* • NLNAC Accreditation: *Not Reported* • CCNE Accreditation: *Yes*

NURSING STUDENT PROFILE

Total Nursing Enrollment: *276* • Total Basic Student Enrollment, Full Time: *190* • Total Basic Student Enrollment, Part Time: *50* • Female Basic Student Enrollment: *222* • Male Basic Student Enrollment: *18* • Total RN Enrollment: *36* • Total New Fall Enrollments: *82* • Total Graduates: *53* • Basic Student Graduates: *38* • RN Student Graduates: *15*

FINANCES

Residential Annual Tuition: *$4,080* • Non-Residential Annual Tuition: *$9,736* • General Institutional Fees: *$70* • Additional Nursing Fees: *$90*

VALPARAISO UNIVERSITY

Address: Le Bien Hall, Valparaiso, IN 46383
Phone: 219-464-5289
Fax: 219-464-5425
Contact: Janet M. Brown, PhD, RN, Dean and Professor
Email: janet.brown@valpo.edu

GENERAL INFORMATION

Type of School: *4-Year College or University, Private (Independent)* • Accreditation: *North Central Association of Colleges and Schools* • Total Enrollment: *3650*

PROGRAM INFORMATION

Two Year Exit Option: *Not Reported* • NLNAC Accreditation: *Yes* • CCNE Accreditation: *Yes*

NURSING STUDENT PROFILE

Total Nursing Enrollment: *123* • Total Basic Student Enrollment, Full Time: *69* • Total Basic Student Enrollment, Part Time: *5* • Female Basic Student Enrollment: *71* • Male Basic Student Enrollment: *3* • Total RN Enrollment: *49* • Total New Fall Enrollments: *21* • Total Graduates: *39* • Basic Student Graduates: *25* • RN Student Graduates: *14*

FINANCES

Residential Annual Tuition: *$17,100* • Non-Residential Annual Tuition: *$17,100* • General Institutional Fees: *$8,550* • Additional Nursing Fees: *Not Reported*

ALLEN COLLEGE

Address: 1825 Logan Ave, Waterloo, IA 50703-1999
Phone: 319-226-2040
Fax: 319-226-2070
Contact: Nancy Kramer, EdD, CPNP, ARNP, BSN
            Department Chair
Email: KramerNA@ihs.org

GENERAL INFORMATION

Type of School: *4-Year College or University, Private (Independent)* • Accreditation: *North Central Association of Colleges and Schools* • Total Enrollment: *257*

PROGRAM INFORMATION

Two Year Exit Option: *No* • NLNAC Accreditation: *Yes* • CCNE Accreditation:

NURSING STUDENT PROFILE

Total Nursing Enrollment: *208* • Total Basic Student Enrollment, Full Time: *160* • Total Basic Student Enrollment, Part Time: *9* • Female Basic Student Enrollment: *158* • Male Basic Student Enrollment: *11* • Total RN Enrollment: *39* • Total New Fall Enrollments: *47* • Total Graduates: *51* • Basic Student Graduates: *37* • RN Student Graduates: *14*

FINANCES

Residential Annual Tuition: *$7,120* • Non-Residential Annual Tuition: *$7,120* • General Institutional Fees: *$650* • Additional Nursing Fees: *$0*

BRIAR CLIFF UNIVERSITY

Address: 3303 Rebecca St, Sioux City, IA 51104
Phone: 712-279-5458
Fax: 712-279-1698
Contact: Ruth Dankanich Daumer, MSN, ARNP, CS, Chairperson
Email: daumer@briarcliff.edu

GENERAL INFORMATION

Type of School: *4-Year College or University, Private (Religious)* • Accreditation: *North Central Association of Colleges and Schools* • Total Enrollment: *969*

PROGRAM INFORMATION

Two Year Exit Option: *Not Reported* • NLNAC Accreditation: *Yes* • CCNE Accreditation:

NURSING STUDENT PROFILE

Total Nursing Enrollment: *161* • Total Basic Student Enrollment, Full Time: *47* • Total Basic Student Enrollment, Part Time: *2* • Female Basic Student Enrollment: *47* • Male Basic Student Enrollment: *2* • Total RN Enrollment: *112* • Total New Fall Enrollments: *9* • Total Graduates: *21* • Basic Student Graduates: *7* • RN Student Graduates: *14*

FINANCES

Residential Annual Tuition: *$12,690* • Non-Residential Annual Tuition: *$12,690* • General Institutional Fees: *$4,230* • Additional Nursing Fees: *$423*

CLARKE COLLEGE

Address: 1550 Clarke Drive, Dubuque, IA 52001
Phone: 319-588-6361
Fax: 319-584-8684
Contact: Mary Margaret Mooney, DNSc, ARNP, FAAN, Professor and Chair
Email: mmooney@clarke.edu

GENERAL INFORMATION

Type of School: *4-Year College or University, Private (Independent)* • Accreditation: *North Central Association of Colleges and Schools* • Total Enrollment: *1249*

PROGRAM INFORMATION

Two Year Exit Option: *Not Reported* • NLNAC Accreditation: *Yes* • CCNE Accreditation:

NURSING STUDENT PROFILE

Total Nursing Enrollment: *88* • Total Basic Student Enrollment, Full Time: *46* • Total Basic Student Enrollment, Part Time: *4* • Female Basic Student Enrollment: *47* • Male Basic Student Enrollment: *3* • Total RN Enrollment: *38* • Total New Fall Enrollments: *16* • Total Graduates: *22* • Basic Student Graduates: *11* • RN Student Graduates: *11*

FINANCES

Residential Annual Tuition: *$14,000* • Non-Residential Annual Tuition: *$14,000* • General Institutional Fees: *$7,000* • Additional Nursing Fees: *$350*

COE COLLEGE

Address: 1220 1st Ave NE, Cedar Rapids, IA 52402
Phone: 319-369-8120
Fax: 319-369-8121
Contact: Jule H. Ohrt, MS, RN, Chair and Associate
          Professor
Email: johrt@coe.edu

GRACELAND UNIVERSITY

Address: 1 University Place, Lamo, IA 50140
Phone: 816-833-0524
Fax: 816-833-2990
Contact: Claudia Horton, MSN, RN, Associate Dean
Email: horton@graceland.edu

GENERAL INFORMATION

Type of School: *4-Year College or University, Private (Independent)* • Accreditation: *North Central Association of Colleges and Schools* • Total Enrollment: *1250*

GENERAL INFORMATION

Type of School: *4-Year College or University, Private (Religious)* • Accreditation: *North Central Association of Colleges and Schools* • Total Enrollment: *2283*

PROGRAM INFORMATION

Two Year Exit Option: *Not Reported* • NLNAC Accreditation: *Yes* • CCNE Accreditation:

PROGRAM INFORMATION

Two Year Exit Option: *No* • NLNAC Accreditation: *Yes* • CCNE Accreditation: *Yes*

NURSING STUDENT PROFILE

Total Nursing Enrollment: *29* • Total Basic Student Enrollment, Full Time: *26* • Total Basic Student Enrollment, Part Time: *2* • Female Basic Student Enrollment: *28* • Male Basic Student Enrollment: *0* • Total RN Enrollment: *1* • Total New Fall Enrollments: *13* • Total Graduates: *10* • Basic Student Graduates: *7* • RN Student Graduates: *3*

NURSING STUDENT PROFILE

Total Nursing Enrollment: *66* • Total Basic Student Enrollment, Full Time: *65* • Total Basic Student Enrollment, Part Time: *1* • Female Basic Student Enrollment: *64* • Male Basic Student Enrollment: *2* • Total RN Enrollment: *0* • Total New Fall Enrollments: *32* • Total Graduates: *30* • Basic Student Graduates: *30* • RN Student Graduates: *0*

FINANCES

Residential Annual Tuition: *$18,240* • Non-Residential Annual Tuition: *$18,240* • General Institutional Fees: *Not Reported* • Additional Nursing Fees: *$925*

FINANCES

Residential Annual Tuition: *$13,025* • Non-Residential Annual Tuition: *Not Reported* • General Institutional Fees: *$0* • Additional Nursing Fees: *$295*

GRAND VIEW COLLEGE

Address: 1204 Grandview Ave, Des Moines, IA 50316
Phone: 515-263-2866
Fax: 515-263-6077
Contact: Jean E. Logan, PhD, RN, Nursing Division Head
Email: jlogan@gvc.edu

GENERAL INFORMATION

Type of School: *4-Year College or University, Private (Religious)* • Accreditation: *North Central Association of Colleges and Schools* • Total Enrollment: *1400*

PROGRAM INFORMATION

Two Year Exit Option: *Not Reported* • NLNAC Accreditation: *Yes* • CCNE Accreditation:

NURSING STUDENT PROFILE

Total Nursing Enrollment: *134* • Total Basic Student Enrollment, Full Time: *98* • Total Basic Student Enrollment, Part Time: *7* • Female Basic Student Enrollment: *94* • Male Basic Student Enrollment: *11* • Total RN Enrollment: *29* • Total New Fall Enrollments: *34* • Total Graduates: *73* • Basic Student Graduates: *46* • RN Student Graduates: *27*

FINANCES

Residential Annual Tuition: *$12,790* • Non-Residential Annual Tuition: *$12,790* • General Institutional Fees: *$6,395* • Additional Nursing Fees: *$380*

IOWA WESLEYAN COLLEGE

Address: 601 N Main Street, Mount Pleasant, IA 52641
Phone: 319-385-6323
Fax: *Not Reported*
Contact: Judith Hausner, PhD, RN, Chair
Email: jhausner@iwc.edu

GENERAL INFORMATION

Type of School: *Independent, Private (Independent)* • Accreditation: *North Central Association of Colleges and Schools* • Total Enrollment: *800*

PROGRAM INFORMATION

Two Year Exit Option: *Not Reported* • NLNAC Accreditation: *Yes* • CCNE Accreditation:

NURSING STUDENT PROFILE

Total Nursing Enrollment: *78* • Total Basic Student Enrollment, Full Time: *5* • Total Basic Student Enrollment, Part Time: *18* • Female Basic Student Enrollment: *18* • Male Basic Student Enrollment: *5* • Total RN Enrollment: *55* • Total New Fall Enrollments: *26* • Total Graduates: *27* • Basic Student Graduates: *14* • RN Student Graduates: *13*

FINANCES

Residential Annual Tuition: *$12,700* • Non-Residential Annual Tuition: *Not Reported* • General Institutional Fees: *$6,350* • Additional Nursing Fees: *$300*

LUTHER COLLEGE

Address: 700 College Dr, Decorah, IA 52101
Phone: 563-387-1057
Fax: 563-387-2149
Contact: Donna Kubesh, PhD, RN, Head
Email: kubeshdt@luther.edu

GENERAL INFORMATION

Type of School: *4-Year College or University, Private (Religious)* • Accreditation: *North Central Association of Colleges and Schools* • Total Enrollment: *2575*

PROGRAM INFORMATION

Two Year Exit Option: *No* • NLNAC Accreditation: *Yes* • CCNE Accreditation:

NURSING STUDENT PROFILE

Total Nursing Enrollment: *111* • Total Basic Student Enrollment, Full Time: *109* • Total Basic Student Enrollment, Part Time: *1* • Female Basic Student Enrollment: *106* • Male Basic Student Enrollment: *4* • Total RN Enrollment: *1* • Total New Fall Enrollments: *34* • Total Graduates: *23* • Basic Student Graduates: *23* • RN Student Graduates: *0*

FINANCES

Residential Annual Tuition: *$19,325* • Non-Residential Annual Tuition: *$19,325* • General Institutional Fees: *$240* • Additional Nursing Fees: *$159*

MARYCREST INTERNATIONAL UNIVERSITY

Address: 1607 West 12th St, Davenport, IA 528044096
Phone: 319-326-9278
Fax: 319-326-9473
Contact: Louise A. Hintze, PhD, RN, Chairperson
Email: LHINTZE@MCREST.EDU

GENERAL INFORMATION

Type of School: *4-Year College or University, Private (Independent)* • Accreditation: *North Central Association of Colleges and Schools* • Total Enrollment: *717*

PROGRAM INFORMATION

Two Year Exit Option: *Not Reported* • NLNAC Accreditation: *Yes* • CCNE Accreditation:

NURSING STUDENT PROFILE

Total Nursing Enrollment: *27* • Total Basic Student Enrollment, Full Time: *11* • Total Basic Student Enrollment, Part Time: *4* • Female Basic Student Enrollment: *15* • Male Basic Student Enrollment: *0* • Total RN Enrollment: *12* • Total New Fall Enrollments: *20* • Total Graduates: *18* • Basic Student Graduates: *5* • RN Student Graduates: *13*

FINANCES

Residential Annual Tuition: *$12,900* • Non-Residential Annual Tuition: *$12,900* • General Institutional Fees: *$6,450* • Additional Nursing Fees: *$430*

MORNINGSIDE COLLEGE

Address: 1501 Morningside Ave, Sioux City, IA 51106-1717
Phone: 712-274-5239
Fax: 712-274-5101
Contact: Richard A. Peterson, EdD, RN, Chair and Associate Professor
Email: peterson@morningside.edu

GENERAL INFORMATION

Type of School: *4-Year College or University, Private (Religious)* • Accreditation: *North Central Association of Colleges and Schools* • Total Enrollment: *850*

PROGRAM INFORMATION

Two Year Exit Option: *Not Reported* • NLNAC Accreditation: *Yes* • CCNE Accreditation:

NURSING STUDENT PROFILE

Total Nursing Enrollment: *50* • Total Basic Student Enrollment, Full Time: *40* • Total Basic Student Enrollment, Part Time: *2* • Female Basic Student Enrollment: *40* • Male Basic Student Enrollment: *2* • Total RN Enrollment: *8* • Total New Fall Enrollments: *6* • Total Graduates: *11* • Basic Student Graduates: *11* • RN Student Graduates: *0*

FINANCES

Residential Annual Tuition: *Not Reported* • Non-Residential Annual Tuition: *Not Reported* • General Institutional Fees: *$6,655* • Additional Nursing Fees: *Not Reported*

MOUNT MERCY COLLEGE

Address: 1330 Elmhurst Dr, NE, Cedar Rapids, IA 52402
Phone: 319-368-6471
Fax: *Not Reported*
Contact: Mary P. Tarbox, EdD, RN, Chair
Email: mtarbox@mmc.mtmercy.edu

GENERAL INFORMATION

Type of School: *4-Year College or University, Private (Religious)* • Accreditation: *North Central Association of Colleges and Schools* • Total Enrollment: *1250*

PROGRAM INFORMATION

Two Year Exit Option: *Not Reported* • NLNAC Accreditation: *Yes* • CCNE Accreditation:

NURSING STUDENT PROFILE

Total Nursing Enrollment: *87* • Total Basic Student Enrollment, Full Time: *46* • Total Basic Student Enrollment, Part Time: *38* • Female Basic Student Enrollment: *80* • Male Basic Student Enrollment: *4* • Total RN Enrollment: *3* • Total New Fall Enrollments: *40* • Total Graduates: *34* • Basic Student Graduates: *32* • RN Student Graduates: *2*

FINANCES

Residential Annual Tuition: *$13,190* • Non-Residential Annual Tuition: *$13,190* • General Institutional Fees: *$6,595* • Additional Nursing Fees: *$365*

UNIVERSITY OF IOWA

Address: Iowa City, IA 52242
Phone: 319-335-7009
Fax: 319-335-7200
Contact: Melanie Dreher, PhD, RN, Dean
Email: *Not Reported*

GENERAL INFORMATION

Type of School: *4-Year College or University, Public* •
Accreditation: *North Central Association of Colleges and Schools* • Total Enrollment: *28840*

PROGRAM INFORMATION

Two Year Exit Option: *Not Reported* • NLNAC
Accreditation: *Not Reported* • CCNE Accreditation:

NURSING STUDENT PROFILE

Total Nursing Enrollment: *470* • Total Basic Student
Enrollment, Full Time: *255* • Total Basic Student
Enrollment, Part Time: *81* • Female Basic Student
Enrollment: *Not Reported* • Male Basic Student Enrollment:
Not Reported • Total RN Enrollment: *134* • Total New Fall
Enrollments: *Not Reported* • Total Graduates: *184* • Basic
Student Graduates: *153* • RN Student Graduates: *31*

FINANCES

Residential Annual Tuition: *Not Reported* • Non-Residential
Annual Tuition: *Not Reported* • General Institutional Fees:
Not Reported • Additional Nursing Fees: *Not Reported*

BAKER UNIVERSITY

Address: 1500 South West 10th Street, Topeka, KS
66604-1301
Phone: 785-354-5853
Fax: 785-354-5832
Contact: Kathleen L. Harr, DNSc, RN, Dean and
Professor
Email: kathleen.harr@bakeru.edu

GENERAL INFORMATION

Type of School: *4-Year College or University, Private
(Religious)* • Accreditation: *North Central Association of
Colleges and Schools* • Total Enrollment: *830*

PROGRAM INFORMATION

Two Year Exit Option: *Not Reported* • NLNAC
Accreditation: *Yes* • CCNE Accreditation:

NURSING STUDENT PROFILE

Total Nursing Enrollment: *95* • Total Basic Student
Enrollment, Full Time: *84* • Total Basic Student Enrollment,
Part Time: *7* • Female Basic Student Enrollment: *84* • Male
Basic Student Enrollment: *7* • Total RN Enrollment: *4* •
Total New Fall Enrollments: *29* • Total Graduates: *40* • Basic
Student Graduates: *34* • RN Student Graduates: *6*

FINANCES

Residential Annual Tuition: *$8,754* • Non-Residential
Annual Tuition: *$8,754* • General Institutional Fees:
$4,377 • Additional Nursing Fees: *$275*

BETHEL COLLEGE

Address: 300 East 27th, North Newton, KS 67117
Phone: 651-638-6368
Fax: 651-635-1965
Contact: Sandra Peterson, PhD, RN, Professor
Email: petsan@bethel.edu

EMPORIA STATE UNIVERSITY

Address: 1127 Chestnut Street, Emporia, KS 66801-2523
Phone: 620-654-7890
Fax: *Not Reported*
Contact: Judith E. Calhoun, PhD, ARNP, Division Chair
Email: *Not Reported*

GENERAL INFORMATION

Type of School: *4-Year College or University, Private (Religious)* • Accreditation: *North Central Association of Colleges and Schools* • Total Enrollment: *502*

GENERAL INFORMATION

Type of School: *4-Year College or University, Public* • Accreditation: *North Central Association of Colleges and Schools* • Total Enrollment: *5823*

PROGRAM INFORMATION

Two Year Exit Option: *No* • NLNAC Accreditation: *Not Reported* • CCNE Accreditation: *Yes*

PROGRAM INFORMATION

Two Year Exit Option: *Not Reported* • NLNAC Accreditation: *Yes* • CCNE Accreditation:

NURSING STUDENT PROFILE

Total Nursing Enrollment: *99* • Total Basic Student Enrollment, Full Time: *99* • Total Basic Student Enrollment, Part Time: *0* • Female Basic Student Enrollment: *95* • Male Basic Student Enrollment: *4* • Total RN Enrollment: *0* • Total New Fall Enrollments: *50* • Total Graduates: *49* • Basic Student Graduates: *49* • RN Student Graduates: *0*

NURSING STUDENT PROFILE

Total Nursing Enrollment: *91* • Total Basic Student Enrollment, Full Time: *91* • Total Basic Student Enrollment, Part Time: *0* • Female Basic Student Enrollment: *85* • Male Basic Student Enrollment: *6* • Total RN Enrollment: *0* • Total New Fall Enrollments: *34* • Total Graduates: *25* • Basic Student Graduates: *23* • RN Student Graduates: *2*

FINANCES

Residential Annual Tuition: *$16,780* • Non-Residential Annual Tuition: *$16,780* • General Institutional Fees: *$0* • Additional Nursing Fees: *$110*

FINANCES

Residential Annual Tuition: *$1,740* • Non-Residential Annual Tuition: *$6,594* • General Institutional Fees: *$544* • Additional Nursing Fees: *$1,650*

FORT HAYS STATE UNIVERSITY

Address: 600 Park Street, Hays, KS 67601-4099
Phone: 785-628-4256
Fax: 785-628-4000
Contact: Dianna Koerner, PhD, RN, Director,
           Undergraduate Nursing Studies
Email: dkoerner@fhsu.edu

GENERAL INFORMATION

Type of School: *Not Reported* • Accreditation: *Not Reported* •
Total Enrollment: *Not Reported*

PROGRAM INFORMATION

Two Year Exit Option: *Not Reported* • NLNAC
Accreditation: *Yes* • CCNE Accreditation:

NURSING STUDENT PROFILE

Total Nursing Enrollment: *151* • Total Basic Student
Enrollment, Full Time: *89* • Total Basic Student Enrollment,
Part Time: *0* • Female Basic Student Enrollment: *80* • Male
Basic Student Enrollment: *9* • Total RN Enrollment: *62* •
Total New Fall Enrollments: *0* • Total Graduates: *61* • Basic
Student Graduates: *37* • RN Student Graduates: *24*

FINANCES

Residential Annual Tuition: *$3,242* • Non-Residential
Annual Tuition: *$10,226* • General Institutional Fees: *Not
Reported* • Additional Nursing Fees: *Not Reported*

MID AMERICA NAZARENE UNIVERSITY

Address: 2030 E College Way, Olathe, KS 66062-1851
Phone: 913-791-3383
Fax: 913-791-3408
Contact: Palma Smith, PhD, RN, Chair, Division of
           Nursing
Email: psmith@mnu.edu

GENERAL INFORMATION

Type of School: *4-Year College or University, Private
(Religious)* • Accreditation: *North Central Association of
Colleges and Schools* • Total Enrollment: *1717*

PROGRAM INFORMATION

Two Year Exit Option: *Not Reported* • NLNAC
Accreditation: *Yes* • CCNE Accreditation:

NURSING STUDENT PROFILE

Total Nursing Enrollment: *92* • Total Basic Student
Enrollment, Full Time: *79* • Total Basic Student Enrollment,
Part Time: *10* • Female Basic Student Enrollment: *87* • Male
Basic Student Enrollment: *2* • Total RN Enrollment: *3* •
Total New Fall Enrollments: *20* • Total Graduates: *31* • Basic
Student Graduates: *31* • RN Student Graduates: *0*

FINANCES

Residential Annual Tuition: *$10,150* • Non-Residential
Annual Tuition: *$10,150* • General Institutional Fees:
$5,075 • Additional Nursing Fees: *$339*

NEWMAN UNIVERSITY

Address: 3100 McCormick Ave, Wichita, KS 67213
Phone: 316-456-7890
Fax: 316-942-4483
Contact: Joan Felt, PhD, RN, Dean
Email: feltsj@newman.edu

GENERAL INFORMATION

Type of School: *Not Reported* • Accreditation: *Not Reported* • Total Enrollment: *Not Reported*

PROGRAM INFORMATION

Two Year Exit Option: *Not Reported* • NLNAC Accreditation: *Yes* • CCNE Accreditation:

NURSING STUDENT PROFILE

Total Nursing Enrollment: *Not Reported* • Total Basic Student Enrollment, Full Time: *Not Reported* • Total Basic Student Enrollment, Part Time: *Not Reported* • Female Basic Student Enrollment: *Not Reported* • Male Basic Student Enrollment: *Not Reported* • Total RN Enrollment: *Not Reported* • Total New Fall Enrollments: *Not Reported* • Total Graduates: *Not Reported* • Basic Student Graduates: *Not Reported* • RN Student Graduates: *Not Reported*

FINANCES

Residential Annual Tuition: *Not Reported* • Non-Residential Annual Tuition: *Not Reported* • General Institutional Fees: *Not Reported* • Additional Nursing Fees: *Not Reported*

PITTSBURG STATE UNIVERSITY

Address: 1701 S. Broadway, Pittsburg, KS 66762
Phone: 316-235-4431
Fax: 316-235-4449
Contact: Barbara Jean McClaskey, PhD, RN, Interim Chair
Email: *Not Reported*

GENERAL INFORMATION

Type of School: *Not Reported* • Accreditation: *Not Reported* • Total Enrollment: *Not Reported*

PROGRAM INFORMATION

Two Year Exit Option: *Not Reported* • NLNAC Accreditation: *Yes* • CCNE Accreditation:

NURSING STUDENT PROFILE

Total Nursing Enrollment: *122* • Total Basic Student Enrollment, Full Time: *107* • Total Basic Student Enrollment, Part Time: *0* • Female Basic Student Enrollment: *Not Reported* • Male Basic Student Enrollment: *Not Reported* • Total RN Enrollment: *15* • Total New Fall Enrollments: *0* • Total Graduates: *82* • Basic Student Graduates: *53* • RN Student Graduates: *29*

FINANCES

Residential Annual Tuition: *$2,100* • Non-Residential Annual Tuition: *$6,464* • General Institutional Fees: *Not Reported* • Additional Nursing Fees: *Not Reported*

UNIVERSITY OF KANSAS

Address: 3901 Rainbow Blvd., Kansas City, KS 66160-7501
Phone: 913-588-1619
Fax: 913-588-1615
Contact: Karen L. Miller, PhD, RN, FAAN, Professor and Dean
Email: soninfo@kumc.edu

GENERAL INFORMATION

Type of School: *4-Year College or University, Public* •
Accreditation: *North Central Association of Colleges and Schools* • Total Enrollment: *25920*

PROGRAM INFORMATION

Two Year Exit Option: *Not Reported* • NLNAC
Accreditation: *Yes* • CCNE Accreditation:

NURSING STUDENT PROFILE

Total Nursing Enrollment: *275* • Total Basic Student Enrollment, Full Time: *222* • Total Basic Student Enrollment, Part Time: *10* • Female Basic Student Enrollment: *205* • Male Basic Student Enrollment: *27* • Total RN Enrollment: *43* • Total New Fall Enrollments: *117* • Total Graduates: *108* • Basic Student Graduates: *99* • RN Student Graduates: *9*

FINANCES

Residential Annual Tuition: *Not Reported* • Non-Residential Annual Tuition: *Not Reported* • General Institutional Fees: *Not Reported* • Additional Nursing Fees: *$7,555*

WASHBURN UNIVERSITY

Address: 1700 SW College Street, Topeka, KS 66621
Phone: 231-785-1010
Fax: 231-785-1032
Contact: Cynthia A. Hornberger, PhD, MBA, RN, Dean
Email: zzhorn@washburn.edu

GENERAL INFORMATION

Type of School: *4-Year College or University, Public* •
Accreditation: *North Central Association of Colleges and Schools* • Total Enrollment: *6500*

PROGRAM INFORMATION

Two Year Exit Option: *Not Reported* • CCNE Accreditation: *Yes*

NURSING STUDENT PROFILE

Total Nursing Enrollment: *185* • Total Basic Student Enrollment, Full Time: *173* • Total Basic Student Enrollment, Part Time: *10* • Female Basic Student Enrollment: *166* • Male Basic Student Enrollment: *17* • Total RN Enrollment: *2* • Total New Fall Enrollments: *50* • Total Graduates: *68* • Basic Student Graduates: *68* • RN Student Graduates: *0*

FINANCES

Residential Annual Tuition: *Not Reported* • Non-Residential Annual Tuition: *Not Reported* • General Institutional Fees: *Not Reported* • Additional Nursing Fees: *$107*

WICHITA STATE UNIVERSITY

Address: 1845 Fairmont, Witchita, KS 67260
Phone: 316-978-5741
Fax: 316-978-3094
Contact: Phyllis Jacobs, MSN, RN, Undergraduate
            Director
Email: phyllis.jacobs@wichita.edu

GENERAL INFORMATION

Type of School: *4-Year College or University, Public* •
Accreditation: *North Central Association of Colleges and
Schools* • Total Enrollment: *15000*

PROGRAM INFORMATION

Two Year Exit Option: *No* • NLNAC Accreditation: *Yes* •
CCNE Accreditation:

NURSING STUDENT PROFILE

Total Nursing Enrollment: *180* • Total Basic Student
Enrollment, Full Time: *146* • Total Basic Student
Enrollment, Part Time: *3* • Female Basic Student
Enrollment: *138* • Male Basic Student Enrollment: *11* • Total
RN Enrollment: *31* • Total New Fall Enrollments: *50* • Total
Graduates: *68* • Basic Student Graduates: *61* • RN Student
Graduates: *7*

FINANCES

Residential Annual Tuition: *$3,704* • Non-Residential
Annual Tuition: *$11,654* • General Institutional Fees: *Not
Reported* • Additional Nursing Fees: *$42*

BELLARMINE COLLEGE

Address: 2001 Newburg Rd, Miles Hall, Louisville, KY
            40205
Phone: 502-452-8414
Fax: *Not Reported*
Contact: Barbara P. Harrison, MSN, RN, C, BSN
            Department Chair
Email: bharrison@bellarmine.edu

GENERAL INFORMATION

Type of School: *Other, Private (Independent)* • Accreditation:
Southern Association of Colleges and Schools • Total
Enrollment: *Not Reported*

PROGRAM INFORMATION

Two Year Exit Option: *Not Reported* • NLNAC
Accreditation: *Yes* • CCNE Accreditation: *Yes*

NURSING STUDENT PROFILE

Total Nursing Enrollment: *190* • Total Basic Student
Enrollment, Full Time: *74* • Total Basic Student Enrollment,
Part Time: *68* • Female Basic Student Enrollment: *126* •
Male Basic Student Enrollment: *16* • Total RN Enrollment:
48 • Total New Fall Enrollments: *79* • Total Graduates: *74* •
Basic Student Graduates: *64* • RN Student Graduates: *10*

FINANCES

Residential Annual Tuition: *$12,480* • Non-Residential
Annual Tuition: *$12,480* • General Institutional Fees:
$6,240 • Additional Nursing Fees: *$330*

BEREA COLLEGE

Address: 2190 College Station, Berea, KY 40404
Phone: 606-985-3384
Fax: *Not Reported*
Contact: Pamela Farley, PhD, RN, Chairperson
Email: pam_farley@berea.edu

GENERAL INFORMATION

Type of School: *4-Year College or University, Private (Independent)* • Accreditation: *Southern Association of Colleges and Schools* • Total Enrollment: *1500*

PROGRAM INFORMATION

Two Year Exit Option: *Not Reported* • NLNAC Accreditation: *Yes* • CCNE Accreditation:

NURSING STUDENT PROFILE

Total Nursing Enrollment: *82* • Total Basic Student Enrollment, Full Time: *82* • Total Basic Student Enrollment, Part Time: *0* • Female Basic Student Enrollment: *73* • Male Basic Student Enrollment: *9* • Total RN Enrollment: *0* • Total New Fall Enrollments: *23* • Total Graduates: *8* • Basic Student Graduates: *8* • RN Student Graduates: *0*

FINANCES

Residential Annual Tuition: *Not Provided* • Non-Residential Annual Tuition: *Not Provided* • General Institutional Fees: *$0* • Additional Nursing Fees: *$0*

BOWLING GREEN TECHNICAL COLLEGE— GLASGOW CAMPUS

Address: 129 State Ave., Glasgow, KY 42141
Phone: 419-383-5859
Fax: 419-383-5894
Contact: Susan Batten, PhD, RN, CNS, Associate Dean, Undergraduate Program
Email: sbatten@mco.edu

GENERAL INFORMATION

Type of School: *Other, Public* • Accreditation: *Not Reported* • Total Enrollment: *1000*

PROGRAM INFORMATION

Two Year Exit Option: *Not Reported* • NLNAC Accreditation: *Not Reported* • CCNE Accreditation: *Yes*

NURSING STUDENT PROFILE

Total Nursing Enrollment: *158* • Total Basic Student Enrollment, Full Time: *114* • Total Basic Student Enrollment, Part Time: *4* • Female Basic Student Enrollment: *111* • Male Basic Student Enrollment: *7* • Total RN Enrollment: *40* • Total New Fall Enrollments: *0* • Total Graduates: *101* • Basic Student Graduates: *55* • RN Student Graduates: *46*

FINANCES

Residential Annual Tuition: *$5,184* • Non-Residential Annual Tuition: *$11,082* • General Institutional Fees: *$427* • Additional Nursing Fees: *$200*

EASTERN KENTUCKY UNIVERSITY

Address: Rowlett Bldg, RM 223, Richmond, KY 40475
Phone: 606-622-1956
Fax: 606-622-1972
Contact: Deborah Whitehouse, PhD, RN, Chair
Email: *Not Reported*

GENERAL INFORMATION

Type of School: *4-Year College or University, Public* •
Accreditation: *Southern Association of Colleges and Schools* •
Total Enrollment: *14997*

PROGRAM INFORMATION

Two Year Exit Option: *Not Reported* • NLNAC
Accreditation: *Yes* • CCNE Accreditation:

NURSING STUDENT PROFILE

Total Nursing Enrollment: *350* • Total Basic Student
Enrollment, Full Time: *204* • Total Basic Student
Enrollment, Part Time: *47* • Female Basic Student
Enrollment: *Not Reported* • Male Basic Student Enrollment:
Not Reported • Total RN Enrollment: *99* • Total New Fall
Enrollments: *0* • Total Graduates: *115* • Basic Student
Graduates: *91* • RN Student Graduates: *24*

FINANCES

Residential Annual Tuition: *$2,190* • Non-Residential
Annual Tuition: *$6,030* • General Institutional Fees: *Not
Reported* • Additional Nursing Fees: *Not Reported*

KENTUCKY WESLEYAN COLLEGE

Address: 3000 Frederica Street, Owensboro, KY 42302-
           1039
Phone: 270-926-3111
Fax: *Not Reported*
Contact: Elizabeth G. Johnson, DSN, RN, Chair,
           Department of Nursing
Email: bethjo@kwc.edu

GENERAL INFORMATION

Type of School: *4-Year College or University, Private
(Religious)* • Accreditation: *Southern Association of Colleges
and Schools* • Total Enrollment: *685*

PROGRAM INFORMATION

Two Year Exit Option: *No* • NLNAC Accreditation: *Not
Reported* • CCNE Accreditation:

NURSING STUDENT PROFILE

Total Nursing Enrollment: *13* • Total Basic Student
Enrollment, Full Time: *13* • Total Basic Student Enrollment,
Part Time: *0* • Female Basic Student Enrollment: *13* • Male
Basic Student Enrollment: *0* • Total RN Enrollment: *0* •
Total New Fall Enrollments: *13* • Total Graduates: *0* • Basic
Student Graduates: *0* • RN Student Graduates: *0*

FINANCES

Residential Annual Tuition: *$3,770* • Non-Residential
Annual Tuition: *$3,770* • General Institutional Fees:
$4,885 • Additional Nursing Fees: *$310*

MOREHEAD STATE UNIVERSITY

Address: 150 University Blvd., Morehead, KY 40351
Phone: 606-783-5173
Fax: 606-783-9104
Contact: Janet J. Gross, DSN, RN, Coordinator, Baccalaureate Nursing Program
Email: j.gross@morehead-st.edu

GENERAL INFORMATION

Type of School: *4-Year College or University, Public* •
Accreditation: *Southern Association of Colleges and Schools* •
Total Enrollment: *8500*

PROGRAM INFORMATION

Two Year Exit Option: *No* • NLNAC Accreditation: *Yes* •
CCNE Accreditation: *Yes*

NURSING STUDENT PROFILE

Total Nursing Enrollment: *79* • Total Basic Student Enrollment, Full Time: *72* • Total Basic Student Enrollment, Part Time: *0* • Female Basic Student Enrollment: *61* • Male Basic Student Enrollment: *11* • Total RN Enrollment: *7* • Total New Fall Enrollments: *27* • Total Graduates: *29* • Basic Student Graduates: *22* • RN Student Graduates: *7*

FINANCES

Residential Annual Tuition: *$1,463* • Non-Residential Annual Tuition: *$3,602* • General Institutional Fees: *$250* • Additional Nursing Fees: *$175*

MURRAY STATE UNIVERSITY

Address: 102 Mason Hall, Murray, KY 42071
Phone: 270-762-2193
Fax: 270-762-6662
Contact: Marcia B. Hobbs, DSN, RN, Chair
Email: marcia.hobbs@murraystate.edu

GENERAL INFORMATION

Type of School: *4-Year College or University, Public* •
Accreditation: *Southern Association of Colleges and Schools* •
Total Enrollment: *8440*

PROGRAM INFORMATION

Two Year Exit Option: *Not Reported* • NLNAC Accreditation: *Yes* • CCNE Accreditation:

NURSING STUDENT PROFILE

Total Nursing Enrollment: *170* • Total Basic Student Enrollment, Full Time: *100* • Total Basic Student Enrollment, Part Time: *22* • Female Basic Student Enrollment: *118* • Male Basic Student Enrollment: *4* • Total RN Enrollment: *48* • Total New Fall Enrollments: *15* • Total Graduates: *79* • Basic Student Graduates: *54* • RN Student Graduates: *25*

FINANCES

Residential Annual Tuition: *$2,556* • Non-Residential Annual Tuition: *$6,990* • General Institutional Fees: *$1,278* • Additional Nursing Fees: *$111*

NORTHERN KENTUCKY UNIVERSITY

Address: Nunn Drive, AHG 303, Highland Heights, KY
            41076
Phone: 859-572-5243
Fax: 859-572-6098
Contact: Ann M. Dollins, PhD, MPH, CNM, Director
            BSN Program
Email: dollinsa@nku.edu

GENERAL INFORMATION

Type of School: *4-Year College or University, Public* •
Accreditation: *Southern Association of Colleges and Schools* •
Total Enrollment: *12000*

PROGRAM INFORMATION

NLNAC Accreditation: *Yes* • CCNE Accreditation:

NURSING STUDENT PROFILE

Total Nursing Enrollment: *63* • Full-Time Enrollment: *40* •
Part-Time Enrollment: *23* • Female Enrollment: *59* • Male
Enrollment: *4* • Total Graduates: *40*

FINANCES

Residential Annual Tuition: *$2,256* • Non-Residential
Annual Tuition: *$6,504* • General Institutional Fees: *$15* •
Additional Nursing Fees: *$35*

SPALDING UNIVERSITY

Address: 851 South Fourth Street, Louisville, KY 40203
Phone: 502-585-7125
Fax: 502-588-7175
Contact: Patricia Spurr, EdD, RN, Director
Email: pspurr@spalding.edu

GENERAL INFORMATION

Type of School: *4-Year College or University, Private
(Religious)* • Accreditation: *Southern Association of Colleges
and Schools* • Total Enrollment: *1700*

PROGRAM INFORMATION

Two Year Exit Option: *Not Reported* • NLNAC
Accreditation: *Yes* • CCNE Accreditation:

NURSING STUDENT PROFILE

Total Nursing Enrollment: *111* • Total Basic Student
Enrollment, Full Time: *101* • Total Basic Student
Enrollment, Part Time: *0* • Female Basic Student
Enrollment: *100* • Male Basic Student Enrollment: *1* • Total
RN Enrollment: *10* • Total New Fall Enrollments: *27* • Total
Graduates: *43* • Basic Student Graduates: *40* • RN Student
Graduates: *3*

FINANCES

Residential Annual Tuition: *$11,400* • Non-Residential
Annual Tuition: *Not Reported* • General Institutional Fees:
$5,700 • Additional Nursing Fees: *$325*

THOMAS MORE COLLEGE

Address: 333 Thomas More Parkway, Ft. Mitchell, KY
41017
Phone: 859-344-3410
Fax: 859-344-3537
Contact: Margaret N. Owens, MSN, RN, Interim
Chairperson
Email: *Not Reported*

GENERAL INFORMATION

Type of School: *4-Year College or University, Private
(Independent)* • Accreditation: *Southern Association of Colleges
and Schools* • Total Enrollment: *1274*

PROGRAM INFORMATION

Two Year Exit Option: *Not Reported* • NLNAC
Accreditation: *Yes* • CCNE Accreditation:

NURSING STUDENT PROFILE

Total Nursing Enrollment: *47* • Total Basic Student
Enrollment, Full Time: *43* • Total Basic Student Enrollment,
Part Time: *4* • Female Basic Student Enrollment: *45* • Male
Basic Student Enrollment: *2* • Total RN Enrollment: *0* •
Total New Fall Enrollments: *11* • Total Graduates: *7* • Basic
Student Graduates: *7* • RN Student Graduates: *0*

FINANCES

Residential Annual Tuition: *$7,775* • Non-Residential
Annual Tuition: *$7,775* • General Institutional Fees: *Not
Reported* • Additional Nursing Fees: *$352*

UNIVERSITY OF KENTUCKY

Address: 760 Rose Street, Rm 315, Lexington, KY 40536
Phone: 859-323-5108
Fax: *Not Reported*
Contact: Dorothy Y. Brockopp, PhD, RN, Assistant Dean
for Undergraduate Studies
Email: dybroc00@pop.uky.edu

GENERAL INFORMATION

Type of School: *4-Year College or University, Public* •
Accreditation: *Southern Association of Colleges and Schools* •
Total Enrollment: *30900*

PROGRAM INFORMATION

Two Year Exit Option: *No* • NLNAC Accreditation: *Yes* •
CCNE Accreditation:

NURSING STUDENT PROFILE

Total Nursing Enrollment: *287* • Total Basic Student
Enrollment, Full Time: *212* • Total Basic Student
Enrollment, Part Time: *23* • Female Basic Student
Enrollment: *220* • Male Basic Student Enrollment: *15* • Total
RN Enrollment: *52* • Total New Fall Enrollments: *91* • Total
Graduates: *108* • Basic Student Graduates: *73* • RN Student
Graduates: *35*

FINANCES

Residential Annual Tuition: *Not Reported* • Non-Residential
Annual Tuition: *Not Reported* • General Institutional Fees:
Not Reported • Additional Nursing Fees: *Not Reported*

UNIVERSITY OF LOUISVILLE

Address: 555 S. Floyd Street, Louisville, KY 40292
Phone: 502-852-8387
Fax: 502-852-8783
Contact: Cynthia McCurren, PhD, RN, Acting Associate
           Dean for Academic Affairs
Email: camccu01@louisville.edu

GENERAL INFORMATION

Type of School: *4-Year College or University, Public* •
Accreditation: *Southern Association of Colleges and Schools* •
Total Enrollment: *20768*

PROGRAM INFORMATION

Two Year Exit Option: *Not Reported* • NLNAC
Accreditation: *Yes* • CCNE Accreditation:

NURSING STUDENT PROFILE

Total Nursing Enrollment: *178* • Total Basic Student
Enrollment, Full Time: *134* • Total Basic Student
Enrollment, Part Time: *8* • Female Basic Student
Enrollment: *122* • Male Basic Student Enrollment: *20* • Total
RN Enrollment: *36* • Total New Fall Enrollments: *33* • Total
Graduates: *116* • Basic Student Graduates: *92* • RN Student
Graduates: *24*

FINANCES

Residential Annual Tuition: *$3,447* • Non-Residential
Annual Tuition: *$9,746* • General Institutional Fees:
$1,723 • Additional Nursing Fees: *$141.50*

WESTERN KENTUCKY UNIVERSITY

Address: 1 Big Red Way, Bowling Green, KY 42101
Phone: 270-745-3579
Fax: 270-745-3392
Contact: Donna Blackburn, PhD, RN, Department Head
Email: donna.blackburn@wku.edu

GENERAL INFORMATION

Type of School: *4-Year College or University, Public* •
Accreditation: *Southern Association of Colleges and Schools* •
Total Enrollment: *15516*

PROGRAM INFORMATION

NLNAC Accreditation: *Yes* • CCNE Accreditation:

NURSING STUDENT PROFILE

Total Nursing Enrollment: *57* • Full-Time Enrollment: *3* •
Part-Time Enrollment: *54* • Female Enrollment: *51* • Male
Enrollment: *6* • Total Graduates: *0*

FINANCES

Residential Annual Tuition: *$5,068* • Non-Residential
Annual Tuition: *$6,834* • General Institutional Fees: *$192* •
Additional Nursing Fees: *$50*

DILLARD UNIVERSITY

Address: 2601 Gentilly Boulevard, New Orleans, LA 70122
Phone: 504-816-4717
Fax: 504-816-4861
Contact: Edwina D. Frank, PhD, EdD, RN, Dean
Email: efrank@dillard.edu

GENERAL INFORMATION

Type of School: *4-Year College or University, Private (Independent)* • Accreditation: *Southern Association of Colleges and Schools* • Total Enrollment: *1953*

PROGRAM INFORMATION

Two Year Exit Option: *Not Reported* • NLNAC Accreditation: *Yes* • CCNE Accreditation:

NURSING STUDENT PROFILE

Total Nursing Enrollment: *75* • Total Basic Student Enrollment, Full Time: *75* • Total Basic Student Enrollment, Part Time: *0* • Female Basic Student Enrollment: *71* • Male Basic Student Enrollment: *4* • Total RN Enrollment: *0* • Total New Fall Enrollments: *14* • Total Graduates: *28* • Basic Student Graduates: *28* • RN Student Graduates: *0*

FINANCES

Residential Annual Tuition: *$9,200* • Non-Residential Annual Tuition: *Not Reported* • General Institutional Fees: *$4,600* • Additional Nursing Fees: *$171*

GRAMBLING STATE UNIVERSITY

Address: 1 Cole Street, Grambling, LA 71245
Phone: 318-274-2672
Fax: 318-274-3491
Contact: Anna Karin Jones, PhD, RN, Director of BSN Program
Email: jonesak@alpha0.gram.edu

GENERAL INFORMATION

Type of School: *4-Year College or University, Public* • Accreditation: *Southern Association of Colleges and Schools* • Total Enrollment: *4716*

PROGRAM INFORMATION

Two Year Exit Option: *Not Reported* • NLNAC Accreditation: *Yes* • CCNE Accreditation:

NURSING STUDENT PROFILE

Total Nursing Enrollment: *315* • Total Basic Student Enrollment, Full Time: *285* • Total Basic Student Enrollment, Part Time: *30* • Female Basic Student Enrollment: *287* • Male Basic Student Enrollment: *28* • Total RN Enrollment: *0* • Total New Fall Enrollments: *19* • Total Graduates: *61* • Basic Student Graduates: *61* • RN Student Graduates: *0*

FINANCES

Residential Annual Tuition: *Not Reported* • Non-Residential Annual Tuition: *Not Reported* • General Institutional Fees: *$1,151* • Additional Nursing Fees: *Not Reported*

LOUISIANA STATE UNIVERSITY

Address: 433 Bolivar Street, New Orleans, LA 70112
Phone: 504-568-4106
Fax: 504-599-0573
Contact: Elizabeth A. Humphrey, EdD, RN, Dean and Professor
Email: ehumph@lsuhsc.edu

GENERAL INFORMATION

Type of School: *Other, Public* • Accreditation: *Southern Association of Colleges and Schools* • Total Enrollment: *2755*

PROGRAM INFORMATION

Two Year Exit Option: *No* • NLNAC Accreditation: *Not Reported* • CCNE Accreditation: *Yes*

NURSING STUDENT PROFILE

Total Nursing Enrollment: *434* • Total Basic Student Enrollment, Full Time: *405* • Total Basic Student Enrollment, Part Time: *14* • Female Basic Student Enrollment: *371* • Male Basic Student Enrollment: *48* • Total RN Enrollment: *15* • Total New Fall Enrollments: *80* • Total Graduates: *114* • Basic Student Graduates: *114* • RN Student Graduates: *0*

FINANCES

Residential Annual Tuition: *$2,196* • Non-Residential Annual Tuition: *$3,896* • General Institutional Fees: *$166* • Additional Nursing Fees: *$0*

MCNEESE STATE UNIVERSITY

Address: P.O.Box 90415, Lake Charles, LA 70609
Phone: 337-475-5987
Fax: 337-475-5924
Contact: Elaine Vallette, PhD, RN, Coordinator, BSN Program
Email: evallete@mail.mcneese.edu

GENERAL INFORMATION

Type of School: *4-Year College or University, Public* • Accreditation: *Southern Association of Colleges and Schools* • Total Enrollment: *7780*

PROGRAM INFORMATION

Two Year Exit Option: *No* • NLNAC Accreditation: *Yes* • CCNE Accreditation:

NURSING STUDENT PROFILE

Total Nursing Enrollment: *301* • Total Basic Student Enrollment, Full Time: *130* • Total Basic Student Enrollment, Part Time: *0* • Female Basic Student Enrollment: *130* • Male Basic Student Enrollment: *0* • Total RN Enrollment: *171* • Total New Fall Enrollments: *19* • Total Graduates: *46* • Basic Student Graduates: *45* • RN Student Graduates: *1*

FINANCES

Residential Annual Tuition: *$1,213* • Non-Residential Annual Tuition: *$3,170* • General Institutional Fees: *$598* • Additional Nursing Fees: *$100*

NICHOLLS STATE UNIVERSITY

Address: P.O. Box 2143, Thibodaux, LA 70310
Phone: 985-448-4694
Fax: 985-448-4932
Contact: Thomas J. Smith, PhD, RN,C, APRN, BSN
           Program Director
Email: nurs-tjs@nicholls.edu

GENERAL INFORMATION

Type of School: *4-Year College or University, Public* •
Accreditation: *Southern Association of Colleges and Schools* •
Total Enrollment: *7400*

PROGRAM INFORMATION

Two Year Exit Option: *Not Reported* • NLNAC
Accreditation: *Yes* • CCNE Accreditation:

NURSING STUDENT PROFILE

Total Nursing Enrollment: *163* • Total Basic Student
Enrollment, Full Time: *157* • Total Basic Student
Enrollment, Part Time: *0* • Female Basic Student
Enrollment: *127* • Male Basic Student Enrollment: *30* • Total
RN Enrollment: *6* • Total New Fall Enrollments: *39* • Total
Graduates: *51* • Basic Student Graduates: *41* • RN Student
Graduates: *10*

FINANCES

Residential Annual Tuition: *Not Reported* • Non-Residential
Annual Tuition: *Not Reported* • General Institutional Fees:
$1,058 • Additional Nursing Fees: *Not Reported*

NORTHWESTERN STATE UNIVERSITY OF LOUISIANA

Address: 1800 Line Avenue, Natchitoches, LA 71497
Phone: 318-677-3100
Fax: 318-677-3127
Contact: Diane Graham Webb, MSN, RN, Director of
           Non-Traditional Studies in Nursing
Email: grahamd@nsula.edu

GENERAL INFORMATION

Type of School: *4-Year College or University, Public* •
Accreditation: *Southern Association of Colleges and Schools* •
Total Enrollment: *9415*

PROGRAM INFORMATION

Two Year Exit Option: *Not Reported* • NLNAC
Accreditation: *Yes* • CCNE Accreditation:

NURSING STUDENT PROFILE

Total Nursing Enrollment: *948* • Total Basic Student
Enrollment, Full Time: *627* • Total Basic Student
Enrollment, Part Time: *207* • Female Basic Student
Enrollment: *716* • Male Basic Student Enrollment: *118* •
Total RN Enrollment: *114* • Total New Fall Enrollments:
69 • Total Graduates: *146* • Basic Student Graduates: *89* •
RN Student Graduates: *57*

FINANCES

Residential Annual Tuition: *$2,250* • Non-Residential
Annual Tuition: *$7,050* • General Institutional Fees: *$128* •
Additional Nursing Fees: *$250*

OUR LADY OF HOLY CROSS COLLEGE

Address: 4123 Woodland Drive, New Orleans, LA 70131
Phone: 504-398-2215
Fax: 504-391-5351
Contact: Margaret T. Shannon, PhD, RN, Dean, Division of Nursing
Email: mshannon@olhcc.edu

GENERAL INFORMATION

Type of School: *4-Year College or University, Private (Independent)* • Accreditation: *Southern Association of Colleges and Schools* • Total Enrollment: *1300*

PROGRAM INFORMATION

Two Year Exit Option: *No* • NLNAC Accreditation: *Yes* • CCNE Accreditation:

NURSING STUDENT PROFILE

Total Nursing Enrollment: *139* • Total Basic Student Enrollment, Full Time: *115* • Total Basic Student Enrollment, Part Time: *24* • Female Basic Student Enrollment: *133* • Male Basic Student Enrollment: *6* • Total RN Enrollment: *0* • Total New Fall Enrollments: *50* • Total Graduates: *37* • Basic Student Graduates: *37* • RN Student Graduates: *0*

FINANCES

Residential Annual Tuition: *$5,800* • Non-Residential Annual Tuition: *Not Reported* • General Institutional Fees: *$500* • Additional Nursing Fees: *$35*

SOUTHEASTERN LOUISIANA UNIVERSITY

Address: SLU 10781, Hammond, LA 70402
Phone: 504-549-3772
Fax: 504-549-5178
Contact: Donnie Booth, PhD, RN, Dean, College of Nursing and Health Sciences
Email: dbooth@selu.edu

GENERAL INFORMATION

Type of School: *4-Year College or University, Public* • Accreditation: *Southern Association of Colleges and Schools* • Total Enrollment: *14500*

PROGRAM INFORMATION

Two Year Exit Option: *Not Reported* • NLNAC Accreditation: *Yes* • CCNE Accreditation:

NURSING STUDENT PROFILE

Total Nursing Enrollment: *1179* • Total Basic Student Enrollment, Full Time: *863* • Total Basic Student Enrollment, Part Time: *300* • Female Basic Student Enrollment: *1052* • Male Basic Student Enrollment: *111* • Total RN Enrollment: *16* • Total New Fall Enrollments: *72* • Total Graduates: *108* • Basic Student Graduates: *108* • RN Student Graduates: *0*

FINANCES

Residential Annual Tuition: *$2,284* • Non-Residential Annual Tuition: *$5,328* • General Institutional Fees: *$1,142* • Additional Nursing Fees: *Not Reported*

SOUTHERN UNIVERSITY AND A&M COLLEGE

Address: PO Box 11784, Baton Rouge, LA 70813
Phone: 225-771-2653
Fax: 225-771-2651
Contact: Mary Abadie, MN, RN, Interim BSN
            Chairperson
Email: maryabadie@suson.subr.edu

GENERAL INFORMATION

Type of School: *4-Year College or University, Public* •
Accreditation: *Southern Association of Colleges and Schools* •
Total Enrollment: *9449*

PROGRAM INFORMATION

Two Year Exit Option: *No* • NLNAC Accreditation: *Yes* •
CCNE Accreditation:

NURSING STUDENT PROFILE

Total Nursing Enrollment: *881* • Total Basic Student
Enrollment, Full Time: *754* • Total Basic Student
Enrollment, Part Time: *127* • Female Basic Student
Enrollment: *783* • Male Basic Student Enrollment: *98* • Total
RN Enrollment: *0* • Total New Fall Enrollments: *358* • Total
Graduates: *74* • Basic Student Graduates: *74* • RN Student
Graduates: *0*

FINANCES

Residential Annual Tuition: *Not Reported* • Non-Residential
Annual Tuition: *Not Reported* • General Institutional Fees:
Not Reported • Additional Nursing Fees: *Not Reported*

UNIVERSITY OF LOUISIANA—LAFAYETTE

Address: PO Box 43810, Lafayette, LA 70504
Phone: 337-482-5609
Fax: 337-482-5649
Contact: Melinda G. Oberleitner, DNS, RN, Acting
            Department Head
Email: mag0712@louisiana.edu

GENERAL INFORMATION

Type of School: *4-Year College or University, Public* •
Accreditation: *Southern Association of Colleges and Schools* •
Total Enrollment: *15740*

PROGRAM INFORMATION

Two Year Exit Option: *Not Reported* • NLNAC
Accreditation: *Yes* • CCNE Accreditation:

NURSING STUDENT PROFILE

Total Nursing Enrollment: *1067* • Total Basic Student
Enrollment, Full Time: *936* • Total Basic Student
Enrollment, Part Time: *124* • Female Basic Student
Enrollment: *851* • Male Basic Student Enrollment: *209* •
Total RN Enrollment: *7* • Total New Fall Enrollments: *204* •
Total Graduates: *127* • Basic Student Graduates: *121* • RN
Student Graduates: *6*

FINANCES

Residential Annual Tuition: *$2,980* • Non-Residential
Annual Tuition: *$9,160* • General Institutional Fees: *$950* •
Additional Nursing Fees: *Not Reported*

HUSSON COLLEGE

Address: 1 College Circle, Bangor, ME 04401
Phone: 207-941-7056
Fax: 207-941-7883
Contact: Anne P. Ellis, EdD, RN, Chair
Email: aultd@husson.edu

GENERAL INFORMATION

Type of School: *4-Year College or University, Private (Independent)* • Accreditation: *Not Reported* • Total Enrollment: *1000*

PROGRAM INFORMATION

Two Year Exit Option: *Not Reported* • NLNAC Accreditation: *Yes* • CCNE Accreditation: *Yes*

NURSING STUDENT PROFILE

Total Nursing Enrollment: *171* • Total Basic Student Enrollment, Full Time: *126* • Total Basic Student Enrollment, Part Time: *28* • Female Basic Student Enrollment: *142* • Male Basic Student Enrollment: *12* • Total RN Enrollment: *17* • Total New Fall Enrollments: *37* • Total Graduates: *43* • Basic Student Graduates: *26* • RN Student Graduates: *17*

FINANCES

Residential Annual Tuition: *$10,140* • Non-Residential Annual Tuition: *$10,140* • General Institutional Fees: *$30* • Additional Nursing Fees: *$30*

UNIVERSITY OF MAINE

Address: Orono, ME 04469
Phone: 207-581-2599
Fax: 207-581-2585
Contact: Therese B. Shipps, DNSc, RN, Director
Email: tshipps@maine.edu

GENERAL INFORMATION

Type of School: *4-Year College or University, Public* • Accreditation: *New England Association of Schools and Colleges* • Total Enrollment: *10698*

PROGRAM INFORMATION

Two Year Exit Option: *No* • NLNAC Accreditation: *Yes* • CCNE Accreditation:

NURSING STUDENT PROFILE

Total Nursing Enrollment: *391* • Total Basic Student Enrollment, Full Time: *319* • Total Basic Student Enrollment, Part Time: *10* • Female Basic Student Enrollment: *301* • Male Basic Student Enrollment: *28* • Total RN Enrollment: *62* • Total New Fall Enrollments: *49* • Total Graduates: *78* • Basic Student Graduates: *57* • RN Student Graduates: *21*

FINANCES

Residential Annual Tuition: *$4,200* • Non-Residential Annual Tuition: *$11,970* • General Institutional Fees: *$860* • Additional Nursing Fees: *$55*

UNIVERSITY OF MAINE— FORT KENT

Address: 25 Pleasant Street, Fort Kent, ME 04743
Phone: 207-834-7584
Fax: *Not Reported*
Contact: Rachel E. Albert, MSN, RN, Director
Email: realbert@maine.edu

GENERAL INFORMATION

Type of School: *4-Year College or University, Public* •
Accreditation: *New England Association of Schools and Colleges* • Total Enrollment: *900*

PROGRAM INFORMATION

Two Year Exit Option: *Not Reported* • NLNAC
Accreditation: *Yes* • CCNE Accreditation:

NURSING STUDENT PROFILE

Total Nursing Enrollment: *169* • Total Basic Student Enrollment, Full Time: *51* • Total Basic Student Enrollment, Part Time: *3* • Female Basic Student Enrollment: *48* • Male Basic Student Enrollment: *6* • Total RN Enrollment: *115* • Total New Fall Enrollments: *14* • Total Graduates: *8* • Basic Student Graduates: *7* • RN Student Graduates: *1*

FINANCES

Residential Annual Tuition: *$3,120* • Non-Residential Annual Tuition: *$7,590* • General Institutional Fees: *$344* • Additional Nursing Fees: *$52*

UNIVERSITY OF NEW ENGLAND

Address: 716 Stevens Avenue, Portland, ME 04103
Phone: 207-797-7261
Fax: *Not Reported*
Contact: Jean Dyer, MSN, RN, Interim Chair
Email: jdyer@mailbox.une.edu

GENERAL INFORMATION

Type of School: *4-Year College or University, Private (Independent)* • Accreditation: *New England Association of Schools and Colleges* • Total Enrollment: *3887*

PROGRAM INFORMATION

Two Year Exit Option: *Not Reported* • NLNAC
Accreditation: *Yes* • CCNE Accreditation:

NURSING STUDENT PROFILE

Total Nursing Enrollment: *Not Reported* • Total Basic Student Enrollment, Full Time: *Not Reported* • Total Basic Student Enrollment, Part Time: *Not Reported* • Female Basic Student Enrollment: *Not Reported* • Male Basic Student Enrollment: *Not Reported* • Total RN Enrollment: *Not Reported* • Total New Fall Enrollments: *Not Reported* • Total Graduates: *Not Reported* • Basic Student Graduates: *Not Reported* • RN Student Graduates: *Not Reported*

FINANCES

Residential Annual Tuition: *Not Reported* • Non-Residential Annual Tuition: *Not Reported* • General Institutional Fees: *Not Reported* • Additional Nursing Fees: *Not Reported*

UNIVERSITY OF SOUTHERN MAINE

Address: 96 Falmouth Street, PO Box 9300, Portland, ME 04104-9300
Phone: 207-780-4404
Fax: 207-780-4997
Contact: Jane Marie Kirschling, DNS, RN, Dean and Professor of Nursing
Email: jane.kirschling@usm.maine.edu

GENERAL INFORMATION

Type of School: *4-Year College or University, Public* • Accreditation: *New England Association of Schools and Colleges* • Total Enrollment: *10966*

PROGRAM INFORMATION

Two Year Exit Option: *No* • NLNAC Accreditation: *Yes* • CCNE Accreditation:

NURSING STUDENT PROFILE

Total Nursing Enrollment: *347* • Total Basic Student Enrollment, Full Time: *196* • Total Basic Student Enrollment, Part Time: *70* • Female Basic Student Enrollment: *247* • Male Basic Student Enrollment: *19* • Total RN Enrollment: *81* • Total New Fall Enrollments: *58* • Total Graduates: *90* • Basic Student Graduates: *60* • RN Student Graduates: *30*

FINANCES

Residential Annual Tuition: *$3,084* • Non-Residential Annual Tuition: *$8,616* • General Institutional Fees: *$500* • Additional Nursing Fees: *$150*

COLUMBIA UNION COLLEGE

Address: 7600 Flower Plaza, Takoma Park, MD 20912
Phone: 301-891-4144
Fax: 301-891-4191
Contact: Gina S. Brown, PhD, RN, Chair
Email: gbrown@cuc.edu

GENERAL INFORMATION

Type of School: *4-Year College or University, Private (Religious)* • Accreditation: *Middle States Association of Colleges and Schools* • Total Enrollment: *Not Reported*

PROGRAM INFORMATION

Two Year Exit Option: *Not Reported* • NLNAC Accreditation: *Yes* • CCNE Accreditation:

NURSING STUDENT PROFILE

Total Nursing Enrollment: *97* • Total Basic Student Enrollment, Full Time: *67* • Total Basic Student Enrollment, Part Time: *20* • Female Basic Student Enrollment: *82* • Male Basic Student Enrollment: *5* • Total RN Enrollment: *10* • Total New Fall Enrollments: *0* • Total Graduates: *22* • Basic Student Graduates: *18* • RN Student Graduates: *4*

FINANCES

Residential Annual Tuition: *$12,810* • Non-Residential Annual Tuition: *$12,810* • General Institutional Fees: *$350* • Additional Nursing Fees: *$400*

COPPIN STATE COLLEGE

Address: 2500 West North Avenue, Baltimore, MD
             21216-3698
Phone: 410-383-5546
Fax: 410-462-3032
Contact: Marcella A. Capes, PhD, RN, Dean and
             Professor
Email: mcopes@wye.coppin.edu

GENERAL INFORMATION

Type of School: *Not Reported* • Accreditation: *Not Reported* •
Total Enrollment: *Not Reported*

PROGRAM INFORMATION

Two Year Exit Option: *No* • NLNAC Accreditation: *Yes* •
CCNE Accreditation:

NURSING STUDENT PROFILE

Total Nursing Enrollment: *195* • Total Basic Student
Enrollment, Full Time: *104* • Total Basic Student
Enrollment, Part Time: *86* • Female Basic Student
Enrollment: *182* • Male Basic Student Enrollment: *8* • Total
RN Enrollment: *5* • Total New Fall Enrollments: *61* • Total
Graduates: *45* • Basic Student Graduates: *40* • RN Student
Graduates: *5*

FINANCES

Residential Annual Tuition: *$3,370* • Non-Residential
Annual Tuition: *$8,347* • General Institutional Fees: *$87* •
Additional Nursing Fees: *$185*

JOHNS HOPKINS UNIVERSITY

Address: 525 N. Wolfe St., Room 501, Baltimore, MD
             21205
Phone: 410-614-4081
Fax: 410-955-7463
Contact: Stella Shiber, PhD, RN, Associate Dean for
             Professional Education Programs
Email: sshiber@son.jhmi.edu

GENERAL INFORMATION

Type of School: *Independent, Private (Independent)* •
Accreditation: *Middle States Association of Colleges and
Schools* • Total Enrollment: *Not Reported*

PROGRAM INFORMATION

Two Year Exit Option: *No* • NLNAC Accreditation: *Yes* •
CCNE Accreditation:

NURSING STUDENT PROFILE

Total Nursing Enrollment: *316* • Total Basic Student
Enrollment, Full Time: *299* • Total Basic Student
Enrollment, Part Time: *9* • Female Basic Student
Enrollment: *289* • Male Basic Student Enrollment: *19* • Total
RN Enrollment: *8* • Total New Fall Enrollments: *98* • Total
Graduates: *174* • Basic Student Graduates: *162* • RN
Student Graduates: *12*

FINANCES

Residential Annual Tuition: *$19,022* • Non-Residential
Annual Tuition: *$19,022* • General Institutional Fees: *$500* •
Additional Nursing Fees: *$0*

SALISBURY STATE UNIVERSITY

Address: 1101 Camden Ave, Salisbury, MD 21801
Phone: 410-543-6413
Fax: 410-548-3313
Contact: Elizabeth A. Seldomridge, PhD, RN, Chair
Email: laseldomridge@salisbury.edu

GENERAL INFORMATION

Type of School: *4-Year College or University, Public* •
Accreditation: *Middle States Association of Colleges and Schools* • Total Enrollment: *Not Reported*

PROGRAM INFORMATION

Two Year Exit Option: *No* • NLNAC Accreditation: *Yes* •
CCNE Accreditation:

NURSING STUDENT PROFILE

Total Nursing Enrollment: *132* • Total Basic Student
Enrollment, Full Time: *118* • Total Basic Student
Enrollment, Part Time: *8* • Female Basic Student
Enrollment: *Not Reported* • Male Basic Student Enrollment:
Not Reported • Total RN Enrollment: *6* • Total New Fall
Enrollments: *68* • Total Graduates: *52* • Basic Student
Graduates: *50* • RN Student Graduates: *2*

FINANCES

Residential Annual Tuition: *$5,538* • Non-Residential
Annual Tuition: *$8,266* • General Institutional Fees: *$50* •
Additional Nursing Fees: *$100*

TOWSON UNIVERSITY

Address: 8000 York Rd, Baltimore, MD 21252-0001
Phone: 410-704-4212
Fax: 410-704-4325
Contact: Cynthia E. Kielinen, EdD, RN, Academic Chair
Email: ckielinen@towson.edu

GENERAL INFORMATION

Type of School: *4-Year College or University, Public* •
Accreditation: *Middle States Association of Colleges and Schools* • Total Enrollment: *Not Reported*

PROGRAM INFORMATION

Two Year Exit Option: *Not Reported* • NLNAC
Accreditation: *Yes* • CCNE Accreditation:

NURSING STUDENT PROFILE

Total Nursing Enrollment: *131* • Total Basic Student
Enrollment, Full Time: *110* • Total Basic Student
Enrollment, Part Time: *11* • Female Basic Student
Enrollment: *109* • Male Basic Student Enrollment: *12* • Total
RN Enrollment: *10* • Total New Fall Enrollments: *42* • Total
Graduates: *64* • Basic Student Graduates: *62* • RN Student
Graduates: *2*

FINANCES

Residential Annual Tuition: *$4,720* • Non-Residential
Annual Tuition: *$11,150* • General Institutional Fees: *$690* •
Additional Nursing Fees: *Not Reported*

UNIVERSITY OF MARYLAND—BALTIMORE

Address: 655 W Lombard St, Baltimore, MD 21210
Phone: 410-706-6741
Fax: 410-706-4231
Contact: Barbara R. Heller, EdD, RN, FAAN, Dean & Professor
Email: heller@son.umaryland.edu

GENERAL INFORMATION

Type of School: *4-Year College or University, Public* • Accreditation: *Middle States Association of Colleges and Schools* • Total Enrollment: *Not Reported*

PROGRAM INFORMATION

Two Year Exit Option: *No* • NLNAC Accreditation: *Yes* • CCNE Accreditation:

NURSING STUDENT PROFILE

Total Nursing Enrollment: *665* • Total Basic Student Enrollment, Full Time: *418* • Total Basic Student Enrollment, Part Time: *65* • Female Basic Student Enrollment: *436* • Male Basic Student Enrollment: *47* • Total RN Enrollment: *182* • Total New Fall Enrollments: *179* • Total Graduates: *254* • Basic Student Graduates: *160* • RN Student Graduates: *94*

FINANCES

Residential Annual Tuition: *$4,767* • Non-Residential Annual Tuition: *$12,092* • General Institutional Fees: *$432* • Additional Nursing Fees: *$357*

VILLA JULIE COLLEGE

Address: 1525 Green Spring Valley Rd, Stevenson, MD 21153
Phone: 410-602-7312
Fax: *Not Reported*
Contact: Judith A. Feustle, ScD, RN, Chair, Nursing Division
Email: fac-feus@mail.vjc.edu

GENERAL INFORMATION

Type of School: *4-Year College or University, Private (Independent)* • Accreditation: *Middle States Association of Colleges and Schools* • Total Enrollment: *Not Reported*

PROGRAM INFORMATION

Two Year Exit Option: *No* • NLNAC Accreditation: *Yes* • CCNE Accreditation:

NURSING STUDENT PROFILE

Total Nursing Enrollment: *256* • Total Basic Student Enrollment, Full Time: *Not Reported* • Total Basic Student Enrollment, Part Time: *Not Reported* • Female Basic Student Enrollment: *Not Reported* • Male Basic Student Enrollment: *Not Reported* • Total RN Enrollment: *21* • Total New Fall Enrollments: *39* • Total Graduates: *78* • Basic Student Graduates: *78* • RN Student Graduates: *0*

FINANCES

Residential Annual Tuition: *Not Reported* • Non-Residential Annual Tuition: *Not Reported* • General Institutional Fees: *Not Reported* • Additional Nursing Fees: *Not Reported*

AMERICAN INTERNATIONAL COLLEGE

Address: 1000 State Street, Box 12L, Springfield, MA
           01109
Phone: 413-205-3519
Fax: 413-205-3957
Contact: Anne R. Glanovsky, PhD, RN, Director,
           Division of Nursing
Email: aglanov@acad.aic.edu

GENERAL INFORMATION

Type of School: *4-Year College or University, Private
(Independent)* • Accreditation: *New England Association of
Schools and Colleges* • Total Enrollment: *1041*

PROGRAM INFORMATION

Two Year Exit Option: *Not Reported* • NLNAC
Accreditation: *Yes* • CCNE Accreditation:

NURSING STUDENT PROFILE

Total Nursing Enrollment: *78* • Total Basic Student
Enrollment, Full Time: *67* • Total Basic Student Enrollment,
Part Time: *0* • Female Basic Student Enrollment: *64* • Male
Basic Student Enrollment: *3* • Total RN Enrollment: *11* •
Total New Fall Enrollments: *35* • Total Graduates: *18* • Basic
Student Graduates: *14* • RN Student Graduates: *4*

FINANCES

Residential Annual Tuition: *$13,600* • Non-Residential
Annual Tuition: *$13,600* • General Institutional Fees:
$6,800 • Additional Nursing Fees: *$330*

BOSTON COLLEGE

Address: 140 Commonwealth Ave., Chestnut Hill, MA
           02467-3812
Phone: 617-552-4274
Fax: 617-552-0931
Contact: Loretta Higgins, EdD, RN, Associate Dean for
           Undergraduate Program
Email: loretta.higgins@bc.edu

GENERAL INFORMATION

Type of School: *4-Year College or University, Private
(Religious)* • Accreditation: *New England Association of Schools
and Colleges* • Total Enrollment: *14000*

PROGRAM INFORMATION

Two Year Exit Option: *No* • NLNAC Accreditation: *Yes* •
CCNE Accreditation:

NURSING STUDENT PROFILE

Total Nursing Enrollment: *229* • Total Basic Student
Enrollment, Full Time: *229* • Total Basic Student
Enrollment, Part Time: *0* • Female Basic Student
Enrollment: *224* • Male Basic Student Enrollment: *5* • Total
RN Enrollment: *0* • Total New Fall Enrollments: *75* • Total
Graduates: *47* • Basic Student Graduates: *47* • RN Student
Graduates: *0*

FINANCES

Residential Annual Tuition: *$24,050* • Non-Residential
Annual Tuition: *$24,050* • General Institutional Fees: *$700* •
Additional Nursing Fees: *$200*

COLLEGE OF OUR LADY OF THE ELMS

Address: 291 Springfield St, Chicopee, MA 01013
Phone: 413-594-2761
Fax: 413-592-4871
Contact: Marjorie Childers, PhD, RN, CS, Interim
            Director of the Nursing Program
Email: childersm@elms.edu

GENERAL INFORMATION

Type of School: *4-Year College or University, Private
(Religious)* • Accreditation: *New England Association of Schools
and Colleges* • Total Enrollment: *Not Reported*

PROGRAM INFORMATION

Two Year Exit Option: *Not Reported* • NLNAC
Accreditation: *Not Reported* • CCNE Accreditation: *Yes*

NURSING STUDENT PROFILE

Total Nursing Enrollment: *83* • Total Basic Student
Enrollment, Full Time: *54* • Total Basic Student Enrollment,
Part Time: *17* • Female Basic Student Enrollment: *68* • Male
Basic Student Enrollment: *3* • Total RN Enrollment: *12* •
Total New Fall Enrollments: *15* • Total Graduates: *25* • Basic
Student Graduates: *16* • RN Student Graduates: *9*

FINANCES

Residential Annual Tuition: *Not Reported* • Non-Residential
Annual Tuition: *Not Reported* • General Institutional Fees:
Not Reported • Additional Nursing Fees: *$450*

CURRY COLLEGE

Address: 1071 Blue Hill Ave, Milton, MA 02186
Phone: 617-333-2281
Fax: 617-333-2335
Contact: Linda Caldwell, DNSc, APRN-BC, Chair
Email: lcaldwel@curry.edu

GENERAL INFORMATION

Type of School: *4-Year College or University, Private
(Independent)* • Accreditation: *New England Association of
Schools and Colleges* • Total Enrollment: *Not Reported*

PROGRAM INFORMATION

Two Year Exit Option: *No* • NLNAC Accreditation: *Not
Reported* • CCNE Accreditation: *Yes*

NURSING STUDENT PROFILE

Total Nursing Enrollment: *Not Reported* • Total Basic Student
Enrollment, Full Time: *Not Reported* • Total Basic Student
Enrollment, Part Time: *Not Reported* • Female Basic Student
Enrollment: *Not Reported* • Male Basic Student Enrollment:
Not Reported • Total RN Enrollment: *Not Reported* • Total
New Fall Enrollments: *57* • Total Graduates: *18* • Basic
Student Graduates: *18* • RN Student Graduates: *0*

FINANCES

Residential Annual Tuition: *$18,595* • Non-Residential
Annual Tuition: *$18,595* • General Institutional Fees: *$575* •
Additional Nursing Fees: *$500*

ENDICOTT COLLEGE

Address: 376 Hale, Beverly, MA 01915
Phone: 978-232-2327
Fax: 978-232-3100
Contact: Sherry Merrow, EdD, RN, Assoc. Dean for Health Sciences
Email: smerrow@endicott.edu

GENERAL INFORMATION

Type of School: *4-Year College or University, Private (Independent)* • Accreditation: *New England Association of Schools and Colleges* • Total Enrollment: *Not Reported*

PROGRAM INFORMATION

Two Year Exit Option: *Not Reported* • NLNAC Accreditation: *Yes* • CCNE Accreditation: *Yes*

NURSING STUDENT PROFILE

Total Nursing Enrollment: *39* • Total Basic Student Enrollment, Full Time: *35* • Total Basic Student Enrollment, Part Time: *1* • Female Basic Student Enrollment: *35* • Male Basic Student Enrollment: *1* • Total RN Enrollment: *3* • Total New Fall Enrollments: *12* • Total Graduates: *6* • Basic Student Graduates: *0* • RN Student Graduates: *6*

FINANCES

Residential Annual Tuition: *$14,550* • Non-Residential Annual Tuition: *$14,550* • General Institutional Fees: *Not Reported* • Additional Nursing Fees: *Not Reported*

FITCHBURG STATE COLLEGE

Address: 160 Pearl St, Fitchburg, MA 01420
Phone: 978-665-3221
Fax: *Not Reported*
Contact: Sophia B. Harrell, PhD, RN, Chairperson
Email: sharrell@fsc.edu

GENERAL INFORMATION

Type of School: *4-Year College or University, Public* • Accreditation: *New England Association of Schools and Colleges* • Total Enrollment: *Not Reported*

PROGRAM INFORMATION

Two Year Exit Option: *Not Reported* • NLNAC Accreditation: *Yes* • CCNE Accreditation:

NURSING STUDENT PROFILE

Total Nursing Enrollment: *292* • Total Basic Student Enrollment, Full Time: *262* • Total Basic Student Enrollment, Part Time: *8* • Female Basic Student Enrollment: *251* • Male Basic Student Enrollment: *19* • Total RN Enrollment: *22* • Total New Fall Enrollments: *54* • Total Graduates: *70* • Basic Student Graduates: *61* • RN Student Graduates: *9*

FINANCES

Residential Annual Tuition: *Not Reported* • Non-Residential Annual Tuition: *Not Reported* • General Institutional Fees: *Not Reported* • Additional Nursing Fees: *Not Reported*

NORTHEASTERN UNIVERSITY

Address: 120 Robinson Hall, Boston, MA 02115
Phone: 617-373-3649
Fax: 617-373-8675
Contact: Eileen Zungolo, EdD, RN, FAAN, Associate
            Professor & Director
Email: ezungolo@lynx.neu.edu

GENERAL INFORMATION

Type of School: *4-Year College or University, Private (Independent)* • Accreditation: *New England Association of Schools and Colleges* • Total Enrollment: *Not Reported*

PROGRAM INFORMATION

Two Year Exit Option: *Not Reported* • NLNAC Accreditation: *Yes* • CCNE Accreditation: *Yes*

NURSING STUDENT PROFILE

Total Nursing Enrollment: *421* • Total Basic Student Enrollment, Full Time: *421* • Total Basic Student Enrollment, Part Time: *0* • Female Basic Student Enrollment: *399* • Male Basic Student Enrollment: *22* • Total RN Enrollment: *0* • Total New Fall Enrollments: *77* • Total Graduates: *119* • Basic Student Graduates: *3* • RN Student Graduates: *116*

FINANCES

Residential Annual Tuition: *$19,395* • Non-Residential Annual Tuition: *Not Reported* • General Institutional Fees: *Not Reported* • Additional Nursing Fees: *Not Reported*

REGIS COLLEGE

Address: 235 Wellesley Street, Weston, MA 00103
Phone: 781-768-7000
Fax: *Not Reported*
Contact: Amy Anderson, EdD, RN, Chairperson
Email: *Not Reported*

GENERAL INFORMATION

Type of School: *Not Reported* • Accreditation: *Not Reported* • Total Enrollment: *Not Reported*

PROGRAM INFORMATION

Two Year Exit Option: *Not Reported* • NLNAC Accreditation: *Not Reported* • CCNE Accreditation:

NURSING STUDENT PROFILE

Total Nursing Enrollment: *Not Reported* • Total Basic Student Enrollment, Full Time: *Not Reported* • Total Basic Student Enrollment, Part Time: *Not Reported* • Female Basic Student Enrollment: *Not Reported* • Male Basic Student Enrollment: *Not Reported* • Total RN Enrollment: *Not Reported* • Total New Fall Enrollments: *Not Reported* • Total Graduates: *Not Reported* • Basic Student Graduates: *Not Reported* • RN Student Graduates: *Not Reported*

FINANCES

Residential Annual Tuition: *Not Reported* • Non-Residential Annual Tuition: *Not Reported* • General Institutional Fees: *Not Reported* • Additional Nursing Fees: *Not Reported*

SALEM STATE COLLEGE

Address: 352 Lafayette, Salem, MA 01970
Phone: 978-542-6649
Fax: 978-542-6818
Contact: Joanne H. Evans, EdD, RN, CCRN, Chairperson
Email: jhe129@mediaone.net

GENERAL INFORMATION

Type of School: *4-Year College or University, Public* • Accreditation: *New England Association of Schools and Colleges* • Total Enrollment: *Not Reported*

PROGRAM INFORMATION

Two Year Exit Option: *Not Reported* • NLNAC Accreditation: *Yes* • CCNE Accreditation:

NURSING STUDENT PROFILE

Total Nursing Enrollment: *480* • Total Basic Student Enrollment, Full Time: *389* • Total Basic Student Enrollment, Part Time: *0* • Female Basic Student Enrollment: *Not Reported* • Male Basic Student Enrollment: *Not Reported* • Total RN Enrollment: *91* • Total New Fall Enrollments: *76* • Total Graduates: *80* • Basic Student Graduates: *65* • RN Student Graduates: *15*

FINANCES

Residential Annual Tuition: *$870* • Non-Residential Annual Tuition: *$7,050* • General Institutional Fees: *$435* • Additional Nursing Fees: *$105*

SIMMONS COLLEGE

Address: 300 The Fenway, Boston, MA 02115
Phone: 617-521-2139
Fax: 617-521-3045
Contact: Judy A. Beal, DNSc, RN, Professor and Assoc. Dean
Email: judy.beal@simmoms.edu

GENERAL INFORMATION

Type of School: *4-Year College or University, Private (Independent)* • Accreditation: *New England Association of Schools and Colleges* • Total Enrollment: *Not Reported*

PROGRAM INFORMATION

Two Year Exit Option: *No* • NLNAC Accreditation: *Yes* • CCNE Accreditation:

NURSING STUDENT PROFILE

Total Nursing Enrollment: *128* • Total Basic Student Enrollment, Full Time: *128* • Total Basic Student Enrollment, Part Time: *0* • Female Basic Student Enrollment: *128* • Male Basic Student Enrollment: *0* • Total RN Enrollment: *0* • Total New Fall Enrollments: *28* • Total Graduates: *32* • Basic Student Graduates: *32* • RN Student Graduates: *0*

FINANCES

Residential Annual Tuition: *$20,260* • Non-Residential Annual Tuition: *$20,260* • General Institutional Fees: *$630* • Additional Nursing Fees: *$1,200*

UNIVERSITY OF MASSACHUSETTS—BOSTON

Address: 100 Morrissy Blvd, Boston, MA 02125-3393
Phone: 617-287-7511
Fax: 617-287-7527
Contact: Brenda S. Cherry, PhD, RN, Dean
Email: brenda.cherry@umb.edu

GENERAL INFORMATION

Type of School: *4-Year College or University, Public* •
Accreditation: *New England Association of Schools and Colleges* • Total Enrollment: *Not Reported*

PROGRAM INFORMATION

Two Year Exit Option: *No* • NLNAC Accreditation: *Yes* •
CCNE Accreditation:

NURSING STUDENT PROFILE

Total Nursing Enrollment: *546* • Total Basic Student
Enrollment, Full Time: *242* • Total Basic Student
Enrollment, Part Time: *192* • Female Basic Student
Enrollment: *388* • Male Basic Student Enrollment: *46* • Total
RN Enrollment: *112* • Total New Fall Enrollments: *107* •
Total Graduates: *141* • Basic Student Graduates: *74* • RN
Student Graduates: *67*

FINANCES

Residential Annual Tuition: *$1,714* • Non-Residential
Annual Tuition: *$9,758* • General Institutional Fees:
$3,218 • Additional Nursing Fees: *$140*

UNIVERSITY OF MASSACHUSETTS—DARTMOUTH

Address: 285 Old Westport Rd, North Dartmouth, MA
02757
Phone: 508-999-8586
Fax: 508-999-9127
Contact: Elisabeth A. Pennington, EdD, RN, Dean and
Professor
Email: epennington@umassd.edu

GENERAL INFORMATION

Type of School: *Not Reported* • Accreditation: *Not Reported* •
Total Enrollment: *Not Reported*

PROGRAM INFORMATION

Two Year Exit Option: *Not Reported* • NLNAC
Accreditation: *Yes* • CCNE Accreditation:

NURSING STUDENT PROFILE

Total Nursing Enrollment: *297* • Total Basic Student
Enrollment, Full Time: *246* • Total Basic Student
Enrollment, Part Time: *30* • Female Basic Student
Enrollment: *257* • Male Basic Student Enrollment: *19* • Total
RN Enrollment: *21* • Total New Fall Enrollments: *65* • Total
Graduates: *78* • Basic Student Graduates: *61* • RN Student
Graduates: *17*

FINANCES

Residential Annual Tuition: *$1,417* • Non-Residential
Annual Tuition: *$7,995* • General Institutional Fees: *$709* •
Additional Nursing Fees: *Not Reported*

Circle 128 on reader card   See in-depth profile for more information

UNIVERSITY OF MASSACHUSETTS—LOWELL

Address: 3 Solomont Way, Suite 2, Lowell, MA 01854-5126
Phone: 978-934-4467
Fax: 978-934-3006
Contact: May Futrell, PhD, RN, FAAN, Professor and Chair, Dept. of Nursing
Email: may-futrell@uml.edu

GENERAL INFORMATION

Type of School: *4-Year College or University, Public* • Accreditation: *New England Association of Schools and Colleges* • Total Enrollment: *Not Reported*

PROGRAM INFORMATION

Two Year Exit Option: *Not Reported* • NLNAC Accreditation: *Yes* • CCNE Accreditation:

NURSING STUDENT PROFILE

Total Nursing Enrollment: *220* • Total Basic Student Enrollment, Full Time: *189* • Total Basic Student Enrollment, Part Time: *0* • Female Basic Student Enrollment: *177* • Male Basic Student Enrollment: *12* • Total RN Enrollment: *31* • Total New Fall Enrollments: *59* • Total Graduates: *71* • Basic Student Graduates: *57* • RN Student Graduates: *14*

FINANCES

Residential Annual Tuition: *$1,454* • Non-Residential Annual Tuition: *$7,870* • General Institutional Fees: *$727* • Additional Nursing Fees: *$126*

UNIVERSITY OF MASSACHUSSETTS—WORCESTER

Address: 55 Lake Ave North, Worcester, MA 01655
Phone: 413-545-2703
Fax: *Not Reported*
Contact: Eileen T. Breslin, PhD, RN, Dean of School Nursing
Email: breslin@nursing.umass.edu

GENERAL INFORMATION

Type of School: *Governmental Agency, Public* • Accreditation: *New England Association of Schools and Colleges* • Total Enrollment: *Not Reported*

PROGRAM INFORMATION

Two Year Exit Option: *Not Reported* • NLNAC Accreditation: *Yes* • CCNE Accreditation:

NURSING STUDENT PROFILE

Total Nursing Enrollment: *217* • Total Basic Student Enrollment, Full Time: *136* • Total Basic Student Enrollment, Part Time: *0* • Female Basic Student Enrollment: *136* • Male Basic Student Enrollment: *0* • Total RN Enrollment: *81* • Total New Fall Enrollments: *59* • Total Graduates: *173* • Basic Student Graduates: *81* • RN Student Graduates: *92*

FINANCES

Residential Annual Tuition: *$1,714* • Non-Residential Annual Tuition: *$9,756* • General Institutional Fees: *$857* • Additional Nursing Fees: *Not Reported*

WORCESTER STATE COLLEGE

Address: 486 Chandler St, Worcester, MA 01602
Phone: 508-929-8129
Fax: 508-929-8168
Contact: Helen M. Rogers, DNSc, RN, Chairperson
Email: hrogers@worcester.edu

GENERAL INFORMATION

Type of School: *4-Year College or University, Public* • Accreditation: *New England Association of Schools and Colleges* • Total Enrollment: *Not Reported*

PROGRAM INFORMATION

Two Year Exit Option: *No* • NLNAC Accreditation: *Yes* • CCNE Accreditation:

NURSING STUDENT PROFILE

Total Nursing Enrollment: *163* • Total Basic Student Enrollment, Full Time: *156* • Total Basic Student Enrollment, Part Time: *0* • Female Basic Student Enrollment: *150* • Male Basic Student Enrollment: *6* • Total RN Enrollment: *7* • Total New Fall Enrollments: *58* • Total Graduates: *49* • Basic Student Graduates: *32* • RN Student Graduates: *17*

FINANCES

Residential Annual Tuition: *$2,573* • Non-Residential Annual Tuition: *$7,050* • General Institutional Fees: *$1,603* • Additional Nursing Fees: *$0*

ANDREWS UNIVERSITY

Address: Marsh Hall Rm 200, Berrien Springs, MI 49104
Phone: 616-471-3366
Fax: *Not Reported*
Contact: Joseph Mucha, PhD, RN, Assoc. Dept. Chair
Email: *Not Reported*

GENERAL INFORMATION

Type of School: *4-Year College or University, Private (Religious)* • Accreditation: *North Central Association of Colleges and Schools* • Total Enrollment: *3000*

PROGRAM INFORMATION

Two Year Exit Option: *Not Reported* • NLNAC Accreditation: *Yes* • CCNE Accreditation:

NURSING STUDENT PROFILE

Total Nursing Enrollment: *142* • Total Basic Student Enrollment, Full Time: *142* • Total Basic Student Enrollment, Part Time: *0* • Female Basic Student Enrollment: *101* • Male Basic Student Enrollment: *41* • Total RN Enrollment: *0* • Total New Fall Enrollments: *Not Reported* • Total Graduates: *Not Reported* • Basic Student Graduates: *Not Reported* • RN Student Graduates: *Not Reported*

FINANCES

Residential Annual Tuition: *Not Reported* • Non-Residential Annual Tuition: *Not Reported* • General Institutional Fees: *$3,895* • Additional Nursing Fees: *$275*

EASTERN MICHIGAN UNIVERSITY

Address: 311 Marshall Blvd., Ypsilanti, MI 48197
Phone: 734-487-2310
Fax: *Not Reported*
Contact: Regina M. Williams, PhD, RN, FAAN, Dept. Head
Email: regina.williams@emich.edu

GENERAL INFORMATION

Type of School: *4-Year College or University, Public* • Accreditation: *North Central Association of Colleges and Schools* • Total Enrollment: *24000*

PROGRAM INFORMATION

Two Year Exit Option: *Not Reported* • NLNAC Accreditation: *Yes* • CCNE Accreditation:

NURSING STUDENT PROFILE

Total Nursing Enrollment: *331* • Total Basic Student Enrollment, Full Time: *60* • Total Basic Student Enrollment, Part Time: *132* • Female Basic Student Enrollment: *140* • Male Basic Student Enrollment: *52* • Total RN Enrollment: *139* • Total New Fall Enrollments: *228* • Total Graduates: *6* • Basic Student Graduates: *4* • RN Student Graduates: *2*

FINANCES

Residential Annual Tuition: *$3,147* • Non-Residential Annual Tuition: *Not Reported* • General Institutional Fees: *$1,573* • Additional Nursing Fees: *$102*

GRAND VALLEY STATE UNIVERSITY

Address: 1 Campus Drive, Allendale, MI 49401
Phone: 616-895-3558
Fax: 616-895-2510
Contact: Kay Setter Kline, PhD, RN, Director, Undergraduate Program
Email: klinek@gvsu.edu

GENERAL INFORMATION

Type of School: *4-Year College or University, Public* • Accreditation: *North Central Association of Colleges and Schools* • Total Enrollment: *19762*

PROGRAM INFORMATION

Two Year Exit Option: *No* • NLNAC Accreditation: *Yes* • CCNE Accreditation:

NURSING STUDENT PROFILE

Total Nursing Enrollment: *672* • Total Basic Student Enrollment, Full Time: *539* • Total Basic Student Enrollment, Part Time: *91* • Female Basic Student Enrollment: *589* • Male Basic Student Enrollment: *41* • Total RN Enrollment: *42* • Total New Fall Enrollments: *149* • Total Graduates: *130* • Basic Student Graduates: *114* • RN Student Graduates: *16*

FINANCES

Residential Annual Tuition: *$4,272* • Non-Residential Annual Tuition: *$9,224* • General Institutional Fees: *$0* • Additional Nursing Fees: *$0*

HOPE-CALVIN COLLEGES

Address: 105 E 14th Street, Holland, MI 49423
Phone: 112-336-5588
Fax: *Not Reported*
Contact: Cheryl Seenstraw, PhD, RN, Chairperson, Dept.
           Head
Email: *Not Reported*

GENERAL INFORMATION

Type of School: *Not Reported* • Accreditation: *Not Reported* •
Total Enrollment: *Not Reported*

PROGRAM INFORMATION

Two Year Exit Option: *Not Reported* • NLNAC
Accreditation: *Yes* • CCNE Accreditation:

NURSING STUDENT PROFILE

Total Nursing Enrollment: *Not Reported* • Total Basic Student
Enrollment, Full Time: *Not Reported* • Total Basic Student
Enrollment, Part Time: *Not Reported* • Female Basic Student
Enrollment: *Not Reported* • Male Basic Student Enrollment:
Not Reported • Total RN Enrollment: *Not Reported* • Total
New Fall Enrollments: *Not Reported* • Total Graduates: *Not
Reported* • Basic Student Graduates: *Not Reported* • RN
Student Graduates: *Not Reported*

FINANCES

Residential Annual Tuition: *Not Reported* • Non-Residential
Annual Tuition: *Not Reported* • General Institutional Fees:
Not Reported • Additional Nursing Fees: *Not Reported*

LAKE SUPERIOR STATE UNIVERSITY

Address: 650 West Easterday Avenue, Sault Sainte Marie,
           MI 49783
Phone: 906-635-2446
Fax: 906-635-2266
Contact: Lynn Conklin, DNSc, RN, Assoc. Dean
Email: lconklin@gw.lssu.edu

GENERAL INFORMATION

Type of School: *4-Year College or University, Public* •
Accreditation: *North Central Association of Colleges and
Schools* • Total Enrollment: *Not Reported*

PROGRAM INFORMATION

Two Year Exit Option: *Not Reported* • NLNAC
Accreditation: *Yes* • CCNE Accreditation:

NURSING STUDENT PROFILE

Total Nursing Enrollment: *142* • Total Basic Student
Enrollment, Full Time: *100* • Total Basic Student
Enrollment, Part Time: *0* • Female Basic Student
Enrollment: *93* • Male Basic Student Enrollment: *7* • Total
RN Enrollment: *42* • Total New Fall Enrollments: *33* • Total
Graduates: *29* • Basic Student Graduates: *15* • RN Student
Graduates: *14*

FINANCES

Residential Annual Tuition: *Not Reported* • Non-Residential
Annual Tuition: *Not Reported* • General Institutional Fees:
$3,726 • Additional Nursing Fees: *Not Reported*

MADONNA UNIVERSITY

Address: 36600 Schoolcraft Road, Livonia, MI 48150
Phone: 734-432-5460
Fax: 734-432-5463
Contact: Sandi Wahtera, PhD, RN, Chair, Undergraduate Nursing Program
Email: swahtera@madonna.edu

GENERAL INFORMATION

Type of School: *4-Year College or University, Private (Religious)* • Accreditation: *North Central Association of Colleges and Schools* • Total Enrollment: *3328*

PROGRAM INFORMATION

Two Year Exit Option: *No* • NLNAC Accreditation: *Not Reported* • CCNE Accreditation:

NURSING STUDENT PROFILE

Total Nursing Enrollment: *300* • Total Basic Student Enrollment, Full Time: *186* • Total Basic Student Enrollment, Part Time: *97* • Female Basic Student Enrollment: *272* • Male Basic Student Enrollment: *11* • Total RN Enrollment: *17* • Total New Fall Enrollments: *44* • Total Graduates: *77* • Basic Student Graduates: *75* • RN Student Graduates: *2*

FINANCES

Residential Annual Tuition: *$3,672* • Non-Residential Annual Tuition: *$3,672* • General Institutional Fees: *$100* • Additional Nursing Fees: *$198*

MICHIGAN STATE UNIVERSITY

Address: A219 Life Sciences, East Lansing, MI 48824-1317
Phone: 517-432-1539
Fax: 517-353-9553
Contact: Geraldine Talarczyk, EdD, RN, Assoc. Professor and Dean of Academic Affairs
Email: talarczy@msu.edu

GENERAL INFORMATION

Type of School: *4-Year College or University, Public* • Accreditation: *North Central Association of Colleges and Schools* • Total Enrollment: *43366*

PROGRAM INFORMATION

Two Year Exit Option: *Not Reported* • NLNAC Accreditation: *Yes* • CCNE Accreditation:

NURSING STUDENT PROFILE

Total Nursing Enrollment: *295* • Total Basic Student Enrollment, Full Time: *232* • Total Basic Student Enrollment, Part Time: *0* • Female Basic Student Enrollment: *207* • Male Basic Student Enrollment: *25* • Total RN Enrollment: *63* • Total New Fall Enrollments: *80* • Total Graduates: *85* • Basic Student Graduates: *70* • RN Student Graduates: *15*

FINANCES

Residential Annual Tuition: *$5,735* • Non-Residential Annual Tuition: *$13,317* • General Institutional Fees: *$2,867* • Additional Nursing Fees: *$170*

NORTHERN MICHIGAN UNIVERSITY

Address: 1401 Presque Isle Ave., New Science Building, Room 2301, Marquette, MI 49855
Phone: 906-227-2834
Fax: 906-227-1658
Contact: Kerri P. Schailing, MSN, RN, CNH, WHNP, Assoc. Director
Email: kschaili@nmu.edu

GENERAL INFORMATION

Type of School: *4-Year College or University, Public* • Accreditation: *North Central Association of Colleges and Schools* • Total Enrollment: *8200*

PROGRAM INFORMATION

Two Year Exit Option: *Not Reported* • NLNAC Accreditation: *Yes* • CCNE Accreditation:

NURSING STUDENT PROFILE

Total Nursing Enrollment: *182* • Total Basic Student Enrollment, Full Time: *101* • Total Basic Student Enrollment, Part Time: *69* • Female Basic Student Enrollment: *136* • Male Basic Student Enrollment: *34* • Total RN Enrollment: *12* • Total New Fall Enrollments: *32* • Total Graduates: *57* • Basic Student Graduates: *45* • RN Student Graduates: *12*

FINANCES

Residential Annual Tuition: *$2,772* • Non-Residential Annual Tuition: *$5,208* • General Institutional Fees: *$1,386* • Additional Nursing Fees: *$77*

OAKLAND UNIVERSITY

Address: 428 O'dowd Hall, Rochester, MI 48309-4401
Phone: 248-370-4081
Fax: 248-370-4279
Contact: Kathleen Emrich, EdD, RN, Interim Dean
Email: emrich@oakland.edu

GENERAL INFORMATION

Type of School: *4-Year College or University, Public* • Accreditation: *North Central Association of Colleges and Schools* • Total Enrollment: *15000*

PROGRAM INFORMATION

Two Year Exit Option: *Not Reported* • NLNAC Accreditation: *Yes* • CCNE Accreditation:

NURSING STUDENT PROFILE

Total Nursing Enrollment: *532* • Total Basic Student Enrollment, Full Time: *235* • Total Basic Student Enrollment, Part Time: *5* • Female Basic Student Enrollment: *216* • Male Basic Student Enrollment: *24* • Total RN Enrollment: *292* • Total New Fall Enrollments: *94* • Total Graduates: *98* • Basic Student Graduates: *66* • RN Student Graduates: *32*

FINANCES

Residential Annual Tuition: *$1,923* • Non-Residential Annual Tuition: *$4,587* • General Institutional Fees: *$243* • Additional Nursing Fees: *Not Reported*

SAGINAW VALLEY STATE UNIVERSITY

Address: 7400 Bay Road, University Center, MI 48603
Phone: 517-790-4145
Fax: *Not Reported*
Contact: Cheryl E. Easley, PhD, RN, Dean
Email: ceasley@svsu.edu

GENERAL INFORMATION

Type of School: *Other* • Accreditation: *Not Reported* • Total Enrollment: *Not Reported*

PROGRAM INFORMATION

Two Year Exit Option: *Not Reported* • NLNAC Accreditation: *Yes* • CCNE Accreditation:

NURSING STUDENT PROFILE

Total Nursing Enrollment: *132* • Total Basic Student Enrollment, Full Time: *72* • Total Basic Student Enrollment, Part Time: *38* • Female Basic Student Enrollment: *100* • Male Basic Student Enrollment: *10* • Total RN Enrollment: *22* • Total New Fall Enrollments: *17* • Total Graduates: *55* • Basic Student Graduates: *32* • RN Student Graduates: *23*

FINANCES

Residential Annual Tuition: *$5,674* • Non-Residential Annual Tuition: *$11,494* • General Institutional Fees: *$552* • Additional Nursing Fees: *Not Reported*

UNIVERSITY OF DETROIT MERCY

Address: 8200 West Outer Drive, PO Box 19900, Detroit, MI 48219
Phone: 313-933-6132
Fax: 313-933-6273
Contact: Suzanne Mellon, PhD, RN, Dean, College of Health Professions and McAuley School of Nursing
Email: mellonsk@udmercy.edu

GENERAL INFORMATION

Type of School: *4-Year College or University, Private (Independent)* • Accreditation: *North Central Association of Colleges and Schools* • Total Enrollment: *6900*

PROGRAM INFORMATION

Two Year Exit Option: *No* • NLNAC Accreditation: *Yes* • CCNE Accreditation:

NURSING STUDENT PROFILE

Total Nursing Enrollment: *553* • Total Basic Student Enrollment, Full Time: *123* • Total Basic Student Enrollment, Part Time: *56* • Female Basic Student Enrollment: *171* • Male Basic Student Enrollment: *8* • Total RN Enrollment: *374* • Total New Fall Enrollments: *15* • Total Graduates: *87* • Basic Student Graduates: *4* • RN Student Graduates: *70*

FINANCES

Residential Annual Tuition: *$1,509* • Non-Residential Annual Tuition: *$1,509* • General Institutional Fees: *$400* • Additional Nursing Fees: *$100*

UNIVERSITY OF MICHIGAN

Address: 400 N. Ingalls, Ann Arbor, MI 48109
Phone: 734-764-2385
Fax: 734-763-6668
Contact: Jan Lee, PhD, RN, Director, Associate Professor
Email: janlee@umich.edu

UNIVERSITY OF MICHIGAN—FLINT

Address: 516 French Hall, 303 East Kearsley Street, Flint, MI 48502-1950
Phone: 810-762-3420
Fax: 810-766-6851
Contact: Ellen Woodman, PhD, RN, Director
Email: eaw@flint.umich.edu

GENERAL INFORMATION

Type of School: *4-Year College or University, Public* •
Accreditation: *North Central Association of Colleges and Schools* • Total Enrollment: *38103*

GENERAL INFORMATION

Type of School: *4-Year College or University, Public* •
Accreditation: *North Central Association of Colleges and Schools* • Total Enrollment: *6320*

PROGRAM INFORMATION

Two Year Exit Option: *No* • NLNAC Accreditation: *Yes* •
CCNE Accreditation: *Yes*

PROGRAM INFORMATION

Two Year Exit Option: *Not Reported* • NLNAC Accreditation: *Yes* • CCNE Accreditation:

NURSING STUDENT PROFILE

Total Nursing Enrollment: *456* • Total Basic Student Enrollment, Full Time: *383* • Total Basic Student Enrollment, Part Time: *12* • Female Basic Student Enrollment: *359* • Male Basic Student Enrollment: *36* • Total RN Enrollment: *61* • Total New Fall Enrollments: *120* • Total Graduates: *109* • Basic Student Graduates: *86* • RN Student Graduates: *23*

NURSING STUDENT PROFILE

Total Nursing Enrollment: *182* • Total Basic Student Enrollment, Full Time: *161* • Total Basic Student Enrollment, Part Time: *0* • Female Basic Student Enrollment: *142* • Male Basic Student Enrollment: *19* • Total RN Enrollment: *21* • Total New Fall Enrollments: *32* • Total Graduates: *90* • Basic Student Graduates: *56* • RN Student Graduates: *34*

FINANCES

Residential Annual Tuition: *Not Reported* • Non-Residential Annual Tuition: *Not Reported* • General Institutional Fees: *Not Reported* • Additional Nursing Fees: *Not Reported*

FINANCES

Residential Annual Tuition: *Not Reported* • Non-Residential Annual Tuition: *Not Reported* • General Institutional Fees: *$2,249* • Additional Nursing Fees: *$489*

WAYNE STATE UNIVERSITY

Address: 5557 Cass Avenue, Detroit, MI 48202
Phone: 313-577-4138
Fax: 313-575-0414
Contact: Marjorie Isenberg, PhD, RN, Associate Dean for
Academic Affairs
Email: misenberg@atlas.nursing.wayne.edu

GENERAL INFORMATION

Type of School: *Not Reported* • Accreditation: *Not Reported* •
Total Enrollment: *Not Reported*

PROGRAM INFORMATION

Two Year Exit Option: *Not Reported* • NLNAC
Accreditation: *Yes* • CCNE Accreditation:

NURSING STUDENT PROFILE

Total Nursing Enrollment: *412* • Total Basic Student
Enrollment, Full Time: *246* • Total Basic Student
Enrollment, Part Time: *51* • Female Basic Student
Enrollment: *Not Reported* • Male Basic Student Enrollment:
Not Reported • Total RN Enrollment: *115* • Total New Fall
Enrollments: *Not Reported* • Total Graduates: *Not Reported* •
Basic Student Graduates: *Not Reported* • RN Student
Graduates: *Not Reported*

FINANCES

Residential Annual Tuition: *Not Reported* • Non-Residential
Annual Tuition: *Not Reported* • General Institutional Fees:
Not Reported • Additional Nursing Fees: *Not Reported*

WESTERN MICHIGAN UNIVERSITY

Address: 1903 West Michigan Avenue, Kalamazoo, MI
49008
Phone: 616-387-8162
Fax: 616-387-8170
Contact: Marie F. Gates, PhD, RN, Professor and Director
Email: marie.gates@wmich.edu

GENERAL INFORMATION

Type of School: *4-Year College or University, Public* •
Accreditation: *North Central Association of Colleges and
Schools* • Total Enrollment: *30000*

PROGRAM INFORMATION

Two Year Exit Option: *No* • NLNAC Accreditation: *Yes* •
CCNE Accreditation:

NURSING STUDENT PROFILE

Total Nursing Enrollment: *236* • Total Basic Student
Enrollment, Full Time: *155* • Total Basic Student
Enrollment, Part Time: *33* • Female Basic Student
Enrollment: *178* • Male Basic Student Enrollment: *10* • Total
RN Enrollment: *48* • Total New Fall Enrollments: *Not
Reported* • Total Graduates: *85* • Basic Student Graduates:
65 • RN Student Graduates: *20*

FINANCES

Residential Annual Tuition: *$5,262* • Non-Residential
Annual Tuition: *$13,276* • General Institutional Fees: *$578* •
Additional Nursing Fees: *$420*

Circle 150 on reader card   See in-depth profile for more information

COLLEGE OF SAINT CATHERINE

Address: 2004 Randolph Ave, St. Paul, MN 55105
Phone: 651-690-6586
Fax: 651-690-6941
Contact: Susan Ellen Campbell, PhD, RN, Director, Baccalaureate Program
Email: secampbell@st.kate.edu

GENERAL INFORMATION

Type of School: *4-Year College or University, Private (Religious)* • Accreditation: *North Central Association of Colleges and Schools* • Total Enrollment: *Not Reported*

PROGRAM INFORMATION

Two Year Exit Option: *No* • NLNAC Accreditation: *Yes* • CCNE Accreditation:

NURSING STUDENT PROFILE

Total Nursing Enrollment: *209* • Total Basic Student Enrollment, Full Time: *178* • Total Basic Student Enrollment, Part Time: *0* • Female Basic Student Enrollment: *178* • Male Basic Student Enrollment: *0* • Total RN Enrollment: *31* • Total New Fall Enrollments: *86* • Total Graduates: *93* • Basic Student Graduates: *63* • RN Student Graduates: *30*

FINANCES

Residential Annual Tuition: *$14,520* • Non-Residential Annual Tuition: *$19,520* • General Institutional Fees: *$125* • Additional Nursing Fees: *Not Reported*

COLLEGE OF SAINT SCHOLASTICA

Address: 1200 Kenwood Ave, Duluth, MN 55811
Phone: 218-723-6020
Fax: 218-723-6472
Contact: Ann Leja, MA, RN, Director, Undergraduate Program
Email: aleja@css.edu

GENERAL INFORMATION

Type of School: *Independent, Private (Independent)* • Accreditation: *North Central Association of Colleges and Schools* • Total Enrollment: *Not Reported*

PROGRAM INFORMATION

Two Year Exit Option: *No* • NLNAC Accreditation: *Yes* • CCNE Accreditation:

NURSING STUDENT PROFILE

Total Nursing Enrollment: *155* • Total Basic Student Enrollment, Full Time: *127* • Total Basic Student Enrollment, Part Time: *1* • Female Basic Student Enrollment: *118* • Male Basic Student Enrollment: *10* • Total RN Enrollment: *27* • Total New Fall Enrollments: *68* • Total Graduates: *66* • Basic Student Graduates: *55* • RN Student Graduates: *11*

FINANCES

Residential Annual Tuition: *$17,080* • Non-Residential Annual Tuition: *$17,080* • General Institutional Fees: *$0* • Additional Nursing Fees: *$300*

COLLEGE OF ST. BENEDICT

Address: 37 College Ave. South, St. Joseph, MN 55105
Phone: 320-363-5249
Fax: 320-363-6099
Contact: Kathleen Twohy, PhD, RN, Professor and Chair
Email: ktwohy@csbsju.edu

GENERAL INFORMATION

Type of School: *4-Year College or University, Private (Religious)* • Accreditation: *North Central Association of Colleges and Schools* • Total Enrollment: *Not Reported*

PROGRAM INFORMATION

Two Year Exit Option: *No* • NLNAC Accreditation: *Yes* • CCNE Accreditation: *Yes*

NURSING STUDENT PROFILE

Total Nursing Enrollment: *120* • Total Basic Student Enrollment, Full Time: *105* • Total Basic Student Enrollment, Part Time: *7* • Female Basic Student Enrollment: *103* • Male Basic Student Enrollment: *9* • Total RN Enrollment: *8* • Total New Fall Enrollments: *56* • Total Graduates: *63* • Basic Student Graduates: *62* • RN Student Graduates: *1*

FINANCES

Residential Annual Tuition: *$18,015* • Non-Residential Annual Tuition: *$18,015* • General Institutional Fees: *$300* • Additional Nursing Fees: *$185*

GUSTAVUS ADOLPHUS COLLEGE/SAINT OLAF COLLEGE INTERCOLLEGIATE NURSING CONSORTIUM

Address: 1520 St. Olaf Avenue, Northfield, MN 55057-1098
Phone: 507-646-3265
Fax: 507-646-3733
Contact: Rita S. Glazebrook, PhD, RN, CNP, Director
Email: glazebr@stolaf.edu

GENERAL INFORMATION

Type of School: *Not Reported* • Accreditation: *North Central Association of Colleges and Schools* • Total Enrollment: *Not Reported*

PROGRAM INFORMATION

Two Year Exit Option: *Not Reported* • NLNAC Accreditation: *Yes* • CCNE Accreditation: *Yes*

NURSING STUDENT PROFILE

Total Nursing Enrollment: *70* • Total Basic Student Enrollment, Full Time: *70* • Total Basic Student Enrollment, Part Time: *0* • Female Basic Student Enrollment: *65* • Male Basic Student Enrollment: *5* • Total RN Enrollment: *0* • Total New Fall Enrollments: *36* • Total Graduates: *34* • Basic Student Graduates: *34* • RN Student Graduates: *0*

FINANCES

Residential Annual Tuition: *$17,970* • Non-Residential Annual Tuition: *Not Reported* • General Institutional Fees: *Not Reported* • Additional Nursing Fees: *Not Reported*

MINNESOTA STATE UNIVERSITY—MANKATO

Address: 360 Wissink Hall, Mankato, MN 56001
Phone: 507-389-6828
Fax: 507-389-6516
Contact: Carol E. Larson, PhD, RN, Undergraduate Program Director
Email: carol.larson@mnsu.edu

GENERAL INFORMATION

Type of School: *4-Year College or University, Public* •
Accreditation: *North Central Association of Colleges and Schools* • Total Enrollment: *Not Reported*

PROGRAM INFORMATION

Two Year Exit Option: *Not Reported* • NLNAC Accreditation: *Yes* • CCNE Accreditation:

NURSING STUDENT PROFILE

Total Nursing Enrollment: *262* • Total Basic Student Enrollment, Full Time: *165* • Total Basic Student Enrollment, Part Time: *27* • Female Basic Student Enrollment: *174* • Male Basic Student Enrollment: *18* • Total RN Enrollment: *70* • Total New Fall Enrollments: *80* • Total Graduates: *92* • Basic Student Graduates: *70* • RN Student Graduates: *22*

FINANCES

Residential Annual Tuition: *$3,208* • Non-Residential Annual Tuition: *$6,232* • General Institutional Fees: *$1,604* • Additional Nursing Fees: *$126*

UNIVERSITY OF MINNESOTA—MINNEAPOLIS

Address: 5-140 WHD, 308 Harvard St SE, Minneapolis, MN 55455-0342
Phone: 612-624-5959
Fax: *Not Reported*
Contact: Sandra R. Edwardson, PhD, RN, Dean
Email: edwardso@mailbox.mail.umn.edu

GENERAL INFORMATION

Type of School: *4-Year College or University, Public* •
Accreditation: *North Central Association of Colleges and Schools* • Total Enrollment: *Not Reported*

PROGRAM INFORMATION

Two Year Exit Option: *Not Reported* • NLNAC Accreditation: *Yes* • CCNE Accreditation:

NURSING STUDENT PROFILE

Total Nursing Enrollment: *205* • Total Basic Student Enrollment, Full Time: *185* • Total Basic Student Enrollment, Part Time: *10* • Female Basic Student Enrollment: *168* • Male Basic Student Enrollment: *27* • Total RN Enrollment: *10* • Total New Fall Enrollments: *96* • Total Graduates: *99* • Basic Student Graduates: *93* • RN Student Graduates: *6*

FINANCES

Residential Annual Tuition: *$4,951* • Non-Residential Annual Tuition: *$11,882* • General Institutional Fees: *$2,085* • Additional Nursing Fees: *$155*

WINONA STATE UNIVERSITY

Address: P O Box 5838, Winona, MN 55987
Phone: 507-457-5127
Fax: 507-457-5550
Contact: Linda Seppanen, PhD, RN, Dept. Chairperson and Professor
Email: lseppanen@winona.edu

GENERAL INFORMATION

Type of School: *4-Year College or University, Public* •
Accreditation: *North Central Association of Colleges and Schools* • Total Enrollment: *6660*

PROGRAM INFORMATION

Two Year Exit Option: *No* • NLNAC Accreditation: *Yes* •
CCNE Accreditation:

NURSING STUDENT PROFILE

Total Nursing Enrollment: *280* • Total Basic Student Enrollment, Full Time: *196* • Total Basic Student Enrollment, Part Time: *11* • Female Basic Student Enrollment: *Not Reported* • Male Basic Student Enrollment: *Not Reported* • Total RN Enrollment: *73* • Total New Fall Enrollments: *110* • Total Graduates: *106* • Basic Student Graduates: *84* • RN Student Graduates: *22*

FINANCES

Residential Annual Tuition: *$2,820* • Non-Residential Annual Tuition: *$6,230* • General Institutional Fees: *$350* • Additional Nursing Fees: *$15*

ALCORN STATE UNIVERSITY

Address: 15 Campus Drive, Alcorn State, MS 39096
Phone: 601-304-4305
Fax: 601-304-4398
Contact: Joyce McManus, PhD, RN, Professor and Chairperson
Email: mcmanus@lorman.alcorn.edu

GENERAL INFORMATION

Type of School: *4-Year College or University, Public* •
Accreditation: *Southern Association of Colleges and Schools* •
Total Enrollment: *3109*

PROGRAM INFORMATION

Two Year Exit Option: *No* • NLNAC Accreditation: *Yes* •
CCNE Accreditation:

NURSING STUDENT PROFILE

Total Nursing Enrollment: *43* • Total Basic Student Enrollment, Full Time: *41* • Total Basic Student Enrollment, Part Time: *1* • Female Basic Student Enrollment: *36* • Male Basic Student Enrollment: *6* • Total RN Enrollment: *1* • Total New Fall Enrollments: *26* • Total Graduates: *17* • Basic Student Graduates: *12* • RN Student Graduates: *5*

FINANCES

Residential Annual Tuition: *$3,202* • Non-Residential Annual Tuition: *$7,375* • General Institutional Fees: *$200* • Additional Nursing Fees: *$30*

DELTA STATE UNIVERSITY

Address: P.O. Box 3343, Cleveland, MS 38733
Phone: 662-846-4255
Fax: 662-846-4267
Contact: Dana T. Lamar, EdD, RNC, Coordinator of
            Academic Programs
Email: dlamar@dsu.deltast.edu

GENERAL INFORMATION

Type of School: *4-Year College or University, Public* •
Accreditation: *Southern Association of Colleges and Schools* •
Total Enrollment: *3746*

PROGRAM INFORMATION

Two Year Exit Option: *No* • NLNAC Accreditation: *Yes* •
CCNE Accreditation: *Yes*

NURSING STUDENT PROFILE

Total Nursing Enrollment: *55* • Total Basic Student
Enrollment, Full Time: *46* • Total Basic Student Enrollment,
Part Time: *4* • Female Basic Student Enrollment: *43* • Male
Basic Student Enrollment: *7* • Total RN Enrollment: *5* •
Total New Fall Enrollments: *19* • Total Graduates: *30* • Basic
Student Graduates: *24* • RN Student Graduates: *6*

FINANCES

Residential Annual Tuition: *$3,100* • Non-Residential
Annual Tuition: *$7,374* • General Institutional Fees: *$0* •
Additional Nursing Fees: *$250*

MISSISSIPPI COLLEGE

Address: 200 South Capitol Street, Clinton, MS 39058
Phone: 601-925-3278
Fax: 601-925-3379
Contact: Mary Jean Padgett, PhD, RN, Dean, School of
            Nursing
Email: padgett@mc.edu

GENERAL INFORMATION

Type of School: *4-Year College or University, Private
(Independent)* • Accreditation: *Southern Association of Colleges
and Schools* • Total Enrollment: *3400*

PROGRAM INFORMATION

Two Year Exit Option: *No* • NLNAC Accreditation: *Yes* •
CCNE Accreditation:

NURSING STUDENT PROFILE

Total Nursing Enrollment: *180* • Total Basic Student
Enrollment, Full Time: *164* • Total Basic Student
Enrollment, Part Time: *11* • Female Basic Student
Enrollment: *154* • Male Basic Student Enrollment: *21* • Total
RN Enrollment: *5* • Total New Fall Enrollments: *38* • Total
Graduates: *47* • Basic Student Graduates: *43* • RN Student
Graduates: *4*

FINANCES

Residential Annual Tuition: *$9,600* • Non-Residential
Annual Tuition: *$9,600* • General Institutional Fees: *$392* •
Additional Nursing Fees: *$500*

MISSISSIPPI UNIVERSITY FOR WOMEN

Address: Taylor Hall, PO Box W910, Columbus, MS
           39701
Phone: 662-329-7301
Fax: *Not Reported*
Contact: Linda Cox, EdD, RN, CNAA, Director,
           Baccalaureate Program
Email: lcox@muw.edu

GENERAL INFORMATION

Type of School: *4-Year College or University, Public* •
Accreditation: *Southern Association of Colleges and Schools* •
Total Enrollment: *3000*

PROGRAM INFORMATION

Two Year Exit Option: *Not Reported* • NLNAC
Accreditation: *Yes* • CCNE Accreditation:

NURSING STUDENT PROFILE

Total Nursing Enrollment: *68* • Total Basic Student
Enrollment, Full Time: *Not Reported* • Total Basic Student
Enrollment, Part Time: *Not Reported* • Female Basic Student
Enrollment: *64* • Male Basic Student Enrollment: *4* • Total
RN Enrollment: *0* • Total New Fall Enrollments: *35* • Total
Graduates: *19* • Basic Student Graduates: *19* • RN Student
Graduates: *0*

FINANCES

Residential Annual Tuition: *$2,556* • Non-Residential
Annual Tuition: *$5,546* • General Institutional Fees:
$1,278 • Additional Nursing Fees: *$107*

UNIVERSITY OF MISSISSIPPI MEDICAL CENTER

Address: 2500 North State Street, Jackson, MS 39216
Phone: 601-984-6200
Fax: 601-815-5958
Contact: Anne Pierce, PhD, RN, Dean
Email: apierce@umsmed.edu

GENERAL INFORMATION

Type of School: *Technical/Specialized Institution, Public* •
Accreditation: *Southern Association of Colleges and Schools* •
Total Enrollment: *1694*

PROGRAM INFORMATION

Two Year Exit Option: *Not Reported* • NLNAC
Accreditation: *Yes* • CCNE Accreditation: *Yes*

NURSING STUDENT PROFILE

Total Nursing Enrollment: *210* • Total Basic Student
Enrollment, Full Time: *172* • Total Basic Student
Enrollment, Part Time: *5* • Female Basic Student
Enrollment: *160* • Male Basic Student Enrollment: *17* • Total
RN Enrollment: *33* • Total New Fall Enrollments: *81* • Total
Graduates: *131* • Basic Student Graduates: *89* • RN Student
Graduates: *42*

FINANCES

Residential Annual Tuition: *$2,378* • Non-Residential
Annual Tuition: *$5,197* • General Institutional Fees:
$1,189 • Additional Nursing Fees: *$99*

THE UNIVERSITY OF SOUTHERN MISSISSIPPI

Address: PO Box 5095, Hattiesburg, MS 39406
Phone: 601-266-5491
Fax: 601-266-5927
Contact: Norma G. Cuellar, DSN, RN, Asst. Dean of Undergraduate Program
Email: norma.cuellar@usm.edu

GENERAL INFORMATION

Type of School: *4-Year College or University, Public* •
Accreditation: *Southern Association of Colleges and Schools* •
Total Enrollment: *14510*

PROGRAM INFORMATION

Two Year Exit Option: *Not Reported* • NLNAC
Accreditation: *Yes* • CCNE Accreditation:

NURSING STUDENT PROFILE

Total Nursing Enrollment: *336* • Total Basic Student
Enrollment, Full Time: *247* • Total Basic Student
Enrollment, Part Time: *5* • Female Basic Student
Enrollment: *206* • Male Basic Student Enrollment: *46* • Total
RN Enrollment: *84* • Total New Fall Enrollments: *95* • Total
Graduates: *178* • Basic Student Graduates: *113* • RN
Student Graduates: *65*

FINANCES

Residential Annual Tuition: *$2,870* • Non-Residential
Annual Tuition: *$5,972* • General Institutional Fees:
$1,435 • Additional Nursing Fees: *$105*

WILLIAM CAREY COLLEGE

Address: 498 Tuscan Avenue, Hattiesburg, MS 39401
Phone: 601-582-6147
Fax: 601-582-6446
Contact: Mary A. Ware, EdD, RN, Dean
Email: mware@wmcarey.edu

GENERAL INFORMATION

Type of School: *4-Year College or University, Private
(Religious)* • Accreditation: *Southern Association of Colleges
and Schools* • Total Enrollment: *2330*

PROGRAM INFORMATION

Two Year Exit Option: *Not Reported* • NLNAC
Accreditation: *Yes* • CCNE Accreditation:

NURSING STUDENT PROFILE

Total Nursing Enrollment: *191* • Total Basic Student
Enrollment, Full Time: *143* • Total Basic Student
Enrollment, Part Time: *16* • Female Basic Student
Enrollment: *139* • Male Basic Student Enrollment: *20* • Total
RN Enrollment: *32* • Total New Fall Enrollments: *61* • Total
Graduates: *96* • Basic Student Graduates: *94* • RN Student
Graduates: *2*

FINANCES

Residential Annual Tuition: *Not Reported* • Non-Residential
Annual Tuition: *Not Reported* • General Institutional Fees:
Not Reported • Additional Nursing Fees: *$220*

AVILA COLLEGE

Address: 11901 Wornall Road, Kansas City, MO 64145
Phone: 816-501-3672
Fax: 816-501-2442
Contact: Susan H. Fetsch, PhD, RN, Professor and
             Chairperson
Email: fetschsh@mail.avila.edu

GENERAL INFORMATION

Type of School: *4-Year College or University, Private (Religious)* • Accreditation: *North Central Association of Colleges and Schools* • Total Enrollment: *1644*

PROGRAM INFORMATION

Two Year Exit Option: *No* • NLNAC Accreditation: *Not Reported* • CCNE Accreditation: *Yes*

NURSING STUDENT PROFILE

Total Nursing Enrollment: *49* • Total Basic Student Enrollment, Full Time: *49* • Total Basic Student Enrollment, Part Time: *0* • Female Basic Student Enrollment: *46* • Male Basic Student Enrollment: *3* • Total RN Enrollment: *0* • Total New Fall Enrollments: *31* • Total Graduates: *18* • Basic Student Graduates: *18* • RN Student Graduates: *0*

FINANCES

Residential Annual Tuition: *$13,150* • Non-Residential Annual Tuition: *$13,150* • General Institutional Fees: *$220* • Additional Nursing Fees: *$290*

CENTRAL METHODIST COLLEGE

Address: 411 Central Methodist Square, Fayette, MO
             65248
Phone: 660-248-6363
Fax: 660-248-6377
Contact: Shirley J. Peterson, PhD, RN, Nursing Division
             Care
Email: speterso@cmc2.cmc.edu

GENERAL INFORMATION

Type of School: *4-Year College or University, Private (Religious)* • Accreditation: *North Central Association of Colleges and Schools* • Total Enrollment: *Not Reported*

PROGRAM INFORMATION

Two Year Exit Option: *Not Reported* • NLNAC Accreditation: *Not Reported* • CCNE Accreditation:

NURSING STUDENT PROFILE

Total Nursing Enrollment: *38* • Total Basic Student Enrollment, Full Time: *38* • Total Basic Student Enrollment, Part Time: *0* • Female Basic Student Enrollment: *33* • Male Basic Student Enrollment: *5* • Total RN Enrollment: *0* • Total New Fall Enrollments: *12* • Total Graduates: *15* • Basic Student Graduates: *15* • RN Student Graduates: *0*

FINANCES

Residential Annual Tuition: *$11,390* • Non-Residential Annual Tuition: *$11,390* • General Institutional Fees: *$5,695* • Additional Nursing Fees: *$470*

CENTRAL MISSOURI STATE UNIVERSITY

Address: HC-106, Warrensburg, MO 64093
Phone: 660-543-4775
Fax: 660-543-8304
Contact: Elaine Frank-Ragan, PhD, RN, Chairperson
Email: frank-ragan@cmsu1.cmsu.edu

GENERAL INFORMATION

Type of School: *Not Reported* • Accreditation: *Not Reported* • Total Enrollment: *Not Reported*

PROGRAM INFORMATION

Two Year Exit Option: *Not Reported* • NLNAC Accreditation: *Yes* • CCNE Accreditation:

NURSING STUDENT PROFILE

Total Nursing Enrollment: *98* • Total Basic Student Enrollment, Full Time: *80* • Total Basic Student Enrollment, Part Time: *6* • Female Basic Student Enrollment: *Not Reported* • Male Basic Student Enrollment: *Not Reported* • Total RN Enrollment: *12* • Total New Fall Enrollments: *90* • Total Graduates: *51* • Basic Student Graduates: *40* • RN Student Graduates: *11*

FINANCES

Residential Annual Tuition: *$2,208* • Non-Residential Annual Tuition: *$4,224* • General Institutional Fees: *$92* • Additional Nursing Fees: *$176*

COLUMBIA COLLEGE

Address: 500 Strawn Road, Columbia, MO 65203
Phone: 787-743-4041
Fax: 787-744-7031
Contact: Myrna Torres, MSN, RN, Coordinator
Email: mvtorre@columbiaco.edu

GENERAL INFORMATION

Type of School: *Independent, Private (Independent)* • Accreditation: *North Central Association of Colleges and Schools* • Total Enrollment: *2000*

PROGRAM INFORMATION

Two Year Exit Option: *Not Reported* • NLNAC Accreditation: *Yes* • CCNE Accreditation:

NURSING STUDENT PROFILE

Total Nursing Enrollment: *Not Reported* • Total Basic Student Enrollment, Full Time: *Not Reported* • Total Basic Student Enrollment, Part Time: *Not Reported* • Female Basic Student Enrollment: *Not Reported* • Male Basic Student Enrollment: *Not Reported* • Total RN Enrollment: *Not Reported* • Total New Fall Enrollments: *Not Reported* • Total Graduates: *Not Reported* • Basic Student Graduates: *Not Reported* • RN Student Graduates: *Not Reported*

FINANCES

Residential Annual Tuition: *Not Reported* • Non-Residential Annual Tuition: *Not Reported* • General Institutional Fees: *Not Reported* • Additional Nursing Fees: *Not Reported*

Circle 32 on reader card

DEACONESS COLLEGE OF NURSING

Address: 6150 Oakland Avenue, Saint Louis, MO 63139
Phone: 314-768-3042
Fax: 314-768-3843
Contact: Janet T. Barrett, PhD, RN, Academic Dean
Email: janet.barrett(college)@tenethhealth.com

GENERAL INFORMATION

Type of School: *4-Year College or University, Other* • Accreditation: *North Central Association of Colleges and Schools* • Total Enrollment: *220*

PROGRAM INFORMATION

Two Year Exit Option: *Not Reported* • NLNAC Accreditation: *Yes* • CCNE Accreditation:

NURSING STUDENT PROFILE

Total Nursing Enrollment: *186* • Total Basic Student Enrollment, Full Time: *98* • Total Basic Student Enrollment, Part Time: *73* • Female Basic Student Enrollment: *162* • Male Basic Student Enrollment: *9* • Total RN Enrollment: *15* • Total New Fall Enrollments: *24* • Total Graduates: *49* • Basic Student Graduates: *49* • RN Student Graduates: *0*

FINANCES

Residential Annual Tuition: *$8,900* • Non-Residential Annual Tuition: *$8,900* • General Institutional Fees: *$4,450* • Additional Nursing Fees: *$350*

MARYVILLE UNIVERSITY— SAINT LOUIS

Address: 13550 Conway Road, Saint Louis, MO 63141-7299
Phone: 314-529-9443
Fax: 314-529-9139
Contact: Karen Balakas, PhD, RN, Interim Director
Email: kab@maryville.edu

GENERAL INFORMATION

Type of School: *4-Year College or University, Private (Independent)* • Accreditation: *North Central Association of Colleges and Schools* • Total Enrollment: *3055*

PROGRAM INFORMATION

Two Year Exit Option: *Not Reported* • NLNAC Accreditation: *Yes* • CCNE Accreditation:

NURSING STUDENT PROFILE

Total Nursing Enrollment: *197* • Total Basic Student Enrollment, Full Time: *75* • Total Basic Student Enrollment, Part Time: *90* • Female Basic Student Enrollment: *157* • Male Basic Student Enrollment: *8* • Total RN Enrollment: *32* • Total New Fall Enrollments: *56* • Total Graduates: *51* • Basic Student Graduates: *48* • RN Student Graduates: *3*

FINANCES

Residential Annual Tuition: *$12,880* • Non-Residential Annual Tuition: *$12,880* • General Institutional Fees: *$6,440* • Additional Nursing Fees: *$367*

MISSOURI SOUTHERN STATE COLLEGE

Address: 3950 East Newman Road, Joplin, MO 64801
Phone: 417-625-9700
Fax: *Not Reported*
Contact: Barbara J. Box, EdD, RN, Director
Email: box-b@mail.mssc.edu

GENERAL INFORMATION

Type of School: *Other* • Accreditation: *Not Reported* • Total Enrollment: *Not Reported*

PROGRAM INFORMATION

Two Year Exit Option: *Not Reported* • NLNAC Accreditation: *Yes* • CCNE Accreditation:

NURSING STUDENT PROFILE

Total Nursing Enrollment: *59* • Total Basic Student Enrollment, Full Time: *Not Reported* • Total Basic Student Enrollment, Part Time: *Not Reported* • Female Basic Student Enrollment: *Not Reported* • Male Basic Student Enrollment: *Not Reported* • Total RN Enrollment: *9* • Total New Fall Enrollments: *31* • Total Graduates: *40* • Basic Student Graduates: *32* • RN Student Graduates: *8*

FINANCES

Residential Annual Tuition: *Not Reported* • Non-Residential Annual Tuition: *Not Reported* • General Institutional Fees: *Not Reported* • Additional Nursing Fees: *Not Reported*

MISSOURI WESTERN STATE COLLEGE

Address: 4525 Downs Drive, Saint Joseph, MO 64507-2246
Phone: 816-271-5910
Fax: 816-271-5849
Contact: Kathleen Andrews, MN, RN, CCRN, Chairperson
Email: andrews@mwsc.edu

GENERAL INFORMATION

Type of School: *4-Year College or University, Public* • Accreditation: *North Central Association of Colleges and Schools* • Total Enrollment: *5100*

PROGRAM INFORMATION

Two Year Exit Option: *Not Reported* • NLNAC Accreditation: *Yes* • CCNE Accreditation:

NURSING STUDENT PROFILE

Total Nursing Enrollment: *172* • Total Basic Student Enrollment, Full Time: *138* • Total Basic Student Enrollment, Part Time: *0* • Female Basic Student Enrollment: *123* • Male Basic Student Enrollment: *15* • Total RN Enrollment: *34* • Total New Fall Enrollments: *35* • Total Graduates: *77* • Basic Student Graduates: *75* • RN Student Graduates: *2*

FINANCES

Residential Annual Tuition: *$3,146* • Non-Residential Annual Tuition: *$5,200* • General Institutional Fees: *$1,573* • Additional Nursing Fees: *$121*

RESEARCH COLLEGE OF NURSING

Address: 2316 East Meyer Boulevard, Kansas City, MO
64132-1199
Phone: 816-276-4721
Fax: 816-276-3526
Contact: Nancy O. DeBasio, PhD, RN, President/Dean
Email: nodebasio@healthmidwest.org

SAINT LOUIS UNIVERSITY

Address: 3525 Caroline Mall, Saint Louis, MO 63104
Phone: 314-577-8931
Fax: 314-577-8949
Contact: Margie Edel, EdD, RN, Director, Baccalaureate
Program
Email: edele@slu.edu

GENERAL INFORMATION

Type of School: *Hospital, Private (Independent)* •
Accreditation: *North Central Association of Colleges and Schools* • Total Enrollment: *156*

GENERAL INFORMATION

Type of School: *4-Year College or University, Private (Religious)* • Accreditation: *North Central Association of Colleges and Schools* • Total Enrollment: *11112*

PROGRAM INFORMATION

Two Year Exit Option: *Not Reported* • NLNAC
Accreditation: *Yes* • CCNE Accreditation:

PROGRAM INFORMATION

Two Year Exit Option: *Not Reported* • NLNAC
Accreditation: *Yes* • CCNE Accreditation:

NURSING STUDENT PROFILE

Total Nursing Enrollment: *143* • Total Basic Student
Enrollment, Full Time: *139* • Total Basic Student
Enrollment, Part Time: *4* • Female Basic Student
Enrollment: *132* • Male Basic Student Enrollment: *11* • Total
RN Enrollment: *0* • Total New Fall Enrollments: *63* • Total
Graduates: *50* • Basic Student Graduates: *50* • RN Student
Graduates: *0*

NURSING STUDENT PROFILE

Total Nursing Enrollment: *271* • Total Basic Student
Enrollment, Full Time: *237* • Total Basic Student
Enrollment, Part Time: *9* • Female Basic Student
Enrollment: *227* • Male Basic Student Enrollment: *19* • Total
RN Enrollment: *25* • Total New Fall Enrollments: *87* • Total
Graduates: *83* • Basic Student Graduates: *80* • RN Student
Graduates: *3*

FINANCES

Residential Annual Tuition: *$13,500* • Non-Residential
Annual Tuition: *$13,500* • General Institutional Fees:
$6,750 • Additional Nursing Fees: *$450*

FINANCES

Residential Annual Tuition: *$22,050* • Non-Residential
Annual Tuition: *$22,050* • General Institutional Fees:
$9,260 • Additional Nursing Fees: *$645*

SAINT LUKES COLLEGE— KANSAS CITY

Address: 4426 Wornall Road, Kansas City, MO 64111
Phone: 816-932-2233
Fax: 816-932-3831
Contact: Helen Anna Jepson, EdD, RN, Dean/Chief Education Officer
Email: hjepson@saint-lukes.org

GENERAL INFORMATION

Type of School: *Hospital, Private (Independent)* • Accreditation: *North Central Association of Colleges and Schools* • Total Enrollment: *110*

PROGRAM INFORMATION

Two Year Exit Option: *Not Reported* • NLNAC Accreditation: *Yes* • CCNE Accreditation: *Yes*

NURSING STUDENT PROFILE

Total Nursing Enrollment: *111* • Total Basic Student Enrollment, Full Time: *Not Reported* • Total Basic Student Enrollment, Part Time: *Not Reported* • Female Basic Student Enrollment: *Not Reported* • Male Basic Student Enrollment: *Not Reported* • Total RN Enrollment: *1* • Total New Fall Enrollments: *Not Reported* • Total Graduates: *47* • Basic Student Graduates: *47* • RN Student Graduates: *0*

FINANCES

Residential Annual Tuition: *Not Reported* • Non-Residential Annual Tuition: *Not Reported* • General Institutional Fees: *Not Reported* • Additional Nursing Fees: *Not Reported*

SOUTHEAST MISSOURI STATE UNIVERSITY

Address: One University Plaza, Cape Girardeau, MO 63701
Phone: 573-651-5961
Fax: 573-651-2142
Contact: Loiuse A. Hart, DNS, RN, Chairperson, Dept. Head
Email: lhart@semorm.semo.edu

GENERAL INFORMATION

Type of School: *Not Reported* • Accreditation: *North Central Association of Colleges and Schools* • Total Enrollment: *Not Reported*

PROGRAM INFORMATION

Two Year Exit Option: *Not Reported* • NLNAC Accreditation: *Yes* • CCNE Accreditation:

NURSING STUDENT PROFILE

Total Nursing Enrollment: *210* • Total Basic Student Enrollment, Full Time: *148* • Total Basic Student Enrollment, Part Time: *0* • Female Basic Student Enrollment: *129* • Male Basic Student Enrollment: *19* • Total RN Enrollment: *62* • Total New Fall Enrollments: *58* • Total Graduates: *55* • Basic Student Graduates: *34* • RN Student Graduates: *21*

FINANCES

Residential Annual Tuition: *Not Reported* • Non-Residential Annual Tuition: *Not Reported* • General Institutional Fees: *Not Reported* • Additional Nursing Fees: *Not Reported*

TRUMAN STATE UNIVERSITY

Address: 100 East Normal Street, Kirkville, MO 63501
Phone: 660-785-4557
Fax: *Not Reported*
Contact: Constance J. Ayers, PhD, RN, Director, Nursing Program
Email: cayers@truman.edu

GENERAL INFORMATION

Type of School: *Not Reported* • Accreditation: *Not Reported* • Total Enrollment: *Not Reported*

PROGRAM INFORMATION

Two Year Exit Option: *Not Reported* • NLNAC Accreditation: *Yes* • CCNE Accreditation:

NURSING STUDENT PROFILE

Total Nursing Enrollment: *170* • Total Basic Student Enrollment, Full Time: *170* • Total Basic Student Enrollment, Part Time: *0* • Female Basic Student Enrollment: *165* • Male Basic Student Enrollment: *5* • Total RN Enrollment: *0* • Total New Fall Enrollments: *38* • Total Graduates: *39* • Basic Student Graduates: *39* • RN Student Graduates: *0*

FINANCES

Residential Annual Tuition: *$1,772* • Non-Residential Annual Tuition: *$3,172* • General Institutional Fees: *$886* • Additional Nursing Fees: *$148*

UNIVERSITY OF MISSOURI— COLUMBIA

Address: S218 Nursing School Bldg, Columbia, MO 65211
Phone: 573-882-0228
Fax: 573-884-4544
Contact: Prisilla LeMone, DSN, RN, FAAN, Director of Undergraduate Studies
Email: plemone@missouri.edu

GENERAL INFORMATION

Type of School: *Not Reported* • Accreditation: *North Central Association of Colleges and Schools* • Total Enrollment: *Not Reported*

PROGRAM INFORMATION

Two Year Exit Option: *Not Reported* • NLNAC Accreditation: *Yes* • CCNE Accreditation:

NURSING STUDENT PROFILE

Total Nursing Enrollment: *316* • Total Basic Student Enrollment, Full Time: *213* • Total Basic Student Enrollment, Part Time: *12* • Female Basic Student Enrollment: *198* • Male Basic Student Enrollment: *27* • Total RN Enrollment: *91* • Total New Fall Enrollments: *225* • Total Graduates: *154* • Basic Student Graduates: *105* • RN Student Graduates: *49*

FINANCES

Residential Annual Tuition: *$6,149* • Non-Residential Annual Tuition: *$14,967* • General Institutional Fees: *$4,436* • Additional Nursing Fees: *$155*

UNIVERSITY OF MISSOURI— ST. LOUIS

Address: 8001 Natural Bridge Road, Saint Louis, MO
             63121
Phone: 314-516-6849
Fax: 314-516-6730
Contact: Teri Murray, PhD, RN, BSN Program Director
Email: murray@umsl.edu

GENERAL INFORMATION

Type of School: *Not Reported* • Accreditation: *North Central Association of Colleges and Schools* • Total Enrollment: *Not Reported*

PROGRAM INFORMATION

Two Year Exit Option: *Not Reported* • NLNAC Accreditation: *Not Reported* • CCNE Accreditation: *Yes*

NURSING STUDENT PROFILE

Total Nursing Enrollment: *258* • Total Basic Student Enrollment, Full Time: *199* • Total Basic Student Enrollment, Part Time: *59* • Female Basic Student Enrollment: *239* • Male Basic Student Enrollment: *19* • Total RN Enrollment: *0* • Total New Fall Enrollments: *86* • Total Graduates: *72* • Basic Student Graduates: *72* • RN Student Graduates: *0*

FINANCES

Residential Annual Tuition: *Not Reported* • Non-Residential Annual Tuition: *Not Reported* • General Institutional Fees: *Not Reported* • Additional Nursing Fees: *$137*

WILLIAM JEWELL COLLEGE

Address: 500 College Hill, Liberty, MO 64068
Phone: 816-781-7700
Fax: 816-415-5024
Contact: Joanne Kersten, EdD, RN, Professor and Chair
Email: kerstenj@william.jewel.edu

GENERAL INFORMATION

Type of School: *4-Year College or University, Private (Religious)* • Accreditation: *North Central Association of Colleges and Schools* • Total Enrollment: *1150*

PROGRAM INFORMATION

Two Year Exit Option: *Not Reported* • NLNAC Accreditation: *Not Reported* • CCNE Accreditation: *Yes*

NURSING STUDENT PROFILE

Total Nursing Enrollment: *76* • Total Basic Student Enrollment, Full Time: *75* • Total Basic Student Enrollment, Part Time: *0* • Female Basic Student Enrollment: *70* • Male Basic Student Enrollment: *5* • Total RN Enrollment: *1* • Total New Fall Enrollments: *0* • Total Graduates: *31* • Basic Student Graduates: *31* • RN Student Graduates: *0*

FINANCES

Residential Annual Tuition: *$13,500* • Non-Residential Annual Tuition: *$13,500* • General Institutional Fees: *$6,750* • Additional Nursing Fees: *$555*

CARROLL COLLEGE

Address: 1601 N. Benton Avenue, Helena, MT 59625
Phone: 406-447-5494
Fax: 406-447-5476
Contact: Cynthia Z. Gustafson, PhD, RN, Chair
Email: cgustafs@carroll.edu

GENERAL INFORMATION

Type of School: *4-Year College or University, Private (Religious)* • Accreditation: *Northwestern Association of Schools and Colleges* • Total Enrollment: *1307*

PROGRAM INFORMATION

Two Year Exit Option: *Not Reported* • NLNAC Accreditation: *Yes* • CCNE Accreditation:

NURSING STUDENT PROFILE

Total Nursing Enrollment: *86* • Total Basic Student Enrollment, Full Time: *86* • Total Basic Student Enrollment, Part Time: *0* • Female Basic Student Enrollment: *84* • Male Basic Student Enrollment: *2* • Total RN Enrollment: *0* • Total New Fall Enrollments: *24* • Total Graduates: *21* • Basic Student Graduates: *21* • RN Student Graduates: *0*

FINANCES

Residential Annual Tuition: *$12,238* • Non-Residential Annual Tuition: *$12,238* • General Institutional Fees: *$6,119* • Additional Nursing Fees: *$408*

MONTANA STATE UNIVERSITY—BOZEMAN

Address: Sherrick Hall, PO Box 173560, Bozeman, MT 59717-3560
Phone: 406-994-3784
Fax: *Not Reported*
Contact: Lea Acord, PhD, RN, Dean and Professor
Email: lacord@montana.edu

GENERAL INFORMATION

Type of School: *4-Year College or University, Public* • Accreditation: *Northwestern Association of Schools and Colleges* • Total Enrollment: *11753*

PROGRAM INFORMATION

Two Year Exit Option: *Not Reported* • NLNAC Accreditation: *Not Reported* • CCNE Accreditation:

NURSING STUDENT PROFILE

Total Nursing Enrollment: *500* • Total Basic Student Enrollment, Full Time: *Not Reported* • Total Basic Student Enrollment, Part Time: *Not Reported* • Female Basic Student Enrollment: *Not Reported* • Male Basic Student Enrollment: *Not Reported* • Total RN Enrollment: *6* • Total New Fall Enrollments: *106* • Total Graduates: *109* • Basic Student Graduates: *106* • RN Student Graduates: *3*

FINANCES

Residential Annual Tuition: *Not Reported* • Non-Residential Annual Tuition: *Not Reported* • General Institutional Fees: *Not Reported* • Additional Nursing Fees: *Not Reported*

CLARKSON COLLEGE

Address: 101 S. 42nd Street, Omaha, NE 68131
Phone: 402-552-3373
Fax: *Not Reported*
Contact: Linda Christensen, MSN, RN, Dean of Nursing
Email: christensen@ucollege.edu

GENERAL INFORMATION

Type of School: *Not Reported* • Accreditation: *North Central Association of Colleges and Schools* • Total Enrollment: *Not Reported*

PROGRAM INFORMATION

Two Year Exit Option: *Not Reported* • NLNAC Accreditation: *Yes* • CCNE Accreditation:

NURSING STUDENT PROFILE

Total Nursing Enrollment: *Not Reported* • Total Basic Student Enrollment, Full Time: *Not Reported* • Total Basic Student Enrollment, Part Time: *Not Reported* • Female Basic Student Enrollment: *Not Reported* • Male Basic Student Enrollment: *Not Reported* • Total RN Enrollment: *Not Reported* • Total New Fall Enrollments: *Not Reported* • Total Graduates: *Not Reported* • Basic Student Graduates: *Not Reported* • RN Student Graduates: *Not Reported*

FINANCES

Residential Annual Tuition: *Not Reported* • Non-Residential Annual Tuition: *Not Reported* • General Institutional Fees: *Not Reported* • Additional Nursing Fees: *Not Reported*

COLLEGE OF SAINT MARY

Address: 1901 S. 72nd St., Omaha, NE 68124
Phone: 402-878-9632
Fax: *Not Reported*
Contact: Mary E. Partusch, Ph.D., RN, Baccalaureate Director
Email: *Not Reported*

GENERAL INFORMATION

Type of School: *4-Year College or University, Private (Religious)* • Accreditation: *North Central Association of Colleges and Schools* • Total Enrollment: *930*

PROGRAM INFORMATION

Two Year Exit Option: *Not Reported* • NLNAC Accreditation: *Yes* • CCNE Accreditation:

NURSING STUDENT PROFILE

Total Nursing Enrollment: *Not Reported* • Total Basic Student Enrollment, Full Time: *Not Reported* • Total Basic Student Enrollment, Part Time: *Not Reported* • Female Basic Student Enrollment: *Not Reported* • Male Basic Student Enrollment: *Not Reported* • Total RN Enrollment: *Not Reported* • Total New Fall Enrollments: *Not Reported* • Total Graduates: *Not Reported* • Basic Student Graduates: *Not Reported* • RN Student Graduates: *Not Reported*

FINANCES

Residential Annual Tuition: *Not Reported* • Non-Residential Annual Tuition: *Not Reported* • General Institutional Fees: *Not Reported* • Additional Nursing Fees: *Not Reported*

CREIGHTON UNIVERSITY

Address: 2500 California Plaza, Omaha, NE 68178
Phone: 402-280-2004
Fax: 402-280-2045
Contact: Edeth K. Kitchens, PhD, RN, Professor and Dean
Email: kitchens@creighton.edu

GENERAL INFORMATION

Type of School: *Not Reported* • Accreditation: *Not Reported* • Total Enrollment: *Not Reported*

PROGRAM INFORMATION

Two Year Exit Option: *Not Reported* • NLNAC Accreditation: *Yes* • CCNE Accreditation:

NURSING STUDENT PROFILE

Total Nursing Enrollment: *356* • Total Basic Student Enrollment, Full Time: *302* • Total Basic Student Enrollment, Part Time: *9* • Female Basic Student Enrollment: *287* • Male Basic Student Enrollment: *24* • Total RN Enrollment: *45* • Total New Fall Enrollments: *120* • Total Graduates: *156* • Basic Student Graduates: *121* • RN Student Graduates: *35*

FINANCES

Residential Annual Tuition: *$14,312* • Non-Residential Annual Tuition: *$22,119* • General Institutional Fees: *$7,156* • Additional Nursing Fees: *$447*

MIDLAND LUTHERAN COLLEGE

Address: 900 N. Clarkson, Fremont, NE 68025
Phone: 402-721-5480
Fax: 402-941-6279
Contact: Nancy Harms, PhD, RN, Chair, Division of Nursing
Email: harms@admin.mlc.edu

GENERAL INFORMATION

Type of School: *4-Year College or University, Private (Independent)* • Accreditation: *North Central Association of Colleges and Schools* • Total Enrollment: *1086*

PROGRAM INFORMATION

Two Year Exit Option: *No* • NLNAC Accreditation: *Yes* • CCNE Accreditation:

NURSING STUDENT PROFILE

Total Nursing Enrollment: *112* • Total Basic Student Enrollment, Full Time: *67* • Total Basic Student Enrollment, Part Time: *0* • Female Basic Student Enrollment: *62* • Male Basic Student Enrollment: *5* • Total RN Enrollment: *45* • Total New Fall Enrollments: *24* • Total Graduates: *14* • Basic Student Graduates: *7* • RN Student Graduates: *7*

FINANCES

Residential Annual Tuition: *$7,300* • Non-Residential Annual Tuition: *$7,300* • General Institutional Fees: *$0* • Additional Nursing Fees: *$200*

UNION COLLEGE

Address: 3800 S 48th St, Lincoln, NE 68506
Phone: 402-488-2331
Fax: *Not Reported*
Contact: Marilyn McArthur, PhD, RN, Chair, Division of
            Health Sciences
Email: mamcarth@ucollege.edu

UNIVERSITY OF NEBRASKA MEDICAL CENTER

Address: 985330 Nebraska Medical Center, Omaha, NE
            68198-5330
Phone: 402-559-4270
Fax: 402-559-6379
Contact: Catherine Todero, PhD, RN, Assoc. Professor
            and Assoc. Dean
Email: ctodero@unmc.edu

GENERAL INFORMATION

Type of School: *4-Year College or University, Private (Independent)* • Accreditation: *North Central Association of Colleges and Schools* • Total Enrollment: *856*

GENERAL INFORMATION

Type of School: *4-Year College or University, Public* • Accreditation: *North Central Association of Colleges and Schools* • Total Enrollment: *2636*

PROGRAM INFORMATION

Two Year Exit Option: *Not Reported* • NLNAC Accreditation: *Yes* • CCNE Accreditation:

PROGRAM INFORMATION

Two Year Exit Option: *No* • NLNAC Accreditation: *Not Reported* • CCNE Accreditation: *Yes*

NURSING STUDENT PROFILE

Total Nursing Enrollment: *91* • Total Basic Student Enrollment, Full Time: *86* • Total Basic Student Enrollment, Part Time: *2* • Female Basic Student Enrollment: *75* • Male Basic Student Enrollment: *13* • Total RN Enrollment: *3* • Total New Fall Enrollments: *22* • Total Graduates: *12* • Basic Student Graduates: *10* • RN Student Graduates: *2*

NURSING STUDENT PROFILE

Total Nursing Enrollment: *541* • Total Basic Student Enrollment, Full Time: *453* • Total Basic Student Enrollment, Part Time: *34* • Female Basic Student Enrollment: *454* • Male Basic Student Enrollment: *33* • Total RN Enrollment: *54* • Total New Fall Enrollments: *111* • Total Graduates: *194* • Basic Student Graduates: *174* • RN Student Graduates: *20*

FINANCES

Residential Annual Tuition: *$10,940* • Non-Residential Annual Tuition: *$10,940* • General Institutional Fees: *$5,470* • Additional Nursing Fees: *$456*

FINANCES

Residential Annual Tuition: *$3,213* • Non-Residential Annual Tuition: *$9,003* • General Institutional Fees: *$1,046* • Additional Nursing Fees: *$1,141*

UNIVERSITY OF NEVADA— LAS VEGAS

Address: 4505 Maryland Pkwy, Las Vegas, NV 89154
Phone: 702-895-3360
Fax: 702-895-4807
Contact: Rosemary Witt, PhD, RN, Chairperson
Email: rwitt@ccmail.nevada.edu

UNIVERSITY OF NEVADA— RENO

Address: P134, Reno, NV 89557
Phone: 775-784-6841
Fax: 775-784-4262
Contact: Julie E. Johnson, PhD, RN, Director
Email: jej@unr.edu

GENERAL INFORMATION

Type of School: *4-Year College or University, Public* •
Accreditation: *Northwestern Association of Schools and Colleges* • Total Enrollment: *23000*

GENERAL INFORMATION

Type of School: *4-Year College or University, Public* •
Accreditation: *Northwestern Association of Schools and Colleges* • Total Enrollment: *12000*

PROGRAM INFORMATION

Two Year Exit Option: *Not Reported* • NLNAC
Accreditation: *Yes* • CCNE Accreditation:

PROGRAM INFORMATION

Two Year Exit Option: *No* • NLNAC Accreditation: *Yes* •
CCNE Accreditation:

NURSING STUDENT PROFILE

Total Nursing Enrollment: *231* • Total Basic Student Enrollment, Full Time: *195* • Total Basic Student Enrollment, Part Time: *14* • Female Basic Student Enrollment: *188* • Male Basic Student Enrollment: *21* • Total RN Enrollment: *22* • Total New Fall Enrollments: *56* • Total Graduates: *74* • Basic Student Graduates: *64* • RN Student Graduates: *10*

NURSING STUDENT PROFILE

Total Nursing Enrollment: *92* • Total Basic Student Enrollment, Full Time: *88* • Total Basic Student Enrollment, Part Time: *0* • Female Basic Student Enrollment: *78* • Male Basic Student Enrollment: *10* • Total RN Enrollment: *4* • Total New Fall Enrollments: *45* • Total Graduates: *44* • Basic Student Graduates: *40* • RN Student Graduates: *4*

FINANCES

Residential Annual Tuition: *Not Reported* • Non-Residential Annual Tuition: *Not Reported* • General Institutional Fees: *$70* • Additional Nursing Fees: *$50*

FINANCES

Residential Annual Tuition: *$2,670* • Non-Residential Annual Tuition: *$11,157* • General Institutional Fees: *Not Reported* • Additional Nursing Fees: *$100*

COLBY-SAWYER COLLEGE

Address: 100 Main Street, New London, NH 03257
Phone: 603-526-3646
Fax: 603-526-3452
Contact: Kathleen M. Thies, PhD, RN, Chairperson
Email: kthies@colby-sawyer.edu

GENERAL INFORMATION

Type of School: *4-Year College or University, Private (Independent)* • Accreditation: *New England Association of Schools and Colleges* • Total Enrollment: *Not Reported*

PROGRAM INFORMATION

Two Year Exit Option: *No* • NLNAC Accreditation: *Yes* • CCNE Accreditation:

NURSING STUDENT PROFILE

Total Nursing Enrollment: *30* • Total Basic Student Enrollment, Full Time: *27* • Total Basic Student Enrollment, Part Time: *1* • Female Basic Student Enrollment: *26* • Male Basic Student Enrollment: *2* • Total RN Enrollment: *2* • Total New Fall Enrollments: *15* • Total Graduates: *12* • Basic Student Graduates: *12* • RN Student Graduates: *0*

FINANCES

Residential Annual Tuition: *$18,960* • Non-Residential Annual Tuition: *$18,960* • General Institutional Fees: *$200* • Additional Nursing Fees: *Not Reported*

SAINT ANSELM COLLEGE

Address: 100 Saint Anselm Drive, Manchester, NH
03102-1310
Phone: 603-641-7084
Fax: 603-641-7377
Contact: Joyce B. Barker, DrPH, RN,
Chairperson/Director, Department of Nursing
Email: jbarker@anselm.edu

GENERAL INFORMATION

Type of School: *4-Year College or University, Private (Religious)* • Accreditation: *New England Association of Schools and Colleges* • Total Enrollment: *Not Reported*

PROGRAM INFORMATION

Two Year Exit Option: *No* • NLNAC Accreditation: *Not Reported* • CCNE Accreditation:

NURSING STUDENT PROFILE

Total Nursing Enrollment: *194* • Total Basic Student Enrollment, Full Time: *49* • Total Basic Student Enrollment, Part Time: *194* • Female Basic Student Enrollment: *0* • Male Basic Student Enrollment: *186* • Total RN Enrollment: *0* • Total New Fall Enrollments: *Not Reported* • Total Graduates: *Not Reported* • Basic Student Graduates: *Not Reported* • RN Student Graduates: *Not Reported*

FINANCES

Residential Annual Tuition: *Not Reported* • Non-Residential Annual Tuition: *Not Reported* • General Institutional Fees: *Not Reported* • Additional Nursing Fees: *Not Reported*

BLOOMFIELD COLLEGE

Address: 467 Franklin Ave, Bloomfield, NJ 07003
Phone: 973-748-9000
Fax: 973-429-3613
Contact: Carolyn R. Tuella, EdD, RN, Chairperson
Email: carolyn-tuella@bloomfield.edu

FAIRLEIGH DICKINSON UNVERSITY

Address: 1000 River Road, Dickinson Hall Rm. 444,
           Teaneck, NJ 07666
Phone: 201-692-2880
Fax: 201-692-2388
Contact: Christine Mihal, MSN, RN, Associate Director,
           Undergraduate Program.
Email: mihal@mailbox.fdu.edu

GENERAL INFORMATION

Type of School: *4-Year College or University, Private (Independent)* • Accreditation: *Middle States Association of Colleges and Schools* • Total Enrollment: *1950*

GENERAL INFORMATION

Type of School: *Not Reported* • Accreditation: *Not Reported* • Total Enrollment: *Not Reported*

PROGRAM INFORMATION

Two Year Exit Option: *No* • NLNAC Accreditation: *Not Reported* • CCNE Accreditation: *Yes*

PROGRAM INFORMATION

Two Year Exit Option: *No* • NLNAC Accreditation: *Not Reported* • CCNE Accreditation: *Yes*

NURSING STUDENT PROFILE

Total Nursing Enrollment: *125* • Total Basic Student Enrollment, Full Time: *52* • Total Basic Student Enrollment, Part Time: *0* • Female Basic Student Enrollment: *48* • Male Basic Student Enrollment: *4* • Total RN Enrollment: *73* • Total New Fall Enrollments: *13* • Total Graduates: *17* • Basic Student Graduates: *11* • RN Student Graduates: *6*

NURSING STUDENT PROFILE

Total Nursing Enrollment: *158* • Total Basic Student Enrollment, Full Time: *95* • Total Basic Student Enrollment, Part Time: *44* • Female Basic Student Enrollment: *126* • Male Basic Student Enrollment: *13* • Total RN Enrollment: *19* • Total New Fall Enrollments: *83* • Total Graduates: *35* • Basic Student Graduates: *35* • RN Student Graduates: *0*

FINANCES

Residential Annual Tuition: *$10,800* • Non-Residential Annual Tuition: *$10,800* • General Institutional Fees: *$5,400* • Additional Nursing Fees: *$273*

FINANCES

Residential Annual Tuition: *$16,346* • Non-Residential Annual Tuition: *$16,346* • General Institutional Fees: *Not Reported* • Additional Nursing Fees: *$525*

FELICIAN COLLEGE

Address: 262 South Main Street, Lodi, NJ 07644-2117
Phone: 201-559-6030
Fax: 201-559-6188
Contact: Rosita Brennan, MSN, RN, Director
Email: brennanr.@inet.felician.edu

GENERAL INFORMATION

Type of School: *4-Year College or University, Private (Religious)* • Accreditation: *Middle States Association of Colleges and Schools* • Total Enrollment: *1374*

PROGRAM INFORMATION

Two Year Exit Option: *No* • NLNAC Accreditation: *Not Reported* • CCNE Accreditation: *Yes*

NURSING STUDENT PROFILE

Total Nursing Enrollment: *91* • Total Basic Student Enrollment, Full Time: *75* • Total Basic Student Enrollment, Part Time: *16* • Female Basic Student Enrollment: *87* • Male Basic Student Enrollment: *4* • Total RN Enrollment: *0* • Total New Fall Enrollments: *57* • Total Graduates: *18* • Basic Student Graduates: *0* • RN Student Graduates: *18*

FINANCES

Residential Annual Tuition: *$10,560* • Non-Residential Annual Tuition: *$10,560* • General Institutional Fees: *$5,280* • Additional Nursing Fees: *$352*

RUTGERS THE STATE UNIVERSITY OF NEW JERSEY

Address: 311 North Fifth Street, Camden, NJ 08102
Phone: 973-353-5293
Fax: *Not Reported*
Contact: Felissa R. Lashley, PhD, RN, FAAN, Dean
Email: greipp@crab.rutgers.edu

GENERAL INFORMATION

Type of School: *4-Year College or University, Public* • Accreditation: *Middle States Association of Colleges and Schools* • Total Enrollment: *48000*

PROGRAM INFORMATION

Two Year Exit Option: *No* • NLNAC Accreditation: *Yes* • CCNE Accreditation:

NURSING STUDENT PROFILE

Total Nursing Enrollment: *466* • Total Basic Student Enrollment, Full Time: *242* • Total Basic Student Enrollment, Part Time: *104* • Female Basic Student Enrollment: *300* • Male Basic Student Enrollment: *46* • Total RN Enrollment: *120* • Total New Fall Enrollments: *172* • Total Graduates: *77* • Basic Student Graduates: *67* • RN Student Graduates: *10*

FINANCES

Residential Annual Tuition: *$4,762* • Non-Residential Annual Tuition: *$9,692* • General Institutional Fees: *$2,381* • Additional Nursing Fees: *$154*

RUTGERS STATE UNIVERSITY

Address: 331 North Fifth St, Camden, NJ 08102
Phone: 856-225-6226
Fax: 856-225-6541
Contact: Mary E. Greipp, EdD, RN, FAAN, Professor and
            Chairperson
Email: *Not Reported*

GENERAL INFORMATION

Type of School: *Not Reported* • Accreditation: *Not Reported* •
Total Enrollment: *Not Reported*

PROGRAM INFORMATION

Two Year Exit Option: *Yes* • NLNAC Accreditation: *Not
Reported* • CCNE Accreditation:

NURSING STUDENT PROFILE

Total Nursing Enrollment: *95* • Total Basic Student
Enrollment, Full Time: *62* • Total Basic Student Enrollment,
Part Time: *5* • Female Basic Student Enrollment: *61* • Male
Basic Student Enrollment: *6* • Total RN Enrollment: *28* •
Total New Fall Enrollments: *67* • Total Graduates: *45* • Basic
Student Graduates: *30* • RN Student Graduates: *15*

FINANCES

Residential Annual Tuition: *$6,290* • Non-Residential
Annual Tuition: *$12,804* • General Institutional Fees: *$219* •
Additional Nursing Fees: *$162*

UNIVERSITY OF MEDICINE AND DENTISTRY OF NEW JERSEY—RAMAPO COLLEGE

Address: 65 Bergen St., Newark, NJ 07430-1680
Phone: 201-684-7737
Fax: 201-684-7954
Contact: Kathleen M. Burke, PhD, RN, Assistant Dean
Email: kmburke@rampo.edu

GENERAL INFORMATION

Type of School: *Not Reported* • Accreditation: *Not Reported* •
Total Enrollment: *Not Reported*

PROGRAM INFORMATION

Two Year Exit Option: *No* • NLNAC Accreditation: *Yes* •
CCNE Accreditation:

NURSING STUDENT PROFILE

Total Nursing Enrollment: *315* • Total Basic Student
Enrollment, Full Time: *98* • Total Basic Student Enrollment,
Part Time: *34* • Female Basic Student Enrollment: *115* •
Male Basic Student Enrollment: *17* • Total RN Enrollment:
183 • Total New Fall Enrollments: *60* • Total Graduates: *43* •
Basic Student Graduates: *12* • RN Student Graduates: *31*

FINANCES

Residential Annual Tuition: *$2,418* • Non-Residential
Annual Tuition: *$4,369* • General Institutional Fees: *$969* •
Additional Nursing Fees: *$13,020*

WILLIAM PATERSON UNIVERSITY

Address: 300 Pomton, Wayne, NJ 7470
Phone: 973-720-2673
Fax: 973-720-2668
Contact: Janet P. Tracy, PhD, RN, Chairperson, Nursing
           Department
Email: tracyj@wpunj.edu

GENERAL INFORMATION

Type of School: *4-Year College or University, Public* •
Accreditation: *Middle States Association of Colleges and
Schools* • Total Enrollment: *11000*

PROGRAM INFORMATION

Two Year Exit Option: *No* • NLNAC Accreditation: *Not
Reported* • CCNE Accreditation: *Yes*

NURSING STUDENT PROFILE

Total Nursing Enrollment: *294* • Total Basic Student
Enrollment, Full Time: *Not Reported* • Total Basic Student
Enrollment, Part Time: *Not Reported* • Female Basic Student
Enrollment: *227* • Male Basic Student Enrollment: *23* • Total
RN Enrollment: *44* • Total New Fall Enrollments: *Not
Reported* • Total Graduates: *64* • Basic Student Graduates:
52 • RN Student Graduates: *12*

FINANCES

Residential Annual Tuition: *Not Reported* • Non-Residential
Annual Tuition: *Not Reported* • General Institutional Fees:
$2,575 • Additional Nursing Fees: *$165*

NEW MEXICO STATE UNIVERSITY

Address: PO Box 30001, Las Cruces, NM 88003-8001
Phone: 505-646-3812
Fax: 505-646-2167
Contact: Wendell W. Oderkirk, PhD, RN, Interim
           Academic Dept. Head
Email: woderkir@nmsu.edu

GENERAL INFORMATION

Type of School: *4-Year College or University, Public* •
Accreditation: *North Central Association of Colleges and
Schools* • Total Enrollment: *Not Reported*

PROGRAM INFORMATION

Two Year Exit Option: *Not Reported* • NLNAC
Accreditation: *Yes* • CCNE Accreditation:

NURSING STUDENT PROFILE

Total Nursing Enrollment: *172* • Total Basic Student
Enrollment, Full Time: *151* • Total Basic Student
Enrollment, Part Time: *3* • Female Basic Student
Enrollment: *125* • Male Basic Student Enrollment: *29* • Total
RN Enrollment: *18* • Total New Fall Enrollments: *62* • Total
Graduates: *58* • Basic Student Graduates: *49* • RN Student
Graduates: *9*

FINANCES

Residential Annual Tuition: *$2,994* • Non-Residential
Annual Tuition: *$9,402* • General Institutional Fees: *Not
Reported* • Additional Nursing Fees: *$280*

UNIVERSITY OF NEW MEXICO

Address: 2502 Marble Northeast, Albuquerque, NM 87131
Phone: 505-272-6284
Fax: 505-272-3970
Contact: Sandra L. Ferketich, PHD, RN, FAAN, Dean and Professor
Email: sferketich@salud.unm.edu

ADELPHI UNIVERSITY

Address: 1 South Ave., Garden City, NY 11530
Phone: 516-877-4568
Fax: 516-877-4558
Contact: Marilyn Klainberg, EdD, RN, Associate Dean
Email: klainberg@adelphi.edu

GENERAL INFORMATION

Type of School: *4-Year College or University, Public* • Accreditation: *North Central Association of Colleges and Schools* • Total Enrollment: *23659*

GENERAL INFORMATION

Type of School: *4-Year College or University, Private (Independent)* • Accreditation: *Middle States Association of Colleges and Schools* • Total Enrollment: *6500*

PROGRAM INFORMATION

Two Year Exit Option: *Not Reported* • NLNAC Accreditation: *Yes* • CCNE Accreditation: *Yes*

PROGRAM INFORMATION

Two Year Exit Option: *No* • NLNAC Accreditation: *Yes* • CCNE Accreditation: *Yes*

NURSING STUDENT PROFILE

Total Nursing Enrollment: *348* • Total Basic Student Enrollment, Full Time: *162* • Total Basic Student Enrollment, Part Time: *18* • Female Basic Student Enrollment: *162* • Male Basic Student Enrollment: *18* • Total RN Enrollment: *168* • Total New Fall Enrollments: *17* • Total Graduates: *191* • Basic Student Graduates: *69* • RN Student Graduates: *122*

NURSING STUDENT PROFILE

Total Nursing Enrollment: *328* • Total Basic Student Enrollment, Full Time: *147* • Total Basic Student Enrollment, Part Time: *17* • Female Basic Student Enrollment: *146* • Male Basic Student Enrollment: *18* • Total RN Enrollment: *164* • Total New Fall Enrollments: *69* • Total Graduates: *60* • Basic Student Graduates: *37* • RN Student Graduates: *23*

FINANCES

Residential Annual Tuition: *$2,430* • Non-Residential Annual Tuition: *$9,171* • General Institutional Fees: *Not Reported* • Additional Nursing Fees: *$150*

FINANCES

Residential Annual Tuition: *$17,000* • Non-Residential Annual Tuition: *$17,000* • General Institutional Fees: *$170* • Additional Nursing Fees: *$407*

COLLEGE OF MOUNT ST. VINCENT

Address: 6301 Riverdale Ave., Riverdale, NY 10471
Phone: 718-405-3362
Fax: *Not Reported*
Contact: Barbara J. Cohen, EdD, RN, Director of
           Division
Email: vistril@aol.com

GENERAL INFORMATION

Type of School: *4-Year College or University, Private
(Independent)* • Accreditation: *Middle States Association of
Colleges and Schools* • Total Enrollment: *1892*

PROGRAM INFORMATION

Two Year Exit Option: *Not Reported* • NLNAC
Accreditation: *Yes* • CCNE Accreditation:

NURSING STUDENT PROFILE

Total Nursing Enrollment: *388* • Total Basic Student
Enrollment, Full Time: *Not Reported* • Total Basic Student
Enrollment, Part Time: *Not Reported* • Female Basic Student
Enrollment: *Not Reported* • Male Basic Student Enrollment:
Not Reported • Total RN Enrollment: *100* • Total New Fall
Enrollments: *84* • Total Graduates: *96* • Basic Student
Graduates: *76* • RN Student Graduates: *20*

FINANCES

Residential Annual Tuition: *$14,510* • Non-Residential
Annual Tuition: *$14,510* • General Institutional Fees: *$100* •
Additional Nursing Fees: *$450*

COLLEGE OF NEW ROCHELLE

Address: 29 Castle Pl., New Rochelle, NY 10801
Phone: 914-654-5493
Fax: 914-654-5994
Contact: Penny Bamford, PhD, RN, Assistant Dean
Email: PBamford@cnr.edu

GENERAL INFORMATION

Type of School: *4-Year College or University, Private
(Independent)* • Accreditation: *Middle States Association of
Colleges and Schools* • Total Enrollment: *6754*

PROGRAM INFORMATION

Two Year Exit Option: *Not Reported* • NLNAC
Accreditation: *Not Reported* • CCNE Accreditation:

NURSING STUDENT PROFILE

Total Nursing Enrollment: *404* • Total Basic Student
Enrollment, Full Time: *138* • Total Basic Student
Enrollment, Part Time: *52* • Female Basic Student
Enrollment: *186* • Male Basic Student Enrollment: *4* • Total
RN Enrollment: *214* • Total New Fall Enrollments: *63* •
Total Graduates: *91* • Basic Student Graduates: *38* • RN
Student Graduates: *53*

FINANCES

Residential Annual Tuition: *$9,600* • Non-Residential
Annual Tuition: *$9,600* • General Institutional Fees: *$150* •
Additional Nursing Fees: *$220*

COLUMBIA UNIVERSITY

Address: 630 West 168th St. Box 6, New York, NY 10032
Phone: 212-305-3582
Fax: 212-305-1116
Contact: Mary O. Mundinger, RN, Dean and Centennial Professor in Health Policy
Email: mm44@columbia.edu

GENERAL INFORMATION

Type of School: *4-Year College or University, Private (Independent)* • Accreditation: *None* • Total Enrollment: *19000*

PROGRAM INFORMATION

Two Year Exit Option: *Not Reported* • NLNAC Accreditation: *Yes* • CCNE Accreditation:

NURSING STUDENT PROFILE

Total Nursing Enrollment: *97* • Total Basic Student Enrollment, Full Time: *82* • Total Basic Student Enrollment, Part Time: *0* • Female Basic Student Enrollment: *Not Reported* • Male Basic Student Enrollment: *Not Reported* • Total RN Enrollment: *15* • Total New Fall Enrollments: *499* • Total Graduates: *Not Reported* • Basic Student Graduates: *Not Reported* • RN Student Graduates: *Not Reported*

FINANCES

Residential Annual Tuition: *Not Reported* • Non-Residential Annual Tuition: *Not Reported* • General Institutional Fees: *$1,726* • Additional Nursing Fees: *Not Reported*

DOMINICAN COLLEGE

Address: 470 Western Highway, Orangeburg, NY 10962
Phone: 914-398-4998
Fax: *Not Reported*
Contact: Maureen C. Creegan, MSN, RN, Director, Division of Nursing
Email: MccDom@aol.com

GENERAL INFORMATION

Type of School: *4-Year College or University, Private (Independent)* • Accreditation: *Middle States Association of Colleges and Schools* • Total Enrollment: *1691*

PROGRAM INFORMATION

Two Year Exit Option: *Not Reported* • NLNAC Accreditation: *Yes* • CCNE Accreditation:

NURSING STUDENT PROFILE

Total Nursing Enrollment: *186* • Total Basic Student Enrollment, Full Time: *Not Reported* • Total Basic Student Enrollment, Part Time: *Not Reported* • Female Basic Student Enrollment: *Not Reported* • Male Basic Student Enrollment: *Not Reported* • Total RN Enrollment: *128* • Total New Fall Enrollments: *242* • Total Graduates: *91* • Basic Student Graduates: *48* • RN Student Graduates: *43*

FINANCES

Residential Annual Tuition: *$11,250* • Non-Residential Annual Tuition: *Not Reported* • General Institutional Fees: *$410* • Additional Nursing Fees: *$300*

D'YOUVILLE COLLEGE

Address: 320 Porter Ave., Buffalo, NY 14201
Phone: 716-881-3200
Fax: 716-881-8159
Contact: Verna Kieffer, DNS, RN, Chair
Email: kiefferv@dyc.edu

ELMIRA COLLEGE

Address: One Park Place, Elmira, NY 14901
Phone: 607-735-1890
Fax: 607-735-1758
Contact: Lois Schoener, DNSc, RN, Acting Director
Email: lschoener@elmira.edu

GENERAL INFORMATION

Type of School: *4-Year College or University, Private (Independent)* • Accreditation: *Middle States Association of Colleges and Schools* • Total Enrollment: *2300*

GENERAL INFORMATION

Type of School: *Not Reported* • Accreditation: *None* • Total Enrollment: *Not Reported*

PROGRAM INFORMATION

Two Year Exit Option: *No* • NLNAC Accreditation: *Not Reported* • CCNE Accreditation:

PROGRAM INFORMATION

Two Year Exit Option: *Not Reported* • NLNAC Accreditation: *Yes* • CCNE Accreditation: *Not Reported*

NURSING STUDENT PROFILE

Total Nursing Enrollment: *162* • Total Basic Student Enrollment, Full Time: *55* • Total Basic Student Enrollment, Part Time: *14* • Female Basic Student Enrollment: *64* • Male Basic Student Enrollment: *5* • Total RN Enrollment: *93* • Total New Fall Enrollments: *21* • Total Graduates: *40* • Basic Student Graduates: *11* • RN Student Graduates: *29*

NURSING STUDENT PROFILE

Total Nursing Enrollment: *160* • Total Basic Student Enrollment, Full Time: *Not Reported* • Total Basic Student Enrollment, Part Time: *Not Reported* • Female Basic Student Enrollment: *Not Reported* • Male Basic Student Enrollment: *Not Reported* • Total RN Enrollment: *80* • Total New Fall Enrollments: *20* • Total Graduates: *Not Reported* • Basic Student Graduates: *Not Reported* • RN Student Graduates: *Not Reported*

FINANCES

Residential Annual Tuition: *$12,350* • Non-Residential Annual Tuition: *$12,350* • General Institutional Fees: *$100* • Additional Nursing Fees: *$120*

FINANCES

Residential Annual Tuition: *Not Reported* • Non-Residential Annual Tuition: *Not Reported* • General Institutional Fees: *Not Reported* • Additional Nursing Fees: *Not Reported*

EXCELSIOR COLLEGE

Address: 7 Columbia Cr., Albany, NY 12203
Phone: 518-464-8661
Fax: 518-464-8777
Contact: Bridget Nettleton, PhD, RN, Associate Dean
Email: bnettleton@excelsiur.edu

GENERAL INFORMATION

Type of School: *4-Year College or University, Private (Independent)* • Accreditation: *Middle States Association of Colleges and Schools* • Total Enrollment: *17250*

PROGRAM INFORMATION

Two Year Exit Option: *Not Reported* • NLNAC Accreditation: *Yes* • CCNE Accreditation:

NURSING STUDENT PROFILE

Total Nursing Enrollment: *2614* • Total Basic Student Enrollment, Full Time: *0* • Total Basic Student Enrollment, Part Time: *509* • Female Basic Student Enrollment: *384* • Male Basic Student Enrollment: *125* • Total RN Enrollment: *2105* • Total New Fall Enrollments: *165* • Total Graduates: *347* • Basic Student Graduates: *52* • RN Student Graduates: *295*

FINANCES

Residential Annual Tuition: *Not Reported* • Non-Residential Annual Tuition: *Not Reported* • General Institutional Fees: *Not Reported* • Additional Nursing Fees: *Not Reported*

HARTWICK COLLEGE

Address: West Street, Oneonta, NY 13820
Phone: 607-431-4785
Fax: 607-431-4850
Contact: Sharon D. Dettenrieder, MSN, RN, Associate Professor and Interim Chair
Email: dettenriedes@hartwick.edu

GENERAL INFORMATION

Type of School: *4-Year College or University, Private (Independent)* • Accreditation: *Middle States Association of Colleges and Schools* • Total Enrollment: *1488*

PROGRAM INFORMATION

Two Year Exit Option: *Not Reported* • NLNAC Accreditation: *Yes* • CCNE Accreditation:

NURSING STUDENT PROFILE

Total Nursing Enrollment: *64* • Total Basic Student Enrollment, Full Time: *57* • Total Basic Student Enrollment, Part Time: *0* • Female Basic Student Enrollment: *55* • Male Basic Student Enrollment: *2* • Total RN Enrollment: *7* • Total New Fall Enrollments: *19* • Total Graduates: *15* • Basic Student Graduates: *13* • RN Student Graduates: *2*

FINANCES

Residential Annual Tuition: *$24,760* • Non-Residential Annual Tuition: *$24,760* • General Institutional Fees: *$325* • Additional Nursing Fees: *$115*

HERBERT H. LEHMAN COLLEGE

Address: 250 Bedford Park Blvd., Bronx, NY 10468
Phone: 718-960-8794
Fax: *Not Reported*
Contact: Ngozi O. Nkongho, MSN, RN, Chairperson
Email: ngozi@alpha.lehman.cuny.edu

GENERAL INFORMATION

Type of School: *4-Year College or University, Public* •
Accreditation: *Middle States Association of Colleges and Schools* • Total Enrollment: *10000*

PROGRAM INFORMATION

Two Year Exit Option: *Not Reported* • NLNAC Accreditation: *Yes* • CCNE Accreditation:

NURSING STUDENT PROFILE

Total Nursing Enrollment: *123* • Total Basic Student Enrollment, Full Time: *73* • Total Basic Student Enrollment, Part Time: *0* • Female Basic Student Enrollment: *Not Reported* • Male Basic Student Enrollment: *Not Reported* • Total RN Enrollment: *50* • Total New Fall Enrollments: *51* • Total Graduates: *64* • Basic Student Graduates: *30* • RN Student Graduates: *34*

FINANCES

Residential Annual Tuition: *$3,000* • Non-Residential Annual Tuition: *$6,600* • General Institutional Fees: *$55* • Additional Nursing Fees: *Not Reported*

HUNTER COLLEGE—CUNY

Address: 425 East 25 Street, New York, NY 10010
Phone: 212-481-7596
Fax: *Not Reported*
Contact: Susan Neville, PhD, RN, Director - Nursing Undergraduate Program
Email: sneville@hunter.cuny.edu

GENERAL INFORMATION

Type of School: *Other* • Accreditation: *Not Reported* • Total Enrollment: *Not Reported*

PROGRAM INFORMATION

Two Year Exit Option: *Not Reported* • NLNAC Accreditation: *Not Reported* • CCNE Accreditation:

NURSING STUDENT PROFILE

Total Nursing Enrollment: *Not Reported* • Total Basic Student Enrollment, Full Time: *Not Reported* • Total Basic Student Enrollment, Part Time: *Not Reported* • Female Basic Student Enrollment: *Not Reported* • Male Basic Student Enrollment: *Not Reported* • Total RN Enrollment: *Not Reported* • Total New Fall Enrollments: *Not Reported* • Total Graduates: *Not Reported* • Basic Student Graduates: *Not Reported* • RN Student Graduates: *Not Reported*

FINANCES

Residential Annual Tuition: *Not Reported* • Non-Residential Annual Tuition: *Not Reported* • General Institutional Fees: *Not Reported* • Additional Nursing Fees: *Not Reported*

KEUKA COLLEGE

Address: Keuka Park, NY 14478
Phone: 315-279-5269
Fax: 315-279-5660
Contact: Linda R. Rossi, EdD, RN, CS, Chair and Professor
Email: lrrossi@mail.keuka.edu

GENERAL INFORMATION

Type of School: *Not Reported* • Accreditation: *No* • Total Enrollment: *Not Reported*

PROGRAM INFORMATION

Two Year Exit Option: *No* • NLNAC Accreditation: *Yes* • CCNE Accreditation:

NURSING STUDENT PROFILE

Total Nursing Enrollment: *44* • Total Basic Student Enrollment, Full Time: *40* • Total Basic Student Enrollment, Part Time: *0* • Female Basic Student Enrollment: *36* • Male Basic Student Enrollment: *4* • Total RN Enrollment: *4* • Total New Fall Enrollments: *14* • Total Graduates: *14* • Basic Student Graduates: *4* • RN Student Graduates: *10*

FINANCES

Residential Annual Tuition: *$14,050* • Non-Residential Annual Tuition: *$14,050* • General Institutional Fees: *Not Reported* • Additional Nursing Fees: *Not Reported*

LONG ISLAND UNIVERSITY—BROOKLYN

Address: 1 University Plaza, Brooklyn, NY 11201
Phone: 718-488-1059
Fax: 718-780-4019
Contact: Esther Levine-Brill, PhD, RN, ANP, Chairperson
Email: ebrill@liu.edu

GENERAL INFORMATION

Type of School: *4-Year College or University, Private (Independent)* • Accreditation: *Middle States Association of Colleges and Schools* • Total Enrollment: *29774*

PROGRAM INFORMATION

Two Year Exit Option: *No* • NLNAC Accreditation: *Yes* • CCNE Accreditation:

NURSING STUDENT PROFILE

Total Nursing Enrollment: *423* • Total Basic Student Enrollment, Full Time: *Not Reported* • Total Basic Student Enrollment, Part Time: *Not Reported* • Female Basic Student Enrollment: *Not Reported* • Male Basic Student Enrollment: *Not Reported* • Total RN Enrollment: *42* • Total New Fall Enrollments: *152* • Total Graduates: *67* • Basic Student Graduates: *57* • RN Student Graduates: *10*

FINANCES

Residential Annual Tuition: *$12,888* • Non-Residential Annual Tuition: *$12,888* • General Institutional Fees: *$955* • Additional Nursing Fees: *$16*

MOUNT SAINT MARY COLLEGE

Address: 330 Powell Ave., Newburgh, NY 12550
Phone: 845-569-3138
Fax: 845-562-6762
Contact: Linda Scheetz, EdD, RN, CS, CEN, Chairperson
Email: scheetz@msmc.edu

GENERAL INFORMATION

Type of School: *Independent, Private (Independent)* • Accreditation: *Middle States Association of Colleges and Schools* • Total Enrollment: *2221*

PROGRAM INFORMATION

Two Year Exit Option: *Not Reported* • NLNAC Accreditation: *Not Reported* • CCNE Accreditation: *Yes*

NURSING STUDENT PROFILE

Total Nursing Enrollment: *159* • Total Basic Student Enrollment, Full Time: *Not Reported* • Total Basic Student Enrollment, Part Time: *Not Reported* • Female Basic Student Enrollment: *Not Reported* • Male Basic Student Enrollment: *Not Reported* • Total RN Enrollment: *47* • Total New Fall Enrollments: *32* • Total Graduates: *35* • Basic Student Graduates: *22* • RN Student Graduates: *13*

FINANCES

Residential Annual Tuition: *$9,264* • Non-Residential Annual Tuition: *$9,264* • General Institutional Fees: *$30* • Additional Nursing Fees: *$200*

NAZARETH COLLEGE

Address: 4245 East Ave, Rochester, NY 14618
Phone: 716-389-2710
Fax: 716-389-2714
Contact: Margaret M. Andrews, PhD, RN, Chairperson and Professor - Nursing Dept.
Email: mmandrew@naz.edu

GENERAL INFORMATION

Type of School: *Not Reported* • Accreditation: *Not Reported* • Total Enrollment: *Not Reported*

PROGRAM INFORMATION

Two Year Exit Option: *Not Reported* • NLNAC Accreditation: *Yes* • CCNE Accreditation:

NURSING STUDENT PROFILE

Total Nursing Enrollment: *Not Reported* • Total Basic Student Enrollment, Full Time: *Not Reported* • Total Basic Student Enrollment, Part Time: *Not Reported* • Female Basic Student Enrollment: *Not Reported* • Male Basic Student Enrollment: *Not Reported* • Total RN Enrollment: *Not Reported* • Total New Fall Enrollments: *Not Reported* • Total Graduates: *Not Reported* • Basic Student Graduates: *Not Reported* • RN Student Graduates: *Not Reported*

FINANCES

Residential Annual Tuition: *Not Reported* • Non-Residential Annual Tuition: *Not Reported* • General Institutional Fees: *Not Reported* • Additional Nursing Fees: *Not Reported*

NEW YORK INSTITUTE OF TECHNOLOGY

Address: P. O. Box 170, Old Westbury, NY 11568
Phone: 516-686-3739
Fax: 516-686-3795
Contact: Linda Soroff, PhD, RN, Chairperson
Email: soroff@nyit.edu

GENERAL INFORMATION

Type of School: *Not Reported* • Accreditation: *Not Reported* • Total Enrollment: *Not Reported*

PROGRAM INFORMATION

Two Year Exit Option: *No* • NLNAC Accreditation: *Not Reported* • CCNE Accreditation:

NURSING STUDENT PROFILE

Total Nursing Enrollment: *85* • Total Basic Student Enrollment, Full Time: *70* • Total Basic Student Enrollment, Part Time: *15* • Female Basic Student Enrollment: *78* • Male Basic Student Enrollment: *7* • Total RN Enrollment: *0* • Total New Fall Enrollments: *26* • Total Graduates: *5* • Basic Student Graduates: *5* • RN Student Graduates: *0*

FINANCES

Residential Annual Tuition: *$13,700* • Non-Residential Annual Tuition: *$13,700* • General Institutional Fees: *Not Reported* • Additional Nursing Fees: *$200*

NEW YORK UNIVERSITY

Address: 246 Greene St., New York, NY 10003
Phone: 212-998-5300
Fax: 212-995-3413
Contact: Diane McGivern, PHD, RN, FAAN, Division Head and Acting Program Director
Email: Diane.McGivern@nyu.edu

GENERAL INFORMATION

Type of School: *4-Year College or University, Private (Independent)* • Accreditation: *Middle States Association of Colleges and Schools* • Total Enrollment: *Not Reported*

PROGRAM INFORMATION

Two Year Exit Option: *Not Reported* • NLNAC Accreditation: *Yes* • CCNE Accreditation: *Yes*

NURSING STUDENT PROFILE

Total Nursing Enrollment: *276* • Total Basic Student Enrollment, Full Time: *170* • Total Basic Student Enrollment, Part Time: *63* • Female Basic Student Enrollment: *217* • Male Basic Student Enrollment: *16* • Total RN Enrollment: *43* • Total New Fall Enrollments: *87* • Total Graduates: *62* • Basic Student Graduates: *54* • RN Student Graduates: *8*

FINANCES

Residential Annual Tuition: *$23,090* • Non-Residential Annual Tuition: *$23,090* • General Institutional Fees: *$793* • Additional Nursing Fees: *Not Reported*

NIAGARA UNIVERSITY

Address: PO 2203, Niagara University, NY 14109
Phone: 716-286-8312
Fax: 716-286-8308
Contact: Dolores A. Bower, PhD, RN, Dean
Email: dab@niagara.edu

GENERAL INFORMATION

Type of School: *4-Year College or University, Private (Religious)* • Accreditation: *Middle States Association of Colleges and Schools* • Total Enrollment: *3000*

PROGRAM INFORMATION

Two Year Exit Option: *Not Reported* • NLNAC Accreditation: *Yes* • CCNE Accreditation:

NURSING STUDENT PROFILE

Total Nursing Enrollment: *126* • Total Basic Student Enrollment, Full Time: *90* • Total Basic Student Enrollment, Part Time: *0* • Female Basic Student Enrollment: *85* • Male Basic Student Enrollment: *5* • Total RN Enrollment: *36* • Total New Fall Enrollments: *0* • Total Graduates: *46* • Basic Student Graduates: *34* • RN Student Graduates: *12*

FINANCES

Residential Annual Tuition: *$14,000* • Non-Residential Annual Tuition: *$14,000* • General Institutional Fees: *$520* • Additional Nursing Fees: *$411*

PACE UNIVERSITY

Address: 861 Bedford Rd. -L28, Pleasentville, NY 10570
Phone: 914-773-3555
Fax: 914-773-3345
Contact: Martha Kelly, EdD, RN, Chairperson, Dept. of Undergraduate Studies
Email: mkelly@pace.edu

GENERAL INFORMATION

Type of School: *4-Year College or University, Private (Independent)* • Accreditation: *Middle States Association of Colleges and Schools* • Total Enrollment: *13000*

PROGRAM INFORMATION

Two Year Exit Option: *Not Reported* • NLNAC Accreditation: *Not Reported* • CCNE Accreditation: *Yes*

NURSING STUDENT PROFILE

Total Nursing Enrollment: *321* • Total Basic Student Enrollment, Full Time: *168* • Total Basic Student Enrollment, Part Time: *41* • Female Basic Student Enrollment: *197* • Male Basic Student Enrollment: *12* • Total RN Enrollment: *112* • Total New Fall Enrollments: *32* • Total Graduates: *135* • Basic Student Graduates: *85* • RN Student Graduates: *50*

FINANCES

Residential Annual Tuition: *Not Reported* • Non-Residential Annual Tuition: *Not Reported* • General Institutional Fees: *Not Reported* • Additional Nursing Fees: *Not Reported*

ROBERTS WESLEYAN COLLEGE

Address: 2301 Westside Dr., Rochester, NY 14624
Phone: 716-594-6330
Fax: 716-594-6592
Contact: Susanne Mohnkern, PhD, RN, Chair, Division
            of Nursing
Email: mohnkerns@roberts.edu

GENERAL INFORMATION

Type of School: *4-Year College or University, Private
(Religious)* • Accreditation: *Middle States Association of
Colleges and Schools* • Total Enrollment: *1697*

PROGRAM INFORMATION

Two Year Exit Option: *No* • NLNAC Accreditation: *Yes* •
CCNE Accreditation:

NURSING STUDENT PROFILE

Total Nursing Enrollment: *97* • Total Basic Student
Enrollment, Full Time: *60* • Total Basic Student Enrollment,
Part Time: *2* • Female Basic Student Enrollment: *60* • Male
Basic Student Enrollment: *2* • Total RN Enrollment: *35* •
Total New Fall Enrollments: *28* • Total Graduates: *7* • Basic
Student Graduates: *7* • RN Student Graduates: *0*

FINANCES

Residential Annual Tuition: *$14,366* • Non-Residential
Annual Tuition: *$14,366* • General Institutional Fees: *$550* •
Additional Nursing Fees: *$75*

THE SAGE COLLEGES

Address: 45 Ferry Street, Troy, NY 12180
Phone: 518-244-2231
Fax: 518-244-2009
Contact: Ann Gothler, PhD, RN, Chairperson
Email: gothla@sage.edu

GENERAL INFORMATION

Type of School: *Not Reported* • Accreditation: *Not Reported* •
Total Enrollment: *Not Reported*

PROGRAM INFORMATION

Two Year Exit Option: *Not Reported* • NLNAC
Accreditation: *Yes* • CCNE Accreditation:

NURSING STUDENT PROFILE

Total Nursing Enrollment: *Not Reported* • Total Basic Student
Enrollment, Full Time: *Not Reported* • Total Basic Student
Enrollment, Part Time: *Not Reported* • Female Basic Student
Enrollment: *Not Reported* • Male Basic Student Enrollment:
Not Reported • Total RN Enrollment: *Not Reported* • Total
New Fall Enrollments: *Not Reported* • Total Graduates: *Not
Reported* • Basic Student Graduates: *Not Reported* • RN
Student Graduates: *Not Reported*

FINANCES

Residential Annual Tuition: *Not Reported* • Non-Residential
Annual Tuition: *Not Reported* • General Institutional Fees:
Not Reported • Additional Nursing Fees: *Not Reported*

SAINT JOHN FISHER COLLEGE

Address: 3690 East Ave., Rochester, NY 14618
Phone: 716-385-8397
Fax: 716-385-7311
Contact: Katherine S. Detherage, PhD, RN, Chairperson and Associate Professor
Email: detherage@sjfc.edu

GENERAL INFORMATION

Type of School: *4-Year College or University, Private (Independent)* • Accreditation: *Middle States Association of Colleges and Schools* • Total Enrollment: *2175*

PROGRAM INFORMATION

Two Year Exit Option: *Not Reported* • NLNAC Accreditation: *Yes* • CCNE Accreditation:

NURSING STUDENT PROFILE

Total Nursing Enrollment: *78* • Total Basic Student Enrollment, Full Time: *47* • Total Basic Student Enrollment, Part Time: *0* • Female Basic Student Enrollment: *Not Reported* • Male Basic Student Enrollment: *Not Reported* • Total RN Enrollment: *31* • Total New Fall Enrollments: *19* • Total Graduates: *33* • Basic Student Graduates: *19* • RN Student Graduates: *14*

FINANCES

Residential Annual Tuition: *$15,200* • Non-Residential Annual Tuition: *$15,200* • General Institutional Fees: *$150* • Additional Nursing Fees: *$0*

SAINT JOSEPH COLLEGE— NEW YORK

Address: 245 Clinton Ave., Brooklyn, NY 11205
Phone: 860-231-5058
Fax: 860-231-8396
Contact: Virginia Knowlden, EdD, RN, Professor and Chairperson
Email: vknowlden@sjc.edu

GENERAL INFORMATION

Type of School: *4-Year College or University, Private (Independent)* • Accreditation: *Middle States Association of Colleges and Schools* • Total Enrollment: *4588*

PROGRAM INFORMATION

Two Year Exit Option: *Not Reported* • NLNAC Accreditation: *Yes* • CCNE Accreditation:

NURSING STUDENT PROFILE

Total Nursing Enrollment: *90* • Total Basic Student Enrollment, Full Time: *45* • Total Basic Student Enrollment, Part Time: *27* • Female Basic Student Enrollment: *72* • Male Basic Student Enrollment: *0* • Total RN Enrollment: *18* • Total New Fall Enrollments: *37* • Total Graduates: *31* • Basic Student Graduates: *26* • RN Student Graduates: *5*

FINANCES

Residential Annual Tuition: *$17,430* • Non-Residential Annual Tuition: *$17,430* • General Institutional Fees: *$8,715* • Additional Nursing Fees: *$430*

STATE UNIVERSITY OF NEW YORK—BINGHAMTON

Address: Decker Sch of Nsg, PO Box 6000, Binghamton, NY 13902-6000
Phone: 607-777-2311
Fax: *Not Reported*
Contact: Mary S. Collins, PhD, RN, Dean and Professor
Email: mcollins@binghamton.edu

STATE UNIVERSITY OF NEW YORK—BROCKPORT

Address: 350 New Campus Dr., Brockport, NY 14420
Phone: 716-395-2355
Fax: 716-395-5312
Contact: Kathryn Wood, PhD, RN, Chairperson
Email: KWood@brockport.edu

GENERAL INFORMATION

Type of School: *Not Reported* • Accreditation: *Not Reported* • Total Enrollment: *Not Reported*

GENERAL INFORMATION

Type of School: *4-Year College or University, Public* • Accreditation: *Middle States Association of Colleges and Schools* • Total Enrollment: *Not Reported*

PROGRAM INFORMATION

Two Year Exit Option: *Not Reported* • NLNAC Accreditation: *Not Reported* • CCNE Accreditation: *Yes*

PROGRAM INFORMATION

Two Year Exit Option: *Not Reported* • NLNAC Accreditation: *Yes* • CCNE Accreditation:

NURSING STUDENT PROFILE

Total Nursing Enrollment: *Not Reported* • Total Basic Student Enrollment, Full Time: *Not Reported* • Total Basic Student Enrollment, Part Time: *Not Reported* • Female Basic Student Enrollment: *Not Reported* • Male Basic Student Enrollment: *Not Reported* • Total RN Enrollment: *Not Reported* • Total New Fall Enrollments: *Not Reported* • Total Graduates: *Not Reported* • Basic Student Graduates: *Not Reported* • RN Student Graduates: *Not Reported*

NURSING STUDENT PROFILE

Total Nursing Enrollment: *109* • Total Basic Student Enrollment, Full Time: *99* • Total Basic Student Enrollment, Part Time: *0* • Female Basic Student Enrollment: *14* • Male Basic Student Enrollment: *85* • Total RN Enrollment: *10* • Total New Fall Enrollments: *55* • Total Graduates: *66* • Basic Student Graduates: *51* • RN Student Graduates: *15*

FINANCES

Residential Annual Tuition: *Not Reported* • Non-Residential Annual Tuition: *Not Reported* • General Institutional Fees: *Not Reported* • Additional Nursing Fees: *Not Reported*

FINANCES

Residential Annual Tuition: *$3,400* • Non-Residential Annual Tuition: *$8,300* • General Institutional Fees: *Not Reported* • Additional Nursing Fees: *$307*

STATE UNIVERSITY OF NEW YORK—BUFFALO

Address: 3435 Main St., 1030 Kimball Tower, Buffalo, NY 14214
Phone: 716-829-2210
Fax: 716-829-2566
Contact: Karen J. Radke, PhD, RN, Associate Dean for Academic Affairs
Email: radke@buffalo.edu

GENERAL INFORMATION

Type of School: *4-Year College or University, Public* •
Accreditation: *Middle States Association of Colleges and Schools* • Total Enrollment: *24830*

PROGRAM INFORMATION

Two Year Exit Option: *Not Reported* • NLNAC
Accreditation: *Not Reported* • CCNE Accreditation: *Yes*

NURSING STUDENT PROFILE

Total Nursing Enrollment: *315* • Total Basic Student
Enrollment, Full Time: *194* • Total Basic Student
Enrollment, Part Time: *17* • Female Basic Student
Enrollment: *190* • Male Basic Student Enrollment: *21* • Total
RN Enrollment: *104* • Total New Fall Enrollments: *70* •
Total Graduates: *94* • Basic Student Graduates: *59* • RN
Student Graduates: *35*

FINANCES

Residential Annual Tuition: *$3,400* • Non-Residential
Annual Tuition: *$8,300* • General Institutional Fees:
$1,255 • Additional Nursing Fees: *Not Reported*

STATE UNIVERSITY OF NEW YORK—PLATTSBURGH

Address: 101 Broad St., Plattsburgh, NY 12901
Phone: 518-564-4225
Fax: 518-564-3100
Contact: Gretchen C. Beebe, PhD, RN, Chairperson
Email: gretchen.beebe@plattsburgh.edu

GENERAL INFORMATION

Type of School: *4-Year College or University, Public* •
Accreditation: *Middle States Association of Colleges and Schools* • Total Enrollment: *6000*

PROGRAM INFORMATION

Two Year Exit Option: *Not Reported* • NLNAC
Accreditation: *Yes* • CCNE Accreditation:

NURSING STUDENT PROFILE

Total Nursing Enrollment: *208* • Total Basic Student
Enrollment, Full Time: *110* • Total Basic Student
Enrollment, Part Time: *3* • Female Basic Student
Enrollment: *107* • Male Basic Student Enrollment: *6* • Total
RN Enrollment: *95* • Total New Fall Enrollments: *28* • Total
Graduates: *49* • Basic Student Graduates: *29* • RN Student
Graduates: *20*

FINANCES

Residential Annual Tuition: *$3,400* • Non-Residential
Annual Tuition: *$8,300* • General Institutional Fees: *$547* •
Additional Nursing Fees: *Not Reported*

STATE UNIVERSITY OF NEW YORK—STONY BROOK

Address: Health Care Center, Level 2, Rm 235, Stony Brook, NY 11794
Phone: 631-444-3260
Fax: 631-444-3136
Contact: Lenora J. McClean, EdD, RN, Dean and Chief Nursing Officer
Email: Lenora.McClean@sunysb.edu

GENERAL INFORMATION

Type of School: *Governmental Agency, Public* • Accreditation: *Middle States Association of Colleges and Schools* • Total Enrollment: *19929*

PROGRAM INFORMATION

Two Year Exit Option: *Not Reported* • NLNAC Accreditation: *Yes* • CCNE Accreditation:

NURSING STUDENT PROFILE

Total Nursing Enrollment: *210* • Total Basic Student Enrollment, Full Time: *94* • Total Basic Student Enrollment, Part Time: *0* • Female Basic Student Enrollment: *81* • Male Basic Student Enrollment: *13* • Total RN Enrollment: *116* • Total New Fall Enrollments: *31* • Total Graduates: *108* • Basic Student Graduates: *47* • RN Student Graduates: *61*

FINANCES

Residential Annual Tuition: *$3,400* • Non-Residential Annual Tuition: *$8,300* • General Institutional Fees: *Not Reported* • Additional Nursing Fees: *$300*

STATE UNIVERSITY OF NEW YORK—UTICA/ROME

Address: PO Box 3050, Utica, NY 13504
Phone: 315-792-7295
Fax: 315-792-7555
Contact: Elizabeth Kellogg Walker, EdD, RN, Dean
Email: aekw@sunyit.edu

GENERAL INFORMATION

Type of School: *Technical/Specialized Institution, Public* • Accreditation: *Middle States Association of Colleges and Schools* • Total Enrollment: *2658*

PROGRAM INFORMATION

Two Year Exit Option: *Not Reported* • NLNAC Accreditation: *Not Reported* • CCNE Accreditation:

NURSING STUDENT PROFILE

Total Nursing Enrollment: *Not Reported* • Total Basic Student Enrollment, Full Time: *Not Reported* • Total Basic Student Enrollment, Part Time: *Not Reported* • Female Basic Student Enrollment: *Not Reported* • Male Basic Student Enrollment: *Not Reported* • Total RN Enrollment: *Not Reported* • Total New Fall Enrollments: *Not Reported* • Total Graduates: *Not Reported* • Basic Student Graduates: *Not Reported* • RN Student Graduates: *Not Reported*

FINANCES

Residential Annual Tuition: *Not Reported* • Non-Residential Annual Tuition: *Not Reported* • General Institutional Fees: *Not Reported* • Additional Nursing Fees: *Not Reported*

SYRACUSE UNIVERSITY

Address: 426 Ostrom Ave., Syracuse, NY 13244
Phone: 315-443-2141
Fax: 315-443-2164
Contact: Cecilia F. Mulvey, PhD, RN, Interim Dean
Email: cfmulvey@nursing.syr.edu

GENERAL INFORMATION

Type of School: *Other* • Accreditation: *Not Reported* • Total Enrollment: *Not Reported*

PROGRAM INFORMATION

Two Year Exit Option: *Not Reported* • NLNAC Accreditation: *Yes* • CCNE Accreditation:

NURSING STUDENT PROFILE

Total Nursing Enrollment: *349* • Total Basic Student Enrollment, Full Time: *Not Reported* • Total Basic Student Enrollment, Part Time: *Not Reported* • Female Basic Student Enrollment: *Not Reported* • Male Basic Student Enrollment: *Not Reported* • Total RN Enrollment: *81* • Total New Fall Enrollments: *78* • Total Graduates: *140* • Basic Student Graduates: *95* • RN Student Graduates: *45*

FINANCES

Residential Annual Tuition: *$19,360* • Non-Residential Annual Tuition: *$19,360* • General Institutional Fees: *$290* • Additional Nursing Fees: *Not Reported*

UNIVERSITY OF ROCHESTER

Address: 601 Elmwood Ave., Box SON, Rochester, NY 14642
Phone: 585-275-8887
Fax: 585-756-8299
Contact: Rita D'Aoust, MS, ACNP, Program Co-Coordinator
Email: Rita_D'Aoust@urmc.rochester.edu

GENERAL INFORMATION

Type of School: *4-Year College or University, Private (Independent)* • Accreditation: *Middle States Association of Colleges and Schools* • Total Enrollment: *8201*

PROGRAM INFORMATION

Two Year Exit Option: *No* • NLNAC Accreditation: *Yes* • CCNE Accreditation:

NURSING STUDENT PROFILE

Total Nursing Enrollment: *138* • Total Basic Student Enrollment, Full Time: *33* • Total Basic Student Enrollment, Part Time: *1* • Female Basic Student Enrollment: *31* • Male Basic Student Enrollment: *3* • Total RN Enrollment: *104* • Total New Fall Enrollments: *Not Reported* • Total Graduates: *57* • Basic Student Graduates: *31* • RN Student Graduates: *26*

FINANCES

Residential Annual Tuition: *$24,150* • Non-Residential Annual Tuition: *$24,150* • General Institutional Fees: *$604* • Additional Nursing Fees: *$75*

UTICA COLLEGE OF SYRACUSE UNIVERSITY

Address: 1600 Burrstone Rd., Utica, NY 13502
Phone: 315-792-3180
Fax: 315-792-3248
Contact: Mary Katherine Maroney, RN, Director of Nursing
Email: mmaroney@utica.ucsu.edu

GENERAL INFORMATION

Type of School: *Other* • Accreditation: *Not Reported* • Total Enrollment: *Not Reported*

PROGRAM INFORMATION

Two Year Exit Option: *Not Reported* • NLNAC Accreditation: *Yes* • CCNE Accreditation:

NURSING STUDENT PROFILE

Total Nursing Enrollment: *100* • Total Basic Student Enrollment, Full Time: *58* • Total Basic Student Enrollment, Part Time: *0* • Female Basic Student Enrollment: *53* • Male Basic Student Enrollment: *5* • Total RN Enrollment: *42* • Total New Fall Enrollments: *15* • Total Graduates: *Not Reported* • Basic Student Graduates: *Not Reported* • RN Student Graduates: *Not Reported*

FINANCES

Residential Annual Tuition: *$15,414* • Non-Residential Annual Tuition: *$15,414* • General Institutional Fees: *$162* • Additional Nursing Fees: *Not Reported*

WAGNER COLLEGE

Address: 1 Campus Road, Staten Island, NY 10301-4428
Phone: 718-390-3452
Fax: *Not Reported*
Contact: Paula Tropello, PhD, RN, Dept. Head
Email: ptropell@wagner.edu

GENERAL INFORMATION

Type of School: *Other* • Accreditation: *Not Reported* • Total Enrollment: *Not Reported*

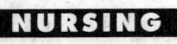

PROGRAM INFORMATION

Two Year Exit Option: *Not Reported* • NLNAC Accreditation: *Yes* • CCNE Accreditation:

NURSING STUDENT PROFILE

Total Nursing Enrollment: *Not Reported* • Total Basic Student Enrollment, Full Time: *Not Reported* • Total Basic Student Enrollment, Part Time: *Not Reported* • Female Basic Student Enrollment: *Not Reported* • Male Basic Student Enrollment: *Not Reported* • Total RN Enrollment: *Not Reported* • Total New Fall Enrollments: *Not Reported* • Total Graduates: *Not Reported* • Basic Student Graduates: *Not Reported* • RN Student Graduates: *Not Reported*

FINANCES

Residential Annual Tuition: *Not Reported* • Non-Residential Annual Tuition: *Not Reported* • General Institutional Fees: *Not Reported* • Additional Nursing Fees: *Not Reported*

BARTON COLLEGE

Address: PO Box 5000, Wilson, NC 27893
Phone: 252-399-6401
Fax: *Not Reported*
Contact: Pet Pruden, PhD, RN, Dean
Email: ppruden@barton.edu

GENERAL INFORMATION

Type of School: *4-Year College or University, Private (Religious)* • Accreditation: *Southern Association of Colleges and Schools* • Total Enrollment: *1300*

PROGRAM INFORMATION

Two Year Exit Option: *Not Reported* • NLNAC Accreditation: *Yes* • CCNE Accreditation:

NURSING STUDENT PROFILE

Total Nursing Enrollment: *124* • Total Basic Student Enrollment, Full Time: *Not Reported* • Total Basic Student Enrollment, Part Time: *Not Reported* • Female Basic Student Enrollment: *Not Reported* • Male Basic Student Enrollment: *Not Reported* • Total RN Enrollment: *11* • Total New Fall Enrollments: *47* • Total Graduates: *36* • Basic Student Graduates: *25* • RN Student Graduates: *11*

FINANCES

Residential Annual Tuition: *$10,030* • Non-Residential Annual Tuition: *$10,030* • General Institutional Fees: *$804* • Additional Nursing Fees: *$15*

EAST CAROLINA UNIVERSITY

Address: 132 Rivers Building, Greenville, NC 27858
Phone: 252-328-6099
Fax: 252-328-4300
Contact: Phyllis N. Horns, DSN, RN, FAAN, Interim Vice Chancellor and Dean
Email: hornsp@mail.ecu.edu

GENERAL INFORMATION

Type of School: *4-Year College or University, Public* • Accreditation: *Southern Association of Colleges and Schools* • Total Enrollment: *19412*

PROGRAM INFORMATION

Two Year Exit Option: *No* • NLNAC Accreditation: *Yes* • CCNE Accreditation:

NURSING STUDENT PROFILE

Total Nursing Enrollment: *420* • Total Basic Student Enrollment, Full Time: *323* • Total Basic Student Enrollment, Part Time: *12* • Female Basic Student Enrollment: *301* • Male Basic Student Enrollment: *34* • Total RN Enrollment: *85* • Total New Fall Enrollments: *90* • Total Graduates: *206* • Basic Student Graduates: *152* • RN Student Graduates: *54*

FINANCES

Residential Annual Tuition: *$1,453* • Non-Residential Annual Tuition: *$9,708* • General Institutional Fees: *$1,113* • Additional Nursing Fees: *$40*

LENOIR-RHYNE COLLEGE

Address: PO Box 7292, Hickory, NC 28603
Phone: 828-328-7282
Fax: 828-328-7284
Contact: Linda W. Reece, PhD, RN, Chair
Email: reecel@lrc.edu

GENERAL INFORMATION

Type of School: *4-Year College or University, Private (Religious)* • Accreditation: *Southern Association of Colleges and Schools* • Total Enrollment: *1500*

PROGRAM INFORMATION

Two Year Exit Option: *Not Reported* • NLNAC Accreditation: *Yes* • CCNE Accreditation:

NURSING STUDENT PROFILE

Total Nursing Enrollment: *98* • Total Basic Student Enrollment, Full Time: *94* • Total Basic Student Enrollment, Part Time: *Not Reported* • Female Basic Student Enrollment: *90* • Male Basic Student Enrollment: *4* • Total RN Enrollment: *4* • Total New Fall Enrollments: *39* • Total Graduates: *32* • Basic Student Graduates: *32* • RN Student Graduates: *0*

FINANCES

Residential Annual Tuition: *$12,870* • Non-Residential Annual Tuition: *$12,870* • General Institutional Fees: *$486* • Additional Nursing Fees: *$160*

NORTH CAROLINA AGRICULTURAL & TECHNICAL UNIVERSITY

Address: 1601 East Market Street-Noble Hall, Greensboro, NC 27411
Phone: 336-334-7752
Fax: *Not Reported*
Contact: Lorna H. Harris, PhD, RN, FAAN, Dean and Professor
Email: Harrisl@ncat.edu

GENERAL INFORMATION

Type of School: *Other* • Accreditation: *Southern Association of Colleges and Schools* • Total Enrollment: *7000*

PROGRAM INFORMATION

Two Year Exit Option: *Not Reported* • NLNAC Accreditation: *Yes* • CCNE Accreditation:

NURSING STUDENT PROFILE

Total Nursing Enrollment: *170* • Total Basic Student Enrollment, Full Time: *Not Reported* • Total Basic Student Enrollment, Part Time: *Not Reported* • Female Basic Student Enrollment: *Not Reported* • Male Basic Student Enrollment: *Not Reported* • Total RN Enrollment: *6* • Total New Fall Enrollments: *13* • Total Graduates: *61* • Basic Student Graduates: *53* • RN Student Graduates: *8*

FINANCES

Residential Annual Tuition: *$2,950* • Non-Residential Annual Tuition: *$6,585* • General Institutional Fees: *$464* • Additional Nursing Fees: *$15*

NORTH CAROLINA CENTRAL UNIVERSITY

Address: P.O. Box 19798-1801, Fayettville St., Durham, NC 27704
Phone: 919-560-6431
Fax: 919-530-5343
Contact: Betty Pierce Dennis, PhD, RN, Interim Chairperson
Email: bpdennis@wpo.nccu.edu

QUEENS COLLEGE

Address: 1900 Selwyn Avenue, Charlotte, NC 28274
Phone: 704-337-2295
Fax: 704-337-2477
Contact: Joan S. McGill, DSN, RN, Professor and Chair
Email: mcgillj@queens.edu

GENERAL INFORMATION

Type of School: *4-Year College or University, Public* •
Accreditation: *Southern Association of Colleges and Schools* •
Total Enrollment: *Not Reported*

GENERAL INFORMATION

Type of School: *4-Year College or University, Private
(Religious)* • Accreditation: *Southern Association of Colleges
and Schools* • Total Enrollment: *1700*

PROGRAM INFORMATION

Two Year Exit Option: *Not Reported* • NLNAC
Accreditation: *Yes* • CCNE Accreditation:

PROGRAM INFORMATION

Two Year Exit Option: *No* • NLNAC Accreditation: *Yes* •
CCNE Accreditation: *Yes*

NURSING STUDENT PROFILE

Total Nursing Enrollment: *139* • Total Basic Student
Enrollment, Full Time: *81* • Total Basic Student Enrollment,
Part Time: *19* • Female Basic Student Enrollment: *94* • Male
Basic Student Enrollment: *6* • Total RN Enrollment: *39* •
Total New Fall Enrollments: *93* • Total Graduates: *52* • Basic
Student Graduates: *34* • RN Student Graduates: *18*

NURSING STUDENT PROFILE

Total Nursing Enrollment: *52* • Total Basic Student
Enrollment, Full Time: *28* • Total Basic Student Enrollment,
Part Time: *9* • Female Basic Student Enrollment: *35* • Male
Basic Student Enrollment: *2* • Total RN Enrollment: *15* •
Total New Fall Enrollments: *Not Reported* • Total Graduates:
30 • Basic Student Graduates: *14* • RN Student Graduates:
16

FINANCES

Residential Annual Tuition: *Not Reported* • Non-Residential
Annual Tuition: *Not Reported* • General Institutional Fees:
Not Reported • Additional Nursing Fees: *$446*

FINANCES

Residential Annual Tuition: *$11,360* • Non-Residential
Annual Tuition: *$11,360* • General Institutional Fees: *$90* •
Additional Nursing Fees: *$20*

UNIVERSITY OF NORTH CAROLINA—CHAPEL HILL

Address: Carrington Hall, Campus Box 7460, Chapel
           Hill, NC 27599
Phone: 919-966-4995
Fax: 919-843-6212
Contact: Beverly Foster, PhD, RN, Associate Professor and
           Director, Undergraduate
Email: bbfoster@email.unc.edu

GENERAL INFORMATION

Type of School: *4-Year College or University, Public* •
Accreditation: *Southern Association of Colleges and Schools* •
Total Enrollment: *24180*

PROGRAM INFORMATION

Two Year Exit Option: *No* • NLNAC Accreditation: *Yes* •
CCNE Accreditation: *Yes*

NURSING STUDENT PROFILE

Total Nursing Enrollment: *335* • Total Basic Student
Enrollment, Full Time: *292* • Total Basic Student
Enrollment, Part Time: *11* • Female Basic Student
Enrollment: *283* • Male Basic Student Enrollment: *20* • Total
RN Enrollment: *32* • Total New Fall Enrollments: *0* • Total
Graduates: *151* • Basic Student Graduates: *135* • RN
Student Graduates: *16*

FINANCES

Residential Annual Tuition: *$1,164* • Non-Residential
Annual Tuition: *$6,160* • General Institutional Fees: *$475* •
Additional Nursing Fees: *$170*

UNIVERSITY OF NORTH CAROLINA—CHARLOTTE

Address: 9201 University City Blvd, Charlotte, NC 28223
Phone: 704-684-4687
Fax: 704-687-3180
Contact: Sue Marquis Bishop, PhD, RN, FAAN, Dean
Email: isbishop@email.uncc.edu

GENERAL INFORMATION

Type of School: *4-Year College or University, Public* •
Accreditation: *Southern Association of Colleges and Schools* •
Total Enrollment: *17000*

PROGRAM INFORMATION

Two Year Exit Option: *No* • NLNAC Accreditation: *Yes* •
CCNE Accreditation:

NURSING STUDENT PROFILE

Total Nursing Enrollment: *216* • Total Basic Student
Enrollment, Full Time: *161* • Total Basic Student
Enrollment, Part Time: *4* • Female Basic Student
Enrollment: *156* • Male Basic Student Enrollment: *9* • Total
RN Enrollment: *51* • Total New Fall Enrollments: *88* • Total
Graduates: *127* • Basic Student Graduates: *92* • RN Student
Graduates: *35*

FINANCES

Residential Annual Tuition: *$1,920* • Non-Residential
Annual Tuition: *$9,190* • General Institutional Fees: *Not
Reported* • Additional Nursing Fees: *$45*

UNIVERSITY OF NORTH CAROLINA—GREENSBORO

Address: PO Box 26172, Greensboro, NC 27402
Phone: 336-334-5177
Fax: 336-334-3628
Contact: Lynne G. Pearcey, PhD, RN, CNAA, Dean
Email: l_pearce@uncg.edu

GENERAL INFORMATION

Type of School: *4-Year College or University, Public* •
Accreditation: *Southern Association of Colleges and Schools* •
Total Enrollment: *12000*

PROGRAM INFORMATION

Two Year Exit Option: *No* • NLNAC Accreditation: *Yes* •
CCNE Accreditation:

NURSING STUDENT PROFILE

Total Nursing Enrollment: *749* • Total Basic Student
Enrollment, Full Time: *520* • Total Basic Student
Enrollment, Part Time: *59* • Female Basic Student
Enrollment: *538* • Male Basic Student Enrollment: *41* • Total
RN Enrollment: *170* • Total New Fall Enrollments: *86* •
Total Graduates: *157* • Basic Student Graduates: *91* • RN
Student Graduates: *66*

FINANCES

Residential Annual Tuition: *$1,108* • Non-Residential
Annual Tuition: *$9,562* • General Institutional Fees:
$1,093 • Additional Nursing Fees: *$90*

UNIVERSITY OF NORTH CAROLINA—WILMINGTON

Address: 601 S. College Road, Wilmington, NC 28403
Phone: 910-962-3784
Fax: 910-962-3723
Contact: Bettie J. Glenn, EdD, RN, Associate Dean
Email: glennb@uncw.edu

GENERAL INFORMATION

Type of School: *4-Year College or University, Public* •
Accreditation: *Southern Association of Colleges and Schools* •
Total Enrollment: *10595*

PROGRAM INFORMATION

Two Year Exit Option: *No* • NLNAC Accreditation: *Yes* •
CCNE Accreditation:

NURSING STUDENT PROFILE

Total Nursing Enrollment: *137* • Total Basic Student
Enrollment, Full Time: *98* • Total Basic Student Enrollment,
Part Time: *0* • Female Basic Student Enrollment: *87* • Male
Basic Student Enrollment: *11* • Total RN Enrollment: *39* •
Total New Fall Enrollments: *46* • Total Graduates: *66* • Basic
Student Graduates: *53* • RN Student Graduates: *13*

FINANCES

Residential Annual Tuition: *$1,102* • Non-Residential
Annual Tuition: *$8,452* • General Institutional Fees:
$1,258 • Additional Nursing Fees: *$129*

WESTERN CAROLINA UNIVERSITY

Address: 207 Moore Building, Cullowhee, NC 28723
Phone: 828-227-7467
Fax: 828-227-7071
Contact: Ann Johnson, PhD, RN, Acting Head
Email: ajohnson@wcu.edu

GENERAL INFORMATION

Type of School: *Not Reported* • Accreditation: *Not Reported* • Total Enrollment: *Not Reported*

PROGRAM INFORMATION

Two Year Exit Option: *Not Reported* • NLNAC Accreditation: *Yes* • CCNE Accreditation:

NURSING STUDENT PROFILE

Total Nursing Enrollment: *157* • Total Basic Student Enrollment, Full Time: *85* • Total Basic Student Enrollment, Part Time: *2* • Female Basic Student Enrollment: *79* • Male Basic Student Enrollment: *8* • Total RN Enrollment: *70* • Total New Fall Enrollments: *Not Reported* • Total Graduates: *Not Reported* • Basic Student Graduates: *Not Reported* • RN Student Graduates: *Not Reported*

FINANCES

Residential Annual Tuition: *$3,076* • Non-Residential Annual Tuition: *$11,991* • General Institutional Fees: *$1,026* • Additional Nursing Fees: *Not Reported*

WINSTON-SALEM STATE UNIVERSITY

Address: 601 Martin Luther King Jr. Dr CB 19523, Winston Salem, NC 27110
Phone: 336-750-2560
Fax: 336-750-2599
Contact: Sylvia A. Flack, EdD, RN, Interim Chair for Nursing/Dean of School of Health Sciences
Email: FlackS@wssu.edu

GENERAL INFORMATION

Type of School: *4-Year College or University, Public* • Accreditation: *Southern Association of Colleges and Schools* • Total Enrollment: *2857*

PROGRAM INFORMATION

Two Year Exit Option: *Not Reported* • NLNAC Accreditation: *Yes* • CCNE Accreditation:

NURSING STUDENT PROFILE

Total Nursing Enrollment: *230* • Total Basic Student Enrollment, Full Time: *120* • Total Basic Student Enrollment, Part Time: *Not Reported* • Female Basic Student Enrollment: *102* • Male Basic Student Enrollment: *18* • Total RN Enrollment: *110* • Total New Fall Enrollments: *0* • Total Graduates: *191* • Basic Student Graduates: *83* • RN Student Graduates: *108*

FINANCES

Residential Annual Tuition: *$1,774* • Non-Residential Annual Tuition: *$8,192* • General Institutional Fees: *$1,177* • Additional Nursing Fees: *$14*

DICKINSON STATE UNIVERSITY

Address: 291 Campus Drive, Dickinson, ND 58601-4896
Phone: 701-483-2480
Fax: 701-483-2524
Contact: Mary Anne Marsh, MSN, RN, Chair,
             Department of Nursing
Email: maryanne_marsh@dsu.nodak.edu

GENERAL INFORMATION

Type of School: *Not Reported* • Accreditation: *North Central Association of Colleges and Schools* • Total Enrollment: *Not Reported*

PROGRAM INFORMATION

Two Year Exit Option: *Not Reported* • NLNAC Accreditation: *Yes* • CCNE Accreditation:

NURSING STUDENT PROFILE

Total Nursing Enrollment: *41* • Total Basic Student Enrollment, Full Time: *30* • Total Basic Student Enrollment, Part Time: *10* • Female Basic Student Enrollment: *38* • Male Basic Student Enrollment: *2* • Total RN Enrollment: *1* • Total New Fall Enrollments: *21* • Total Graduates: *26* • Basic Student Graduates: *0* • RN Student Graduates: *26*

FINANCES

Residential Annual Tuition: *$2,067* • Non-Residential Annual Tuition: *$2,316* • General Institutional Fees: *$396* • Additional Nursing Fees: *$300*

JAMESTOWN COLLEGE

Address: 6010 College Lane, Jamestown, ND 58405
Phone: 701-252-3467
Fax: 701-253-4318
Contact: Geneal E. Hall, PhD, RN, Chairperson
Email: hall@jc.edu

GENERAL INFORMATION

Type of School: *4-Year College or University, Private (Religious)* • Accreditation: *North Central Association of Colleges and Schools* • Total Enrollment: *Not Reported*

PROGRAM INFORMATION

Two Year Exit Option: *No* • NLNAC Accreditation: *Yes* • CCNE Accreditation:

NURSING STUDENT PROFILE

Total Nursing Enrollment: *45* • Total Basic Student Enrollment, Full Time: *42* • Total Basic Student Enrollment, Part Time: *3* • Female Basic Student Enrollment: *44* • Male Basic Student Enrollment: *1* • Total RN Enrollment: *0* • Total New Fall Enrollments: *0* • Total Graduates: *25* • Basic Student Graduates: *25* • RN Student Graduates: *0*

FINANCES

Residential Annual Tuition: *$7,926* • Non-Residential Annual Tuition: *$7,925* • General Institutional Fees: *$3,386* • Additional Nursing Fees: *$600*

MEDCENTER ONE COLLEGE OF NURSING

Address: 512 N 7th Street, Bismarck, ND 58501
Phone: 701-325-6734
Fax: 701-323-6967
Contact: Karen Latham, PhD, RN, Provost and
            Department Head
Email: klatham@mohs.org

GENERAL INFORMATION

Type of School: *Independent, Private (Independent)* •
Accreditation: *North Central Association of Colleges and
Schools* • Total Enrollment: *Not Reported*

PROGRAM INFORMATION

Two Year Exit Option: *Not Reported* • NLNAC
Accreditation: *Yes* • CCNE Accreditation:

NURSING STUDENT PROFILE

Total Nursing Enrollment: *91* • Total Basic Student
Enrollment, Full Time: *82* • Total Basic Student Enrollment,
Part Time: *6* • Female Basic Student Enrollment: *80* • Male
Basic Student Enrollment: *8* • Total RN Enrollment: *3* •
Total New Fall Enrollments: *48* • Total Graduates: *38* • Basic
Student Graduates: *36* • RN Student Graduates: *2*

FINANCES

Residential Annual Tuition: *$3,258* • Non-Residential
Annual Tuition: *$3,258* • General Institutional Fees: *$320* •
Additional Nursing Fees: *Not Reported*

MINOT STATE UNIVERSITY

Address: 500 University Ave West, Minot, ND 58707
Phone: 701-858-3101
Fax: 701-858-4309
Contact: Linda Pettersen, MS, RN, Department
            Chairperson
Email: petterse@minotstateu.edu

GENERAL INFORMATION

Type of School: *4-Year College or University, Public* •
Accreditation: *North Central Association of Colleges and
Schools* • Total Enrollment: *Not Reported*

PROGRAM INFORMATION

Two Year Exit Option: *No* • NLNAC Accreditation: *Yes* •
CCNE Accreditation:

NURSING STUDENT PROFILE

Total Nursing Enrollment: *112* • Total Basic Student
Enrollment, Full Time: *82* • Total Basic Student Enrollment,
Part Time: *22* • Female Basic Student Enrollment: *94* • Male
Basic Student Enrollment: *10* • Total RN Enrollment: *8* •
Total New Fall Enrollments: *16* • Total Graduates: *33* • Basic
Student Graduates: *30* • RN Student Graduates: *3*

FINANCES

Residential Annual Tuition: *$2,244* • Non-Residential
Annual Tuition: *$5,991* • General Institutional Fees: *$310* •
Additional Nursing Fees: *$218*

TRI-COLLEGE UNIVERSITY NURSING CONSORTIUM

Address: Engineering & Technology 209, PO Box 5630,
            Fargo, ND 58105-5630
Phone: 218-299-3883
Fax: 218-299-4309
Contact: Lois F. Nelson, EdD, RN, CNS, Chair and
            Professor
Email: Lois.Nelson@ndsu.nodak.edu

GENERAL INFORMATION

Type of School: *Other* • Accreditation: *North Central Association of Colleges and Schools* • Total Enrollment: *Not Reported*

PROGRAM INFORMATION

Two Year Exit Option: *No* • NLNAC Accreditation: *Yes* • CCNE Accreditation:

NURSING STUDENT PROFILE

Total Nursing Enrollment: *105* • Total Basic Student Enrollment, Full Time: *104* • Total Basic Student Enrollment, Part Time: *1* • Female Basic Student Enrollment: *99* • Male Basic Student Enrollment: *6* • Total RN Enrollment: *0* • Total New Fall Enrollments: *0* • Total Graduates: *48* • Basic Student Graduates: *48* • RN Student Graduates: *0*

FINANCES

Residential Annual Tuition: *$3,317* • Non-Residential Annual Tuition: *$7,916* • General Institutional Fees: *Not Reported* • Additional Nursing Fees: *$300*

UNIVERSITY OF MARY

Address: 7500 University Dr, Bismarck, ND 58504
Phone: 701-255-7500
Fax: *Not Reported*
Contact: Betty Rambur, DNSc, RN, Chairperson,
            Division of Nursing
Email: barambur@umary.edu

GENERAL INFORMATION

Type of School: *4-Year College or University, Private (Religious)* • Accreditation: *North Central Association of Colleges and Schools* • Total Enrollment: *Not Reported*

PROGRAM INFORMATION

Two Year Exit Option: *Not Reported* • NLNAC Accreditation: *Yes* • CCNE Accreditation:

NURSING STUDENT PROFILE

Total Nursing Enrollment: *109* • Total Basic Student Enrollment, Full Time: *96* • Total Basic Student Enrollment, Part Time: *10* • Female Basic Student Enrollment: *Not Reported* • Male Basic Student Enrollment: *Not Reported* • Total RN Enrollment: *3* • Total New Fall Enrollments: *40* • Total Graduates: *60* • Basic Student Graduates: *53* • RN Student Graduates: *7*

FINANCES

Residential Annual Tuition: *$8,200* • Non-Residential Annual Tuition: *$8,200* • General Institutional Fees: *$100* • Additional Nursing Fees: *$75*

UNIVERSITY OF NORTH DAKOTA

Address: PO Box 9025, Grand Forks, ND 58202-9025
Phone: 701-777-4555
Fax: 701-777-4096
Contact: Elizabeth Nichols, DNS, RN, FAAN, Dean and
             Professor
Email: elizabeth_nichols@mail.und.nodak.edu

GENERAL INFORMATION

Type of School: *4-Year College or University, Public* •
Accreditation: *North Central Association of Colleges and
Schools* • Total Enrollment: *Not Reported*

PROGRAM INFORMATION

Two Year Exit Option: *No* • NLNAC Accreditation: *Yes* •
CCNE Accreditation: *Yes*

NURSING STUDENT PROFILE

Total Nursing Enrollment: *266* • Total Basic Student
Enrollment, Full Time: *224* • Total Basic Student
Enrollment, Part Time: *34* • Female Basic Student
Enrollment: *219* • Male Basic Student Enrollment: *39* • Total
RN Enrollment: *8* • Total New Fall Enrollments: *49* • Total
Graduates: *82* • Basic Student Graduates: *79* • RN Student
Graduates: *3*

FINANCES

Residential Annual Tuition: *$2,754* • Non-Residential
Annual Tuition: *$7,354* • General Institutional Fees: *$508* •
Additional Nursing Fees: *$300*

CAPITAL UNIVERSITY

Address: 2199 E. Main St., Columbus, OH 43209-2394
Phone: 614-236-6703
Fax: *Not Reported*
Contact: Doris S. Edwards, EdD, RN, Dean and Professor
Email: dedwards@capital.edu

GENERAL INFORMATION

Type of School: *4-Year College or University, Private
(Religious)* • Accreditation: *North Central Association of
Colleges and Schools* • Total Enrollment: *4000*

PROGRAM INFORMATION

Two Year Exit Option: *Not Reported* • NLNAC
Accreditation: *Yes* • CCNE Accreditation: *Yes*

NURSING STUDENT PROFILE

Total Nursing Enrollment: *237* • Total Basic Student
Enrollment, Full Time: *Not Reported* • Total Basic Student
Enrollment, Part Time: *Not Reported* • Female Basic Student
Enrollment: *Not Reported* • Male Basic Student Enrollment:
Not Reported • Total RN Enrollment: *81* • Total New Fall
Enrollments: *78* • Total Graduates: *83* • Basic Student
Graduates: *65* • RN Student Graduates: *18*

FINANCES

Residential Annual Tuition: *$16,000* • Non-Residential
Annual Tuition: *$16,000* • General Institutional Fees: *$200* •
Additional Nursing Fees: *$720*

CASE WESTERN RESERVE UNIVERSITY

Address: 10900 Euclid Avenue, Cleveland, OH 44106-
           4904
Phone: 216-368-2541
Fax: 216-368-5050
Contact: Marilyn J. Lotas, PhD, RN, Director, BSN
           Program
Email: mjl25@po.cwru.edu

GENERAL INFORMATION

Type of School: *4-Year College or University, Private
(Independent)* • Accreditation: *North Central Association of
Colleges and Schools* • Total Enrollment: *Not Reported*

PROGRAM INFORMATION

Two Year Exit Option: *No* • NLNAC Accreditation: *Yes* •
CCNE Accreditation:

NURSING STUDENT PROFILE

Total Nursing Enrollment: *126* • Total Basic Student
Enrollment, Full Time: *124* • Total Basic Student
Enrollment, Part Time: *2* • Female Basic Student
Enrollment: *118* • Male Basic Student Enrollment: *8* • Total
RN Enrollment: *0* • Total New Fall Enrollments: *Not
Reported* • Total Graduates: *45* • Basic Student Graduates:
43 • RN Student Graduates: *2*

FINANCES

Residential Annual Tuition: *$21,000* • Non-Residential
Annual Tuition: *$21,000* • General Institutional Fees: *$218* •
Additional Nursing Fees: *$165*

CEDARVILLE UNIVERSITY

Address: 251 North Main St., PO Box 601, Cedarville,
           OH 45314
Phone: 937-766-7716
Fax: 937-766-7754
Contact: Irene B. Alyn, PhD, RN, Chair
Email: Alyni@cedarville.edu

GENERAL INFORMATION

Type of School: *4-Year College or University, Private
(Religious)* • Accreditation: *North Central Association of
Colleges and Schools* • Total Enrollment: *2987*

PROGRAM INFORMATION

Two Year Exit Option: *Not Reported* • NLNAC
Accreditation: *Yes* • CCNE Accreditation:

NURSING STUDENT PROFILE

Total Nursing Enrollment: *235* • Total Basic Student
Enrollment, Full Time: *235* • Total Basic Student
Enrollment, Part Time: *0* • Female Basic Student
Enrollment: *221* • Male Basic Student Enrollment: *14* • Total
RN Enrollment: *0* • Total New Fall Enrollments: *70* • Total
Graduates: *55* • Basic Student Graduates: *55* • RN Student
Graduates: *0*

FINANCES

Residential Annual Tuition: *$11,424* • Non-Residential
Annual Tuition: *$11,424* • General Institutional Fees: *$424* •
Additional Nursing Fees: *$240*

| Circle 25 on reader card | See in-depth profile for more information |

CLEVELAND STATE UNIVERSITY

Address: 1860 East 22 Street, Cleveland, OH 44115-2407
Phone: 216-523-7237
Fax: 216-687-3556
Contact: Noreen Frisch, PhD, RN, FAAN, Professor and Chairperson
Email: n.frisch@csuohio.edu

GENERAL INFORMATION

Type of School: *Not Reported* • Accreditation: *North Central Association of Colleges and Schools* • Total Enrollment: *Not Reported*

PROGRAM INFORMATION

Two Year Exit Option: *Not Reported* • NLNAC Accreditation: *Yes* • CCNE Accreditation:

NURSING STUDENT PROFILE

Total Nursing Enrollment: *223* • Total Basic Student Enrollment, Full Time: *154* • Total Basic Student Enrollment, Part Time: *10* • Female Basic Student Enrollment: *144* • Male Basic Student Enrollment: *20* • Total RN Enrollment: *59* • Total New Fall Enrollments: *69* • Total Graduates: *50* • Basic Student Graduates: *36* • RN Student Graduates: *14*

FINANCES

Residential Annual Tuition: *$3,864* • Non-Residential Annual Tuition: *$7,608* • General Institutional Fees: *$276* • Additional Nursing Fees: *$140*

COLLEGE OF MOUNT ST. JOSEPH

Address: 5701 Delphi Road, Cincinnati, OH 45233-1672
Phone: 513-244-4511
Fax: 513-451-2547
Contact: Darla Vale, DNSc, CCRN, RN, Chairperson and Associate Professor
Email: darla_vale@mail.msj.edu

GENERAL INFORMATION

Type of School: *4-Year College or University, Private (Religious)* • Accreditation: *North Central Association of Colleges and Schools* • Total Enrollment: *2300*

PROGRAM INFORMATION

Two Year Exit Option: *No* • NLNAC Accreditation: *Yes* • CCNE Accreditation:

NURSING STUDENT PROFILE

Total Nursing Enrollment: *211* • Total Basic Student Enrollment, Full Time: *117* • Total Basic Student Enrollment, Part Time: *0* • Female Basic Student Enrollment: *109* • Male Basic Student Enrollment: *8* • Total RN Enrollment: *94* • Total New Fall Enrollments: *33* • Total Graduates: *34* • Basic Student Graduates: *15* • RN Student Graduates: *19*

FINANCES

Residential Annual Tuition: *$14,200* • Non-Residential Annual Tuition: *$14,200* • General Institutional Fees: *Not Reported* • Additional Nursing Fees: *$840*

Circle 30 on reader card   **See in-depth profile for more information**

FRANCISCAN UNIVERSITY— STEUBENVILLE

Address: 1235 University Boulevard, Steubenville, OH 43952
Phone: 740-283-6324
Fax: 740-283-6449
Contact: Carolyn S. Miller, PhD, MPH, RN, Professor, Chairman
Email: cmiller@franuniv.edu

GENERAL INFORMATION

Type of School: *4-Year College or University, Private (Religious)* • Accreditation: *North Central Association of Colleges and Schools* • Total Enrollment: *2000*

PROGRAM INFORMATION

Two Year Exit Option: *Not Reported* • NLNAC Accreditation: *Yes* • CCNE Accreditation: *Yes*

NURSING STUDENT PROFILE

Total Nursing Enrollment: *118* • Total Basic Student Enrollment, Full Time: *86* • Total Basic Student Enrollment, Part Time: *2* • Female Basic Student Enrollment: *79* • Male Basic Student Enrollment: *9* • Total RN Enrollment: *30* • Total New Fall Enrollments: *19* • Total Graduates: *29* • Basic Student Graduates: *19* • RN Student Graduates: *10*

FINANCES

Residential Annual Tuition: *$11,990* • Non-Residential Annual Tuition: *$11,990* • General Institutional Fees: *$280* • Additional Nursing Fees: *Not Reported*

KENT STATE UNIVERSITY

Address: 113 Henderson Hall Box 5190, Kent, OH 44242-0001
Phone: 330-672-3777
Fax: 330-672-2433
Contact: Davina J. Gosnell, PhD, RN, Dean and Professor
Email: *Not Reported*

GENERAL INFORMATION

Type of School: *Not Reported* • Accreditation: *Not Reported* • Total Enrollment: *Not Reported*

PROGRAM INFORMATION

Two Year Exit Option: *Not Reported* • NLNAC Accreditation: *Yes* • CCNE Accreditation:

NURSING STUDENT PROFILE

Total Nursing Enrollment: *734* • Total Basic Student Enrollment, Full Time: *603* • Total Basic Student Enrollment, Part Time: *104* • Female Basic Student Enrollment: *Not Reported* • Male Basic Student Enrollment: *Not Reported* • Total RN Enrollment: *27* • Total New Fall Enrollments: *207* • Total Graduates: *Not Reported* • Basic Student Graduates: *Not Reported* • RN Student Graduates: *Not Reported*

FINANCES

Residential Annual Tuition: *$4,288* • Non-Residential Annual Tuition: *$8,576* • General Institutional Fees: *Not Reported* • Additional Nursing Fees: *Not Reported*

LOURDES COLLEGE

Address: 6832 Convent Boulevard, Sylvania, OH 43560
Phone: 419-824-3794
Fax: 419-824-3513
Contact: Elizabeth Cain, MS, RN, Dean of the School of Nursing and Allied Health
Email: ecain@lourdes.edu

GENERAL INFORMATION

Type of School: *4-Year College or University, Private (Religious)* • Accreditation: *North Central Association of Colleges and Schools* • Total Enrollment: *1300*

PROGRAM INFORMATION

Two Year Exit Option: *No* • NLNAC Accreditation: *Yes* • CCNE Accreditation:

NURSING STUDENT PROFILE

Total Nursing Enrollment: *186* • Total Basic Student Enrollment, Full Time: *57* • Total Basic Student Enrollment, Part Time: *52* • Female Basic Student Enrollment: *Not Reported* • Male Basic Student Enrollment: *Not Reported* • Total RN Enrollment: *77* • Total New Fall Enrollments: *23* • Total Graduates: *42* • Basic Student Graduates: *13* • RN Student Graduates: *29*

FINANCES

Residential Annual Tuition: *$12,600* • Non-Residential Annual Tuition: *Not Reported* • General Institutional Fees: *$300* • Additional Nursing Fees: *$0*

MALONE COLLEGE

Address: 515 25th St., NW, Canton, OH 44709
Phone: 330-471-8366
Fax: 330-471-8478
Contact: Loretta Reinhart, PhD, RN, Chair, Dean
Email: lornhart@malone.edu

GENERAL INFORMATION

Type of School: *4-Year College or University, Private (Religious)* • Accreditation: *North Central Association of Colleges and Schools* • Total Enrollment: *2168*

PROGRAM INFORMATION

Two Year Exit Option: *Not Reported* • NLNAC Accreditation: *Yes* • CCNE Accreditation:

NURSING STUDENT PROFILE

Total Nursing Enrollment: *154* • Total Basic Student Enrollment, Full Time: *96* • Total Basic Student Enrollment, Part Time: *10* • Female Basic Student Enrollment: *100* • Male Basic Student Enrollment: *6* • Total RN Enrollment: *48* • Total New Fall Enrollments: *32* • Total Graduates: *52* • Basic Student Graduates: *25* • RN Student Graduates: *27*

FINANCES

Residential Annual Tuition: *$12,800* • Non-Residential Annual Tuition: *$12,800* • General Institutional Fees: *$230* • Additional Nursing Fees: *$270*

MEDCENTRAL HEALTH SYSTEM

Address: 335 Glessner Avenue, Mansfield, OH 44903-2265
Phone: 419-520-2600
Fax: 419-520-2610
Contact: Patrice McCarthy, PhD, RN, President / Dean
Email: mccarthy@osu.edu

GENERAL INFORMATION

Type of School: *Hospital, Private (Independent)* •
Accreditation: *Not Reported* • Total Enrollment: *20*

PROGRAM INFORMATION

Two Year Exit Option: *Not Reported* • NLNAC
Accreditation: *Not Reported* • CCNE Accreditation:

NURSING STUDENT PROFILE

Total Nursing Enrollment: *31* • Total Basic Student
Enrollment, Full Time: *22* • Total Basic Student Enrollment,
Part Time: *8* • Female Basic Student Enrollment: *27* • Male
Basic Student Enrollment: *3* • Total RN Enrollment: *1* •
Total New Fall Enrollments: *17* • Total Graduates: *0* • Basic
Student Graduates: *0* • RN Student Graduates: *0*

FINANCES

Residential Annual Tuition: *Not Reported* • Non-Residential
Annual Tuition: *Not Reported* • General Institutional Fees:
Not Reported • Additional Nursing Fees: *Not Reported*

MEDICAL COLLEGE OF OHIO

Address: 3015 Arlington Avenue, Toledo, OH 43614-5803
Phone: 419-383-5859
Fax: 419-383-5894
Contact: Susan Batten, PhD, RN, CNS, Associate Dean, Undergraduate Program
Email: sbatten@mco.edu

GENERAL INFORMATION

Type of School: *Other, Public* • Accreditation: *North Central
Association of Colleges and Schools* • Total Enrollment: *89*

PROGRAM INFORMATION

Two Year Exit Option: *No* • NLNAC Accreditation: *Not
Reported* • CCNE Accreditation: *Yes*

NURSING STUDENT PROFILE

Total Nursing Enrollment: *111* • Total Basic Student
Enrollment, Full Time: *111* • Total Basic Student
Enrollment, Part Time: *0* • Female Basic Student
Enrollment: *99* • Male Basic Student Enrollment: *12* • Total
RN Enrollment: *0* • Total New Fall Enrollments: *93* • Total
Graduates: *42* • Basic Student Graduates: *42* • RN Student
Graduates: *0*

FINANCES

Residential Annual Tuition: *$3,832* • Non-Residential
Annual Tuition: *$10,578* • General Institutional Fees: *$852* •
Additional Nursing Fees: *$150*

MERCY COLLEGE OF NORTHWEST OHIO

Address: 2221 Madison Avenue, Toledo, OH 43624-1132
Phone: 419-251-1583
Fax: 419-251-1570
Contact: Maria E. Nowicki, PhD, RN, Director of Nursing
Email: Maria.Nowicki@mercycollege.edu

GENERAL INFORMATION

Type of School: *4-Year College or University, Private (Religious)* • Accreditation: *North Central Association of Colleges and Schools* • Total Enrollment: *222*

PROGRAM INFORMATION

Two Year Exit Option: *Not Reported* • NLNAC Accreditation: *Not Reported* • CCNE Accreditation:

NURSING STUDENT PROFILE

Total Nursing Enrollment: *150* • Total Basic Student Enrollment, Full Time: *36* • Total Basic Student Enrollment, Part Time: *9* • Female Basic Student Enrollment: *41* • Male Basic Student Enrollment: *4* • Total RN Enrollment: *105* • Total New Fall Enrollments: *27* • Total Graduates: *0* • Basic Student Graduates: *0* • RN Student Graduates: *0*

FINANCES

Residential Annual Tuition: *$4,000* • Non-Residential Annual Tuition: *$4,000* • General Institutional Fees: *$65* • Additional Nursing Fees: *$250*

MOUNT CARMEL COLLEGE OF NURSING

Address: 127 S Davis Ave, Columbus, OH 43222-1504
Phone: 614-234-5032
Fax: *Not Reported*
Contact: Ann E. Schiele, PhD, RN, President / Dean
Email: aschiele@mchs.com

GENERAL INFORMATION

Type of School: *Not Reported* • Accreditation: *Not Reported* • Total Enrollment: *Not Reported*

PROGRAM INFORMATION

Two Year Exit Option: *Not Reported* • NLNAC Accreditation: *Yes* • CCNE Accreditation:

NURSING STUDENT PROFILE

Total Nursing Enrollment: *305* • Total Basic Student Enrollment, Full Time: *Not Reported* • Total Basic Student Enrollment, Part Time: *Not Reported* • Female Basic Student Enrollment: *Not Reported* • Male Basic Student Enrollment: *Not Reported* • Total RN Enrollment: *28* • Total New Fall Enrollments: *98* • Total Graduates: *85* • Basic Student Graduates: *75* • RN Student Graduates: *10*

FINANCES

Residential Annual Tuition: *Not Reported* • Non-Residential Annual Tuition: *Not Reported* • General Institutional Fees: *Not Reported* • Additional Nursing Fees: *Not Reported*

Circle 86 on reader card   See in-depth profile for more information

THE OHIO STATE UNIVERSITY

Address: 1585 Neil Avenue, Columbus, OH 43210
Phone: 614-292-8900
Fax: *Not Reported*
Contact: Carole A. Anderson, PhD, RN, FAAN, Dean and Professor; Asst. VP for Health Sciences
Email: Anderson.32@osu.edu

GENERAL INFORMATION

Type of School: *4-Year College or University, Public* • Accreditation: *North Central Association of Colleges and Schools* • Total Enrollment: 55233

PROGRAM INFORMATION

Two Year Exit Option: *Not Reported* • NLNAC Accreditation: *Not Reported* • CCNE Accreditation: *Yes*

NURSING STUDENT PROFILE

Total Nursing Enrollment: *407* • Total Basic Student Enrollment, Full Time: *Not Reported* • Total Basic Student Enrollment, Part Time: *Not Reported* • Female Basic Student Enrollment: *Not Reported* • Male Basic Student Enrollment: *Not Reported* • Total RN Enrollment: *16* • Total New Fall Enrollments: *148* • Total Graduates: *137* • Basic Student Graduates: *133* • RN Student Graduates: *4*

FINANCES

Residential Annual Tuition: *$4,137* • Non-Residential Annual Tuition: *$12,087* • General Institutional Fees: *Not Reported* • Additional Nursing Fees: *Not Reported*

OTTERBEIN COLLEGE

Address: One Otterbein College, Westerville, OH 43081
Phone: 614-823-1614
Fax: *Not Reported*
Contact: Judy Strayer, PhD, RN, CNS, Chair, Dept. of Nursing
Email: JStrayer@otterbein.edu

GENERAL INFORMATION

Type of School: *Other* • Accreditation: *Not Reported* • Total Enrollment: *Not Reported*

PROGRAM INFORMATION

Two Year Exit Option: *Not Reported* • NLNAC Accreditation: *Yes* • CCNE Accreditation:

NURSING STUDENT PROFILE

Total Nursing Enrollment: *173* • Total Basic Student Enrollment, Full Time: *Not Reported* • Total Basic Student Enrollment, Part Time: *Not Reported* • Female Basic Student Enrollment: *Not Reported* • Male Basic Student Enrollment: *Not Reported* • Total RN Enrollment: *8* • Total New Fall Enrollments: *35* • Total Graduates: *37* • Basic Student Graduates: *30* • RN Student Graduates: *7*

FINANCES

Residential Annual Tuition: *Not Reported* • Non-Residential Annual Tuition: *Not Reported* • General Institutional Fees: *Not Reported* • Additional Nursing Fees: *Not Reported*

THE UNIVERSITY OF AKRON

Address: 209 Carroll Street, Akron, OH 44325-3701
Phone: 330-972-7465
Fax: 330-972-5737
Contact: Cheryl Buchanan, MSN, RN, Coordinator, Baccalaureate Programs
Email: CB12@uakron.edu

GENERAL INFORMATION

Type of School: *Not Reported* • Accreditation: *Not Reported* • Total Enrollment: *Not Reported*

PROGRAM INFORMATION

Two Year Exit Option: *Not Reported* • NLNAC Accreditation: *Yes* • CCNE Accreditation:

NURSING STUDENT PROFILE

Total Nursing Enrollment: *391* • Total Basic Student Enrollment, Full Time: *346* • Total Basic Student Enrollment, Part Time: *0* • Female Basic Student Enrollment: *303* • Male Basic Student Enrollment: *43* • Total RN Enrollment: *45* • Total New Fall Enrollments: *122* • Total Graduates: *153* • Basic Student Graduates: *114* • RN Student Graduates: *39*

FINANCES

Residential Annual Tuition: *$3,755* • Non-Residential Annual Tuition: *$8,716* • General Institutional Fees: *$198* • Additional Nursing Fees: *$60*

UNIVERSITY OF CINCINNATI—RAYMOND WALTERS COLLEGE

Address: 9555 Plainfield Road, Cincinnati, OH 45236
Phone: 513-558-0310
Fax: 513-558-5054
Contact: Susan Kennerly, PhD, RN, Associate Dean for Academic Affairs
Email: Susan.Kennerly@uc.edu

GENERAL INFORMATION

Type of School: *2-Year College or University, Public* • Accreditation: *North Central Association of Colleges and Schools* • Total Enrollment: *3500*

PROGRAM INFORMATION

Two Year Exit Option: *Not Reported* • NLNAC Accreditation: *Yes* • CCNE Accreditation:

NURSING STUDENT PROFILE

Total Nursing Enrollment: *356* • Total Basic Student Enrollment, Full Time: *227* • Total Basic Student Enrollment, Part Time: *11* • Female Basic Student Enrollment: *221* • Male Basic Student Enrollment: *17* • Total RN Enrollment: *118* • Total New Fall Enrollments: *90* • Total Graduates: *140* • Basic Student Graduates: *86* • RN Student Graduates: *54*

FINANCES

Residential Annual Tuition: *$4,467* • Non-Residential Annual Tuition: *$12,744* • General Institutional Fees: *$870* • Additional Nursing Fees: *Not Reported*

URSULINE COLLEGE

Address: 2550 Lander Rd, Pepper Pike, OH 44124-4398
Phone: 440-646-8168
Fax: 440-449-4267
Contact: Kathleen Mary Flanagan, MSN, MA, RN,
             Associate Professor, Dir. Undergraduate Program
Email: kflanaga@ursuline.edu

WALSH UNIVERSITY

Address: 2020 Easton Street NW, North Canton, OH
             44720-3396
Phone: 330-490-7250
Fax: 330-490-7206
Contact: Mary E. Meeker, DNSc, RN, CNS, Chair,
             Nursing Division
Email: mmeeker@walsh.edu

GENERAL INFORMATION

Type of School: *Not Reported* • Accreditation: *Not Reported* •
Total Enrollment: *Not Reported*

GENERAL INFORMATION

Type of School: *4-Year College or University, Private
(Religious)* • Accreditation: *North Central Association of
Colleges and Schools* • Total Enrollment: *4500*

PROGRAM INFORMATION

Two Year Exit Option: *Not Reported* • NLNAC
Accreditation: *Not Reported* • CCNE Accreditation: *Yes*

PROGRAM INFORMATION

Two Year Exit Option: *Not Reported* • NLNAC
Accreditation: *Yes* • CCNE Accreditation:

NURSING STUDENT PROFILE

Total Nursing Enrollment: *242* • Total Basic Student
Enrollment, Full Time: *120* • Total Basic Student
Enrollment, Part Time: *30* • Female Basic Student
Enrollment: *139* • Male Basic Student Enrollment: *11* • Total
RN Enrollment: *92* • Total New Fall Enrollments: *33* • Total
Graduates: *72* • Basic Student Graduates: *37* • RN Student
Graduates: *35*

NURSING STUDENT PROFILE

Total Nursing Enrollment: *33* • Total Basic Student
Enrollment, Full Time: *Not Reported* • Total Basic Student
Enrollment, Part Time: *Not Reported* • Female Basic Student
Enrollment: *29* • Male Basic Student Enrollment: *4* • Total
RN Enrollment: *0* • Total New Fall Enrollments: *Not
Reported* • Total Graduates: *Not Reported* • Basic Student
Graduates: *Not Reported* • RN Student Graduates: *Not
Reported*

FINANCES

Residential Annual Tuition: *$10,800* • Non-Residential
Annual Tuition: *$10,800* • General Institutional Fees: *Not
Reported* • Additional Nursing Fees: *$40*

FINANCES

Residential Annual Tuition: *$12,050* • Non-Residential
Annual Tuition: *$12,050* • General Institutional Fees: *$288* •
Additional Nursing Fees: *$65*

WRIGHT STATE UNIVERSITY

Address: 3640 Colonel Glenn Highway, Dayton, OH 45435
Phone: 937-775-3133
Fax: 937-775-4571
Contact: Patricia A. Martin, PhD, RN, Dean
Email: patricia.martin@wright.edu

GENERAL INFORMATION

Type of School: *4-Year College or University, Public* • Accreditation: *North Central Association of Colleges and Schools* • Total Enrollment: *15810*

PROGRAM INFORMATION

Two Year Exit Option: *No* • NLNAC Accreditation: *Yes* • CCNE Accreditation:

NURSING STUDENT PROFILE

Total Nursing Enrollment: *343* • Total Basic Student Enrollment, Full Time: *200* • Total Basic Student Enrollment, Part Time: *49* • Female Basic Student Enrollment: *238* • Male Basic Student Enrollment: *11* • Total RN Enrollment: *94* • Total New Fall Enrollments: *50* • Total Graduates: *104* • Basic Student Graduates: *90* • RN Student Graduates: *14*

FINANCES

Residential Annual Tuition: *$3,751* • Non-Residential Annual Tuition: *$9,315* • General Institutional Fees: *$906* • Additional Nursing Fees: *$90*

XAVIER UNIVERSITY

Address: 3800 Victory Parkway, Cincinnati, OH 45207-7351
Phone: 513-745-3815
Fax: 513-745-1987
Contact: Susan M. Schmidt, PhD, RN, COHN-S, CNS, Chair
Email: schmidts@xu.edu

GENERAL INFORMATION

Type of School: *4-Year College or University, Private (Religious)* • Accreditation: *North Central Association of Colleges and Schools* • Total Enrollment: *6523*

PROGRAM INFORMATION

Two Year Exit Option: *Not Reported* • NLNAC Accreditation: *Yes* • CCNE Accreditation:

NURSING STUDENT PROFILE

Total Nursing Enrollment: *96* • Total Basic Student Enrollment, Full Time: *75* • Total Basic Student Enrollment, Part Time: *6* • Female Basic Student Enrollment: *78* • Male Basic Student Enrollment: *3* • Total RN Enrollment: *15* • Total New Fall Enrollments: *17* • Total Graduates: *34* • Basic Student Graduates: *24* • RN Student Graduates: *10*

FINANCES

Residential Annual Tuition: *Not Reported* • Non-Residential Annual Tuition: *Not Reported* • General Institutional Fees: *$100* • Additional Nursing Fees: *$55*

YOUNGSTOWN STATE UNIVERSITY

Address:　One University Place, Youngstown, OH 44555
Phone:　330-742-3292
Fax:　*Not Reported*
Contact:　Patricia A. McCarthy, PhD, RN, CS, Chairperson and Professor
Email:　nursing@ysu.cc.edu

EAST CENTRAL UNIVERSITY

Address:　1000 East 14th St, Ada, OK 74820-6229
Phone:　580-774-3261
Fax:　*Not Reported*
Contact:　Elizabeth Schmelling, PhD, RN, Professor and Chair
Email:　eschmlng@mailclerk.ecok.edu

GENERAL INFORMATION

Type of School: *4-Year College or University, Public* •
Accreditation: *North Central Association of Colleges and Schools* • Total Enrollment: *11800*

GENERAL INFORMATION

Type of School: *4-Year College or University, Public* •
Accreditation: *North Central Association of Colleges and Schools* • Total Enrollment: *4800*

PROGRAM INFORMATION

Two Year Exit Option: *Not Reported* • NLNAC
Accreditation: *Yes* • CCNE Accreditation:

PROGRAM INFORMATION

Two Year Exit Option: *Not Reported* • NLNAC
Accreditation: *Yes* • CCNE Accreditation:

NURSING STUDENT PROFILE

Total Nursing Enrollment: *70* • Total Basic Student Enrollment, Full Time: *49* • Total Basic Student Enrollment, Part Time: *0* • Female Basic Student Enrollment: *43* • Male Basic Student Enrollment: *6* • Total RN Enrollment: *21* • Total New Fall Enrollments: *17* • Total Graduates: *63* • Basic Student Graduates: *47* • RN Student Graduates: *16*

NURSING STUDENT PROFILE

Total Nursing Enrollment: *90* • Total Basic Student Enrollment, Full Time: *Not Reported* • Total Basic Student Enrollment, Part Time: *Not Reported* • Female Basic Student Enrollment: *65* • Male Basic Student Enrollment: *6* • Total RN Enrollment: *19* • Total New Fall Enrollments: *50* • Total Graduates: *Not Reported* • Basic Student Graduates: *Not Reported* • RN Student Graduates: *Not Reported*

FINANCES

Residential Annual Tuition: *$4,320* • Non-Residential Annual Tuition: *$6,648* • General Institutional Fees: *$768* • Additional Nursing Fees: *$200*

FINANCES

Residential Annual Tuition: *Not Reported* • Non-Residential Annual Tuition: *Not Reported* • General Institutional Fees: *Not Reported* • Additional Nursing Fees: *Not Reported*

LANGSTON UNIVERSITY

Address: P.O. Box 1500, Langston, OK 73050
Phone: 405-466-3411
Fax: *Not Reported*
Contact: Carolyn T. Cornegay, PhD, RN, Director
Email: ctkornegay@lunet.edu

GENERAL INFORMATION

Type of School: *Governmental Agency, Public* • Accreditation: *North Central Association of Colleges and Schools* • Total Enrollment: *4200*

PROGRAM INFORMATION

Two Year Exit Option: *Not Reported* • NLNAC Accreditation: *Yes* • CCNE Accreditation:

NURSING STUDENT PROFILE

Total Nursing Enrollment: *126* • Total Basic Student Enrollment, Full Time: *115* • Total Basic Student Enrollment, Part Time: *11* • Female Basic Student Enrollment: *111* • Male Basic Student Enrollment: *15* • Total RN Enrollment: *0* • Total New Fall Enrollments: *49* • Total Graduates: *52* • Basic Student Graduates: *49* • RN Student Graduates: *3*

FINANCES

Residential Annual Tuition: *$1,744* • Non-Residential Annual Tuition: *$2,784* • General Institutional Fees: *$470* • Additional Nursing Fees: *$130*

NORTHERN OKLAHOMA COLLEGE

Address: 1220 E Grand Ave # 310, Tonkawa, OK 74653-4022
Phone: 580-327-8489
Fax: 580-327-8434
Contact: Lannie Buechner, EdD, RN, Director
Email: flbuechner@nwosu.edu

GENERAL INFORMATION

Type of School: *2-Year College or University, Public* • Accreditation: *North Central Association of Colleges and Schools* • Total Enrollment: *2000*

PROGRAM INFORMATION

Two Year Exit Option: *No* • NLNAC Accreditation: *Yes* • CCNE Accreditation:

NURSING STUDENT PROFILE

Total Nursing Enrollment: *40* • Total Basic Student Enrollment, Full Time: *19* • Total Basic Student Enrollment, Part Time: *13* • Female Basic Student Enrollment: *27* • Male Basic Student Enrollment: *5* • Total RN Enrollment: *8* • Total New Fall Enrollments: *14* • Total Graduates: *11* • Basic Student Graduates: *10* • RN Student Graduates: *1*

FINANCES

Residential Annual Tuition: *$1,572* • Non-Residential Annual Tuition: *$5,636* • General Institutional Fees: *$420* • Additional Nursing Fees: *$81*

NORTHWESTERN OKLAHOMA STATE UNIVERSITY

Address: 709 Oklahoma Blvd, Alva, OK 73717
Phone: 580-327-8489
Fax: 580-327-8434
Contact: Janice E. Stephen, PhD, RN, Dean
Email: jestephns@rwosu.edu

GENERAL INFORMATION

Type of School: *4-Year College or University, Public* • Accreditation: *North Central Association of Colleges and Schools* • Total Enrollment: *2000*

PROGRAM INFORMATION

Two Year Exit Option: *Not Reported* • NLNAC Accreditation: *Yes* • CCNE Accreditation:

NURSING STUDENT PROFILE

Total Nursing Enrollment: *Not Reported* • Total Basic Student Enrollment, Full Time: *Not Reported* • Total Basic Student Enrollment, Part Time: *Not Reported* • Female Basic Student Enrollment: *Not Reported* • Male Basic Student Enrollment: *Not Reported* • Total RN Enrollment: *Not Reported* • Total New Fall Enrollments: *Not Reported* • Total Graduates: *Not Reported* • Basic Student Graduates: *Not Reported* • RN Student Graduates: *Not Reported*

FINANCES

Residential Annual Tuition: *Not Reported* • Non-Residential Annual Tuition: *Not Reported* • General Institutional Fees: *Not Reported* • Additional Nursing Fees: *Not Reported*

OKLAHOMA BAPTIST UNIVERSITY

Address: 500 W. University, Shawnee, OK 74804
Phone: 405-878-2081
Fax: 405-878-2083
Contact: Lana Bolhouse, PhD, RN, Dean, School of Nursing
Email: lana_bolhouse@mail.okbu.edu

GENERAL INFORMATION

Type of School: *4-Year College or University, Private (Independent)* • Accreditation: *North Central Association of Colleges and Schools* • Total Enrollment: *1933*

PROGRAM INFORMATION

Two Year Exit Option: *No* • NLNAC Accreditation: *Yes* • CCNE Accreditation:

NURSING STUDENT PROFILE

Total Nursing Enrollment: *112* • Total Basic Student Enrollment, Full Time: *111* • Total Basic Student Enrollment, Part Time: *1* • Female Basic Student Enrollment: *111* • Male Basic Student Enrollment: *1* • Total RN Enrollment: *0* • Total New Fall Enrollments: *16* • Total Graduates: *26* • Basic Student Graduates: *26* • RN Student Graduates: *0*

FINANCES

Residential Annual Tuition: *$10,800* • Non-Residential Annual Tuition: *$10,800* • General Institutional Fees: *$369* • Additional Nursing Fees: *$560*

OKLAHOMA CITY UNIVERSITY

Address: 2501 N Blackwelder, Oklahoma City, OK
            73106-1402
Phone: 405-521-5900
Fax: 405-521-5914
Contact: Andrea M. West, PhD, RN, Dean
Email: awest@okcu.edu

GENERAL INFORMATION

Type of School: *4-Year College or University, Private
(Religious)* • Accreditation: *North Central Association of
Colleges and Schools* • Total Enrollment: *Not Reported*

PROGRAM INFORMATION

Two Year Exit Option: *Not Reported* • NLNAC
Accreditation: *Yes* • CCNE Accreditation:

NURSING STUDENT PROFILE

Total Nursing Enrollment: *73* • Total Basic Student
Enrollment, Full Time: *69* • Total Basic Student Enrollment,
Part Time: *2* • Female Basic Student Enrollment: *63* • Male
Basic Student Enrollment: *8* • Total RN Enrollment: *2* •
Total New Fall Enrollments: *24* • Total Graduates: *16* • Basic
Student Graduates: *15* • RN Student Graduates: *1*

FINANCES

Residential Annual Tuition: *$9,880* • Non-Residential
Annual Tuition: *$9,880* • General Institutional Fees: *$40* •
Additional Nursing Fees: *$88*

ORAL ROBERTS UNIVERSITY

Address: 7777 South Lewis Ave, Tulsa, OK 74171-0003
Phone: 918-495-6198
Fax: 918-495-6020
Contact: Kenda Jezek, PhD, RN, Dean
Email: kjezek@oru.edu

GENERAL INFORMATION

Type of School: *4-Year College or University, Private
(Religious)* • Accreditation: *North Central Association of
Colleges and Schools* • Total Enrollment: *5368*

PROGRAM INFORMATION

Two Year Exit Option: *Not Reported* • NLNAC
Accreditation: *Yes* • CCNE Accreditation:

NURSING STUDENT PROFILE

Total Nursing Enrollment: *40* • Total Basic Student
Enrollment, Full Time: *40* • Total Basic Student Enrollment,
Part Time: *0* • Female Basic Student Enrollment: *39* • Male
Basic Student Enrollment: *1* • Total RN Enrollment: *0* •
Total New Fall Enrollments: *29* • Total Graduates: *25* • Basic
Student Graduates: *25* • RN Student Graduates: *0*

FINANCES

Residential Annual Tuition: *$11,300* • Non-Residential
Annual Tuition: *$11,300* • General Institutional Fees: *$350* •
Additional Nursing Fees: *$200*

SOUTHERN NAZARENE UNIVERISTY

Address: 6729 NW 39th Expressway, Bethany, OK 73008
Phone: 405-491-6365
Fax: *Not Reported*
Contact: Ann Ferguson, PhD, RN, Chairperson
Email: afergus9o@snu.edu

GENERAL INFORMATION

Type of School: *4-Year College or University, Private (Religious)* • Accreditation: *North Central Association of Colleges and Schools* • Total Enrollment: *2013*

PROGRAM INFORMATION

Two Year Exit Option: *No* • NLNAC Accreditation: *Yes* • CCNE Accreditation:

NURSING STUDENT PROFILE

Total Nursing Enrollment: *81* • Total Basic Student Enrollment, Full Time: *Not Reported* • Total Basic Student Enrollment, Part Time: *Not Reported* • Female Basic Student Enrollment: *Not Reported* • Male Basic Student Enrollment: *Not Reported* • Total RN Enrollment: *50* • Total New Fall Enrollments: *34* • Total Graduates: *18* • Basic Student Graduates: *16* • RN Student Graduates: *2*

FINANCES

Residential Annual Tuition: *$8,850* • Non-Residential Annual Tuition: *$8,850* • General Institutional Fees: *$390* • Additional Nursing Fees: *$150*

SOUTHWESTERN OKLAHOMA STATE UNIVERSITY

Address: 100 Campus Drive, Weatherford, OK 73096
Phone: 580-774-3261
Fax: 580-774-7075
Contact: Patricia Meyer, PhD, RN, Associate Dean
Email: meyerp@swosu.edu

GENERAL INFORMATION

Type of School: *4-Year College or University, Public* • Accreditation: *North Central Association of Colleges and Schools* • Total Enrollment: *4468*

PROGRAM INFORMATION

Two Year Exit Option: *No* • NLNAC Accreditation: *Yes* • CCNE Accreditation:

NURSING STUDENT PROFILE

Total Nursing Enrollment: *65* • Total Basic Student Enrollment, Full Time: *53* • Total Basic Student Enrollment, Part Time: *Not Reported* • Female Basic Student Enrollment: *44* • Male Basic Student Enrollment: *9* • Total RN Enrollment: *12* • Total New Fall Enrollments: *29* • Total Graduates: *33* • Basic Student Graduates: *16* • RN Student Graduates: *17*

FINANCES

Residential Annual Tuition: *$54* • Non-Residential Annual Tuition: *$155* • General Institutional Fees: *$18* • Additional Nursing Fees: *$50*

UNIVERSITY OF CENTRAL OKLAHOMA

Address: 100 N University Dr, Edmond, OK 73034-5207
Phone: 405-974-5176
Fax: 405-974-3848
Contact: Pat Lagrow, PhD, RN, Chairperson
Email: plagrow@ucok.edu

THE UNIVERSITY OF TULSA

Address: 600 S College Ave, Tulsa, OK 74104-3126
Phone: 918-631-3116
Fax: 918-631-2068
Contact: Susan Gaston, PhD, RN, Director, School of Nursing
Email: susan-gaston@utulsa.edu

GENERAL INFORMATION

Type of School: *4-Year College or University, Public* • Accreditation: *North Central Association of Colleges and Schools* • Total Enrollment: *14195*

GENERAL INFORMATION

Type of School: *Not Reported* • Accreditation: *North Central Association of Colleges and Schools* • Total Enrollment: *Not Reported*

PROGRAM INFORMATION

Two Year Exit Option: *Not Reported* • NLNAC Accreditation: *Yes* • CCNE Accreditation:

PROGRAM INFORMATION

Two Year Exit Option: *No* • NLNAC Accreditation: *Yes* • CCNE Accreditation:

NURSING STUDENT PROFILE

Total Nursing Enrollment: *139* • Total Basic Student Enrollment, Full Time: *127* • Total Basic Student Enrollment, Part Time: *1* • Female Basic Student Enrollment: *114* • Male Basic Student Enrollment: *14* • Total RN Enrollment: *11* • Total New Fall Enrollments: *82* • Total Graduates: *62* • Basic Student Graduates: *59* • RN Student Graduates: *3*

NURSING STUDENT PROFILE

Total Nursing Enrollment: *Not Reported* • Total Basic Student Enrollment, Full Time: *Not Reported* • Total Basic Student Enrollment, Part Time: *Not Reported* • Female Basic Student Enrollment: *Not Reported* • Male Basic Student Enrollment: *Not Reported* • Total RN Enrollment: *Not Reported* • Total New Fall Enrollments: *Not Reported* • Total Graduates: *Not Reported* • Basic Student Graduates: *Not Reported* • RN Student Graduates: *Not Reported*

FINANCES

Residential Annual Tuition: *Not Reported* • Non-Residential Annual Tuition: *Not Reported* • General Institutional Fees: *Not Reported* • Additional Nursing Fees: *Not Reported*

FINANCES

Residential Annual Tuition: *Not Reported* • Non-Residential Annual Tuition: *Not Reported* • General Institutional Fees: *Not Reported* • Additional Nursing Fees: *Not Reported*

UNIVERSITY OF OKLAHOMA

Address: PO Box 26901, Oklahoma City, OK 73190-
             0001
Phone: 405-271-2420
Fax: 405-271-3443
Contact: Patricia R. Forni, PhD, RN, FAAN, Dean and
             Professor
Email: Patricia-Forni@ouhsc.edu

GENERAL INFORMATION

Type of School: *4-Year College or University, Public* •
Accreditation: *North Central Association of Colleges and
Schools* • Total Enrollment: *27000*

PROGRAM INFORMATION

Two Year Exit Option: *Not Reported* • NLNAC
Accreditation: *Yes* • CCNE Accreditation:

NURSING STUDENT PROFILE

Total Nursing Enrollment: *334* • Total Basic Student
Enrollment, Full Time: *236* • Total Basic Student
Enrollment, Part Time: *34* • Female Basic Student
Enrollment: *242* • Male Basic Student Enrollment: *28* • Total
RN Enrollment: *64* • Total New Fall Enrollments: *171* •
Total Graduates: *182* • Basic Student Graduates: *129* • RN
Student Graduates: *53*

FINANCES

Residential Annual Tuition: *$1,935* • Non-Residential
Annual Tuition: *$6,540* • General Institutional Fees: *$254* •
Additional Nursing Fees: *$428*

LINFIELD COLLEGE

Address: 2255 North West Northrup Street, Portland, OR
             97210
Phone: 503-413-7694
Fax: *Not Reported*
Contact: Pamela Harris, PhD, RN, Dean
Email: pharris@linfield.edu

GENERAL INFORMATION

Type of School: *4-Year College or University, Private
(Religious)* • Accreditation: *Northwestern Association of Schools
and Colleges* • Total Enrollment: *1500*

PROGRAM INFORMATION

Two Year Exit Option: *Not Reported* • NLNAC
Accreditation: *Yes* • CCNE Accreditation:

NURSING STUDENT PROFILE

Total Nursing Enrollment: *329* • Total Basic Student
Enrollment, Full Time: *297* • Total Basic Student
Enrollment, Part Time: *22* • Female Basic Student
Enrollment: *302* • Male Basic Student Enrollment: *17* • Total
RN Enrollment: *10* • Total New Fall Enrollments: *116* •
Total Graduates: *71* • Basic Student Graduates: *71* • RN
Student Graduates: *0*

FINANCES

Residential Annual Tuition: *$19,380* • Non-Residential
Annual Tuition: *$19,380* • General Institutional Fees: *$225* •
Additional Nursing Fees: *Not Reported*

OREGON HEALTH SCIENCES UNIVERSITY

Address: 3181 South West Sam Jackson Park Road,
            Portland, OR 97201
Phone: 503-494-3894
Fax: 503-494-4350
Contact: Beverly Hoeffer, DNSc, RN, FAAN, Assoc.
            Dean for Academic Affairs
Email: hoefferb@ohsu.edu

GENERAL INFORMATION

Type of School: *Other, Public* • Accreditation: *Northwestern Association of Schools and Colleges* • Total Enrollment: *2679*

PROGRAM INFORMATION

Two Year Exit Option: *Not Reported* • NLNAC Accreditation: *Yes* • CCNE Accreditation: *Yes*

NURSING STUDENT PROFILE

Total Nursing Enrollment: *497* • Total Basic Student Enrollment, Full Time: *354* • Total Basic Student Enrollment, Part Time: *11* • Female Basic Student Enrollment: *336* • Male Basic Student Enrollment: *29* • Total RN Enrollment: *132* • Total New Fall Enrollments: *205* • Total Graduates: *198* • Basic Student Graduates: *146* • RN Student Graduates: *52*

FINANCES

Residential Annual Tuition: *$14,946* • Non-Residential Annual Tuition: *$26,496* • General Institutional Fees: *$4,005* • Additional Nursing Fees: *Not Reported*

UNIVERSITY OF PORTLAND

Address: 5000 North Willamette Boulevard, Portland, OR
            97203
Phone: 503-943-7211
Fax: 503-943-7729
Contact: Terry R. Misener, PhD, RN, FAAN, Dean and
            Professor
Email: misener@up.edu

GENERAL INFORMATION

Type of School: *4-Year College or University, Private (Religious)* • Accreditation: *Northwestern Association of Schools and Colleges* • Total Enrollment: *2464*

PROGRAM INFORMATION

Two Year Exit Option: *No* • NLNAC Accreditation: *Yes* • CCNE Accreditation:

NURSING STUDENT PROFILE

Total Nursing Enrollment: *Not Reported* • Total Basic Student Enrollment, Full Time: *Not Reported* • Total Basic Student Enrollment, Part Time: *Not Reported* • Female Basic Student Enrollment: *Not Reported* • Male Basic Student Enrollment: *Not Reported* • Total RN Enrollment: *Not Reported* • Total New Fall Enrollments: *Not Reported* • Total Graduates: *Not Reported* • Basic Student Graduates: *Not Reported* • RN Student Graduates: *Not Reported*

FINANCES

Residential Annual Tuition: *Not Reported* • Non-Residential Annual Tuition: *Not Reported* • General Institutional Fees: *Not Reported* • Additional Nursing Fees: *Not Reported*

WALLA WALLA COLLEGE

Address: 10345 SE Market, Portland, OR 97216
Phone: 503-251-6115
Fax: 503-251-6249
Contact: Lucille Krull, PhD, RN, FNP, Dean, School of Nursing
Email: krullu@wwc.edu

GENERAL INFORMATION

Type of School: *4-Year College or University, Private (Religious)* • Accreditation: *Northwestern Association of Schools and Colleges* • Total Enrollment: *1792*

PROGRAM INFORMATION

Two Year Exit Option: *No* • NLNAC Accreditation: *Yes* • CCNE Accreditation:

NURSING STUDENT PROFILE

Total Nursing Enrollment: *101* • Total Basic Student Enrollment, Full Time: *98* • Total Basic Student Enrollment, Part Time: *1* • Female Basic Student Enrollment: *93* • Male Basic Student Enrollment: *6* • Total RN Enrollment: *2* • Total New Fall Enrollments: *22* • Total Graduates: *36* • Basic Student Graduates: *35* • RN Student Graduates: *1*

FINANCES

Residential Annual Tuition: *$15,222* • Non-Residential Annual Tuition: *$0* • General Institutional Fees: *$150* • Additional Nursing Fees: *$480*

ALLENTOWN COLLEGE OF ST. FRANCIS DE SALES

Address: 2755 Station Avenue, Center Valley, PA 18034
Phone: 610-282-1100
Fax: *Not Reported*
Contact: Kerry H. Cheever, PhD, RN, CCRN, CEN, Chair
Email: khc@email-allencol.edu

GENERAL INFORMATION

Type of School: *Not Reported* • Accreditation: *Not Reported* • Total Enrollment: *Not Reported*

PROGRAM INFORMATION

Two Year Exit Option: *Not Reported* • NLNAC Accreditation: *Yes* • CCNE Accreditation:

NURSING STUDENT PROFILE

Total Nursing Enrollment: *89* • Total Basic Student Enrollment, Full Time: *Not Reported* • Total Basic Student Enrollment, Part Time: *Not Reported* • Female Basic Student Enrollment: *Not Reported* • Male Basic Student Enrollment: *Not Reported* • Total RN Enrollment: *21* • Total New Fall Enrollments: *Not Reported* • Total Graduates: *Not Reported* • Basic Student Graduates: *Not Reported* • RN Student Graduates: *Not Reported*

FINANCES

Residential Annual Tuition: *$13,350* • Non-Residential Annual Tuition: *Not Reported* • General Institutional Fees: *Not Reported* • Additional Nursing Fees: *Not Reported*

ALVERNIA COLLEGE

Address: 400 St. Bernadine Street, Reading, PA 19607
Phone: 610-796-8306
Fax: 610-796-8464
Contact: Karen S. Thacker, MSN, RN, CS, Assistant Professor
Email: karen.thacker@alvernia.edu

GENERAL INFORMATION

Type of School: *4-Year College or University, Private (Religious)* • Accreditation: *Middle States Association of Colleges and Schools* • Total Enrollment: *1400*

PROGRAM INFORMATION

Two Year Exit Option: *No* • NLNAC Accreditation: *Not Reported* • CCNE Accreditation: *Yes*

NURSING STUDENT PROFILE

Total Nursing Enrollment: *57* • Total Basic Student Enrollment, Full Time: *31* • Total Basic Student Enrollment, Part Time: *2* • Female Basic Student Enrollment: *32* • Male Basic Student Enrollment: *1* • Total RN Enrollment: *24* • Total New Fall Enrollments: *16* • Total Graduates: *5* • Basic Student Graduates: *0* • RN Student Graduates: *5*

FINANCES

Residential Annual Tuition: *$1,400* • Non-Residential Annual Tuition: *$1,400* • General Institutional Fees: *$500* • Additional Nursing Fees: *$400*

BLOOMSBURG UNIVERSITY

Address: 400 E. 2nd Street, RM 3109, MCHS, Bloomsburg, PA 17815
Phone: 570-389-4426
Fax: 570-389-5008
Contact: Christine Alichnie, PhD, RN, Chairperson and Professor
Email: cmalic@husky.bloomu.edu

GENERAL INFORMATION

Type of School: *4-Year College or University, Public* • Accreditation: *Middle States Association of Colleges and Schools* • Total Enrollment: *7916*

PROGRAM INFORMATION

Two Year Exit Option: *No* • NLNAC Accreditation: *Not Reported* • CCNE Accreditation:

NURSING STUDENT PROFILE

Total Nursing Enrollment: *256* • Total Basic Student Enrollment, Full Time: *232* • Total Basic Student Enrollment, Part Time: *12* • Female Basic Student Enrollment: *227* • Male Basic Student Enrollment: *17* • Total RN Enrollment: *12* • Total New Fall Enrollments: *70* • Total Graduates: *37* • Basic Student Graduates: *35* • RN Student Graduates: *2*

FINANCES

Residential Annual Tuition: *$4,016* • Non-Residential Annual Tuition: *$10,040* • General Institutional Fees: *$976* • Additional Nursing Fees: *$0*

CARLOW COLLEGE

Address: 3333 5th Avenue, Pittsburg, PA 15213
Phone: 412-578-6115
Fax: 412-578-6114
Contact: Mary Louise Bost, DrPH, RN, Chair
Email: bost@carlow.edu

GENERAL INFORMATION

Type of School: *4-Year College or University, Private (Religious)* • Accreditation: *Middle States Association of Colleges and Schools* • Total Enrollment: *1933*

PROGRAM INFORMATION

Two Year Exit Option: *Not Reported* • NLNAC Accreditation: *Yes* • CCNE Accreditation: *Yes*

NURSING STUDENT PROFILE

Total Nursing Enrollment: *323* • Total Basic Student Enrollment, Full Time: *88* • Total Basic Student Enrollment, Part Time: *4* • Female Basic Student Enrollment: *90* • Male Basic Student Enrollment: *2* • Total RN Enrollment: *231* • Total New Fall Enrollments: *21* • Total Graduates: *101* • Basic Student Graduates: *22* • RN Student Graduates: *79*

FINANCES

Residential Annual Tuition: *$11,970* • Non-Residential Annual Tuition: *$11,970* • General Institutional Fees: *$181* • Additional Nursing Fees: *Not Reported*

CEDAR CREST COLLEGE

Address: 100 College Drive, Allentown, PA 18104
Phone: 610-606-4606
Fax: 610-606-4615
Contact: Laurie R. Murray, DSN, RN, Chair and
            Associate Professor
Email: lrmurray@cedarcrest.edu

GENERAL INFORMATION

Type of School: *4-Year College or University, Private (Independent)* • Accreditation: *Middle States Association of Colleges and Schools* • Total Enrollment: *1600*

PROGRAM INFORMATION

Two Year Exit Option: *Not Reported* • NLNAC Accreditation: *Yes* • CCNE Accreditation:

NURSING STUDENT PROFILE

Total Nursing Enrollment: *132* • Total Basic Student Enrollment, Full Time: *Not Reported* • Total Basic Student Enrollment, Part Time: *Not Reported* • Female Basic Student Enrollment: *73* • Male Basic Student Enrollment: *5* • Total RN Enrollment: *54* • Total New Fall Enrollments: *53* • Total Graduates: *44* • Basic Student Graduates: *26* • RN Student Graduates: *18*

FINANCES

Residential Annual Tuition: *$17,790* • Non-Residential Annual Tuition: *$17,790* • General Institutional Fees: *$150* • Additional Nursing Fees: *Not Reported*

COLLEGE MISERICORDIA

Address: 301 Lake Street, Dallas, PA 18612
Phone: 570-674-6357
Fax: 570-674-3052
Contact: Donna Ayers Snelson, MSN, RN, CS, Associate
          Professor and Active Chairperson
Email: dsnelson@miseri.edu

GENERAL INFORMATION

Type of School: *4-Year College or University, Private (Religious)* • Accreditation: *Middle States Association of Colleges and Schools* • Total Enrollment: *1765*

PROGRAM INFORMATION

Two Year Exit Option: *Not Reported* • NLNAC Accreditation: *Yes* • CCNE Accreditation:

NURSING STUDENT PROFILE

Total Nursing Enrollment: *55* • Total Basic Student Enrollment, Full Time: *45* • Total Basic Student Enrollment, Part Time: *10* • Female Basic Student Enrollment: *43* • Male Basic Student Enrollment: *12* • Total RN Enrollment: *0* • Total New Fall Enrollments: *13* • Total Graduates: *22* • Basic Student Graduates: *20* • RN Student Graduates: *2*

FINANCES

Residential Annual Tuition: *$15,190* • Non-Residential Annual Tuition: *$15,190* • General Institutional Fees: *$760* • Additional Nursing Fees: *$105*

DUQUESNE UNIVERSITY

Address: 600 Forbes Ave., Pittsburgh, PA 15282
Phone: 412-396-6540
Fax: 412-396-1821
Contact: Joan Such Lockhart, PhD, RN, CORN, Assoc.
          Dean BSN Program and Professor
Email: lockhart@duq.edu

GENERAL INFORMATION

Type of School: *4-Year College or University, Private (Religious)* • Accreditation: *Middle States Association of Colleges and Schools* • Total Enrollment: *9555*

PROGRAM INFORMATION

Two Year Exit Option: *No* • NLNAC Accreditation: *Yes* • CCNE Accreditation:

NURSING STUDENT PROFILE

Total Nursing Enrollment: *162* • Total Basic Student Enrollment, Full Time: *Not Reported* • Total Basic Student Enrollment, Part Time: *Not Reported* • Female Basic Student Enrollment: *138* • Male Basic Student Enrollment: *10* • Total RN Enrollment: *14* • Total New Fall Enrollments: *43* • Total Graduates: *31* • Basic Student Graduates: *21* • RN Student Graduates: *10*

FINANCES

Residential Annual Tuition: *$15,169* • Non-Residential Annual Tuition: *$15,169* • General Institutional Fees: *$1,351* • Additional Nursing Fees: *$50*

EAST STROUDSBURG UNIVERSITY

Address: 200 Prospect St., East Stroudsburg, PA 18353
Phone: 570-422-3566
Fax: 570-422-3838
Contact: Karen Johnson Kramer, EdD, RN, CS, Chairperson
Email: karner@po-box.esu.edu

GENERAL INFORMATION

Type of School: *Other, Public* • Accreditation: *Middle States Association of Colleges and Schools* • Total Enrollment: *5079*

PROGRAM INFORMATION

Two Year Exit Option: *No* • NLNAC Accreditation: *Yes* • CCNE Accreditation:

NURSING STUDENT PROFILE

Total Nursing Enrollment: *137* • Total Basic Student Enrollment, Full Time: *Not Reported* • Total Basic Student Enrollment, Part Time: *Not Reported* • Female Basic Student Enrollment: *Not Reported* • Male Basic Student Enrollment: *Not Reported* • Total RN Enrollment: *19* • Total New Fall Enrollments: *Not Reported* • Total Graduates: *25* • Basic Student Graduates: *19* • RN Student Graduates: *6*

FINANCES

Residential Annual Tuition: *$3,792* • Non-Residential Annual Tuition: *$9,480* • General Institutional Fees: *$1,000* • Additional Nursing Fees: *$0*

EDINBORO UNIVERSITY OF PENNSYLVANIA

Address: 135 Centennial Hall, Edinboro, PA 16444
Phone: 814-732-2900
Fax: 814-732-2536
Contact: Patricia L. Nosel, MN, RN, Chairperson
Email: nosel@edinboro.edu

GENERAL INFORMATION

Type of School: *4-Year College or University, Public* • Accreditation: *Middle States Association of Colleges and Schools* • Total Enrollment: *7079*

PROGRAM INFORMATION

Two Year Exit Option: *Not Reported* • NLNAC Accreditation: *Not Reported* • CCNE Accreditation: *Yes*

NURSING STUDENT PROFILE

Total Nursing Enrollment: *205* • Total Basic Student Enrollment, Full Time: *Not Reported* • Total Basic Student Enrollment, Part Time: *Not Reported* • Female Basic Student Enrollment: *Not Reported* • Male Basic Student Enrollment: *Not Reported* • Total RN Enrollment: *20* • Total New Fall Enrollments: *73* • Total Graduates: *41* • Basic Student Graduates: *36* • RN Student Graduates: *5*

FINANCES

Residential Annual Tuition: *$3,792* • Non-Residential Annual Tuition: *$5,688* • General Institutional Fees: *$526* • Additional Nursing Fees: *$0*

GANNON UNIVERSITY

Address: 109 University Ave., Erie, PA 16541
Phone: 814-871-5470
Fax: 814-871-5662
Contact: Patricia Marshall, MSN, RN, CCRN, Assistant
            Professor
Email: marshall001@gannon.edu

GENERAL INFORMATION

Type of School: *4-Year College or University, Private (Religious)* • Accreditation: *Middle States Association of Colleges and Schools* • Total Enrollment: *3400*

PROGRAM INFORMATION

Two Year Exit Option: *Not Reported* • NLNAC Accreditation: *Yes* • CCNE Accreditation:

NURSING STUDENT PROFILE

Total Nursing Enrollment: *138* • Total Basic Student Enrollment, Full Time: *86* • Total Basic Student Enrollment, Part Time: *2* • Female Basic Student Enrollment: *Not Reported* • Male Basic Student Enrollment: *Not Reported* • Total RN Enrollment: *50* • Total New Fall Enrollments: *Not Reported* • Total Graduates: *Not Reported* • Basic Student Graduates: *Not Reported* • RN Student Graduates: *Not Reported*

FINANCES

Residential Annual Tuition: *$7,690* • Non-Residential Annual Tuition: *$7,690* • General Institutional Fees: *Not Reported* • Additional Nursing Fees: *Not Reported*

HOLY FAMILY COLLEGE

Address: Frankford and Grant Aves., Philadelphia, PA
            19114
Phone: 215-637-7700
Fax: 215-637-6598
Contact: Kathleen McMullen, PhD, RN, BSN Chair
Email: McMullen@hfc.edu

GENERAL INFORMATION

Type of School: *4-Year College or University, Private (Religious)* • Accreditation: *Middle States Association of Colleges and Schools* • Total Enrollment: *2800*

PROGRAM INFORMATION

Two Year Exit Option: *Not Reported* • NLNAC Accreditation: *Yes* • CCNE Accreditation:

NURSING STUDENT PROFILE

Total Nursing Enrollment: *103* • Total Basic Student Enrollment, Full Time: *51* • Total Basic Student Enrollment, Part Time: *23* • Female Basic Student Enrollment: *65* • Male Basic Student Enrollment: *9* • Total RN Enrollment: *29* • Total New Fall Enrollments: *26* • Total Graduates: *32* • Basic Student Graduates: *21* • RN Student Graduates: *11*

FINANCES

Residential Annual Tuition: *$11,500* • Non-Residential Annual Tuition: *$11,500* • General Institutional Fees: *$180* • Additional Nursing Fees: *$140*

INDIANA UNIVERSITY OF PENNSYLVANIA

Address: 1010 Oakland Avenue, Indiana, PA 45623
Phone: 724-357-2557
Fax: *Not Reported*
Contact: Jodell Kuzneski, MNEd, RN, Chairperson
Email: kuzneski@group.iup.edu

LA SALLE UNIVERSITY

Address: 1900 West Olney Ave., Philadelphia, PA 19141
Phone: 215-951-1902
Fax: 215-951-1896
Contact: Joanne Farley Serembus, EdD, RN, CCRN, Director
Email: serembus@lasalle.edu

GENERAL INFORMATION

Type of School: *Not Reported* • Accreditation: *Not Reported* • Total Enrollment: *Not Reported*

GENERAL INFORMATION

Type of School: *4-Year College or University, Private (Religious)* • Accreditation: *Middle States Association of Colleges and Schools* • Total Enrollment: *Not Reported*

PROGRAM INFORMATION

Two Year Exit Option: *Not Reported* • NLNAC Accreditation: *Not Reported* • CCNE Accreditation:

PROGRAM INFORMATION

Two Year Exit Option: *Not Reported* • NLNAC Accreditation: *Yes* • CCNE Accreditation:

NURSING STUDENT PROFILE

Total Nursing Enrollment: *273* • Total Basic Student Enrollment, Full Time: *Not Reported* • Total Basic Student Enrollment, Part Time: *Not Reported* • Female Basic Student Enrollment: *Not Reported* • Male Basic Student Enrollment: *Not Reported* • Total RN Enrollment: *1* • Total New Fall Enrollments: *55* • Total Graduates: *59* • Basic Student Graduates: *57* • RN Student Graduates: *2*

NURSING STUDENT PROFILE

Total Nursing Enrollment: *286* • Total Basic Student Enrollment, Full Time: *124* • Total Basic Student Enrollment, Part Time: *5* • Female Basic Student Enrollment: *118* • Male Basic Student Enrollment: *11* • Total RN Enrollment: *157* • Total New Fall Enrollments: *37* • Total Graduates: *68* • Basic Student Graduates: *25* • RN Student Graduates: *43*

FINANCES

Residential Annual Tuition: *Not Reported* • Non-Residential Annual Tuition: *Not Reported* • General Institutional Fees: *Not Reported* • Additional Nursing Fees: *Not Reported*

FINANCES

Residential Annual Tuition: *$18,020* • Non-Residential Annual Tuition: *$18,020* • General Institutional Fees: *$40* • Additional Nursing Fees: *Not Reported*

Circle 70 on reader card   **See in-depth profile for more information**

LYCOMING COLLEGE

Address: 700 College Pl., Box 21, Williamsport, PA
          17701
Phone: 570-321-4224
Fax: 570-321-4389
Contact: Doris P. Parrish, PhD, RN, Chair and Assoc.
          Professor
Email: parrish@lycoming.edu

GENERAL INFORMATION

Type of School: *4-Year College or University, Private
(Religious)* • Accreditation: *Middle States Association of
Colleges and Schools* • Total Enrollment: *1500*

PROGRAM INFORMATION

Two Year Exit Option: *Not Reported* • NLNAC
Accreditation: *Yes* • CCNE Accreditation:

NURSING STUDENT PROFILE

Total Nursing Enrollment: *50* • Total Basic Student
Enrollment, Full Time: *50* • Total Basic Student Enrollment,
Part Time: *0* • Female Basic Student Enrollment: *45* • Male
Basic Student Enrollment: *5* • Total RN Enrollment: *0* •
Total New Fall Enrollments: *3* • Total Graduates: *16* • Basic
Student Graduates: *15* • RN Student Graduates: *1*

FINANCES

Residential Annual Tuition: *$17,440* • Non-Residential
Annual Tuition: *$17,440* • General Institutional Fees: *$80* •
Additional Nursing Fees: *$50*

MANSFIELD UNIVERSITY

Address: 203 A Elliot Hall, Mansfield, PA 16933
Phone: 570-662-4522
Fax: 570-662-4137
Contact: Janeen Bartlett Sheehe, DNSc, RN, Dept. Chair
Email: Jsheehe@mnfld.edu

GENERAL INFORMATION

Type of School: *4-Year College or University, Public* •
Accreditation: *Middle States Association of Colleges and
Schools* • Total Enrollment: *1857*

PROGRAM INFORMATION

Two Year Exit Option: *Not Reported* • NLNAC
Accreditation: *Yes* • CCNE Accreditation:

NURSING STUDENT PROFILE

Total Nursing Enrollment: *133* • Total Basic Student
Enrollment, Full Time: *77* • Total Basic Student Enrollment,
Part Time: *2* • Female Basic Student Enrollment: *70* • Male
Basic Student Enrollment: *9* • Total RN Enrollment: *54* •
Total New Fall Enrollments: *Not Reported* • Total Graduates:
Not Reported • Basic Student Graduates: *Not Reported* • RN
Student Graduates: *Not Reported*

FINANCES

Residential Annual Tuition: *$3,792* • Non-Residential
Annual Tuition: *$9,480* • General Institutional Fees: *$974* •
Additional Nursing Fees: *$0*

MARYWOOD UNIVERSITY

Address: 2300 Adams Avenue, Scranton, PA 18509-1514
Phone: 570-348-6275
Fax: 570-961-4761
Contact: Mary Alice Golden, PhD, RN, Associate Professor, Chairperson
Email: golden@ac.marywood.edu

GENERAL INFORMATION

Type of School: *4-Year College or University, Private (Religious)* • Accreditation: *Middle States Association of Colleges and Schools* • Total Enrollment: *2859*

PROGRAM INFORMATION

Two Year Exit Option: *Not Reported* • NLNAC Accreditation: *Yes* • CCNE Accreditation:

NURSING STUDENT PROFILE

Total Nursing Enrollment: *46* • Total Basic Student Enrollment, Full Time: *29* • Total Basic Student Enrollment, Part Time: *11* • Female Basic Student Enrollment: *33* • Male Basic Student Enrollment: *7* • Total RN Enrollment: *6* • Total New Fall Enrollments: *7* • Total Graduates: *12* • Basic Student Graduates: *10* • RN Student Graduates: *2*

FINANCES

Residential Annual Tuition: *$15,840* • Non-Residential Annual Tuition: *$15,840* • General Institutional Fees: *$558* • Additional Nursing Fees: *$1,347*

MCP HAHNEMANN UNIVERSITY

Address: 245 North 15th Street, Mail Stop 501, Philadelphia, PA 19102
Phone: 215-762-7483
Fax: 215-762-1259
Contact: Mary Ellen Smith, MSN, RN, CS, Program Director
Email: ms55@drexel.edu

GENERAL INFORMATION

Type of School: *4-Year College or University, Private (Independent)* • Accreditation: *Middle States Association of Colleges and Schools* • Total Enrollment: *3000*

PROGRAM INFORMATION

Two Year Exit Option: *No* • NLNAC Accreditation: *Yes* • CCNE Accreditation: *Yes*

NURSING STUDENT PROFILE

Total Nursing Enrollment: *138* • Total Basic Student Enrollment, Full Time: *69* • Total Basic Student Enrollment, Part Time: *0* • Female Basic Student Enrollment: *58* • Male Basic Student Enrollment: *11* • Total RN Enrollment: *69* • Total New Fall Enrollments: *59* • Total Graduates: *0* • Basic Student Graduates: *0* • RN Student Graduates: *0*

FINANCES

Residential Annual Tuition: *$20,000* • Non-Residential Annual Tuition: *$20,000* • General Institutional Fees: *Not Reported* • Additional Nursing Fees: *$150*

MESSIAH COLLEGE

Address: 1 College Avenue, Grantham, PA 17027
Phone: 717-691-6029
Fax: *Not Reported*
Contact: Sandra L. Jamison, DNS, RN, Chair
Email: sjamison@messiah.edu

GENERAL INFORMATION

Type of School: *4-Year College or University, Private (Religious)* • Accreditation: *Middle States Association of Colleges and Schools* • Total Enrollment: *2735*

PROGRAM INFORMATION

Two Year Exit Option: *Not Reported* • NLNAC Accreditation: *Yes* • CCNE Accreditation:

NURSING STUDENT PROFILE

Total Nursing Enrollment: *168* • Total Basic Student Enrollment, Full Time: *146* • Total Basic Student Enrollment, Part Time: *21* • Female Basic Student Enrollment: *160* • Male Basic Student Enrollment: *7* • Total RN Enrollment: *1* • Total New Fall Enrollments: *43* • Total Graduates: *54* • Basic Student Graduates: *54* • RN Student Graduates: *0*

FINANCES

Residential Annual Tuition: *$15,000* • Non-Residential Annual Tuition: *$15,000* • General Institutional Fees: *$270* • Additional Nursing Fees: *Not Reported*

MORAVIAN COLLEGE

Address: 1200 Main Street, Bethlehem, PA 18018
Phone: 610-861-1608
Fax: 610-625-7861
Contact: Janet A. Sipple, EdD, RN, Professor and
            Chairperson
Email: sipplej@moravian.edu

GENERAL INFORMATION

Type of School: *4-Year College or University, Private (Independent)* • Accreditation: *Middle States Association of Colleges and Schools* • Total Enrollment: *1300*

PROGRAM INFORMATION

Two Year Exit Option: *No* • NLNAC Accreditation: *Not Reported* • CCNE Accreditation:

NURSING STUDENT PROFILE

Total Nursing Enrollment: *43* • Total Basic Student Enrollment, Full Time: *35* • Total Basic Student Enrollment, Part Time: *0* • Female Basic Student Enrollment: *34* • Male Basic Student Enrollment: *1* • Total RN Enrollment: *8* • Total New Fall Enrollments: *12* • Total Graduates: *0* • Basic Student Graduates: *0* • RN Student Graduates: *0*

FINANCES

Residential Annual Tuition: *$19,070* • Non-Residential Annual Tuition: *$19,070* • General Institutional Fees: *$330* • Additional Nursing Fees: *$450*

NEUMANN COLLEGE

Address: One Neumann Drive, Aston, PA 19014-1298
Phone: 610-558-5561
Fax: 610-361-5265
Contact: Gregg E. Newschwander, PhD, RN, Professor and Chair
Email: newschwg@neuman.edu

PENNSYLVANIA STATE UNIVERSITY

Address: 201 Health and Human Development E., University Park, PA 16802-6508
Phone: 814-863-0245
Fax: 814-865-3779
Contact: Sarah Hall Guelder, DSN, RN, FAAN, Director
Email: shg9@psu.edu

GENERAL INFORMATION

Type of School: *4-Year College or University, Private (Religious)* • Accreditation: *Middle States Association of Colleges and Schools* • Total Enrollment: *1658*

GENERAL INFORMATION

Type of School: *4-Year College or University, Public* • Accreditation: *Middle States Association of Colleges and Schools* • Total Enrollment: *15582*

PROGRAM INFORMATION

Two Year Exit Option: *Not Reported* • NLNAC Accreditation: *Yes* • CCNE Accreditation:

PROGRAM INFORMATION

Two Year Exit Option: *Not Reported* • NLNAC Accreditation: *Yes* • CCNE Accreditation: *Yes*

NURSING STUDENT PROFILE

Total Nursing Enrollment: *125* • Total Basic Student Enrollment, Full Time: *94* • Total Basic Student Enrollment, Part Time: *30* • Female Basic Student Enrollment: *118* • Male Basic Student Enrollment: *6* • Total RN Enrollment: *1* • Total New Fall Enrollments: *23* • Total Graduates: *34* • Basic Student Graduates: *34* • RN Student Graduates: *0*

NURSING STUDENT PROFILE

Total Nursing Enrollment: *656* • Total Basic Student Enrollment, Full Time: *335* • Total Basic Student Enrollment, Part Time: *13* • Female Basic Student Enrollment: *322* • Male Basic Student Enrollment: *26* • Total RN Enrollment: *308* • Total New Fall Enrollments: *98* • Total Graduates: *204* • Basic Student Graduates: *69* • RN Student Graduates: *135*

FINANCES

Residential Annual Tuition: *$13,750* • Non-Residential Annual Tuition: *$13,750* • General Institutional Fees: *$250* • Additional Nursing Fees: *$570*

FINANCES

Residential Annual Tuition: *$6,546* • Non-Residential Annual Tuition: *$14,088* • General Institutional Fees: *$286* • Additional Nursing Fees: *$1,708*

TEMPLE UNIVERSITY

Address: Jones Hall 3307 North Broad Street,
           Philadelphia, PA 19140
Phone: 215-707-8327
Fax: 215-707-3758
Contact: Jill B. Derstine, EdD, RN, Chair
Email: jderst01@unix.temple.edu

GENERAL INFORMATION

Type of School: *4-Year College or University, Public* •
Accreditation: *Middle States Association of Colleges and
Schools* • Total Enrollment: *Not Reported*

PROGRAM INFORMATION

Two Year Exit Option: *Not Reported* • NLNAC
Accreditation: *Yes* • CCNE Accreditation:

NURSING STUDENT PROFILE

Total Nursing Enrollment: *260* • Total Basic Student
Enrollment, Full Time: *107* • Total Basic Student
Enrollment, Part Time: *13* • Female Basic Student
Enrollment: *107* • Male Basic Student Enrollment: *13* • Total
RN Enrollment: *140* • Total New Fall Enrollments: *56* •
Total Graduates: *99* • Basic Student Graduates: *61* • RN
Student Graduates: *38*

FINANCES

Residential Annual Tuition: *$8,034* • Non-Residential
Annual Tuition: *$14,164* • General Institutional Fees: *$340* •
Additional Nursing Fees: *$160*

THIEL COLLEGE

Address: 75 College Avenue, Greenville, PA 16125-2181
Phone: 724-589-2053
Fax: 724-589-2021
Contact: Evelyn E. Ramming, PhD, RN, Director and
           Chairperson
Email: *Not Reported*

GENERAL INFORMATION

Type of School: *4-Year College or University, Private
(Religious)* • Accreditation: *Middle States Association of
Colleges and Schools* • Total Enrollment: *1000*

PROGRAM INFORMATION

Two Year Exit Option: *Not Reported* • NLNAC
Accreditation: *Yes* • CCNE Accreditation:

NURSING STUDENT PROFILE

Total Nursing Enrollment: *11* • Total Basic Student
Enrollment, Full Time: *10* • Total Basic Student Enrollment,
Part Time: *0* • Female Basic Student Enrollment: *9* • Male
Basic Student Enrollment: *1* • Total RN Enrollment: *1* •
Total New Fall Enrollments: *Not Reported* • Total Graduates:
7 • Basic Student Graduates: *7* • RN Student Graduates: *0*

FINANCES

Residential Annual Tuition: *$14,958* • Non-Residential
Annual Tuition: *$14,958* • General Institutional Fees:
$1,700 • Additional Nursing Fees: *$45*

THOMAS JEFFERSON UNIVERSITY

Address: 130 S 9th Street, 12th Floor, Philadelphia, PA 19107
Phone: 215-503-8104
Fax: 215-503-0376
Contact: Anne E. Belcher, PhD, RN, AOCN, FAAN, Director
Email: Anne.Belcher@mail.tji.edu

GENERAL INFORMATION

Type of School: *Not Reported* • Accreditation: *Middle States Association of Colleges and Schools* • Total Enrollment: *Not Reported*

PROGRAM INFORMATION

Two Year Exit Option: *Not Reported* • NLNAC Accreditation: *Yes* • CCNE Accreditation:

NURSING STUDENT PROFILE

Total Nursing Enrollment: *247* • Total Basic Student Enrollment, Full Time: *93* • Total Basic Student Enrollment, Part Time: *13* • Female Basic Student Enrollment: *84* • Male Basic Student Enrollment: *22* • Total RN Enrollment: *141* • Total New Fall Enrollments: *50* • Total Graduates: *146* • Basic Student Graduates: *44* • RN Student Graduates: *102*

FINANCES

Residential Annual Tuition: *$17,500* • Non-Residential Annual Tuition: *$17,500* • General Institutional Fees: *Not Reported* • Additional Nursing Fees: *Not Reported*

UNIVERSITY OF PENNSYLVANIA

Address: 420 Guardian Drive, Philadelphia, PA 19104
Phone: 215-898-2995
Fax: *Not Reported*
Contact: Kathleen McCualey, PhD, CRNP, FAAN, Interim Associate and Director
Email: *Not Reported*

GENERAL INFORMATION

Type of School: *4-Year College or University, Private (Independent)* • Accreditation: *Middle States Association of Colleges and Schools* • Total Enrollment: *21800*

PROGRAM INFORMATION

Two Year Exit Option: *No* • NLNAC Accreditation: *Yes* • CCNE Accreditation: *Yes*

NURSING STUDENT PROFILE

Total Nursing Enrollment: *365* • Total Basic Student Enrollment, Full Time: *347* • Total Basic Student Enrollment, Part Time: *18* • Female Basic Student Enrollment: *339* • Male Basic Student Enrollment: *26* • Total RN Enrollment: *0* • Total New Fall Enrollments: *108* • Total Graduates: *89* • Basic Student Graduates: *89* • RN Student Graduates: *0*

FINANCES

Residential Annual Tuition: *$23,998* • Non-Residential Annual Tuition: *$23,998* • General Institutional Fees: *$2,144* • Additional Nursing Fees: *$488*

UNIVERSITY OF PITTSBURGH

Address: 300 Victoria Street, Room 350, Pittsburgh, PA 15261
Phone: 912-624-1291
Fax: *Not Reported*
Contact: Kathy Lucke, PhD, RN, Assistant Dean, Student Services
Email: luck01+@pitt.edu

GENERAL INFORMATION

Type of School: *4-Year College or University, Public* • Accreditation: *Middle States Association of Colleges and Schools* • Total Enrollment: *25461*

PROGRAM INFORMATION

Two Year Exit Option: *Not Reported* • NLNAC Accreditation: *Yes* • CCNE Accreditation: *Yes*

NURSING STUDENT PROFILE

Total Nursing Enrollment: *572* • Total Basic Student Enrollment, Full Time: *Not Reported* • Total Basic Student Enrollment, Part Time: *Not Reported* • Female Basic Student Enrollment: *Not Reported* • Male Basic Student Enrollment: *Not Reported* • Total RN Enrollment: *189* • Total New Fall Enrollments: *187* • Total Graduates: *Not Reported* • Basic Student Graduates: *Not Reported* • RN Student Graduates: *Not Reported*

FINANCES

Residential Annual Tuition: *$7,872* • Non-Residential Annual Tuition: *$17,168* • General Institutional Fees: *$290* • Additional Nursing Fees: *$11*

UNIVERSITY OF SCRANTON

Address: 800 Linden Street, Scranton, PA 18510
Phone: 570-941-7673
Fax: 570-941-7903
Contact: Patricia Harrington, EdD, RN, Chairperson
Email: harringtonpi@scranton.edu

GENERAL INFORMATION

Type of School: *4-Year College or University, Private (Religious)* • Accreditation: *Middle States Association of Colleges and Schools* • Total Enrollment: *5000*

PROGRAM INFORMATION

Two Year Exit Option: *Not Reported* • NLNAC Accreditation: *Yes* • CCNE Accreditation:

NURSING STUDENT PROFILE

Total Nursing Enrollment: *182* • Total Basic Student Enrollment, Full Time: *116* • Total Basic Student Enrollment, Part Time: *4* • Female Basic Student Enrollment: *112* • Male Basic Student Enrollment: *8* • Total RN Enrollment: *62* • Total New Fall Enrollments: *34* • Total Graduates: *28* • Basic Student Graduates: *25* • RN Student Graduates: *3*

FINANCES

Residential Annual Tuition: *$18,500* • Non-Residential Annual Tuition: *$18,500* • General Institutional Fees: *$330* • Additional Nursing Fees: *Not Reported*

VILLANOVA UNIVERSITY

Address:　800 Lancaster Avenue, Villanova, PA 19085
Phone:　　610-519-4923
Fax:　　　610-519-7650
Contact:　M Frances Keen, PhD, RN, Director,
　　　　　Undergraduate Program
Email:　　frances.keen@villanova.edu

GENERAL INFORMATION

Type of School: *Not Reported* • Accreditation: *Middle States Association of Colleges and Schools* • Total Enrollment: *Not Reported*

PROGRAM INFORMATION

Two Year Exit Option: *No* • NLNAC Accreditation: *Yes* • CCNE Accreditation: *Yes*

NURSING STUDENT PROFILE

Total Nursing Enrollment: *347* • Total Basic Student Enrollment, Full Time: *310* • Total Basic Student Enrollment, Part Time: *5* • Female Basic Student Enrollment: *306* • Male Basic Student Enrollment: *9* • Total RN Enrollment: *32* • Total New Fall Enrollments: *88* • Total Graduates: *96* • Basic Student Graduates: *71* • RN Student Graduates: *25*

FINANCES

Residential Annual Tuition: *$23,210* • Non-Residential Annual Tuition: *$23,210* • General Institutional Fees: *$300* • Additional Nursing Fees: *$150*

WAYNESBURG COLLEGE

Address:　51 West College Street, Waynesburg, PA 15370
Phone:　　724-852-3356
Fax:　　　724-852-3220
Contact:　Patty Kraft, EdD, RN, CFNP, Chairperson and
　　　　　Director
Email:　　pkraft@waynesburg.edu

GENERAL INFORMATION

Type of School: *Not Reported* • Accreditation: *Middle States Association of Colleges and Schools* • Total Enrollment: *Not Reported*

PROGRAM INFORMATION

Two Year Exit Option: *Not Reported* • NLNAC Accreditation: *Yes* • CCNE Accreditation:

NURSING STUDENT PROFILE

Total Nursing Enrollment: *186* • Total Basic Student Enrollment, Full Time: *96* • Total Basic Student Enrollment, Part Time: *0* • Female Basic Student Enrollment: *76* • Male Basic Student Enrollment: *20* • Total RN Enrollment: *90* • Total New Fall Enrollments: *36* • Total Graduates: *30* • Basic Student Graduates: *30* • RN Student Graduates: *0*

FINANCES

Residential Annual Tuition: *$11,670* • Non-Residential Annual Tuition: *$11,670* • General Institutional Fees: *$280* • Additional Nursing Fees: *$210*

WEST CHESTER UNIVERSITY

Address: South Church Street, West Chester, PA 19383
Phone: 610-436-2331
Fax: 610-436-3083
Contact: Ann Coghlan Stowe, DNSc, RN, C, Chairperson
Email: Astowe@WCUPA.edu

GENERAL INFORMATION

Type of School: *Not Reported* • Accreditation: *Middle States Association of Colleges and Schools* • Total Enrollment: *Not Reported*

PROGRAM INFORMATION

Two Year Exit Option: *Not Reported* • NLNAC Accreditation: *Yes* • CCNE Accreditation:

NURSING STUDENT PROFILE

Total Nursing Enrollment: *245* • Total Basic Student Enrollment, Full Time: *Not Reported* • Total Basic Student Enrollment, Part Time: *Not Reported* • Female Basic Student Enrollment: *196* • Male Basic Student Enrollment: *11* • Total RN Enrollment: *38* • Total New Fall Enrollments: *45* • Total Graduates: *38* • Basic Student Graduates: *38* • RN Student Graduates: *0*

FINANCES

Residential Annual Tuition: *$3,618* • Non-Residential Annual Tuition: *$9,046* • General Institutional Fees: *Not Reported* • Additional Nursing Fees: *Not Reported*

WIDENER UNIVERSITY

Address: One University Place, Chester, PA 19013
Phone: 610-499-4210
Fax: 610-499-4216
Contact: Jane Brennan, DNSc, RN, Assistant Dean Undergraduate Studies
Email: jane.m.brennan@widener.edu

GENERAL INFORMATION

Type of School: *Not Reported* • Accreditation: *Middle States Association of Colleges and Schools* • Total Enrollment: *Not Reported*

PROGRAM INFORMATION

Two Year Exit Option: *No* • NLNAC Accreditation: *Yes* • CCNE Accreditation:

NURSING STUDENT PROFILE

Total Nursing Enrollment: *246* • Total Basic Student Enrollment, Full Time: *132* • Total Basic Student Enrollment, Part Time: *34* • Female Basic Student Enrollment: *153* • Male Basic Student Enrollment: *13* • Total RN Enrollment: *80* • Total New Fall Enrollments: *38* • Total Graduates: *70* • Basic Student Graduates: *43* • RN Student Graduates: *27*

FINANCES

Residential Annual Tuition: *Not Reported* • Non-Residential Annual Tuition: *Not Reported* • General Institutional Fees: *Not Reported* • Additional Nursing Fees: *Not Reported*

WILKES UNIVERSITY

Address: 109 South Franklin Street Pearsall Hall,
            Wilkes, PA 18766
Phone: 717-408-4074
Fax: 717-408-7807
Contact: Mary Ann Merrigan, PhD, RN, Chairperson
Email: merrigan@wilkes1.wilkes.edu

YORK COLLEGE OF PENNSYLVANIA

Address: Country Club Road, York, PA 17405
Phone: 717-815-1420
Fax: 717-849-1651
Contact: Jacquelin H. Harrington, DEd, RN, Assoc.
            Professor and Chairperson
Email: jharring@ycp.edu

GENERAL INFORMATION

Type of School: *Not Reported* • Accreditation: *Middle States Association of Colleges and Schools* • Total Enrollment: *Not Reported*

GENERAL INFORMATION

Type of School: *Not Reported* • Accreditation: *Middle States Association of Colleges and Schools* • Total Enrollment: *Not Reported*

PROGRAM INFORMATION

Two Year Exit Option: *Not Reported* • NLNAC Accreditation: *Yes* • CCNE Accreditation:

PROGRAM INFORMATION

Two Year Exit Option: *No* • NLNAC Accreditation: *Yes* • CCNE Accreditation:

NURSING STUDENT PROFILE

Total Nursing Enrollment: *83* • Total Basic Student Enrollment, Full Time: *51* • Total Basic Student Enrollment, Part Time: *27* • Female Basic Student Enrollment: *Not Reported* • Male Basic Student Enrollment: *Not Reported* • Total RN Enrollment: *5* • Total New Fall Enrollments: *Not Reported* • Total Graduates: *Not Reported* • Basic Student Graduates: *Not Reported* • RN Student Graduates: *Not Reported*

NURSING STUDENT PROFILE

Total Nursing Enrollment: *391* • Total Basic Student Enrollment, Full Time: *256* • Total Basic Student Enrollment, Part Time: *77* • Female Basic Student Enrollment: *318* • Male Basic Student Enrollment: *15* • Total RN Enrollment: *58* • Total New Fall Enrollments: *85* • Total Graduates: *88* • Basic Student Graduates: *76* • RN Student Graduates: *12*

FINANCES

Residential Annual Tuition: *$15,050* • Non-Residential Annual Tuition: *$15,050* • General Institutional Fees: *$652* • Additional Nursing Fees: *Not Reported*

FINANCES

Residential Annual Tuition: *$7,000* • Non-Residential Annual Tuition: *$7,000* • General Institutional Fees: *$422* • Additional Nursing Fees: *$0*

ANTILLEAN ADVENTIST UNIVERSITY

Address: PO Box 118, Mayaguez, PR 00681
Phone: 787-834-9595
Fax: *Not Reported*
Contact: Maria L. Cruz, MSN, RN, Director of Nursing Dept.
Email: *Not Reported*

GENERAL INFORMATION

Type of School: *4-Year College or University, Private (Religious)* • Accreditation: *Middle States Association of Colleges and Schools* • Total Enrollment: *719*

PROGRAM INFORMATION

Two Year Exit Option: *Not Reported* • NLNAC Accreditation: *Yes* • CCNE Accreditation:

NURSING STUDENT PROFILE

Total Nursing Enrollment: *202* • Total Basic Student Enrollment, Full Time: *Not Reported* • Total Basic Student Enrollment, Part Time: *Not Reported* • Female Basic Student Enrollment: *Not Reported* • Male Basic Student Enrollment: *Not Reported* • Total RN Enrollment: *45* • Total New Fall Enrollments: *69* • Total Graduates: *62* • Basic Student Graduates: *41* • RN Student Graduates: *21*

FINANCES

Residential Annual Tuition: *$4,060* • Non-Residential Annual Tuition: *$4,060* • General Institutional Fees: *$760* • Additional Nursing Fees: *$380*

BAYAMON CENTRAL UNIVERSITY

Address: Box 1725, Bayamon, PR 00960-1725
Phone: 787-786-3030
Fax: 787-740-2200
Contact: Norma L. Rodriguez, EdD, RN, Nursing Coordinator
Email: nmoctezuma@ucb.edu.pr

GENERAL INFORMATION

Type of School: *4-Year College or University, Private (Religious)* • Accreditation: *Middle States Association of Colleges and Schools* • Total Enrollment: *Not Reported*

PROGRAM INFORMATION

Two Year Exit Option: *Not Reported* • NLNAC Accreditation: *Not Reported* • CCNE Accreditation:

NURSING STUDENT PROFILE

Total Nursing Enrollment: *167* • Total Basic Student Enrollment, Full Time: *150* • Total Basic Student Enrollment, Part Time: *17* • Female Basic Student Enrollment: *152* • Male Basic Student Enrollment: *15* • Total RN Enrollment: *0* • Total New Fall Enrollments: *29* • Total Graduates: *19* • Basic Student Graduates: *19* • RN Student Graduates: *0*

FINANCES

Residential Annual Tuition: *Not Reported* • Non-Residential Annual Tuition: *Not Reported* • General Institutional Fees: *Not Reported* • Additional Nursing Fees: *Not Reported*

CARRIBBEAN UNIVERSITY

Address: Box 493, Bayamon, PR 00960
Phone: 787-780-0070
Fax: 787-785-0101
Contact: Sara Cruz, MSN, RN, Director
Email: *Not Reported*

GENERAL INFORMATION

Type of School: *Not Reported* • Accreditation: *Not Reported* • Total Enrollment: *Not Reported*

PROGRAM INFORMATION

Two Year Exit Option: *Not Reported* • NLNAC Accreditation: *Not Reported* • CCNE Accreditation:

NURSING STUDENT PROFILE

Total Nursing Enrollment: *50* • Total Basic Student Enrollment, Full Time: *10* • Total Basic Student Enrollment, Part Time: *15* • Female Basic Student Enrollment: *Not Reported* • Male Basic Student Enrollment: *Not Reported* • Total RN Enrollment: *25* • Total New Fall Enrollments: *Not Reported* • Total Graduates: *20* • Basic Student Graduates: *20* • RN Student Graduates: *0*

FINANCES

Residential Annual Tuition: *Not Reported* • Non-Residential Annual Tuition: *Not Reported* • General Institutional Fees: *Not Reported* • Additional Nursing Fees: *Not Reported*

INTERAMERICAN UNIVERSITY—SAN GERMAN

Address: Box 5106, San German, PR 00683
Phone: 787-264-1912
Fax: 787-892-6380
Contact: Leida Madera, MSN, RN, Director
Email: lmadera@sg.inter.edu

GENERAL INFORMATION

Type of School: *Not Reported* • Accreditation: *Not Reported* • Total Enrollment: *Not Reported*

PROGRAM INFORMATION

Two Year Exit Option: *Yes* • NLNAC Accreditation: *Not Reported* • CCNE Accreditation: *Yes*

NURSING STUDENT PROFILE

Total Nursing Enrollment: *86* • Total Basic Student Enrollment, Full Time: *43* • Total Basic Student Enrollment, Part Time: *0* • Female Basic Student Enrollment: *37* • Male Basic Student Enrollment: *6* • Total RN Enrollment: *43* • Total New Fall Enrollments: *24* • Total Graduates: *12* • Basic Student Graduates: *6* • RN Student Graduates: *6*

FINANCES

Residential Annual Tuition: *Not Reported* • Non-Residential Annual Tuition: *Not Reported* • General Institutional Fees: *Not Reported* • Additional Nursing Fees: *Not Reported*

INTERAMERICAN UNIVERSITY—SAN JUAN

Address: PO Box 191293, San Juan, PR 00919
Phone: 787-763-3066
Fax: 787-250-1242
Contact: Gloria E. Ortiz, EdD, RN, Director
Email: glortiz@inter.edu

GENERAL INFORMATION

Type of School: *4-Year College or University, Private (Independent)* • Accreditation: *Middle States Association of Colleges and Schools* • Total Enrollment: *Not Reported*

PROGRAM INFORMATION

Two Year Exit Option: *Yes* • NLNAC Accreditation: *Yes* • CCNE Accreditation:

NURSING STUDENT PROFILE

Total Nursing Enrollment: *162* • Total Basic Student Enrollment, Full Time: *125* • Total Basic Student Enrollment, Part Time: *7* • Female Basic Student Enrollment: *100* • Male Basic Student Enrollment: *32* • Total RN Enrollment: *30* • Total New Fall Enrollments: *82* • Total Graduates: *83* • Basic Student Graduates: *61* • RN Student Graduates: *22*

FINANCES

Residential Annual Tuition: *$5,000* • Non-Residential Annual Tuition: *Not Reported* • General Institutional Fees: *$2,500* • Additional Nursing Fees: *$110*

INTERAMERICAN UNIVERSITY OF PUERTO RICO

Address: P. O. Box 10004, Guayama, PR 00785
Phone: 787-864-2222
Fax: 787-866-4986
Contact: Carlos Cobeo, MSN, RN, CNS, Director
Email: ccobeo@ns.inter.edu

GENERAL INFORMATION

Type of School: *4-Year College or University, Private (Independent)* • Accreditation: *Middle States Association of Colleges and Schools* • Total Enrollment: *Not Reported*

PROGRAM INFORMATION

Two Year Exit Option: *Yes* • NLNAC Accreditation: *Not Reported* • CCNE Accreditation:

NURSING STUDENT PROFILE

Total Nursing Enrollment: *115* • Total Basic Student Enrollment, Full Time: *115* • Total Basic Student Enrollment, Part Time: *0* • Female Basic Student Enrollment: *109* • Male Basic Student Enrollment: *6* • Total RN Enrollment: *0* • Total New Fall Enrollments: *20* • Total Graduates: *24* • Basic Student Graduates: *15* • RN Student Graduates: *9*

FINANCES

Residential Annual Tuition: *$2,640* • Non-Residential Annual Tuition: *Not Reported* • General Institutional Fees: *$580* • Additional Nursing Fees: *$580*

PONTIFICAL CATHOLIC UNIVERSITY—PUERTO RICO

Address: 2250 Ave Las Americas, Ponce, PR 00717-0777
Phone: 787-841-2000
Fax: *Not Reported*
Contact: Carmen L. Madera, MSN, RN, Chairperson
Email: clmadera@pucpr.edu

GENERAL INFORMATION

Type of School: *4-Year College or University, Private (Religious)* • Accreditation: *Middle States Association of Colleges and Schools* • Total Enrollment: *330*

PROGRAM INFORMATION

Two Year Exit Option: *Not Reported* • NLNAC Accreditation: *Yes* • CCNE Accreditation:

NURSING STUDENT PROFILE

Total Nursing Enrollment: *475* • Total Basic Student Enrollment, Full Time: *436* • Total Basic Student Enrollment, Part Time: *38* • Female Basic Student Enrollment: *396* • Male Basic Student Enrollment: *78* • Total RN Enrollment: *1* • Total New Fall Enrollments: *88* • Total Graduates: *121* • Basic Student Graduates: *121* • RN Student Graduates: *0*

FINANCES

Residential Annual Tuition: *$3,660* • Non-Residential Annual Tuition: *$3,660* • General Institutional Fees: *$210* • Additional Nursing Fees: *$125*

UNIVERSIDAD DEL SAGRADO CORAZÓN

Address: PO Box 12383, Loiza Street, Santurce, PR 00914
Phone: 787-728-1515
Fax: 787-727-1250
Contact: Gloria E. Rivas, MSN, RN, Director
Email: grivas@sagrado.edu

GENERAL INFORMATION

Type of School: *4-Year College or University, Private (Independent)* • Accreditation: *Middle States Association of Colleges and Schools* • Total Enrollment: *5500*

PROGRAM INFORMATION

Two Year Exit Option: *Not Reported* • NLNAC Accreditation: *Yes* • CCNE Accreditation:

NURSING STUDENT PROFILE

Total Nursing Enrollment: *98* • Total Basic Student Enrollment, Full Time: *98* • Total Basic Student Enrollment, Part Time: *0* • Female Basic Student Enrollment: *95* • Male Basic Student Enrollment: *3* • Total RN Enrollment: *0* • Total New Fall Enrollments: *98* • Total Graduates: *25* • Basic Student Graduates: *25* • RN Student Graduates: *0*

FINANCES

Residential Annual Tuition: *Not Reported* • Non-Residential Annual Tuition: *Not Reported* • General Institutional Fees: *Not Reported* • Additional Nursing Fees: *Not Reported*

UNIVERSIDAD INTERAMERICANA DE PUERTO RICO

Address: Universidad Interamericana De Puerto Rico, Apartado 20000, Aguadilla, PR 00605
Phone: 787-891-0925
Fax: *Not Reported*
Contact: Rosa M. Mercado, MPH, RN, Nursing Program Coordinator
Email: *Not Reported*

GENERAL INFORMATION

Type of School: *4-Year College or University, Private (Independent)* • Accreditation: *Middle States Association of Colleges and Schools* • Total Enrollment: *3564*

PROGRAM INFORMATION

Two Year Exit Option: *Not Reported* • NLNAC Accreditation: *Not Reported* • CCNE Accreditation:

NURSING STUDENT PROFILE

Total Nursing Enrollment: *126* • Total Basic Student Enrollment, Full Time: *Not Reported* • Total Basic Student Enrollment, Part Time: *Not Reported* • Female Basic Student Enrollment: *Not Reported* • Male Basic Student Enrollment: *Not Reported* • Total RN Enrollment: *16* • Total New Fall Enrollments: *20* • Total Graduates: *40* • Basic Student Graduates: *33* • RN Student Graduates: *7*

FINANCES

Residential Annual Tuition: *$3,520* • Non-Residential Annual Tuition: *Not Reported* • General Institutional Fees: *$554* • Additional Nursing Fees: *$156*

UNIVERSIDAD METROPOLITANA

Address: PO Box 21150, San Juan, PR 00928-1150
Phone: 787-766-1717
Fax: 787-766-1717
Contact: Mayra Pedroza Lopez, MSN, MA, RN, Director
Email: um_mpedroza@suagm.edu

GENERAL INFORMATION

Type of School: *4-Year College or University, Private (Independent)* • Accreditation: *Middle States Association of Colleges and Schools* • Total Enrollment: *6501*

PROGRAM INFORMATION

Two Year Exit Option: *Not Reported* • NLNAC Accreditation: *Yes* • CCNE Accreditation:

NURSING STUDENT PROFILE

Total Nursing Enrollment: *269* • Total Basic Student Enrollment, Full Time: *Not Reported* • Total Basic Student Enrollment, Part Time: *Not Reported* • Female Basic Student Enrollment: *217* • Male Basic Student Enrollment: *52* • Total RN Enrollment: *0* • Total New Fall Enrollments: *0* • Total Graduates: *48* • Basic Student Graduates: *48* • RN Student Graduates: *0*

FINANCES

Residential Annual Tuition: *Not Reported* • Non-Residential Annual Tuition: *Not Reported* • General Institutional Fees: *Not Reported* • Additional Nursing Fees: *Not Reported*

UNIVERSITY OF PUERTO RICO

Address: GPO Box 365067, San Juan, PR 00936-5067
Phone: 787-758-2525
Fax: *Not Reported*
Contact: Irma R. Ortiz, PhD, RN, Director BSN Dept.
Email: i-ortiz@rcmaca.upr.cu.edu

GENERAL INFORMATION

Type of School: *Independent, Public* • Accreditation: *Middle States Association of Colleges and Schools* • Total Enrollment: *3154*

PROGRAM INFORMATION

Two Year Exit Option: *Not Reported* • NLNAC Accreditation: *Yes* • CCNE Accreditation:

NURSING STUDENT PROFILE

Total Nursing Enrollment: *352* • Total Basic Student Enrollment, Full Time: *Not Reported* • Total Basic Student Enrollment, Part Time: *Not Reported* • Female Basic Student Enrollment: *Not Reported* • Male Basic Student Enrollment: *Not Reported* • Total RN Enrollment: *134* • Total New Fall Enrollments: *50* • Total Graduates: *95* • Basic Student Graduates: *69* • RN Student Graduates: *26*

FINANCES

Residential Annual Tuition: *$1,600* • Non-Residential Annual Tuition: *$1,600* • General Institutional Fees: *$1,130* • Additional Nursing Fees: *$453*

UNIVERSITY OF PUERTO RICO—ARECIBO

Address: Box 4010, Arecibo, PR 00613-4010
Phone: 787-878-2830
Fax: 787-880-6277
Contact: Miqdalia Lopez Forty, PhD, RN, Director
Email: *Not Reported*

GENERAL INFORMATION

Type of School: *Not Reported* • Accreditation: *Not Reported* • Total Enrollment: *Not Reported*

PROGRAM INFORMATION

Two Year Exit Option: *Not Reported* • NLNAC Accreditation: *Not Reported* • CCNE Accreditation:

NURSING STUDENT PROFILE

Total Nursing Enrollment: *Not Reported* • Total Basic Student Enrollment, Full Time: *Not Reported* • Total Basic Student Enrollment, Part Time: *Not Reported* • Female Basic Student Enrollment: *Not Reported* • Male Basic Student Enrollment: *Not Reported* • Total RN Enrollment: *Not Reported* • Total New Fall Enrollments: *Not Reported* • Total Graduates: *Not Reported* • Basic Student Graduates: *Not Reported* • RN Student Graduates: *Not Reported*

FINANCES

Residential Annual Tuition: *Not Reported* • Non-Residential Annual Tuition: *Not Reported* • General Institutional Fees: *Not Reported* • Additional Nursing Fees: *Not Reported*

UNIVERSITY OF PUERTO RICO—HUMACAO

Address: CUH Station 100 Road 1908, Humacao, PR
00791-4300
Phone: 787-850-9346
Fax: 787-850-9411
Contact: Francisca Trinidad, EdD, RN, Director
Email: f_rodriguez@cuhac.upr.clu.edu

GENERAL INFORMATION

Type of School: *4-Year College or University, Public* •
Accreditation: *Middle States Association of Colleges and
Schools* • Total Enrollment: *4592*

PROGRAM INFORMATION

Two Year Exit Option: *Not Reported* • NLNAC
Accreditation: *Yes* • CCNE Accreditation:

NURSING STUDENT PROFILE

Total Nursing Enrollment: *158* • Total Basic Student
Enrollment, Full Time: *153* • Total Basic Student
Enrollment, Part Time: *0* • Female Basic Student
Enrollment: *134* • Male Basic Student Enrollment: *19* • Total
RN Enrollment: *5* • Total New Fall Enrollments: *62* • Total
Graduates: *29* • Basic Student Graduates: *28* • RN Student
Graduates: *1*

FINANCES

Residential Annual Tuition: *$1,245* • Non-Residential
Annual Tuition: *$2,400* • General Institutional Fees: *$75* •
Additional Nursing Fees: *Not Reported*

UNIVERSITY OF PUERTO RICO—MAYAGUEZ

Address: PO Box 9015, Mayaguez, PR 00681-9015
Phone: 787-265-3842
Fax: 787-832-3875
Contact: Zaida Lina Torres, MSN, RN, Assoc. Professor
Email: Ztorres@rumad.uprm.edu

GENERAL INFORMATION

Type of School: *Governmental Agency, Public* • Accreditation:
Middle States Association of Colleges and Schools • Total
Enrollment: *12000*

PROGRAM INFORMATION

Two Year Exit Option: *Not Reported* • NLNAC
Accreditation: *Yes* • CCNE Accreditation:

NURSING STUDENT PROFILE

Total Nursing Enrollment: *238* • Total Basic Student
Enrollment, Full Time: *238* • Total Basic Student
Enrollment, Part Time: *0* • Female Basic Student
Enrollment: *201* • Male Basic Student Enrollment: *37* • Total
RN Enrollment: *0* • Total New Fall Enrollments: *44* • Total
Graduates: *30* • Basic Student Graduates: *30* • RN Student
Graduates: *0*

FINANCES

Residential Annual Tuition: *$1,245* • Non-Residential
Annual Tuition: *$1,245* • General Institutional Fees: *$70* •
Additional Nursing Fees: *$50*

RHODE ISLAND COLLEGE

Address: 600 Mount Pleasant Avenue, Providence, RI
02908-1991
Phone: 401-456-8014
Fax: *Not Reported*
Contact: Patricia A. Thomas, PhD, RNC, Chair
Email: pthomas@ric.edu

GENERAL INFORMATION

Type of School: *New England Association of Schools and Colleges, 4-Year College or University, Public* • Accreditation: *1854* • Total Enrollment: *Not Provided*

PROGRAM INFORMATION

Two Year Exit Option: *Not Reported* • NLNAC Accreditation: *Yes* • CCNE Accreditation:

NURSING STUDENT PROFILE

Total Nursing Enrollment: *339* • Total Basic Student Enrollment, Full Time: *198* • Total Basic Student Enrollment, Part Time: *120* • Female Basic Student Enrollment: *267* • Male Basic Student Enrollment: *51* • Total RN Enrollment: *21* • Total New Fall Enrollments: *96* • Total Graduates: *129* • Basic Student Graduates: *112* • RN Student Graduates: *17*

FINANCES

Residential Annual Tuition: *$2,676* • Non-Residential Annual Tuition: *$7,600* • General Institutional Fees: *$1,338* • Additional Nursing Fees: *$120*

SALVE REGINA UNIVERSITY

Address: 100 Ochre Point Avenue, Newport, RI 02840
Phone: 401-847-6650
Fax: 401-847-6658
Contact: Louise L. Mundock, PhD, RN, Co. Chair Person
Email: mundockl@salve.edu

GENERAL INFORMATION

Type of School: *4-Year College or University, Private (Religious)* • Accreditation: *New England Association of Schools and Colleges* • Total Enrollment: *2200*

PROGRAM INFORMATION

Two Year Exit Option: *Not Reported* • NLNAC Accreditation: *Yes* • CCNE Accreditation:

NURSING STUDENT PROFILE

Total Nursing Enrollment: *122* • Total Basic Student Enrollment, Full Time: *57* • Total Basic Student Enrollment, Part Time: *0* • Female Basic Student Enrollment: *57* • Male Basic Student Enrollment: *0* • Total RN Enrollment: *65* • Total New Fall Enrollments: *17* • Total Graduates: *17* • Basic Student Graduates: *14* • RN Student Graduates: *3*

FINANCES

Residential Annual Tuition: *Not Reported* • Non-Residential Annual Tuition: *Not Reported* • General Institutional Fees: *Not Reported* • Additional Nursing Fees: *Not Reported*

UNIVERSITY OF RHODE ISLAND

Address: White Hall, 2 Heathman Road, Kingston, RI
             02881
Phone: 401-874-2766
Fax: 401-874-3811
Contact: Dayle Joseph, EdD, RN, Dean
Email: dayle@uri.edu

GENERAL INFORMATION

Type of School: *4-Year College or University, Public* •
Accreditation: *New England Association of Schools and
Colleges* • Total Enrollment: *14362*

PROGRAM INFORMATION

Two Year Exit Option: *Not Reported* • NLNAC
Accreditation: *Yes* • CCNE Accreditation:

NURSING STUDENT PROFILE

Total Nursing Enrollment: *428* • Total Basic Student
Enrollment, Full Time: *335* • Total Basic Student
Enrollment, Part Time: *35* • Female Basic Student
Enrollment: *328* • Male Basic Student Enrollment: *42* • Total
RN Enrollment: *58* • Total New Fall Enrollments: *60* • Total
Graduates: *84* • Basic Student Graduates: *72* • RN Student
Graduates: *12*

FINANCES

Residential Annual Tuition: *$3,464* • Non-Residential
Annual Tuition: *$11,906* • General Institutional Fees:
$1,732 • Additional Nursing Fees: *$145*

BOB JONES UNIVERSITY

Address: 1700 Wade Hampton Blvd, Greenville, SC
             29614
Phone: 864-242-5100
Fax: 864-242-1858
Contact: Kathleen M. Crispin, EdD, RN, Chairman,
             Division of Nursing
Email: kcrispin@bju.edu

GENERAL INFORMATION

Type of School: *4-Year College or University, Private
(Religious)* • Accreditation: *Not Reported* • Total Enrollment:
Not Reported

PROGRAM INFORMATION

Two Year Exit Option: *No* • NLNAC Accreditation: *Not
Reported* • CCNE Accreditation:

NURSING STUDENT PROFILE

Total Nursing Enrollment: *140* • Total Basic Student
Enrollment, Full Time: *139* • Total Basic Student
Enrollment, Part Time: *0* • Female Basic Student
Enrollment: *134* • Male Basic Student Enrollment: *5* • Total
RN Enrollment: *1* • Total New Fall Enrollments: *30* • Total
Graduates: *26* • Basic Student Graduates: *26* • RN Student
Graduates: *0*

FINANCES

Residential Annual Tuition: *$6,060* • Non-Residential
Annual Tuition: *$6,060* • General Institutional Fees:
$3,030 • Additional Nursing Fees: *Not Reported*

CHARLESTON SOUTHERN UNIVERSITY

Address: PO Box 118087, Charleston, SC 29423
Phone: 803-863-7032
Fax: 803-863-7540
Contact: Marian Larisey, PhD, RN, Dean
Email: mlarisey@csuniv.edu

GENERAL INFORMATION

Type of School: *4-Year College or University, Private (Religious)* • Accreditation: *Southern Association of Colleges and Schools* • Total Enrollment: *Not Reported*

PROGRAM INFORMATION

Two Year Exit Option: *No* • NLNAC Accreditation: *Yes* • CCNE Accreditation:

NURSING STUDENT PROFILE

Total Nursing Enrollment: *57* • Total Basic Student Enrollment, Full Time: *57* • Total Basic Student Enrollment, Part Time: *0* • Female Basic Student Enrollment: *54* • Male Basic Student Enrollment: *3* • Total RN Enrollment: *0* • Total New Fall Enrollments: *32* • Total Graduates: *13* • Basic Student Graduates: *13* • RN Student Graduates: *0*

FINANCES

Residential Annual Tuition: *$11,346* • Non-Residential Annual Tuition: *$11,346* • General Institutional Fees: *$5,673* • Additional Nursing Fees: *$185*

CLEMSON UNIVERSITY

Address: 508 Edwards Hall, Clemson, SC 29634-0743
Phone: 864-656-5489
Fax: 864-656-5488
Contact: Juanite E. Lee, EdD, RN, PNP, Professor
Email: leee@clemson.edu

GENERAL INFORMATION

Type of School: *4-Year College or University, Public* • Accreditation: *Southern Association of Colleges and Schools* • Total Enrollment: *Not Reported*

PROGRAM INFORMATION

Two Year Exit Option: *No* • NLNAC Accreditation: *Yes* • CCNE Accreditation:

NURSING STUDENT PROFILE

Total Nursing Enrollment: *393* • Total Basic Student Enrollment, Full Time: *357* • Total Basic Student Enrollment, Part Time: *11* • Female Basic Student Enrollment: *348* • Male Basic Student Enrollment: *20* • Total RN Enrollment: *25* • Total New Fall Enrollments: *91* • Total Graduates: *82* • Basic Student Graduates: *72* • RN Student Graduates: *10*

FINANCES

Residential Annual Tuition: *$3,470* • Non-Residential Annual Tuition: *$9,456* • General Institutional Fees: *$1,735* • Additional Nursing Fees: *$138*

LANDER UNIVERSITY

Address: 320 Stanley Street, Greenwood, SC 29649
Phone: 864-388-8337
Fax: 864-388-8221
Contact: Carol J. Scales, PhD, RN, Assoc. Professor and
            Dean
Email: cscales@lander.edu

GENERAL INFORMATION

Type of School: *4-Year College or University, Public* •
Accreditation: *Southern Association of Colleges and Schools* •
Total Enrollment: *Not Reported*

PROGRAM INFORMATION

Two Year Exit Option: *No* • NLNAC Accreditation: *Yes* •
CCNE Accreditation:

NURSING STUDENT PROFILE

Total Nursing Enrollment: *93* • Total Basic Student
Enrollment, Full Time: *71* • Total Basic Student Enrollment,
Part Time: *6* • Female Basic Student Enrollment: *72* • Male
Basic Student Enrollment: *5* • Total RN Enrollment: *16* •
Total New Fall Enrollments: *24* • Total Graduates: *28* • Basic
Student Graduates: *27* • RN Student Graduates: *1*

FINANCES

Residential Annual Tuition: *$3,888* • Non-Residential
Annual Tuition: *$7,776* • General Institutional Fees:
$1,944 • Additional Nursing Fees: *$162*

MEDICAL UNIVERSITY OF SOUTH CAROLINA

Address: 99 Johnathan Lucas St, Charleston, SC 29425
Phone: 843-792-3815
Fax: 843-792-9258
Contact: Jean D. Leuner, PhD, RN, Assoc. Dean
Email: leunerj@musc.edu

GENERAL INFORMATION

Type of School: *4-Year College or University, Public* •
Accreditation: *Southern Association of Colleges and Schools* •
Total Enrollment: *Not Reported*

PROGRAM INFORMATION

Two Year Exit Option: *No* • NLNAC Accreditation: *Yes* •
CCNE Accreditation:

NURSING STUDENT PROFILE

Total Nursing Enrollment: *246* • Total Basic Student
Enrollment, Full Time: *192* • Total Basic Student
Enrollment, Part Time: *8* • Female Basic Student
Enrollment: *187* • Male Basic Student Enrollment: *13* • Total
RN Enrollment: *46* • Total New Fall Enrollments: *72* • Total
Graduates: *129* • Basic Student Graduates: *93* • RN Student
Graduates: *36*

FINANCES

Residential Annual Tuition: *$5,024* • Non-Residential
Annual Tuition: *$13,754* • General Institutional Fees:
$2,512 • Additional Nursing Fees: *$208*

SOUTH CAROLINA STATE UNIVERSITY

Address:　PO Box 7158, 300 College St, Orangeburg, SC 29117
Phone:　803-536-8605
Fax:　*Not Reported*
Contact:　Ruth W. Johnson, EdD, RN, FAAN, Chair
Email:　rwjohnson@scsu.edu

GENERAL INFORMATION

Type of School: *Not Reported* • Accreditation: *Southern Association of Colleges and Schools* • Total Enrollment: *Not Reported*

PROGRAM INFORMATION

Two Year Exit Option: *Not Reported* • NLNAC Accreditation: *Not Reported* • CCNE Accreditation:

NURSING STUDENT PROFILE

Total Nursing Enrollment: *145* • Total Basic Student Enrollment, Full Time: *131* • Total Basic Student Enrollment, Part Time: *7* • Female Basic Student Enrollment: *135* • Male Basic Student Enrollment: *3* • Total RN Enrollment: *7* • Total New Fall Enrollments: *Not Reported* • Total Graduates: *3* • Basic Student Graduates: *1* • RN Student Graduates: *2*

FINANCES

Residential Annual Tuition: *Not Reported* • Non-Residential Annual Tuition: *Not Reported* • General Institutional Fees: *Not Reported* • Additional Nursing Fees: *Not Reported*

UNIVERSITY OF SOUTH CAROLINA—AIKEN

Address:　471 University Parkway, Aiken, SC 29801
Phone:　803-641-3508
Fax:　803-641-3725
Contact:　Patricia R. Cook, PhD, RN, BSN Program Coordinator.
Email:　pattic@aikensc.edu

GENERAL INFORMATION

Type of School: *4-Year College or University, Public* • Accreditation: *Southern Association of Colleges and Schools* • Total Enrollment: *Not Reported*

PROGRAM INFORMATION

Two Year Exit Option: *Not Reported* • NLNAC Accreditation: *Yes* • CCNE Accreditation:

NURSING STUDENT PROFILE

Total Nursing Enrollment: *Not Reported* • Total Basic Student Enrollment, Full Time: *Not Reported* • Total Basic Student Enrollment, Part Time: *Not Reported* • Female Basic Student Enrollment: *Not Reported* • Male Basic Student Enrollment: *Not Reported* • Total RN Enrollment: *Not Reported* • Total New Fall Enrollments: *Not Reported* • Total Graduates: *Not Reported* • Basic Student Graduates: *Not Reported* • RN Student Graduates: *Not Reported*

FINANCES

Residential Annual Tuition: *Not Reported* • Non-Residential Annual Tuition: *Not Reported* • General Institutional Fees: *Not Reported* • Additional Nursing Fees: *Not Reported*

UNIVERSITY OF SOUTH CAROLINA—COLUMBIA

Address: 1601 Greene Street, William Brice Bldg., Columbia, SC 29208
Phone: 803-777-3862
Fax: 803-777-2027
Contact: Mary Ann Parsons, PhD, RN, Dean
Email: maryann.parsons@sc.edu

GENERAL INFORMATION

Type of School: *4-Year College or University, Public* •
Accreditation: *Southern Association of Colleges and Schools* •
Total Enrollment: *Not Reported*

PROGRAM INFORMATION

Two Year Exit Option: *No* • NLNAC Accreditation: *Not Reported* • CCNE Accreditation: *Yes*

NURSING STUDENT PROFILE

Total Nursing Enrollment: *525* • Total Basic Student Enrollment, Full Time: *461* • Total Basic Student Enrollment, Part Time: *22* • Female Basic Student Enrollment: *459* • Male Basic Student Enrollment: *24* • Total RN Enrollment: *42* • Total New Fall Enrollments: *48* • Total Graduates: *106* • Basic Student Graduates: *83* • RN Student Graduates: *23*

FINANCES

Residential Annual Tuition: *$5,040* • Non-Residential Annual Tuition: *$12,764* • General Institutional Fees: *$100* • Additional Nursing Fees: *$50*

UNIVERSITY OF SOUTH CAROLINA—SPARTANBURG

Address: 800 University Way, Spartanburg, SC 29303
Phone: 864-503-5469
Fax: 864-503-5411
Contact: Angelise L. Davis, DSN, RN, BSN Program Division Chair
Email: adavis@gw.uscs.edu

GENERAL INFORMATION

Type of School: *4-Year College or University, Public* •
Accreditation: *Southern Association of Colleges and Schools* •
Total Enrollment: *Not Reported*

PROGRAM INFORMATION

Two Year Exit Option: *No* • NLNAC Accreditation: *Yes* • CCNE Accreditation:

NURSING STUDENT PROFILE

Total Nursing Enrollment: *167* • Total Basic Student Enrollment, Full Time: *104* • Total Basic Student Enrollment, Part Time: *12* • Female Basic Student Enrollment: *105* • Male Basic Student Enrollment: *11* • Total RN Enrollment: *51* • Total New Fall Enrollments: *35* • Total Graduates: *94* • Basic Student Graduates: *53* • RN Student Graduates: *41*

FINANCES

Residential Annual Tuition: *$3,844* • Non-Residential Annual Tuition: *$8,736* • General Institutional Fees: *$220* • Additional Nursing Fees: *$114*

AUGUSTANA COLLEGE

Address: 2001 South Summit Avenue, Souix Falls, SD
            57197
Phone: 605-336-4726
Fax: *Not Reported*
Contact: Sandra Bunkers, PhD, RN, FAAN, Department
            Chair and Associate Professor
Email: bunkers@inst.augie.edu

GENERAL INFORMATION

Type of School: *4-Year College or University, Private
(Religious)* • Accreditation: *North Central Association of
Colleges and Schools* • Total Enrollment: *1783*

PROGRAM INFORMATION

Two Year Exit Option: *Not Reported* • NLNAC
Accreditation: *Yes* • CCNE Accreditation:

NURSING STUDENT PROFILE

Total Nursing Enrollment: *120* • Total Basic Student
Enrollment, Full Time: *Not Reported* • Total Basic Student
Enrollment, Part Time: *Not Reported* • Female Basic Student
Enrollment: *Not Reported* • Male Basic Student Enrollment:
Not Reported • Total RN Enrollment: *2* • Total New Fall
Enrollments: *30* • Total Graduates: *42* • Basic Student
Graduates: *39* • RN Student Graduates: *3*

FINANCES

Residential Annual Tuition: *$13,960* • Non-Residential
Annual Tuition: *$13,960* • General Institutional Fees: *$154* •
Additional Nursing Fees: *$200*

HURON UNIVERSITY

Address: 333 9th Street South West, Huron, SD 57350
Phone: 605-352-8721
Fax: *Not Reported*
Contact: Ella Brooks, PhD, RN, Dean of Nursing and
            Health Science
Email: *Not Reported*

GENERAL INFORMATION

Type of School: *4-Year College or University, Private
(Independent)* • Accreditation: *North Central Association of
Colleges and Schools* • Total Enrollment: *598*

PROGRAM INFORMATION

Two Year Exit Option: *Yes* • NLNAC Accreditation: *Not
Reported* • CCNE Accreditation:

NURSING STUDENT PROFILE

Total Nursing Enrollment: *13* • Total Basic Student
Enrollment, Full Time: *Not Reported* • Total Basic Student
Enrollment, Part Time: *Not Reported* • Female Basic Student
Enrollment: *Not Reported* • Male Basic Student Enrollment:
Not Reported • Total RN Enrollment: *13* • Total New Fall
Enrollments: *13* • Total Graduates: *4* • Basic Student
Graduates: *0* • RN Student Graduates: *4*

FINANCES

Residential Annual Tuition: *Not Reported* • Non-Residential
Annual Tuition: *Not Reported* • General Institutional Fees:
Not Reported • Additional Nursing Fees: *Not Reported*

MOUNT MARTY COLLEGE

Address: 1105 West 8th Street, Yankton, SD 57078-3724
Phone: 605-668-1594
Fax: 605-668-1607
Contact: Janice E. Stephens, PhD, RN, Division of Nursing Chair
Email: jstephens@mtmc.edu

GENERAL INFORMATION

Type of School: *4-Year College or University, Private (Religious)* • Accreditation: *North Central Association of Colleges and Schools* • Total Enrollment: *567*

PROGRAM INFORMATION

Two Year Exit Option: *No* • NLNAC Accreditation: *Yes* • CCNE Accreditation:

NURSING STUDENT PROFILE

Total Nursing Enrollment: *72* • Total Basic Student Enrollment, Full Time: *62* • Total Basic Student Enrollment, Part Time: *1* • Female Basic Student Enrollment: *54* • Male Basic Student Enrollment: *9* • Total RN Enrollment: *9* • Total New Fall Enrollments: *17* • Total Graduates: *22* • Basic Student Graduates: *21* • RN Student Graduates: *1*

FINANCES

Residential Annual Tuition: *$12,000* • Non-Residential Annual Tuition: *$12,000* • General Institutional Fees: *$75* • Additional Nursing Fees: *$257*

PRESENTATION COLLEGE

Address: 1500 North Main, Aberdeen, SD 57401
Phone: 605-229-8473
Fax: 605-229-8489
Contact: Janice S. Williams, ND, MSN, RN, CS, CDE, Chair and Associate Professor
Email: janicesw@presentation.edu

GENERAL INFORMATION

Type of School: *4-Year College or University, Private (Religious)* • Accreditation: *North Central Association of Colleges and Schools* • Total Enrollment: *615*

PROGRAM INFORMATION

Two Year Exit Option: *No* • NLNAC Accreditation: *Yes* • CCNE Accreditation:

NURSING STUDENT PROFILE

Total Nursing Enrollment: *112* • Total Basic Student Enrollment, Full Time: *Not Reported* • Total Basic Student Enrollment, Part Time: *Not Reported* • Female Basic Student Enrollment: *Not Reported* • Male Basic Student Enrollment: *Not Reported* • Total RN Enrollment: *10* • Total New Fall Enrollments: *33* • Total Graduates: *34* • Basic Student Graduates: *28* • RN Student Graduates: *6*

FINANCES

Residential Annual Tuition: *$8,500* • Non-Residential Annual Tuition: *$8,500* • General Institutional Fees: *$300* • Additional Nursing Fees: *$500*

SOUTH DAKOTA STATE UNIVERSITY

Address: Box 2275, Brookings, SD 57007-0098
Phone: 605-688-6153
Fax: *Not Reported*
Contact: Judith Vinson, PhD, RN, Department Head,
Undergraduate Nursing
Email: Judith_Vinson@sdstate.edu

GENERAL INFORMATION

Type of School: *4-Year College or University, Public* •
Accreditation: *North Central Association of Colleges and Schools* • Total Enrollment: *8720*

PROGRAM INFORMATION

Two Year Exit Option: *Not Reported* • NLNAC
Accreditation: *Yes* • CCNE Accreditation:

NURSING STUDENT PROFILE

Total Nursing Enrollment: *381* • Total Basic Student
Enrollment, Full Time: *Not Reported* • Total Basic Student
Enrollment, Part Time: *Not Reported* • Female Basic Student
Enrollment: *Not Reported* • Male Basic Student Enrollment:
Not Reported • Total RN Enrollment: *59* • Total New Fall
Enrollments: *48* • Total Graduates: *157* • Basic Student
Graduates: *122* • RN Student Graduates: *35*

FINANCES

Residential Annual Tuition: *$1,348* • Non-Residential
Annual Tuition: *$4,288* • General Institutional Fees: *Not
Reported* • Additional Nursing Fees: *$605*

AUSTIN PEAY STATE UNIVERSITY

Address: 601 College Street, Clarksville, TN 37044
Phone: 931-221-7737
Fax: 931-221-7595
Contact: Kathy L. Martin, PhD, RN, CNAA, Professor
and Director, School of Nursing
Email: martinl@apsu.edu

GENERAL INFORMATION

Type of School: *4-Year College or University, Public* •
Accreditation: *Southern Association of Colleges and Schools* •
Total Enrollment: *7033*

PROGRAM INFORMATION

Two Year Exit Option: *No* • NLNAC Accreditation: *Yes* •
CCNE Accreditation:

NURSING STUDENT PROFILE

Total Nursing Enrollment: *157* • Total Basic Student
Enrollment, Full Time: *153* • Total Basic Student
Enrollment, Part Time: *0* • Female Basic Student
Enrollment: *136* • Male Basic Student Enrollment: *17* • Total
RN Enrollment: *4* • Total New Fall Enrollments: *79* • Total
Graduates: *67* • Basic Student Graduates: *62* • RN Student
Graduates: *5*

FINANCES

Residential Annual Tuition: *$3,208* • Non-Residential
Annual Tuition: *$9,680* • General Institutional Fees: *$224* •
Additional Nursing Fees: *$100*

BAPTIST MEMORIAL COLLEGE OF HEALTH SCIENCES

Address: 1003 Monroe Avenue, Memphis, TN 38104
Phone: 901-227-6912
Fax: 901-227-5533
Contact: Veta Massey, PhD, RN, Dean
Email: veta.massey@bchs.edu

GENERAL INFORMATION

Type of School: *4-Year College or University, Private (Religious)* • Accreditation: *Southern Association of Colleges and Schools* • Total Enrollment: *462*

PROGRAM INFORMATION

Two Year Exit Option: *No* • NLNAC Accreditation: *Not Reported* • CCNE Accreditation: *Yes*

NURSING STUDENT PROFILE

Total Nursing Enrollment: *128* • Total Basic Student Enrollment, Full Time: *104* • Total Basic Student Enrollment, Part Time: *6* • Female Basic Student Enrollment: *103* • Male Basic Student Enrollment: *7* • Total RN Enrollment: *18* • Total New Fall Enrollments: *58* • Total Graduates: *109* • Basic Student Graduates: *60* • RN Student Graduates: *49*

FINANCES

Residential Annual Tuition: *Not Reported* • Non-Residential Annual Tuition: *Not Reported* • General Institutional Fees: *Not Reported* • Additional Nursing Fees: *$140*

CARSON NEWMAN COLLEGE

Address: 1646 Russell Avenue, Jefferson City, TN 37760
Phone: 865-471-3463
Fax: 865-471-4574
Contact: Tippie Pollard, EdD, RN, Chair
Email: tpollard@cn.edu

GENERAL INFORMATION

Type of School: *4-Year College or University, Private (Religious)* • Accreditation: *Southern Association of Colleges and Schools* • Total Enrollment: *2230*

PROGRAM INFORMATION

Two Year Exit Option: *No* • NLNAC Accreditation: *Yes* • CCNE Accreditation:

NURSING STUDENT PROFILE

Total Nursing Enrollment: *117* • Total Basic Student Enrollment, Full Time: *108* • Total Basic Student Enrollment, Part Time: *5* • Female Basic Student Enrollment: *106* • Male Basic Student Enrollment: *7* • Total RN Enrollment: *4* • Total New Fall Enrollments: *Not Reported* • Total Graduates: *22* • Basic Student Graduates: *20* • RN Student Graduates: *2*

FINANCES

Residential Annual Tuition: *$11,240* • Non-Residential Annual Tuition: *$11,240* • General Institutional Fees: *$5,620* • Additional Nursing Fees: *$460*

CUMBERLAND UNIVERSITY

Address: One Cumberland Square, Lebanon, TN 37087
Phone: 615-444-2562
Fax: 615-443-8427
Contact: Leanne C. Busby, DSN, RNC, FAAN, Professor
           and Dean
Email: lbusby@cumberland.edu

GENERAL INFORMATION

Type of School: *4-Year College or University, Private (Independent)* • Accreditation: *Southern Association of Colleges and Schools* • Total Enrollment: *Not Reported*

PROGRAM INFORMATION

Two Year Exit Option: *No* • NLNAC Accreditation: *Yes* • CCNE Accreditation:

NURSING STUDENT PROFILE

Total Nursing Enrollment: *72* • Total Basic Student Enrollment, Full Time: *68* • Total Basic Student Enrollment, Part Time: *2* • Female Basic Student Enrollment: *66* • Male Basic Student Enrollment: *4* • Total RN Enrollment: *2* • Total New Fall Enrollments: *Not Reported* • Total Graduates: *26* • Basic Student Graduates: *23* • RN Student Graduates: *3*

FINANCES

Residential Annual Tuition: *$10,500* • Non-Residential Annual Tuition: *$10,500* • General Institutional Fees: *$60* • Additional Nursing Fees: *$30*

EAST TENNESSEE STATE UNIVERSITY

Address: 807 University Parkway, Johnson City, TN
           37614
Phone: 423-439-4624
Fax: 423-439-4522
Contact: Patricia Smith, EdD, RN, Assoc. Dean,
           Academic Programs
Email: smithp@etsu.edu

GENERAL INFORMATION

Type of School: *4-Year College or University, Public* • Accreditation: *Southern Association of Colleges and Schools* • Total Enrollment: *11000*

PROGRAM INFORMATION

Two Year Exit Option: *No* • NLNAC Accreditation: *Yes* • CCNE Accreditation:

NURSING STUDENT PROFILE

Total Nursing Enrollment: *380* • Total Basic Student Enrollment, Full Time: *276* • Total Basic Student Enrollment, Part Time: *61* • Female Basic Student Enrollment: *287* • Male Basic Student Enrollment: *50* • Total RN Enrollment: *43* • Total New Fall Enrollments: *53* • Total Graduates: *119* • Basic Student Graduates: *106* • RN Student Graduates: *13*

FINANCES

Residential Annual Tuition: *$2,716* • Non-Residential Annual Tuition: *$9,188* • General Institutional Fees: *$203* • Additional Nursing Fees: *$750*

KING COLLEGE

Address: 1350 King College Road, Bristol, TN 38620
Phone: 423-652-4748
Fax: 423-652-4833
Contact: Johanne A. Quinn, PhD, RN, HNC, Professor and Director
Email: jaquinn@king.edu

GENERAL INFORMATION

Type of School: *4-Year College or University, Private (Religious)* • Accreditation: *Southern Association of Colleges and Schools* • Total Enrollment: *Not Reported*

PROGRAM INFORMATION

Two Year Exit Option: *No* • NLNAC Accreditation: *Not Reported* • CCNE Accreditation: *Yes*

NURSING STUDENT PROFILE

Total Nursing Enrollment: *42* • Total Basic Student Enrollment, Full Time: *26* • Total Basic Student Enrollment, Part Time: *7* • Female Basic Student Enrollment: *32* • Male Basic Student Enrollment: *1* • Total RN Enrollment: *9* • Total New Fall Enrollments: *9* • Total Graduates: *5* • Basic Student Graduates: *4* • RN Student Graduates: *1*

FINANCES

Residential Annual Tuition: *$12,390* • Non-Residential Annual Tuition: *$12,390* • General Institutional Fees: *$950* • Additional Nursing Fees: *$350*

LINCOLN MEMORIAL UNIVERSITY

Address: Cumberland Gap Parkway, Harrogate, TN 37752
Phone: 423-865-6326
Fax: *Not Reported*
Contact: Mary Anne Talbott, PhD, RN, Chair
Email: *Not Reported*

GENERAL INFORMATION

Type of School: *4-Year College or University, Private (Independent)* • Accreditation: *Southern Association of Colleges and Schools* • Total Enrollment: *1753*

PROGRAM INFORMATION

Two Year Exit Option: *Not Reported* • NLNAC Accreditation: *Yes* • CCNE Accreditation:

NURSING STUDENT PROFILE

Total Nursing Enrollment: *Not Reported* • Total Basic Student Enrollment, Full Time: *Not Reported* • Total Basic Student Enrollment, Part Time: *Not Reported* • Female Basic Student Enrollment: *Not Reported* • Male Basic Student Enrollment: *Not Reported* • Total RN Enrollment: *Not Reported* • Total New Fall Enrollments: *Not Reported* • Total Graduates: *Not Reported* • Basic Student Graduates: *Not Reported* • RN Student Graduates: *Not Reported*

FINANCES

Residential Annual Tuition: *Not Reported* • Non-Residential Annual Tuition: *Not Reported* • General Institutional Fees: *Not Reported* • Additional Nursing Fees: *Not Reported*

MIDDLE TENNESSEE STATE UNIVERSITY

Address: Box 81-1301 East Main Street, Murfreesboro, TN 37132
Phone: 615-898-2437
Fax: *Not Reported*
Contact: Pamela G. Holder, DSN, RN, Director
Email: *Not Reported*

GENERAL INFORMATION

Type of School: *Not Reported* • Accreditation: *Southern Association of Colleges and Schools* • Total Enrollment: *18000*

PROGRAM INFORMATION

Two Year Exit Option: *Not Reported* • NLNAC Accreditation: *Yes* • CCNE Accreditation:

NURSING STUDENT PROFILE

Total Nursing Enrollment: *Not Reported* • Total Basic Student Enrollment, Full Time: *Not Reported* • Total Basic Student Enrollment, Part Time: *Not Reported* • Female Basic Student Enrollment: *Not Reported* • Male Basic Student Enrollment: *Not Reported* • Total RN Enrollment: *Not Reported* • Total New Fall Enrollments: *Not Reported* • Total Graduates: *Not Reported* • Basic Student Graduates: *Not Reported* • RN Student Graduates: *Not Reported*

FINANCES

Residential Annual Tuition: *Not Reported* • Non-Residential Annual Tuition: *Not Reported* • General Institutional Fees: *Not Reported* • Additional Nursing Fees: *Not Reported*

MILLIGAN COLLEGE

Address: PO Box 500, Milligan College, TN 37682
Phone: 423-461-8655
Fax: 423-461-3328
Contact: Melinda Collins, MSN, RN, Interim Chair
Email: mcollins@milligan.edu

GENERAL INFORMATION

Type of School: *4-Year College or University, Private (Religious)* • Accreditation: *Southern Association of Colleges and Schools* • Total Enrollment: *899*

PROGRAM INFORMATION

Two Year Exit Option: *No* • NLNAC Accreditation: *Not Reported* • CCNE Accreditation:

NURSING STUDENT PROFILE

Total Nursing Enrollment: *51* • Total Basic Student Enrollment, Full Time: *51* • Total Basic Student Enrollment, Part Time: *0* • Female Basic Student Enrollment: *51* • Male Basic Student Enrollment: *0* • Total RN Enrollment: *0* • Total New Fall Enrollments: *12* • Total Graduates: *5* • Basic Student Graduates: *5* • RN Student Graduates: *0*

FINANCES

Residential Annual Tuition: *$12,750* • Non-Residential Annual Tuition: *$12,750* • General Institutional Fees: *$500* • Additional Nursing Fees: *$250*

TENNESSEE STATE UNIVERSITY

Address: 3500 John A. Merritt Boulevard, Box 9596, Nashville, TN 37209
Phone: 615-963-7615
Fax: 615-963-5593
Contact: Yvonne N. Stringfield, EdD, RN, BSN Program Director
Email: ystringfield@tnstate.edu

GENERAL INFORMATION

Type of School: *4-Year College or University, Public* • Accreditation: *Southern Association of Colleges and Schools* • Total Enrollment: *10000*

PROGRAM INFORMATION

Two Year Exit Option: *No* • NLNAC Accreditation: *Yes* • CCNE Accreditation:

NURSING STUDENT PROFILE

Total Nursing Enrollment: *111* • Total Basic Student Enrollment, Full Time: *93* • Total Basic Student Enrollment, Part Time: *1* • Female Basic Student Enrollment: *80* • Male Basic Student Enrollment: *14* • Total RN Enrollment: *17* • Total New Fall Enrollments: *0* • Total Graduates: *33* • Basic Student Graduates: *23* • RN Student Graduates: *10*

FINANCES

Residential Annual Tuition: *$1,672* • Non-Residential Annual Tuition: *$8,300* • General Institutional Fees: *$1,336* • Additional Nursing Fees: *$152*

TENNESSEE TECHNOLOGICAL UNIVERSITY

Address: Box 5001, Cookeville, TN 38505
Phone: 931-372-3213
Fax: 931-372-6244
Contact: Marilyn J. Musacchio, PhD, RN, CNM, FAAN, Dean and Professor
Email: mmusacchio@tntech.edu

GENERAL INFORMATION

Type of School: *Other, Public* • Accreditation: *Southern Association of Colleges and Schools* • Total Enrollment: *8653*

PROGRAM INFORMATION

Two Year Exit Option: *No* • NLNAC Accreditation: *Yes* • CCNE Accreditation:

NURSING STUDENT PROFILE

Total Nursing Enrollment: *93* • Total Basic Student Enrollment, Full Time: *75* • Total Basic Student Enrollment, Part Time: *6* • Female Basic Student Enrollment: *77* • Male Basic Student Enrollment: *4* • Total RN Enrollment: *12* • Total New Fall Enrollments: *39* • Total Graduates: *39* • Basic Student Graduates: *36* • RN Student Graduates: *3*

FINANCES

Residential Annual Tuition: *$2,555* • Non-Residential Annual Tuition: *$9,149* • General Institutional Fees: *$511* • Additional Nursing Fees: *$207*

TENNESSEE WESLEYAN COLLEGE

Address: 9821 Cogdill Road, Knoxville, TN 37932
Phone: 865-777-5100
Fax: 865-777-5114
Contact: Margaret Heins, EdD, RN, FAAN, Chair and Professor
Email: mheins@twcnet.edu

GENERAL INFORMATION

Type of School: *4-Year College or University, Private (Religious)* • Accreditation: *Southern Association of Colleges and Schools* • Total Enrollment: *795*

PROGRAM INFORMATION

Two Year Exit Option: *No* • NLNAC Accreditation: *Not Reported* • CCNE Accreditation:

NURSING STUDENT PROFILE

Total Nursing Enrollment: *20* • Total Basic Student Enrollment, Full Time: *18* • Total Basic Student Enrollment, Part Time: *0* • Female Basic Student Enrollment: *15* • Male Basic Student Enrollment: *3* • Total RN Enrollment: *2* • Total New Fall Enrollments: *18* • Total Graduates: *Not Reported* • Basic Student Graduates: *Not Reported* • RN Student Graduates: *Not Reported*

FINANCES

Residential Annual Tuition: *$11,000* • Non-Residential Annual Tuition: *$11,000* • General Institutional Fees: *$366* • Additional Nursing Fees: *Not Reported*

UNION UNIVERSITY

Address: 1050 Union University Drive, Jackson, TN 39305-9901
Phone: 901-661-5200
Fax: 731-661-5504
Contact: Susan R. Jacob, PhD, RN, Dean and Professor
Email: sjacob@uu.edu

GENERAL INFORMATION

Type of School: *4-Year College or University, Private (Independent)* • Accreditation: *Southern Association of Colleges and Schools* • Total Enrollment: *2800*

PROGRAM INFORMATION

Two Year Exit Option: *No* • NLNAC Accreditation: *Yes* • CCNE Accreditation:

NURSING STUDENT PROFILE

Total Nursing Enrollment: *168* • Total Basic Student Enrollment, Full Time: *46* • Total Basic Student Enrollment, Part Time: *2* • Female Basic Student Enrollment: *45* • Male Basic Student Enrollment: *3* • Total RN Enrollment: *120* • Total New Fall Enrollments: *20* • Total Graduates: *65* • Basic Student Graduates: *36* • RN Student Graduates: *29*

FINANCES

Residential Annual Tuition: *Not Reported* • Non-Residential Annual Tuition: *Not Reported* • General Institutional Fees: *Not Reported* • Additional Nursing Fees: *Not Reported*

THE UNIVERSITY OF MEMPHIS

Address: 102 Newport Hall, 610 Goodman Avenue,
            Memphis, TN 38152
Phone: 901-678-2020
Fax: 901-678-4906
Contact: Toni Bargagliotti, DNSc, RN, Dean
Email: tbargag1@memphis.edu

GENERAL INFORMATION

Type of School: *4-Year College or University, Public* •
Accreditation: *Southern Association of Colleges and Schools* •
Total Enrollment: *20000*

PROGRAM INFORMATION

Two Year Exit Option: *No* • NLNAC Accreditation: *Yes* •
CCNE Accreditation:

NURSING STUDENT PROFILE

Total Nursing Enrollment: *226* • Total Basic Student
Enrollment, Full Time: *137* • Total Basic Student
Enrollment, Part Time: *48* • Female Basic Student
Enrollment: *166* • Male Basic Student Enrollment: *19* • Total
RN Enrollment: *41* • Total New Fall Enrollments: *51* • Total
Graduates: *114* • Basic Student Graduates: *84* • RN Student
Graduates: *30*

FINANCES

Residential Annual Tuition: *$3,087* • Non-Residential
Annual Tuition: *$8,873* • General Institutional Fees:
$1,544 • Additional Nursing Fees: *$149*

UNIVERSITY OF TENNESSEE— CHATTANOOGA

Address: 615 McCallie Avenue, Chattanooga, TN 37403
Phone: 423-755-4724
Fax: 423-755-4668
Contact: Dana Hames Wertenberger, PhD, RN, Director
            and Professor
Email: dana-wertenberger@utc.edu

GENERAL INFORMATION

Type of School: *4-Year College or University, Public* •
Accreditation: *Southern Association of Colleges and Schools* •
Total Enrollment: *8485*

PROGRAM INFORMATION

Two Year Exit Option: *No* • NLNAC Accreditation: *Not
Reported* • CCNE Accreditation: *Yes*

NURSING STUDENT PROFILE

Total Nursing Enrollment: *179* • Total Basic Student
Enrollment, Full Time: *133* • Total Basic Student
Enrollment, Part Time: *0* • Female Basic Student
Enrollment: *120* • Male Basic Student Enrollment: *13* • Total
RN Enrollment: *46* • Total New Fall Enrollments: *34* • Total
Graduates: *58* • Basic Student Graduates: *44* • RN Student
Graduates: *14*

FINANCES

Residential Annual Tuition: *$2,698* • Non-Residential
Annual Tuition: *$9,228* • General Institutional Fees: *$538* •
Additional Nursing Fees: *$142*

THE UNIVERSITY OF TENNESSEE—MARTIN

Address: 136 Gooch Hall, Martin, TN 38238
Phone: 901-587-7131
Fax: 901-587-7939
Contact: Nancy A. Warren, PhD, RN, Associate Professor and Interim Chair
Email: nwarren@utm.edu

GENERAL INFORMATION

Type of School: *4-Year College or University, Public* • Accreditation: *Southern Association of Colleges and Schools* • Total Enrollment: *5877*

PROGRAM INFORMATION

Two Year Exit Option: *No* • NLNAC Accreditation: *Yes* • CCNE Accreditation:

NURSING STUDENT PROFILE

Total Nursing Enrollment: *147* • Total Basic Student Enrollment, Full Time: *117* • Total Basic Student Enrollment, Part Time: *1* • Female Basic Student Enrollment: *114* • Male Basic Student Enrollment: *4* • Total RN Enrollment: *29* • Total New Fall Enrollments: *42* • Total Graduates: *34* • Basic Student Graduates: *26* • RN Student Graduates: *8*

FINANCES

Residential Annual Tuition: *$2,346* • Non-Residential Annual Tuition: *$8,026* • General Institutional Fees: *$1,173* • Additional Nursing Fees: *$91*

UNIVERSITY OF TENNESSEE COLLEGE OF NURSING—KNOXVILLE

Address: 1200 Volunteer Blvd, Knoxville, TN 37996-4110
Phone: 865-974-7583
Fax: 865-974-3569
Contact: Joan L. Creasia, PhD, RN, Dean
Email: jcreasia@utk.edu

GENERAL INFORMATION

Type of School: *4-Year College or University, Public* • Accreditation: *Southern Association of Colleges and Schools* • Total Enrollment: *26000*

PROGRAM INFORMATION

Two Year Exit Option: *Not Reported* • NLNAC Accreditation: *Yes* • CCNE Accreditation:

NURSING STUDENT PROFILE

Total Nursing Enrollment: *233* • Total Basic Student Enrollment, Full Time: *202* • Total Basic Student Enrollment, Part Time: *9* • Female Basic Student Enrollment: *198* • Male Basic Student Enrollment: *13* • Total RN Enrollment: *22* • Total New Fall Enrollments: *103* • Total Graduates: *125* • Basic Student Graduates: *107* • RN Student Graduates: *18*

FINANCES

Residential Annual Tuition: *$3,362* • Non-Residential Annual Tuition: *$10,166* • General Institutional Fees: *$1,681* • Additional Nursing Fees: *$118*

ACU-HSU-MCM CONSORTIUM

Address: 2149 Hickory, Abilene, TX 79601
Phone: 915-672-2441
Fax: 915-672-5026
Contact: Cecilia Tiller, DSN, RN, WHNP, Dean and
            Professor
Email: ctiller.aisn@hsutx.edu

GENERAL INFORMATION

Type of School: *Not Reported* • Accreditation: *Southern Association of Colleges and Schools* • Total Enrollment: *Not Reported*

PROGRAM INFORMATION

Two Year Exit Option: *No* • NLNAC Accreditation: *Not Reported* • CCNE Accreditation: *Yes*

NURSING STUDENT PROFILE

Total Nursing Enrollment: *101* • Total Basic Student Enrollment, Full Time: *101* • Total Basic Student Enrollment, Part Time: *0* • Female Basic Student Enrollment: *Not Reported* • Male Basic Student Enrollment: *Not Reported* • Total RN Enrollment: *0* • Total New Fall Enrollments: *58* • Total Graduates: *34* • Basic Student Graduates: *31* • RN Student Graduates: *3*

FINANCES

Residential Annual Tuition: *Not Reported* • Non-Residential Annual Tuition: *Not Reported* • General Institutional Fees: *Not Reported* • Additional Nursing Fees: *$305*

EAST TEXAS BAPTIST UNIVERSITY

Address: 1209 N. Grove, Marshall, TX 75670
Phone: 903-923-2211
Fax: 903-938-9225
Contact: Celeste K. Hammock, DrPH, RN, CNS, Dean
            and Professor, School of Nursing
Email: chammock@etbu.edu

GENERAL INFORMATION

Type of School: *4-Year College or University, Private (Religious)* • Accreditation: *Southern Association of Colleges and Schools* • Total Enrollment: *1401*

PROGRAM INFORMATION

Two Year Exit Option: *No* • NLNAC Accreditation: *Not Reported* • CCNE Accreditation: *Yes*

NURSING STUDENT PROFILE

Total Nursing Enrollment: *46* • Total Basic Student Enrollment, Full Time: *46* • Total Basic Student Enrollment, Part Time: *Not Reported* • Female Basic Student Enrollment: *45* • Male Basic Student Enrollment: *1* • Total RN Enrollment: *0* • Total New Fall Enrollments: *24* • Total Graduates: *12* • Basic Student Graduates: *12* • RN Student Graduates: *0*

FINANCES

Residential Annual Tuition: *$8,800* • Non-Residential Annual Tuition: *$8,800* • General Institutional Fees: *$800* • Additional Nursing Fees: *$271*

HOUSTON BAPTIST UNIVERSITY

Address: 7502 Fondren, Houston, TX 77074
Phone: 281-649-3300
Fax: 281-649-3340
Contact: Nancy Yuill, PhD, RN, Dean
Email: nyuill@hbu.edu

GENERAL INFORMATION

Type of School: *4-Year College or University, Private (Independent)* • Accreditation: *Southern Association of Colleges and Schools* • Total Enrollment: *2300*

PROGRAM INFORMATION

Two Year Exit Option: *Not Reported* • NLNAC Accreditation: *Yes* • CCNE Accreditation:

NURSING STUDENT PROFILE

Total Nursing Enrollment: *103* • Total Basic Student Enrollment, Full Time: *103* • Total Basic Student Enrollment, Part Time: *Not Reported* • Female Basic Student Enrollment: *97* • Male Basic Student Enrollment: *6* • Total RN Enrollment: *0* • Total New Fall Enrollments: *45* • Total Graduates: *22* • Basic Student Graduates: *21* • RN Student Graduates: *1*

FINANCES

Residential Annual Tuition: *$10,048* • Non-Residential Annual Tuition: *$10,048* • General Institutional Fees: *$1,040* • Additional Nursing Fees: *$100*

LAMAR UNIVERSITY

Address: PO Box 10081, Beaumont, TX 77710
Phone: 409-880-8817
Fax: *Not Reported*
Contact: Alexia Green, PhD, RN, Chair, Department of Nursing
Email: greenau@hal.lamar.edu

GENERAL INFORMATION

Type of School: *4-Year College or University, Public* • Accreditation: *Southern Association of Colleges and Schools* • Total Enrollment: *8149*

PROGRAM INFORMATION

Two Year Exit Option: *Not Reported* • NLNAC Accreditation: *Yes* • CCNE Accreditation:

NURSING STUDENT PROFILE

Total Nursing Enrollment: *166* • Total Basic Student Enrollment, Full Time: *Not Reported* • Total Basic Student Enrollment, Part Time: *Not Reported* • Female Basic Student Enrollment: *Not Reported* • Male Basic Student Enrollment: *Not Reported* • Total RN Enrollment: *27* • Total New Fall Enrollments: *92* • Total Graduates: *53* • Basic Student Graduates: *28* • RN Student Graduates: *25*

FINANCES

Residential Annual Tuition: *$2,024* • Non-Residential Annual Tuition: *$7,208* • General Institutional Fees: *$536* • Additional Nursing Fees: *$280*

MIDWESTERN STATE UNIVERSITY

Address: 3410 Taft Blvd, Wichita Falls, TX 76308
Phone: 940-397-4598
Fax: *Not Reported*
Contact: Sandra J. Church, MS, RN (Retired), Chair,
          Undergraduate Nursing Program
Email: fchurchs@nexus.mwsu.edu

GENERAL INFORMATION

Type of School: *4-Year College or University, Public* •
Accreditation: *Southern Association of Colleges and Schools* •
Total Enrollment: *5800*

PROGRAM INFORMATION

Two Year Exit Option: *Not Reported* • NLNAC
Accreditation: *Yes* • CCNE Accreditation:

NURSING STUDENT PROFILE

Total Nursing Enrollment: *167* • Total Basic Student
Enrollment, Full Time: *Not Reported* • Total Basic Student
Enrollment, Part Time: *Not Reported* • Female Basic Student
Enrollment: *Not Reported* • Male Basic Student Enrollment:
Not Reported • Total RN Enrollment: *16* • Total New Fall
Enrollments: *60* • Total Graduates: *60* • Basic Student
Graduates: *53* • RN Student Graduates: *7*

FINANCES

Residential Annual Tuition: *$2,096* • Non-Residential
Annual Tuition: *$8,456* • General Institutional Fees: *$61* •
Additional Nursing Fees: *$63*

PRAIRIE VIEW A&M UNIVERSITY

Address: P.O. Box 519, Prarie View, TX 77446
Phone: 713-797-7009
Fax: 713-797-7013
Contact: Betty N. Adams, PhD, RN, Dean and Professor,
          College of Nursing
Email: Betty_Adams@pvamu.edu

GENERAL INFORMATION

Type of School: *4-Year College or University, Public* •
Accreditation: *Southern Association of Colleges and Schools* •
Total Enrollment: *6500*

PROGRAM INFORMATION

Two Year Exit Option: *No* • NLNAC Accreditation: *Yes* •
CCNE Accreditation:

NURSING STUDENT PROFILE

Total Nursing Enrollment: *230* • Total Basic Student
Enrollment, Full Time: *188* • Total Basic Student
Enrollment, Part Time: *23* • Female Basic Student
Enrollment: *192* • Male Basic Student Enrollment: *19* • Total
RN Enrollment: *19* • Total New Fall Enrollments: *38* • Total
Graduates: *80* • Basic Student Graduates: *62* • RN Student
Graduates: *18*

FINANCES

Residential Annual Tuition: *$1,320* • Non-Residential
Annual Tuition: *$7,860* • General Institutional Fees:
$2,000 • Additional Nursing Fees: *$200*

STEPHEN F. AUSTIN STATE UNIVERSITY

Address: PO Box 6156, Nacogdoches, TX 75962
Phone: 936-468-3604
Fax: 936-468-1696
Contact: Glenda C. Walker, DSN, RN, Director of Nursing
Email: gwalker@sfasu.edu

GENERAL INFORMATION

Type of School: *Not Reported* • Accreditation: *Not Reported* • Total Enrollment: *Not Reported*

PROGRAM INFORMATION

Two Year Exit Option: *No* • NLNAC Accreditation: *Yes* • CCNE Accreditation:

NURSING STUDENT PROFILE

Total Nursing Enrollment: *89* • Total Basic Student Enrollment, Full Time: *82* • Total Basic Student Enrollment, Part Time: *7* • Female Basic Student Enrollment: *81* • Male Basic Student Enrollment: *8* • Total RN Enrollment: *0* • Total New Fall Enrollments: *29* • Total Graduates: *42* • Basic Student Graduates: *36* • RN Student Graduates: *6*

FINANCES

Residential Annual Tuition: *$5,278* • Non-Residential Annual Tuition: *$16,614* • General Institutional Fees: *$548* • Additional Nursing Fees: *Not Reported*

TEXAS A&M INTERNATIONAL UNIVERSITY

Address: 5201 University Boulevard, Laredo, TX 78041-1900
Phone: 956-326-2450
Fax: 956-326-2449
Contact: Susan Scoville Baker, PhD, RN, CS, Director
Email: sbaker@tamiu.edu

GENERAL INFORMATION

Type of School: *4-Year College or University, Public* • Accreditation: *Southern Association of Colleges and Schools* • Total Enrollment: *3200*

PROGRAM INFORMATION

Two Year Exit Option: *No* • NLNAC Accreditation: *Yes* • CCNE Accreditation:

NURSING STUDENT PROFILE

Total Nursing Enrollment: *88* • Total Basic Student Enrollment, Full Time: *51* • Total Basic Student Enrollment, Part Time: *2* • Female Basic Student Enrollment: *Not Reported* • Male Basic Student Enrollment: *Not Reported* • Total RN Enrollment: *35* • Total New Fall Enrollments: *1* • Total Graduates: *32* • Basic Student Graduates: *21* • RN Student Graduates: *11*

FINANCES

Residential Annual Tuition: *$1,408* • Non-Residential Annual Tuition: *$8,096* • General Institutional Fees: *$291* • Additional Nursing Fees: *$0*

TEXAS A&M UNIVERSITY— CORPUS CHRISTI

Address: 6300 Ocean Drive, Corpus Christi, TX 78412
Phone: 361-825-3439
Fax: 361-825-2484
Contact: Rebecca L. Stephens, PhD, RN, Assistant Director and Associate Professor
Email: stephens@falcon.tamucc.edu

GENERAL INFORMATION

Type of School: *4-Year College or University, Public* • Accreditation: *Southern Association of Colleges and Schools* • Total Enrollment: *6823*

PROGRAM INFORMATION

Two Year Exit Option: *Not Reported* • NLNAC Accreditation: *Not Reported* • CCNE Accreditation:

NURSING STUDENT PROFILE

Total Nursing Enrollment: *315* • Total Basic Student Enrollment, Full Time: *251* • Total Basic Student Enrollment, Part Time: *31* • Female Basic Student Enrollment: *233* • Male Basic Student Enrollment: *49* • Total RN Enrollment: *33* • Total New Fall Enrollments: *44* • Total Graduates: *64* • Basic Student Graduates: *47* • RN Student Graduates: *17*

FINANCES

Residential Annual Tuition: *Not Reported* • Non-Residential Annual Tuition: *Not Reported* • General Institutional Fees: *Not Reported* • Additional Nursing Fees: *Not Reported*

TEXAS CHRISTIAN UNIVERSITY

Address: TCU Box 2988620, Fort Worth, TX 76129
Phone: 817-257-7650
Fax: 817-257-7944
Contact: Rhonda Keen-Payne, PhD, RN, Rankin Professor and Dean, College of Health and Human Sciences
Email: *Not Reported*

GENERAL INFORMATION

Type of School: *Not Reported* • Accreditation: *Not Reported* • Total Enrollment: *Not Reported*

PROGRAM INFORMATION

Two Year Exit Option: *Not Reported* • NLNAC Accreditation: *Yes* • CCNE Accreditation:

NURSING STUDENT PROFILE

Total Nursing Enrollment: *301* • Total Basic Student Enrollment, Full Time: *Not Reported* • Total Basic Student Enrollment, Part Time: *Not Reported* • Female Basic Student Enrollment: *Not Reported* • Male Basic Student Enrollment: *Not Reported* • Total RN Enrollment: *0* • Total New Fall Enrollments: *0* • Total Graduates: *87* • Basic Student Graduates: *87* • RN Student Graduates: *0*

FINANCES

Residential Annual Tuition: *Not Reported* • Non-Residential Annual Tuition: *Not Reported* • General Institutional Fees: *Not Reported* • Additional Nursing Fees: *Not Reported*

TEXAS TECH UNIVERSITY HEALTH SCIENCES CENTER

Address: 3601-4th Street, Lubbock, TX 79430
Phone: 806-743-2279
Fax: 806-743-1622
Contact: Ana Valadez, EdD, RN, Associate Dean,
           Undergraduate Program
Email: ana.valadez@ttmc.ttuhsc.edu

TEXAS WOMAN'S UNIVERSITY

Address: Box 425498 TWU Station, Denton, TX 76204-
           5498
Phone: 940-898-2401
Fax: *Not Reported*
Contact: Carolyn S. Gunning, PhD, RN, Dean
Email: CGunning@twu.edu

GENERAL INFORMATION

Type of School: *Other, Public* • Accreditation: *Southern Association of Colleges and Schools* • Total Enrollment: *1788*

GENERAL INFORMATION

Type of School: *4-Year College or University, Public* • Accreditation: *Southern Association of Colleges and Schools* • Total Enrollment: *8500*

PROGRAM INFORMATION

Two Year Exit Option: *No* • NLNAC Accreditation: *Yes* • CCNE Accreditation: *Yes*

PROGRAM INFORMATION

Two Year Exit Option: *Not Reported* • NLNAC Accreditation: *Yes* • CCNE Accreditation:

NURSING STUDENT PROFILE

Total Nursing Enrollment: *418* • Total Basic Student Enrollment, Full Time: *Not Reported* • Total Basic Student Enrollment, Part Time: *Not Reported* • Female Basic Student Enrollment: *Not Reported* • Male Basic Student Enrollment: *Not Reported* • Total RN Enrollment: *63* • Total New Fall Enrollments: *28* • Total Graduates: *108* • Basic Student Graduates: *75* • RN Student Graduates: *33*

NURSING STUDENT PROFILE

Total Nursing Enrollment: *670* • Total Basic Student Enrollment, Full Time: *Not Reported* • Total Basic Student Enrollment, Part Time: *Not Reported* • Female Basic Student Enrollment: *Not Reported* • Male Basic Student Enrollment: *Not Reported* • Total RN Enrollment: *116* • Total New Fall Enrollments: *Not Reported* • Total Graduates: *264* • Basic Student Graduates: *225* • RN Student Graduates: *39*

FINANCES

Residential Annual Tuition: *$1,260* • Non-Residential Annual Tuition: *$7,590* • General Institutional Fees: *$1,952* • Additional Nursing Fees: *$300*

FINANCES

Residential Annual Tuition: *Not Reported* • Non-Residential Annual Tuition: *Not Reported* • General Institutional Fees: *Not Reported* • Additional Nursing Fees: *Not Reported*

UNIVERSITY OF MARY HARDIN—BAYLOR

Address: 900 College Street, Belton, TX 76513
Phone: 254-295-4662
Fax: 254-295-4141
Contact: Grace Labaj, PhD, RN, Dean, School of Nursing
Email: glabaj@umhb.edu

GENERAL INFORMATION

Type of School: *4-Year College or University, Private (Religious)* • Accreditation: *Southern Association of Colleges and Schools* • Total Enrollment: *2600*

PROGRAM INFORMATION

Two Year Exit Option: *No* • NLNAC Accreditation: *Yes* • CCNE Accreditation:

NURSING STUDENT PROFILE

Total Nursing Enrollment: *105* • Total Basic Student Enrollment, Full Time: *97* • Total Basic Student Enrollment, Part Time: *1* • Female Basic Student Enrollment: *91* • Male Basic Student Enrollment: *7* • Total RN Enrollment: *7* • Total New Fall Enrollments: *29* • Total Graduates: *35* • Basic Student Graduates: *29* • RN Student Graduates: *6*

FINANCES

Residential Annual Tuition: *$8,700* • Non-Residential Annual Tuition: *Not Reported* • General Institutional Fees: *$22* • Additional Nursing Fees: *$300*

UNIVERSITY OF TEXAS— ARLINGTON

Address: 411 S Nedderman Drive, Arlington, TX 76019
Phone: 817-272-2776
Fax: 817-272-5006
Contact: Elizabeth C. Poster, PhD, RN, Dean
Email: poster@uta.edu

GENERAL INFORMATION

Type of School: *4-Year College or University, Public* • Accreditation: *Southern Association of Colleges and Schools* • Total Enrollment: *20424*

PROGRAM INFORMATION

Two Year Exit Option: *Not Reported* • NLNAC Accreditation: *Yes* • CCNE Accreditation:

NURSING STUDENT PROFILE

Total Nursing Enrollment: *528* • Total Basic Student Enrollment, Full Time: *303* • Total Basic Student Enrollment, Part Time: *91* • Female Basic Student Enrollment: *361* • Male Basic Student Enrollment: *33* • Total RN Enrollment: *134* • Total New Fall Enrollments: *134* • Total Graduates: *274* • Basic Student Graduates: *153* • RN Student Graduates: *121*

FINANCES

Residential Annual Tuition: *$2,560* • Non-Residential Annual Tuition: *$9,440* • General Institutional Fees: *$1,102* • Additional Nursing Fees: *$15*

UNIVERSITY OF TEXAS— AUSTIN

Address: 1700 Red River, Austin, TX 78701
Phone: 512-471-4100
Fax: 512-471-4910
Contact: Dolores Sands, PhD, RN, Dean
Email: *Not Reported*

UNIVERSITY OF TEXAS— EL PASO

Address: 1101 N. Campbell, El Paso, TX 79902
Phone: 915-747-8217
Fax: *Not Reported*
Contact: Leticia Lantican, PhD, RN, Associate Professor
           and Director, School of Nursing
Email: llantica@utep.edu

GENERAL INFORMATION

Type of School: *Not Reported* • Accreditation: *Not Reported* • Total Enrollment: *Not Reported*

GENERAL INFORMATION

Type of School: *Other* • Accreditation: *Not Reported* • Total Enrollment: *Not Reported*

PROGRAM INFORMATION

Two Year Exit Option: *Not Reported* • NLNAC Accreditation: *Not Reported* • CCNE Accreditation:

PROGRAM INFORMATION

Two Year Exit Option: *Not Reported* • NLNAC Accreditation: *Not Reported* • CCNE Accreditation:

NURSING STUDENT PROFILE

Total Nursing Enrollment: *Not Reported* • Total Basic Student Enrollment, Full Time: *Not Reported* • Total Basic Student Enrollment, Part Time: *Not Reported* • Female Basic Student Enrollment: *Not Reported* • Male Basic Student Enrollment: *Not Reported* • Total RN Enrollment: *Not Reported* • Total New Fall Enrollments: *Not Reported* • Total Graduates: *Not Reported* • Basic Student Graduates: *Not Reported* • RN Student Graduates: *Not Reported*

NURSING STUDENT PROFILE

Total Nursing Enrollment: *296* • Total Basic Student Enrollment, Full Time: *Not Reported* • Total Basic Student Enrollment, Part Time: *Not Reported* • Female Basic Student Enrollment: *Not Reported* • Male Basic Student Enrollment: *Not Reported* • Total RN Enrollment: *13* • Total New Fall Enrollments: *63* • Total Graduates: *86* • Basic Student Graduates: *79* • RN Student Graduates: *7*

FINANCES

Residential Annual Tuition: *Not Reported* • Non-Residential Annual Tuition: *Not Reported* • General Institutional Fees: *Not Reported* • Additional Nursing Fees: *Not Reported*

FINANCES

Residential Annual Tuition: *Not Reported* • Non-Residential Annual Tuition: *Not Reported* • General Institutional Fees: *Not Reported* • Additional Nursing Fees: *Not Reported*

UNIVERSITY OF TEXAS—PAN AMERICAN

Address: 1201 W. University Drive, Edinburg, TX 78539
Phone: 956-381-3491
Fax: 356-381-2384
Contact: Sandy Sanchez, PhD, RN, BSN Program Coordinator
Email: ssanchez@panam.edu

GENERAL INFORMATION

Type of School: *4-Year College or University, Public* •
Accreditation: *Southern Association of Colleges and Schools* •
Total Enrollment: *12500*

PROGRAM INFORMATION

Two Year Exit Option: *No* • NLNAC Accreditation: *Yes* •
CCNE Accreditation:

NURSING STUDENT PROFILE

Total Nursing Enrollment: *127* • Total Basic Student
Enrollment, Full Time: *99* • Total Basic Student Enrollment,
Part Time: *Not Reported* • Female Basic Student Enrollment:
66 • Male Basic Student Enrollment: *33* • Total RN
Enrollment: *28* • Total New Fall Enrollments: *0* • Total
Graduates: *51* • Basic Student Graduates: *45* • RN Student
Graduates: *6*

FINANCES

Residential Annual Tuition: *$1,985* • Non-Residential
Annual Tuition: *$7,145* • General Institutional Fees: *$497* •
Additional Nursing Fees: *$30*

UNIVERSITY OF TEXAS— TYLER

Address: 3900 University Blvd., Tyler, TX 75799
Phone: 903-565-7043
Fax: 903-565-5533
Contact: Pamela Martin, PhD, RN, Assistant Dean for Undergraduate Nursing Programs
Email: pmartin@mail.uttyl.edu

GENERAL INFORMATION

Type of School: *4-Year College or University, Public* •
Accreditation: *Southern Association of Colleges and Schools* •
Total Enrollment: *3742*

PROGRAM INFORMATION

Two Year Exit Option: *No* • NLNAC Accreditation: *Yes* •
CCNE Accreditation:

NURSING STUDENT PROFILE

Total Nursing Enrollment: *414* • Total Basic Student
Enrollment, Full Time: *313* • Total Basic Student
Enrollment, Part Time: *50* • Female Basic Student
Enrollment: *315* • Male Basic Student Enrollment: *48* • Total
RN Enrollment: *51* • Total New Fall Enrollments: *100* •
Total Graduates: *182* • Basic Student Graduates: *151* • RN
Student Graduates: *31*

FINANCES

Residential Annual Tuition: *$1,168* • Non-Residential
Annual Tuition: *$3,760* • General Institutional Fees: *$127* •
Additional Nursing Fees: *$114*

UNIVERSITY OF TEXAS HEALTH SCIENCE CENTER—HOUSTON

Address: 1100 Holcombe Blvd. #5504, Houston, TX
            77030
Phone: 713-500-2002
Fax: *Not Reported*
Contact: Patricia L. Starck, DSN, RN, FAAN, Dean and
           John P. McGovern Professor
Email: pstarck@sonl.nur.uth.tmc.edu

GENERAL INFORMATION

Type of School: *Not Reported* • Accreditation: *Southern Association of Colleges and Schools* • Total Enrollment: *Not Reported*

PROGRAM INFORMATION

Two Year Exit Option: *Not Reported* • NLNAC Accreditation: *Yes* • CCNE Accreditation:

NURSING STUDENT PROFILE

Total Nursing Enrollment: *185* • Total Basic Student Enrollment, Full Time: *Not Reported* • Total Basic Student Enrollment, Part Time: *Not Reported* • Female Basic Student Enrollment: *Not Reported* • Male Basic Student Enrollment: *Not Reported* • Total RN Enrollment: *29* • Total New Fall Enrollments: *80* • Total Graduates: *91* • Basic Student Graduates: *68* • RN Student Graduates: *23*

FINANCES

Residential Annual Tuition: *$2,088* • Non-Residential Annual Tuition: *$9,864* • General Institutional Fees: *$233* • Additional Nursing Fees: *$201*

UNIVERSITY OF TEXAS HEALTH SCIENCE CENTER— SAN ANTONIO

Address: 7703 Floyd Curl Drive - MSC 7942, San
            Antonio, TX 78229-3900
Phone: 210-567-5810
Fax: 210-567-3813
Contact: Brenda S. Jackson, PhD, RN, Interim Associate
           Dean, Undergraduate Nursing Program
Email: jacksonbg@uthscsa.edu

GENERAL INFORMATION

Type of School: *4-Year College or University, Public* • Accreditation: *Southern Association of Colleges and Schools* • Total Enrollment: *2544*

PROGRAM INFORMATION

Two Year Exit Option: *Not Reported* • NLNAC Accreditation: *Yes* • CCNE Accreditation:

NURSING STUDENT PROFILE

Total Nursing Enrollment: *421* • Total Basic Student Enrollment, Full Time: *298* • Total Basic Student Enrollment, Part Time: *58* • Female Basic Student Enrollment: *287* • Male Basic Student Enrollment: *69* • Total RN Enrollment: *65* • Total New Fall Enrollments: *156* • Total Graduates: *207* • Basic Student Graduates: *153* • RN Student Graduates: *54*

FINANCES

Residential Annual Tuition: *$1,008* • Non-Residential Annual Tuition: *$6,124* • General Institutional Fees: *$493* • Additional Nursing Fees: *$100*

UNIVERSITY OF TEXAS MEDICAL BRANCH— GALVESTON

Address: 1100 Mechanic, Galveston, TX 77555
Phone: 409-772-8205
Fax: 709-772-5118
Contact: Poldi Tschirch, PhD, RN, Director, Undergraduate Program
Email: ptschir@utmb.edu

GENERAL INFORMATION

Type of School: *4-Year College or University, Public* • Accreditation: *Southern Association of Colleges and Schools* • Total Enrollment: *1927*

PROGRAM INFORMATION

Two Year Exit Option: *Not Reported* • NLNAC Accreditation: *Yes* • CCNE Accreditation: *Yes*

NURSING STUDENT PROFILE

Total Nursing Enrollment: *385* • Total Basic Student Enrollment, Full Time: *171* • Total Basic Student Enrollment, Part Time: *36* • Female Basic Student Enrollment: *192* • Male Basic Student Enrollment: *15* • Total RN Enrollment: *178* • Total New Fall Enrollments: *117* • Total Graduates: *156* • Basic Student Graduates: *68* • RN Student Graduates: *88*

FINANCES

Residential Annual Tuition: *Not Reported* • Non-Residential Annual Tuition: *Not Reported* • General Institutional Fees: *Not Reported* • Additional Nursing Fees: *Not Reported*

UNIVERSITY OF THE INCARNATE WORD

Address: 4301 Broadway, San Antonio, TX 78209
Phone: 210-829-3987
Fax: 210-829-3174
Contact: Caroline Spana, PhD, MSW, RN, Assistant Professor/Chair, BSN Program
Email: cspan@universe.uiwtx.edu

GENERAL INFORMATION

Type of School: *4-Year College or University, Private (Independent)* • Accreditation: *Southern Association of Colleges and Schools* • Total Enrollment: *4289*

PROGRAM INFORMATION

Two Year Exit Option: *No* • NLNAC Accreditation: *Yes* • CCNE Accreditation: *Yes*

NURSING STUDENT PROFILE

Total Nursing Enrollment: *156* • Total Basic Student Enrollment, Full Time: *137* • Total Basic Student Enrollment, Part Time: *Not Reported* • Female Basic Student Enrollment: *127* • Male Basic Student Enrollment: *10* • Total RN Enrollment: *19* • Total New Fall Enrollments: *34* • Total Graduates: *43* • Basic Student Graduates: *39* • RN Student Graduates: *4*

FINANCES

Residential Annual Tuition: *$7,400* • Non-Residential Annual Tuition: *$7,400* • General Institutional Fees: *Not Reported* • Additional Nursing Fees: *Not Reported*

Circle 125 on reader card   See in-depth profile for more information

WEST TEXAS A&M UNIVERSITY

Address: 2501 Fourth Avenue, Canyon, TX 79016
Phone: 806-651-2659
Fax: 806-651-2632
Contact: Jeanette Embrey, PhD, RNC, Undergraduate
             Coordinator and Assistant Professor
Email: jembrey@mail.wtamu.edu

GENERAL INFORMATION

Type of School: *4-Year College or University, Public* •
Accreditation: *Southern Association of Colleges and Schools* •
Total Enrollment: *6678*

PROGRAM INFORMATION

Two Year Exit Option: *No* • NLNAC Accreditation: *Not
Reported* • CCNE Accreditation: *Yes*

NURSING STUDENT PROFILE

Total Nursing Enrollment: *331* • Total Basic Student
Enrollment, Full Time: *264* • Total Basic Student
Enrollment, Part Time: *5* • Female Basic Student
Enrollment: *229* • Male Basic Student Enrollment: *40* • Total
RN Enrollment: *62* • Total New Fall Enrollments: *42* • Total
Graduates: *87* • Basic Student Graduates: *58* • RN Student
Graduates: *29*

FINANCES

Residential Annual Tuition: *$2,085* • Non-Residential
Annual Tuition: *$8,415* • General Institutional Fees: *$681* •
Additional Nursing Fees: *$200*

BRIGHAM YOUNG UNIVERSITY

Address: 500 SWKT, B-130 ASB, Provo, UT 84602
Phone: 801-378-7210
Fax: 801-422-0536
Contact: Rae Jeanne Memmott, MS, RN, Associate Dean
Email: rae_jeanne_memmott@byu.edu

GENERAL INFORMATION

Type of School: *4-Year College or University, Private
(Religious)* • Accreditation: *Northwestern Association of Schools
and Colleges* • Total Enrollment: *32771*

PROGRAM INFORMATION

Two Year Exit Option: *No* • NLNAC Accreditation: *Yes* •
CCNE Accreditation: *Yes*

NURSING STUDENT PROFILE

Total Nursing Enrollment: *228* • Total Basic Student
Enrollment, Full Time: *146* • Total Basic Student
Enrollment, Part Time: *58* • Female Basic Student
Enrollment: *187* • Male Basic Student Enrollment: *17* • Total
RN Enrollment: *24* • Total New Fall Enrollments: *48* • Total
Graduates: *101* • Basic Student Graduates: *97* • RN Student
Graduates: *4*

FINANCES

Residential Annual Tuition: *$1,530* • Non-Residential
Annual Tuition: *$2,300* • General Institutional Fees: *$400* •
Additional Nursing Fees: *Not Reported*

Circle 19 on reader card   See in-depth profile for more information

UNIVERSITY OF UTAH

Address: 10 S. 2000 E. Front, Salt Lake City, UT 84112
Phone: 801-581-8480
Fax: *Not Reported*
Contact: B. Lee Walker, PhD, RN, Interim Associate Dean
for Academic Affairs
Email: lee.walker@nurse.utah.edu

GENERAL INFORMATION

Type of School: *4-Year College or University, Public* •
Accreditation: *Northwestern Association of Schools and
Colleges* • Total Enrollment: *1494*

PROGRAM INFORMATION

Two Year Exit Option: *Not Reported* • NLNAC
Accreditation: *Yes* • CCNE Accreditation: *Yes*

NURSING STUDENT PROFILE

Total Nursing Enrollment: *304* • Total Basic Student
Enrollment, Full Time: *Not Reported* • Total Basic Student
Enrollment, Part Time: *Not Reported* • Female Basic Student
Enrollment: *216* • Male Basic Student Enrollment: *41* • Total
RN Enrollment: *47* • Total New Fall Enrollments: *60* • Total
Graduates: *116* • Basic Student Graduates: *99* • RN Student
Graduates: *17*

FINANCES

Residential Annual Tuition: *$2,350* • Non-Residential
Annual Tuition: *$7,118* • General Institutional Fees: *Not
Reported* • Additional Nursing Fees: *Not Reported*

WEBER STATE UNIVERSITY

Address: 3903 University Circle, Ogden, UT 84408
Phone: 801-626-7305
Fax: 801-626-6397
Contact: Evelyn Draper, MA, RN, Coordinator,
Baccalaureate Nursing Program
Email: edraper1@weber.edu

GENERAL INFORMATION

Type of School: *4-Year College or University, Public* •
Accreditation: *Northwestern Association of Schools and
Colleges* • Total Enrollment: *Not Reported*

PROGRAM INFORMATION

Two Year Exit Option: *No* • NLNAC Accreditation: *Yes* •
CCNE Accreditation:

NURSING STUDENT PROFILE

Total Nursing Enrollment: *123* • Total Basic Student
Enrollment, Full Time: *Not Reported* • Total Basic Student
Enrollment, Part Time: *Not Reported* • Female Basic Student
Enrollment: *Not Reported* • Male Basic Student Enrollment:
Not Reported • Total RN Enrollment: *123* • Total New Fall
Enrollments: *Not Reported* • Total Graduates: *75* • Basic
Student Graduates: *0* • RN Student Graduates: *75*

FINANCES

Residential Annual Tuition: *$2,118* • Non-Residential
Annual Tuition: *$6,294* • General Institutional Fees: *Not
Reported* • Additional Nursing Fees: *Not Reported*

| WESTMINSTER COLLEGE— ST. MARKS | NORWICH UNIVERSITY |

Address: 1840 South 13th Street, East, Salt Lake City, UT 84105
Phone: 801-488-4234
Fax: 801-467-8601
Contact: Gretchen McNeely, PhD, RN, Dean
Email: g-mcneel@wcslc.edu

Address: 65 S. Main St., Northfield, VT 05663
Phone: 802-485-2609
Fax: 802-485-2607
Contact: Marilyn Rinker, MSN, RN, OCN, Program Chair
Email: mrinker@norwich.edu

GENERAL INFORMATION

Type of School: *Not Reported* • Accreditation: *Not Reported* • Total Enrollment: *Not Reported*

GENERAL INFORMATION

Type of School: *Not Reported, Private (Independent)* • Accreditation: *New England Association of Schools and Colleges* • Total Enrollment: *Not Reported*

PROGRAM INFORMATION

Two Year Exit Option: *Not Reported* • NLNAC Accreditation: *Not Reported* • CCNE Accreditation:

PROGRAM INFORMATION

Two Year Exit Option: *No* • NLNAC Accreditation: *Yes* • CCNE Accreditation:

NURSING STUDENT PROFILE

Total Nursing Enrollment: *42* • Total Basic Student Enrollment, Full Time: *37* • Total Basic Student Enrollment, Part Time: *3* • Female Basic Student Enrollment: *Not Reported* • Male Basic Student Enrollment: *Not Reported* • Total RN Enrollment: *2* • Total New Fall Enrollments: *Not Reported* • Total Graduates: *Not Reported* • Basic Student Graduates: *Not Reported* • RN Student Graduates: *Not Reported*

NURSING STUDENT PROFILE

Total Nursing Enrollment: *Not Reported* • Total Basic Student Enrollment, Full Time: *Not Reported* • Total Basic Student Enrollment, Part Time: *Not Reported* • Female Basic Student Enrollment: *Not Reported* • Male Basic Student Enrollment: *Not Reported* • Total RN Enrollment: *Not Reported* • Total New Fall Enrollments: *35* • Total Graduates: *Not Reported* • Basic Student Graduates: *Not Reported* • RN Student Graduates: *Not Reported*

FINANCES

Residential Annual Tuition: *Not Reported* • Non-Residential Annual Tuition: *Not Reported* • General Institutional Fees: *Not Reported* • Additional Nursing Fees: *Not Reported*

FINANCES

Residential Annual Tuition: *$8,355* • Non-Residential Annual Tuition: *$8,355* • General Institutional Fees: *$225* • Additional Nursing Fees: *Not Reported*

THE UNIVERSITY OF VERMONT

Address: 216 Rowell Building, Burlington, VT 05405
Phone: 802-656-3051
Fax: 802-656-8306
Contact: Gail Ann DeLuca-Havens, PhD, APRN, BC,
           Associate Professor and Chair
Email: Gail.Havens@uvm.edu

GENERAL INFORMATION

Type of School: *4-Year College or University, Public* •
Accreditation: *New England Association of Schools and
Colleges* • Total Enrollment: *Not Reported*

PROGRAM INFORMATION

Two Year Exit Option: *No* • NLNAC Accreditation: *Yes* •
CCNE Accreditation:

NURSING STUDENT PROFILE

Total Nursing Enrollment: *251* • Total Basic Student
Enrollment, Full Time: *204* • Total Basic Student
Enrollment, Part Time: *29* • Female Basic Student
Enrollment: *218* • Male Basic Student Enrollment: *15* • Total
RN Enrollment: *18* • Total New Fall Enrollments: *72* • Total
Graduates: *56* • Basic Student Graduates: *53* • RN Student
Graduates: *3*

FINANCES

Residential Annual Tuition: *$8,040* • Non-Residential
Annual Tuition: *$20,100* • General Institutional Fees: *$605* •
Additional Nursing Fees: *$39*

UNIVERSITY OF THE VIRGIN ISLANDS

Address: #2 John Brewers Bay, Saint Thomas, VI 00802
Phone: 340-693-1291
Fax: 340-693-1285
Contact: Gloria B. Callwood, PhD, RN, Associate
           Professor and Chair
Email: gcallwo@uvi.edu

GENERAL INFORMATION

Type of School: *4-Year College or University, Public* •
Accreditation: *Middle States Association of Colleges and
Schools* • Total Enrollment: *Not Reported*

PROGRAM INFORMATION

Two Year Exit Option: *No* • NLNAC Accreditation: *Yes* •
CCNE Accreditation:

NURSING STUDENT PROFILE

Total Nursing Enrollment: *53* • Total Basic Student
Enrollment, Full Time: *41* • Total Basic Student Enrollment,
Part Time: *1* • Female Basic Student Enrollment: *41* • Male
Basic Student Enrollment: *1* • Total RN Enrollment: *11* •
Total New Fall Enrollments: *0* • Total Graduates: *13* • Basic
Student Graduates: *11* • RN Student Graduates: *2*

FINANCES

Residential Annual Tuition: *$1,365* • Non-Residential
Annual Tuition: *$4,095* • General Institutional Fees: *$128* •
Additional Nursing Fees: *$30*

EASTERN MENNONITE UNIVERSITY

Address: 1200 Park Road, Harrisonburg, VA 22802-2462
Phone: 540-432-4187
Fax: 540-432-4444
Contact: Arlene G. Wiens, PhD, RN, Department Chair
Email: wiensag@emu.edu

GEORGE MASON UNIVERSITY

Address: 4400 University Drive/3C4, Fairfax, VA 22030-4444
Phone: 703-993-1904
Fax: 703-993-1964
Contact: Christena Langley, PhD, RN, Assistant Dean
Email: clangley@gmu.edu

GENERAL INFORMATION

Type of School: *4-Year College or University, Private (Religious)* • Accreditation: *Southern Association of Colleges and Schools* • Total Enrollment: *1496*

GENERAL INFORMATION

Type of School: *4-Year College or University, Public* • Accreditation: *Southern Association of Colleges and Schools* • Total Enrollment: *24897*

PROGRAM INFORMATION

Two Year Exit Option: *Not Reported* • NLNAC Accreditation: *Yes* • CCNE Accreditation:

PROGRAM INFORMATION

Two Year Exit Option: *No* • NLNAC Accreditation: *Yes* • CCNE Accreditation: *Yes*

NURSING STUDENT PROFILE

Total Nursing Enrollment: *92* • Total Basic Student Enrollment, Full Time: *72* • Total Basic Student Enrollment, Part Time: *Not Reported* • Female Basic Student Enrollment: *71* • Male Basic Student Enrollment: *1* • Total RN Enrollment: *20* • Total New Fall Enrollments: *19* • Total Graduates: *Not Reported* • Basic Student Graduates: *Not Reported* • RN Student Graduates: *Not Reported*

NURSING STUDENT PROFILE

Total Nursing Enrollment: *649* • Total Basic Student Enrollment, Full Time: *529* • Total Basic Student Enrollment, Part Time: *120* • Female Basic Student Enrollment: *624* • Male Basic Student Enrollment: *25* • Total RN Enrollment: *0* • Total New Fall Enrollments: *110* • Total Graduates: *158* • Basic Student Graduates: *101* • RN Student Graduates: *57*

FINANCES

Residential Annual Tuition: *$14,115* • Non-Residential Annual Tuition: *$14,150* • General Institutional Fees: *$46* • Additional Nursing Fees: *Not Reported*

FINANCES

Residential Annual Tuition: *$1,896* • Non-Residential Annual Tuition: *$6,348* • General Institutional Fees: *$0* • Additional Nursing Fees: *$100*

HAMPTON UNIVERSITY

Address: Hampton University, Hampton, VA 23668
Phone: 757-727-5252
Fax: 757-727-5423
Contact: Pamela V. Hammond, PhD, RN, FAAN, Dean, School of Nursing
Email: pamela.hammond@hamptonu.edu

GENERAL INFORMATION

Type of School: *4-Year College or University, Private (Independent)* • Accreditation: *Southern Association of Colleges and Schools* • Total Enrollment: *5743*

PROGRAM INFORMATION

Two Year Exit Option: *Not Reported* • NLNAC Accreditation: *Yes* • CCNE Accreditation: *Yes*

NURSING STUDENT PROFILE

Total Nursing Enrollment: *219* • Total Basic Student Enrollment, Full Time: *184* • Total Basic Student Enrollment, Part Time: *10* • Female Basic Student Enrollment: *175* • Male Basic Student Enrollment: *19* • Total RN Enrollment: *25* • Total New Fall Enrollments: *48* • Total Graduates: *101* • Basic Student Graduates: *83* • RN Student Graduates: *18*

FINANCES

Residential Annual Tuition: *$16,200* • Non-Residential Annual Tuition: *$16,200* • General Institutional Fees: *$600* • Additional Nursing Fees: *$130*

JAMES MADISON UNIVERSITY

Address: Department of Nursing, MSC 4305, Harrisonburg, VA 22807
Phone: 540-568-6314
Fax: 540-568-7896
Contact: Merle E. Mast, PhD, RN, ANP, Interim Department Head
Email: mastme@aol.com

GENERAL INFORMATION

Type of School: *4-Year College or University, Public* • Accreditation: *Southern Association of Colleges and Schools* • Total Enrollment: *15000*

PROGRAM INFORMATION

Two Year Exit Option: *Not Reported* • NLNAC Accreditation: *Not Reported* • CCNE Accreditation: *Yes*

NURSING STUDENT PROFILE

Total Nursing Enrollment: *223* • Total Basic Student Enrollment, Full Time: *202* • Total Basic Student Enrollment, Part Time: *21* • Female Basic Student Enrollment: *217* • Male Basic Student Enrollment: *6* • Total RN Enrollment: *0* • Total New Fall Enrollments: *52* • Total Graduates: *41* • Basic Student Graduates: *0* • RN Student Graduates: *41*

FINANCES

Residential Annual Tuition: *$4,000* • Non-Residential Annual Tuition: *$9,850* • General Institutional Fees: *Not Reported* • Additional Nursing Fees: *$100*

LIBERTY UNIVERSITY

Address: 1971 University Boulevard, Lynchburg, VA
24502
Phone: 804-582-2521
Fax: 804-582-7035
Contact: Deanna Britt, PhD, RN, Chair
Email: dbritt@liberty.edu

GENERAL INFORMATION

Type of School: *4-Year College or University, Private
(Independent)* • Accreditation: *Southern Association of Colleges
and Schools* • Total Enrollment: *5000*

PROGRAM INFORMATION

Two Year Exit Option: *Not Reported* • NLNAC
Accreditation: *Yes* • CCNE Accreditation:

NURSING STUDENT PROFILE

Total Nursing Enrollment: *132* • Total Basic Student
Enrollment, Full Time: *123* • Total Basic Student
Enrollment, Part Time: *Not Reported* • Female Basic Student
Enrollment: *114* • Male Basic Student Enrollment: *9* • Total
RN Enrollment: *9* • Total New Fall Enrollments: *41* • Total
Graduates: *52* • Basic Student Graduates: *47* • RN Student
Graduates: *5*

FINANCES

Residential Annual Tuition: *Not Reported* • Non-Residential
Annual Tuition: *Not Reported* • General Institutional Fees:
$440 • Additional Nursing Fees: *$160*

LYNCHBURG COLLEGE

Address: 1501 Lakeside Drive, Lynchburg, VA 24501
Phone: 434-544-8324
Fax: 434-544-8323
Contact: Nancy L. Whitman, PhD, RN, Dean, School of
Health Sciences and Human Performance
Email: whitman@lynchburg.edu

GENERAL INFORMATION

Type of School: *4-Year College or University, Private
(Independent)* • Accreditation: *Southern Association of Colleges
and Schools* • Total Enrollment: *1982*

PROGRAM INFORMATION

Two Year Exit Option: *No* • NLNAC Accreditation: *Yes* •
CCNE Accreditation:

NURSING STUDENT PROFILE

Total Nursing Enrollment: *98* • Total Basic Student
Enrollment, Full Time: *92* • Total Basic Student Enrollment,
Part Time: *6* • Female Basic Student Enrollment: *95* • Male
Basic Student Enrollment: *3* • Total RN Enrollment: *0* •
Total New Fall Enrollments: *0* • Total Graduates: *24* • Basic
Student Graduates: *24* • RN Student Graduates: *0*

FINANCES

Residential Annual Tuition: *$18,880* • Non-Residential
Annual Tuition: *$18,880* • General Institutional Fees: *$125* •
Additional Nursing Fees: *$1,251*

NORFOLK STATE UNIVERSITY

Address: 700 Park Avenue, Norfolk, VA 23504
Phone: 757-823-9013
Fax: *Not Reported*
Contact: Willar F. White-Parson, PhD, RNCS, FAAN, Department Head
Email: wfwhiteparson@nsu.edu

GENERAL INFORMATION

Type of School: *4-Year College or University, Public* •
Accreditation: *Southern Association of Colleges and Schools* •
Total Enrollment: *6000*

PROGRAM INFORMATION

Two Year Exit Option: *Not Reported* • NLNAC
Accreditation: *Yes* • CCNE Accreditation:

NURSING STUDENT PROFILE

Total Nursing Enrollment: *167* • Total Basic Student Enrollment, Full Time: *136* • Total Basic Student Enrollment, Part Time: *31* • Female Basic Student Enrollment: *151* • Male Basic Student Enrollment: *16* • Total RN Enrollment: *0* • Total New Fall Enrollments: *Not Reported* • Total Graduates: *9* • Basic Student Graduates: *9* • RN Student Graduates: *0*

FINANCES

Residential Annual Tuition: *$2,856* • Non-Residential Annual Tuition: *$8,056* • General Institutional Fees: *Not Reported* • Additional Nursing Fees: *$60*

OLD DOMINION UNIVERSITY

Address: 355 Technology Building, Norfolk, VA 23529
Phone: 757-683-5261
Fax: 757-683-5253
Contact: Brenda Nichols, DNS, RN, Chairperson
Email: bnichols@odu.edu

GENERAL INFORMATION

Type of School: *4-Year College or University, Public* •
Accreditation: *Southern Association of Colleges and Schools* •
Total Enrollment: *18500*

PROGRAM INFORMATION

Two Year Exit Option: *Not Reported* • NLNAC
Accreditation: *Yes* • CCNE Accreditation: *Yes*

NURSING STUDENT PROFILE

Total Nursing Enrollment: *476* • Total Basic Student Enrollment, Full Time: *Not Reported* • Total Basic Student Enrollment, Part Time: *Not Reported* • Female Basic Student Enrollment: *Not Reported* • Male Basic Student Enrollment: *Not Reported* • Total RN Enrollment: *271* • Total New Fall Enrollments: *181* • Total Graduates: *98* • Basic Student Graduates: *70* • RN Student Graduates: *28*

FINANCES

Residential Annual Tuition: *Not Reported* • Non-Residential Annual Tuition: *Not Reported* • General Institutional Fees: *Not Reported* • Additional Nursing Fees: *Not Reported*

RADFORD UNIVERSITY

Address: Box 6964, RU Station, Radford, VA 24142
Phone: 540-831-7700
Fax: 540-831-7716
Contact: Lisa Onega, PhD, RN, Coordinator
Email: lonega@radford.edu

GENERAL INFORMATION

Type of School: *4-Year College or University, Public* •
Accreditation: *Southern Association of Colleges and Schools* •
Total Enrollment: *8500*

PROGRAM INFORMATION

Two Year Exit Option: *Not Reported* • NLNAC
Accreditation: *Yes* • CCNE Accreditation: *Yes*

NURSING STUDENT PROFILE

Total Nursing Enrollment: *324* • Total Basic Student
Enrollment, Full Time: *290* • Total Basic Student
Enrollment, Part Time: *16* • Female Basic Student
Enrollment: *293* • Male Basic Student Enrollment: *13* • Total
RN Enrollment: *18* • Total New Fall Enrollments: *69* • Total
Graduates: *43* • Basic Student Graduates: *30* • RN Student
Graduates: *13*

FINANCES

Residential Annual Tuition: *Not Reported* • Non-Residential
Annual Tuition: *Not Reported* • General Institutional Fees:
Not Reported • Additional Nursing Fees: *Not Reported*

SHENANDOAH UNIVERSITY

Address: 1460 University Drive, Winchester, VA 22601
Phone: 540-678-4381
Fax: 540-665-5519
Contact: Sheila M. Sparks, DNSc, RN, CS, Interim
            Director
Email: ssparks@su.edu

GENERAL INFORMATION

Type of School: *4-Year College or University, Private
(Independent)* • Accreditation: *Southern Association of Colleges
and Schools* • Total Enrollment: *2428*

PROGRAM INFORMATION

Two Year Exit Option: *Not Reported* • NLNAC
Accreditation: *Yes* • CCNE Accreditation:

NURSING STUDENT PROFILE

Total Nursing Enrollment: *26* • Total Basic Student
Enrollment, Full Time: *25* • Total Basic Student Enrollment,
Part Time: *1* • Female Basic Student Enrollment: *26* • Male
Basic Student Enrollment: *Not Reported* • Total RN
Enrollment: *0* • Total New Fall Enrollments: *26* • Total
Graduates: *Not Reported* • Basic Student Graduates: *Not
Reported* • RN Student Graduates: *Not Reported*

FINANCES

Residential Annual Tuition: *$16,300* • Non-Residential
Annual Tuition: *$16,600* • General Institutional Fees: *$400* •
Additional Nursing Fees: *Not Reported*

UNIVERSITY OF VIRGINIA

Address: PO Box 800782, Charlottesville, VA 22908-0782
Phone: 434-924-0096
Fax: 434-924-2787
Contact: Judith K. Sands, EdD, RN, Associate Professor
Email: jks@virginia.edu

GENERAL INFORMATION

Type of School: *4-Year College or University, Public* •
Accreditation: *Southern Association of Colleges and Schools* •
Total Enrollment: *23717*

PROGRAM INFORMATION

Two Year Exit Option: *No* • NLNAC Accreditation: *Yes* •
CCNE Accreditation:

NURSING STUDENT PROFILE

Total Nursing Enrollment: *319* • Total Basic Student
Enrollment, Full Time: *293* • Total Basic Student
Enrollment, Part Time: *3* • Female Basic Student
Enrollment: *285* • Male Basic Student Enrollment: *11* • Total
RN Enrollment: *23* • Total New Fall Enrollments: *54* • Total
Graduates: *89* • Basic Student Graduates: *78* • RN Student
Graduates: *11*

FINANCES

Residential Annual Tuition: *$3,046* • Non-Residential
Annual Tuition: *$17,078* • General Institutional Fees:
$1,430 • Additional Nursing Fees: *Not Reported*

VIRGINIA COMMONWEALTH UNIVERSITY

Address: P.O. Box 980567, 1220 E Broad St., Richmond, VA 23284
Phone: 804-828-3968
Fax: 804-828-7743
Contact: Janet B. Younger, PhD, RN, CPNP, Associate Dean and Professor
Email: younger@hsc.vsc.edu

GENERAL INFORMATION

Type of School: *4-Year College or University, Public* •
Accreditation: *Southern Association of Colleges and Schools* •
Total Enrollment: *25000*

PROGRAM INFORMATION

Two Year Exit Option: *No* • NLNAC Accreditation: *Yes* •
CCNE Accreditation:

NURSING STUDENT PROFILE

Total Nursing Enrollment: *247* • Total Basic Student
Enrollment, Full Time: *224* • Total Basic Student
Enrollment, Part Time: *23* • Female Basic Student
Enrollment: *229* • Male Basic Student Enrollment: *18* • Total
RN Enrollment: *0* • Total New Fall Enrollments: *107* • Total
Graduates: *69* • Basic Student Graduates: *69* • RN Student
Graduates: *0*

FINANCES

Residential Annual Tuition: *$2,494* • Non-Residential
Annual Tuition: *$12,672* • General Institutional Fees: *$967* •
Additional Nursing Fees: *$0*

NORTHWEST COLLEGE

Address: 231 West 6th Street, Powell, WA 82435
Phone: 425-889-7837
Fax: 425-889-7815
Contact: Carl Christensen, PhD, RN, Dean of the
            Buntain School of Nursing
Email: carl.christensen@ncag.edu

GENERAL INFORMATION

Type of School: *2-Year College or University, Public* •
Accreditation: *North Central Association of Colleges and
Schools* • Total Enrollment: *1900*

PROGRAM INFORMATION

Two Year Exit Option: *Not Reported* • NLNAC
Accreditation: *Not Reported* • CCNE Accreditation: *Yes*

NURSING STUDENT PROFILE

Total Nursing Enrollment: *15* • Total Basic Student
Enrollment, Full Time: *15* • Total Basic Student Enrollment,
Part Time: *0* • Female Basic Student Enrollment: *14* • Male
Basic Student Enrollment: *1* • Total RN Enrollment: *0* •
Total New Fall Enrollments: *15* • Total Graduates: *Not
Reported* • Basic Student Graduates: *Not Reported* • RN
Student Graduates: *Not Reported*

FINANCES

Residential Annual Tuition: *$10,550* • Non-Residential
Annual Tuition: *$10,550* • General Institutional Fees: *$198* •
Additional Nursing Fees: *$900*

PACIFIC LUTHERAN UNIVERSITY

Address: 121 and Park Ave., School of Nursing, Tacoma,
            WA 98447-0003
Phone: 253-535-7674
Fax: 253-535-7590
Contact: Terry W. Miller, PhD, RN, Dean and Professor
Email: millertw@plu.edu

GENERAL INFORMATION

Type of School: *4-Year College or University, Private
(Religious)* • Accreditation: *Western Association of Schools and
Colleges* • Total Enrollment: *3515*

PROGRAM INFORMATION

Two Year Exit Option: *Not Reported* • NLNAC
Accreditation: *Yes* • CCNE Accreditation:

NURSING STUDENT PROFILE

Total Nursing Enrollment: *234* • Total Basic Student
Enrollment, Full Time: *234* • Total Basic Student
Enrollment, Part Time: *0* • Female Basic Student
Enrollment: *213* • Male Basic Student Enrollment: *21* • Total
RN Enrollment: *0* • Total New Fall Enrollments: *49* • Total
Graduates: *69* • Basic Student Graduates: *66* • RN Student
Graduates: *3*

FINANCES

Residential Annual Tuition: *$16,800* • Non-Residential
Annual Tuition: *$16,800* • General Institutional Fees: *Not
Reported* • Additional Nursing Fees: *$1,200*

SEATTLE UNIVERSITY

Address: 900 Broadway and Madison, Seattle, WA 98122
Phone: 206-296-5672
Fax: 206-296-5544
Contact: Maureen Niland, PhD, RN, Director
Email: nilandm@seattleu.edu

UNIVERSITY OF WASHINGTON

Address: Box 357260, Seattle, WA 98195
Phone: 206-618-8407
Fax: *Not Reported*
Contact: Susan L. Woods, PhD, RN, Associate Dean for Academic Program
Email: slwoods@washnigton.edu

GENERAL INFORMATION

Type of School: *4-Year College or University, Private (Religious)* • Accreditation: *Western Association of Schools and Colleges* • Total Enrollment: *6000*

GENERAL INFORMATION

Type of School: *Not Reported* • Accreditation: *Not Reported* • Total Enrollment: *Not Reported*

PROGRAM INFORMATION

Two Year Exit Option: *Not Reported* • NLNAC Accreditation: *Yes* • CCNE Accreditation:

PROGRAM INFORMATION

Two Year Exit Option: *Not Reported* • NLNAC Accreditation: *Yes* • CCNE Accreditation:

NURSING STUDENT PROFILE

Total Nursing Enrollment: *281* • Total Basic Student Enrollment, Full Time: *Not Reported* • Total Basic Student Enrollment, Part Time: *Not Reported* • Female Basic Student Enrollment: *256* • Male Basic Student Enrollment: *25* • Total RN Enrollment: *0* • Total New Fall Enrollments: *49* • Total Graduates: *67* • Basic Student Graduates: *67* • RN Student Graduates: *0*

NURSING STUDENT PROFILE

Total Nursing Enrollment: *Not Reported* • Total Basic Student Enrollment, Full Time: *Not Reported* • Total Basic Student Enrollment, Part Time: *Not Reported* • Female Basic Student Enrollment: *Not Reported* • Male Basic Student Enrollment: *Not Reported* • Total RN Enrollment: *Not Reported* • Total New Fall Enrollments: *206* • Total Graduates: *187* • Basic Student Graduates: *61* • RN Student Graduates: *126*

FINANCES

Residential Annual Tuition: *$17,010* • Non-Residential Annual Tuition: *$17,010* • General Institutional Fees: *Not Reported* • Additional Nursing Fees: *Not Reported*

FINANCES

Residential Annual Tuition: *$3,639* • Non-Residential Annual Tuition: *$12,030* • General Institutional Fees: *$80* • Additional Nursing Fees: *Not Reported*

WASHINGTON STATE UNIVERSITY

Address: 2917 W Ft. George Wright Drive, Spokane, WA 99224
Phone: 509-324-7335
Fax: 509-324-7336
Contact: Anne M. Hirsch, DNS, ARNP, Assoc. Dean for Academic Affairs
Email: hirsch@wsu.edu

GENERAL INFORMATION

Type of School: *4-Year College or University, Public* •
Accreditation: *Northwestern Association of Schools and Colleges* • Total Enrollment: *20984*

PROGRAM INFORMATION

Two Year Exit Option: *Not Reported* • NLNAC
Accreditation: *Yes* • CCNE Accreditation:

NURSING STUDENT PROFILE

Total Nursing Enrollment: *464* • Total Basic Student Enrollment, Full Time: *320* • Total Basic Student Enrollment, Part Time: *4* • Female Basic Student Enrollment: *293* • Male Basic Student Enrollment: *31* • Total RN Enrollment: *140* • Total New Fall Enrollments: *90* • Total Graduates: *168* • Basic Student Graduates: *130* • RN Student Graduates: *38*

FINANCES

Residential Annual Tuition: *$3,898* • Non-Residential Annual Tuition: *$11,258* • General Institutional Fees: *$142* • Additional Nursing Fees: *$300*

ALDERSON-BROADDUS COLLEGE

Address: PO Box 2033, Philippi, WV 26416
Phone: 304-457-6261
Fax: 304-457-6308
Contact: M Sharon Boni, DNSc, RN, Chair, Division of Health Sciences
Email: boni@ab.edu

GENERAL INFORMATION

Type of School: *4-Year College or University, Private (Religious)* • Accreditation: *North Central Association of Colleges and Schools* • Total Enrollment: *751*

PROGRAM INFORMATION

Two Year Exit Option: *Not Reported* • NLNAC
Accreditation: *Yes* • CCNE Accreditation:

NURSING STUDENT PROFILE

Total Nursing Enrollment: *91* • Total Basic Student Enrollment, Full Time: *69* • Total Basic Student Enrollment, Part Time: *0* • Female Basic Student Enrollment: *62* • Male Basic Student Enrollment: *7* • Total RN Enrollment: *22* • Total New Fall Enrollments: *14* • Total Graduates: *17* • Basic Student Graduates: *17* • RN Student Graduates: *0*

FINANCES

Residential Annual Tuition: *$13,719* • Non-Residential Annual Tuition: *$13,719* • General Institutional Fees: *$200* • Additional Nursing Fees: *$200*

MARSHALL UNIVERSITY

Address: 1 John Marshall Drive, Huntington, WV 25755-9500
Phone: 304-696-2633
Fax: 304-696-6739
Contact: Linda M. Scott, PhD, RN, C-FNP, Associate Dean
Email: scott@marshall.edu

GENERAL INFORMATION

Type of School: *4-Year College or University, Public* • Accreditation: *North Central Association of Colleges and Schools* • Total Enrollment: *16000*

PROGRAM INFORMATION

Two Year Exit Option: *Not Reported* • NLNAC Accreditation: *Yes* • CCNE Accreditation:

NURSING STUDENT PROFILE

Total Nursing Enrollment: *314* • Total Basic Student Enrollment, Full Time: *211* • Total Basic Student Enrollment, Part Time: *20* • Female Basic Student Enrollment: *201* • Male Basic Student Enrollment: *30* • Total RN Enrollment: *83* • Total New Fall Enrollments: *66* • Total Graduates: *58* • Basic Student Graduates: *41* • RN Student Graduates: *17*

FINANCES

Residential Annual Tuition: *$2,238* • Non-Residential Annual Tuition: *$6,810* • General Institutional Fees: *$488* • Additional Nursing Fees: *$250*

MOUNTAIN STATE UNIVERSITY

Address: 609 S Kanawha St, Beckley, WV 25801
Phone: 304-929-1327
Fax: 304-929-1600
Contact: Patsy Haslay, EdD, RN, Program Director
Email: phaslam@mountainstate.edu

GENERAL INFORMATION

Type of School: *4-Year College or University, Private (Independent)* • Accreditation: *North Central Association of Colleges and Schools* • Total Enrollment: *1783*

PROGRAM INFORMATION

Two Year Exit Option: *No* • NLNAC Accreditation: *Yes* • CCNE Accreditation:

NURSING STUDENT PROFILE

Total Nursing Enrollment: *166* • Total Basic Student Enrollment, Full Time: *106* • Total Basic Student Enrollment, Part Time: *0* • Female Basic Student Enrollment: *101* • Male Basic Student Enrollment: *5* • Total RN Enrollment: *60* • Total New Fall Enrollments: *0* • Total Graduates: *32* • Basic Student Graduates: *28* • RN Student Graduates: *4*

FINANCES

Residential Annual Tuition: *$3,600* • Non-Residential Annual Tuition: *$3,600* • General Institutional Fees: *$720* • Additional Nursing Fees: *$2,400*

Circle 87 on reader card   See in-depth profile for more information

SHEPHERD COLLEGE

Address: PO Box 3210, Shepherdstown, WV 25443
Phone: 304-876-5341
Fax: 304-876-5169
Contact: Lynn Hanson, MSN, RN, Chair, Department of
           Nursing
Email: lhanson@shepherd.edu

UNIVERSITY OF CHARLESTON

Address: 2300 McCorkle Avenue, SE, Charleston, WV
           25304
Phone: 304-357-4846
Fax: 304-357-4965
Contact: Martha Sue Forsbrey, EdD, RN, BSN Program
           Coordinator
Email: mforsbrey@uchaswv.edu

GENERAL INFORMATION

Type of School: *4-Year College or University, Public* •
Accreditation: *North Central Association of Colleges and
Schools* • Total Enrollment: *4600*

GENERAL INFORMATION

Type of School: *4-Year College or University, Private
(Independent)* • Accreditation: *North Central Association of
Colleges and Schools* • Total Enrollment: *955*

PROGRAM INFORMATION

Two Year Exit Option: *No* • NLNAC Accreditation: *Yes* •
CCNE Accreditation:

PROGRAM INFORMATION

Two Year Exit Option: *Not Reported* • NLNAC
Accreditation: *Yes* • CCNE Accreditation:

NURSING STUDENT PROFILE

Total Nursing Enrollment: *61* • Total Basic Student
Enrollment, Full Time: *57* • Total Basic Student Enrollment,
Part Time: *0* • Female Basic Student Enrollment: *54* • Male
Basic Student Enrollment: *3* • Total RN Enrollment: *4* •
Total New Fall Enrollments: *33* • Total Graduates: *26* • Basic
Student Graduates: *20* • RN Student Graduates: *6*

NURSING STUDENT PROFILE

Total Nursing Enrollment: *144* • Total Basic Student
Enrollment, Full Time: *133* • Total Basic Student
Enrollment, Part Time: *7* • Female Basic Student
Enrollment: *129* • Male Basic Student Enrollment: *11* • Total
RN Enrollment: *4* • Total New Fall Enrollments: *18* • Total
Graduates: *30* • Basic Student Graduates: *30* • RN Student
Graduates: *0*

FINANCES

Residential Annual Tuition: *$2,608* • Non-Residential
Annual Tuition: *$6,294* • General Institutional Fees: *$40* •
Additional Nursing Fees: *$140*

FINANCES

Residential Annual Tuition: *$13,200* • Non-Residential
Annual Tuition: *$13,200* • General Institutional Fees: *Not
Reported* • Additional Nursing Fees: *$140*

WEST LIBERTY STATE COLLEGE

Address: PO Box 295, Route 88 N, West Liberty, WV
            26074
Phone: 304-336-8175
Fax: 304-336-5104
Contact: Donna Lukich, EdD, RN, Program Director,
            Nursing
Email: lukichda@wlsc.wvnet.edu

GENERAL INFORMATION

Type of School: *4-Year College or University, Public* •
Accreditation: *North Central Association of Colleges and
Schools* • Total Enrollment: *2450*

PROGRAM INFORMATION

Two Year Exit Option: *Not Reported* • NLNAC
Accreditation: *Yes* • CCNE Accreditation:

NURSING STUDENT PROFILE

Total Nursing Enrollment: *114* • Total Basic Student
Enrollment, Full Time: *56* • Total Basic Student Enrollment,
Part Time: *1* • Female Basic Student Enrollment: *49* • Male
Basic Student Enrollment: *8* • Total RN Enrollment: *57* •
Total New Fall Enrollments: *13* • Total Graduates: *14* • Basic
Student Graduates: *8* • RN Student Graduates: *6*

FINANCES

Residential Annual Tuition: *$2,420* • Non-Residential
Annual Tuition: *$5,860* • General Institutional Fees: *$590* •
Additional Nursing Fees: *$50*

WEST VIRGINIA WESLEYAN COLLEGE

Address: 59 College Avenue, Buckhannon, WV 26201
Phone: 304-473-8224
Fax: 304-473-8435
Contact: Shauna Aurelio, MSN, RN, Chairperson
Email: aurelio_s@wvwc.edu

GENERAL INFORMATION

Type of School: *4-Year College or University, Private
(Religious)* • Accreditation: *North Central Association of
Colleges and Schools* • Total Enrollment: *1550*

PROGRAM INFORMATION

Two Year Exit Option: *Not Reported* • NLNAC
Accreditation: *Yes* • CCNE Accreditation: *Yes*

NURSING STUDENT PROFILE

Total Nursing Enrollment: *90* • Total Basic Student
Enrollment, Full Time: *51* • Total Basic Student Enrollment,
Part Time: *0* • Female Basic Student Enrollment: *48* • Male
Basic Student Enrollment: *3* • Total RN Enrollment: *39* •
Total New Fall Enrollments: *20* • Total Graduates: *26* • Basic
Student Graduates: *19* • RN Student Graduates: *7*

FINANCES

Residential Annual Tuition: *$16,800* • Non-Residential
Annual Tuition: *Not Reported* • General Institutional Fees:
$1,250 • Additional Nursing Fees: *Not Reported*

Circle 157 on reader card   See in-depth profile for more information

WHEELING JESUIT UNIVERSITY

Address:　316 Washington Avenue, Wheeling, WV 26003
Phone:　304-243-2227
Fax:　304-243-4441
Contact:　Rose Kuthenios, PhD, RN, CS, Chair and Professor
Email:　rosekut@wju.edu

GENERAL INFORMATION

Type of School: *4-Year College or University, Private (Religious)* • Accreditation: *North Central Association of Colleges and Schools* • Total Enrollment: *1280*

PROGRAM INFORMATION

Two Year Exit Option: *Not Reported* • NLNAC Accreditation: *Yes* • CCNE Accreditation:

NURSING STUDENT PROFILE

Total Nursing Enrollment: *124* • Total Basic Student Enrollment, Full Time: *42* • Total Basic Student Enrollment, Part Time: *0* • Female Basic Student Enrollment: *36* • Male Basic Student Enrollment: *6* • Total RN Enrollment: *82* • Total New Fall Enrollments: *21* • Total Graduates: *23* • Basic Student Graduates: *7* • RN Student Graduates: *16*

FINANCES

Residential Annual Tuition: *$16,000* • Non-Residential Annual Tuition: *$16,000* • General Institutional Fees: *$600* • Additional Nursing Fees: *$36*

ALVERNO COLLEGE

Address:　3400 South 43rd Street, PO Box 343922, Milwaukee, WI 53234-3922
Phone:　414-382-6284
Fax:　414-382-6279
Contact:　Judeen Schulte, PhD, RN, Chairperson
Email:　judeen.schulte@alverno.edu

GENERAL INFORMATION

Type of School: *4-Year College or University, Private (Religious)* • Accreditation: *North Central Association of Colleges and Schools* • Total Enrollment: *1950*

PROGRAM INFORMATION

Two Year Exit Option: *No* • NLNAC Accreditation: *Not Reported* • CCNE Accreditation: *Yes*

NURSING STUDENT PROFILE

Total Nursing Enrollment: *270* • Total Basic Student Enrollment, Full Time: *183* • Total Basic Student Enrollment, Part Time: *70* • Female Basic Student Enrollment: *253* • Male Basic Student Enrollment: *Not Reported* • Total RN Enrollment: *17* • Total New Fall Enrollments: *Not Reported* • Total Graduates: *41* • Basic Student Graduates: *35* • RN Student Graduates: *6*

FINANCES

Residential Annual Tuition: *$12,744* • Non-Residential Annual Tuition: *$12,744* • General Institutional Fees: *Not Reported* • Additional Nursing Fees: *Not Reported*

BELLIN COLLEGE OF NURSING

Address: 725 South Webster Avenue, PO Box 23400,
           Green Bay, WI 54305-3400
Phone: 920-433-7849
Fax: 920-433-7416
Contact: Patricia Swinford, PhD, RN, Dean
Email: swinford@bcon.edu

GENERAL INFORMATION

Type of School: *Hospital, Private (Independent)* •
Accreditation: *North Central Association of Colleges and
Schools* • Total Enrollment: *Not Reported*

PROGRAM INFORMATION

Two Year Exit Option: *No* • NLNAC Accreditation: *Yes* •
CCNE Accreditation:

NURSING STUDENT PROFILE

Total Nursing Enrollment: *151* • Total Basic Student
Enrollment, Full Time: *141* • Total Basic Student
Enrollment, Part Time: *10* • Female Basic Student
Enrollment: *141* • Male Basic Student Enrollment: *10* • Total
RN Enrollment: *0* • Total New Fall Enrollments: *61* • Total
Graduates: *51* • Basic Student Graduates: *51* • RN Student
Graduates: *0*

FINANCES

Residential Annual Tuition: *$9,753* • Non-Residential
Annual Tuition: *$9,753* • General Institutional Fees:
$4,877 • Additional Nursing Fees: *$487*

CARDINAL STRITCH UNIVERSITY

Address: 6801 North Yates Road, Milwaukee, WI 53217
Phone: 414-410-4390
Fax: *Not Reported*
Contact: Zaiga G.P. Kalnins, EdD, RN, Dean, College of
           Nursing
Email: *Not Reported*

GENERAL INFORMATION

Type of School: *4-Year College or University, Private
(Religious)* • Accreditation: *North Central Association of
Colleges and Schools* • Total Enrollment: *5700*

PROGRAM INFORMATION

Two Year Exit Option: *Not Reported* • NLNAC
Accreditation: *Yes* • CCNE Accreditation: *Yes*

NURSING STUDENT PROFILE

Total Nursing Enrollment: *Not Reported* • Total Basic Student
Enrollment, Full Time: *Not Reported* • Total Basic Student
Enrollment, Part Time: *Not Reported* • Female Basic Student
Enrollment: *Not Reported* • Male Basic Student Enrollment:
Not Reported • Total RN Enrollment: *Not Reported* • Total
New Fall Enrollments: *10* • Total Graduates: *14* • Basic
Student Graduates: *0* • RN Student Graduates: *14*

FINANCES

Residential Annual Tuition: *$11,000* • Non-Residential
Annual Tuition: *$11,000* • General Institutional Fees: *$100* •
Additional Nursing Fees: *Not Reported*

COLUMBIA COLLEGE OF NURSING

Address: 2121 East Newport Avenue, Milwaukee, WI 53211
Phone: 414-961-3531
Fax: 414-961-4121
Contact: Marian H. Snyder, PhD, RN, Dean and CEO
Email: msnyder@ccon.edu

GENERAL INFORMATION

Type of School: *4-Year College or University, Private (Independent)* • Accreditation: *North Central Association of Colleges and Schools* • Total Enrollment: *194*

PROGRAM INFORMATION

Two Year Exit Option: *Not Reported* • NLNAC Accreditation: *Yes* • CCNE Accreditation:

NURSING STUDENT PROFILE

Total Nursing Enrollment: *194* • Total Basic Student Enrollment, Full Time: *150* • Total Basic Student Enrollment, Part Time: *28* • Female Basic Student Enrollment: *168* • Male Basic Student Enrollment: *10* • Total RN Enrollment: *16* • Total New Fall Enrollments: *25* • Total Graduates: *61* • Basic Student Graduates: *54* • RN Student Graduates: *7*

FINANCES

Residential Annual Tuition: *$15,250* • Non-Residential Annual Tuition: *$15,250* • General Institutional Fees: *$330* • Additional Nursing Fees: *$325*

CONCORDIA UNIVERSITY WISCONSIN (LCMS)

Address: 12800 North Lake Shore Drive, Mequon, WI 53097
Phone: 262-243-4205
Fax: 262-243-4466
Contact: Grace A. Peterson, PhD, MSN, RN, Chairperson, Nursing Division
Email: grace.peterson@cuw.edu

GENERAL INFORMATION

Type of School: *4-Year College or University, Private (Religious)* • Accreditation: *North Central Association of Colleges and Schools* • Total Enrollment: *4810*

PROGRAM INFORMATION

Two Year Exit Option: *No* • NLNAC Accreditation: *Yes* • CCNE Accreditation: *Yes*

NURSING STUDENT PROFILE

Total Nursing Enrollment: *142* • Total Basic Student Enrollment, Full Time: *82* • Total Basic Student Enrollment, Part Time: *4* • Female Basic Student Enrollment: *85* • Male Basic Student Enrollment: *1* • Total RN Enrollment: *56* • Total New Fall Enrollments: *34* • Total Graduates: *Not Reported* • Basic Student Graduates: *Not Reported* • RN Student Graduates: *Not Reported*

FINANCES

Residential Annual Tuition: *$13,500* • Non-Residential Annual Tuition: *Not Reported* • General Institutional Fees: *Not Reported* • Additional Nursing Fees: *$35*

EDGEWOOD COLLEGE

Address: 1000 Edgewood College Drive, Madison, WI
            53711
Phone: 608-663-2292
Fax: 608-663-2863
Contact: Mary Kelly-Powell, PhD, RN, Chair
Email: mkellypowell@edgewood.edu

GENERAL INFORMATION

Type of School: *4-Year College or University, Private
(Religious)* • Accreditation: *North Central Association of
Colleges and Schools* • Total Enrollment: *1900*

PROGRAM INFORMATION

Two Year Exit Option: *Not Reported* • NLNAC
Accreditation: *Not Reported* • CCNE Accreditation: *Yes*

NURSING STUDENT PROFILE

Total Nursing Enrollment: *91* • Total Basic Student
Enrollment, Full Time: *71* • Total Basic Student Enrollment,
Part Time: *10* • Female Basic Student Enrollment: *79* • Male
Basic Student Enrollment: *2* • Total RN Enrollment: *10* •
Total New Fall Enrollments: *22* • Total Graduates: *34* • Basic
Student Graduates: *31* • RN Student Graduates: *3*

FINANCES

Residential Annual Tuition: *$12,250* • Non-Residential
Annual Tuition: *$12,250* • General Institutional Fees: *Not
Reported* • Additional Nursing Fees: *$726*

MARIAN COLLEGE OF FOND DU LAC

Address: 45 South National Avenue, Fond du Lac, WI
            54935
Phone: 920-923-8094
Fax: 920-923-8770
Contact: Elizabeth A. Parato, PhD, RN, Chairperson,
            Nursing Studies Division
Email: eparato@mariancollege.edu

GENERAL INFORMATION

Type of School: *Independent, Private (Religious)* •
Accreditation: *North Central Association of Colleges and
Schools* • Total Enrollment: *2555*

PROGRAM INFORMATION

Two Year Exit Option: *Not Reported* • NLNAC
Accreditation: *Yes* • CCNE Accreditation:

NURSING STUDENT PROFILE

Total Nursing Enrollment: *348* • Total Basic Student
Enrollment, Full Time: *137* • Total Basic Student
Enrollment, Part Time: *6* • Female Basic Student
Enrollment: *138* • Male Basic Student Enrollment: *5* • Total
RN Enrollment: *205* • Total New Fall Enrollments: *Not
Reported* • Total Graduates: *72* • Basic Student Graduates:
31 • RN Student Graduates: *41*

FINANCES

Residential Annual Tuition: *$12,624* • Non-Residential
Annual Tuition: *$12,624* • General Institutional Fees:
$4,290 • Additional Nursing Fees: *Not Reported*

MARQUETTE UNIVERSITY

Address:　PO Box 1881, Milwaukee, WI 53201-1881
Phone:　　414-288-3812
Fax:　　　414-288-1597
Contact:　Madeline Wake, PhD, RN, FAAN, Dean and
　　　　　Professor
Email:　　madeline.wake@marquette.edu

GENERAL INFORMATION

Type of School: *4-Year College or University, Private (Religious)* • Accreditation: *North Central Association of Colleges and Schools* • Total Enrollment: *10832*

PROGRAM INFORMATION

Two Year Exit Option: *No* • NLNAC Accreditation: *Yes* • CCNE Accreditation: *Yes*

NURSING STUDENT PROFILE

Total Nursing Enrollment: *334* • Total Basic Student Enrollment, Full Time: *278* • Total Basic Student Enrollment, Part Time: *3* • Female Basic Student Enrollment: *263* • Male Basic Student Enrollment: *18* • Total RN Enrollment: *53* • Total New Fall Enrollments: *78* • Total Graduates: *83* • Basic Student Graduates: *68* • RN Student Graduates: *15*

FINANCES

Residential Annual Tuition: *$18,680* • Non-Residential Annual Tuition: *$18,680* • General Institutional Fees: *$116* • Additional Nursing Fees: *$50*

MILWAUKEE SCHOOL OF ENGINEERING

Address:　1025 North Broadway, Milwaukee, WI 53202
Phone:　　414-277-4516
Fax:　　　414-277-4540
Contact:　Mary Louise Brown, PhD, RN, Professor,
　　　　　Interim Chair
Email:　　brown@msoc.edu

GENERAL INFORMATION

Type of School: *Not Reported* • Accreditation: *Not Reported* • Total Enrollment: *Not Reported*

PROGRAM INFORMATION

Two Year Exit Option: *Not Reported* • NLNAC Accreditation: *Not Reported* • CCNE Accreditation: *Yes*

NURSING STUDENT PROFILE

Total Nursing Enrollment: *Not Reported* • Total Basic Student Enrollment, Full Time: *Not Reported* • Total Basic Student Enrollment, Part Time: *Not Reported* • Female Basic Student Enrollment: *Not Reported* • Male Basic Student Enrollment: *Not Reported* • Total RN Enrollment: *Not Reported* • Total New Fall Enrollments: *19* • Total Graduates: *5* • Basic Student Graduates: *5* • RN Student Graduates: *0*

FINANCES

Residential Annual Tuition: *$19,845* • Non-Residential Annual Tuition: *$19,845* • General Institutional Fees: *Not Reported* • Additional Nursing Fees: *$75*

UNIVERSITY OF WISCONSIN— EAU CLAIRE

Address: PO Box 4004, Eau Claire, WI 54702
Phone: 715-836-5287
Fax: 715-836-5925
Contact: Rita Kisting Sparks, PhD, RN, Interim Associate; Dean and Educational Administrator
Email: sparksrk@vwec.edu

GENERAL INFORMATION

Type of School: *4-Year College or University, Public* • Accreditation: *North Central Association of Colleges and Schools* • Total Enrollment: *10559*

PROGRAM INFORMATION

Two Year Exit Option: *No* • NLNAC Accreditation: *Yes* • CCNE Accreditation: *Yes*

NURSING STUDENT PROFILE

Total Nursing Enrollment: *314* • Total Basic Student Enrollment, Full Time: *253* • Total Basic Student Enrollment, Part Time: *33* • Female Basic Student Enrollment: *275* • Male Basic Student Enrollment: *11* • Total RN Enrollment: *28* • Total New Fall Enrollments: *40* • Total Graduates: *94* • Basic Student Graduates: *86* • RN Student Graduates: *8*

FINANCES

Residential Annual Tuition: *$3,476* • Non-Residential Annual Tuition: *$11,946* • General Institutional Fees: *$596* • Additional Nursing Fees: *$25*

UNIVERSITY OF WISCONSIN—MADISON

Address: 600 Highland Avenue, H6/150, Madison, WI 53792-2455
Phone: 608-263-5155
Fax: 608-263-5323
Contact: Katharyn A. May, DNSc, RN, FAAN, Dean and Professor
Email: kamay@facstaff.wisc.edu

GENERAL INFORMATION

Type of School: *4-Year College or University, Public* • Accreditation: *North Central Association of Colleges and Schools* • Total Enrollment: *Not Reported*

PROGRAM INFORMATION

Two Year Exit Option: *Not Reported* • NLNAC Accreditation: *Not Reported* • CCNE Accreditation: *Yes*

NURSING STUDENT PROFILE

Total Nursing Enrollment: *Not Reported* • Total Basic Student Enrollment, Full Time: *Not Reported* • Total Basic Student Enrollment, Part Time: *Not Reported* • Female Basic Student Enrollment: *Not Reported* • Male Basic Student Enrollment: *Not Reported* • Total RN Enrollment: *Not Reported* • Total New Fall Enrollments: *110* • Total Graduates: *Not Reported* • Basic Student Graduates: *Not Reported* • RN Student Graduates: *Not Reported*

FINANCES

Residential Annual Tuition: *Not Reported* • Non-Residential Annual Tuition: *Not Reported* • General Institutional Fees: *Not Reported* • Additional Nursing Fees: *Not Reported*

UNIVERSITY OF WISCONSIN—MILWAUKEE

Address: PO Box 413, Milwaukee, WI 53201
Phone: 414-229-5468
Fax: 414-229-2640
Contact: Susan Dean-Baar, PhD, RN, FAAN, Associate Dean of Academic Affairs
Email: deanbaar@uwm.edu

GENERAL INFORMATION

Type of School: *4-Year College or University, Public* • Accreditation: *North Central Association of Colleges and Schools* • Total Enrollment: *24223*

PROGRAM INFORMATION

Two Year Exit Option: *Not Reported* • NLNAC Accreditation: *Not Reported* • CCNE Accreditation: *Yes*

NURSING STUDENT PROFILE

Total Nursing Enrollment: *852* • Total Basic Student Enrollment, Full Time: *510* • Total Basic Student Enrollment, Part Time: *304* • Female Basic Student Enrollment: *746* • Male Basic Student Enrollment: *68* • Total RN Enrollment: *38* • Total New Fall Enrollments: *71* • Total Graduates: *133* • Basic Student Graduates: *126* • RN Student Graduates: *7*

FINANCES

Residential Annual Tuition: *$3,445* • Non-Residential Annual Tuition: *$12,893* • General Institutional Fees: *$318* • Additional Nursing Fees: *Not Reported*

UNIVERSITY OF WISCONSIN—OSHKOSH

Address: 800 Algoma Boulevard, Oshkosh, WI 54901
Phone: 920-424-2121
Fax: 920-424-0123
Contact: Stephanie Stewart, PhD, RN, Undergraduate Program Director
Email: stewart@uwash.edu

GENERAL INFORMATION

Type of School: *4-Year College or University, Public* • Accreditation: *North Central Association of Colleges and Schools* • Total Enrollment: *11000*

PROGRAM INFORMATION

Two Year Exit Option: *No* • NLNAC Accreditation: *Not Reported* • CCNE Accreditation: *Yes*

NURSING STUDENT PROFILE

Total Nursing Enrollment: *831* • Total Basic Student Enrollment, Full Time: *608* • Total Basic Student Enrollment, Part Time: *145* • Female Basic Student Enrollment: *Not Reported* • Male Basic Student Enrollment: *Not Reported* • Total RN Enrollment: *78* • Total New Fall Enrollments: *Not Reported* • Total Graduates: *120* • Basic Student Graduates: *115* • RN Student Graduates: *5*

FINANCES

Residential Annual Tuition: *$2,776* • Non-Residential Annual Tuition: *$9,920* • General Institutional Fees: *$449* • Additional Nursing Fees: *$122*

VITERBO COLLEGE

Address: 815 South 9th Street, La Crosse, WI 54601
Phone: 608-796-3687
Fax: 608-796-3050
Contact: Silvana F. Richardson, PhD, RN, Dean
Email: sfrichardson@viterbo.edu

GENERAL INFORMATION

Type of School: *4-Year College or University, Private (Independent)* • Accreditation: *North Central Association of Colleges and Schools* • Total Enrollment: *1750*

PROGRAM INFORMATION

Two Year Exit Option: *Not Reported* • NLNAC Accreditation: *Yes* • CCNE Accreditation:

NURSING STUDENT PROFILE

Total Nursing Enrollment: *467* • Total Basic Student Enrollment, Full Time: *Not Reported* • Total Basic Student Enrollment, Part Time: *Not Reported* • Female Basic Student Enrollment: *273* • Male Basic Student Enrollment: *21* • Total RN Enrollment: *173* • Total New Fall Enrollments: *69* • Total Graduates: *136* • Basic Student Graduates: *49* • RN Student Graduates: *87*

FINANCES

Residential Annual Tuition: *$12,220* • Non-Residential Annual Tuition: *$12,220* • General Institutional Fees: *$290* • Additional Nursing Fees: *Not Reported*

UNIVERSITY OF WYOMING

Address: PO Box 3434, Laramie, WY 82071
Phone: 307-766-6569
Fax: 307-766-4294
Contact: Marcia L. Dale, EdD, RN, FAAN, Dean, School of Nursing
Email: marcia@owyo.edu

GENERAL INFORMATION

Type of School: *4-Year College or University, Public* • Accreditation: *North Central Association of Colleges and Schools* • Total Enrollment: *11057*

PROGRAM INFORMATION

Two Year Exit Option: *No* • NLNAC Accreditation: *Not Reported* • CCNE Accreditation: *Yes*

NURSING STUDENT PROFILE

Total Nursing Enrollment: *277* • Total Basic Student Enrollment, Full Time: *204* • Total Basic Student Enrollment, Part Time: *31* • Female Basic Student Enrollment: *203* • Male Basic Student Enrollment: *32* • Total RN Enrollment: *42* • Total New Fall Enrollments: *52* • Total Graduates: *44* • Basic Student Graduates: *30* • RN Student Graduates: *14*

FINANCES

Residential Annual Tuition: *$2,316* • Non-Residential Annual Tuition: *$7,788* • General Institutional Fees: *$491* • Additional Nursing Fees: *$200*

BSRN DEGREE PROGRAMS

AUBURN UNIVERSITY

Address: 107 Samford Hall, Auburn University, AL 36849
Phone: 334-844-6759
Fax: 334-844-5654
Contact: Glenda Avery, PhD, RN, Associate Professor
Email: averygp@auburn.edu

GENERAL INFORMATION

Type of School: *4-Year College or University, Public* •
Accreditation: *Southern Association of Colleges and Schools* •
Total Enrollment: *22000*

PROGRAM INFORMATION

NLNAC Accreditation: *Yes* • CCNE Accreditation:

NURSING STUDENT PROFILE

Total Nursing Enrollment: *4* • Full-Time Enrollment: *4* •
Part-Time Enrollment: *0* • Female Enrollment: *4* • Male
Enrollment: *0* • Total Graduates: *6*

FINANCES

Residential Annual Tuition: *$3,050* • Non-Residential
Annual Tuition: *$9,150* • General Institutional Fees: *$288* •
Additional Nursing Fees: *$15*

THE UNIVERSITY OF ALABAMA

Address: 504 University Blvd PO Box 870358,
          Tuscaloosa, AL 35487-0358
Phone: 205-348-1044
Fax: 205-348-5559
Contact: Donna R. Packa, DSN, RN, Associate Dean
Email: dpacka@bama.ua.edu

GENERAL INFORMATION

Type of School: *4-Year College or University, Public* •
Accreditation: *Southern Association of Colleges and Schools* •
Total Enrollment: *19171*

PROGRAM INFORMATION

NLNAC Accreditation: *Not Reported* • CCNE Accreditation:
Yes

NURSING STUDENT PROFILE

Total Nursing Enrollment: *18* • Full-Time Enrollment: *16* •
Part-Time Enrollment: *2* • Female Enrollment: *15* • Male
Enrollment: *3* • Total Graduates: *11*

FINANCES

Residential Annual Tuition: *$1,646* • Non-Residential
Annual Tuition: *$4,456* • General Institutional Fees: *$132* •
Additional Nursing Fees: *$20*

TROY STATE UNIVERSITY

Address: Collegeview Building, Troy, AL 36082
Phone: 334-241-8650
Fax: 334-241-8627
Contact: Lillian Wise, DSN, RN, Associate Professor
Email: lwise@troyst.edu

GENERAL INFORMATION

Type of School: *4-Year College or University, Public* •
Accreditation: *Southern Association of Colleges and Schools* •
Total Enrollment: *6777*

PROGRAM INFORMATION

NLNAC Accreditation: *Yes* • CCNE Accreditation:

NURSING STUDENT PROFILE

Total Nursing Enrollment: *17* • Full-Time Enrollment: *16* •
Part-Time Enrollment: *1* • Female Enrollment: *16* • Male
Enrollment: *1* • Total Graduates: *17*

FINANCES

Residential Annual Tuition: *$3,020* • Non-Residential
Annual Tuition: *$6,040* • General Institutional Fees: *$276* •
Additional Nursing Fees: *$200*

ARIZONA STATE UNIVERSITY

Address: Tempe, AZ 85287-2602
Phone: 602-965-6431
Fax: 602-965-6488
Contact: Barbara Durand, PhD, RN, Dean
Email: mwatters@asuvm.inre.asu.edu

GENERAL INFORMATION

Type of School: *Not Reported, Not Reported* • Accreditation:
Not Reported • Total Enrollment: *Not Reported*

PROGRAM INFORMATION

NLNAC Accreditation: *Not Reported* • CCNE Accreditation:

NURSING STUDENT PROFILE

Total Nursing Enrollment: *Not Reported* • Full-Time
Enrollment: *Not Reported* • Part-Time Enrollment: *Not
Reported* • Female Enrollment: *Not Reported* • Male
Enrollment: *Not Reported* • Total Graduates: *154*

FINANCES

Residential Annual Tuition: *$1,044* • Non-Residential
Annual Tuition: *$4,520* • General Institutional Fees:
$1,050 • Additional Nursing Fees: *Not Reported*

UNIVERSITY OF PHOENIX

Address: 4614 East Elwood, Phoenix, AZ 85040
Phone: 480-966-9577
Fax: 480-929-7164
Contact: Catherine Garner, DrPH, RNC, FAAN, Dean,
   College of Health Sciences and Nursing
Email: catherine.garner@phoenix.edu

GENERAL INFORMATION

Type of School: *Independent, Private (Independent)* •
Accreditation: *North Central Association of Colleges and
Schools* • Total Enrollment: *Not Reported*

PROGRAM INFORMATION

NLNAC Accreditation: *Yes* • CCNE Accreditation:

NURSING STUDENT PROFILE

Total Nursing Enrollment: *2155* • Full-Time Enrollment:
2155 • Part-Time Enrollment: *0* • Female Enrollment:
1939 • Male Enrollment: *216* • Total Graduates: *661*

FINANCES

Residential Annual Tuition: *Not Reported* • Non-Residential
Annual Tuition: *Not Reported* • General Institutional Fees:
Not Reported • Additional Nursing Fees: *Not Reported*

SOUTHERN ARKANSAS UNIVERSITY

Address: 100 East University, Magnolia, AR 71754
Phone: 870-235-4331
Fax: 870-235-5058
Contact: Vonda Dees, MSN, RN, Interim Chairperson
Email: vjdees@saumag.edu

GENERAL INFORMATION

Type of School: *4-Year College or University, Public* •
Accreditation: *North Central Association of Colleges and
Schools* • Total Enrollment: *3127*

PROGRAM INFORMATION

NLNAC Accreditation: *Not Reported* • CCNE Accreditation:

NURSING STUDENT PROFILE

Total Nursing Enrollment: *6* • Full-Time Enrollment: *0* •
Part-Time Enrollment: *6* • Female Enrollment: *6* • Male
Enrollment: *0* • Total Graduates: *3*

FINANCES

Residential Annual Tuition: *$1,625* • Non-Residential
Annual Tuition: *$2,470* • General Institutional Fees: *$75* •
Additional Nursing Fees: *$90*

UNIVERSITY OF ARKANSAS—FAYETTEVILLE

Address: 1 University of Arkansas, Fayetteville, AR 72701
Phone: 479-575-3907
Fax: 479-575-3218
Contact: Barbara Conrad, PhD, RN, Director and Associate Professor
Email: bsconrad@uark.edu

GENERAL INFORMATION

Type of School: *4-Year College or University, Public* • Accreditation: *North Central Association of Colleges and Schools* • Total Enrollment: *14600*

PROGRAM INFORMATION

NLNAC Accreditation: *Yes* • CCNE Accreditation: *Yes*

NURSING STUDENT PROFILE

Total Nursing Enrollment: *4* • Full-Time Enrollment: *0* • Part-Time Enrollment: *4* • Female Enrollment: *4* • Male Enrollment: *0* • Total Graduates: *3*

FINANCES

Residential Annual Tuition: *$3,810* • Non-Residential Annual Tuition: *$10,560* • General Institutional Fees: *$716* • Additional Nursing Fees: *$30*

CALIFORNIA STATE UNIVERSITY—BAKERSFIELD

Address: 9001 Stockdale Highway, Bakersfield, CA 93311-1099
Phone: 661-664-2093
Fax: 661-665-6903
Contact: Candace J. Meares, PhD, RN, CNAA, Professor and Chair
Email: cmeares@csub.edu

GENERAL INFORMATION

Type of School: *4-Year College or University, Public* • Accreditation: *Western Association of Schools and Colleges* • Total Enrollment: *6000*

PROGRAM INFORMATION

NLNAC Accreditation: *Yes* • CCNE Accreditation:

NURSING STUDENT PROFILE

Total Nursing Enrollment: *14* • Full-Time Enrollment: *10* • Part-Time Enrollment: *4* • Female Enrollment: *11* • Male Enrollment: *3* • Total Graduates: *3*

FINANCES

Residential Annual Tuition: *Not Reported* • Non-Residential Annual Tuition: *Not Reported* • General Institutional Fees: *$599* • Additional Nursing Fees: *$1*

CALIFORNIA STATE UNIVERSITY—FULLERTON

Address: 800 North State College Boulvard, Fullerton, CA 92834
Phone: 714-278-2291
Fax: 714-278-3338
Contact: Christine Latham, DNSc, RN, Chair
Email: clatham@fullerton.edu

GENERAL INFORMATION

Type of School: *4-Year College or University, Public* •
Accreditation: *Western Association of Schools and Colleges* •
Total Enrollment: *30357*

PROGRAM INFORMATION

NLNAC Accreditation: *Yes* • CCNE Accreditation:

NURSING STUDENT PROFILE

Total Nursing Enrollment: *253* • Full-Time Enrollment: *42* •
Part-Time Enrollment: *211* • Female Enrollment: *226* • Male
Enrollment: *27* • Total Graduates: *31*

FINANCES

Residential Annual Tuition: *$1,258* • Non-Residential
Annual Tuition: *$10,282* • General Institutional Fees: *Not
Reported* • Additional Nursing Fees: *Not Reported*

CALIFORNIA STATE UNIVERSITY—SACRAMENTO

Address: 6000 J Street, Sacramento, CA 95819-6096
Phone: 916-278-7258
Fax: 916-278-6311
Contact: Mary Braham, PhD, RN, Professor
Email: brahamm@scus.edu

GENERAL INFORMATION

Type of School: *4-Year College or University, Public* •
Accreditation: *Western Association of Schools and Colleges* •
Total Enrollment: *26923*

PROGRAM INFORMATION

NLNAC Accreditation: *Not Reported* • CCNE Accreditation:
Yes

NURSING STUDENT PROFILE

Total Nursing Enrollment: *26* • Full-Time Enrollment: *0* •
Part-Time Enrollment: *26* • Female Enrollment: *24* • Male
Enrollment: *2* • Total Graduates: *12*

FINANCES

Residential Annual Tuition: *$714* • Non-Residential Annual
Tuition: *Not Reported* • General Institutional Fees: *$220* •
Additional Nursing Fees: *$0*

CALIFORNIA STATE UNIVERSITY—STANISLAUS

Address: 801 W. Nonte Vista Avenue, Turkock, CA 95382
Phone: 209-667-3142
Fax: 209-667-3690
Contact: Nancy Clark, EdD, RN, Chair and Professor
Email: nclark@csustan.edu

HOLY NAMES COLLEGE

Address: 3500 Mountain Blvd., Oakland, CA 94619
Phone: 510-436-1024
Fax: 510-436-1376
Contact: Fay L. Bower, DNSc, RN, FAAN, Chair
Email: bower@hnc.edu

GENERAL INFORMATION

Type of School: *Governmental Agency, Public* • Accreditation: *Western Association of Schools and Colleges* • Total Enrollment: *7534*

GENERAL INFORMATION

Type of School: *4-Year College or University, Private (Religious)* • Accreditation: *Western Association of Schools and Colleges* • Total Enrollment: *832*

PROGRAM INFORMATION

NLNAC Accreditation: *Yes* • CCNE Accreditation:

PROGRAM INFORMATION

NLNAC Accreditation: *Yes* • CCNE Accreditation:

NURSING STUDENT PROFILE

Total Nursing Enrollment: *101* • Full-Time Enrollment: *23* • Part-Time Enrollment: *78* • Female Enrollment: *93* • Male Enrollment: *8* • Total Graduates: *17*

NURSING STUDENT PROFILE

Total Nursing Enrollment: *46* • Full-Time Enrollment: *14* • Part-Time Enrollment: *32* • Female Enrollment: *45* • Male Enrollment: *1* • Total Graduates: *22*

FINANCES

Residential Annual Tuition: *$1,323* • Non-Residential Annual Tuition: *Not Reported* • General Institutional Fees: *Not Reported* • Additional Nursing Fees: *$25*

FINANCES

Residential Annual Tuition: *$10,050* • Non-Residential Annual Tuition: *$10,050* • General Institutional Fees: *$120* • Additional Nursing Fees: *$75*

LOMA LINDA UNIVERSITY

Address: 11234 Anderson Street, Loma Linda, CA 92350
Phone: 909-558-8060
Fax: 909-558-0643
Contact: Marilyn Herrmann, PhD, RN, Associate Dean, Undergradute Program
Email: mhermann@sn.iiu.edu

GENERAL INFORMATION

Type of School: *4-Year College or University, Private (Religious)* • Accreditation: *Western Association of Schools and Colleges* • Total Enrollment: *3338*

PROGRAM INFORMATION

NLNAC Accreditation: *Not Reported* • CCNE Accreditation: *Yes*

NURSING STUDENT PROFILE

Total Nursing Enrollment: *18* • Full-Time Enrollment: *2* • Part-Time Enrollment: *16* • Female Enrollment: *15* • Male Enrollment: *3* • Total Graduates: *6*

FINANCES

Residential Annual Tuition: *$17,640* • Non-Residential Annual Tuition: *$17,640* • General Institutional Fees: *$0* • Additional Nursing Fees: *$30*

UNIVERSITY OF CALIFORNIA—LOS ANGELES

Address: 700 Tiverton Avenue Box 951702, Los Angeles, CA 90095-1702
Phone: 310-825-9621
Fax: 910-206-7433
Contact: Marie J. Cowan, PhD, RN, FAAN, Dean and Professor
Email: mcowan@sonnet.ucla.edu

GENERAL INFORMATION

Type of School: *4-Year College or University, Public* • Accreditation: *Western Association of Schools and Colleges* • Total Enrollment: *34000*

PROGRAM INFORMATION

NLNAC Accreditation: *Yes* • CCNE Accreditation:

NURSING STUDENT PROFILE

Total Nursing Enrollment: *8* • Full-Time Enrollment: *8* • Part-Time Enrollment: *0* • Female Enrollment: *6* • Male Enrollment: *2* • Total Graduates: *4*

FINANCES

Residential Annual Tuition: *$5,820* • Non-Residential Annual Tuition: *$20,030* • General Institutional Fees: *Not Reported* • Additional Nursing Fees: *$0*

METROPOLITAN STATE COLLEGE OF DENVER

Address: Box 173362, Denver, CO 80217-3362
Phone: 303-556-8425
Fax: 303-556-3430
Contact: Roberta Hills, PhD, RN, Coordinator
Email: hillsro@mscd.edu

GENERAL INFORMATION

Type of School: *Governmental Agency, Public* • Accreditation: *Northwestern Association of Schools and Colleges* • Total Enrollment: *18432*

PROGRAM INFORMATION

NLNAC Accreditation: *Yes* • CCNE Accreditation:

NURSING STUDENT PROFILE

Total Nursing Enrollment: *74* • Full-Time Enrollment: *19* • Part-Time Enrollment: *55* • Female Enrollment: *65* • Male Enrollment: *9* • Total Graduates: *26*

FINANCES

Residential Annual Tuition: *$1,840* • Non-Residential Annual Tuition: *$7,686* • General Institutional Fees: *$250* • Additional Nursing Fees: *$10*

UNIVERSITY OF COLORADO— COLORADO SPRINGS–BETH-EL COLLEGE OF NURSING

Address: PO Box 7150, Colorado Springs, CO 80933
Phone: 719-262-4429
Fax: 719-262-4416
Contact: Cindy Roach, DSN, RN, Chair, Undergraduate Nursing
Email: croach@mail.uccs.edu

GENERAL INFORMATION

Type of School: *4-Year College or University, Public* • Accreditation: *North Central Association of Colleges and Schools* • Total Enrollment: *Not Reported*

PROGRAM INFORMATION

NLNAC Accreditation: *Yes* • CCNE Accreditation:

NURSING STUDENT PROFILE

Total Nursing Enrollment: *57* • Full-Time Enrollment: *0* • Part-Time Enrollment: *57* • Female Enrollment: *51* • Male Enrollment: *6* • Total Graduates: *8*

FINANCES

Residential Annual Tuition: *$1,814* • Non-Residential Annual Tuition: *$6,846* • General Institutional Fees: *$147* • Additional Nursing Fees: *Not Reported*

SACRED HEART UNIVERSITY

Address: 5151 Park Avenue, Fairfield, CT 06432
Phone: 203-371-7715
Fax: 203-365-7662
Contact: Constance Young, EdD, RN, Associate Professor
Email: youngc@sacredheart.edu

GENERAL INFORMATION

Type of School: *4-Year College or University, Private (Religious)* • Accreditation: *New England Association of Schools and Colleges* • Total Enrollment: *6000*

PROGRAM INFORMATION

NLNAC Accreditation: *Yes* • CCNE Accreditation:

NURSING STUDENT PROFILE

Total Nursing Enrollment: *76* • Full-Time Enrollment: *0* • Part-Time Enrollment: *76* • Female Enrollment: *73* • Male Enrollment: *3* • Total Graduates: *19*

FINANCES

Residential Annual Tuition: *$16,328* • Non-Residential Annual Tuition: *Not Reported* • General Institutional Fees: *$1,460* • Additional Nursing Fees: *$0*

UNIVERSITY OF HARTFORD

Address: 200 Bloomfield Avenue, West Hartford, CT 06117-1545
Phone: 860-768-4217
Fax: 860-768-5346
Contact: Mary Beth Mathews, PhD, RN, C, Chair, Division of Nursing
Email: mbmathews@hartford.edu

GENERAL INFORMATION

Type of School: *4-Year College or University, Private (Religious)* • Accreditation: *New England Association of Schools and Colleges* • Total Enrollment: *7300*

PROGRAM INFORMATION

NLNAC Accreditation: *Yes* • CCNE Accreditation:

NURSING STUDENT PROFILE

Total Nursing Enrollment: *92* • Full-Time Enrollment: *0* • Part-Time Enrollment: *92* • Female Enrollment: *90* • Male Enrollment: *2* • Total Graduates: *28*

FINANCES

Residential Annual Tuition: *$5,130* • Non-Residential Annual Tuition: *$5,130* • General Institutional Fees: *$55* • Additional Nursing Fees: *$0*

UNIVERSITY OF DELAWARE

Address: School of Nursing, Newark, DE 19716
Phone: 302-831-4549
Fax: 302-831-4550
Contact: Madeline E Lambrecht, EdD, RN, Director
Email: madeline@ude1.edu

GENERAL INFORMATION

Type of School: *4-Year College or University, Private (Independent)* • Accreditation: *Middle States Association of Colleges and Schools* • Total Enrollment: *20888*

PROGRAM INFORMATION

NLNAC Accreditation: *Yes* • CCNE Accreditation: *Yes*

NURSING STUDENT PROFILE

Total Nursing Enrollment: *271* • Full-Time Enrollment: *0* • Part-Time Enrollment: *271* • Female Enrollment: *252* • Male Enrollment: *19* • Total Graduates: *48*

FINANCES

Residential Annual Tuition: *$4,511* • Non-Residential Annual Tuition: *$13,260* • General Institutional Fees: *Not Reported* • Additional Nursing Fees: *Not Reported*

WILMINGTON COLLEGE

Address: 320 N. Dupont Highway, New Castle, DE 19720
Phone: 302-328-9401
Fax: 302-322-7081
Contact: Tish Gallagher, MS, RN, Chair
Email: tgall@wilmcoll.edu

GENERAL INFORMATION

Type of School: *4-Year College or University, Private (Independent)* • Accreditation: *Middle States Association of Colleges and Schools* • Total Enrollment: *7500*

PROGRAM INFORMATION

NLNAC Accreditation: *Yes* • CCNE Accreditation: *Yes*

NURSING STUDENT PROFILE

Total Nursing Enrollment: *226* • Full-Time Enrollment: *22* • Part-Time Enrollment: *204* • Female Enrollment: *213* • Male Enrollment: *13* • Total Graduates: *78*

FINANCES

Residential Annual Tuition: *$6,480* • Non-Residential Annual Tuition: *$6,480* • General Institutional Fees: *$75* • Additional Nursing Fees: *$0*

THE CATHOLIC UNIVERSITY OF AMERICA

Address: 620 Michigan Avenue, North East, Washington, DC 20064
Phone: 202-319-6458
Fax: 202-319-6485
Contact: Shirley Jarecki, PhD, RN, Director, Baccalaureate Program
Email: jarceki@cua.du

GENERAL INFORMATION

Type of School: *4-Year College or University, Private (Independent)* • Accreditation: *Middle States Association of Colleges and Schools* • Total Enrollment: *5500*

PROGRAM INFORMATION

NLNAC Accreditation: *Yes* • CCNE Accreditation:

NURSING STUDENT PROFILE

Total Nursing Enrollment: *6* • Full-Time Enrollment: *0* • Part-Time Enrollment: *6* • Female Enrollment: *6* • Male Enrollment: *0* • Total Graduates: *6*

FINANCES

Residential Annual Tuition: *$10,025* • Non-Residential Annual Tuition: *$10,025* • General Institutional Fees: *Not Reported* • Additional Nursing Fees: *$500*

UNIVERSITY OF CENTRAL FLORIDA

Address: PO Box 162210, Orlando, FL 32816-2210
Phone: 407-823-5848
Fax: 407-823-5675
Contact: Linda M Hennig, EdD, RN, RN-BSN Program Coordinator
Email: lindah@mail.ucf.edu

GENERAL INFORMATION

Type of School: *4-Year College or University, Public* • Accreditation: *Southern Association of Colleges and Schools* • Total Enrollment: *36000*

PROGRAM INFORMATION

NLNAC Accreditation: *Yes* • CCNE Accreditation:

NURSING STUDENT PROFILE

Total Nursing Enrollment: *158* • Full-Time Enrollment: *0* • Part-Time Enrollment: *158* • Female Enrollment: *138* • Male Enrollment: *20* • Total Graduates: *93*

FINANCES

Residential Annual Tuition: *Not Reported* • Non-Residential Annual Tuition: *Not Reported* • General Institutional Fees: *$180* • Additional Nursing Fees: *$50*

UNIVERSITY OF SOUTH FLORIDA

Address: 4202 East Fowler Avenue, Tampa, FL 33620
Phone: 813-974-9091
Fax: 813-974-5418
Contact: Patricia A. Burns, PhD, RN, FAAN, Dean and Professor
Email: pburns@hsc.usf.edu

GENERAL INFORMATION

Type of School: *4-Year College or University, Public* •
Accreditation: *Southern Association of Colleges and Schools* •
Total Enrollment: *37814*

PROGRAM INFORMATION

NLNAC Accreditation: *Yes* • CCNE Accreditation: *Yes*

NURSING STUDENT PROFILE

Total Nursing Enrollment: *208* • Full-Time Enrollment: *21* •
Part-Time Enrollment: *187* • Female Enrollment: *174* • Male
Enrollment: *34* • Total Graduates: *62*

FINANCES

Residential Annual Tuition: *$2,350* • Non-Residential
Annual Tuition: *$9,690* • General Institutional Fees: *$34* •
Additional Nursing Fees: *Not Reported*

UNIVERSITY OF TAMPA

Address: School of Nursing, Tampa, FL 33606
Phone: 813-253-3333
Fax: 813-258-7214
Contact: Nancy Ross, PhD, ARNP, Director
Email: nross@alpha.utampa.edu

GENERAL INFORMATION

Type of School: *4-Year College or University, Private
(Independent)* • Accreditation: *Southern Association of Colleges
and Schools* • Total Enrollment: *3474*

PROGRAM INFORMATION

NLNAC Accreditation: *Yes* • CCNE Accreditation:

NURSING STUDENT PROFILE

Total Nursing Enrollment: *53* • Full-Time Enrollment: *15* •
Part-Time Enrollment: *38* • Female Enrollment: *48* • Male
Enrollment: *5* • Total Graduates: *37*

FINANCES

Residential Annual Tuition: *$5,850* • Non-Residential
Annual Tuition: *$5,850* • General Institutional Fees: *$70* •
Additional Nursing Fees: *$0*

UNIVERSITY OF WEST FLORIDA

Address: 11000 University Parkway, Pensacola, FL 332514
Phone: 850-474-2884
Fax: 850-857-6390
Contact: Marilyn L Lamborn, PhD, RN, Chair and Associate Professor
Email: mlamborn@uwf.edu

GENERAL INFORMATION

Type of School: *4-Year College or University, Public* •
Accreditation: *Southern Association of Colleges and Schools* •
Total Enrollment: *9500*

PROGRAM INFORMATION

NLNAC Accreditation: *Yes* • CCNE Accreditation:

NURSING STUDENT PROFILE

Total Nursing Enrollment: *95* • Full-Time Enrollment: *10* •
Part-Time Enrollment: *85* • Female Enrollment: *80* • Male
Enrollment: *15* • Total Graduates: *8*

FINANCES

Residential Annual Tuition: *Not Reported* • Non-Residential
Annual Tuition: *Not Reported* • General Institutional Fees:
$50 • Additional Nursing Fees: *$0*

COLUMBUS STATE UNIVERSITY

Address: 4225 University Avenue, Columbus, GA 31907-5645
Phone: 706-568-2243
Fax: 706-569-3101
Contact: Peggy H. Batastini, MSN, Program Coordinator
Email: batastini_peggy@colstate.edu

GENERAL INFORMATION

Type of School: *4-Year College or University, Public* •
Accreditation: *Southern Association of Colleges and Schools* •
Total Enrollment: *5522*

PROGRAM INFORMATION

NLNAC Accreditation: *Yes* • CCNE Accreditation:

NURSING STUDENT PROFILE

Total Nursing Enrollment: *5* • Full-Time Enrollment: *0* •
Part-Time Enrollment: *5* • Female Enrollment: *4* • Male
Enrollment: *1* • Total Graduates: *Not Reported*

FINANCES

Residential Annual Tuition: *$1,338* • Non-Residential
Annual Tuition: *$4,656* • General Institutional Fees:
$2,352 • Additional Nursing Fees: *Not Reported*

EMORY UNIVERSITY—NELL HODGSON WOODRUFF

Address: 1520 Clifton Road, Suite 40, Atlanta, GA 30322
Phone: 404-727-7967
Fax: 404-727-8514
Contact: Helen O'Shera, PhD, RN, Professor and
           Chairperson
Email: hoshea@nurse.emory.edu

GENERAL INFORMATION

Type of School: *4-Year College or University, Private
(Religious)* • Accreditation: *Southern Association of Colleges
and Schools* • Total Enrollment: *11400*

PROGRAM INFORMATION

NLNAC Accreditation: *Not Reported* • CCNE Accreditation:
Yes

NURSING STUDENT PROFILE

Total Nursing Enrollment: *3* • Full-Time Enrollment: *1* •
Part-Time Enrollment: *2* • Female Enrollment: *2* • Male
Enrollment: *1* • Total Graduates: *Not Reported*

FINANCES

Residential Annual Tuition: *$24,240* • Non-Residential
Annual Tuition: *$24,240* • General Institutional Fees: *$312* •
Additional Nursing Fees: *$35*

GEORGIA SOUTHWESTERN STATE UNIVERSITY

Address: 800 Wheatley Street, Americus, GA 31709
Phone: 229-931-2275
Fax: 229-931-2288
Contact: JM Malachowski, PhD, RN, Interim Dean
Email: jmm@canes.gsw.edu

GENERAL INFORMATION

Type of School: *4-Year College or University, Public* •
Accreditation: *Southern Association of Colleges and Schools* •
Total Enrollment: *2622*

PROGRAM INFORMATION

NLNAC Accreditation: *Yes* • CCNE Accreditation: *Yes*

NURSING STUDENT PROFILE

Total Nursing Enrollment: *29* • Full-Time Enrollment: *0* •
Part-Time Enrollment: *29* • Female Enrollment: *26* • Male
Enrollment: *3* • Total Graduates: *41*

FINANCES

Residential Annual Tuition: *$3,752* • Non-Residential
Annual Tuition: *$15,012* • General Institutional Fees: *$268* •
Additional Nursing Fees: *$30*

MEDICAL COLLEGE OF GEORGIA

Address: 997 St. Sebastian Way, Augusta, GA 30912
Phone: 706-721-2787
Fax: 706-721-7390
Contact: Katherine E. Nugent, PhD, RN, Professor and Associate Dean, Academic Program
Email: knugent@mail.mcg.edu

GENERAL INFORMATION

Type of School: *4-Year College or University, Public* •
Accreditation: *Southern Association of Colleges and Schools* •
Total Enrollment: *1939*

PROGRAM INFORMATION

NLNAC Accreditation: *Yes* • CCNE Accreditation:

NURSING STUDENT PROFILE

Total Nursing Enrollment: *42* • Full-Time Enrollment: *20* •
Part-Time Enrollment: *22* • Female Enrollment: *38* • Male
Enrollment: *4* • Total Graduates: *22*

FINANCES

Residential Annual Tuition: *$3,083* • Non-Residential
Annual Tuition: *$10,829* • General Institutional Fees: *Not
Reported* • Additional Nursing Fees: *$15*

NORTH GEORGIA COLLEGE AND STATE UNIVERSITY

Address: School of Nursing, Dahlonega, GA 30597
Phone: 706-864-1930
Fax: 706-864-1845
Contact: Jill Hayes, PhD, RN, Department Head
Email: jhayes@ngcsu.edu

GENERAL INFORMATION

Type of School: *4-Year College or University, Public* •
Accreditation: *Southern Association of Colleges and Schools* •
Total Enrollment: *3400*

PROGRAM INFORMATION

NLNAC Accreditation: *Yes* • CCNE Accreditation:

NURSING STUDENT PROFILE

Total Nursing Enrollment: *37* • Full-Time Enrollment: *13* •
Part-Time Enrollment: *24* • Female Enrollment: *35* • Male
Enrollment: *2* • Total Graduates: *16*

FINANCES

Residential Annual Tuition: *$1,876* • Non-Residential
Annual Tuition: *$8,840* • General Institutional Fees: *$239* •
Additional Nursing Fees: *$76*

HAWAII PACIFIC UNIVERSITY

Address: 45-045 Kamehameha Highway, Kaneohe, HI
            96744
Phone: 808-236-5829
Fax: 808-236-5818
Contact: Linda Beechinor, MS, APRN-Rx, BC, FNP,
            Assistant Professor and RN-BSN Program
            Coordinator
Email: lbeechinor@hpu.edu

GENERAL INFORMATION

Type of School: *4-Year College or University, Private (Independent)* • Accreditation: *Western Association of Schools and Colleges* • Total Enrollment: *768*

PROGRAM INFORMATION

NLNAC Accreditation: *Yes* • CCNE Accreditation:

NURSING STUDENT PROFILE

Total Nursing Enrollment: *20* • Full-Time Enrollment: *6* • Part-Time Enrollment: *14* • Female Enrollment: *15* • Male Enrollment: *5* • Total Graduates: *3*

FINANCES

Residential Annual Tuition: *$10,368* • Non-Residential Annual Tuition: *$10,368* • General Institutional Fees: *Not Reported* • Additional Nursing Fees: *Not Reported*

BENEDICTINE UNIVERSITY

Address: 5700 College Road, Lisle, IL 60532
Phone: 630-829-6583
Fax: 630-829-6551
Contact: Ethel C. Ragland, EdD, MN, RN, Department
            Chair
Email: wragland@ben.edu

GENERAL INFORMATION

Type of School: *4-Year College or University, Private (Religious)* • Accreditation: *North Central Association of Colleges and Schools* • Total Enrollment: *2900*

PROGRAM INFORMATION

NLNAC Accreditation: *Yes* • CCNE Accreditation:

NURSING STUDENT PROFILE

Total Nursing Enrollment: *49* • Full-Time Enrollment: *6* • Part-Time Enrollment: *43* • Female Enrollment: *46* • Male Enrollment: *3* • Total Graduates: *18*

FINANCES

Residential Annual Tuition: *$9,600* • Non-Residential Annual Tuition: *$9,600* • General Institutional Fees: *Not Reported* • Additional Nursing Fees: *Not Reported*

GOVERNORS STATE UNIVERSITY

Address: Division of Nursing, University Park, IL 60466
Phone: 708-534-4040
Fax: 708-235-2197
Contact: June Krawczak, EdD, RN, Program Director
Email: j-krawczak@govst.edu

GENERAL INFORMATION

Type of School: *Other, Public* • Accreditation: *North Central Association of Colleges and Schools* • Total Enrollment: *Not Reported*

PROGRAM INFORMATION

NLNAC Accreditation: *Yes* • CCNE Accreditation:

NURSING STUDENT PROFILE

Total Nursing Enrollment: *Not Reported* • Full-Time Enrollment: *Not Reported* • Part-Time Enrollment: *Not Reported* • Female Enrollment: *Not Reported* • Male Enrollment: *Not Reported* • Total Graduates: *Not Reported*

FINANCES

Residential Annual Tuition: *Not Reported* • Non-Residential Annual Tuition: *Not Reported* • General Institutional Fees: $85 • Additional Nursing Fees: $0

MCKENDREE COLLEGE

Address: 701 College Road, Lebanon, IL 62254
Phone: 618-537-6841
Fax: 618-537-6402
Contact: Karen Muench, PhD, RN, Chairperson
Email: kmuench@mckendree.edu

GENERAL INFORMATION

Type of School: *4-Year College or University, Private (Independent)* • Accreditation: *North Central Association of Colleges and Schools* • Total Enrollment: *Not Reported*

PROGRAM INFORMATION

NLNAC Accreditation: *Yes* • CCNE Accreditation:

NURSING STUDENT PROFILE

Total Nursing Enrollment: *261* • Full-Time Enrollment: *41* • Part-Time Enrollment: *220* • Female Enrollment: *235* • Male Enrollment: *26* • Total Graduates: *87*

FINANCES

Residential Annual Tuition: *$9,840* • Non-Residential Annual Tuition: *$9,840* • General Institutional Fees: *Not Reported* • Additional Nursing Fees: *Not Reported*

SAINT ANTHONY COLLEGE OF NURSING

Address: 5658 East State Street, Rockford, IL 61108
Phone: 815-395-5090
Fax: 815-395-2275
Contact: Terese Ann Burch, PhD, RN, Dean and CEO
Email: terriburch@sacn.edu

GENERAL INFORMATION

Type of School: *Other, Private (Religious)* • Accreditation: *North Central Association of Colleges and Schools* • Total Enrollment: *66*

PROGRAM INFORMATION

NLNAC Accreditation: *Yes* • CCNE Accreditation:

NURSING STUDENT PROFILE

Total Nursing Enrollment: *2* • Full-Time Enrollment: *0* • Part-Time Enrollment: *2* • Female Enrollment: *2* • Male Enrollment: *0* • Total Graduates: *0*

FINANCES

Residential Annual Tuition: *$12,000* • Non-Residential Annual Tuition: *$12,000* • General Institutional Fees: *$100* • Additional Nursing Fees: *$13*

SAINT XAVIER UNIVERSITY

Address: 3700 West 103 Street, Chicago, IL 60655
Phone: 773-298-3700
Fax: 773-298-3704
Contact: Mary M. Lebold, EdD, RN, Dean
Email: lebold@sxu.edu

GENERAL INFORMATION

Type of School: *4-Year College or University, Private (Religious)* • Accreditation: *North Central Association of Colleges and Schools* • Total Enrollment: *4867*

PROGRAM INFORMATION

NLNAC Accreditation: *Yes* • CCNE Accreditation:

NURSING STUDENT PROFILE

Total Nursing Enrollment: *99* • Full-Time Enrollment: *2* • Part-Time Enrollment: *97* • Female Enrollment: *95* • Male Enrollment: *4* • Total Graduates: *7*

FINANCES

Residential Annual Tuition: *$15,000* • Non-Residential Annual Tuition: *$15,000* • General Institutional Fees: *$130* • Additional Nursing Fees: *$90*

UNIVERSITY OF ST. FRANCIS— JOLIET

Address: 500 Wilcox Street, Joliet, IL 60435
Phone: 815-773-7820
Fax: 815-741-7131
Contact: Sharon Abbate, MSN, RN, Coordinator
Email: sabbate@stfrancis.edu

GENERAL INFORMATION

Type of School: *4-Year College or University, Private (Religious)* • Accreditation: *North Central Association of Colleges and Schools* • Total Enrollment: *1650*

PROGRAM INFORMATION

NLNAC Accreditation: *Yes* • CCNE Accreditation:

NURSING STUDENT PROFILE

Total Nursing Enrollment: *71* • Full-Time Enrollment: *0* • Part-Time Enrollment: *71* • Female Enrollment: *64* • Male Enrollment: *7* • Total Graduates: *26*

FINANCES

Residential Annual Tuition: *Not Reported* • Non-Residential Annual Tuition: *Not Reported* • General Institutional Fees: *Not Reported* • Additional Nursing Fees: *Not Reported*

BALL STATE UNIVERSITY

Address: 2000 West University Avenue, Muncie, IN 47306
Phone: 765-285-2169
Fax: 765-285-2169
Contact: Linda Skitberg, PhD, RN, Director
Email: lskitberg@bsu.edu

GENERAL INFORMATION

Type of School: *4-Year College or University, Public* • Accreditation: *North Central Association of Colleges and Schools* • Total Enrollment: *18000*

PROGRAM INFORMATION

NLNAC Accreditation: *Yes* • CCNE Accreditation:

NURSING STUDENT PROFILE

Total Nursing Enrollment: *23* • Full-Time Enrollment: *0* • Part-Time Enrollment: *23* • Female Enrollment: *21* • Male Enrollment: *2* • Total Graduates: *9*

FINANCES

Residential Annual Tuition: *Not Reported* • Non-Residential Annual Tuition: *Not Reported* • General Institutional Fees: *Not Reported* • Additional Nursing Fees: *$85*

GOSHEN COLLEGE

Address: 1700 South Main Street, Goshen, IN 46526
Phone: 574-535-7376
Fax: 574-535-7609
Contact: Vicky S. Kirkton, MA, BSN, RN, Director
Email: vickysk@goshen.edu

GENERAL INFORMATION

Type of School: *4-Year College or University, Private (Religious)* • Accreditation: *North Central Association of Colleges and Schools* • Total Enrollment: *970*

PROGRAM INFORMATION

NLNAC Accreditation: *Yes* • CCNE Accreditation:

NURSING STUDENT PROFILE

Total Nursing Enrollment: *10* • Full-Time Enrollment: *10* • Part-Time Enrollment: *0* • Female Enrollment: *10* • Male Enrollment: *0* • Total Graduates: *8*

FINANCES

Residential Annual Tuition: *$12,000* • Non-Residential Annual Tuition: *$12,000* • General Institutional Fees: *$100* • Additional Nursing Fees: *$0*

INDIANA STATE UNIVERSITY

Address: 210 North 7th Street, Terre Haute, IN 47809
Phone: 812-237-3688
Fax: 812-237-4000
Contact: Suzy Fletcher, DNS, RN, Interim Chair
Email: s-fletcher@indstate.edu

GENERAL INFORMATION

Type of School: *4-Year College or University, Public* • Accreditation: *North Central Association of Colleges and Schools* • Total Enrollment: *11321*

PROGRAM INFORMATION

NLNAC Accreditation: *Yes* • CCNE Accreditation:

NURSING STUDENT PROFILE

Total Nursing Enrollment: *44* • Full-Time Enrollment: *14* • Part-Time Enrollment: *30* • Female Enrollment: *40* • Male Enrollment: *4* • Total Graduates: *10*

FINANCES

Residential Annual Tuition: *$3,744* • Non-Residential Annual Tuition: *$4,673* • General Institutional Fees: *$0* • Additional Nursing Fees: *$766*

INDIANA UNIVERSITY— PURDUE UNIVERSITY

Address: 3551 Lansing Street, Indianapolis, IN 46202-
             2896
Phone: 317-274-8010
Fax: 317-274-2996
Contact: Donna L. Boland, PhD, RN, Associate Dean for
            Undergraduate Programs
Email: dboland@iupui.edu

GENERAL INFORMATION

Type of School: *4-Year College or University, Public* •
Accreditation: *North Central Association of Colleges and
Schools* • Total Enrollment: *27500*

PROGRAM INFORMATION

NLNAC Accreditation: *Yes* • CCNE Accreditation: *Yes*

NURSING STUDENT PROFILE

Total Nursing Enrollment: *56* • Full-Time Enrollment: *1* •
Part-Time Enrollment: *55* • Female Enrollment: *49* • Male
Enrollment: *7* • Total Graduates: *15*

FINANCES

Residential Annual Tuition: *$5,494* • Non-Residential
Annual Tuition: *$15,290* • General Institutional Fees: *$350* •
Additional Nursing Fees: *$450*

INDIANA UNIVERSITY— PURDUE UNIVERSITY— FORT WAYNE

Address: 2101 East Coliseum Boulevard, Fort Wayne, IN
             46805
Phone: 219-481-6216
Fax: 219-481-5767
Contact: Linda Meyer, PhD, RN, Director of
            Undergraduate Nursing and Associate Professor
Email: meye@ipfw.edu

GENERAL INFORMATION

Type of School: *4-Year College or University, Public* •
Accreditation: *North Central Association of Colleges and
Schools* • Total Enrollment: *11129*

PROGRAM INFORMATION

NLNAC Accreditation: *Yes* • CCNE Accreditation:

NURSING STUDENT PROFILE

Total Nursing Enrollment: *56* • Full-Time Enrollment: *1* •
Part-Time Enrollment: *55* • Female Enrollment: *49* • Male
Enrollment: *7* • Total Graduates: *15*

FINANCES

Residential Annual Tuition: *$2,303* • Non-Residential
Annual Tuition: *$7,164* • General Institutional Fees: *$350* •
Additional Nursing Fees: *$450*

MARIAN COLLEGE

Address: 3200 Cold Spring Road, Indianapolis, IN 46222
Phone: 317-955-6155
Fax: 317-955-6135
Contact: Marian Pettengill, PhD, RN, Professor and Chair
Email: mpettengill@marian.edu

GENERAL INFORMATION

Type of School: *4-Year College or University, Private (Religious)* • Accreditation: *North Central Association of Colleges and Schools* • Total Enrollment: *1260*

PROGRAM INFORMATION

NLNAC Accreditation: *Yes* • CCNE Accreditation:

NURSING STUDENT PROFILE

Total Nursing Enrollment: *10* • Full-Time Enrollment: *0* • Part-Time Enrollment: *10* • Female Enrollment: *9* • Male Enrollment: *1* • Total Graduates: *0*

FINANCES

Residential Annual Tuition: *$14,499* • Non-Residential Annual Tuition: *$14,499* • General Institutional Fees: *$100* • Additional Nursing Fees: *$950*

PURDUE UNIVERSITY— CALUMET CAMPUS

Address: 2233 171st Street, Hammond, IN 46323
Phone: 219-989-2814
Fax: 219-989-2848
Contact: Gail D. Wegner, MSN, RN, Coordinator, Undergraduate Program
Email: wegner@calumet.purdue.edu

GENERAL INFORMATION

Type of School: *4-Year College or University, Public* • Accreditation: *North Central Association of Colleges and Schools* • Total Enrollment: *9100*

PROGRAM INFORMATION

NLNAC Accreditation: *Yes* • CCNE Accreditation:

NURSING STUDENT PROFILE

Total Nursing Enrollment: *88* • Full-Time Enrollment: *14* • Part-Time Enrollment: *74* • Female Enrollment: *79* • Male Enrollment: *9* • Total Graduates: *16*

FINANCES

Residential Annual Tuition: *$3,450* • Non-Residential Annual Tuition: *$8,674* • General Institutional Fees: *Not Reported* • Additional Nursing Fees: *$34*

UNIVERSITY OF INDIANPOLIS

Address: 1400 East Hanna Avenue, Indianapolis, IN 46227
Phone: 317-788-3324
Fax: 317-788-3542
Contact: Karla Backer, PhD, RN, BSN Program Director
Email: backer@iindy.edu

UNIVERSITY OF ST. FRANCIS—FORT WAYNE

Address: 2701 Spring Street, Fort Wayne, IN 46808
Phone: 260-434-3284
Fax: 260-434-7404
Contact: Stephanie Oetting, MSN, RN, BSN Program Director
Email: soetting@sf.edu

GENERAL INFORMATION

Type of School: *4-Year College or University, Private (Religious)* • Accreditation: *North Central Association of Colleges and Schools* • Total Enrollment: *2839*

GENERAL INFORMATION

Type of School: *Not Reported* • Accreditation: *Not Reported* • Total Enrollment: *Not Reported*

PROGRAM INFORMATION

NLNAC Accreditation: *Yes* • CCNE Accreditation:

PROGRAM INFORMATION

NLNAC Accreditation: *Not Reported* • CCNE Accreditation: *Yes*

NURSING STUDENT PROFILE

Total Nursing Enrollment: *14* • Full-Time Enrollment: *0* • Part-Time Enrollment: *14* • Female Enrollment: *14* • Male Enrollment: *0* • Total Graduates: *4*

NURSING STUDENT PROFILE

Total Nursing Enrollment: *18* • Full-Time Enrollment: *10* • Part-Time Enrollment: *8* • Female Enrollment: *18* • Male Enrollment: *0* • Total Graduates: *11*

FINANCES

Residential Annual Tuition: *$5,640* • Non-Residential Annual Tuition: *$5,640* • General Institutional Fees: *$0* • Additional Nursing Fees: *Not Reported*

FINANCES

Residential Annual Tuition: *$13,100* • Non-Residential Annual Tuition: *$13,100* • General Institutional Fees: *$470* • Additional Nursing Fees: *$200*

GRACELAND UNIVERSITY

Address: One University Place, Lamoni, IA 50140
Phone: 816-833-0524
Fax: 816-833-2990
Contact: Patricia Trachsel, PhD, RN, Associate Dean
Email: trachsel@graceland.edu

GENERAL INFORMATION

Type of School: *4-Year College or University, Private (Religious)* • Accreditation: *North Central Association of Colleges and Schools* • Total Enrollment: *2283*

PROGRAM INFORMATION

NLNAC Accreditation: *Yes* • CCNE Accreditation: *Yes*

NURSING STUDENT PROFILE

Total Nursing Enrollment: *392* • Full-Time Enrollment: *2* • Part-Time Enrollment: *390* • Female Enrollment: *368* • Male Enrollment: *24* • Total Graduates: *111*

FINANCES

Residential Annual Tuition: *$5,984* • Non-Residential Annual Tuition: *$5,984* • General Institutional Fees: *$560* • Additional Nursing Fees: *$897*

MERCY COLLEGE OF HEALTH SCIENCES

Address: 928 6th Avnue, Des Moines, IA 50309
Phone: 515-643-6615
Fax: 515-643-6698
Contact: Mary Kelly, PhD, RN, Chair
Email: mkelly@mercydesmoines.org

GENERAL INFORMATION

Type of School: *4-Year College or University, Private (Religious)* • Accreditation: *North Central Association of Colleges and Schools* • Total Enrollment: *420*

PROGRAM INFORMATION

NLNAC Accreditation: *Not Reported* • CCNE Accreditation:

NURSING STUDENT PROFILE

Total Nursing Enrollment: *72* • Full-Time Enrollment: *9* • Part-Time Enrollment: *63* • Female Enrollment: *67* • Male Enrollment: *5* • Total Graduates: *22*

FINANCES

Residential Annual Tuition: *$7,800* • Non-Residential Annual Tuition: *$7,800* • General Institutional Fees: *$0* • Additional Nursing Fees: *$0*

KANSAS WESLEYAN UNIVERSITY

Address: 100 Clafin, Salina, KS 67402
Phone: 785-827-5541
Fax: 785-827-0927
Contact: Patricia D. Kissell, PhD, RN, Chair
Email: pkissell@kwu.edu

GENERAL INFORMATION

Type of School: *4-Year College or University, Private (Religious)* • Accreditation: *North Central Association of Colleges and Schools* • Total Enrollment: *755*

PROGRAM INFORMATION

NLNAC Accreditation: *Yes* • CCNE Accreditation: *Yes*

NURSING STUDENT PROFILE

Total Nursing Enrollment: *16* • Full-Time Enrollment: *1* • Part-Time Enrollment: *15* • Female Enrollment: *16* • Male Enrollment: *0* • Total Graduates: *3*

FINANCES

Residential Annual Tuition: *Not Reported* • Non-Residential Annual Tuition: *Not Reported* • General Institutional Fees: *Not Reported* • Additional Nursing Fees: *Not Reported*

TABOR COLLEGE OF WICHITA

Address: 7348 21st, Wichita, KS 57205
Phone: 620-947-3120
Fax: Not Reported
Contact: Jane Perkins, MSN, RN, Chair Department of Nursing Education
Email: janep@tabor.edu

GENERAL INFORMATION

Type of School: *4-Year College or University, Private (Religious)* • Accreditation: *North Central Association of Colleges and Schools* • Total Enrollment: *518*

PROGRAM INFORMATION

NLNAC Accreditation: *Not Reported* • CCNE Accreditation:

NURSING STUDENT PROFILE

Total Nursing Enrollment: *15* • Full-Time Enrollment: *0* • Part-Time Enrollment: *15* • Female Enrollment: *15* • Male Enrollment: *0* • Total Graduates: *0*

FINANCES

Residential Annual Tuition: *$5,220* • Non-Residential Annual Tuition: *$5,220* • General Institutional Fees: *$0* • Additional Nursing Fees: *$0*

WICHITA STATE UNIVERSITY

Address: 1845 Fairmount, Wichita, KS 67260
Phone: 316-978-5741
Fax: 316-978-3094
Contact: Phyllis Jacobs, MSN, RN, Undergraduate
            Director
Email: phyllis.jacobs@wichita.edu

GENERAL INFORMATION

Type of School: *4-Year College or University, Public* •
Accreditation: *North Central Association of Colleges and
Schools* • Total Enrollment: *15000*

PROGRAM INFORMATION

NLNAC Accreditation: *Yes* • CCNE Accreditation:

NURSING STUDENT PROFILE

Total Nursing Enrollment: *31* • Full-Time Enrollment: *6* •
Part-Time Enrollment: *25* • Female Enrollment: *26* • Male
Enrollment: *5* • Total Graduates: *7*

FINANCES

Residential Annual Tuition: *$1,770* • Non-Residential
Annual Tuition: *$7,191* • General Institutional Fees: *$835* •
Additional Nursing Fees: *Not Reported*

MIDWAY COLLEGE

Address: 512 E. Stephens Street, Midway, KY 40347
Phone: 859-846-5335
Fax: 859-846-5876
Contact: Diana Weaver, DNS, RN, Chair
Email: dweaver@midway.edu

GENERAL INFORMATION

Type of School: *Independent, Private (Religious)* •
Accreditation: *Southern Association of Colleges and Schools* •
Total Enrollment: *900*

PROGRAM INFORMATION

NLNAC Accreditation: *Yes* • CCNE Accreditation:

NURSING STUDENT PROFILE

Total Nursing Enrollment: *10* • Full-Time Enrollment: *1* •
Part-Time Enrollment: *9* • Female Enrollment: *10* • Male
Enrollment: *0* • Total Graduates: *9*

FINANCES

Residential Annual Tuition: *$10,200* • Non-Residential
Annual Tuition: *$10,200* • General Institutional Fees: *Not
Reported* • Additional Nursing Fees: *$35*

NORTHERN KENTUCKY UNIVERSITY

Address: School of Nursing, Highland Heights, KY 41076
Phone: 859-572-5243
Fax: 859-572-6098
Contact: Ann M. Dollins, PhD, MPH, CNM, Director
            BSN Program
Email: dollinsa@nku.edu

GENERAL INFORMATION

Type of School: *4-Year College or University, Public* •
Accreditation: *Southern Association of Colleges and Schools* •
Total Enrollment: *12000*

PROGRAM INFORMATION

NLNAC Accreditation: *Yes* • CCNE Accreditation:

NURSING STUDENT PROFILE

Total Nursing Enrollment: *63* • Full-Time Enrollment: *40* •
Part-Time Enrollment: *23* • Female Enrollment: *59* • Male
Enrollment: *4* • Total Graduates: *40*

FINANCES

Residential Annual Tuition: *$2,256* • Non-Residential
Annual Tuition: *$6,504* • General Institutional Fees: *$15* •
Additional Nursing Fees: *$35*

WESTERN KENTUCKY UNIVERSITY

Address: 1 Big Red Way, Bowling Green, KY 42101
Phone: 270-745-3579
Fax: 270-745-3392
Contact: Donna Blackburn, PhD, RN, Department Head
Email: donna.blackburn@wku.edu

GENERAL INFORMATION

Type of School: *4-Year College or University, Public* •
Accreditation: *Southern Association of Colleges and Schools* •
Total Enrollment: *15516*

PROGRAM INFORMATION

NLNAC Accreditation: *Yes* • CCNE Accreditation:

NURSING STUDENT PROFILE

Total Nursing Enrollment: *57* • Full-Time Enrollment: *3* •
Part-Time Enrollment: *54* • Female Enrollment: *51* • Male
Enrollment: *6* • Total Graduates: *0*

FINANCES

Residential Annual Tuition: *$5,068* • Non-Residential
Annual Tuition: *$6,834* • General Institutional Fees: *$192* •
Additional Nursing Fees: *$50*

LOUISIANA STATE UNIVERSITY

Address: 433 Bolivar St, New Orleans, LA 70112
Phone: 504-568-4106
Fax: 504-599-0573
Contact: Elizabeth A Humphrey, EdD, RN, Dean and Professor
Email: ehumph@lsuhsc.edu

GENERAL INFORMATION

Type of School: *Other, Public* • Accreditation: *Southern Association of Colleges and Schools* • Total Enrollment: *2755*

PROGRAM INFORMATION

NLNAC Accreditation: *Not Reported* • CCNE Accreditation: *Yes*

NURSING STUDENT PROFILE

Total Nursing Enrollment: *15* • Full-Time Enrollment: *3* • Part-Time Enrollment: *12* • Female Enrollment: *12* • Male Enrollment: *3* • Total Graduates: *0*

FINANCES

Residential Annual Tuition: *$2,196* • Non-Residential Annual Tuition: *$3,896* • General Institutional Fees: *$166* • Additional Nursing Fees: *$0*

NORTHWESTERN STATE UNIVERSITY OF LOUISIANA

Address: Natchitoches, LA 71497
Phone: 318-677-3100
Fax: 318-677-3127
Contact: Diane Graham Webb, MSN, RN, Director of Non-Traditional Studies in Nursing
Email: grahamd@nsula.edu

GENERAL INFORMATION

Type of School: *4-Year College or University, Public* • Accreditation: *Southern Association of Colleges and Schools* • Total Enrollment: *9415*

PROGRAM INFORMATION

NLNAC Accreditation: *Yes* • CCNE Accreditation:

NURSING STUDENT PROFILE

Total Nursing Enrollment: *114* • Full-Time Enrollment: *31* • Part-Time Enrollment: *83* • Female Enrollment: *97* • Male Enrollment: *17* • Total Graduates: *57*

FINANCES

Residential Annual Tuition: *$2,250* • Non-Residential Annual Tuition: *$7,050* • General Institutional Fees: *$128* • Additional Nursing Fees: *$180*

OUR LADY OF THE LAKE COLLEGE

Address: 7500 Hennessy Blvd, Baton Rouge, LA 70808
Phone: 225-768-1709
Fax: 225-768-1760
Contact: Lousie Plaisance, DNS, RN, Acting Dean
Email: lplaisan@ololcollege.edu

GENERAL INFORMATION

Type of School: *4-Year College or University, Private (Religious)* • Accreditation: *Southern Association of Colleges and Schools* • Total Enrollment: *1200*

PROGRAM INFORMATION

NLNAC Accreditation: *Not Reported* • CCNE Accreditation:

NURSING STUDENT PROFILE

Total Nursing Enrollment: *30* • Full-Time Enrollment: *1* • Part-Time Enrollment: *29* • Female Enrollment: *27* • Male Enrollment: *3* • Total Graduates: *1*

FINANCES

Residential Annual Tuition: *$4,320* • Non-Residential Annual Tuition: *Not Reported* • General Institutional Fees: *$5* • Additional Nursing Fees: *$80*

UNIVERSITY OF NEW ENGLAND

Address: 716 Stevens Avenue, Portland, ME 04103
Phone: 207-797-7688
Fax: 807-878-4895
Contact: Jean Dyer, MSN, BSN, RN, Chair
Email: jdyer@une.edu

GENERAL INFORMATION

Type of School: *4-Year College or University, Private (Independent)* • Accreditation: *New England Association of Schools and Colleges* • Total Enrollment: *3887*

PROGRAM INFORMATION

NLNAC Accreditation: *Yes* • CCNE Accreditation:

NURSING STUDENT PROFILE

Total Nursing Enrollment: *14* • Full-Time Enrollment: *7* • Part-Time Enrollment: *7* • Female Enrollment: *13* • Male Enrollment: *1* • Total Graduates: *16*

FINANCES

Residential Annual Tuition: *$15,740* • Non-Residential Annual Tuition: *$15,740* • General Institutional Fees: *$210* • Additional Nursing Fees: *$50*

COLLEGE OF NOTRE DAME

Address: 4701 North Charles St., Baltimore, MD 21210
Phone: 410-532-5509
Fax: 410-532-5795
Contact: Sandra Dunnington, PhD, RN, Chair
Email: sdunning@ndm.edu

GENERAL INFORMATION

Type of School: *4-Year College or University, Private (Religious)* • Accreditation: *Middle States Association of Colleges and Schools* • Total Enrollment: *Not Reported*

PROGRAM INFORMATION

NLNAC Accreditation: *Not Reported* • CCNE Accreditation:

NURSING STUDENT PROFILE

Total Nursing Enrollment: *Not Reported* • Full-Time Enrollment: *Not Reported* • Part-Time Enrollment: *Not Reported* • Female Enrollment: *Not Reported* • Male Enrollment: *Not Reported* • Total Graduates: 39

FINANCES

Residential Annual Tuition: *$5,160* • Non-Residential Annual Tuition: *Not Reported* • General Institutional Fees: *$60* • Additional Nursing Fees: *Not Reported*

UNIVERSITY OF MARYLAND—BALTIMORE

Address: 655 West Lombard Street, Baltimore, MD 21210
Phone: 410-706-6741
Fax: 410-706-4231
Contact: Barbara R. Heller, EdD, RN, FAAN, Dean and Professor
Email: heller@son.umaryland.edu

GENERAL INFORMATION

Type of School: *4-Year College or University, Public* • Accreditation: *Middle States Association of Colleges and Schools* • Total Enrollment: *Not Reported*

PROGRAM INFORMATION

NLNAC Accreditation: *Yes* • CCNE Accreditation:

NURSING STUDENT PROFILE

Total Nursing Enrollment: *182* • Full-Time Enrollment: *35* • Part-Time Enrollment: *147* • Female Enrollment: *157* • Male Enrollment: *25* • Total Graduates: 66

FINANCES

Residential Annual Tuition: *$4,767* • Non-Residential Annual Tuition: *$12,092* • General Institutional Fees: *$432* • Additional Nursing Fees: *$357*

Circle 127 on reader card   See in-depth profile for more information

ANNA MARIA COLLEGE

Address: 50 Sunset Lane, Paxton, MA 01612-1198
Phone: 508-849-3316
Fax: 508-849-3362
Contact: Audrey M. Silveri, EdD, RN, Director
Email: asilveri@annamaria.edu

GENERAL INFORMATION

Type of School: *4-Year College or University, Private (Religious)* • Accreditation: *New England Association of Schools and Colleges* • Total Enrollment: *1255*

PROGRAM INFORMATION

NLNAC Accreditation: *Yes* • CCNE Accreditation:

NURSING STUDENT PROFILE

Total Nursing Enrollment: *71* • Full-Time Enrollment: *1* • Part-Time Enrollment: *70* • Female Enrollment: *70* • Male Enrollment: *1* • Total Graduates: *19*

FINANCES

Residential Annual Tuition: *$5,880* • Non-Residential Annual Tuition: *$5,880* • General Institutional Fees: *$0* • Additional Nursing Fees: *$0*

ATLANTIC UNION COLLEGE

Address: 338 Main Street P.O. Box 1000, South Lancaster, MA 01561
Phone: 978-368-2404
Fax: 978-368-2518
Contact: Ninon P. Amertil, PhD, RN, FNP, Chairperson
Email: namertil@atlanticuc.edu

GENERAL INFORMATION

Type of School: *4-Year College or University, Private (Religious)* • Accreditation: *New England Association of Schools and Colleges* • Total Enrollment: *720*

PROGRAM INFORMATION

NLNAC Accreditation: *Yes* • CCNE Accreditation:

NURSING STUDENT PROFILE

Total Nursing Enrollment: *22* • Full-Time Enrollment: *8* • Part-Time Enrollment: *14* • Female Enrollment: *19* • Male Enrollment: *3* • Total Graduates: *27*

FINANCES

Residential Annual Tuition: *Not Reported* • Non-Residential Annual Tuition: *Not Reported* • General Institutional Fees: *$650* • Additional Nursing Fees: *$360*

EMMANUEL COLLEGE

Address: 400 The Fenway, Boston, MA 02118
Phone: 617-735-9935
Fax: 617-735-9708
Contact: Joan M. Riley, EdD, RN, Professor and Chair
Email: riley@emmanuel.edu

GENERAL INFORMATION

Type of School: *4-Year College or University, Private (Religious)* • Accreditation: *New England Association of Schools and Colleges* • Total Enrollment: *Not Reported*

PROGRAM INFORMATION

NLNAC Accreditation: *Yes* • CCNE Accreditation:

NURSING STUDENT PROFILE

Total Nursing Enrollment: *111* • Full-Time Enrollment: *10* • Part-Time Enrollment: *101* • Female Enrollment: *110* • Male Enrollment: *1* • Total Graduates: *36*

FINANCES

Residential Annual Tuition: *$1,937* • Non-Residential Annual Tuition: *$1,937* • General Institutional Fees: *$495* • Additional Nursing Fees: *$0*

FRAMINGHAM STATE COLLEGE

Address: 100 State Street, Framingham, MA 01701
Phone: 508-626-4713
Fax: 508-626-4746
Contact: Dolores Rojas Torti, DNSc, RN, Professor and Chairperson
Email: dtorti@frc.mass.edu

GENERAL INFORMATION

Type of School: *4-Year College or University, Public* • Accreditation: *New England Association of Schools and Colleges* • Total Enrollment: *Not Reported*

PROGRAM INFORMATION

NLNAC Accreditation: *Not Reported* • CCNE Accreditation:

NURSING STUDENT PROFILE

Total Nursing Enrollment: *43* • Full-Time Enrollment: *4* • Part-Time Enrollment: *39* • Female Enrollment: *41* • Male Enrollment: *2* • Total Graduates: *18*

FINANCES

Residential Annual Tuition: *$970* • Non-Residential Annual Tuition: *$7,050* • General Institutional Fees: *$3,440* • Additional Nursing Fees: *$0*

MASSACHUSETTS COLLEGE OF PHARMACY

Address: 179 Longwood Avenue, Boston, MA 02115
Phone: 617-732-2882
Fax: 617-732-2236
Contact: Sandra Gibson, EdD, ARNP, Program Chair
Email: sgibson@mcp.edu

REGIS COLLEGE

Address: 235 Wellesley St, Weston, MA 02193
Phone: 781-768-7090
Fax: 781-768-7089
Contact: Amy Anderson, EdD, RN, Chair, Division of Nursing
Email: amy.anderson@regiscollege.edu

GENERAL INFORMATION

Type of School: *4-Year College or University, Private (Independent)* • Accreditation: *Not Reported* • Total Enrollment: *Not Reported*

GENERAL INFORMATION

Type of School: *Not Reported, Not Reported* • Accreditation: *Not Reported* • Total Enrollment: *Not Reported*

PROGRAM INFORMATION

NLNAC Accreditation: *Yes* • CCNE Accreditation:

PROGRAM INFORMATION

NLNAC Accreditation: *Yes* • CCNE Accreditation:

NURSING STUDENT PROFILE

Total Nursing Enrollment: *15* • Full-Time Enrollment: *4* • Part-Time Enrollment: *11* • Female Enrollment: *13* • Male Enrollment: *2* • Total Graduates: *6*

NURSING STUDENT PROFILE

Total Nursing Enrollment: *66* • Full-Time Enrollment: *17* • Part-Time Enrollment: *49* • Female Enrollment: *60* • Male Enrollment: *6* • Total Graduates: *5*

FINANCES

Residential Annual Tuition: *$16,863* • Non-Residential Annual Tuition: *$16,863* • General Institutional Fees: *$240* • Additional Nursing Fees: *$0*

FINANCES

Residential Annual Tuition: *$17,500* • Non-Residential Annual Tuition: *$17,500* • General Institutional Fees: *$70* • Additional Nursing Fees: *$50*

Circle 99 on reader card   See in-depth profile for more information

FERRIS STATE UNIVERSITY

Address: 200 Ferris Drive, Big Rapids, MI 49307-2740
Phone: 231-591-2267
Fax: 231-591-2325
Contact: Sally K Johnson, EdD, MN, BS, RN,
          Department Head
Email: johnsons@ferris.edu

GENERAL INFORMATION

Type of School: *4-Year College or University, Public* •
Accreditation: *North Central Association of Colleges and Schools* • Total Enrollment: *9000*

PROGRAM INFORMATION

NLNAC Accreditation: *Yes* • CCNE Accreditation:

NURSING STUDENT PROFILE

Total Nursing Enrollment: *314* • Full-Time Enrollment: *10* •
Part-Time Enrollment: *304* • Female Enrollment: *309* • Male
Enrollment: *5* • Total Graduates: *74*

FINANCES

Residential Annual Tuition: *$4,284* • Non-Residential
Annual Tuition: *$9,076* • General Institutional Fees: *Not
Reported* • Additional Nursing Fees: *$125*

GRAND VALLEY STATE UNIVERSITY

Address: 401 West Fulton, 388c DeVos, Grand Rapids,
          MI 49504
Phone: 616-336-7167
Fax: 616-336-7362
Contact: Jean Martin, DNSc, RNc, PNP, Associate
          Professor and Director of RN/BSN and
          Graduate Programs
Email: martinj@gvsu.edu

GENERAL INFORMATION

Type of School: *4-Year College or University, Public* •
Accreditation: *North Central Association of Colleges and Schools* • Total Enrollment: *19762*

PROGRAM INFORMATION

NLNAC Accreditation: *Yes* • CCNE Accreditation:

NURSING STUDENT PROFILE

Total Nursing Enrollment: *42* • Full-Time Enrollment: *1* •
Part-Time Enrollment: *41* • Female Enrollment: *40* • Male
Enrollment: *2* • Total Graduates: *16*

FINANCES

Residential Annual Tuition: *$4,430* • Non-Residential
Annual Tuition: *$9,556* • General Institutional Fees: *Not
Reported* • Additional Nursing Fees: *Not Reported*

MADONNA UNIVERSITY

Address: 36600 Schoolcraft Road, Livonia, MI 48150
Phone: 734-432-5482
Fax: 734-432-5463
Contact: Marilyn Harton, MSN, RN, Degree Completion
Coordinator
Email: mharton@madonna.edu

GENERAL INFORMATION

Type of School: *4-Year College or University, Private (Religious)* • Accreditation: *North Central Association of Colleges and Schools* • Total Enrollment: *3328*

PROGRAM INFORMATION

NLNAC Accreditation: *Yes* • CCNE Accreditation:

NURSING STUDENT PROFILE

Total Nursing Enrollment: *20* • Full-Time Enrollment: *2* • Part-Time Enrollment: *18* • Female Enrollment: *20* • Male Enrollment: *0* • Total Graduates: *1*

FINANCES

Residential Annual Tuition: *$3,672* • Non-Residential Annual Tuition: *$3,672* • General Institutional Fees: *$100* • Additional Nursing Fees: *$80*

SPRING ARBOR UNIVERSITY

Address: 106 E. Main St., Spring Arbor, MI 49228-9799
Phone: 517-750-6344
Fax: 517-750-6602
Contact: Cindy E. Meredith, MSN, RN, Director of
Nursing
Email: cemered@arbor.edu

GENERAL INFORMATION

Type of School: *Not Reported, Not Reported* • Accreditation: *Not Reported* • Total Enrollment: *Not Reported*

PROGRAM INFORMATION

NLNAC Accreditation: *Not Reported* • CCNE Accreditation:

NURSING STUDENT PROFILE

Total Nursing Enrollment: *12* • Full-Time Enrollment: *12* • Part-Time Enrollment: *0* • Female Enrollment: *12* • Male Enrollment: *0* • Total Graduates: *Not Reported*

FINANCES

Residential Annual Tuition: *$10,050* • Non-Residential Annual Tuition: *Not Reported* • General Institutional Fees: *$115* • Additional Nursing Fees: *$1,200*

UNIVERSITY OF DETROIT MERCY

Address: 8200 West Outer Drive, PO Box 19900, Detroit, MI 48219
Phone: 313-993-6132
Fax: 313-993-6273
Contact: Suzanne Mellon, PhD, RN, Dean
Email: mellonsk@udmercy.edu

GENERAL INFORMATION

Type of School: *4-Year College or University, Private (Independent)* • Accreditation: *North Central Association of Colleges and Schools* • Total Enrollment: *6900*

PROGRAM INFORMATION

NLNAC Accreditation: *Yes* • CCNE Accreditation:

NURSING STUDENT PROFILE

Total Nursing Enrollment: *374* • Full-Time Enrollment: *4* • Part-Time Enrollment: *370* • Female Enrollment: *344* • Male Enrollment: *30* • Total Graduates: *17*

FINANCES

Residential Annual Tuition: *$7,950* • Non-Residential Annual Tuition: *$7,950* • General Institutional Fees: *$400* • Additional Nursing Fees: *$100*

UNIVERSITY OF MICHIGAN

Address: 400 N. Ingalls, Ann Arbor, MI 48109
Phone: 734-765-8490
Fax: 734-647-1419
Contact: Jan Lee, PhD, RN, Director
Email: janlee@umich.edu

GENERAL INFORMATION

Type of School: *4-Year College or University, Public* • Accreditation: *North Central Association of Colleges and Schools* • Total Enrollment: *38103*

PROGRAM INFORMATION

NLNAC Accreditation: *Yes* • CCNE Accreditation:

NURSING STUDENT PROFILE

Total Nursing Enrollment: *61* • Full-Time Enrollment: *5* • Part-Time Enrollment: *56* • Female Enrollment: *53* • Male Enrollment: *8* • Total Graduates: *23*

FINANCES

Residential Annual Tuition: *$3,596* • Non-Residential Annual Tuition: *$11,271* • General Institutional Fees: *$555* • Additional Nursing Fees: *$15*

AUGSBURG COLLEGE	BEMIDJI STATE UNIVERSITY

Address: 2211 Riverside Ave S, Minneapolis, MN 55454
Phone: 612-330-1211
Fax: 612-330-1676
Contact: Beverly Nilsson, PhD, RN, Department Chair
Email: nilsson@augsburg.edu

Address: 105 Deputy Hall, 1500 Birchmont Drive NE,
Bemidji, MN 56601
Phone: 218-755-3892
Fax: 218-755-4402
Contact: Rochelle Scheela, PhD, RN, CS, Professor,
Department of Nursing
Email: rscheela@bemidji@state.edu

GENERAL INFORMATION

Type of School: *4-Year College or University, Private (Religious)* • Accreditation: *North Central Association of Colleges and Schools* • Total Enrollment: *Not Reported*

GENERAL INFORMATION

Type of School: *4-Year College or University, Public* • Accreditation: *North Central Association of Colleges and Schools* • Total Enrollment: *Not Reported*

PROGRAM INFORMATION

NLNAC Accreditation: *Yes* • CCNE Accreditation:

PROGRAM INFORMATION

NLNAC Accreditation: *Yes* • CCNE Accreditation:

NURSING STUDENT PROFILE

Total Nursing Enrollment: *132* • Full-Time Enrollment: *62* • Part-Time Enrollment: *70* • Female Enrollment: *124* • Male Enrollment: *8* • Total Graduates: *6*

NURSING STUDENT PROFILE

Total Nursing Enrollment: *75* • Full-Time Enrollment: *0* • Part-Time Enrollment: *75* • Female Enrollment: *72* • Male Enrollment: *3* • Total Graduates: *15*

FINANCES

Residential Annual Tuition: *$7,548* • Non-Residential Annual Tuition: *$7,548* • General Institutional Fees: *Not Reported* • Additional Nursing Fees: *$214*

FINANCES

Residential Annual Tuition: *$2,954* • Non-Residential Annual Tuition: *$5,908* • General Institutional Fees: *$311* • Additional Nursing Fees: *$30*

BETHEL COLLEGE

Address: 3900 Bethel Drive, St. Paul, MN 55112
Phone: 651-638-6335
Fax: 651-635-1965
Contact: Ann Jones, DNSc, RN, Associate Professor and
    Program Director
Email: ajones@bethell.edu

GENERAL INFORMATION

Type of School: *4-Year College or University, Private (Religious)* • Accreditation: *North Central Association of Colleges and Schools* • Total Enrollment: *3500*

PROGRAM INFORMATION

NLNAC Accreditation: *Not Reported* • CCNE Accreditation: *Yes*

NURSING STUDENT PROFILE

Total Nursing Enrollment: *108* • Full-Time Enrollment: *108* • Part-Time Enrollment: *0* • Female Enrollment: *95* • Male Enrollment: *13* • Total Graduates: *44*

FINANCES

Residential Annual Tuition: *$6,360* • Non-Residential Annual Tuition: *Not Reported* • General Institutional Fees: *Not Reported* • Additional Nursing Fees: *$60*

METROPOLITAN STATE UNIVERSITY

Address: 700 East Seventh Street, St. Paul, MN 55106-
    5000
Phone: 651-772-7705
Fax: 651-772-6130
Contact: Marilyn Loen, PhD, RN, GNP, HNP, Executive
    Director
Email: marilyn.loen@metrostate.edu

GENERAL INFORMATION

Type of School: *4-Year College or University, Public* • Accreditation: *North Central Association of Colleges and Schools* • Total Enrollment: *Not Reported*

PROGRAM INFORMATION

NLNAC Accreditation: *Yes* • CCNE Accreditation:

NURSING STUDENT PROFILE

Total Nursing Enrollment: *167* • Full-Time Enrollment: *3* • Part-Time Enrollment: *164* • Female Enrollment: *149* • Male Enrollment: *18* • Total Graduates: *41*

FINANCES

Residential Annual Tuition: *$2,054* • Non-Residential Annual Tuition: *$4,390* • General Institutional Fees: *$15* • Additional Nursing Fees: *$0*

WINONA STATE UNIVERSITY

Address: PO Box 5838, Winona, MN 55987
Phone: 507-457-5127
Fax: 507-457-5550
Contact: Linda Seppanen, PhD, RN, Department
           Chairperson and Professor
Email: lsppanen@winona.edu

GENERAL INFORMATION

Type of School: *4-Year College or University, Public •*
Accreditation: *North Central Association of Colleges and
Schools •* Total Enrollment: *6660*

PROGRAM INFORMATION

NLNAC Accreditation: *Yes •* CCNE Accreditation:

NURSING STUDENT PROFILE

Total Nursing Enrollment: *73 •* Full-Time Enrollment: *11 •*
Part-Time Enrollment: *62 •* Female Enrollment: *64 •* Male
Enrollment: *9 •* Total Graduates: *22*

FINANCES

Residential Annual Tuition: *$2,820 •* Non-Residential
Annual Tuition: *$6,230 •* General Institutional Fees: *Not
Reported •* Additional Nursing Fees: *Not Reported*

DELTA STATE UNIVERSITY

Address: Highway 8 West, Cleveland, MS 38733
Phone: 662-846-4255
Fax: 662-846-4267
Contact: Dana Lamar, EdD, RNC, Coordinator of
           Academic Program
Email: dlamar@dsu.deltast.edu

GENERAL INFORMATION

Type of School: *4-Year College or University, Public •*
Accreditation: *Southern Association of Colleges and Schools •*
Total Enrollment: *3746*

PROGRAM INFORMATION

NLNAC Accreditation: *Yes •* CCNE Accreditation: *Yes*

NURSING STUDENT PROFILE

Total Nursing Enrollment: *5 •* Full-Time Enrollment: *4 •*
Part-Time Enrollment: *1 •* Female Enrollment: *2 •* Male
Enrollment: *3 •* Total Graduates: *6*

FINANCES

Residential Annual Tuition: *$3,100 •* Non-Residential
Annual Tuition: *$7,374 •* General Institutional Fees: *$0 •*
Additional Nursing Fees: *$30*

CENTRAL METHODIST COLLEGE

Address: 411 Central Methodist Square, Fayette, MO 65248
Phone: 660-248-6363
Fax: 660-248-6377
Contact: Shirley J Peterson, PhD, RN, Nursing Division Chair
Email: speterson@cmc2.cmc.edu

GENERAL INFORMATION

Type of School: *4-Year College or University, Private (Religious)* • Accreditation: *North Central Association of Colleges and Schools* • Total Enrollment: *Not Reported*

PROGRAM INFORMATION

NLNAC Accreditation: *Not Reported* • CCNE Accreditation:

NURSING STUDENT PROFILE

Total Nursing Enrollment: *23* • Full-Time Enrollment: *20* • Part-Time Enrollment: *3* • Female Enrollment: *22* • Male Enrollment: *1* • Total Graduates: *6*

FINANCES

Residential Annual Tuition: *$11,390* • Non-Residential Annual Tuition: *$11,390* • General Institutional Fees: *Not Reported* • Additional Nursing Fees: *$570*

HANNIBAL LAGRANGE COLLEGE

Address: 2800 Palmyra Road, Hannibal, MO 63401
Phone: 573-221-3675
Fax: 573-248-0294
Contact: Senda Guertzgen, MS, RN, Director
Email: sguertzg@hlg.edu

GENERAL INFORMATION

Type of School: *4-Year College or University, Private (Religious)* • Accreditation: *North Central Association of Colleges and Schools* • Total Enrollment: *1152*

PROGRAM INFORMATION

NLNAC Accreditation: *Not Reported* • CCNE Accreditation:

NURSING STUDENT PROFILE

Total Nursing Enrollment: *4* • Full-Time Enrollment: *0* • Part-Time Enrollment: *4* • Female Enrollment: *4* • Male Enrollment: *0* • Total Graduates: *3*

FINANCES

Residential Annual Tuition: *$8,550* • Non-Residential Annual Tuition: *$8,550* • General Institutional Fees: *$260* • Additional Nursing Fees: *$240*

JEWISH HOSPITAL

Address: 306 South Kings Highway Blvd, St. Louis, MO 63110
Phone: 314-454-8416
Fax: 314-454-5239
Contact: Elizabeth A Buck, PhD, RN, Academic Dean
Email: eab1458@bjc.org

GENERAL INFORMATION

Type of School: *Hospital, Private (Independent)* •
Accreditation: *North Central Association of Colleges and Schools* • Total Enrollment: *Not Reported*

PROGRAM INFORMATION

NLNAC Accreditation: *Yes* • CCNE Accreditation: *Yes*

NURSING STUDENT PROFILE

Total Nursing Enrollment: *97* • Full-Time Enrollment: *15* •
Part-Time Enrollment: *82* • Female Enrollment: *90* • Male Enrollment: *7* • Total Graduates: *46*

FINANCES

Residential Annual Tuition: *$11,360* • Non-Residential Annual Tuition: *$11,360* • General Institutional Fees: *$200* • Additional Nursing Fees: *$0*

LINCOLN UNIVERSITY

Address: Nursing Science Department, Jefferson City, MO 65102-0029
Phone: 573-681-5421
Fax: 573-681-5422
Contact: Connie Hamacher, PhD, RN, Department Head
Email: hamacher@lincoln.edu

GENERAL INFORMATION

Type of School: *4-Year College or University, Public* •
Accreditation: *North Central Association of Colleges and Schools* • Total Enrollment: *3347*

PROGRAM INFORMATION

NLNAC Accreditation: *Not Reported* • CCNE Accreditation:

NURSING STUDENT PROFILE

Total Nursing Enrollment: *40* • Full-Time Enrollment: *4* •
Part-Time Enrollment: *36* • Female Enrollment: *38* • Male Enrollment: *2* • Total Graduates: *8*

FINANCES

Residential Annual Tuition: *$1,818* • Non-Residential Annual Tuition: *$3,636* • General Institutional Fees: *$374* • Additional Nursing Fees: *$50*

SOUTHWEST BAPTIST UNIVERSITY

Address: Springfield Center-4431 South Fremont,
           Springfield, MO 65804
Phone: 417-885-3262
Fax: 417-887-4847
Contact: Paula Garner, MS, RN, Chair
Email: pgarner@sbuniv.edu

GENERAL INFORMATION

Type of School: *4-Year College or University, Private (Religious)* • Accreditation: *North Central Association of Colleges and Schools* • Total Enrollment: *3593*

PROGRAM INFORMATION

NLNAC Accreditation: *Yes* • CCNE Accreditation:

NURSING STUDENT PROFILE

Total Nursing Enrollment: *120* • Full-Time Enrollment: *25* • Part-Time Enrollment: *95* • Female Enrollment: *110* • Male Enrollment: *10* • Total Graduates: *Not Reported*

FINANCES

Residential Annual Tuition: *$2,070* • Non-Residential Annual Tuition: *$2,070* • General Institutional Fees: *$20* • Additional Nursing Fees: *Not Reported*

SOUTHWEST MISSOURI STATE UNIVERSITY

Address: 907 South National, Springfield, MO 65804
Phone: 417-836-5310
Fax: 417-836-5484
Contact: Kathryn Hope, PhD, RN, CS, FNP, Head
Email: klh895f@smsu.edu

GENERAL INFORMATION

Type of School: *4-Year College or University, Public* • Accreditation: *North Central Association of Colleges and Schools* • Total Enrollment: *13796*

PROGRAM INFORMATION

NLNAC Accreditation: *Yes* • CCNE Accreditation:

NURSING STUDENT PROFILE

Total Nursing Enrollment: *79* • Full-Time Enrollment: *75* • Part-Time Enrollment: *4* • Female Enrollment: *69* • Male Enrollment: *10* • Total Graduates: *19*

FINANCES

Residential Annual Tuition: *$2,544* • Non-Residential Annual Tuition: *$5,088* • General Institutional Fees: *$384* • Additional Nursing Fees: *$0*

UNIVERSITY OF MISSOURI— KANSAS CITY

Address: 2220 Holmes, Kansas City, MO 64108
Phone: 816-235-5965
Fax: 816-235-1701
Contact: Cordelia Esry, PhD, RN, Assistant Dean
Email: esryd@umkc.edu

GENERAL INFORMATION

Type of School: *Not Reported, Public* • Accreditation: *North Central Association of Colleges and Schools* • Total Enrollment: *Not Reported*

PROGRAM INFORMATION

NLNAC Accreditation: *Not Reported* • CCNE Accreditation: *Yes*

NURSING STUDENT PROFILE

Total Nursing Enrollment: *49* • Full-Time Enrollment: *14* • Part-Time Enrollment: *35* • Female Enrollment: *41* • Male Enrollment: *8* • Total Graduates: *9*

FINANCES

Residential Annual Tuition: *$2,866* • Non-Residential Annual Tuition: *$7,767* • General Institutional Fees: *$60* • Additional Nursing Fees: *$0*

UNIVERSITY OF MISSOURI— ST. LOUIS

Address: 8001 Natural Bridge, St. Louis, MO 63121
Phone: 314-516-6849
Fax: 314-516-6730
Contact: Teri Murray, PhD, RN, BSN Program Director
Email: murray@umsl.edu

GENERAL INFORMATION

Type of School: *Not Reported, Public* • Accreditation: *North Central Association of Colleges and Schools* • Total Enrollment: *Not Reported*

PROGRAM INFORMATION

NLNAC Accreditation: *Not Reported* • CCNE Accreditation: *Yes*

NURSING STUDENT PROFILE

Total Nursing Enrollment: *101* • Full-Time Enrollment: *3* • Part-Time Enrollment: *98* • Female Enrollment: *100* • Male Enrollment: *1* • Total Graduates: *42*

FINANCES

Residential Annual Tuition: *$2,466* • Non-Residential Annual Tuition: *$7,362* • General Institutional Fees: *Not Reported* • Additional Nursing Fees: *Not Reported*

WEBSTER UNIVERSITY

Address: 470 East Lockwood, Saint Louis, MO 63119
Phone: 314-968-7483
Fax: 314-963-6101
Contact: Anne Schappe, PhD, RN, Acting Chair
Email: schappan@webster.edu

GENERAL INFORMATION

Type of School: *4-Year College or University, Private (Independent)* • Accreditation: *North Central Association of Colleges and Schools* • Total Enrollment: *16000*

PROGRAM INFORMATION

NLNAC Accreditation: *Yes* • CCNE Accreditation:

NURSING STUDENT PROFILE

Total Nursing Enrollment: *242* • Full-Time Enrollment: *38* • Part-Time Enrollment: *204* • Female Enrollment: *225* • Male Enrollment: *17* • Total Graduates: *100*

FINANCES

Residential Annual Tuition: *$12,880* • Non-Residential Annual Tuition: *$12,880* • General Institutional Fees: *$150* • Additional Nursing Fees: *$0*

COLLEGE OF SAINT MARY

Address: 1901 S. 72nd St., Omaha, NE 68124
Phone: 402-399-2653
Fax: 402-399-2654
Contact: Mary E. Partusch, PhD, RN, BSN Program Director
Email: mpartusch@csm.edu

GENERAL INFORMATION

Type of School: *4-Year College or University, Private (Religious)* • Accreditation: *North Central Association of Colleges and Schools* • Total Enrollment: *930*

PROGRAM INFORMATION

NLNAC Accreditation: *Not Reported* • CCNE Accreditation:

NURSING STUDENT PROFILE

Total Nursing Enrollment: *18* • Full-Time Enrollment: *8* • Part-Time Enrollment: *10* • Female Enrollment: *18* • Male Enrollment: *0* • Total Graduates: *9*

FINANCES

Residential Annual Tuition: *$13,350* • Non-Residential Annual Tuition: *$13,350* • General Institutional Fees: *$0* • Additional Nursing Fees: *$215*

CREIGHTON UNIVERSITY

Address: 2500 California Plaza, Omaha, NE 68178
Phone: 402-280-2049
Fax: 402-280-2045
Contact: Mary Parsons, MSN, RN, Program Chair
Email: parsonsm@creighton.edu

GENERAL INFORMATION

Type of School: *Not Reported* • Accreditation: *Not Reported* •
Total Enrollment: *Not Reported*

PROGRAM INFORMATION

NLNAC Accreditation: *Yes* • CCNE Accreditation:

NURSING STUDENT PROFILE

Total Nursing Enrollment: *Not Reported* • Full-Time
Enrollment: *Not Reported* • Part-Time Enrollment: *Not
Reported* • Female Enrollment: *Not Reported* • Male
Enrollment: *Not Reported* • Total Graduates: *37*

FINANCES

Residential Annual Tuition: *$21,468* • Non-Residential
Annual Tuition: *$21,468* • General Institutional Fees: *$566* •
Additional Nursing Fees: *$112*

UNIVERSITY OF NEBRASKA MEDICAL CENTER

Address: Box 985330, Omaha, NE 68198
Phone: 402-559-4270
Fax: 402-559-6379
Contact: Catherine Todero, PhD, RN, Associate Professor
and Associate Dean
Email: ctodero@unmc.edu

GENERAL INFORMATION

Type of School: *4-Year College or University, Public* •
Accreditation: *North Central Association of Colleges and
Schools* • Total Enrollment: *2636*

PROGRAM INFORMATION

NLNAC Accreditation: *Not Reported* • CCNE Accreditation:
Yes

NURSING STUDENT PROFILE

Total Nursing Enrollment: *54* • Full-Time Enrollment: *2* •
Part-Time Enrollment: *52* • Female Enrollment: *49* • Male
Enrollment: *5* • Total Graduates: *18*

FINANCES

Residential Annual Tuition: *$4,489* • Non-Residential
Annual Tuition: *$13,335* • General Institutional Fees: *$598* •
Additional Nursing Fees: *$652*

COLLEGE OF SAINT ELIZABETH

Address: 2 Convent Road, Morristown, NJ 07960
Phone: 973-290-4072
Fax: 973-290-4177
Contact: Janet Lehmann, PhD, RN, Chairperson
Email: jlehmann@liza.st-elizabeth.edu

FELICIAN COLLEGE

Address: 262 South Main Street, Lodi, NJ 07644
Phone: 201-559-6099
Fax: 201-559-6188
Contact: Maureen Murphy-Ruocco, EdD, RN, APC, BC,
           Chairperson
Email: ruoccom@inet.felician.edu

GENERAL INFORMATION

Type of School: *4-Year College or University, Private (Religious)* • Accreditation: *Middle States Association of Colleges and Schools* • Total Enrollment: *1741*

GENERAL INFORMATION

Type of School: *4-Year College or University, Private (Religious)* • Accreditation: *Middle States Association of Colleges and Schools* • Total Enrollment: *1374*

PROGRAM INFORMATION

NLNAC Accreditation: *Yes* • CCNE Accreditation:

PROGRAM INFORMATION

NLNAC Accreditation: *Not Reported* • CCNE Accreditation: *Yes*

NURSING STUDENT PROFILE

Total Nursing Enrollment: *86* • Full-Time Enrollment: *2* • Part-Time Enrollment: *84* • Female Enrollment: *83* • Male Enrollment: *3* • Total Graduates: *15*

NURSING STUDENT PROFILE

Total Nursing Enrollment: *59* • Full-Time Enrollment: *9* • Part-Time Enrollment: *50* • Female Enrollment: *55* • Male Enrollment: *4* • Total Graduates: *10*

FINANCES

Residential Annual Tuition: *$7,650* • Non-Residential Annual Tuition: *Not Reported* • General Institutional Fees: *$186* • Additional Nursing Fees: *$25*

FINANCES

Residential Annual Tuition: *$11,460* • Non-Residential Annual Tuition: *Not Reported* • General Institutional Fees: *$382* • Additional Nursing Fees: *$300*

Circle 49 on reader card   See in-depth profile for more information

KEAN UNIVERSITY

Address: Morris Ave., Union, NJ 07083
Phone: 908-527-2608
Fax: 908-352-6427
Contact: Susan Salmond, EdD, RN, Chairperson
Email: ssalmond@kean.edu

GENERAL INFORMATION

Type of School: *4-Year College or University, Public* • Accreditation: *Middle States Association of Colleges and Schools* • Total Enrollment: *10000*

PROGRAM INFORMATION

NLNAC Accreditation: *Yes* • CCNE Accreditation:

NURSING STUDENT PROFILE

Total Nursing Enrollment: *203* • Full-Time Enrollment: *19* • Part-Time Enrollment: *184* • Female Enrollment: *189* • Male Enrollment: *14* • Total Graduates: *55*

FINANCES

Residential Annual Tuition: *$1,875* • Non-Residential Annual Tuition: *$2,835* • General Institutional Fees: *$685* • Additional Nursing Fees: *Not Reported*

MONMOUTH UNIVERSITY

Address: Cedar Avenue, West Long Branch, NJ 07764
Phone: 732-571-3692
Fax: 732-263-5131
Contact: Linda Rosen, DNSc, RN, Coordinator BSN
          Program
Email: lrosen@monmouth.edu

GENERAL INFORMATION

Type of School: *4-Year College or University, Private (Independent)* • Accreditation: *Middle States Association of Colleges and Schools* • Total Enrollment: *5753*

PROGRAM INFORMATION

NLNAC Accreditation: *Not Reported* • CCNE Accreditation: *Yes*

NURSING STUDENT PROFILE

Total Nursing Enrollment: *63* • Full-Time Enrollment: *2* • Part-Time Enrollment: *61* • Female Enrollment: *62* • Male Enrollment: *1* • Total Graduates: *24*

FINANCES

Residential Annual Tuition: *$16,506* • Non-Residential Annual Tuition: *$16,506* • General Institutional Fees: *$66* • Additional Nursing Fees: *Not Reported*

Circle 85 on reader card   See in-depth profile for more information

NEW JERSEY CITY UNIVERSITY

Address: 2039 Kennedy Blvd, Jersey City, NJ 07305
Phone: 201-200-3157
Fax: 201-200-3141
Contact: Gloria Boseman, PhD, RN, Chairperson
Email: gboseman@njcu.edu

GENERAL INFORMATION

Type of School: *4-Year College or University, Public* •
Accreditation: *Middle States Association of Colleges and
Schools* • Total Enrollment: *9450*

PROGRAM INFORMATION

NLNAC Accreditation: *Yes* • CCNE Accreditation:

NURSING STUDENT PROFILE

Total Nursing Enrollment: *156* • Full-Time Enrollment: *45* •
Part-Time Enrollment: *111* • Female Enrollment: *147* • Male
Enrollment: *9* • Total Graduates: *69*

FINANCES

Residential Annual Tuition: *$3,540* • Non-Residential
Annual Tuition: *$6,900* • General Institutional Fees: *$154* •
Additional Nursing Fees: *Not Reported*

RICHARD STOCKTON COLLEGE OF NEW JERSEY

Address: Jim Leads Road, Pomona, NJ 08240
Phone: 609-652-4496
Fax: 609-652-4496
Contact: Cheryle Fisher Eisele, EdD, RN, Coordinator
Email: ceisele@stockton.edu

GENERAL INFORMATION

Type of School: *4-Year College or University, Public* •
Accreditation: *Middle States Association of Colleges and
Schools* • Total Enrollment: *206*

PROGRAM INFORMATION

NLNAC Accreditation: *Yes* • CCNE Accreditation:

NURSING STUDENT PROFILE

Total Nursing Enrollment: *44* • Full-Time Enrollment: *9* •
Part-Time Enrollment: *35* • Female Enrollment: *41* • Male
Enrollment: *3* • Total Graduates: *22*

FINANCES

Residential Annual Tuition: *$2,025* • Non-Residential
Annual Tuition: *$3,285* • General Institutional Fees: *$74* •
Additional Nursing Fees: *$0*

SAINT PETER'S COLLEGE

Address: Kennedy Boulevard, Jersey City, NJ 07306
Phone: 201-915-9412
Fax: 201-915-9062
Contact: Marylou Yam, PhD, RN, CS, Chairperson
Email: yam_m@spcvxa.spc.edu

GENERAL INFORMATION

Type of School: *4-Year College or University, Private (Religious)* • Accreditation: *Middle States Association of Colleges and Schools* • Total Enrollment: *3300*

PROGRAM INFORMATION

NLNAC Accreditation: *Yes* • CCNE Accreditation: *Yes*

NURSING STUDENT PROFILE

Total Nursing Enrollment: *109* • Full-Time Enrollment: *0* • Part-Time Enrollment: *109* • Female Enrollment: *106* • Male Enrollment: *3* • Total Graduates: *42*

FINANCES

Residential Annual Tuition: *$6,840* • Non-Residential Annual Tuition: *$6,840* • General Institutional Fees: *$20* • Additional Nursing Fees: *Not Reported*

SETON HALL UNIVERSITY

Address: 400 South Orange Avenue, South Orange, NJ 07079
Phone: 973-761-9276
Fax: 973-761-9607
Contact: Linda J Ulak, EdD, RN, Chair, Undergraduate Nursing Department
Email: ulaklind@shu.edu

GENERAL INFORMATION

Type of School: *4-Year College or University, Private (Religious)* • Accreditation: *Middle States Association of Colleges and Schools* • Total Enrollment: *9600*

PROGRAM INFORMATION

NLNAC Accreditation: *Yes* • CCNE Accreditation: *Yes*

NURSING STUDENT PROFILE

Total Nursing Enrollment: *24* • Full-Time Enrollment: *22* • Part-Time Enrollment: *2* • Female Enrollment: *23* • Male Enrollment: *1* • Total Graduates: *11*

FINANCES

Residential Annual Tuition: *$9,846* • Non-Residential Annual Tuition: *Not Reported* • General Institutional Fees: *$980* • Additional Nursing Fees: *$0*

THOMAS EDISON STATE COLLEGE

Address: 101 West State Street, Trenton, NJ 08608
Phone: 609-633-6460
Fax: 609-777-3003
Contact: Susan McMullen O'Brien, EdD, RN, Associate Dean
Email: Sobrien@tesc.edu

GENERAL INFORMATION

Type of School: *4-Year College or University, Public* • Accreditation: *Middle States Association of Colleges and Schools* • Total Enrollment: *8137*

PROGRAM INFORMATION

NLNAC Accreditation: *Yes* • CCNE Accreditation:

NURSING STUDENT PROFILE

Total Nursing Enrollment: *125* • Full-Time Enrollment: *Not Reported* • Part-Time Enrollment: *Not Reported* • Female Enrollment: *116* • Male Enrollment: *9* • Total Graduates: *23*

FINANCES

Residential Annual Tuition: *Not Reported* • Non-Residential Annual Tuition: *Not Reported* • General Institutional Fees: *$75* • Additional Nursing Fees: *Not Reported*

UNIVERSITY OF MEDICAL DENTISTRY OF NEW JERSEY/NJIT JOINT BSN PROGRAM

Address: 3331 Route 38 and Hartford Road, Mt. Laurel, NJ 08054
Phone: 856-222-9311
Fax: 856-222-1537
Contact: Barbara A Benjamin, EdD, RNC, On-Site Faculty Administrator
Email: barbara.a.benjamin@njit.edu

GENERAL INFORMATION

Type of School: *Other, Public* • Accreditation: *Middle States Association of Colleges and Schools* • Total Enrollment: *600*

PROGRAM INFORMATION

NLNAC Accreditation: *Yes* • CCNE Accreditation:

NURSING STUDENT PROFILE

Total Nursing Enrollment: *79* • Full-Time Enrollment: *79* • Part-Time Enrollment: *0* • Female Enrollment: *72* • Male Enrollment: *7* • Total Graduates: *5*

FINANCES

Residential Annual Tuition: *$5,758* • Non-Residential Annual Tuition: *$10,102* • General Institutional Fees: *$972* • Additional Nursing Fees: *Not Reported*

UNIVERSITY OF MEDICINE AND DENTISTRY OF NEW JERSEY—RAMAPO COLLEGE

Address: 505 Ramapo Valley Road, Mahwah, NJ 07430-1680
Phone: 201-684-7737
Fax: 201-684-7954
Contact: Kathleen M. Burke, PhD, RN, Assistant Dean
Email: burkkm@umdnj.edu

GENERAL INFORMATION

Type of School: *Not Reported, Not Reported* • Accreditation: *Not Reported* • Total Enrollment: *Not Reported*

PROGRAM INFORMATION

NLNAC Accreditation: *Yes* • CCNE Accreditation:

NURSING STUDENT PROFILE

Total Nursing Enrollment: *315* • Full-Time Enrollment: *128* • Part-Time Enrollment: *187* • Female Enrollment: *280* • Male Enrollment: *35* • Total Graduates: *43*

FINANCES

Residential Annual Tuition: *$4,166* • Non-Residential Annual Tuition: *$7,291* • General Institutional Fees: *$80* • Additional Nursing Fees: *$50*

EASTERN NEW MEXICO UNIVERSITY—PORTALES

Address: Portales, NM 88130
Phone: 505-562-2403
Fax: 505-562-2293
Contact: Ginny Guido, PhD, RN, Professor and Chair, Department of Nursing
Email: ginny.guido@enmu.edu

GENERAL INFORMATION

Type of School: *4-Year College or University, Public* • Accreditation: *North Central Association of Colleges and Schools* • Total Enrollment: *3577*

PROGRAM INFORMATION

NLNAC Accreditation: *Not Reported* • CCNE Accreditation:

NURSING STUDENT PROFILE

Total Nursing Enrollment: *Not Reported* • Full-Time Enrollment: *Not Reported* • Part-Time Enrollment: *Not Reported* • Female Enrollment: *Not Reported* • Male Enrollment: *Not Reported* • Total Graduates: *21*

FINANCES

Residential Annual Tuition: *$1,752* • Non-Residential Annual Tuition: *$6,504* • General Institutional Fees: *Not Reported* • Additional Nursing Fees: *Not Reported*

ADELPHI UNIVERSITY

Address: School of Nursing, Garden City, NY 11530
Phone: 516-877-4530
Fax: 516-877-4558
Contact: Jean Winter, EdD, Associate Dean
Email: winter@adelphi.edu

GENERAL INFORMATION

Type of School: *4-Year College or University, Private (Independent)* • Accreditation: *Middle States Association of Colleges and Schools* • Total Enrollment: *6500*

PROGRAM INFORMATION

NLNAC Accreditation: *Yes* • CCNE Accreditation: *Yes*

NURSING STUDENT PROFILE

Total Nursing Enrollment: *116* • Full-Time Enrollment: *13* • Part-Time Enrollment: *103* • Female Enrollment: *107* • Male Enrollment: *9* • Total Graduates: *37*

FINANCES

Residential Annual Tuition: *$15,750* • Non-Residential Annual Tuition: *$15,750* • General Institutional Fees: *$770* • Additional Nursing Fees: *$6*

CITY UNIVERSITY OF NEW YORK—JAMAICA

Address: Science Building, Room 10, Jamaica, NY 11451
Phone: 718-262-2054
Fax: 718-262-2002
Contact: Reuphenia James, EdD, RN, Director
Email: james_r@york.cuny.edu

GENERAL INFORMATION

Type of School: *4-Year College or University, Public* • Accreditation: *Middle States Association of Colleges and Schools* • Total Enrollment: *5389*

PROGRAM INFORMATION

NLNAC Accreditation: *Yes* • CCNE Accreditation:

NURSING STUDENT PROFILE

Total Nursing Enrollment: *58* • Full-Time Enrollment: *58* • Part-Time Enrollment: *0* • Female Enrollment: *55* • Male Enrollment: *3* • Total Graduates: *25*

FINANCES

Residential Annual Tuition: *$3,200* • Non-Residential Annual Tuition: *$6,800* • General Institutional Fees: *$85* • Additional Nursing Fees: *$0*

THE COLLEGE OF STATEN ISLAND

Address: 2800 Victory Boulevard, Staten Island, NY 10314
Phone: 718-982-3810
Fax: 718-982-3813
Contact: Linda E. Reese, MA, RN, Chairperson
Email: reese@postbox.csi.cuny.edu

GENERAL INFORMATION

Type of School: *Not Reported, Not Reported* • Accreditation: *Not Reported* • Total Enrollment: *Not Reported*

PROGRAM INFORMATION

NLNAC Accreditation: *Yes* • CCNE Accreditation:

NURSING STUDENT PROFILE

Total Nursing Enrollment: *166* • Full-Time Enrollment: *33* • Part-Time Enrollment: *133* • Female Enrollment: *150* • Male Enrollment: *16* • Total Graduates: *52*

FINANCES

Residential Annual Tuition: *$3,200* • Non-Residential Annual Tuition: *$6,800* • General Institutional Fees: *$158* • Additional Nursing Fees: *$20*

DAEMEN COLLEGE

Address: 4380 Main Street, Amherst, NY 14226
Phone: 716-839-8387
Fax: 716-839-8516
Contact: Mary Lou Rusin, EdD, RN, Professor and Chair
Email: mrusin@daemen.edu

GENERAL INFORMATION

Type of School: *4-Year College or University, Private (Independent)* • Accreditation: *Middle States Association of Colleges and Schools* • Total Enrollment: *2000*

PROGRAM INFORMATION

NLNAC Accreditation: *Yes* • CCNE Accreditation:

NURSING STUDENT PROFILE

Total Nursing Enrollment: *218* • Full-Time Enrollment: *35* • Part-Time Enrollment: *183* • Female Enrollment: *202* • Male Enrollment: *16* • Total Graduates: *73*

FINANCES

Residential Annual Tuition: *$7,470* • Non-Residential Annual Tuition: *$7,470* • General Institutional Fees: *$200* • Additional Nursing Fees: *$50*

LONG ISLAND UNIVERSITY

Address: CW Post Campus, Brookville, NY 11548
Phone: 516-299-4158
Fax: 516-299-2352
Contact: Loretta Knapp, PhD, RN, Chairperson
Email: lknapp@liu.edu

GENERAL INFORMATION

Type of School: *4-Year College or University, Private (Independent)* • Accreditation: *Middle States Association of Colleges and Schools* • Total Enrollment: *28000*

PROGRAM INFORMATION

NLNAC Accreditation: *Yes* • CCNE Accreditation:

NURSING STUDENT PROFILE

Total Nursing Enrollment: *70* • Full-Time Enrollment: *0* • Part-Time Enrollment: *70* • Female Enrollment: *66* • Male Enrollment: *4* • Total Graduates: *15*

FINANCES

Residential Annual Tuition: *$13,920* • Non-Residential Annual Tuition: *$13,920* • General Institutional Fees: *$240* • Additional Nursing Fees: *$30*

NAZARETH COLLEGE

Address: 4245 East Avenue, Rochester, NY 14618
Phone: 716-389-2710
Fax: 716-389-2714
Contact: Margaret M. Andrews, PhD, RN, Chairperson and Professor
Email: mmandrew@naz.edu

GENERAL INFORMATION

Type of School: *Not Reported, Not Reported* • Accreditation: *Not Reported* • Total Enrollment: *Not Reported*

PROGRAM INFORMATION

NLNAC Accreditation: *Not Reported* • CCNE Accreditation: *Yes*

NURSING STUDENT PROFILE

Total Nursing Enrollment: *101* • Full-Time Enrollment: *6* • Part-Time Enrollment: *95* • Female Enrollment: *97* • Male Enrollment: *4* • Total Graduates: *22*

FINANCES

Residential Annual Tuition: *$14,680* • Non-Residential Annual Tuition: *$14,680* • General Institutional Fees: *$440* • Additional Nursing Fees: *Not Reported*

PACE UNIVERSITY

Address: 861 Bedford Road, Pleasantville, NY 10570
Phone: 914-773-3555
Fax: 914-773-3345
Contact: Martha Kelly, EdD, RN, Chairperson
Email: mkelly@pace.edu

GENERAL INFORMATION

Type of School: *4-Year College or University, Private (Independent)* • Accreditation: *Middle States Association of Colleges and Schools* • Total Enrollment: *13000*

PROGRAM INFORMATION

NLNAC Accreditation: *Not Reported* • CCNE Accreditation: *Yes*

NURSING STUDENT PROFILE

Total Nursing Enrollment: *112* • Full-Time Enrollment: *18* • Part-Time Enrollment: *94* • Female Enrollment: *105* • Male Enrollment: *7* • Total Graduates: *50*

FINANCES

Residential Annual Tuition: *Not Reported* • Non-Residential Annual Tuition: *Not Reported* • General Institutional Fees: *Not Reported* • Additional Nursing Fees: *Not Reported*

SAINT JOHN FISHER COLLEGE

Address: 3990 East Avenue, Rochester, NY 14618
Phone: 716-385-8395
Fax: 716-385-7311
Contact: Audrey Bopp, MS, RN, Director RN/BSN Program
Email: bopp@sjfc.edu

GENERAL INFORMATION

Type of School: *4-Year College or University, Private (Independent)* • Accreditation: *Middle States Association of Colleges and Schools* • Total Enrollment: *2175*

PROGRAM INFORMATION

NLNAC Accreditation: *Yes* • CCNE Accreditation:

NURSING STUDENT PROFILE

Total Nursing Enrollment: *31* • Full-Time Enrollment: *0* • Part-Time Enrollment: *31* • Female Enrollment: *27* • Male Enrollment: *4* • Total Graduates: *14*

FINANCES

Residential Annual Tuition: *$14,690* • Non-Residential Annual Tuition: *$14,690* • General Institutional Fees: *Not Reported* • Additional Nursing Fees: *Not Reported*

SAINT JOSEPH'S COLLEGE

Address: 245 Clinton Avenue, Brooklyn, NY 11205
Phone: 718-399-0185
Fax: 718-638-8839
Contact: Barbara L Sands, PhD, RN, Director
Email: bsands@sjcny.edu

GENERAL INFORMATION

Type of School: *4-Year College or University, Private (Independent)* • Accreditation: *Middle States Association of Colleges and Schools* • Total Enrollment: *4588*

PROGRAM INFORMATION

NLNAC Accreditation: *Yes* • CCNE Accreditation:

NURSING STUDENT PROFILE

Total Nursing Enrollment: *229* • Full-Time Enrollment: *12* • Part-Time Enrollment: *217* • Female Enrollment: *218* • Male Enrollment: *11* • Total Graduates: *42*

FINANCES

Residential Annual Tuition: *$4,875* • Non-Residential Annual Tuition: *$4,875* • General Institutional Fees: *$166* • Additional Nursing Fees: *$60*

SUNY HEALTH SCIENCE CENTER—BROOKLYN

Address: 450 Clackson Avenue, Box 22, Brooklyn, NY 11203
Phone: 718-370-7644
Fax: Not Reported
Contact: Yvonne Nathan, EdD, RN, RN Coordinator
Email: YNathan@netmail.HSCBklyn.edu

GENERAL INFORMATION

Type of School: *4-Year College or University, Public* • Accreditation: *Middle States Association of Colleges and Schools* • Total Enrollment: *1451*

PROGRAM INFORMATION

NLNAC Accreditation: *Yes* • CCNE Accreditation:

NURSING STUDENT PROFILE

Total Nursing Enrollment: *192* • Full-Time Enrollment: *19* • Part-Time Enrollment: *173* • Female Enrollment: *181* • Male Enrollment: *11* • Total Graduates: *94*

FINANCES

Residential Annual Tuition: *$3,400* • Non-Residential Annual Tuition: *$8,300* • General Institutional Fees: *Not Reported* • Additional Nursing Fees: *Not Reported*

GARDNER-WEBB UNIVERSITY

Address: PO Box 7268, Boiling Springs, NC 28017
Phone: 704-406-4364
Fax: 704-406-3919
Contact: Marcia M. Miller, PhD, RN, Co-Chair
Email: mlmiller@gardner-webb.edu

GENERAL INFORMATION

Type of School: *4-Year College or University, Private (Religious)* • Accreditation: *Southern Association of Colleges and Schools* • Total Enrollment: *3400*

PROGRAM INFORMATION

NLNAC Accreditation: *Yes* • CCNE Accreditation:

NURSING STUDENT PROFILE

Total Nursing Enrollment: *153* • Full-Time Enrollment: *45* • Part-Time Enrollment: *108* • Female Enrollment: *147* • Male Enrollment: *6* • Total Graduates: *49*

FINANCES

Residential Annual Tuition: *$3,780* • Non-Residential Annual Tuition: *$3,780* • General Institutional Fees: *$0* • Additional Nursing Fees: *$14*

TRI-COLLEGE UNIVERSITY NURSING CONSORTIUM

Address: Engineering and Technology 209, PO Box 5630, Fargo, ND 58105
Phone: 218-236-4696
Fax: 218-299-5990
Contact: Barbara Vellenga, PhD, RN, CNS, Director and Professor of RN/BSN track
Email: vellenga@mnstate.edu

GENERAL INFORMATION

Type of School: *Other* • Accreditation: *North Central Association of Colleges and Schools* • Total Enrollment: *Not Reported*

PROGRAM INFORMATION

NLNAC Accreditation: *Yes* • CCNE Accreditation:

NURSING STUDENT PROFILE

Total Nursing Enrollment: *99* • Full-Time Enrollment: *21* • Part-Time Enrollment: *78* • Female Enrollment: *95* • Male Enrollment: *4* • Total Graduates: *29*

FINANCES

Residential Annual Tuition: *$2,300* • Non-Residential Annual Tuition: *$5,156* • General Institutional Fees: *$511* • Additional Nursing Fees: *$0*

ASHLAND UNIVERSITY

Address: Department of Nursing, Ashland, OH 44805
Phone: 419-289-5244
Fax: 419-289-5989
Contact: Dorothy Stitzlein, PhD, RN, Chair
Email: dstitzle@ashland.edu

GENERAL INFORMATION

Type of School: *4-Year College or University, Private (Religious)* • Accreditation: *North Central Association of Colleges and Schools* • Total Enrollment: *5500*

PROGRAM INFORMATION

NLNAC Accreditation: *Yes* • CCNE Accreditation:

NURSING STUDENT PROFILE

Total Nursing Enrollment: *101* • Full-Time Enrollment: *1* • Part-Time Enrollment: *100* • Female Enrollment: *96* • Male Enrollment: *5* • Total Graduates: *35*

FINANCES

Residential Annual Tuition: *$5,400* • Non-Residential Annual Tuition: *Not Reported* • General Institutional Fees: *$300* • Additional Nursing Fees: *$170*

CASE WESTERN RESERVE UNIVERSITY

Address: 10900 Euclid Avenue, Cleveland, OH 44106
Phone: 216-368-5129
Fax: 216-368-5050
Contact: Marilyn B Lotas, PhD, RN, Director
Email: mjl25@po.cwru.edu

GENERAL INFORMATION

Type of School: *4-Year College or University, Private (Independent)* • Accreditation: *North Central Association of Colleges and Schools* • Total Enrollment: *Not Reported*

PROGRAM INFORMATION

NLNAC Accreditation: *Yes* • CCNE Accreditation:

NURSING STUDENT PROFILE

Total Nursing Enrollment: *5* • Full-Time Enrollment: *3* • Part-Time Enrollment: *2* • Female Enrollment: *5* • Male Enrollment: *0* • Total Graduates: *2*

FINANCES

Residential Annual Tuition: *$20,100* • Non-Residential Annual Tuition: *$20,100* • General Institutional Fees: *$115* • Additional Nursing Fees: *$150*

MIAMI UNIVERSITY

Address: 501 E. High Street, Oxford, OH 45056
Phone: 513-785-3280
Fax: 513-785-3284
Contact: Eugenia M Mills, PhD, RN, Chair
Email: millsem@muohio.edu

GENERAL INFORMATION

Type of School: *4-Year College or University, Public* •
Accreditation: *North Central Association of Colleges and Schools* • Total Enrollment: *19600*

PROGRAM INFORMATION

NLNAC Accreditation: *Yes* • CCNE Accreditation:

NURSING STUDENT PROFILE

Total Nursing Enrollment: *77* • Full-Time Enrollment: *21* •
Part-Time Enrollment: *56* • Female Enrollment: *73* • Male
Enrollment: *4* • Total Graduates: *33*

FINANCES

Residential Annual Tuition: *$4,137* • Non-Residential
Annual Tuition: *$11,811* • General Institutional Fees: *$166* •
Additional Nursing Fees: *$0*

OHIO UNIVERSITY

Address: 312 McCracken Hall, Athens, OH 45701
Phone: 740-593-4494
Fax: 740-593-0286
Contact: Emily Harman, MSN, MA, RN, Interim Director
Email: harman@ohio.edu

GENERAL INFORMATION

Type of School: *4-Year College or University, Public* •
Accreditation: *North Central Association of Colleges and Schools* • Total Enrollment: *17000*

PROGRAM INFORMATION

NLNAC Accreditation: *Yes* • CCNE Accreditation: *Yes*

NURSING STUDENT PROFILE

Total Nursing Enrollment: *130* • Full-Time Enrollment: *30* •
Part-Time Enrollment: *100* • Female Enrollment: *118* • Male
Enrollment: *12* • Total Graduates: *56*

FINANCES

Residential Annual Tuition: *$1,401* • Non-Residential
Annual Tuition: *$3,424* • General Institutional Fees: *$430* •
Additional Nursing Fees: *$0*

WALSH UNIVERSITY

Address: 2020 Easton Street, NW, North Canton, OH
          44720
Phone: 330-490-7250
Fax: 330-490-7206
Contact: Mary E Meeker, DNSc, RN, CNS, Chair
Email: mmeeker@walsh.edu

XAVIER UNIVERSITY

Address: 3800 Victory Parkway, Cincinnati, OH 45207
Phone: 513-745-3815
Fax: 513-745-1087
Contact: Susan M Schmidt, PhD, RN, COHN-S, CNS,
          Chair
Email: schmidts@xu.edu

GENERAL INFORMATION

Type of School: *4-Year College or University, Private
(Religious)* • Accreditation: *North Central Association of
Colleges and Schools* • Total Enrollment: *4500*

GENERAL INFORMATION

Type of School: *4-Year College or University, Private
(Religious)* • Accreditation: *North Central Association of
Colleges and Schools* • Total Enrollment: *6523*

PROGRAM INFORMATION

NLNAC Accreditation: *Yes* • CCNE Accreditation:

PROGRAM INFORMATION

NLNAC Accreditation: *Yes* • CCNE Accreditation:

NURSING STUDENT PROFILE

Total Nursing Enrollment: *29* • Full-Time Enrollment: *0* •
Part-Time Enrollment: *29* • Female Enrollment: *26* • Male
Enrollment: *3* • Total Graduates: *19*

NURSING STUDENT PROFILE

Total Nursing Enrollment: *22* • Full-Time Enrollment: *0* •
Part-Time Enrollment: *22* • Female Enrollment: *21* • Male
Enrollment: *1* • Total Graduates: *10*

FINANCES

Residential Annual Tuition: *$12,050* • Non-Residential
Annual Tuition: *$12,050* • General Institutional Fees: *Not
Reported* • Additional Nursing Fees: *Not Reported*

FINANCES

Residential Annual Tuition: *$9,090* • Non-Residential
Annual Tuition: *Not Reported* • General Institutional Fees:
$200 • Additional Nursing Fees: *$140*

Circle 144 on reader card   See in-depth profile for more information

BARTLESVILLE WESLEYAN COLLEGE

Address: 2201 Saline Lake Road, Bartlesville, OK 74006-6299
Phone: 918-335-6254
Fax: 918-335-6204
Contact: Pamela Giles, MS, RN, Director
Email: tpgiles@bwc.edu

GENERAL INFORMATION

Type of School: *4-Year College or University, Private (Religious)* • Accreditation: *North Central Association of Colleges and Schools* • Total Enrollment: *23*

PROGRAM INFORMATION

NLNAC Accreditation: *Not Reported* • CCNE Accreditation: *Yes*

NURSING STUDENT PROFILE

Total Nursing Enrollment: *156* • Full-Time Enrollment: *156* • Part-Time Enrollment: *0* • Female Enrollment: *151* • Male Enrollment: *5* • Total Graduates: *59*

FINANCES

Residential Annual Tuition: *Not Reported* • Non-Residential Annual Tuition: *Not Reported* • General Institutional Fees: *Not Reported* • Additional Nursing Fees: *$60*

NORTHEASTERN STATE UNIVERSITY

Address: 705 North Grand Avenue, Tahlequah, OK 74464-2300
Phone: 918-458-2087
Fax: 918-458-2349
Contact: Joyce A. Van Nostrand, PhD, RN, Chair
Email: vannostr@nsuok.edu

GENERAL INFORMATION

Type of School: *4-Year College or University, Public* • Accreditation: *North Central Association of Colleges and Schools* • Total Enrollment: *8100*

PROGRAM INFORMATION

NLNAC Accreditation: *Yes* • CCNE Accreditation:

NURSING STUDENT PROFILE

Total Nursing Enrollment: *27* • Full-Time Enrollment: *3* • Part-Time Enrollment: *24* • Female Enrollment: *26* • Male Enrollment: *1* • Total Graduates: *8*

FINANCES

Residential Annual Tuition: *$2,011* • Non-Residential Annual Tuition: *$4,804* • General Institutional Fees: *$5* • Additional Nursing Fees: *Not Reported*

OKLAHOMA PANHANDLE

Address: PO Box 430, Goodwell, OK 73939
Phone: 580-349-2611
Fax: 580-349-2302
Contact: Connie Carpenter, EdD, RN, Director
Email: conniec@opsu.edu

GENERAL INFORMATION

Type of School: *4-Year College or University, Public* •
Accreditation: *North Central Association of Colleges and
Schools* • Total Enrollment: *1175*

PROGRAM INFORMATION

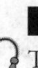

NLNAC Accreditation: *Yes* • CCNE Accreditation:

NURSING STUDENT PROFILE

Total Nursing Enrollment: *Not Reported* • Full-Time
Enrollment: *Not Reported* • Part-Time Enrollment: *Not
Reported* • Female Enrollment: *Not Reported* • Male
Enrollment: *Not Reported* • Total Graduates: *Not Reported*

FINANCES

Residential Annual Tuition: *$1,500* • Non-Residential
Annual Tuition: *$3,732* • General Institutional Fees: *$33* •
Additional Nursing Fees: *$100*

OREGON HEALTH SCIENCES UNIVERSITY

Address: 3181 Sam Tacks Park Road, Portland, OR 97201
Phone: 503-494-3558
Fax: 503-494-4350
Contact: Catherine Salveson, PhD, RN, Director of
Statewide RN-to-BS Program
Email: salveson@ohsu.edu

GENERAL INFORMATION

Type of School: *Other, Public* • Accreditation: *Northwestern
Association of Schools and Colleges* • Total Enrollment: *2679*

PROGRAM INFORMATION

NLNAC Accreditation: *Yes* • CCNE Accreditation: *Yes*

NURSING STUDENT PROFILE

Total Nursing Enrollment: *132* • Full-Time Enrollment: *42* •
Part-Time Enrollment: *90* • Female Enrollment: *111* • Male
Enrollment: *21* • Total Graduates: *47*

FINANCES

Residential Annual Tuition: *$2,175* • Non-Residential
Annual Tuition: *$2,175* • General Institutional Fees: *$868* •
Additional Nursing Fees: *Not Reported*

ALVERNIA COLLEGE

Address: 400 St. Bernardine Street, Reading, PA 19607
Phone: 610-796-8306
Fax: 610-796-8464
Contact: Karen S. Thacker, MSN, RN, CS, Assistant
Professor and Nursing Department Chair
Email: karen.thacker@alvernia.edu

GENERAL INFORMATION

Type of School: *4-Year College or University, Private (Religious)* • Accreditation: *Middle States Association of Colleges and Schools* • Total Enrollment: *1400*

PROGRAM INFORMATION

NLNAC Accreditation: *Not Reported* • CCNE Accreditation: *Yes*

NURSING STUDENT PROFILE

Total Nursing Enrollment: *24* • Full-Time Enrollment: *3* • Part-Time Enrollment: *21* • Female Enrollment: *23* • Male Enrollment: *1* • Total Graduates: *5*

FINANCES

Residential Annual Tuition: *$1,400* • Non-Residential Annual Tuition: *$1,400* • General Institutional Fees: *$500* • Additional Nursing Fees: *Not Reported*

BLOOMSBURG UNIVERSITY

Address: 400 East Second Street, Rm 3109, MCHS,
Bloomsburg, PA 17815
Phone: 570-389-4426
Fax: 570-389-5008
Contact: Christine Alichnie, PhD, RN, Chairperson and
Professor
Email: cmalic@husky.bloom.edu

GENERAL INFORMATION

Type of School: *4-Year College or University, Public* • Accreditation: *Middle States Association of Colleges and Schools* • Total Enrollment: *7916*

PROGRAM INFORMATION

NLNAC Accreditation: *Not Reported* • CCNE Accreditation:

NURSING STUDENT PROFILE

Total Nursing Enrollment: *12* • Full-Time Enrollment: *0* • Part-Time Enrollment: *12* • Female Enrollment: *11* • Male Enrollment: *1* • Total Graduates: *1*

FINANCES

Residential Annual Tuition: *$4,016* • Non-Residential Annual Tuition: *$10,040* • General Institutional Fees: *$976* • Additional Nursing Fees: *$0*

CALIFORNIA UNIVERSITY OF PENNSYLVANIA

Address: School of Nursing, California, PA 15419
Phone: 724-938-4130
Fax: 724-938-1612
Contact: Margaret Marcinek, EdD, RN, Chair,
          Department of Nursing
Email: marcinek@cup.edu

GENERAL INFORMATION

Type of School: *4-Year College or University, Public* •
Accreditation: *Middle States Association of Colleges and
Schools* • Total Enrollment: *5000*

PROGRAM INFORMATION

NLNAC Accreditation: *Yes* • CCNE Accreditation: *Yes*

NURSING STUDENT PROFILE

Total Nursing Enrollment: *81* • Full-Time Enrollment: *7* •
Part-Time Enrollment: *74* • Female Enrollment: *75* • Male
Enrollment: *6* • Total Graduates: *42*

FINANCES

Residential Annual Tuition: *$3,792* • Non-Residential
Annual Tuition: *$9,480* • General Institutional Fees: *$572* •
Additional Nursing Fees: *Not Reported*

CLARION UNIVERSITY

Address: 1801 West First Street, Oil City, PA 16301
Phone: 814-676-6591
Fax: 814-676-0251
Contact: T. Audean Duespohl, PhD, RN, Dean
Email: aduespohl@clarion.edu

GENERAL INFORMATION

Type of School: *4-Year College or University, Public* •
Accreditation: *Middle States Association of Colleges and
Schools* • Total Enrollment: *6192*

PROGRAM INFORMATION

NLNAC Accreditation: *Yes* • CCNE Accreditation:

NURSING STUDENT PROFILE

Total Nursing Enrollment: *96* • Full-Time Enrollment: *8* •
Part-Time Enrollment: *88* • Female Enrollment: *82* • Male
Enrollment: *14* • Total Graduates: *29*

FINANCES

Residential Annual Tuition: *$7,584* • Non-Residential
Annual Tuition: *$11,376* • General Institutional Fees: *$378* •
Additional Nursing Fees: *$100*

DUQUESNE UNIVERSITY

Address: 600 Fobes Avenue, Pittsburgh, PA 15282
Phone: 412-396-6383
Fax: 412-396-6346
Contact: Leah Cunningham, MNEd, RN, Director
Email: cunningh@duq.edu

GENERAL INFORMATION

Type of School: *4-Year College or University, Private (Religious)* • Accreditation: *Middle States Association of Colleges and Schools* • Total Enrollment: *9555*

PROGRAM INFORMATION

NLNAC Accreditation: *Yes* • CCNE Accreditation:

NURSING STUDENT PROFILE

Total Nursing Enrollment: *26* • Full-Time Enrollment: *1* • Part-Time Enrollment: *25* • Female Enrollment: *23* • Male Enrollment: *3* • Total Graduates: *6*

FINANCES

Residential Annual Tuition: *$15,169* • Non-Residential Annual Tuition: *$15,169* • General Institutional Fees: *$1,351* • Additional Nursing Fees: *$50*

EASTERN COLLEGE

Address: 1300 Eagle Road, St Davids, PA 19087
Phone: 610-341-5834
Fax: 610-225-5016
Contact: Margaret Lacey, PhD, RN, AOCN, Chair, Division of Nursing
Email: mlacey@eastern.edu

GENERAL INFORMATION

Type of School: *Not Reported* • Accreditation: *Middle States Association of Colleges and Schools* • Total Enrollment: *Not Reported*

PROGRAM INFORMATION

NLNAC Accreditation: *Yes* • CCNE Accreditation:

NURSING STUDENT PROFILE

Total Nursing Enrollment: *103* • Full-Time Enrollment: *2* • Part-Time Enrollment: *101* • Female Enrollment: *97* • Male Enrollment: *6* • Total Graduates: *26*

FINANCES

Residential Annual Tuition: *$8,160* • Non-Residential Annual Tuition: *$8,160* • General Institutional Fees: *Not Reported* • Additional Nursing Fees: *Not Reported*

GANNON UNIVERSITY

Address: 109 University Square, Erie, PA 16541
Phone: 814-871-5470
Fax: 814-871-5662
Contact: Patricia Marshall, MSN, RN, CCRN, Assistant
           Professor
Email: marshall001@gannon.edu

GENERAL INFORMATION

Type of School: *4-Year College or University, Private
(Religious)* • Accreditation: *Middle States Association of
Colleges and Schools* • Total Enrollment: *3400*

PROGRAM INFORMATION

NLNAC Accreditation: *Yes* • CCNE Accreditation:

NURSING STUDENT PROFILE

Total Nursing Enrollment: *50* • Full-Time Enrollment: *Not
Reported* • Part-Time Enrollment: *50* • Female Enrollment:
48 • Male Enrollment: *2* • Total Graduates: *8*

FINANCES

Residential Annual Tuition: *Not Reported* • Non-Residential
Annual Tuition: *Not Reported* • General Institutional Fees:
Not Reported • Additional Nursing Fees: *Not Reported*

IMMACULATA COLLEGE

Address: School of Nursing, Immaculata, PA 19345
Phone: 610-647-4400
Fax: Not Reported
Contact: Janice Cranmer, EdD, RN, Chairperson
Email: jcranmer@immaculata.edu

GENERAL INFORMATION

Type of School: *4-Year College or University, Private
(Religious)* • Accreditation: *Middle States Association of
Colleges and Schools* • Total Enrollment: *Not Reported*

PROGRAM INFORMATION

NLNAC Accreditation: *Yes* • CCNE Accreditation:

NURSING STUDENT PROFILE

Total Nursing Enrollment: *375* • Full-Time Enrollment: *0* •
Part-Time Enrollment: *375* • Female Enrollment: *300* • Male
Enrollment: *75* • Total Graduates: *Not Reported*

FINANCES

Residential Annual Tuition: *$6,720* • Non-Residential
Annual Tuition: *$6,720* • General Institutional Fees: *Not
Reported* • Additional Nursing Fees: *Not Reported*

KUTZTOWN UNIVERSITY

Address: 219 Beekey Building, Kutztown, PA 19530
Phone: 610-683-4328
Fax: 610-683-4708
Contact: Kimberly Johnston, EdD, RNC, Chairperson
Email: Kjohnston@kutztown.edu

GENERAL INFORMATION

Type of School: *4-Year College or University, Public* •
Accreditation: *Middle States Association of Colleges and Schools* • Total Enrollment: *7700*

PROGRAM INFORMATION

NLNAC Accreditation: *Yes* • CCNE Accreditation:

NURSING STUDENT PROFILE

Total Nursing Enrollment: *197* • Full-Time Enrollment: *7* •
Part-Time Enrollment: *190* • Female Enrollment: *183* • Male
Enrollment: *14* • Total Graduates: *34*

FINANCES

Residential Annual Tuition: *$2,008* • Non-Residential
Annual Tuition: *$5,020* • General Institutional Fees: *$544* •
Additional Nursing Fees: *$100*

LA ROCHE COLLEGE

Address: 9000 Babcock Blvd, Pittsburgh, PA 15237
Phone: 412-536-1166
Fax: 412-536-1175
Contact: Diane D Cox, PhD, RN, Chair, Division of
Nursing
Email: coxd1@laroche.edu

GENERAL INFORMATION

Type of School: *4-Year College or University, Private
(Religious)* • Accreditation: *Middle States Association of
Colleges and Schools* • Total Enrollment: *1875*

PROGRAM INFORMATION

NLNAC Accreditation: *Yes* • CCNE Accreditation:

NURSING STUDENT PROFILE

Total Nursing Enrollment: *87* • Full-Time Enrollment: *4* •
Part-Time Enrollment: *83* • Female Enrollment: *82* • Male
Enrollment: *5* • Total Graduates: *14*

FINANCES

Residential Annual Tuition: *$11,600* • Non-Residential
Annual Tuition: *$11,600* • General Institutional Fees: *$100* •
Additional Nursing Fees: *Not Reported*

LA SALLE UNIVERSITY

Address: 1900 West Olney Avenue, Philadelphia, PA 19141
Phone: 215-951-1902
Fax: 215-951-1896
Contact: Joanne Serembus, EdD, RN, CCRN, Director and Assistant Professor
Email: serembus@lasalle.edu

GENERAL INFORMATION

Type of School: *4-Year College or University, Private (Religious)* • Accreditation: *Middle States Association of Colleges and Schools* • Total Enrollment: *Not Reported*

PROGRAM INFORMATION

NLNAC Accreditation: *Yes* • CCNE Accreditation:

NURSING STUDENT PROFILE

Total Nursing Enrollment: *157* • Full-Time Enrollment: *3* • Part-Time Enrollment: *154* • Female Enrollment: *141* • Male Enrollment: *16* • Total Graduates: *43*

FINANCES

Residential Annual Tuition: *$7,800* • Non-Residential Annual Tuition: *$7,800* • General Institutional Fees: *$40* • Additional Nursing Fees: *$40*

MCP HAHNEMANN UNIVERSITY

Address: 345 North 15th Street, Mail Stop 501, Philadelphia, PA 19102
Phone: 215-762-7483
Fax: 215-762-1259
Contact: Mary Ellen Smith, MSN, RN, Program Director
Email: ms55@drexel.edu

GENERAL INFORMATION

Type of School: *4-Year College or University, Private (Independent)* • Accreditation: *Middle States Association of Colleges and Schools* • Total Enrollment: *3000*

PROGRAM INFORMATION

NLNAC Accreditation: *Yes* • CCNE Accreditation: *Yes*

NURSING STUDENT PROFILE

Total Nursing Enrollment: *123* • Full-Time Enrollment: *0* • Part-Time Enrollment: *123* • Female Enrollment: *104* • Male Enrollment: *19* • Total Graduates: *45*

FINANCES

Residential Annual Tuition: *$21,400* • Non-Residential Annual Tuition: *$21,400* • General Institutional Fees: *Not Reported* • Additional Nursing Fees: *Not Reported*

MILLERSVILLE UNIVERSITY

Address: PO Box 1002, Millersville, PA 17551
Phone: 717-871-2183
Fax: 717-871-4877
Contact: Ruth E. Davis, EdD, RNC, CRNP, NP-C,
            Chairperson and Associate Professor
Email: ruth.davis@millersville.edu

GENERAL INFORMATION

Type of School: *4-Year College or University, Public* •
Accreditation: *Middle States Association of Colleges and
Schools* • Total Enrollment: *7378*

PROGRAM INFORMATION

NLNAC Accreditation: *Yes* • CCNE Accreditation:

NURSING STUDENT PROFILE

Total Nursing Enrollment: *60* • Full-Time Enrollment: *15* •
Part-Time Enrollment: *45* • Female Enrollment: *55* • Male
Enrollment: *5* • Total Graduates: *13*

FINANCES

Residential Annual Tuition: *$5,053* • Non-Residential
Annual Tuition: *$11,077* • General Institutional Fees: *Not
Reported* • Additional Nursing Fees: *Not Reported*

MOUNT ALOYSIUS COLLEGE

Address: 7373 Admiral Peary Highway, Cresson, PA
            16630
Phone: 814-886-6401
Fax: 814-886-4906
Contact: Cheryl A. Webb, PhD, RN, CS, Chariperson
Email: cwebb@mtaloy.edu

GENERAL INFORMATION

Type of School: *4-Year College or University, Private
(Religious)* • Accreditation: *Middle States Association of
Colleges and Schools* • Total Enrollment: *900*

PROGRAM INFORMATION

NLNAC Accreditation: *Yes* • CCNE Accreditation:

NURSING STUDENT PROFILE

Total Nursing Enrollment: *45* • Full-Time Enrollment: *6* •
Part-Time Enrollment: *39* • Female Enrollment: *44* • Male
Enrollment: *1* • Total Graduates: *10*

FINANCES

Residential Annual Tuition: *$12,430* • Non-Residential
Annual Tuition: *$12,430* • General Institutional Fees: *$100* •
Additional Nursing Fees: *$0*

PENNSYLVANIA COLLEGE OF TECHNOLOGY

Address: One College Avenue, Williamsport, PA 17701
Phone: 570-327-4525
Fax: 570-321-5556
Contact: Pamela L. Starcher, PhD(c), MN, RN, Director
Email: pstarche@pct.edu

GENERAL INFORMATION

Type of School: *4-Year College or University, Public* •
Accreditation: *Middle States Association of Colleges and Schools* • Total Enrollment: *5320*

PROGRAM INFORMATION

NLNAC Accreditation: *Not Reported* • CCNE Accreditation:

NURSING STUDENT PROFILE

Total Nursing Enrollment: *52* • Full-Time Enrollment: *2* • Part-Time Enrollment: *50* • Female Enrollment: *50* • Male Enrollment: *2* • Total Graduates: *11*

FINANCES

Residential Annual Tuition: *$5,928* • Non-Residential Annual Tuition: *$7,008* • General Institutional Fees: *Not Reported* • Additional Nursing Fees: *$17*

SLIPPERY ROCK UNIVERSITY

Address: Behavioral Science Building 119, Slippery Rock, PA 16057
Phone: 724-738-2326
Fax: 724-728-2881
Contact: Kit Kellinger, PhD, CRNP, Chairperson
Email: kathleen.kellinger@sru.edu

GENERAL INFORMATION

Type of School: *4-Year College or University, Public* •
Accreditation: *Middle States Association of Colleges and Schools* • Total Enrollment: *7000*

PROGRAM INFORMATION

NLNAC Accreditation: *Yes* • CCNE Accreditation:

NURSING STUDENT PROFILE

Total Nursing Enrollment: *75* • Full-Time Enrollment: *12* • Part-Time Enrollment: *63* • Female Enrollment: *3* • Male Enrollment: *72* • Total Graduates: *24*

FINANCES

Residential Annual Tuition: *$3,618* • Non-Residential Annual Tuition: *$9,046* • General Institutional Fees: *Not Reported* • Additional Nursing Fees: *Not Reported*

UNIVERSITY OF PITTSBURGH

Address: 300 Campus Dr, Bradford, PA 16701
Phone: 814-362-7640
Fax: 814-362-0919
Contact: Lisa M Fiorentino, PhD, RN, Director
Email: lmfl+@pitt.edu

GENERAL INFORMATION

Type of School: *4-Year College or University, Public* • Accreditation: *Middle States Association of Colleges and Schools* • Total Enrollment: *25461*

PROGRAM INFORMATION

NLNAC Accreditation: *Yes* • CCNE Accreditation:

NURSING STUDENT PROFILE

Total Nursing Enrollment: *7* • Full-Time Enrollment: *3* • Part-Time Enrollment: *4* • Female Enrollment: *6* • Male Enrollment: *1* • Total Graduates: *6*

FINANCES

Residential Annual Tuition: *$8,264* • Non-Residential Annual Tuition: *$18,026* • General Institutional Fees: *$227* • Additional Nursing Fees: *$11*

VILLANOVA UNIVERSITY

Address: 800 Lancaster Avenue, Villanova, PA 19085
Phone: 610-519-6832
Fax: 610-519-7650
Contact: Joyce S. Willens, PhD, RN, Coordinator
Email: joyce.willens@villanova.edu

GENERAL INFORMATION

Type of School: *Not Reported* • Accreditation: *Middle States Association of Colleges and Schools* • Total Enrollment: *Not Reported*

PROGRAM INFORMATION

NLNAC Accreditation: *Yes* • CCNE Accreditation: *Yes*

NURSING STUDENT PROFILE

Total Nursing Enrollment: *32* • Full-Time Enrollment: *22* • Part-Time Enrollment: *10* • Female Enrollment: *27* • Male Enrollment: *5* • Total Graduates: *30*

FINANCES

Residential Annual Tuition: *$26,300* • Non-Residential Annual Tuition: *$26,300* • General Institutional Fees: *$300* • Additional Nursing Fees: *$440*

WIDENER UNIVERSITY

Address: One University Place, Chester, PA 19013
Phone: 610-499-4209
Fax: 610-499-4216
Contact: Ann Birney, MSN, RN, Director of Special
Programs
Email: ann.m.birney@widener.edu

GENERAL INFORMATION

Type of School: *Not Reported* • Accreditation: *Middle States Association of Colleges and Schools* • Total Enrollment: *Not Reported*

PROGRAM INFORMATION

NLNAC Accreditation: *Yes* • CCNE Accreditation:

NURSING STUDENT PROFILE

Total Nursing Enrollment: *80* • Full-Time Enrollment: *0* • Part-Time Enrollment: *80* • Female Enrollment: *74* • Male Enrollment: *6* • Total Graduates: *27*

FINANCES

Residential Annual Tuition: *$21,400* • Non-Residential Annual Tuition: *$21,400* • General Institutional Fees: *$100* • Additional Nursing Fees: *Not Reported*

YORK COLLEGE OF PENNSYLVANIA

Address: Country Club Road, York, PA 17405-7199
Phone: 717-815-1355
Fax: 717-849-1651
Contact: Marian Condon, EdD, RN, Assistant Professor
Email: mcondon@ycp.edu

GENERAL INFORMATION

Type of School: *Not Reported* • Accreditation: *Middle States Association of Colleges and Schools* • Total Enrollment: *Not Reported*

PROGRAM INFORMATION

NLNAC Accreditation: *Yes* • CCNE Accreditation: *Yes*

NURSING STUDENT PROFILE

Total Nursing Enrollment: *58* • Full-Time Enrollment: *0* • Part-Time Enrollment: *58* • Female Enrollment: *54* • Male Enrollment: *4* • Total Graduates: *12*

FINANCES

Residential Annual Tuition: *$7,000* • Non-Residential Annual Tuition: *$7,000* • General Institutional Fees: *$422* • Additional Nursing Fees: *$0*

UNIVERSITY OF SOUTH CAROLINA—AIKEN

Address: 171 University Parkway, Aiken, SC 29801
Phone: 803-641-3508
Fax: 803-641-3725
Contact: Patricia R. Cook, PhD, RN, Assistant Head, BSN Program
Email: pattic@aiken.sc.edu

GENERAL INFORMATION

Type of School: *4-Year College or University, Public* •
Accreditation: *Southern Association of Colleges and Schools* •
Total Enrollment: *Not Reported*

PROGRAM INFORMATION

NLNAC Accreditation: *Yes* • CCNE Accreditation:

NURSING STUDENT PROFILE

Total Nursing Enrollment: *96* • Full-Time Enrollment: *90* •
Part-Time Enrollment: *6* • Female Enrollment: *90* • Male
Enrollment: *6* • Total Graduates: *45*

FINANCES

Residential Annual Tuition: *$3,638* • Non-Residential
Annual Tuition: *$8,164* • General Institutional Fees: *$140* •
Additional Nursing Fees: *$200*

UNIVERSITY OF SOUTH CAROLINA—COLUMBIA

Address: 1601 Greene Street, Columbia, SC 29208
Phone: 803-777-3862
Fax: 803-777-2027
Contact: Mary Ann Parsons, PhD, RN, Dean
Email: maryann.parsons@sc.edu

GENERAL INFORMATION

Type of School: *4-Year College or University, Public* •
Accreditation: *Southern Association of Colleges and Schools* •
Total Enrollment: *Not Reported*

PROGRAM INFORMATION

NLNAC Accreditation: *Not Reported* • CCNE Accreditation: *Yes*

NURSING STUDENT PROFILE

Total Nursing Enrollment: *42* • Full-Time Enrollment: *8* •
Part-Time Enrollment: *34* • Female Enrollment: *37* • Male
Enrollment: *5* • Total Graduates: *23*

FINANCES

Residential Annual Tuition: *$5,040* • Non-Residential
Annual Tuition: *$12,764* • General Institutional Fees: *$100* •
Additional Nursing Fees: *$16*

HURON UNIVERSITY

Address: 333 9th St. S.W., Huron, SD 57350
Phone: 605-352-8721
Fax: 605-352-7421
Contact: Ella M. Brooks, PhD, RN, Dean
Email: ebrooks@huron.edu

GENERAL INFORMATION

Type of School: *4-Year College or University, Private (Independent)* • Accreditation: *North Central Association of Colleges and Schools* • Total Enrollment: *598*

PROGRAM INFORMATION

NLNAC Accreditation: *Not Reported* • CCNE Accreditation:

NURSING STUDENT PROFILE

Total Nursing Enrollment: *12* • Full-Time Enrollment: *5* • Part-Time Enrollment: *7* • Female Enrollment: *9* • Male Enrollment: *3* • Total Graduates: *3*

FINANCES

Residential Annual Tuition: *$4,800* • Non-Residential Annual Tuition: *$4,800* • General Institutional Fees: *$400* • Additional Nursing Fees: *$200*

MOUNT MARTY COLLEGE

Address: 1105 W. 8th Street, Yankton, SD 57078
Phone: 605-668-1594
Fax: 605-668-1607
Contact: Janice E. Stephens, PhD, RN, Division of Nursing Chair
Email: jstephens@mtmc.edu

GENERAL INFORMATION

Type of School: *4-Year College or University, Private (Religious)* • Accreditation: *North Central Association of Colleges and Schools* • Total Enrollment: *567*

PROGRAM INFORMATION

NLNAC Accreditation: *Yes* • CCNE Accreditation:

NURSING STUDENT PROFILE

Total Nursing Enrollment: *9* • Full-Time Enrollment: *0* • Part-Time Enrollment: *9* • Female Enrollment: *7* • Male Enrollment: *2* • Total Graduates: *1*

FINANCES

Residential Annual Tuition: *$12,506* • Non-Residential Annual Tuition: *$12,506* • General Institutional Fees: *$1,720* • Additional Nursing Fees: *$257*

PRESENTATION COLLEGE

Address: 1500 North Main St., Aberdeen, SD 57401
Phone: 605-229-8473
Fax: 605-229-8489
Contact: Janice S. Williams, ND, MSN, CS, CDE, Chair
           and Associate Professor
Email: janicesw@presentation.edu

GENERAL INFORMATION

Type of School: *4-Year College or University, Private (Religious)* • Accreditation: *North Central Association of Colleges and Schools* • Total Enrollment: *615*

PROGRAM INFORMATION

NLNAC Accreditation: *Yes* • CCNE Accreditation:

NURSING STUDENT PROFILE

Total Nursing Enrollment: *8* • Full-Time Enrollment: *5* • Part-Time Enrollment: *3* • Female Enrollment: *8* • Male Enrollment: *0* • Total Graduates: *6*

FINANCES

Residential Annual Tuition: *$8,000* • Non-Residential Annual Tuition: *$8,000* • General Institutional Fees: *$110* • Additional Nursing Fees: *$75*

AQUINAS COLLEGE

Address: 4210 Harding Avenue, Nashville, TN 37205
Phone: 615-222-4038
Fax: 615-222-4008
Contact: Linda W Watlington, MSN, RN, Director
Email: watlingtonl@aquinas-tn.edu

GENERAL INFORMATION

Type of School: *4-Year College or University, Private (Religious)* • Accreditation: *Southern Association of Colleges and Schools* • Total Enrollment: *Not Reported*

PROGRAM INFORMATION

NLNAC Accreditation: *Not Reported* • CCNE Accreditation:

NURSING STUDENT PROFILE

Total Nursing Enrollment: *22* • Full-Time Enrollment: *0* • Part-Time Enrollment: *22* • Female Enrollment: *22* • Male Enrollment: *0* • Total Graduates: *8*

FINANCES

Residential Annual Tuition: *$7,800* • Non-Residential Annual Tuition: *$7,800* • General Institutional Fees: *$100* • Additional Nursing Fees: *$40*

KING COLLEGE

Address: 1350 King College Road, Bristol, TN 37620
Phone: 423-652-4748
Fax: 423-652-4833
Contact: Johanne A. Quinn, PhD, RN, HNC, Professor
and Director
Email: jaquinn@king.edu

GENERAL INFORMATION

Type of School: *4-Year College or University, Private (Religious)* • Accreditation: *Southern Association of Colleges and Schools* • Total Enrollment: *Not Reported*

PROGRAM INFORMATION

NLNAC Accreditation: *Not Reported* • CCNE Accreditation: *Yes*

NURSING STUDENT PROFILE

Total Nursing Enrollment: *9* • Full-Time Enrollment: *0* • Part-Time Enrollment: *9* • Female Enrollment: *9* • Male Enrollment: *0* • Total Graduates: *1*

FINANCES

Residential Annual Tuition: *$12,390* • Non-Residential Annual Tuition: *$12,390* • General Institutional Fees: *$950* • Additional Nursing Fees: *$350*

LINCOLN MEMORIAL UNIVERSITY

Address: Cumberland Gap Parkway, Harrogate, TN
37752-0901
Phone: 423-869-6319
Fax: 423-869-6244
Contact: Mary Anne Madrcin-Talbott, PhD, RN, Chair
Email: DrTalbott@aol.com

GENERAL INFORMATION

Type of School: *4-Year College or University, Private (Independent)* • Accreditation: *Southern Association of Colleges and Schools* • Total Enrollment: *1753*

PROGRAM INFORMATION

NLNAC Accreditation: *Yes* • CCNE Accreditation:

NURSING STUDENT PROFILE

Total Nursing Enrollment: *7* • Full-Time Enrollment: *5* • Part-Time Enrollment: *2* • Female Enrollment: *4* • Male Enrollment: *3* • Total Graduates: *8*

FINANCES

Residential Annual Tuition: *$5,400* • Non-Residential Annual Tuition: *$5,400* • General Institutional Fees: *$30* • Additional Nursing Fees: *$0*

SOUTHERN ADVENTIST UNIVERSITY

Address: PO Box 370, Collegadale, TN 37315
Phone: 423-238-2942
Fax: 423-238-3004
Contact: L. Phil Hunt, EdD, RN, Dean and Professor
Email: phunt@southern.edu

UNIVERSITY OF TENNESSEE—CHATTANOOGA

Address: 615 McCallie Avenue, Chattanooga, TN 37403
Phone: 423-755-4724
Fax: 423-755-4668
Contact: Dana Hames Wertenberger, PhD, RN, Director and Professor
Email: dana-wertenberger@utc.edu

GENERAL INFORMATION

Type of School: *4-Year College or University, Private (Religious)* • Accreditation: *Southern Association of Colleges and Schools* • Total Enrollment: *1900*

GENERAL INFORMATION

Type of School: *4-Year College or University, Public* • Accreditation: *Southern Association of Colleges and Schools* • Total Enrollment: *8485*

PROGRAM INFORMATION

NLNAC Accreditation: *Yes* • CCNE Accreditation:

PROGRAM INFORMATION

NLNAC Accreditation: *Not Reported* • CCNE Accreditation: *Yes*|

NURSING STUDENT PROFILE

Total Nursing Enrollment: *67* • Full-Time Enrollment: *29* • Part-Time Enrollment: *38* • Female Enrollment: *53* • Male Enrollment: *14* • Total Graduates: *35*

NURSING STUDENT PROFILE

Total Nursing Enrollment: *46* • Full-Time Enrollment: *0* • Part-Time Enrollment: *46* • Female Enrollment: *43* • Male Enrollment: *3* • Total Graduates: *14*

FINANCES

Residential Annual Tuition: *$11,250* • Non-Residential Annual Tuition: *$11,250* • General Institutional Fees: *$360* • Additional Nursing Fees: *$496*

FINANCES

Residential Annual Tuition: *$2,698* • Non-Residential Annual Tuition: *$9,228* • General Institutional Fees: *$538* • Additional Nursing Fees: *$42*

ACU-HSU-MCM CONSORTIUM

Address: 2149 Hickory, Abeline, TX 79601
Phone: 915-672-2441
Fax: 915-672-5026
Contact: Cecilia Tiller, DSN, RNC, WHNP, Dean and
          Professor
Email: ctiller@aisn.hsutx.edu

GENERAL INFORMATION

Type of School: *Not Reported* • Accreditation: *Southern Association of Colleges and Schools* • Total Enrollment: *Not Reported*

PROGRAM INFORMATION

NLNAC Accreditation: *Not Reported* • CCNE Accreditation: *Yes*

NURSING STUDENT PROFILE

Total Nursing Enrollment: *Not Reported* • Full-Time Enrollment: *Not Reported* • Part-Time Enrollment: *Not Reported* • Female Enrollment: *Not Reported* • Male Enrollment: *Not Reported* • Total Graduates: *3*

FINANCES

Residential Annual Tuition: *$5,490* • Non-Residential Annual Tuition: *$5,490* • General Institutional Fees: *$150* • Additional Nursing Fees: *$300*

ANGELO STATE UNIVERSITY

Address: 2601 W. Avenue North, San Angelo, TX 76904
Phone: 915-942-2224
Fax: 915-942-2236
Contact: Edward L. Russell, PhD, RNCS, CNS, Program
          Director and Head of the Department of
          Nursing
Email: edward.russell@angelo.edu

GENERAL INFORMATION

Type of School: *4-Year College or University, Public* • Accreditation: *Southern Association of Colleges and Schools* • Total Enrollment: *6000*

PROGRAM INFORMATION

NLNAC Accreditation: *Yes* • CCNE Accreditation:

NURSING STUDENT PROFILE

Total Nursing Enrollment: *78* • Full-Time Enrollment: *10* • Part-Time Enrollment: *68* • Female Enrollment: *66* • Male Enrollment: *12* • Total Graduates: *17*

FINANCES

Residential Annual Tuition: *$1,043* • Non-Residential Annual Tuition: *$3,623* • General Institutional Fees: *$563* • Additional Nursing Fees: *$30*

TEXAS A&M INTERNATIONAL UNIVERSITY

Address:　5201 University Blvd, Laredo, TX 78041
Phone:　956-326-2450
Fax:　956-326-2449
Contact:　Susan Scoville Baker, PhD, RN, CS, Director
Email:　sbaker@tamiu.edu

THE UNIVERSITY OF TEXAS— BROWNSVILLE AND TEXAS SOUTHMOST COLLEGE

Address:　80 Fort Brown, Brownsville, TX 78520
Phone:　956-544-8270
Fax:　956-544-8881
Contact:　Katherine B Dougherty, EdD, RN, Director
Email:　kdougherty@utbl.utb.edu

GENERAL INFORMATION

Type of School: *4-Year College or University, Public* •
Accreditation: *Southern Association of Colleges and Schools* •
Total Enrollment: *3200*

GENERAL INFORMATION

Type of School: *Not Reported, Not Reported* • Accreditation: *Not Reported* • Total Enrollment: *Not Reported*

PROGRAM INFORMATION

NLNAC Accreditation: *Yes* • CCNE Accreditation:

PROGRAM INFORMATION

NLNAC Accreditation: *Yes* • CCNE Accreditation:

NURSING STUDENT PROFILE

Total Nursing Enrollment: *42* • Full-Time Enrollment: *3* •
Part-Time Enrollment: *39* • Female Enrollment: *22* • Male
Enrollment: *20* • Total Graduates: *15*

NURSING STUDENT PROFILE

Total Nursing Enrollment: *26* • Full-Time Enrollment: *19* •
Part-Time Enrollment: *7* • Female Enrollment: *21* • Male
Enrollment: *5* • Total Graduates: *18*

FINANCES

Residential Annual Tuition: *$1,860* • Non-Residential
Annual Tuition: *$8,310* • General Institutional Fees:
$1,094 • Additional Nursing Fees: *Not Reported*

FINANCES

Residential Annual Tuition: *$1,876* • Non-Residential
Annual Tuition: *$7,036* • General Institutional Fees: *Not Reported* • Additional Nursing Fees: *Not Reported*

WEBER STATE UNIVERSITY

Address: 3903 University Circle, Ogden, UT 84408
Phone: 801-626-6833
Fax: 801-626-6397
Contact: Evelyn Draper, MA, RN, Level Manager
Email: edraper@weber.edu

GENERAL INFORMATION

Type of School: *4-Year College or University, Public* •
Accreditation: *Northwestern Association of Schools and
Colleges* • Total Enrollment: *Not Reported*

PROGRAM INFORMATION

NLNAC Accreditation: *Yes* • CCNE Accreditation:

NURSING STUDENT PROFILE

Total Nursing Enrollment: *177* • Full-Time Enrollment:
171 • Part-Time Enrollment: *6* • Female Enrollment: *150* •
Male Enrollment: *27* • Total Graduates: *88*

FINANCES

Residential Annual Tuition: *$2,118* • Non-Residential
Annual Tuition: *$6,294* • General Institutional Fees: *Not
Reported* • Additional Nursing Fees: *$70*

NORWICH UNIVERSITY

Address: 158 Harmon Drive, Northfield, VT 05663
Phone: 802-485-2609
Fax: 802-485-2607
Contact: Marilyn Rinker, RN, MSN, OCN, Program
           Chair
Email: mrinker@norwich.edu

GENERAL INFORMATION

Type of School: *Not Reported, Private (Independent)* •
Accreditation: *New England Association of Schools and
Colleges* • Total Enrollment: *Not Reported*

PROGRAM INFORMATION

NLNAC Accreditation: *Yes* • CCNE Accreditation:

NURSING STUDENT PROFILE

Total Nursing Enrollment: *23* • Full-Time Enrollment: *0* •
Part-Time Enrollment: *23* • Female Enrollment: *22* • Male
Enrollment: *1* • Total Graduates: *5*

FINANCES

Residential Annual Tuition: *$8,355* • Non-Residential
Annual Tuition: *$8,355* • General Institutional Fees: *$255* •
Additional Nursing Fees: *$0*

SOUTHERN VERMONT COLLEGE

Address: 982 Mansion, Bennington, VT 05201
Phone: 802-447-4661
Fax: 802-447-4695
Contact: Holly Evans Madison, RN, MSN, Nursing Division Chairperson
Email: hmadison@svc.edu

GENERAL INFORMATION

Type of School: *4-Year College or University, Private (Independent)* • Accreditation: *New England Association of Schools and Colleges* • Total Enrollment: *Not Reported*

PROGRAM INFORMATION

NLNAC Accreditation: *Yes* • CCNE Accreditation:

NURSING STUDENT PROFILE

Total Nursing Enrollment: *22* • Full-Time Enrollment: *0* • Part-Time Enrollment: *22* • Female Enrollment: *21* • Male Enrollment: *1* • Total Graduates: *5*

FINANCES

Residential Annual Tuition: *$10,999* • Non-Residential Annual Tuition: *Not Reported* • General Institutional Fees: *Not Reported* • Additional Nursing Fees: *$190*

FAIRMONT STATE COLLEGE

Address: 1201 Locust Avenue, Fairmont, VA 26554
Phone: 304-367-4767
Fax: 304-367-4268
Contact: Deborah M Kisner, EdD, RN, Chairperson
Email: dkisner@mail.fscwv.edu

GENERAL INFORMATION

Type of School: *Not Reported, Not Reported* • Accreditation: *Not Reported* • Total Enrollment: *Not Reported*

PROGRAM INFORMATION

NLNAC Accreditation: *Not Reported* • CCNE Accreditation: *Yes*

NURSING STUDENT PROFILE

Total Nursing Enrollment: *49* • Full-Time Enrollment: *11* • Part-Time Enrollment: *38* • Female Enrollment: *42* • Male Enrollment: *7* • Total Graduates: *18*

FINANCES

Residential Annual Tuition: *$2,408* • Non-Residential Annual Tuition: *$5,672* • General Institutional Fees: *$200* • Additional Nursing Fees: *$200*

MARYMOUNT UNIVERSITY

Address: 2807 North Glebe Road, Arlington, VA 22207
Phone: 703-526-6881
Fax: 703-284-3819
Contact: Rajamma V George, EdD, RNC, Chair
Email: rajamma.george@marymount.edu

GENERAL INFORMATION

Type of School: *4-Year College or University, Private (Religious)* • Accreditation: *Southern Association of Colleges and Schools* • Total Enrollment: *3600*

PROGRAM INFORMATION

NLNAC Accreditation: *Yes* • CCNE Accreditation:

NURSING STUDENT PROFILE

Total Nursing Enrollment: *47* • Full-Time Enrollment: *17* • Part-Time Enrollment: *30* • Female Enrollment: *37* • Male Enrollment: *10* • Total Graduates: *26*

FINANCES

Residential Annual Tuition: *$14,850* • Non-Residential Annual Tuition: *Not Reported* • General Institutional Fees: *$400* • Additional Nursing Fees: *$115*

UNIVERSITY OF VIRGINIA'S-COLLEGE AT WISE

Address: One College Avenue, Wise, VA 24293
Phone: 540-328-0275
Fax: 540-328-0247
Contact: Kathleen W. Huttlinger, PhD, RN, Professor and
            Chairperson
Email: kwh3c@uvawise.edu

GENERAL INFORMATION

Type of School: *4-Year College or University, Public* • Accreditation: *Southern Association of Colleges and Schools* • Total Enrollment: *1490*

PROGRAM INFORMATION

NLNAC Accreditation: *Not Reported* • CCNE Accreditation:

NURSING STUDENT PROFILE

Total Nursing Enrollment: *62* • Full-Time Enrollment: *Not Reported* • Part-Time Enrollment: *Not Reported* • Female Enrollment: *Not Reported* • Male Enrollment: *Not Reported* • Total Graduates: *Not Reported*

FINANCES

Residential Annual Tuition: *$3,192* • Non-Residential Annual Tuition: *$9,286* • General Institutional Fees: *$1,262* • Additional Nursing Fees: *Not Reported*

VIRGINIA COMMONWEALTH UNIVERSITY

Address: 910 W. Franklin, Richmond, VA 23284
Phone: 804-828-3968
Fax: 804-828-7743
Contact: Janet B Younger, PhD, RN, CPNP, Associate Dean and Professor
Email: younger@hsc.vcu.edu

GENERAL INFORMATION

Type of School: *4-Year College or University, Public* •
Accreditation: *Southern Association of Colleges and Schools* •
Total Enrollment: *25000*

PROGRAM INFORMATION

NLNAC Accreditation: *Yes* • CCNE Accreditation:

NURSING STUDENT PROFILE

Total Nursing Enrollment: *292* • Full-Time Enrollment: *8* •
Part-Time Enrollment: *284* • Female Enrollment: *283* • Male
Enrollment: *9* • Total Graduates: *74*

FINANCES

Residential Annual Tuition: *$2,494* • Non-Residential
Annual Tuition: *$12,672* • General Institutional Fees: *$967* •
Additional Nursing Fees: *Not Reported*

BLUEFIELD STATE COLLEGE

Address: 219 Rock St., Bluefield, WV 24701
Phone: 304-327-4139
Fax: 304-327-4219
Contact: Beth Pritchett, MN, RN, CS, Director
Email: BPritchett@bluefield.wvnet.edu

GENERAL INFORMATION

Type of School: *4-Year College or University, Public* •
Accreditation: *North Central Association of Colleges and Schools* • Total Enrollment: *2648*

PROGRAM INFORMATION

NLNAC Accreditation: *Yes* • CCNE Accreditation: *Yes*

NURSING STUDENT PROFILE

Total Nursing Enrollment: *54* • Full-Time Enrollment: *50* •
Part-Time Enrollment: *4* • Female Enrollment: *52* • Male
Enrollment: *2* • Total Graduates: *16*

FINANCES

Residential Annual Tuition: *$2,288* • Non-Residential
Annual Tuition: *$5,554* • General Institutional Fees: *$0* •
Additional Nursing Fees: *$60*

ALVERNO COLLEGE

Address: 3400 South 43rd St, Milwaukee, WI 53234
Phone: 414-382-6284
Fax: 414-382-6279
Contact: Judeen Schulte, PhD, RN, Chairperson
Email: judeen.schulte@alverno.edu

CARDINAL STRITCH UNIVERSITY

Address: 6801 North Yates Road, Milwaukee, WI 53217
Phone: 414-410-4387
Fax: Not Reported
Contact: Kristen Bachman, MSN, RN, Chair
Email: Not Reported

GENERAL INFORMATION

Type of School: *4-Year College or University, Private (Religious)* • Accreditation: *North Central Association of Colleges and Schools* • Total Enrollment: *1950*

GENERAL INFORMATION

Type of School: *4-Year College or University, Private (Religious)* • Accreditation: *North Central Association of Colleges and Schools* • Total Enrollment: *5700*

PROGRAM INFORMATION

NLNAC Accreditation: *Not Reported* • CCNE Accreditation: *Yes*

PROGRAM INFORMATION

NLNAC Accreditation: *Yes* • CCNE Accreditation:

NURSING STUDENT PROFILE

Total Nursing Enrollment: *17* • Full-Time Enrollment: *4* • Part-Time Enrollment: *13* • Female Enrollment: *17* • Male Enrollment: *Not Reported* • Total Graduates: *6*

NURSING STUDENT PROFILE

Total Nursing Enrollment: *42* • Full-Time Enrollment: *42* • Part-Time Enrollment: *0* • Female Enrollment: *40* • Male Enrollment: *2* • Total Graduates: *14*

FINANCES

Residential Annual Tuition: *$12,744* • Non-Residential Annual Tuition: *$12,744* • General Institutional Fees: *$0* • Additional Nursing Fees: *$0*

FINANCES

Residential Annual Tuition: *$10,000* • Non-Residential Annual Tuition: *$10,000* • General Institutional Fees: *$200* • Additional Nursing Fees: *Not Reported*

Circle 23 on reader card   See in-depth profile for more information

UNIVERSITY OF WISCONSIN—GREEN BAY

Address: 2420 Nicolet Drive, Green Bay, WI 54311-7001
Phone: 920-465-2365
Fax: 920-465-2854
Contact: V. Jane Muhl, PhD, RN, Associate Professor and Chair
Email: muhlj@uwgb.edu

GENERAL INFORMATION

Type of School: *4-Year College or University, Public* • Accreditation: *North Central Association of Colleges and Schools* • Total Enrollment: *5506*

PROGRAM INFORMATION

NLNAC Accreditation: *Yes* • CCNE Accreditation:

NURSING STUDENT PROFILE

Total Nursing Enrollment: *134* • Full-Time Enrollment: *4* • Part-Time Enrollment: *130* • Female Enrollment: *118* • Male Enrollment: *16* • Total Graduates: *26*

FINANCES

Residential Annual Tuition: *$3,305* • Non-Residential Annual Tuition: *$10,833* • General Institutional Fees: *Not Reported* • Additional Nursing Fees: *Not Reported*

UNIVERSITY OF WYOMING

Address: P.O. Box 3434, Laramie, WY 82071-3434
Phone: 307-766-6565
Fax: 307-766-4294
Contact: Karen Ouzts, MS, RN, Coordinator, Outreach Nursing Programs
Email: kouzts@uwyo.edu

GENERAL INFORMATION

Type of School: *Not Reported, Not Reported* • Accreditation: *Not Reported* • Total Enrollment: *Not Reported*

PROGRAM INFORMATION

NLNAC Accreditation: *Not Reported* • CCNE Accreditation:

NURSING STUDENT PROFILE

Total Nursing Enrollment: *42* • Full-Time Enrollment: *5* • Part-Time Enrollment: *37* • Female Enrollment: *38* • Male Enrollment: *4* • Total Graduates: *14*

FINANCES

Residential Annual Tuition: *$2,316* • Non-Residential Annual Tuition: *$2,316* • General Institutional Fees: *$960* • Additional Nursing Fees: *$200*

DIPLOMA PROGRAMS

BAPTIST HEALTH SCHOOLS OF NURSING AND ALLIED HEALTH

Address: 11900 Colonel Glenn Road, Suite 1000, Little Rock, AR, 72210-2820
Phone: 501-202-7415
Fax: 501-202-7406
Contact: Shirlene Harris, PhD, RN, Director
Email: swharris@baptist-health.org
Web: www.baptist-health.com

GENERAL INFORMATION

Type of School: *Hospital, Private (Religious)* • Accreditation: *None* • Total Enrollment: *Not Reported*

PROGRAM INFORMATION

NLNAC Accreditation: *Yes*

NURSING STUDENT PROFILE

Total Nursing Enrollment: *401* • Full-Time Enrollment: *341* • Part-Time Enrollment: *60* • Female Enrollment: *364* • Male Enrollment: *37* • Total New Fall Enrollments: *328* • Total Graduates: *79*

FINANCES

Residential Annual Tuition: *$2,720* • Non-Residential Annual Tuition: *$5,440* • General Institutional Fees: *$150* • Additional Nursing Fees: *Not Reported*

JEFFERSON REGIONAL MEDICAL CENTER

Address: 1600 West 40th Avenue, Pine Bluff, AR 71603
Phone: 870-541-7853
Fax: 870-541-7807
Contact: Jessie M. Clemmons, MNSc, RN, Director
Email: jefferso@cei.net

GENERAL INFORMATION

Type of School: *Hospital, Private (Independent)* • Accreditation: *None* • Total Enrollment: *117*

PROGRAM INFORMATION

NLNAC Accreditation: *Yes*

NURSING STUDENT PROFILE

Total Nursing Enrollment: *117* • Full-Time Enrollment: *117* • Part-Time Enrollment: *0* • Female Enrollment: *105* • Male Enrollment: *12* • Total New Fall Enrollments: *41* • Total Graduates: *49*

FINANCES

Residential Annual Tuition: *$2,375* • Non-Residential Annual Tuition: *$2,375* • General Institutional Fees: *37 per semester* • Additional Nursing Fees: *Not Reported*

NORTHWEST HEALTH SYSTEM

Address: 610 East Emma Avenue, Springdale, AR 72764
Phone: 501-750-6200
Fax: 501-750-6205
Contact: Ellen Odell, MSN, RN, Director
Email: ellenodell@hotmail.com

GENERAL INFORMATION

Type of School: *Hospital, Private (Independent)* •
Accreditation: *None* • Total Enrollment: *87*

PROGRAM INFORMATION

NLNAC Accreditation: *Yes*

NURSING STUDENT PROFILE

Total Nursing Enrollment: *73* • Full-Time Enrollment: *73* •
Part-Time Enrollment: *0* • Female Enrollment: *67* • Male
Enrollment: *6* • Total New Fall Enrollments: *30* • Total
Graduates: *28*

FINANCES

Residential Annual Tuition: *$4,400* • Non-Residential
Annual Tuition: *$4,400* • General Institutional Fees: *$0* •
Additional Nursing Fees: *Not Reported*

BRIDGEPORT HOSPITAL

Address: 267 Grant Street, Bridgeport, CT 06610
Phone: 203-384-3205
Fax: 203-384-3046
Contact: Carol deBlois, MA, CNOR, Director
Email: ncdebl@bpthosp.org

GENERAL INFORMATION

Type of School: *Other, Private (Independent)* • Accreditation:
None • Total Enrollment: *Not Reported*

PROGRAM INFORMATION

NLNAC Accreditation: *Yes*

NURSING STUDENT PROFILE

Total Nursing Enrollment: *130* • Full-Time Enrollment: *73* •
Part-Time Enrollment: *57* • Female Enrollment: *119* • Male
Enrollment: *11* • Total New Fall Enrollments: *73* • Total
Graduates: *44*

FINANCES

Residential Annual Tuition: *$5,400* • Non-Residential
Annual Tuition: *$5,400* • General Institutional Fees: *$580* •
Additional Nursing Fees: *Not Reported*

BEEBE MEDICAL CENTER

Address: 424 Savannah Road, Lewes, DE 19958
Phone: 302-645-3251
Fax: 302-645-3488
Contact: Constance E. Bushey, MEd,RN, Director
Email: cbushey@bbmc.org

GENERAL INFORMATION

Type of School: *Hospital, Private (Independent)* •
Accreditation: *None* • Total Enrollment: *Not Provided*

PROGRAM INFORMATION

NLNAC Accreditation: *Yes*

NURSING STUDENT PROFILE

Total Nursing Enrollment: *38* • Full-Time Enrollment: *38* •
Part-Time Enrollment: *0* • Female Enrollment: *35* • Male
Enrollment: *3* • Total New Fall Enrollments: *20* • Total
Graduates: *12*

FINANCES

Residential Annual Tuition: *$2,950* • Non-Residential
Annual Tuition: *$2,950* • General Institutional Fees: *$270* •
Additional Nursing Fees: *Not Reported*

GRAHAM HOSPITAL

Address: 210 West Walnut Street, Canton, IL 61520
Phone: 309-647-4086
Fax: 309-649-5127
Contact: Susan Livingston, MSN, RNC, Director
Email: sondir@winco.net

GENERAL INFORMATION

Type of School: *Hospital, Public* • Accreditation: *None* • Total
Enrollment: *Not Provided*

PROGRAM INFORMATION

NLNAC Accreditation: *Yes*

NURSING STUDENT PROFILE

Total Nursing Enrollment: *69* • Full-Time Enrollment: *51* •
Part-Time Enrollment: *18* • Female Enrollment: *62* • Male
Enrollment: *7* • Total New Fall Enrollments: *64* • Total
Graduates: *15*

FINANCES

Residential Annual Tuition: *$4,150* • Non-Residential
Annual Tuition: *$4,150* • General Institutional Fees: *$630* •
Additional Nursing Fees: *$0*

METHODIST MEDICAL CENTER OF ILLINOIS

Address: 221 North East Glen Oak, Peoria, IL 61636
Phone: 309-672-5511
Fax: 309-671-5383
Contact: Martha Brodkorb, MSN, RN, Director
Email: mbrodkorb@mmci.org

GENERAL INFORMATION

Type of School: *Hospital, Private (Independent)* •
Accreditation: *None* • Total Enrollment: *Not Provided*

PROGRAM INFORMATION

NLNAC Accreditation: *Yes*

NURSING STUDENT PROFILE

Total Nursing Enrollment: *Not Provided* • Full-Time
Enrollment: *Not Provided* • Part-Time Enrollment: *Not
Provided* • Female Enrollment: *Not Provided* • Male
Enrollment: *Not Provided* • Total New Fall Enrollments: *Not
Provided* • Total Graduates: *Not Provided*

FINANCES

Residential Annual Tuition: *Not Reported* • Non-Residential
Annual Tuition: *Not Reported* • General Institutional Fees:
Not Reported • Additional Nursing Fees: *Not Reported*

BATON ROUGE GENERAL MEDICAL CENTER

Address: PO Box 2511, Baton Rouge, LA 70821
Phone: 225-387-7623
Fax: 225-381-6168
Contact: Carol A. Tingle, MSN, RN, Director
Email: carol_tingle@generalhealth.org

GENERAL INFORMATION

Type of School: *Hospital, Private (Independent)* •
Accreditation: *None* • Total Enrollment: *57*

PROGRAM INFORMATION

NLNAC Accreditation: *Yes*

NURSING STUDENT PROFILE

Total Nursing Enrollment: *37* • Full-Time Enrollment: *30* •
Part-Time Enrollment: *7* • Female Enrollment: *36* • Male
Enrollment: *1* • Total New Fall Enrollments: *22* • Total
Graduates: *8*

FINANCES

Residential Annual Tuition: *$5,770* • Non-Residential
Annual Tuition: *$11,918* • General Institutional Fees: *$0* •
Additional Nursing Fees: *$100*

BROCKTON HOSPITAL INC.

Address: 680 Centre Street, Brockton, MA 02302-3395
Phone: 508-941-7056
Fax: 508-941-6302
Contact: Carol Bortman, EdD, RN, Dean
Email: Not Reported

GENERAL INFORMATION

Type of School: *Hospital, Private (Independent)* •
Accreditation: *None* • Total Enrollment: *Not Provided*

PROGRAM INFORMATION

NLNAC Accreditation: *Yes*

NURSING STUDENT PROFILE

Total Nursing Enrollment: *297* • Full-Time Enrollment:
136 • Part-Time Enrollment: *161* • Female Enrollment:
272 • Male Enrollment: *25* • Total New Fall Enrollments:
109 • Total Graduates: *89*

FINANCES

Residential Annual Tuition: *$23,000* • Non-Residential
Annual Tuition: *Not Reported* • General Institutional Fees:
$151 • Additional Nursing Fees: *Not Reported*

LAWRENCE MEMORIAL/ REGIS COLLEGE

Address: 170 Governor Avenue, Medford, MA 02155-1643
Phone: 781-306-6000
Fax: 781-306-6655
Contact: Marie B. McCarthy, MSN, RN, Vice President for Education
Email: mmcam2@hhs.lmh.edu

GENERAL INFORMATION

Type of School: *Not Provided, Other* • Accreditation: *None* •
Total Enrollment: *Not Provided*

PROGRAM INFORMATION

NLNAC Accreditation: *Yes*

NURSING STUDENT PROFILE

Total Nursing Enrollment: *12* • Full-Time Enrollment: *0* •
Part-Time Enrollment: *12* • Female Enrollment: *12* • Male
Enrollment: *0* • Total New Fall Enrollments: *0* • Total
Graduates: *16*

FINANCES

Residential Annual Tuition: *$3,470* • Non-Residential
Annual Tuition: *Not Reported* • General Institutional Fees:
$180 • Additional Nursing Fees: *Not Reported*

ST. ALEXIUS HOSPITAL

Address: 2611 Miami Street, Saint Louis, MO 63118
Phone: 314-268-6000
Fax: 314-268-6160
Contact: Regina Cundall, MSN, RN, Director of Nursing Education
Email: regina.cundall@tenetstl.com

GENERAL INFORMATION

Type of School: *Hospital, Other* • Accreditation: *None* • Total Enrollment: *Not Provided*

PROGRAM INFORMATION

NLNAC Accreditation: *Yes*

NURSING STUDENT PROFILE

Total Nursing Enrollment: *Not Provided* • Full-Time Enrollment: *Not Provided* • Part-Time Enrollment: *Not Provided* • Female Enrollment: *Not Provided* • Male Enrollment: *Not Provided* • Total New Fall Enrollments: *Not Provided* • Total Graduates: *Not Provided*

FINANCES

Residential Annual Tuition: *Not Reported* • Non-Residential Annual Tuition: *Not Reported* • General Institutional Fees: *Not Reported* • Additional Nursing Fees: *Not Reported*

BRYAN LGH MEDICAL CENTER

Address: 1600 South 48th Street, Lincoln, NE 68506
Phone: 402-481-3867
Fax: 402-481-8421
Contact: Phylis Hollamon, MSN, MA, RN, Director
Email: phollamon@bryanlgh.org

GENERAL INFORMATION

Type of School: *Hospital, Private (Independent)* • Accreditation: *None* • Total Enrollment: *158*

PROGRAM INFORMATION

NLNAC Accreditation: *Yes*

NURSING STUDENT PROFILE

Total Nursing Enrollment: *Not Provided* • Full-Time Enrollment: *Not Provided* • Part-Time Enrollment: *Not Provided* • Female Enrollment: *Not Provided* • Male Enrollment: *Not Provided* • Total New Fall Enrollments: *Not Provided* • Total Graduates: *Not Provided*

FINANCES

Residential Annual Tuition: *Not Reported* • Non-Residential Annual Tuition: *Not Reported* • General Institutional Fees: *Not Reported* • Additional Nursing Fees: *Not Reported*

ATLANTIC HEALTH SYSTEM

Address: 1 Bay Avenue, Montclair, NJ 07042
Phone: 973-429-6060
Fax: 973-429-6068
Contact: Louise M. DeBlois, MEd, RN, Director
Email: louise.deblois@ahsys.org

GENERAL INFORMATION

Type of School: *Not Provided* • Accreditation: *Not Provided* •
Total Enrollment: *Not Provided*

PROGRAM INFORMATION

NLNAC Accreditation: *Yes*

NURSING STUDENT PROFILE

Total Nursing Enrollment: *Not Provided* • Full-Time
Enrollment: *Not Provided* • Part-Time Enrollment: *Not
Provided* • Female Enrollment: *Not Provided* • Male
Enrollment: *Not Provided* • Total New Fall Enrollments: *Not
Provided* • Total Graduates: *Not Provided*

FINANCES

Residential Annual Tuition: *Not Reported* • Non-Residential
Annual Tuition: *Not Reported* • General Institutional Fees:
Not Reported • Additional Nursing Fees: *Not Reported*

BAYONNE HOSPITAL

Address: 69-71 New Hook Road, Bayonne, NJ 07002
Phone: 201-339-9656
Fax: 201-339-9157
Contact: Donna Stankiewicz, MSN, RN, Director
Email: dstankiewicz@bayonnemedicalcenter.org

GENERAL INFORMATION

Type of School: *Hospital, Private (Independent)* •
Accreditation: *None* • Total Enrollment: *37*

PROGRAM INFORMATION

NLNAC Accreditation: *Yes*

NURSING STUDENT PROFILE

Total Nursing Enrollment: *37* • Full-Time Enrollment: *30* •
Part-Time Enrollment: *7* • Female Enrollment: *36* • Male
Enrollment: *1* • Total New Fall Enrollments: *22* • Total
Graduates: *8*

FINANCES

Residential Annual Tuition: *$2,950* • Non-Residential
Annual Tuition: *$2,950* • General Institutional Fees: *$0* •
Additional Nursing Fees: *$110*

BON SECOURS NEW JERSEY

Address: 1 McWilliams Place, Jersey City, NJ 07302
Phone: 201-418-2204
Fax: 201-418-2207
Contact: Sharon Zaucha, MSN, RNC, Interim Director
Email: szaucha@fhsnj.org

GENERAL INFORMATION

Type of School: *Hospital, Private (Religious)* • Accreditation: *None* • Total Enrollment: *22*

PROGRAM INFORMATION

NLNAC Accreditation: *Yes*

NURSING STUDENT PROFILE

Total Nursing Enrollment: *22* • Full-Time Enrollment: *22* • Part-Time Enrollment: *0* • Female Enrollment: *21* • Male Enrollment: *1* • Total New Fall Enrollments: *Not Provided* • Total Graduates: *24*

FINANCES

Residential Annual Tuition: *$7,443* • Non-Residential Annual Tuition: *$7,443* • General Institutional Fees: *$1,104* • Additional Nursing Fees: *Not Reported*

CAPITAL HEALTH SYSTEM

Address: 446 Bellevue Avenue, Trenton, NJ 08618
Phone: 609-394-4281
Fax: 609-394-4354
Contact: Nancy M. Murray, EdD, RN, Chairperson
Email: nmurray@chsnj.org

GENERAL INFORMATION

Type of School: *Hospital, Private (Independent)* • Accreditation: *Middle States Association of Colleges and Schools* • Total Enrollment: *Not Provided*

PROGRAM INFORMATION

NLNAC Accreditation: *Yes*

NURSING STUDENT PROFILE

Total Nursing Enrollment: *87* • Full-Time Enrollment: *15* • Part-Time Enrollment: *72* • Female Enrollment: *79* • Male Enrollment: *8* • Total New Fall Enrollments: *52* • Total Graduates: *18*

FINANCES

Residential Annual Tuition: *$2,261* • Non-Residential Annual Tuition: *$2,261* • General Institutional Fees: *$491* • Additional Nursing Fees: *Not Reported*

CHRIST HOSPITAL

Address: 176 Palisade Avenue, Jersey City, NJ 07306
Phone: 201-795-8365
Fax: 201-795-8737
Contact: Carol A. Fasano, MA, RN, NP, C, Director of Organizational Education
Email: cfasano@christhospital.org

HELENE FULD SCHOOL OF NURSING IN CAMDEN COUNTY

Address: 1669 College Drive, Blackwood, NJ 08012
Phone: 856-374-0100
Fax: 856-374-0710
Contact: Regina M. Mastrangelo, EdD, RN, Dean
Email: RMASTRANGELO@VIRTUA.ORG

GENERAL INFORMATION

Type of School: *Hospital, Private (Religious)* • Accreditation: *None* • Total Enrollment: *163*

GENERAL INFORMATION

Type of School: *Independent, Private (Independent)* • Accreditation: *None* • Total Enrollment: *285*

PROGRAM INFORMATION

NLNAC Accreditation: *Yes*

PROGRAM INFORMATION

NLNAC Accreditation: *Yes*

NURSING STUDENT PROFILE

Total Nursing Enrollment: *163* • Full-Time Enrollment: *69* • Part-Time Enrollment: *94* • Female Enrollment: *141* • Male Enrollment: *22* • Total New Fall Enrollments: *52* • Total Graduates: *17*

NURSING STUDENT PROFILE

Total Nursing Enrollment: *298* • Full-Time Enrollment: *298* • Part-Time Enrollment: *0* • Female Enrollment: *272* • Male Enrollment: *26* • Total New Fall Enrollments: *122* • Total Graduates: *53*

FINANCES

Residential Annual Tuition: *$16,928* • Non-Residential Annual Tuition: *$16,928* • General Institutional Fees: *$175* • Additional Nursing Fees: *Not Reported*

FINANCES

Residential Annual Tuition: *$6,888* • Non-Residential Annual Tuition: *Not Reported* • General Institutional Fees: *$343* • Additional Nursing Fees: *Not Reported*

HOLY NAME HOSPITAL

Address: 609 Teaneck Road, Teaneck, NJ 07666
Phone: 201-833-3008
Fax: 201-833-7209
Contact: Claire Tynan, EdD, RN, Senior Vice President
           and Director
Email: sr-tynan@mail.holyname.org

GENERAL INFORMATION

Type of School: *Hospital, Private (Religious)* • Accreditation: *None* • Total Enrollment: *Not Provided*

PROGRAM INFORMATION

NLNAC Accreditation: *Yes*

NURSING STUDENT PROFILE

Total Nursing Enrollment: *96* • Full-Time Enrollment: *80* • Part-Time Enrollment: *16* • Female Enrollment: *88* • Male Enrollment: *8* • Total New Fall Enrollments: *57* • Total Graduates: *30*

FINANCES

Residential Annual Tuition: *$18,368* • Non-Residential Annual Tuition: *$18,368* • General Institutional Fees: *$650* • Additional Nursing Fees: *Not Reported*

MUHLENBERG REGIONAL MEDICAL CENTER

Address: Park Avenue and Randolph Road, Plainfield, NJ
           07061
Phone: 908-668-2400
Fax: 908-226-4568
Contact: Judith Mathews, PhD, RN, Dean
Email: Mayerski@solarishs.org

GENERAL INFORMATION

Type of School: *Hospital, Other* • Accreditation: *None* • Total Enrollment: *273*

PROGRAM INFORMATION

NLNAC Accreditation: *Yes*

NURSING STUDENT PROFILE

Total Nursing Enrollment: *273* • Full-Time Enrollment: *45* • Part-Time Enrollment: *228* • Female Enrollment: *258* • Male Enrollment: *15* • Total New Fall Enrollments: *116* • Total Graduates: *75*

FINANCES

Residential Annual Tuition: *$2,502* • Non-Residential Annual Tuition: *$2,502* • General Institutional Fees: *$406* • Additional Nursing Fees: *Not Reported*

| Circle 88 on reader card | See in-depth profile for more information |

OUR LADY OF LOURDES SCHOOL OF NURSING

Address: 340 East Evesham Avenue, Magnolia, NJ 08049
Phone: 856-782-2104
Fax: 856-782-9551
Contact: Dorothy Letizia, EdD, RN, Dean
Email: letiziad@lourdesnet.org

GENERAL INFORMATION

Type of School: *Independent, Private (Independent)* •
Accreditation: *None* • Total Enrollment: *Not Provided*

PROGRAM INFORMATION

NLNAC Accreditation: *Yes*

NURSING STUDENT PROFILE

Total Nursing Enrollment: *87* • Full-Time Enrollment: *18* •
Part-Time Enrollment: *61* • Female Enrollment: *78* • Male
Enrollment: *9* • Total New Fall Enrollments: *62* • Total
Graduates: *32*

FINANCES

Residential Annual Tuition: *$600* • Non-Residential Annual
Tuition: *$640* • General Institutional Fees: *$901* • Additional
Nursing Fees: *Not Reported*

RARITAN BAY MEDICAL CENTER

Address: 530 New Brunswick Avenue, Perth Amboy, NJ 08861
Phone: 732-607-6500
Fax: 732-607-6516
Contact: Cathleen M. McCormack, MA, RN, Director Nursing Education
Email: Not Reported

GENERAL INFORMATION

Type of School: *Hospital, Private (Independent)* •
Accreditation: *None* • Total Enrollment: *Not Provided*

PROGRAM INFORMATION

NLNAC Accreditation: *Yes*

NURSING STUDENT PROFILE

Total Nursing Enrollment: *79* • Full-Time Enrollment: *79* •
Part-Time Enrollment: *0* • Female Enrollment: *71* • Male
Enrollment: *8* • Total New Fall Enrollments: *51* • Total
Graduates: *37*

FINANCES

Residential Annual Tuition: *$6,000* • Non-Residential
Annual Tuition: *$7,000* • General Institutional Fees: *$454* •
Additional Nursing Fees: *Not Reported*

SAINT FRANCIS MEDICAL CENTER

Address: 601 Hamilton Avenue, Trenton, NJ 08629
Phone: 609-599-5192
Fax: 609-599-5799
Contact: Bonny Ross, EdD, RN, Director
Email: bross@che-east.org

GENERAL INFORMATION

Type of School: *Not Provided* • Accreditation: *Not Provided* •
Total Enrollment: *Not Provided*

PROGRAM INFORMATION

NLNAC Accreditation: *Yes*

NURSING STUDENT PROFILE

Total Nursing Enrollment: *34* • Full-Time Enrollment: *4* •
Part-Time Enrollment: *32* • Female Enrollment: *35* • Male
Enrollment: *1* • Total New Fall Enrollments: *16* • Total
Graduates: *13*

FINANCES

Residential Annual Tuition: *$7,225* • Non-Residential
Annual Tuition: *$7,225* • General Institutional Fees: *$500* •
Additional Nursing Fees: *Not Reported*

TRINITAS HEALTH SCHOOL OF NURSING

Address: 925 East Jersey Street, Elizabeth, NJ 07206
Phone: 908-994-8600
Fax: Not Provided
Contact: Mary E. Kelley, MEd, MSN, RN, Dean
Email: mkelley@trinitashospital.org

GENERAL INFORMATION

Type of School: *Hospital, Private (Religious)* • Accreditation:
None • Total Enrollment: *Not Provided*

PROGRAM INFORMATION

NLNAC Accreditation: *Yes*

NURSING STUDENT PROFILE

Total Nursing Enrollment: *449* • Full-Time Enrollment:
188 • Part-Time Enrollment: *261* • Female Enrollment:
404 • Male Enrollment: *45* • Total New Fall Enrollments:
110 • Total Graduates: *52*

FINANCES

Residential Annual Tuition: *$1,668* • Non-Residential
Annual Tuition: *$3,336* • General Institutional Fees: *$240* •
Additional Nursing Fees: *Not Reported*

Circle 120 on reader card   See in-depth profile for more information

ARNOT OGDEN MEDICAL CENTER

Address: 600 Roe Avenue, Elmira, NY 14905
Phone: 607-737-4263
Fax: 607-737-4116
Contact: Linda MacAuslan, MS, RN, Director School Nursing
Email: lmacauslan@aomc.org

GENERAL INFORMATION

Type of School: *Hospital, Public* • Accreditation: *None* • Total Enrollment: *39*

PROGRAM INFORMATION

NLNAC Accreditation: *Yes*

NURSING STUDENT PROFILE

Total Nursing Enrollment: *39* • Full-Time Enrollment: *34* • Part-Time Enrollment: *5* • Female Enrollment: *34* • Male Enrollment: *5* • Total New Fall Enrollments: *16* • Total Graduates: *4*

FINANCES

Residential Annual Tuition: *$6,400* • Non-Residential Annual Tuition: *$6,400* • General Institutional Fees: *$190* • Additional Nursing Fees: *Not Reported*

MERCY HOSPITAL INC.

Address: 1921 Vail Avenue, Charlotte, NC 28207
Phone: 704-379-5842
Fax: 704-379-5141
Contact: Claire B. Corbin, MN, RN, Dean
Email: ccorbin@carolinas.org

GENERAL INFORMATION

Type of School: *Hospital, Private (Religious)* • Accreditation: *None* • Total Enrollment: *Not Provided*

PROGRAM INFORMATION

NLNAC Accreditation: *Yes*

NURSING STUDENT PROFILE

Total Nursing Enrollment: *113* • Full-Time Enrollment: *113* • Part-Time Enrollment: *0* • Female Enrollment: *102* • Male Enrollment: *11* • Total New Fall Enrollments: *72* • Total Graduates: *51*

FINANCES

Residential Annual Tuition: *$2,880* • Non-Residential Annual Tuition: *$2,880* • General Institutional Fees: *$140* • Additional Nursing Fees: *Not Reported*

PRESBYTERIAN HOSPITAL

Address: 1901 East 5th Street, Charlotte, NC 28233-3549
Phone: 704-384-4143
Fax: 704-384-5628
Contact: Judith C. Trexler, PhD, RN, Director
Email: jctrexler@novanthealth.org

GENERAL INFORMATION

Type of School: *Hospital, Private (Independent)* •
Accreditation: *None* • Total Enrollment: *179*

PROGRAM INFORMATION

NLNAC Accreditation: *Yes*

NURSING STUDENT PROFILE

Total Nursing Enrollment: *165* • Full-Time Enrollment: *96* •
Part-Time Enrollment: *69* • Female Enrollment: *155* • Male
Enrollment: *10* • Total New Fall Enrollments: *84* • Total
Graduates: *51*

FINANCES

Residential Annual Tuition: *$3,000* • Non-Residential
Annual Tuition: *$3,000* • General Institutional Fees: *$252* •
Additional Nursing Fees: *Not Reported*

WATTS SCHOOL OF NURSING

Address: 3643 North Roxboro Street, Durham, NC 27704
Phone: 919-470-7348
Fax: 919-470-7346
Contact: Peggy C. Burke, EdD, RN, Director of Nursing Education
Email: bakerpec@drh.duhs.duke.edu

GENERAL INFORMATION

Type of School: *Not Provided* • Accreditation: *Not Provided* •
Total Enrollment: *Not Provided*

PROGRAM INFORMATION

NLNAC Accreditation: *Yes*

NURSING STUDENT PROFILE

Total Nursing Enrollment: *48* • Full-Time Enrollment: *48* •
Part-Time Enrollment: *0* • Female Enrollment: *46* • Male
Enrollment: *2* • Total New Fall Enrollments: *28* • Total
Graduates: *18*

FINANCES

Residential Annual Tuition: *$2,800* • Non-Residential
Annual Tuition: *$2,800* • General Institutional Fees: *Not
Reported* • Additional Nursing Fees: *Not Reported*

Circle 145 on reader card　　　　　　　**See in-depth profile for more information**

AULTMAN HEALTH FOUNDATION

Address: 2600 Sixth Street SW, Canton, OH 44710
Phone: 330-363-6347
Fax: 330-580-6654
Contact: Joan L. Frey, MSN, RN, Director
Email: jfrey@aultman.com

GENERAL INFORMATION

Type of School: *Other, Private (Independent)* • Accreditation: *None* • Total Enrollment: *Not Provided*

PROGRAM INFORMATION

NLNAC Accreditation: *Yes*

NURSING STUDENT PROFILE

Total Nursing Enrollment: *142* • Full-Time Enrollment: *101* • Part-Time Enrollment: *41* • Female Enrollment: *88* • Male Enrollment: *13* • Total New Fall Enrollments: *50* • Total Graduates: *12*

FINANCES

Residential Annual Tuition: *$8,600* • Non-Residential Annual Tuition: *$8,600* • General Institutional Fees: *$200* • Additional Nursing Fees: *Not Reported*

THE CHRIST HOSPITAL

Address: 2139 Auburn Avenue, Cincinnati, OH 45219-2988
Phone: 513-585-2051
Fax: 513-585-3540
Contact: Teresa E. Goodwin, MEd, RN, Executive Director
Email: Goodwite@healthall.com

GENERAL INFORMATION

Type of School: *Hospital, Private (Independent)* • Accreditation: *None* • Total Enrollment: *Not Provided*

PROGRAM INFORMATION

NLNAC Accreditation: *Yes*

NURSING STUDENT PROFILE

Total Nursing Enrollment: *99* • Full-Time Enrollment: *99* • Part-Time Enrollment: *0* • Female Enrollment: *94* • Male Enrollment: *5* • Total New Fall Enrollments: *58* • Total Graduates: *73*

FINANCES

Residential Annual Tuition: *$4,200* • Non-Residential Annual Tuition: *$4,200* • General Institutional Fees: *$460* • Additional Nursing Fees: *Not Reported*

COMMUNITY HOSPITAL

Address: 2615 East High Street, PO Box 1226,
           Springfield, OH 45505
Phone: 937-328-8901
Fax: 937-328-8668
Contact: Dala J. DeWitt, MSN, RN, Director
Email: dala.dewitt@communityhospital.com

FIRELANDS REGIONAL MEDICAL CENTER

Address: 1912 Hayes Avenue, Sandusky, OH 44870-4788
Phone: 419-621-7114
Fax: 419-621-7116
Contact: Holly J. Price, MSN, RN, Director
Email: hprice@providencehealth.org

GENERAL INFORMATION

Type of School: *Hospital, Private (Independent)* •
Accreditation: *North Central Association of Colleges and Schools* • Total Enrollment: *78*

GENERAL INFORMATION

Type of School: *Hospital, Private (Religious)* • Accreditation: *None* • Total Enrollment: *Not Provided*

PROGRAM INFORMATION

NLNAC Accreditation: *Yes*

PROGRAM INFORMATION

NLNAC Accreditation: *Yes*

NURSING STUDENT PROFILE

Total Nursing Enrollment: *78* • Full-Time Enrollment: *69* •
Part-Time Enrollment: *9* • Female Enrollment: *76* • Male
Enrollment; *2* • Total New Fall Enrollments: *46* • Total
Graduates: *13*

NURSING STUDENT PROFILE

Total Nursing Enrollment: *Not Provided* • Full-Time
Enrollment: *Not Provided* • Part-Time Enrollment: *Not Provided* • Female Enrollment: *Not Provided* • Male
Enrollment: *Not Provided* • Total New Fall Enrollments: *Not Provided* • Total Graduates: *Not Provided*

FINANCES

Residential Annual Tuition: *$9,760* • Non-Residential
Annual Tuition: *$9,760* • General Institutional Fees: *$80* •
Additional Nursing Fees: *Not Reported*

FINANCES

Residential Annual Tuition: *Not Reported* • Non-Residential
Annual Tuition: *Not Reported* • General Institutional Fees:
Not Reported • Additional Nursing Fees: *Not Reported*

GOOD SAMARITAN HOSPITAL

Address: 375 Dixmyth Avenue, Cincinnati, OH 45220-2489
Phone: 513-872-2491
Fax: 513-872-3572
Contact: Morris Cohen, MA, RN, Director
Email: morris_cohen@trihealth.com

GENERAL INFORMATION

Type of School: *Independent, Private (Religious)* •
Accreditation: *None* • Total Enrollment: *263*

PROGRAM INFORMATION

NLNAC Accreditation: *Yes*

NURSING STUDENT PROFILE

Total Nursing Enrollment: *230* • Full-Time Enrollment:
104 • Part-Time Enrollment: *126* • Female Enrollment:
223 • Male Enrollment: *7* • Total New Fall Enrollments:
147 • Total Graduates: *67*

FINANCES

Residential Annual Tuition: *$9,011* • Non-Residential
Annual Tuition: *Not Reported* • General Institutional Fees:
$170 • Additional Nursing Fees: *Not Reported*

HURON SCHOOL OF NURSING

Address: 13951 Terrace Road, East Cleveland, OH 44112
Phone: 216-761-6939
Fax: 216-761-7541
Contact: Kathleen Knittel, MSN, RN, Director
Email: kknittek@meridia.org

GENERAL INFORMATION

Type of School: *Other, Private (Independent)* • Accreditation:
None • Total Enrollment: *239*

PROGRAM INFORMATION

NLNAC Accreditation: *Yes*

NURSING STUDENT PROFILE

Total Nursing Enrollment: *137* • Full-Time Enrollment:
137 • Part-Time Enrollment: *0* • Female Enrollment: *117* •
Male Enrollment: *20* • Total New Fall Enrollments: *90* •
Total Graduates: *60*

FINANCES

Residential Annual Tuition: *$4,982* • Non-Residential
Annual Tuition: *Not Reported* • General Institutional Fees:
$50 • Additional Nursing Fees: *Not Reported*

Circle 62 on reader card   See in-depth profile for more information

MANSFIELD GENERAL HOSPITAL SCHOOL OF NURSING

Address: 335 Glessner Avenue, Mansfield, OH 44903-
           2265
Phone: 419-526-8606
Fax: 419-526-8694
Contact: Nancy Collier, MS, RN, Director
Email: collier.69@postbox.acs.ohio-state.edu

TRINITY HEALTH SYSTEMS

Address: 380 Summit Avenue, Steubenville, OH 43952
Phone: 740-283-7273
Fax: 740-283-7461
Contact: Patricia Gerlando, PhD, RN, Director
Email: pgerland@trinityhealtch.com

GENERAL INFORMATION

Type of School: *Hospital, Private (Independent)* •
Accreditation: *None* • Total Enrollment: *20*

GENERAL INFORMATION

Type of School: *Hospital, Private (Religious)* • Accreditation:
None • Total Enrollment: *Not Provided*

PROGRAM INFORMATION

NLNAC Accreditation: *Yes*

PROGRAM INFORMATION

NLNAC Accreditation: *Yes*

NURSING STUDENT PROFILE

Total Nursing Enrollment: *20* • Full-Time Enrollment: *20* •
Part-Time Enrollment: *0* • Female Enrollment: *16* • Male
Enrollment: *4* • Total New Fall Enrollments: *6* • Total
Graduates: *21*

NURSING STUDENT PROFILE

Total Nursing Enrollment: *90* • Full-Time Enrollment: *90* •
Part-Time Enrollment: *0* • Female Enrollment: *76* • Male
Enrollment: *14* • Total New Fall Enrollments: *55* • Total
Graduates: *13*

FINANCES

Residential Annual Tuition: *$8,526* • Non-Residential
Annual Tuition: *$8,526* • General Institutional Fees: *Not
Reported* • Additional Nursing Fees: *Not Reported*

FINANCES

Residential Annual Tuition: *$7,341* • Non-Residential
Annual Tuition: *$7,760* • General Institutional Fees: *$500* •
Additional Nursing Fees: *Not Reported*

ABINGTON MEMORIAL HOSPITAL

Address: 2500 Maryland Road, Suite 200, Willow Grove, PA 19090
Phone: 215-481-5514
Fax: 215-481-5597
Contact: Eileen Van Parys, EdD, RN, Chairman
Email: evanparys@amh.org

GENERAL INFORMATION

Type of School: *Hospital, Private (Independent)* •
Accreditation: *None* • Total Enrollment: *52*

PROGRAM INFORMATION

NLNAC Accreditation: *Yes*

NURSING STUDENT PROFILE

Total Nursing Enrollment: *52* • Full-Time Enrollment: *52* •
Part-Time Enrollment: *0* • Female Enrollment: *45* • Male
Enrollment: *7* • Total New Fall Enrollments: *39* • Total
Graduates: *15*

FINANCES

Residential Annual Tuition: *$6,000* • Non-Residential
Annual Tuition: *$6,000* • General Institutional Fees: *$0* •
Additional Nursing Fees: *$100*

BRANDYWINE SCHOOL OF NURSING

Address: 215 Reeceville Road, Coatsville, PA 19320
Phone: 610-383-8216
Fax: 610-383-8325
Contact: Sharon L. Wolf, MSN, MEd, RN, Director
Email: sharon_wolf@hg.chs.net

GENERAL INFORMATION

Type of School: *Hospital, Private (Independent)* •
Accreditation: *None* • Total Enrollment: *Not Provided*

PROGRAM INFORMATION

NLNAC Accreditation: *Yes*

NURSING STUDENT PROFILE

Total Nursing Enrollment: *59* • Full-Time Enrollment: *32* •
Part-Time Enrollment: *23* • Female Enrollment: *55* • Male
Enrollment: *4* • Total New Fall Enrollments: *68* • Total
Graduates: *31*

FINANCES

Residential Annual Tuition: *$6,000* • Non-Residential
Annual Tuition: *$6,000* • General Institutional Fees:
$1,375 • Additional Nursing Fees: *Not Reported*

CITIZENS SCHOOL OF NURSING

Address:　200 Freeport Road, New Kesington, PA 15068
Phone:　724-337-5090
Fax:　724-334-7708
Contact:　Mary Lynne Rugh, MSN, RN, Director
Email:　Not Reported

GENERAL INFORMATION

Type of School: *Hospital, Private (Independent)* • Accreditation: *None* • Total Enrollment: *Not Provided*

PROGRAM INFORMATION

NLNAC Accreditation: *Yes*

NURSING STUDENT PROFILE

Total Nursing Enrollment: *45* • Full-Time Enrollment: *45* • Part-Time Enrollment: *0* • Female Enrollment: *42* • Male Enrollment: *3* • Total New Fall Enrollments: *39* • Total Graduates: *20*

FINANCES

Residential Annual Tuition: *$6,540* • Non-Residential Annual Tuition: *$6,540* • General Institutional Fees: *$40* • Additional Nursing Fees: *Not Reported*

CONEMAUGH VALLEY MEMORIAL HOSPITAL

Address:　1086 Franklin Street, Johnstown, PA 15905
Phone:　814-534-9118
Fax:　814-534-3354
Contact:　Louise Pugliese, MSN, RN, Director
Email:　lpuglie@conemaugh.org

GENERAL INFORMATION

Type of School: *Public* • Accreditation: *None* • Total Enrollment: *86*

PROGRAM INFORMATION

NLNAC Accreditation: *Yes*

NURSING STUDENT PROFILE

Total Nursing Enrollment: *53* • Full-Time Enrollment: *52* • Part-Time Enrollment: *1* • Female Enrollment: *49* • Male Enrollment: *4* • Total New Fall Enrollments: *35* • Total Graduates: *15*

FINANCES

Residential Annual Tuition: *$7,800* • Non-Residential Annual Tuition: *$10,500* • General Institutional Fees: *$280* • Additional Nursing Fees: *Not Reported*

EPISCOPAL SCHOOL OF NURSING

Address: 100 East Lehigh Avenue, Philadelphia, PA 19125
Phone: 215-707-0010
Fax: Not Provided
Contact: Dolores Alabrodzinski, MSN, RN, Director
Email: alabrod@eh.temple.edu

SEWICKLEY VALLEY HOSPITAL SCHOOL OF NURSING

Address: 720 Blackburn Road, Sewickley, PA 15143-1498
Phone: 412-749-7089
Fax: 412-749-4241
Contact: Marilu Piotrowski, MSN, RN, Director
Email: mpiotrowski@hvhs.org

GENERAL INFORMATION

Type of School: *Hospital, Public* • Accreditation: *None* • Total Enrollment: *109*

GENERAL INFORMATION

Type of School: *Hospital, Public* • Accreditation: *None* • Total Enrollment: *69*

PROGRAM INFORMATION

NLNAC Accreditation: *Yes*

PROGRAM INFORMATION

NLNAC Accreditation: *Yes*

NURSING STUDENT PROFILE

Total Nursing Enrollment: *81* • Full-Time Enrollment: *5* • Part-Time Enrollment: *76* • Female Enrollment: *79* • Male Enrollment: *2* • Total New Fall Enrollments: *46* • Total Graduates: *20*

NURSING STUDENT PROFILE

Total Nursing Enrollment: *Not Provided* • Full-Time Enrollment: *Not Provided* • Part-Time Enrollment: *Not Provided* • Female Enrollment: *Not Provided* • Male Enrollment: *Not Provided* • Total New Fall Enrollments: *Not Provided* • Total Graduates: *Not Provided*

FINANCES

Residential Annual Tuition: *$4,800* • Non-Residential Annual Tuition: *$4,800* • General Institutional Fees: *$60* • Additional Nursing Fees: *Not Reported*

FINANCES

Residential Annual Tuition: *Not Reported* • Non-Residential Annual Tuition: *Not Reported* • General Institutional Fees: *Not Reported* • Additional Nursing Fees: *Not Reported*

JAMESON HEALTH SYSTEM

Address: 1211 Wilmington Avenue, New Castle, PA
16105
Phone: 724-656-4052
Fax: 724-656-4179
Contact: Jayne Sheehan, MSN, RN, CRNP, Director
Email: jsheehan@jamesonhealthsystem.com

LANCASTER INSTITUTE FOR HEALTH EDUCATION

Address: 410 North Lime Street, PO Box 3555, Lancaster,
PA 17602
Phone: 717-290-4912
Fax: 717-290-5970
Contact: Mary Grace Simcox, EdD, RN, Director
Email: mrsimcox@lha.org

GENERAL INFORMATION

Type of School: *Hospital, Public* • Accreditation: *None* • Total
Enrollment: *71*

GENERAL INFORMATION

Type of School: *Hospital, Private (Independent)* •
Accreditation: *None* • Total Enrollment: *205*

PROGRAM INFORMATION

NLNAC Accreditation: *Yes*

PROGRAM INFORMATION

NLNAC Accreditation: *Yes*

NURSING STUDENT PROFILE

Total Nursing Enrollment: *67* • Full-Time Enrollment: *38* •
Part-Time Enrollment: *29* • Female Enrollment: *59* • Male
Enrollment: *8* • Total New Fall Enrollments: *37* • Total
Graduates: *32*

NURSING STUDENT PROFILE

Total Nursing Enrollment: *125* • Full-Time Enrollment: *79* •
Part-Time Enrollment: *46* • Female Enrollment: *114* • Male
Enrollment: *11* • Total New Fall Enrollments: *50* • Total
Graduates: *50*

FINANCES

Residential Annual Tuition: *$7,512* • Non-Residential
Annual Tuition: *$7,512* • General Institutional Fees: *$445* •
Additional Nursing Fees: *Not Reported*

FINANCES

Residential Annual Tuition: *$4,800* • Non-Residential
Annual Tuition: *$10,488* • General Institutional Fees: *Not
Reported* • Additional Nursing Fees: *Not Reported*

Circle 69 on reader card   **See in-depth profile for more information**

METHODIST HOSPITAL

Address: 2301 South Broad Street, Philadelphia, PA
           19148
Phone: 215-952-9411
Fax: 215-952-9407
Contact: Maria Henninger Toth, EdD, CRNP, Director
Email: maria.toth@mail.tju.edu

GENERAL INFORMATION

Type of School: *Hospital, Public* • Accreditation: *None* • Total
Enrollment: *113*

PROGRAM INFORMATION

NLNAC Accreditation: *Yes*

NURSING STUDENT PROFILE

Total Nursing Enrollment: *113* • Full-Time Enrollment:
113 • Part-Time Enrollment: *0* • Female Enrollment: *96* •
Male Enrollment: *7* • Total New Fall Enrollments: *78* • Total
Graduates: *24*

FINANCES

Residential Annual Tuition: *$5,200* • Non-Residential
Annual Tuition: *Not Reported* • General Institutional Fees:
$390 • Additional Nursing Fees: *Not Reported*

NORTHEASTERN HOSPITAL

Address: 2301 East Allegheny Avenue, Philadelphia, PA
           19134-4499
Phone: 215-291-3140
Fax: 215-291-3146
Contact: Mary E. Wombwell, EdD, RN, Director
Email: wombwem@te.temple.edu

GENERAL INFORMATION

Type of School: *Not Provided* • Accreditation: *Not Provided* •
Total Enrollment: *Not Provided*

PROGRAM INFORMATION

NLNAC Accreditation: *Yes*

NURSING STUDENT PROFILE

Total Nursing Enrollment: *50* • Full-Time Enrollment: *50* •
Part-Time Enrollment: *0* • Female Enrollment: *47* • Male
Enrollment: *3* • Total New Fall Enrollments: *30* • Total
Graduates: *19*

FINANCES

Residential Annual Tuition: *$3,000* • Non-Residential
Annual Tuition: *Not Reported* • General Institutional Fees:
$50 • Additional Nursing Fees: *Not Reported*

OHIO VALLEY GENERAL HOSPITAL

Address: 25 Heckel Road, McKees Rocks, PA 15136
Phone: 412-777-6234
Fax: Not Reported
Contact: Ann M. Pitassi, MSN, RN, CRNP, Chairperson
Email: Not Reported

GENERAL INFORMATION

Type of School: *Hospital, Private (Independent)* •
Accreditation: *None* • Total Enrollment: *Not Provided*

PROGRAM INFORMATION

NLNAC Accreditation: *Yes*

NURSING STUDENT PROFILE

Total Nursing Enrollment: *19* • Full-Time Enrollment: *19* •
Part-Time Enrollment: *0* • Female Enrollment: *19* • Male
Enrollment: *Not Provided* • Total New Fall Enrollments: *9* •
Total Graduates: *10*

FINANCES

Residential Annual Tuition: *$6,840* • Non-Residential
Annual Tuition: *Not Reported* • General Institutional Fees:
Not Reported • Additional Nursing Fees: *Not Reported*

PITTSBURGH MERCY HEALTH SYSTEM

Address: 1401 Boulevard of the Allies, Pittsburgh, PA
15219
Phone: 412-232-7964
Fax: 412-232-7951
Contact: Joanne Sperry, MN, RN, Director
Email: jsperry@mercy.pmhs.org

GENERAL INFORMATION

Type of School: *Hospital, Private (Religious)* • Accreditation:
None • Total Enrollment: *Not Provided*

PROGRAM INFORMATION

NLNAC Accreditation: *Yes*

NURSING STUDENT PROFILE

Total Nursing Enrollment: *42* • Full-Time Enrollment: *42* •
Part-Time Enrollment: *0* • Female Enrollment: *37* • Male
Enrollment: *5* • Total New Fall Enrollments: *25* • Total
Graduates: *24*

FINANCES

Residential Annual Tuition: *$7,685* • Non-Residential
Annual Tuition: *$7,685* • General Institutional Fees: *Not
Reported* • Additional Nursing Fees: *Not Reported*

POTTSVILLE HOSPITAL AND WARNE CLINIC

Address: 420 South Jackson Street, Pottsville, PA 17901
Phone: 570-621-5032
Fax: 570-621-5113
Contact: Angela A. Pasco, MSN, RN, Director
Email: phson@pothosp.com

GENERAL INFORMATION

Type of School: *Hospital, Private (Independent)* •
Accreditation: *None* • Total Enrollment: *108*

PROGRAM INFORMATION

NLNAC Accreditation: *Yes*

NURSING STUDENT PROFILE

Total Nursing Enrollment: *108* • Full-Time Enrollment:
108 • Part-Time Enrollment: *0* • Female Enrollment: *98* •
Male Enrollment: *10* • Total New Fall Enrollments: *43* •
Total Graduates: *26*

FINANCES

Residential Annual Tuition: *$6,200* • Non-Residential
Annual Tuition: *$6,200* • General Institutional Fees: *$50* •
Additional Nursing Fees: *Not Reported*

THE READING HOSPITAL SCHOOL OF NURSING

Address: 6th and Spruce Streets, West Reading, PA 19611
Phone: 610-988-8331
Fax: 610-988-5246
Contact: Joanne Kovach, MSN, MEd, RN, Director
Email: kovachj@readinghospital.org

GENERAL INFORMATION

Type of School: *Hospital, Private (Independent)* •
Accreditation: *None* • Total Enrollment: *Not Provided*

PROGRAM INFORMATION

NLNAC Accreditation: *Yes*

NURSING STUDENT PROFILE

Total Nursing Enrollment: *106* • Full-Time Enrollment:
106 • Part-Time Enrollment: *0* • Female Enrollment: *95* •
Male Enrollment: *11* • Total New Fall Enrollments: *50* •
Total Graduates: *36*

FINANCES

Residential Annual Tuition: *$6,759* • Non-Residential
Annual Tuition: *$11,258* • General Institutional Fees: *$295* •
Additional Nursing Fees: *Not Reported*

ROXBOROUGH MEMORIAL HOSPITAL

Address: 5800 Ridge Avenue, Philadelphia, PA 19128
Phone: 215-487-4458
Fax: 215-487-4591
Contact: Paulina M. Marra-Powers, MSN, RN, Director
Email: happynurse1@juno.com

GENERAL INFORMATION

Type of School: *Not Provided* • Accreditation: *Not Provided* •
Total Enrollment: *Not Provided*

PROGRAM INFORMATION

NLNAC Accreditation: *Yes*

NURSING STUDENT PROFILE

Total Nursing Enrollment: *86* • Full-Time Enrollment: *86* •
Part-Time Enrollment: *0* • Female Enrollment: *79* • Male
Enrollment: *7* • Total New Fall Enrollments: *49* • Total
Graduates: *23*

FINANCES

Residential Annual Tuition: *$7,973* • Non-Residential
Annual Tuition: *$7,973* • General Institutional Fees: *$225* •
Additional Nursing Fees: *Not Reported*

Circle 104 on reader card   See in-depth profile for more information

SAINT LUKE'S HOSPITAL

Address: 801 Ostrum Street, Bethlehem, PA 18105
Phone: 610-954-3441
Fax: 610-954-3412
Contact: Janet A. Sipple, EdD, RN, Dean
Email: sipplej@slhn.org

GENERAL INFORMATION

Type of School: *4-Year College or University, Private
(Independent)* • Accreditation: *Middle States Association of
Colleges and Schools* • Total Enrollment: *1,300*

PROGRAM INFORMATION

NLNAC Accreditation: *Yes*

NURSING STUDENT PROFILE

Total Nursing Enrollment: *135* • Full-Time Enrollment: *82* •
Part-Time Enrollment: *53* • Female Enrollment: *121* • Male
Enrollment: *14* • Total New Fall Enrollments: *54* • Total
Graduates: *45*

FINANCES

Residential Annual Tuition: *$12,476* • Non-Residential
Annual Tuition: *$12,476* • General Institutional Fees: *$600* •
Additional Nursing Fees: *Not Reported*

Circle 112 on reader card   See in-depth profile for more information

SHARON REGIONAL HEALTH SYSTEM

Address: 740 East State Street, Sharon, PA 16146
Phone: 724-983-3971
Fax: 724-983-5621
Contact: Nora E. Bennett, MSN, RN, Director
Email: Not Reported

GENERAL INFORMATION

Type of School: *Hospital, Public* • Accreditation: *None* • Total Enrollment: *Not Provided*

PROGRAM INFORMATION

NLNAC Accreditation: *Yes*

NURSING STUDENT PROFILE

Total Nursing Enrollment: *20* • Full-Time Enrollment: *20* • Part-Time Enrollment: *0* • Female Enrollment: *18* • Male Enrollment: *2* • Total New Fall Enrollments: *25* • Total Graduates: *15*

FINANCES

Residential Annual Tuition: *Not Reported* • Non-Residential Annual Tuition: *Not Reported* • General Institutional Fees: *Not Reported* • Additional Nursing Fees: *Not Reported*

ST. FRANCIS HOSPITAL OF NEW CASTLE

Address: 1000 South Mercer Street, New Castle, PA 16101
Phone: 724-656-6001
Fax: 724-656-6167
Contact: Linda B. Werner, MSN, MSEd, RN, Executive Director
Email: werner1@sfhs.edu

GENERAL INFORMATION

Type of School: *Hospital, Private (Religious)* • Accreditation: *None* • Total Enrollment: *Not Provided*

PROGRAM INFORMATION

NLNAC Accreditation: *Yes*

NURSING STUDENT PROFILE

Total Nursing Enrollment: *79* • Full-Time Enrollment: *79* • Part-Time Enrollment: *0* • Female Enrollment: *66* • Male Enrollment: *13* • Total New Fall Enrollments: *48* • Total Graduates: *29*

FINANCES

Residential Annual Tuition: *$6,805* • Non-Residential Annual Tuition: *$6,805* • General Institutional Fees: *$155* • Additional Nursing Fees: *Not Reported*

ST. FRANCIS MEDICAL CENTER

Address: 400 45th Street, Pittsburgh, PA 15201
Phone: 412-622-4749
Fax: 412-622-6770
Contact: Alexis K. Weber, MSN, RN, Director
Email: webera@sfhs.edu

GENERAL INFORMATION

Type of School: *Hospital, Public* • Accreditation: *None* • Total Enrollment: *75*

PROGRAM INFORMATION

NLNAC Accreditation: *Yes*

NURSING STUDENT PROFILE

Total Nursing Enrollment: *51* • Full-Time Enrollment: *40* • Part-Time Enrollment: *11* • Female Enrollment: *45* • Male Enrollment: *6* • Total New Fall Enrollments: *31* • Total Graduates: *13*

FINANCES

Residential Annual Tuition: *$7,675* • Non-Residential Annual Tuition: *$7,675* • General Institutional Fees: *Not Reported* • Additional Nursing Fees: *Not Reported*

UPMC—SHADYSIDE

Address: 5230 Centre Avenue, Pittsburgh, PA 15232
Phone: 412-623-2983
Fax: 412-623-1134
Contact: Mary E. Aukerman, PhD, RN, Director
Email: aukermanme@msx.upmc.edu

GENERAL INFORMATION

Type of School: *Other* • Accreditation: *None* • Total Enrollment: *Not Provided*

PROGRAM INFORMATION

NLNAC Accreditation: *Yes*

NURSING STUDENT PROFILE

Total Nursing Enrollment: *157* • Full-Time Enrollment: *126* • Part-Time Enrollment: *31* • Female Enrollment: *127* • Male Enrollment: *30* • Total New Fall Enrollments: *136* • Total Graduates: *20*

FINANCES

Residential Annual Tuition: *$7,200* • Non-Residential Annual Tuition: *$7,200* • General Institutional Fees: *$450* • Additional Nursing Fees: *Not Reported*

UPMC—ST. MARGARET MEMORIAL HOSPITAL

Address: 815 Freeport Road, Pittsburgh, PA 15215-3301
Phone: 412-784-4992
Fax: 412-784-4994
Contact: Ann D. Ciak, PhD, RN, Director
Email: ciakad@msx.upmc.edu

GENERAL INFORMATION

Type of School: *Other* • Accreditation: *None* • Total Enrollment: *Not Provided*

PROGRAM INFORMATION

NLNAC Accreditation: *Yes*

NURSING STUDENT PROFILE

Total Nursing Enrollment: *28* • Full-Time Enrollment: *28* • Part-Time Enrollment: *0* • Female Enrollment: *20* • Male Enrollment: *8* • Total New Fall Enrollments: *16* • Total Graduates: *13*

FINANCES

Residential Annual Tuition: *$8,680* • Non-Residential Annual Tuition: *$8,680* • General Institutional Fees: *Not Reported* • Additional Nursing Fees: *Not Reported*

THE WASHINGTON HOSPITAL

Address: 155 Wilson Avenue, Washington, PA 15301-3398
Phone: 724-223-3272
Fax: 724-223-4083
Contact: Kathryn M. Yecko, MSN, RN, Director
Email: kyecko@washingtonhospital.org

GENERAL INFORMATION

Type of School: *Hospital, Public* • Accreditation: *None* • Total Enrollment: *70*

PROGRAM INFORMATION

NLNAC Accreditation: *Yes*

NURSING STUDENT PROFILE

Total Nursing Enrollment: *70* • Full-Time Enrollment: *69* • Part-Time Enrollment: *1* • Female Enrollment: *55* • Male Enrollment: *15* • Total New Fall Enrollments: *30* • Total Graduates: *21*

FINANCES

Residential Annual Tuition: *$6,500* • Non-Residential Annual Tuition: *$6,500* • General Institutional Fees: *$785* • Additional Nursing Fees: *Not Reported*

THE WESTERN PENNSYLVANIA HOSPITAL

Address: 4900 Friendship Avenue, Pittsburgh, PA 15224
Phone: 412-578-5531
Fax: 412-578-1837
Contact: Nancy Cobb, MSN, RN, Director
Email: necobb@wpahs.org

GENERAL INFORMATION

Type of School: *Hospital, Private (Independent)* •
Accreditation: *None* • Total Enrollment: *46*

PROGRAM INFORMATION

NLNAC Accreditation: *Yes*

NURSING STUDENT PROFILE

Total Nursing Enrollment: *49* • Full-Time Enrollment: *49* •
Part-Time Enrollment: *0* • Female Enrollment: *42* • Male
Enrollment: *7* • Total New Fall Enrollments: *26* • Total
Graduates: *23*

FINANCES

Residential Annual Tuition: *$7,257* • Non-Residential
Annual Tuition: *Not Reported* • General Institutional Fees:
$607 • Additional Nursing Fees: *Not Reported*

ST. JOSEPH HEALTH SERVICES OF RHODE ISLAND

Address: 200 High Service Avenue, N Providence, RI
           02904
Phone: 401-456-3050
Fax: 401-456-3640
Contact: Elizabeth H. DeCosta, MSN, RN, Director
Email: edecosta@saintjosephri.com

GENERAL INFORMATION

Type of School: *Other* • Accreditation: *None* • Total
Enrollment: *Not Provided*

PROGRAM INFORMATION

NLNAC Accreditation: *Yes*

NURSING STUDENT PROFILE

Total Nursing Enrollment: *51* • Full-Time Enrollment: *51* •
Part-Time Enrollment: *0* • Female Enrollment: *44* • Male
Enrollment: *7* • Total New Fall Enrollments: *11* • Total
Graduates: *15*

FINANCES

Residential Annual Tuition: *$5,500* • Non-Residential
Annual Tuition: *Not Reported* • General Institutional Fees:
Not Reported • Additional Nursing Fees: *Not Reported*

CENTRAL CAROLINA TECHNICAL COLLEGE

Address: 506 North Guignard Drive, Sumter, SC 29150
Phone: 803-778-7822
Fax: 803-778-7868
Contact: Beverly Gulledge, MN, RN, Chairperson
Email: gulledgebh@cctc6.sum.tec.sc.us

GENERAL INFORMATION

Type of School: *2-Year College or University, Public* •
Accreditation: *Southern Association of Colleges and Schools* •
Total Enrollment: *Not Provided*

PROGRAM INFORMATION

NLNAC Accreditation: *Yes*

NURSING STUDENT PROFILE

Total Nursing Enrollment: *18* • Full-Time Enrollment: *0* •
Part-Time Enrollment: *18* • Female Enrollment: *18* • Male
Enrollment: *Not Provided* • Total New Fall Enrollments: *23* •
Total Graduates: *10*

FINANCES

Residential Annual Tuition: *$850* • Non-Residential Annual
Tuition: *$1,922* • General Institutional Fees: *Not Reported* •
Additional Nursing Fees: *Not Reported*

METHODIST HEALTHCARE

Address: 251 S. Claybrook, Memphis, TN 38104
Phone: 901-726-8516
Fax: 901-726-8524
Contact: Elizabeth D. Clarke, MSN, RN, Assistant Vice
President, Nursing Education
Email: clarke@methodisthealth.org

GENERAL INFORMATION

Type of School: *Hospital, Private (Religious)* • Accreditation:
None • Total Enrollment: *Not Provided*

PROGRAM INFORMATION

NLNAC Accreditation: *Yes*

NURSING STUDENT PROFILE

Total Nursing Enrollment: *Not Provided* • Full-Time
Enrollment: *Not Provided* • Part-Time Enrollment: *Not
Provided* • Female Enrollment: *Not Provided* • Male
Enrollment: *Not Provided* • Total New Fall Enrollments: *Not
Provided* • Total Graduates: *Not Provided*

FINANCES

Residential Annual Tuition: *Not Reported* • Non-Residential
Annual Tuition: *Not Reported* • General Institutional Fees:
Not Reported • Additional Nursing Fees: *Not Reported*

BAPTIST HEALTH SYSTEM

Address: 111 Dallas Street, San Antonio, TX 78205-1230
Phone: 210-297-9102
Fax: 210-297-0915
Contact: Darlene Nebel Cantu, MSN, RNC, Director
Email: dcantu@baptisthealthsystem.org

GENERAL INFORMATION

Type of School: *Hospital, Other* • Accreditation: *None* • Total Enrollment: *218*

PROGRAM INFORMATION

NLNAC Accreditation: *Yes*

NURSING STUDENT PROFILE

Total Nursing Enrollment: *129* • Full-Time Enrollment: *129* • Part-Time Enrollment: *0* • Female Enrollment: *112* • Male Enrollment: *17* • Total New Fall Enrollments: *45* • Total Graduates: *68*

FINANCES

Residential Annual Tuition: *$1,440* • Non-Residential Annual Tuition: *$1,440* • General Institutional Fees: *$40* • Additional Nursing Fees: *Not Reported*

COVENANT HEALTH SYSTEM

Address: 2002 Miami Avenue, Lubbock, TX 79410
Phone: 806-797-0955
Fax: Not Reported
Contact: Irene S. Wilson, MSN, RN, Dean
Email: iwilson@covhs.org

GENERAL INFORMATION

Type of School: *Hospital, Private (Religious)* • Accreditation: *None* • Total Enrollment: *Not Provided*

PROGRAM INFORMATION

NLNAC Accreditation: *Yes*

NURSING STUDENT PROFILE

Total Nursing Enrollment: *128* • Full-Time Enrollment: *128* • Part-Time Enrollment: *0* • Female Enrollment: *108* • Male Enrollment: *20* • Total New Fall Enrollments: *76* • Total Graduates: *63*

FINANCES

Residential Annual Tuition: *$5,000* • Non-Residential Annual Tuition: *$5,000* • General Institutional Fees: *Not Reported* • Additional Nursing Fees: *Not Reported*

Circle 37 on reader card   **See in-depth profile for more information**

BON SECOURS MEMORIAL

Address: 8550 Magellan Parkway, Suite 1100, Richmond, VA 23227
Phone: 804-915-8025
Fax: 804-915-8281
Contact: Mary Ruth Fox, MSN, RN, Dean
Email: mary-fox@bshsi.com

GENERAL INFORMATION

Type of School: *Hospital, Private (Religious)* • Accreditation: *None* • Total Enrollment: *99*

PROGRAM INFORMATION

NLNAC Accreditation: *Yes*

NURSING STUDENT PROFILE

Total Nursing Enrollment: *99* • Full-Time Enrollment: *99* • Part-Time Enrollment: *0* • Female Enrollment: *93* • Male Enrollment: *6* • Total New Fall Enrollments: *51* • Total Graduates: *21*

FINANCES

Residential Annual Tuition: *$1,800* • Non-Residential Annual Tuition: *$1,800* • General Institutional Fees: *$600* • Additional Nursing Fees: *Not Reported*

CENTRA HEALTH

Address: 1901 Tate Springs Road, Lynchburgh, VA 24501
Phone: 434-947-3070
Fax: 434-947-5239
Contact: Patricia J. Uzsoy, EdS, RN, Dean
Email: pat.uzsoy@centrahealth.com

GENERAL INFORMATION

Type of School: *Hospital, Private (Independent)* • Accreditation: *None* • Total Enrollment: *Not Provided*

PROGRAM INFORMATION

NLNAC Accreditation: *Yes*

NURSING STUDENT PROFILE

Total Nursing Enrollment: *Not Provided* • Full-Time Enrollment: *Not Provided* • Part-Time Enrollment: *Not Provided* • Female Enrollment: *Not Provided* • Male Enrollment: *Not Provided* • Total New Fall Enrollments: *Not Provided* • Total Graduates: *Not Provided*

FINANCES

Residential Annual Tuition: *Not Reported* • Non-Residential Annual Tuition: *Not Reported* • General Institutional Fees: *Not Reported* • Additional Nursing Fees: *Not Reported*

DANVILLE REGIONAL MEDICAL CENTER

Address: 142 South Main Street, Danville, VA 24541
Phone: 434-799-4510
Fax: 434-799-3718
Contact: Darnelle H. Cockram-Cox, EdD, RN, Director
Email: cockramd@drhsi.org

GENERAL INFORMATION

Type of School: *Hospital, Private (Independent)* •
Accreditation: *None* • Total Enrollment: *Not Provided*

PROGRAM INFORMATION

NLNAC Accreditation: *Yes*

NURSING STUDENT PROFILE

Total Nursing Enrollment: *68* • Full-Time Enrollment: *68* •
Part-Time Enrollment: *0* • Female Enrollment: *64* • Male
Enrollment: *4* • Total New Fall Enrollments: *43* • Total
Graduates: *33*

FINANCES

Residential Annual Tuition: *$4,700* • Non-Residential
Annual Tuition: *$4,700* • General Institutional Fees: *$455* •
Additional Nursing Fees: *Not Reported*

RIVERSIDE HEALTH SYSTEM

Address: 500 J. Clyde Morris Blvd, Newport News, VA
            23601
Phone: 757-594-2714
Fax: 757-594-3713
Contact: Deborah Sullivan-Yates, MSN, RN, Director
Email: debbie.sullivan-yates@rivhs.com

GENERAL INFORMATION

Type of School: *Other, Private (Independent)* • Accreditation:
None • Total Enrollment: *136*

PROGRAM INFORMATION

NLNAC Accreditation: *Yes*

NURSING STUDENT PROFILE

Total Nursing Enrollment: *Not Provided* • Full-Time
Enrollment: *Not Provided* • Part-Time Enrollment: *Not
Provided* • Female Enrollment: *Not Provided* • Male
Enrollment: *Not Provided* • Total New Fall Enrollments: *Not
Provided* • Total Graduates: *Not Provided*

FINANCES

Residential Annual Tuition: *Not Reported* • Non-Residential
Annual Tuition: *Not Reported* • General Institutional Fees:
Not Reported • Additional Nursing Fees: *Not Reported*

SENTARA NORFOLK GENERAL HOSPITAL

Address: 600 Gresham Drive, Norfolk, VA 23507
Phone: 757-668-2900
Fax: 757-668-2905
Contact: Shelly Vinson, MSN, MS, RN, Director
Email: sgvinson@sentara.com

GENERAL INFORMATION

Type of School: *Hospital, Private (Independent)* •
Accreditation: *None* • Total Enrollment: *150*

PROGRAM INFORMATION

NLNAC Accreditation: *Yes*

NURSING STUDENT PROFILE

Total Nursing Enrollment: *54* • Full-Time Enrollment: *51* •
Part-Time Enrollment: *3* • Female Enrollment: *51* • Male
Enrollment: *3* • Total New Fall Enrollments: *27* • Total
Graduates: *26*

FINANCES

Residential Annual Tuition: *$4,500* • Non-Residential
Annual Tuition: *Not Reported* • General Institutional Fees:
$800 • Additional Nursing Fees: *Not Reported*

SOUTHSIDE REGIONAL MEDICAL CENTER

Address: 801 South Adams Street, Petersburg, VA 23803
Phone: 804-862-5801
Fax: 804-862-5937
Contact: Rose Saunders, MN, RN, Vice President and
Director
Email: rsaunders@ssrmc.org

GENERAL INFORMATION

Type of School: *Hospital, Public* • Accreditation: *None* • Total
Enrollment: *54*

PROGRAM INFORMATION

NLNAC Accreditation: *Yes*

NURSING STUDENT PROFILE

Total Nursing Enrollment: *54* • Full-Time Enrollment: *54* •
Part-Time Enrollment: *0* • Female Enrollment: *53* • Male
Enrollment: *1* • Total New Fall Enrollments: *25* • Total
Graduates: *20*

FINANCES

Residential Annual Tuition: *$1,080* • Non-Residential
Annual Tuition: *$1,080* • General Institutional Fees: *Not
Reported* • Additional Nursing Fees: *Not Reported*

SUFFOLK PUBLIC SCHOOL LOUISE OBICI MEMORIAL HOSPITAL

Address: 1900 North Main Street, Suffolk, VA 23439-
          1100
Phone: 757-934-4741
Fax: 757-934-4760
Contact: Sondra Y. Statzer, EdS, RN, Director
Email: sstatzer@obici.com

GENERAL INFORMATION

Type of School: *Hospital, Other* • Accreditation: *None* • Total
Enrollment: *Not Provided*

PROGRAM INFORMATION

NLNAC Accreditation: *Yes*

NURSING STUDENT PROFILE

Total Nursing Enrollment: *51* • Full-Time Enrollment: *51* •
Part-Time Enrollment: *0* • Female Enrollment: *50* • Male
Enrollment: *1* • Total New Fall Enrollments: *18* • Total
Graduates: *2243*

FINANCES

Residential Annual Tuition: *$2,500* • Non-Residential
Annual Tuition: *$360* • General Institutional Fees: *Not
Reported* • Additional Nursing Fees: *Not Reported*

Section 3

MASTER'S PROGRAMS

IDA V. MOFFETT SCHOOL— SAMFORD UNIVERSITY

Address: 800 Lake Shore Drive, Birmingham, AL 35229
Phone: 205-726-2760
Fax: 205-726-4179
Contact: Jane S. Martin, PhD, RN, CS, NP-C, FNP,
Assistant Dean of Graduate Studies
Email: jsmartin@samford.edu

GENERAL INFORMATION

Type of School: *4-Year College or University, Public* •
Accreditation: *Southern Association of Colleges and Schools* •
Total Enrollment: *1000*

PROGRAM INFORMATION

NLNAC Accreditation: *Not Reported* • CCNE Accreditation:
Yes

_____

For specialty program listings, refer to the index.

NURSING STUDENT PROFILE

Total Nursing Enrollments: *69* • Full-Time Enrollment: *60* •
Part-Time Enrollment: *9* • Female Enrollment: *61* • Male
Enrollment: *8* • Total Graduates: *25*

FINANCES

Residental Annual Tuition: *$6,894* • Non-Residential
Annual Tuition: *$6,894* • General Institutional Fees: *$25* •
Additional Nursing Fees: *$35*

JACKSONVILLE STATE UNIVERSITY

Address: 700 Pelham Road North, Jacksonville, AL 30230
Phone: 256-782-5431
Fax: 256-782-5406
Contact: Beth S. Hembree, DSN, RN, Professor and
Director of Graduate Studies
Email: bhembree@jsucc.jsu.edu

GENERAL INFORMATION

Type of School: *4-Year College or University, Public* •
Accreditation: *Southern Association of Colleges and Schools* •
Total Enrollment: *Not Provided*

PROGRAM INFORMATION

NLNAC Accreditation: *Not Reported* • CCNE Accreditation:
Yes

_____

For specialty program listings, refer to the index.

NURSING STUDENT PROFILE

Total Nursing Enrollments: *27* • Full-Time Enrollment: *8* •
Part-Time Enrollment: *19* • Female Enrollment: *27* • Male
Enrollment: *0* • Total Graduates: *10*

FINANCES

Residental Annual Tuition: *$2,940* • Non-Residential
Annual Tuition: *$5,880* • General Institutional Fees: *$0* •
Additional Nursing Fees: *$15*

TROY STATE UNIVERSITY

Address: P.O. Box 967, Troy, AL 36082
Phone: 334-241-8656
Fax: 334-241-8627
Contact: Charlene H. Schwab, RN, PhD, Director of
             MSN Program
Email: cschwab@troyst.edu

GENERAL INFORMATION

Type of School: *Not Provided* • Accreditation: *Southern Association of Colleges and Schools* • Total Enrollment: *19374*

PROGRAM INFORMATION

NLNAC Accreditation: *Yes* • CCNE Accreditation:

For specialty program listings, refer to the index.

NURSING STUDENT PROFILE

Total Nursing Enrollments: *93* • Full-Time Enrollment: *38* • Part-Time Enrollment: *55* • Female Enrollment: *89* • Male Enrollment: *4* • Total Graduates: *41*

FINANCES

Residental Annual Tuition: *$5,152* • Non-Residential Annual Tuition: *$10,304* • General Institutional Fees: *$156* • Additional Nursing Fees: *$150*

UNIVERSITY OF ALABAMA

Address: 1530 Third Avenue, South, Birmingham, AL
             35294-1210
Phone: 205-348-1044
Fax: 205-348-5559
Contact: Donna R. Packa, RN, DSN, Associate Dean for
             Academic Programs
Email: dpacka@bama.ua.edu

GENERAL INFORMATION

Type of School: *4-Year College or University, Public* • Accreditation: *Southern Association of Colleges and Schools* • Total Enrollment: *Not Provided*

PROGRAM INFORMATION

NLNAC Accreditation: *Not Reported* • CCNE Accreditation: *Yes*

For specialty program listings, refer to the index.

NURSING STUDENT PROFILE

Total Nursing Enrollments: *39* • Full-Time Enrollment: *11* • Part-Time Enrollment: *28* • Female Enrollment: *35* • Male Enrollment: *4* • Total Graduates: *17*

FINANCES

Residental Annual Tuition: *$1,646* • Non-Residential Annual Tuition: *$4,456* • General Institutional Fees: *$140* • Additional Nursing Fees: *$20*

UNIVERSITY OF ALABAMA— HUNTSVILLE

Address: 301 Sparkman Drive, Huntsville, AL 35899-0001
Phone: 256-824-6345
Fax: Not Provided
Contact: Fay Raines, PhD, Dean
Email: nursing@uah.edu

GENERAL INFORMATION

Type of School: *Other* • Accreditation: *Southern Association of Colleges and Schools* • Total Enrollment: *19171*

PROGRAM INFORMATION

NLNAC Accreditation: *Yes* • CCNE Accreditation:

_____

For specialty program listings, refer to the index.

NURSING STUDENT PROFILE

Total Nursing Enrollments: *176* • Full-Time Enrollment: *89* • Part-Time Enrollment: *87* • Female Enrollment: *Not Provided* • Male Enrollment: *Not Provided* • Total Graduates: *57*

FINANCES

Residental Annual Tuition: *Not Reported* • Non-Residential Annual Tuition: *Not Reported* • General Institutional Fees: *Not Reported* • Additional Nursing Fees: *Not Reported*

UNIVERSITY OF ALABAMA— TUSCALOOA

Address: PO Box 870358, Tuscaloosa, AL 35487-0358
Phone: 205-348-4404
Fax: 205-348-5559
Contact: Donna R Packa, DSN, RN, Associate Dean for Academic Programs
Email: dpacka@bama.ua.edu

GENERAL INFORMATION

Type of School: *4-Year College or University, Other* • Accreditation: *Southern Association of Colleges and Schools* • Total Enrollment: *6501*

PROGRAM INFORMATION

NLNAC Accreditation: *Not Reported* • CCNE Accreditation:

_____

For specialty program listings, refer to the index.

NURSING STUDENT PROFILE

Total Nursing Enrollments: *Not Provided* • Full-Time Enrollment: *Not Provided* • Part-Time Enrollment: *Not Provided* • Female Enrollment: *Not Provided* • Male Enrollment: *Not Provided* • Total Graduates: *Not Provided*

FINANCES

Residental Annual Tuition: *Not Reported* • Non-Residential Annual Tuition: *Not Reported* • General Institutional Fees: *Not Reported* • Additional Nursing Fees: *Not Reported*

UNIVERSITY OF SOUTH ALABAMA

Address: 471 University Parkway, Mobile, AL 36688
Phone: 334-434-3425
Fax: Not Provided
Contact: Rosemary Rhodes, DNS, RN, Associate Dean for Academic Affairs
Email: rrhodes@usamail.usouthal.edu

GENERAL INFORMATION

Type of School: *4-Year College or University, Private (Religious)* • Accreditation: *Southern Association of Colleges and Schools* • Total Enrollment: *7366*

PROGRAM INFORMATION

NLNAC Accreditation: *Yes* • CCNE Accreditation:

_____

For specialty program listings, refer to the index.

NURSING STUDENT PROFILE

Total Nursing Enrollments: *255* • Full-Time Enrollment: *190* • Part-Time Enrollment: *65* • Female Enrollment: *223* • Male Enrollment: *32* • Total Graduates: *114*

FINANCES

Residental Annual Tuition: *$2,070* • Non-Residential Annual Tuition: *$4,140* • General Institutional Fees: *$240* • Additional Nursing Fees: *$180*

UNIVERSITY OF ALASKA— ANCHORAGE

Address: 3211 Providence Drive, Anchorage, AK 99508-8030
Phone: 907-786-4571
Fax: 907-786-4574
Contact: Tina D. DeLapp, RN, EdD, Director, School of Nursing
Email: aftdd@uaa.alaska.edu

GENERAL INFORMATION

Type of School: *4-Year College or University, Public* • Accreditation: *Northwestern Association of Schools and Colleges* • Total Enrollment: *10420*

PROGRAM INFORMATION

NLNAC Accreditation: *Yes* • CCNE Accreditation:

_____

For specialty program listings, refer to the index.

NURSING STUDENT PROFILE

Total Nursing Enrollments: *68* • Full-Time Enrollment: *12* • Part-Time Enrollment: *56* • Female Enrollment: *65* • Male Enrollment: *3* • Total Graduates: *13*

FINANCES

Residental Annual Tuition: *Not Reported* • Non-Residential Annual Tuition: *Not Reported* • General Institutional Fees: *Not Reported* • Additional Nursing Fees: *Not Reported*

UNIVERSITY OF ARIZONA

Address: 1 Bruce St., Tucson, AZ 72110
Phone: 520-626-6151
Fax: Not Provided
Contact: Pamela G. Reed, RN, PhD, FAAN, Associate
             Dean for Academic Affairs
Email: preed@nursing.arizona.edu

GENERAL INFORMATION

Type of School: *4-Year College or University, Public •*
Accreditation: *North Central Association of Colleges and
Schools •* Total Enrollment: *6500*

PROGRAM INFORMATION

NLNAC Accreditation: *Yes •* CCNE Accreditation:

_____

For specialty program listings, refer to the index.

NURSING STUDENT PROFILE

Total Nursing Enrollments: *81 •* Full-Time Enrollment: *31 •*
Part-Time Enrollment: *50 •* Female Enrollment: *75 •* Male
Enrollment: *6 •* Total Graduates: *40*

FINANCES

Residental Annual Tuition: *$2,264 •* Non-Residential
Annual Tuition: *$7,078 •* General Institutional Fees: *$76 •*
Additional Nursing Fees: *$150*

UNIVERSITY OF PHOENIX

Address: 4615 East Elwood, Phoenix, AZ 85040
Phone: 480-966-9577
Fax: 480-929-7164
Contact: Catherine Garner, DrPH, RNC, FAAN, Dean,
             College of Health Sciences and Nursing
Email: catherine.garner@phoenix.edu

GENERAL INFORMATION

Type of School: *4-Year College or University, Private
(Independent) •* Accreditation: *North Central Association of
Colleges and Schools •* Total Enrollment: *27000*

PROGRAM INFORMATION

NLNAC Accreditation: *Yes •* CCNE Accreditation:

_____

For specialty program listings, refer to the index.

NURSING STUDENT PROFILE

Total Nursing Enrollments: *1613 •* Full-Time Enrollment:
1613 • Part-Time Enrollment: *0 •* Female Enrollment: *Not
Provided •* Male Enrollment: *Not Provided •* Total Graduates:
669

FINANCES

Residental Annual Tuition: *Not Reported •* Non-Residential
Annual Tuition: *Not Reported •* General Institutional Fees:
Not Reported • Additional Nursing Fees: *Not Reported*

ARKANSAS STATE UNIVERSITY

Address:　P.O.Box 910, State University, AR 72467
Phone:　　870-972-3074
Fax:　　　870-972-2954
Contact:　Elizabeth N. Stokes, Ed, RN, Director, MSN
　　　　　Program
Email:　　estokes@astate.edu

GENERAL INFORMATION

Type of School: *4-Year College or University, Public* •
Accreditation: *North Central Association of Colleges and
Schools* • Total Enrollment: *10000*

PROGRAM INFORMATION

NLNAC Accreditation: *Yes* • CCNE Accreditation:

_____

For specialty program listings, refer to the index.

NURSING STUDENT PROFILE

Total Nursing Enrollments: *56* • Full-Time Enrollment: *18* •
Part-Time Enrollment: *38* • Female Enrollment: *51* • Male
Enrollment: *5* • Total Graduates: *25*

FINANCES

Residental Annual Tuition: *$2,976* • Non-Residential
Annual Tuition: *$7,488* • General Institutional Fees: *$186* •
Additional Nursing Fees: *$110*

HARDING UNIVERSITY

Address:　PO Box 12265, Searcy, AR 72149-0001
Phone:　　501-279-4476
Fax:　　　501-279-4669
Contact:　Cathleen M. Schultz, PhD, RN, FAAN,
　　　　　Professor and Dean
Email:　　shultz@harding.edu

GENERAL INFORMATION

Type of School: *Not Provided* • Accreditation: *North Central
Association of Colleges and Schools* • Total Enrollment: *1152*

PROGRAM INFORMATION

NLNAC Accreditation: *Not Reported* • CCNE Accreditation:

_____

For specialty program listings, refer to the index.

NURSING STUDENT PROFILE

Total Nursing Enrollments: *8* • Full-Time Enrollment: *0* •
Part-Time Enrollment: *8* • Female Enrollment: *8* • Male
Enrollment: *0* • Total Graduates: *2*

FINANCES

Residental Annual Tuition: *$6,138* • Non-Residential
Annual Tuition: *Not Reported* • General Institutional Fees:
$150 • Additional Nursing Fees: *Not Reported*

UNIVERSITY OF ARKANSAS FOR MEDICAL SCIENCES

Address: 1200 University Drive, Little Rock, AR 71601
Phone: 501-686-7997
Fax: Not Provided
Contact: Pegge L. Bell, RN, Interim Associate Dean
Email: bellpegge1@exchange.uams.edu

GENERAL INFORMATION

Type of School: *4-Year College or University, Public* •
Accreditation: *North Central Association of Colleges and Schools* • Total Enrollment: *1056*

PROGRAM INFORMATION

NLNAC Accreditation: *Yes* • CCNE Accreditation:

———————

For specialty program listings, refer to the index.

NURSING STUDENT PROFILE

Total Nursing Enrollments: *201* • Full-Time Enrollment: *23* • Part-Time Enrollment: *178* • Female Enrollment: *180* • Male Enrollment: *21* • Total Graduates: *44*

FINANCES

Residental Annual Tuition: *$3,360* • Non-Residential Annual Tuition: *$7,200* • General Institutional Fees: *$75* • Additional Nursing Fees: *$212*

UNIVERSITY OF CENTRAL ARKANSAS

Address: 201 Donaghey Avenue, Conway, AR 72035-0001
Phone: 501-450-3119
Fax: 501-450-5560
Contact: Barbara G. Williams, RN, PhD, Professor and Chair
Email: barbaraw@mail.uca.edu

GENERAL INFORMATION

Type of School: *4-Year College or University, Public* •
Accreditation: *North Central Association of Colleges and Schools* • Total Enrollment: *2500*

PROGRAM INFORMATION

NLNAC Accreditation: *Yes* • CCNE Accreditation: *Provisional*

———————

For specialty program listings, refer to the index.

NURSING STUDENT PROFILE

Total Nursing Enrollments: *58* • Full-Time Enrollment: *5* • Part-Time Enrollment: *53* • Female Enrollment: *54* • Male Enrollment: *4* • Total Graduates: *16*

FINANCES

Residental Annual Tuition: *$3,812* • Non-Residential Annual Tuition: *$7,896* • General Institutional Fees: *$58* • Additional Nursing Fees: *$11*

AZUSA PACIFIC UNIVERSITY

Address: 901 East Alosta Avenue, Azusa, CA 91702-7000
Phone: 626-815-5386
Fax: 626-815-5414
Contact: Leslie Van Dover, RN, MScN, PhD, Chair, Graduate Program
Email: lvandover@apu.edu

GENERAL INFORMATION

Type of School: *4-Year College or University, Private (Religious)* • Accreditation: *Western Association of Schools and Colleges* • Total Enrollment: *7000*

PROGRAM INFORMATION

NLNAC Accreditation: *Yes* • CCNE Accreditation:

_____

For specialty program listings, refer to the index.

NURSING STUDENT PROFILE

Total Nursing Enrollments: *74* • Full-Time Enrollment: *74* • Part-Time Enrollment: *0* • Female Enrollment: *71* • Male Enrollment: *3* • Total Graduates: *15*

FINANCES

Residental Annual Tuition: *$4,560* • Non-Residential Annual Tuition: *$4,560* • General Institutional Fees: *$70* • Additional Nursing Fees: *$270*

CALIFORNIA STATE UNIVERSITY—BAKERSFIELD

Address: 9001 Stockdale Highway, Hazard, CA 93311-1099
Phone: 661-664-2093
Fax: Not Provided
Contact: Candace Meares, PhD, RN, CNAA, Department Chair
Email: cmeares@csubak.edu

GENERAL INFORMATION

Type of School: *4-Year College or University, Public* • Accreditation: *Western Association of Schools and Colleges* • Total Enrollment: *6000*

PROGRAM INFORMATION

NLNAC Accreditation: *Yes* • CCNE Accreditation:

_____

For specialty program listings, refer to the index.

NURSING STUDENT PROFILE

Total Nursing Enrollments: *32* • Full-Time Enrollment: *0* • Part-Time Enrollment: *32* • Female Enrollment: *28* • Male Enrollment: *4* • Total Graduates: *8*

FINANCES

Residental Annual Tuition: *Not Reported* • Non-Residential Annual Tuition: *Not Reported* • General Institutional Fees: *Not Reported* • Additional Nursing Fees: *Not Reported*

CALIFORNIA STATE UNIVERSITY—CHICO

Address: 1st and Orange Street, Highland Springs, CA 95929
Phone: 530-898-5891
Fax: 230-898-4363
Contact: Shelley Young, RN, EdD, Graduate Coordinator
Email: syoung@csuchico.edu

GENERAL INFORMATION

Type of School: *4-Year College or University, Public* •
Accreditation: *Western Association of Schools and Colleges* •
Total Enrollment: *14000*

PROGRAM INFORMATION

NLNAC Accreditation: *Yes* • CCNE Accreditation:

For specialty program listings, refer to the index.

NURSING STUDENT PROFILE

Total Nursing Enrollments: *19* • Full-Time Enrollment: *0* •
Part-Time Enrollment: *19* • Female Enrollment: *18* • Male
Enrollment: *1* • Total Graduates: *Not Provided*

FINANCES

Residental Annual Tuition: *$1,128* • Non-Residential
Annual Tuition: *$10,152* • General Institutional Fees: *$750* •
Additional Nursing Fees: *$30*

CALIFORNIA STATE UNIVERSITY—DOMINGUEZ HILLS

Address: LaCorte Hall, 1000 East Victoria Street, Carson, CA 90747
Phone: 310-243-2059
Fax: Not Provided
Contact: Carole Shea, PhD, RN, FAAN, Professor and Chair
Email: cshea@soh.csudh.edu

GENERAL INFORMATION

Type of School: *4-Year College or University, Public* •
Accreditation: *Western Association of Schools and Colleges* •
Total Enrollment: *10000*

PROGRAM INFORMATION

NLNAC Accreditation: *Yes* • CCNE Accreditation:

For specialty program listings, refer to the index.

NURSING STUDENT PROFILE

Total Nursing Enrollments: *436* • Full-Time Enrollment:
84 • Part-Time Enrollment: *352* • Female Enrollment: *410* •
Male Enrollment: *26* • Total Graduates: *128*

FINANCES

Residental Annual Tuition: *Not Reported* • Non-Residential
Annual Tuition: *Not Reported* • General Institutional Fees:
Not Reported • Additional Nursing Fees: *Not Reported*

Circle 21 on reader card   See in-depth profile for more information

CALIFORNIA STATE UNIVERSITY—FRESNO

Address: 2345 East San Ramon M/s MH25, Arkadelphia, CA 93727
Phone: 559-278-2429
Fax: Not Provided
Contact: Michael Russler, RN, EdD, CFNP, Professor, Graduate Coordinator
Email: michaelr@csufresno.edu

GENERAL INFORMATION

Type of School: *4-Year College or University, Public* •
Accreditation: *Western Association of Schools and Colleges* •
Total Enrollment: *19000*

PROGRAM INFORMATION

NLNAC Accreditation: *Not Reported* • CCNE Accreditation:

_____

For specialty program listings, refer to the index.

NURSING STUDENT PROFILE

Total Nursing Enrollments: *66* • Full-Time Enrollment: *42* •
Part-Time Enrollment: *24* • Female Enrollment: *57* • Male
Enrollment: *9* • Total Graduates: *29*

FINANCES

Residental Annual Tuition: *$1,194* • Non-Residential
Annual Tuition: *$4,146* • General Institutional Fees: *Not
Reported* • Additional Nursing Fees: *$100*

CALIFORNIA STATE UNIVERSITY—FULLERTON

Address: 800 North State College Boulevard, Fullerton, CA 92834
Phone: 714-278-2291
Fax: 714-278-3338
Contact: Christine Latham, RN,DNSc, Nursing Department Chair
Email: clatham@fullerton.edu

GENERAL INFORMATION

Type of School: *4-Year College or University, Public* •
Accreditation: *Western Association of Schools and Colleges* •
Total Enrollment: *30357*

PROGRAM INFORMATION

NLNAC Accreditation: *Not Reported* • CCNE Accreditation:

_____

For specialty program listings, refer to the index.

NURSING STUDENT PROFILE

Total Nursing Enrollments: *66* • Full-Time Enrollment: *51* •
Part-Time Enrollment: *15* • Female Enrollment: *33* • Male
Enrollment: *33* • Total Graduates: *21*

FINANCES

Residental Annual Tuition: *$1,363* • Non-Residential
Annual Tuition: *$8,460* • General Institutional Fees: *Not
Reported* • Additional Nursing Fees: *$1,610*

CALIFORNIA STATE UNIVERSITY—HAYWARD

Address: 25800 Carlos Bee Boulevard, Hayward, CA 94542
Phone: 510-885-2797
Fax: 510-885-2156
Contact: Bette Felton, PhD, RN, Professor/Graduate Coordinator
Email: bfelton@csuhayward.edu

GENERAL INFORMATION

Type of School: *4-Year College or University, Public* •
Accreditation: *Western Association of Schools and Colleges* •
Total Enrollment: *13000*

PROGRAM INFORMATION

NLNAC Accreditation: *Not Reported* • CCNE Accreditation:

———

For specialty program listings, refer to the index.

NURSING STUDENT PROFILE

Total Nursing Enrollments: *7* • Full-Time Enrollment: *0* •
Part-Time Enrollment: *7* • Female Enrollment: *3* • Male
Enrollment: *4* • Total Graduates: *Not Provided*

FINANCES

Residental Annual Tuition: *$1,156* • Non-Residential
Annual Tuition: *$3,710* • General Institutional Fees: *$124* •
Additional Nursing Fees: *Not Reported*

CALIFORNIA STATE UNIVERSITY—LOS ANGELES

Address: 5151 State Univ. Drive, Los Angeles, CA 90032-4226
Phone: 323-343-4700
Fax: 323-343-6454
Contact: Judith L. Papenhausen, PhD, RN, Chairperson and Professor
Email: jpapenh@cslanet.calstatela.edu

GENERAL INFORMATION

Type of School: *Not Provided* • Accreditation: *Not Provided* •
Total Enrollment: *Not Provided*

PROGRAM INFORMATION

NLNAC Accreditation: *Yes* • CCNE Accreditation:

———

For specialty program listings, refer to the index.

NURSING STUDENT PROFILE

Total Nursing Enrollments: *111* • Full-Time Enrollment:
73 • Part-Time Enrollment: *38* • Female Enrollment: *94* •
Male Enrollment: *17* • Total Graduates: *24*

FINANCES

Residental Annual Tuition: *$1,770* • Non-Residential
Annual Tuition: *$7,786* • General Institutional Fees: *$357* •
Additional Nursing Fees: *Not Reported*

CALIFORNIA STATE UNIVERSITY—SACRAMENTO

Address: 6000 J. Street, Hilo, CA 95819-6096
Phone: 916-278-6525
Fax: 916-278-6311
Contact: Susan Proctor, RN, MPH, DNS, Acting
            Graduate Coordinator, School Nurse
            Coordinator and Professor
Email: proctors@csus.edu

GENERAL INFORMATION

Type of School: *4-Year College or University, Public* •
Accreditation: *Western Association of Schools and Colleges* •
Total Enrollment: *26923*

PROGRAM INFORMATION

NLNAC Accreditation: *Not Reported* • CCNE Accreditation:
Yes

———

For specialty program listings, refer to the index.

NURSING STUDENT PROFILE

Total Nursing Enrollments: *Not Provided* • Full-Time
Enrollment: *Not Provided* • Part-Time Enrollment: *Not
Provided* • Female Enrollment: *Not Provided* • Male
Enrollment: *Not Provided* • Total Graduates: *Not Provided*

FINANCES

Residental Annual Tuition: *Not Reported* • Non-Residential
Annual Tuition: *Not Reported* • General Institutional Fees:
Not Reported • Additional Nursing Fees: *Not Reported*

CALIFORNIA STATE UNIVERSITY—SAN BERNARDINO

Address: 5500 University Parkway, Washington, CA
            92407
Phone: 909-880-5382
Fax: 909-880-7089
Contact: Susan L. Lloyd, PhD, RN, Director, MSN,
            Professor
Email: slloyd@csusb.edu

GENERAL INFORMATION

Type of School: *4-Year College or University, Public* •
Accreditation: *Western Association of Schools and Colleges* •
Total Enrollment: *15000*

PROGRAM INFORMATION

NLNAC Accreditation: *Not Reported* • CCNE Accreditation:

———

For specialty program listings, refer to the index.

NURSING STUDENT PROFILE

Total Nursing Enrollments: *38* • Full-Time Enrollment: *22* •
Part-Time Enrollment: *16* • Female Enrollment: *35* • Male
Enrollment: *3* • Total Graduates: *Not Provided*

FINANCES

Residental Annual Tuition: *$937* • Non-Residential Annual
Tuition: *$6,953* • General Institutional Fees: *Not Reported* •
Additional Nursing Fees: *Not Reported*

HOLY NAMES COLLEGE

Address: 3500 Montains Blvd, Oakland, CA 29440-9620
Phone: 510-436-1024
Fax: 510-436-1376
Contact: Fay L. Bower, DNSc,FAAN, Chair
Email: bower@hnc.edu

GENERAL INFORMATION

Type of School: *4-Year College or University, Private (Religious)* • Accreditation: *Not Provided* • Total Enrollment: *2800*

PROGRAM INFORMATION

NLNAC Accreditation: *Not Reported* • CCNE Accreditation: *Yes*

_____

For specialty program listings, refer to the index.

NURSING STUDENT PROFILE

Total Nursing Enrollments: *40* • Full-Time Enrollment: *37* • Part-Time Enrollment: *3* • Female Enrollment: *37* • Male Enrollment: *3* • Total Graduates: *17*

FINANCES

Residental Annual Tuition: *$8,280* • Non-Residential Annual Tuition: *$8,280* • General Institutional Fees: *$120* • Additional Nursing Fees: *$75*

LOMA LINDA UNIVERSITY

Address: 11262 Campus Street, Loma Linda, CA 92350
Phone: 909-558-8061
Fax: 909-558-0719
Contact: Loise Van Cleve, PhD, RN, Associate Dean, Graduate Program
Email: lvancleve@sn.llu.edu

GENERAL INFORMATION

Type of School: *4-Year College or University, Public* • Accreditation: *Western Association of Schools and Colleges* • Total Enrollment: *1174*

PROGRAM INFORMATION

NLNAC Accreditation: *Not Reported* • CCNE Accreditation:

_____

For specialty program listings, refer to the index.

NURSING STUDENT PROFILE

Total Nursing Enrollments: *62* • Full-Time Enrollment: *20* • Part-Time Enrollment: *42* • Female Enrollment: *60* • Male Enrollment: *2* • Total Graduates: *27*

FINANCES

Residental Annual Tuition: *$14,240* • Non-Residential Annual Tuition: *$14,240* • General Institutional Fees: *$0* • Additional Nursing Fees: *$0*

MOUNT ST. MARY'S COLLEGE

Address: 10 Chester Place, Los Angeles, CA 90007
Phone: 213-477-2676
Fax: Not Provided
Contact: Colette R. York, DNSC, RN, Chairperson
Email: cyork@msmc.la.edu

SAMUEL MERRITT COLLEGE

Address: 1313-12th Avenue, Oakland, CA 92101
Phone: 510-869-6129
Fax: Not Provided
Contact: Sarah B. Keating, EdD, FAAN, Dean
Email: skeating@samuelmerritt.edu

GENERAL INFORMATION

Type of School: *Not Reported, Other* • Accreditation: *None* •
Total Enrollment: *Not Reported*

GENERAL INFORMATION

Type of School: *4-Year College or University, Public* •
Accreditation: *Western Association of Schools and Colleges* •
Total Enrollment: *2200*

PROGRAM INFORMATION

NLNAC Accreditation: *Not Reported* • CCNE Accreditation: *Yes*

_____

For specialty program listings, refer to the index.

PROGRAM INFORMATION

NLNAC Accreditation: *Not Reported* • CCNE Accreditation:

_____

For specialty program listings, refer to the index.

NURSING STUDENT PROFILE

Total Nursing Enrollments: *33* • Full-Time Enrollment: *6* •
Part-Time Enrollment: *27* • Female Enrollment: *31* • Male
Enrollment: *2* • Total Graduates: *4*

NURSING STUDENT PROFILE

Total Nursing Enrollments: *186* • Full-Time Enrollment:
156 • Part-Time Enrollment: *30* • Female Enrollment: *Not
Provided* • Male Enrollment: *Not Provided* • Total Graduates:
49

FINANCES

Residental Annual Tuition: *$7,002* • Non-Residential
Annual Tuition: *$7,002* • General Institutional Fees: *$40* •
Additional Nursing Fees: *$50*

FINANCES

Residental Annual Tuition: *Not Reported* • Non-Residential
Annual Tuition: *Not Reported* • General Institutional Fees:
Not Reported • Additional Nursing Fees: *Not Reported*

SAN DIEGO STATE UNIVERSITY

Address: 5300 Campantle Drive, San Diego, CA 92182-4158
Phone: 619-594-6384
Fax: Not Provided
Contact: Patricia R. Wahl, PhD, RN, FAAN, Professor and Director, School of Nursing
Email: pwahl@mail.sdsu.edu

GENERAL INFORMATION

Type of School: *4-Year College or University, Public* •
Accreditation: *Western Association of Schools and Colleges* •
Total Enrollment: *12000*

PROGRAM INFORMATION

NLNAC Accreditation: *Yes* • CCNE Accreditation:

_____

For specialty program listings, refer to the index.

NURSING STUDENT PROFILE

Total Nursing Enrollments: *109* • Full-Time Enrollment: *52* • Part-Time Enrollment: *57* • Female Enrollment: *101* • Male Enrollment: *8* • Total Graduates: *20*

FINANCES

Residental Annual Tuition: *$1,932* • Non-Residential Annual Tuition: *$4,428* • General Institutional Fees: *$0* • Additional Nursing Fees: *$0*

SAN FRANCISCO STATE UNIVERSITY

Address: 8400 West Mineral King Avenue, San Francisco, CA 93291-9283
Phone: 415-338-3465
Fax: 415-338-0555
Contact: Frank E. McLaughlin, BS, MA, PhD, FAAN, Professor and Associate Director, School of Nursing
Email: femc@sfsu.edu

GENERAL INFORMATION

Type of School: *4-Year College or University, Public* •
Accreditation: *Western Association of Schools and Colleges* •
Total Enrollment: *14135*

PROGRAM INFORMATION

NLNAC Accreditation: *Yes* • CCNE Accreditation: *Yes*

_____

For specialty program listings, refer to the index.

NURSING STUDENT PROFILE

Total Nursing Enrollments: *40* • Full-Time Enrollment: *40* • Part-Time Enrollment: *0* • Female Enrollment: *36* • Male Enrollment: *4* • Total Graduates: *56*

FINANCES

Residental Annual Tuition: *$1,982* • Non-Residential Annual Tuition: *$7,380* • General Institutional Fees: *$140* • Additional Nursing Fees: *$200*

SAN JOSE STATE UNIVERSITY

Address: 3307 3rd Avenue W at Nickerson, San Jose, CA
            95192-0057
Phone: 408-924-3144
Fax: 408-924-3135
Contact: Phyllis M Connolly, PhD, RN, CS, Professor
Email: connollydr@aol.com

SONOMA STATE UNIVERSITY

Address: 7011 Koll Center Parkway, Suite 200, Rohnert
            Park, CA 94566
Phone: 707-664-2654
Fax: 707-664-2653
Contact: Liz Close, PhD, MSN, RN, Chair
Email: liz.close@sonoma.edu

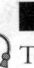

GENERAL INFORMATION

Type of School: *4-Year College or University, Private
(Independent)* • Accreditation: *Western Association of Schools
and Colleges* • Total Enrollment: *18546*

GENERAL INFORMATION

Type of School: *4-Year College or University, Public* •
Accreditation: *Not Provided* • Total Enrollment: *50*

PROGRAM INFORMATION

NLNAC Accreditation: *Yes* • CCNE Accreditation:

———————

For specialty program listings, refer to the index.

PROGRAM INFORMATION

NLNAC Accreditation: *Yes* • CCNE Accreditation:

———————

For specialty program listings, refer to the index.

NURSING STUDENT PROFILE

Total Nursing Enrollments: *113* • Full-Time Enrollment:
23 • Part-Time Enrollment: *90* • Female Enrollment: *107* •
Male Enrollment: *6* • Total Graduates: *22*

NURSING STUDENT PROFILE

Total Nursing Enrollments: *58* • Full-Time Enrollment: *32* •
Part-Time Enrollment: *26* • Female Enrollment: *54* • Male
Enrollment: *4* • Total Graduates: *34*

FINANCES

Residental Annual Tuition: *Not Reported* • Non-Residential
Annual Tuition: *Not Reported* • General Institutional Fees:
Not Reported • Additional Nursing Fees: *Not Reported*

FINANCES

Residental Annual Tuition: *$2,080* • Non-Residential
Annual Tuition: *$7,000* • General Institutional Fees: *Not
Reported* • Additional Nursing Fees: *$10*

UNIVERSITY OF CALIFORNIA—LOS ANGELES

Address: Box 951702, Los Angeles, CA 90095-1702
Phone: 310-825-9621
Fax: Not Provided
Contact: Marie Cowan, RN, PhD, FAAN, Dean and Professor
Email: mcowan@sonnet.ucla.edu

UNIVERSITY OF CALIFORNIA— SAN FRANCISCO

Address: 500 Parnassus Avenue, San Francisco, CA 94143
Phone: 415-476-9710
Fax: 415-476-9707
Contact: Dorrie Fontaine, RN, DNSc, FAAN, Associate Dean, Academic Programs
Email: dorrie.fontaine@nursing.ucsf.edu

GENERAL INFORMATION

Type of School: *4-Year College or University, Public* •
Accreditation: *Western Association of Schools and Colleges* •
Total Enrollment: *3030*

GENERAL INFORMATION

Type of School: *4-Year College or University, Public* •
Accreditation: *Western Association of Schools and Colleges* •
Total Enrollment: *1600*

PROGRAM INFORMATION

NLNAC Accreditation: *Yes* • CCNE Accreditation:

For specialty program listings, refer to the index.

PROGRAM INFORMATION

NLNAC Accreditation: *Not Reported* • CCNE Accreditation: *Yes*

For specialty program listings, refer to the index.

NURSING STUDENT PROFILE

Total Nursing Enrollments: *263* • Full-Time Enrollment: *263* • Part-Time Enrollment: *0* • Female Enrollment: *247* • Male Enrollment: *16* • Total Graduates: *110*

NURSING STUDENT PROFILE

Total Nursing Enrollments: *350* • Full-Time Enrollment: *346* • Part-Time Enrollment: *4* • Female Enrollment: *328* • Male Enrollment: *22* • Total Graduates: *148*

FINANCES

Residental Annual Tuition: *$6,394* • Non-Residential Annual Tuition: *$16,198* • General Institutional Fees: *$1,265* • Additional Nursing Fees: *$600*

FINANCES

Residental Annual Tuition: *$5,599* • Non-Residential Annual Tuition: *$16,731* • General Institutional Fees: *$1,219* • Additional Nursing Fees: *Not Reported*

UNIVERSITY OF SAN FRANCISCO

Address: 2130 Fulton Street, San Francisco, CA 94117-1080
Phone: 415-422-2959
Fax: 415-422-6877
Contact: John M. Lantz, PhD, RN, Dean
Email: lantzj@usfca.edu

GENERAL INFORMATION

Type of School: *4-Year College or University, Private (Religious)* • Accreditation: *Western Association of Schools and Colleges* • Total Enrollment: *8201*

PROGRAM INFORMATION

NLNAC Accreditation: *Yes* • CCNE Accreditation:

_____

For specialty program listings, refer to the index.

NURSING STUDENT PROFILE

Total Nursing Enrollments: *56* • Full-Time Enrollment: *39* • Part-Time Enrollment: *17* • Female Enrollment: *51* • Male Enrollment: *5* • Total Graduates: *9*

FINANCES

Residental Annual Tuition: *$28,160* • Non-Residential Annual Tuition: *$28,160* • General Institutional Fees: *Not Reported* • Additional Nursing Fees: *$150*

REGIS UNIVERSITY

Address: 3333 Regis Boulevard, Denver, CO 80221-1099
Phone: 303-458-4347
Fax: Not Provided
Contact: Nancy Kiernan Case, RN, PhD, Associate Dean, School for Health Care Professions
Email: ncase@regis.edu

GENERAL INFORMATION

Type of School: *4-Year College* • Accreditation: *North Central Association of Colleges* • Total Enrollment: *12,000*

PROGRAM INFORMATION

NLNAC Accreditation: *Yes* • CCNE Accreditation: *Yes*

_____

For specialty program listings, refer to the index.

NURSING STUDENT PROFILE

Total Nursing Enrollments: *54* • Full-Time Enrollment: *52* • Part-Time Enrollment: *2* • Female Enrollment: *52* • Male Enrollment: *2* • Total Graduates: *26*

FINANCES

Residental Annual Tuition: *$4,644* • Non-Residential Annual Tuition: *$4,644* • General Institutional Fees: *$80* • Additional Nursing Fees: *$265*

UNIVERSITY OF COLORADO—DENVER

Address: 4200 East 9th Avenue, Box C288, Denver, CO 80262
Phone: 303-315-4241
Fax: Not Provided
Contact: Marlaine C. Smith, PhD, RN, Director
Email: Marlaine.Smith@uchsc.edu

GENERAL INFORMATION

Type of School: *4-Year College or University, Public* • Accreditation: *North Central Association of Colleges and Schools* • Total Enrollment: *3130*

PROGRAM INFORMATION

NLNAC Accreditation: *Yes* • CCNE Accreditation:

_____

For specialty program listings, refer to the index.

NURSING STUDENT PROFILE

Total Nursing Enrollments: *194* • Full-Time Enrollment: *153* • Part-Time Enrollment: *41* • Female Enrollment: *186* • Male Enrollment: *8* • Total Graduates: *75*

FINANCES

Residental Annual Tuition: *$2,756* • Non-Residential Annual Tuition: *$9,503* • General Institutional Fees: *$146* • Additional Nursing Fees: *$30*

UNIVERSITY OF COLORADO HEALTH SCIENCES CENTER

Address: 4200 East 9th Avenue, Denver, CO 80262
Phone: 303-315-4246
Fax: 303-315-8660
Contact: Kathy Magilvy, PhD, RN, Interim Assistant Dean
Email: Kathy.Magilvy@uchsc.edu

GENERAL INFORMATION

Type of School: *4-Year College or University, Public* • Accreditation: *North Central Association of Colleges and Schools* • Total Enrollment: *955*

PROGRAM INFORMATION

NLNAC Accreditation: *Yes* • CCNE Accreditation:

_____

For specialty program listings, refer to the index.

NURSING STUDENT PROFILE

Total Nursing Enrollments: *190* • Full-Time Enrollment: *143* • Part-Time Enrollment: *47* • Female Enrollment: *178* • Male Enrollment: *12* • Total Graduates: *64*

FINANCES

Residental Annual Tuition: *$2,756* • Non-Residential Annual Tuition: *$9,503* • General Institutional Fees: *$146* • Additional Nursing Fees: *$3,014*

UNIVERSITY OF COLORADO—COLORADO SPRINGS–BETH-EL COLLEGE OF NURSING

Address: 1420 Austin Bluffs Parkway, P. O. Box 7150,
          Colorado Springs, CO 80933-7150
Phone: 719-262-4430
Fax: Not Provided
Contact: Barbara Joyce-Nagata, PhD, RN, Director of
          Graduate Nursing
Email: bnagata@mail.ucs.edu

GENERAL INFORMATION

Type of School: *4-Year College or University, Public* •
Accreditation: *North Central Association of Colleges and
Schools* • Total Enrollment: *3500*

PROGRAM INFORMATION

NLNAC Accreditation: *Yes* • CCNE Accreditation:

_____

For specialty program listings, refer to the index.

NURSING STUDENT PROFILE

Total Nursing Enrollments: *61* • Full-Time Enrollment: *33* •
Part-Time Enrollment: *28* • Female Enrollment: *53* • Male
Enrollment: *8* • Total Graduates: *21*

FINANCES

Residental Annual Tuition: *$3,564* • Non-Residential
Annual Tuition: *$7,740* • General Institutional Fees: *$268* •
Additional Nursing Fees: *$200*

UNIVERSITY OF NORTHERN COLORADO

Address: Gunte Hall 3080, Greeley, CO 80639
Phone: 970-351-2663
Fax: Not Provided
Contact: Judith M. Richter, RN, MS Program
          Coordinator
Email: jrichter@hhs.unco.edu

GENERAL INFORMATION

Type of School: *4-Year College or University, Public* •
Accreditation: *North Central Association of Colleges and
Schools* • Total Enrollment: *Not Provided*

PROGRAM INFORMATION

NLNAC Accreditation: *Yes* • CCNE Accreditation:

_____

For specialty program listings, refer to the index.

NURSING STUDENT PROFILE

Total Nursing Enrollments: *61* • Full-Time Enrollment: *30* •
Part-Time Enrollment: *31* • Female Enrollment: *55* • Male
Enrollment: *6* • Total Graduates: *24*

FINANCES

Residental Annual Tuition: *$2,382* • Non-Residential
Annual Tuition: *$9,578* • General Institutional Fees: *$220* •
Additional Nursing Fees: *$200*

UNIVERSITY OF SOUTHERN COLORADO

Address: 2200 Bonforte Boulevard, Pueblo, CO 81001
Phone: 323-442-2058
Fax: 323-442-2090
Contact: Wynne R. Waugaman, PhD, CRNA, FAAN, Interim Chairperson
Email: waugaman@usc.edu

GENERAL INFORMATION

Type of School: *4-Year College or University, Public* • Accreditation: *North Central Association of Colleges and Schools* • Total Enrollment: *4000*

PROGRAM INFORMATION

NLNAC Accreditation: *Yes* • CCNE Accreditation:

_____

For specialty program listings, refer to the index.

NURSING STUDENT PROFILE

Total Nursing Enrollments: *47* • Full-Time Enrollment: *20* • Part-Time Enrollment: *27* • Female Enrollment: *39* • Male Enrollment: *8* • Total Graduates: *15*

FINANCES

Residental Annual Tuition: *$23,664* • Non-Residential Annual Tuition: *$23,664* • General Institutional Fees: *Not Reported* • Additional Nursing Fees: *Not Reported*

FAIRFIELD UNIVERSITY

Address: North Benson Road, Fairfield, CT 06430
Phone: 203-254-4000
Fax: Not Provided
Contact: Kathleen Wheeler, PhD, APRN, Associate Professor and Director
Email: kwheeler@fair1.fairfield.edu

GENERAL INFORMATION

Type of School: *4-Year College or University, Private (Religious)* • Accreditation: *New England Association of Schools and Colleges* • Total Enrollment: *5188*

PROGRAM INFORMATION

NLNAC Accreditation: *Yes* • CCNE Accreditation:

_____

For specialty program listings, refer to the index.

NURSING STUDENT PROFILE

Total Nursing Enrollments: *52* • Full-Time Enrollment: *16* • Part-Time Enrollment: *36* • Female Enrollment: *51* • Male Enrollment: *1* • Total Graduates: *7*

FINANCES

Residental Annual Tuition: *$6,570* • Non-Residential Annual Tuition: *$6,570* • General Institutional Fees: *$25* • Additional Nursing Fees: *$360*

QUINNIPIAC UNIVERSITY

Address: 275 Mount Carmel Avenue, Hamden, CT 06518
Phone: 203-582-5366
Fax: Not Provided
Contact: Joy Ruth Cohen, RN, Director of Nursing Program
Email: joyruth.cohen@quinnipiac.edu

GENERAL INFORMATION

Type of School: *4-Year College or University, Other* • Accreditation: *New England Association of Schools and Colleges* • Total Enrollment: *Not Reported*

PROGRAM INFORMATION

NLNAC Accreditation: *Not Reported* • CCNE Accreditation:

_____

For specialty program listings, refer to the index.

NURSING STUDENT PROFILE

Total Nursing Enrollments: *15* • Full-Time Enrollment: *2* • Part-Time Enrollment: *13* • Female Enrollment: *15* • Male Enrollment: *0* • Total Graduates: *Not Provided*

FINANCES

Residental Annual Tuition: *Not Reported* • Non-Residential Annual Tuition: *Not Reported* • General Institutional Fees: *Not Reported* • Additional Nursing Fees: *Not Reported*

SACRED HEART UNIVERSITY

Address: 5151 Park Avenue, Fairfield, CT 06432
Phone: 203-371-7715
Fax: 203-365-7662
Contact: Dori Taylor Sullivan, PhD, RNC, Director, Nursing Programs
Email: sullivand@sacredhealth.edu

GENERAL INFORMATION

Type of School: *4-Year College or University, Private (Religious)* • Accreditation: *New England Association of Schools and Colleges* • Total Enrollment: *6000*

PROGRAM INFORMATION

NLNAC Accreditation: *Yes* • CCNE Accreditation:

_____

For specialty program listings, refer to the index.

NURSING STUDENT PROFILE

Total Nursing Enrollments: *34* • Full-Time Enrollment: *5* • Part-Time Enrollment: *29* • Female Enrollment: *27* • Male Enrollment: *7* • Total Graduates: *10*

FINANCES

Residental Annual Tuition: *$9,480* • Non-Residential Annual Tuition: *$9,480* • General Institutional Fees: *$200* • Additional Nursing Fees: *$100*

SAINT JOSEPH COLLEGE

Address: 1678 Asylum Ave, West Hartford, CT 06117
Phone: 860-232-4571
Fax: 860-231-8396
Contact: Virginia Knowlden, PhD, Director
Email: vknowlden@sjc.edu

GENERAL INFORMATION

Type of School: *Not Provided* • Accreditation: *Not Provided* •
Total Enrollment: *Not Provided*

PROGRAM INFORMATION

NLNAC Accreditation: *Yes* • CCNE Accreditation:

_____

For specialty program listings, refer to the index.

NURSING STUDENT PROFILE

Total Nursing Enrollments: *50* • Full-Time Enrollment: *7* •
Part-Time Enrollment: *43* • Female Enrollment: *47* • Male
Enrollment: *3* • Total Graduates: *21*

FINANCES

Residental Annual Tuition: *$7,110* • Non-Residential
Annual Tuition: *$7,110* • General Institutional Fees: *$100* •
Additional Nursing Fees: *Not Reported*

SOUTHERN CONNECTICUT STATE UNIVERSITY

Address: 501 Crescent Street, New Haven, CT 06515
Phone: 203-392-6482
Fax: Not Provided
Contact: Susan Killion, PhD, RN, Coordinator, Graduate
Programs
Email: killion@scsu.ctstateu.edu

GENERAL INFORMATION

Type of School: *Not Provided* • Accreditation: *Not Provided* •
Total Enrollment: *896*

PROGRAM INFORMATION

NLNAC Accreditation: *Yes* • CCNE Accreditation:

_____

For specialty program listings, refer to the index.

NURSING STUDENT PROFILE

Total Nursing Enrollments: *37* • Full-Time Enrollment: *2* •
Part-Time Enrollment: *35* • Female Enrollment: *32* • Male
Enrollment: *5* • Total Graduates: *14*

FINANCES

Residental Annual Tuition: *$4,498* • Non-Residential
Annual Tuition: *$10,153* • General Institutional Fees: *$478* •
Additional Nursing Fees: *Not Reported*

UNIVERSITY OF CONNECTICUT

Address: 231 Glenbrook Road, Storrs Mansfield, CT 06269
Phone: 860-486-3716
Fax: Not Provided
Contact: Kathleen Bruttomerso, RN, Interim Dean
Email: bruttome@uconnvm.uconn.edu

GENERAL INFORMATION

Type of School: *4-Year College or University, Public* • Accreditation: *New England Association of Schools and Colleges* • Total Enrollment: *16696*

PROGRAM INFORMATION

NLNAC Accreditation: *Yes* • CCNE Accreditation: *Yes*

_____

For specialty program listings, refer to the index.

NURSING STUDENT PROFILE

Total Nursing Enrollments: *93* • Full-Time Enrollment: *31* • Part-Time Enrollment: *62* • Female Enrollment: *82* • Male Enrollment: *11* • Total Graduates: *48*

FINANCES

Residental Annual Tuition: *$5,272* • Non-Residential Annual Tuition: *$13,696* • General Institutional Fees: *$506* • Additional Nursing Fees: *$0*

UNIVERSITY OF HARTFORD

Address: 200 Bloomfield Avenue, W Hartford, CT 06117
Phone: 860-768-4217
Fax: 860-768-5346
Contact: Mary Beth Mathews, PhD, RN, BC, Chair, Division of Nursing
Email: mbmathews@hartford.edu

GENERAL INFORMATION

Type of School: *Not Provided* • Accreditation: *Not Provided* • Total Enrollment: *7300*

PROGRAM INFORMATION

NLNAC Accreditation: *Yes* • CCNE Accreditation:

_____

For specialty program listings, refer to the index.

NURSING STUDENT PROFILE

Total Nursing Enrollments: *109* • Full-Time Enrollment: *0* • Part-Time Enrollment: *109* • Female Enrollment: *102* • Male Enrollment: *7* • Total Graduates: *30*

FINANCES

Residental Annual Tuition: *Not Reported* • Non-Residential Annual Tuition: *Not Reported* • General Institutional Fees: *Not Reported* • Additional Nursing Fees: *Not Reported*

WESTERN CONNECTICUT STATE UNIVERSITY

Address: 4647 Stone Ave PO Box 265, Danbury, CT 06810
Phone: 203-837-9411
Fax: 203-837-8526
Contact: Barbara Piscone, RN, Chair
Email: piscopob@wscu.edu

GENERAL INFORMATION

Type of School: *Not Provided* • Accreditation: *Not Provided* • Total Enrollment: *1000*

PROGRAM INFORMATION

NLNAC Accreditation: *Yes* • CCNE Accreditation:
_____

For specialty program listings, refer to the index.

NURSING STUDENT PROFILE

Total Nursing Enrollments: *47* • Full-Time Enrollment: *Not Provided* • Part-Time Enrollment: *Not Provided* • Female Enrollment: *Not Provided* • Male Enrollment: *Not Provided* • Total Graduates: *9*

FINANCES

Residental Annual Tuition: *Not Reported* • Non-Residential Annual Tuition: *Not Reported* • General Institutional Fees: *Not Reported* • Additional Nursing Fees: *Not Reported*

YALE UNIVERSITY

Address: 100 Church Street South, PO Box 9740, New Haven, CT 06536-0740
Phone: 203-785-2399
Fax: Not Provided
Contact: Paula Milone-Nuzzo, RN, PhD, FAAN, Associate Dean for Academic Affairs
Email: paula.milone-nuzzo@yale.edu

GENERAL INFORMATION

Type of School: *4-Year College or University, Public* • Accreditation: *New England Association of Schools and Colleges* • Total Enrollment: *6523*

PROGRAM INFORMATION

NLNAC Accreditation: *Yes* • CCNE Accreditation:
_____

For specialty program listings, refer to the index.

NURSING STUDENT PROFILE

Total Nursing Enrollments: *220* • Full-Time Enrollment: *187* • Part-Time Enrollment: *33* • Female Enrollment: *203* • Male Enrollment: *17* • Total Graduates: *75*

FINANCES

Residental Annual Tuition: *$20,570* • Non-Residential Annual Tuition: *$20,570* • General Institutional Fees: *Not Reported* • Additional Nursing Fees: *$150*

UNIVERSITY OF DELAWARE

Address: McDowell Hall, Newark, DE 19716
Phone: 302-831-2193
Fax: Not Provided
Contact: Janice Selekman, DNSc, RN, Chairperson,
    Department of Nursing
Email: selekman@udel.edu

GENERAL INFORMATION

Type of School: *4-Year College or University, Public* •
Accreditation: *Middle States Association of Colleges and
Schools* • Total Enrollment: *Not Provided*

PROGRAM INFORMATION

NLNAC Accreditation: *Yes* • CCNE Accreditation:

_____

For specialty program listings, refer to the index.

NURSING STUDENT PROFILE

Total Nursing Enrollments: *100* • Full-Time Enrollment:
16 • Part-Time Enrollment: *84* • Female Enrollment: *96* •
Male Enrollment: *4* • Total Graduates: *36*

FINANCES

Residental Annual Tuition: *$4,380* • Non-Residential
Annual Tuition: *$12,750* • General Institutional Fees: *Not
Reported* • Additional Nursing Fees: *Not Reported*

WESLEY COLLEGE

Address: 120 North State Street, Denver, DE 30116
Phone: 302-736-2512
Fax: 302-736-2548
Contact: Lucille C. Gambardella, PhD, RN, CS, APN,
    Chair
Email: gambarlu@mail.wesley.edu

GENERAL INFORMATION

Type of School: *4-Year College or University, Public* •
Accreditation: *Not Provided* • Total Enrollment: *2150*

PROGRAM INFORMATION

NLNAC Accreditation: *Yes* • CCNE Accreditation:

_____

For specialty program listings, refer to the index.

NURSING STUDENT PROFILE

Total Nursing Enrollments: *42* • Full-Time Enrollment: *32* •
Part-Time Enrollment: *10* • Female Enrollment: *40* • Male
Enrollment: *2* • Total Graduates: *12*

FINANCES

Residental Annual Tuition: *$13,000* • Non-Residential
Annual Tuition: *$13,000* • General Institutional Fees: *$705* •
Additional Nursing Fees: *$0*

WILMINGTON COLLEGE

Address: 320 North, Dupont Highway, New Castle, DE 19720
Phone: 302-328-9401
Fax: 302-322-7081
Contact: Tish Gallagher, RN, MS, DNSc (abd), Chair, Division of Nursing
Email: tgall@wilmcoll.edu

GENERAL INFORMATION

Type of School: *4-Year College or University, Public* • Accreditation: *Middle States Association of Colleges and Schools* • Total Enrollment: *7500*

PROGRAM INFORMATION

NLNAC Accreditation: *Yes* • CCNE Accreditation: *Yes*

_____

For specialty program listings, refer to the index.

NURSING STUDENT PROFILE

Total Nursing Enrollments: *129* • Full-Time Enrollment: *105* • Part-Time Enrollment: *24* • Female Enrollment: *115* • Male Enrollment: *14* • Total Graduates: *41*

FINANCES

Residental Annual Tuition: *$4,788* • Non-Residential Annual Tuition: *$4,788* • General Institutional Fees: *$75* • Additional Nursing Fees: *$0*

THE CATHOLIC UNIVERSITY OF AMERICA

Address: 3800 Brookland Avenue NE, Washington, DC 20064
Phone: 202-319-5400
Fax: 202-319-6485
Contact: Ann Marie T. Brooks, RN, DNSc, FAAN, FACHE, Dean
Email: brooks@cua.edu

GENERAL INFORMATION

Type of School: *4-Year College or University, Private (Independent)* • Accreditation: *Middle States Association of Colleges and Schools* • Total Enrollment: *5500*

PROGRAM INFORMATION

NLNAC Accreditation: *Yes* • CCNE Accreditation:

_____

For specialty program listings, refer to the index.

NURSING STUDENT PROFILE

Total Nursing Enrollments: *55* • Full-Time Enrollment: *22* • Part-Time Enrollment: *33* • Female Enrollment: *54* • Male Enrollment: *1* • Total Graduates: *21*

FINANCES

Residental Annual Tuition: *$10,025* • Non-Residential Annual Tuition: *$10,025* • General Institutional Fees: *$550* • Additional Nursing Fees: *$200*

GEORGETOWN UNIVERSITY

Address: 3700 Reservoir Rd NW, Washington, DC 20007
Phone: 202-687-3118
Fax: Not Provided
Contact: Bette Keltner, PhD, RN, FAAN, Dean
Email: Keltnerb@gunet.georgetown.edu

GENERAL INFORMATION

Type of School: *4-Year College or University, Public* •
Accreditation: *Middle States Association of Colleges and
Schools* • Total Enrollment: *Not Provided*

PROGRAM INFORMATION

NLNAC Accreditation: *Yes* • CCNE Accreditation:

_____

For specialty program listings, refer to the index.

NURSING STUDENT PROFILE

Total Nursing Enrollments: *182* • Full-Time Enrollment:
99 • Part-Time Enrollment: *83* • Female Enrollment: *136* •
Male Enrollment: *46* • Total Graduates: *62*

FINANCES

Residental Annual Tuition: *$15,210* • Non-Residential
Annual Tuition: *Not Reported* • General Institutional Fees:
Not Reported • Additional Nursing Fees: *Not Reported*

HOWARD UNIVERSITY

Address: Box 552, Washington, DC 57350
Phone: 202-806-5581
Fax: 202-806-5958
Contact: Beatrice Adderley-Kelly, PhD, RN, Assistant
Dean, Graduate Program
Email: bkelly@howard.edu

GENERAL INFORMATION

Type of School: *4-Year College or University, Public* •
Accreditation: *Middle States Association of Colleges and
Schools* • Total Enrollment: *1100*

PROGRAM INFORMATION

NLNAC Accreditation: *Yes* • CCNE Accreditation:

_____

For specialty program listings, refer to the index.

NURSING STUDENT PROFILE

Total Nursing Enrollments: *26* • Full-Time Enrollment: *6* •
Part-Time Enrollment: *20* • Female Enrollment: *22* • Male
Enrollment: *4* • Total Graduates: *9*

FINANCES

Residental Annual Tuition: *$10,816* • Non-Residential
Annual Tuition: *$10,816* • General Institutional Fees: *$278* •
Additional Nursing Fees: *$50*

BARRY UNIVERSITY

Address: 11300 North East Second Avenue, Miami
           Shores, FL 33161-6695
Phone: 305-899-3800
Fax: 305-899-3831
Contact: Janyce G. Dyer, DNSc, CS, FNP, C, Associate
           Dean Graduate Program
Email: jdyer@mail.barry.edu

GENERAL INFORMATION

Type of School: *4-Year College or University, Private
(Religious)* • Accreditation: *Southern Association of Colleges
and Schools* • Total Enrollment: *8700*

PROGRAM INFORMATION

NLNAC Accreditation: *Not Reported* • CCNE Accreditation:
Yes

———

For specialty program listings, refer to the index.

NURSING STUDENT PROFILE

Total Nursing Enrollments: *75* • Full-Time Enrollment: *20* •
Part-Time Enrollment: *55* • Female Enrollment: *68* • Male
Enrollment: *7* • Total Graduates: *50*

FINANCES

Residental Annual Tuition: *$12,000* • Non-Residential
Annual Tuition: *$12,000* • General Institutional Fees: *$0* •
Additional Nursing Fees: *$30*

FLORIDA A & M UNIVERSITY

Address: P.O. Box 136, Tallahassee, FL 32307
Phone: 850-412-7067
Fax: Not Provided
Contact: Doris E. Ballard-Ferguson, RN, Associate Dean
Email: dballard@famu.edu

GENERAL INFORMATION

Type of School: *4-Year College, Public* • Accreditation:
Southern Association of Colleges • Total Enrollment: *12000*

PROGRAM INFORMATION

NLNAC Accreditation: *No* • CCNE Accreditation:

———

For specialty program listings, refer to the index.

NURSING STUDENT PROFILE

Total Nursing Enrollments: *25* • Full-Time Enrollment: *22* •
Part-Time Enrollment: *3* • Female Enrollment: *22* • Male
Enrollment: *3* • Total Graduates: *Not Provided*

FINANCES

Residental Annual Tuition: *$2,643* • Non-Residential
Annual Tuition: *$9,136* • General Institutional Fees: *Not
Reported* • Additional Nursing Fees: *Not Reported*

FLORIDA ATLANTIC UNIVERSITY

Address: 4501 Capper Road, Boca Raton, FL 32218
Phone: 561-297-3384
Fax: Not Provided
Contact: Ellis Quinn Youngkin, PhD, ARNP, Professor and Graduate Program Coordinator
Email: eyoungkin@fau.edu

GENERAL INFORMATION

Type of School: *4-Year College or University, Public* •
Accreditation: *Southern Association of Colleges and Schools* •
Total Enrollment: *Not Provided*

PROGRAM INFORMATION

NLNAC Accreditation: *Yes* • CCNE Accreditation:

_____

For specialty program listings, refer to the index.

NURSING STUDENT PROFILE

Total Nursing Enrollments: *133* • Full-Time Enrollment: *39* • Part-Time Enrollment: *94* • Female Enrollment: *123* • Male Enrollment: *10* • Total Graduates: *40*

FINANCES

Residental Annual Tuition: *$3,550* • Non-Residential Annual Tuition: *$12,207* • General Institutional Fees: *Not Reported* • Additional Nursing Fees: *$30*

FLORIDA GULF COAST UNIVERSITY

Address: 10501 FGCU Boulevard South, Fort Myers, FL 33965
Phone: 941-590-7454
Fax: 941-590-7474
Contact: Karen E. Miles, EdD, MSN, RN, Associate Director Academic Programs
Email: kmiles@fgcu.edu

GENERAL INFORMATION

Type of School: *4-Year College or University, Public* •
Accreditation: *Southern Association of Colleges and Schools* •
Total Enrollment: *7500*

PROGRAM INFORMATION

NLNAC Accreditation: *No* • CCNE Accreditation:

_____

For specialty program listings, refer to the index.

NURSING STUDENT PROFILE

Total Nursing Enrollments: *82* • Full-Time Enrollment: *60* • Part-Time Enrollment: *22* • Female Enrollment: *55* • Male Enrollment: *27* • Total Graduates: *Not Provided*

FINANCES

Residental Annual Tuition: *$5,246* • Non-Residential Annual Tuition: *$18,275* • General Institutional Fees: *$221* • Additional Nursing Fees: *$200*

Circle 51 on reader card   See in-depth profile for more information

FLORIDA STATE UNIVERSITY

Address: 102 Vivian M. Duxbury Hall, Tallahasee, FL
32306
Phone: 850-644-5974
Fax: Not Provided
Contact: Deborah I. Frank, PhD, Graduate Program
Coordinator
Email: dfrank@mailer.fsu.edu

GENERAL INFORMATION

Type of School: *Not Provided* • Accreditation: *Not Provided* •
Total Enrollment: *58*

PROGRAM INFORMATION

NLNAC Accreditation: *Yes* • CCNE Accreditation:

_____

For specialty program listings, refer to the index.

NURSING STUDENT PROFILE

Total Nursing Enrollments: *67* • Full-Time Enrollment: *20* •
Part-Time Enrollment: *47* • Female Enrollment: *59* • Male
Enrollment: *8* • Total Graduates: *26*

FINANCES

Residental Annual Tuition: *$2,628* • Non-Residential
Annual Tuition: *$9,108* • General Institutional Fees: *Not
Reported* • Additional Nursing Fees: *$20*

UNIVERSITY OF CENTRAL FLORIDA

Address: 2300 McCorkle Avenue, SE, Orlando, FL
32816-2210
Phone: 407-823-2744
Fax: 407-823-5675
Contact: Jean C. Kijek, PhD, RN, Graduate
Coordinator/Associate Professor
Email: kijek@mail.ucf.edu

GENERAL INFORMATION

Type of School: *4-Year College or University, Public* •
Accreditation: *Southern Association of Colleges and Schools* •
Total Enrollment: *34000*

PROGRAM INFORMATION

NLNAC Accreditation: *Yes* • CCNE Accreditation:

_____

For specialty program listings, refer to the index.

NURSING STUDENT PROFILE

Total Nursing Enrollments: *84* • Full-Time Enrollment: *26* •
Part-Time Enrollment: *58* • Female Enrollment: *77* • Male
Enrollment: *7* • Total Graduates: *29*

FINANCES

Residental Annual Tuition: *$3,215* • Non-Residential
Annual Tuition: *$12,522* • General Institutional Fees: *$180* •
Additional Nursing Fees: *$50*

UNIVERSITY OF FLORIDA

Address: Health Science Bldg. Rm 100, Gainesville, FL
32601
Phone: 352-392-3752
Fax: Not Provided
Contact: Kathleen Ann Long, PhD, RNCS, FAAN, Dean
and Professor
Email: longka@nursing.ufl.edu

GENERAL INFORMATION

Type of School: *Not Provided, Private (Religious)* •
Accreditation: *Southern Association of Colleges and Schools* •
Total Enrollment: *6900*

PROGRAM INFORMATION

NLNAC Accreditation: *Yes* • CCNE Accreditation:

_____

For specialty program listings, refer to the index.

NURSING STUDENT PROFILE

Total Nursing Enrollments: *258* • Full-Time Enrollment:
101 • Part-Time Enrollment: *157* • Female Enrollment:
235 • Male Enrollment: *23* • Total Graduates: *93*

FINANCES

Residental Annual Tuition: *$3,605* • Non-Residential
Annual Tuition: *$12,623* • General Institutional Fees: *$0* •
Additional Nursing Fees: *$0*

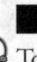

UNIVERSITY OF MIAMI

Address: 58010 Red Road, Coral Gables, FL 33143
Phone: 305
Fax: Not Provided
Contact: Diane Horner, EdD, RN, Dean
Email: dhorner@miami.edu

GENERAL INFORMATION

Type of School: *Independent, Private Independent* •
Accreditation: *Southern Association of Colleges and Schools* •
Total Enrollment: *13963*

PROGRAM INFORMATION

NLNAC Accreditation: *Yes* • CCNE Accreditation:

_____

For specialty program listings, refer to the index.

NURSING STUDENT PROFILE

Total Nursing Enrollments: *62* • Full-Time Enrollment: *20* •
Part-Time Enrollment: *42* • Female Enrollment: *54* • Male
Enrollment: *8* • Total Graduates: *22*

FINANCES

Residental Annual Tuition: *$16,179* • Non-Residential
Annual Tuition: *$16,179* • General Institutional Fees: *$97* •
Additional Nursing Fees: *$50*

UNIVERSITY OF NORTH FLORIDA

Address: 4567 Saint Johns Bluff Road South, Jacksonville, FL 32224-2673
Phone: 701-777-4552
Fax: 701-777-4096
Contact: Ginny W. Guido, RN, MSN, JD, Associate Dean and Director of Graduate Studies
Email: Ginny_Guido@mail.und.nodak.edu

GENERAL INFORMATION

Type of School: *4-Year College or University, Public* •
Accreditation: *Southern Association of Colleges and Schools* •
Total Enrollment: *12000*

PROGRAM INFORMATION

NLNAC Accreditation: *No* • CCNE Accreditation:

For specialty program listings, refer to the index.

NURSING STUDENT PROFILE

Total Nursing Enrollments: *64* • Full-Time Enrollment: *35* • Part-Time Enrollment: *29* • Female Enrollment: *51* • Male Enrollment: *13* • Total Graduates: *30*

FINANCES

Residental Annual Tuition: *$4,947* • Non-Residential Annual Tuition: *$11,997* • General Institutional Fees: *$242* • Additional Nursing Fees: *$1,000*

UNIVERSITY OF SOUTH FLORIDA

Address: 4202 East Fowler Avenue, Tampa, FL 33620
Phone: 813-974-9091
Fax: 813-974-5418
Contact: Patricia A. Burns, PhD, RN, FAAN, Dean and Professor
Email: pburns@hsc.usf.ledu

GENERAL INFORMATION

Type of School: *4-Year College or University, Public* •
Accreditation: *Southern Association of Colleges and Schools* •
Total Enrollment: *Not Provided*

PROGRAM INFORMATION

NLNAC Accreditation: *Yes* • CCNE Accreditation: *Yes*

For specialty program listings, refer to the index.

NURSING STUDENT PROFILE

Total Nursing Enrollments: *215* • Full-Time Enrollment: *69* • Part-Time Enrollment: *146* • Female Enrollment: *189* • Male Enrollment: *26* • Total Graduates: *85*

FINANCES

Residental Annual Tuition: *$3,823* • Non-Residential Annual Tuition: *$13,188* • General Institutional Fees: *Not Reported* • Additional Nursing Fees: *Not Reported*

UNIVERSITY OF TAMPA

Address: 401 West Kennedy Boulevard, Tampa, FL 33606
Phone: 813-253-3333
Fax: 813-258-7214
Contact: Nancy Ross, ARNP, PhD, Director/Chair,
           Department of Nursing
Email: nross@alpha.utampa.edu

GENERAL INFORMATION

Type of School: *4-Year College or University, Public* •
Accreditation: *Southern Association of Colleges and Schools* •
Total Enrollment: *10966*

PROGRAM INFORMATION

NLNAC Accreditation: *Yes* • CCNE Accreditation:

_____

For specialty program listings, refer to the index.

NURSING STUDENT PROFILE

Total Nursing Enrollments: *102* • Full-Time Enrollment:
27 • Part-Time Enrollment: *75* • Female Enrollment: *92* •
Male Enrollment: *10* • Total Graduates: *33*

FINANCES

Residental Annual Tuition: *Not Reported* • Non-Residential
Annual Tuition: *Not Reported* • General Institutional Fees:
Not Reported • Additional Nursing Fees: *Not Reported*

ALBANY STATE UNIVERSITY

Address: 504 College Drive, Albany, GA 31705
Phone: 229-430-4731
Fax: 229-430-3937
Contact: Adebisi Fabayo, PhD, RN, MSN Coordinator
Email: afabayo@asurams.edu

GENERAL INFORMATION

Type of School: *4-Year College or University, Public* •
Accreditation: *Southern Association of Colleges and Schools* •
Total Enrollment: *3456*

PROGRAM INFORMATION

NLNAC Accreditation: *Yes* • CCNE Accreditation:

_____

For specialty program listings, refer to the index.

NURSING STUDENT PROFILE

Total Nursing Enrollments: *37* • Full-Time Enrollment: *31* •
Part-Time Enrollment: *6* • Female Enrollment: *37* • Male
Enrollment: *0* • Total Graduates: *12*

FINANCES

Residental Annual Tuition: *$1,432* • Non-Residential
Annual Tuition: *$4,912* • General Institutional Fees: *$272* •
Additional Nursing Fees: *$0*

ARMSTRONG ATLANTIC STATE UNIVERSITY

Address: 11935 Abercorn Street, Savannah, GA 31419
Phone: 912-927-5311
Fax: Not Provided
Contact: Sue W. Young, PhD, Department Head
Email: youngsue@mail.armstrong.edu

GENERAL INFORMATION

Type of School: *4-Year College or University, Public* •
Accreditation: *Southern Association of Colleges and Schools* •
Total Enrollment: *5700*

PROGRAM INFORMATION

NLNAC Accreditation: *Yes* • CCNE Accreditation:

─────────

For specialty program listings, refer to the index.

NURSING STUDENT PROFILE

Total Nursing Enrollments: *57* • Full-Time Enrollment: *50* •
Part-Time Enrollment: *7* • Female Enrollment: *53* • Male
Enrollment: *4* • Total Graduates: *20*

FINANCES

Residental Annual Tuition: *$2,170* • Non-Residential
Annual Tuition: *$8,680* • General Institutional Fees: *$170* •
Additional Nursing Fees: *Not Reported*

BRENAU UNIVERSITY

Address: One Centenial Circle, Gainesville, GA 39501
Phone: 770-534-6210
Fax: 770-538-4666
Contact: Ginny Kemp, PhD, FNP, Graduate Coordinator
Email: gkemp@lib.brenau.edu

GENERAL INFORMATION

Type of School: *4-Year College or University, Private
(Independent)* • Accreditation: *Southern Association of Colleges
and Schools* • Total Enrollment: *22139*

PROGRAM INFORMATION

NLNAC Accreditation: *Yes* • CCNE Accreditation:

─────────

For specialty program listings, refer to the index.

NURSING STUDENT PROFILE

Total Nursing Enrollments: *32* • Full-Time Enrollment: *0* •
Part-Time Enrollment: *32* • Female Enrollment: *28* • Male
Enrollment: *4* • Total Graduates: *Not Provided*

FINANCES

Residental Annual Tuition: *Not Reported* • Non-Residential
Annual Tuition: *Not Reported* • General Institutional Fees:
Not Reported • Additional Nursing Fees: *Not Reported*

EMORY UNIVERSITY

Address: 1520 Clifton Road, Atlanta, GA 30322
Phone: 404-727-6961
Fax: 404-727-0536
Contact: Maureen A. Kelley, PhD, CNM, RN, Associate
          Professor (Clinical) and Interim Coordinator of
          the MSN program
Email: makelle@emory.edu

GENERAL INFORMATION

Type of School: *4-Year College or University, Private
(Religious)* • Accreditation: *Southern Association of Colleges
and Schools* • Total Enrollment: *11400*

PROGRAM INFORMATION

NLNAC Accreditation: *Not Reported* • CCNE Accreditation:
Yes

_____

For specialty program listings, refer to the index.

NURSING STUDENT PROFILE

Total Nursing Enrollments: *164* • Full-Time Enrollment:
76 • Part-Time Enrollment: *88* • Female Enrollment: *157* •
Male Enrollment: *7* • Total Graduates: *86*

FINANCES

Residental Annual Tuition: *$24,240* • Non-Residential
Annual Tuition: *$24,240* • General Institutional Fees: *$468* •
Additional Nursing Fees: *$0*

GEORGIA COLLEGE AND STATE UNIVERSITY

Address: 555 N Indian Creek Dr, Milledgeville, GA
          30021-2361
Phone: 912-445-2633
Fax: Not Provided
Contact: Cheryl Pope Kish, RN, Professor and
          Coordinator Graduate Programs in Health
          Sciences
Email: ckish@mail.gcsu.edu

GENERAL INFORMATION

Type of School: *Not Provided* • Accreditation: *Not Provided* •
Total Enrollment: *3174*

PROGRAM INFORMATION

NLNAC Accreditation: *Yes* • CCNE Accreditation:

_____

For specialty program listings, refer to the index.

NURSING STUDENT PROFILE

Total Nursing Enrollments: *47* • Full-Time Enrollment: *0* •
Part-Time Enrollment: *47* • Female Enrollment: *38* • Male
Enrollment: *9* • Total Graduates: *23*

FINANCES

Residental Annual Tuition: *$1,638* • Non-Residential
Annual Tuition: *$3,690* • General Institutional Fees: *Not
Reported* • Additional Nursing Fees: *Not Reported*

GEORGIA SOUTHERN UNIVERSITY

Address: 800 Wheatley Street, Statesboro, GA 31709
Phone: 912-681-0017
Fax: Not Provided
Contact: Donna Hadnicki, MSN, RN, Director MSN program
Email: dhodnick@gsaix2.cc.gasou.edu

GENERAL INFORMATION

Type of School: *4-Year College or University, Public* •
Accreditation: *Southern Association of Colleges and Schools* •
Total Enrollment: *5400*

PROGRAM INFORMATION

NLNAC Accreditation: *Yes* • CCNE Accreditation: *Yes*

_____

For specialty program listings, refer to the index.

NURSING STUDENT PROFILE

Total Nursing Enrollments: *38* • Full-Time Enrollment: *38* •
Part-Time Enrollment: *0* • Female Enrollment: *31* • Male
Enrollment: *7* • Total Graduates: *18*

FINANCES

Residental Annual Tuition: *$2,443* • Non-Residential
Annual Tuition: *$8,680* • General Institutional Fees: *$312* •
Additional Nursing Fees: *$0*

GEORGIA STATE UNIVERSITY

Address: University Plaza, Room 983 Urban Life, Atlanta, GA 30303
Phone: 404-463-9284
Fax: Not Provided
Contact: Sherry Gaines, PhD, RN, Interim Director of Graduate Program
Email: nurskg@langate.gsu.edu

GENERAL INFORMATION

Type of School: *4-Year College or University, Public* •
Accreditation: *Southern Association of Colleges and Schools* •
Total Enrollment: *15000*

PROGRAM INFORMATION

NLNAC Accreditation: *Yes* • CCNE Accreditation: *Yes*

_____

For specialty program listings, refer to the index.

NURSING STUDENT PROFILE

Total Nursing Enrollments: *174* • Full-Time Enrollment:
66 • Part-Time Enrollment: *108* • Female Enrollment: *172* •
Male Enrollment: *2* • Total Graduates: *54*

FINANCES

Residental Annual Tuition: *$3,100* • Non-Residential
Annual Tuition: *$12,400* • General Institutional Fees: *$236* •
Additional Nursing Fees: *$62*

KENNESAW STATE UNIVERSITY

Address: 604 Broad Street, Kennesaw, GA 30240-2999
Phone: 770-423-6172
Fax: 770-423-6627
Contact: Regina E. Dorman, RN, PhD, CS, FNP,
            Program Director
Email: gdorman@kennesaw.edu

GENERAL INFORMATION

Type of School: *4-Year College or University, Public* •
Accreditation: *Southern Association of Colleges and Schools* •
Total Enrollment: *1135*

PROGRAM INFORMATION

NLNAC Accreditation: *Yes* • CCNE Accreditation:

————

For specialty program listings, refer to the index.

NURSING STUDENT PROFILE

Total Nursing Enrollments: *68* • Full-Time Enrollment: *65* •
Part-Time Enrollment: *3* • Female Enrollment: *64* • Male
Enrollment: *4* • Total Graduates: *32*

FINANCES

Residental Annual Tuition: *$3,480* • Non-Residential
Annual Tuition: *$13,932* • General Institutional Fees: *$744* •
Additional Nursing Fees: *$105*

MEDICAL COLLEGE OF GEORGIA

Address: 997 St. Sebastian Way, Augusta, GA 19901
Phone: 706-721-2787
Fax: 706-721-7390
Contact: Katherine E. Nugent, PhD, RN, Professor and
            Associate Dean for Academic Programs
Email: knugent@mail.mcg.edu

GENERAL INFORMATION

Type of School: *4-Year College or University, Private
(Independent)* • Accreditation: *Southern Association of
Colleges* • Total Enrollment: *1939*

PROGRAM INFORMATION

NLNAC Accreditation: *Yes* • CCNE Accreditation:
Provisional

————

For specialty program listings, refer to the index.

NURSING STUDENT PROFILE

Total Nursing Enrollments: *79* • Full-Time Enrollment: *45* •
Part-Time Enrollment: *34* • Female Enrollment: *56* • Male
Enrollment: *23* • Total Graduates: *33*

FINANCES

Residental Annual Tuition: *$1,578* • Non-Residential
Annual Tuition: *$6,312* • General Institutional Fees: *$218* •
Additional Nursing Fees: *$0*

VALDOSTA STATE UNIVERSITY

Address: 1300 N Patterson Street, Valdosta, GA 31698
Phone: 912-333-5959
Fax: Not Provided
Contact: MaryAnn B Reichenbach, PhD, RN, Dean
Email: mreichen@valdosta.edu

GENERAL INFORMATION

Type of School: *Other* • Accreditation: *Not Provided* • Total Enrollment: *21000*

PROGRAM INFORMATION

NLNAC Accreditation: *Yes* • CCNE Accreditation:

_____

For specialty program listings, refer to the index.

NURSING STUDENT PROFILE

Total Nursing Enrollments: *39* • Full-Time Enrollment: *22* • Part-Time Enrollment: *17* • Female Enrollment: *35* • Male Enrollment: *4* • Total Graduates: *12*

FINANCES

Residental Annual Tuition: *Not Reported* • Non-Residential Annual Tuition: *Not Reported* • General Institutional Fees: *Not Reported* • Additional Nursing Fees: *Not Reported*

HAWAII PACIFIC UNIVERSITY

Address: 5101 Evergreen Road, Kaneohe, HI 96744
Phone: 808-236-5850
Fax: 808-236-5818
Contact: Patricia Lange-Otsuka, EdD, MSN, APRN, BC, Associate Professor of Nursing/Coordinator MSN Program
Email: potsuka@hpu.edu

GENERAL INFORMATION

Type of School: *4-Year College or University, Private Independent* • Accreditation: *Western Association of Schools and Colleges* • Total Enrollment: *768*

PROGRAM INFORMATION

NLNAC Accreditation: *Yes* • CCNE Accreditation:

_____

For specialty program listings, refer to the index.

NURSING STUDENT PROFILE

Total Nursing Enrollments: *46* • Full-Time Enrollment: *21* • Part-Time Enrollment: *25* • Female Enrollment: *40* • Male Enrollment: *6* • Total Graduates: *4*

FINANCES

Residental Annual Tuition: *Not Reported* • Non-Residential Annual Tuition: *Not Reported* • General Institutional Fees: *Not Reported* • Additional Nursing Fees: *Not Reported*

UNIVERSITY OF HAWAII AT MANOA

Address: 3-1901 Kaumualii Highway, Honolulu, HI
            96766
Phone: 808-956-8522
Fax: 808-956-3257
Contact: Rosanne C. Harrigan, EdD, APRNRx, FAAN,
            Dean
Email: harrigan@hawaii.edu

GENERAL INFORMATION

Type of School: *4-Year College or University, Private
Independent* • Accreditation: *Western Association of Schools
and Colleges* • Total Enrollment: *Not Provided*

PROGRAM INFORMATION

NLNAC Accreditation: *Yes* • CCNE Accreditation: *Yes*

_____

For specialty program listings, refer to the index.

NURSING STUDENT PROFILE

Total Nursing Enrollments: *58* • Full-Time Enrollment: *17* •
Part-Time Enrollment: *41* • Female Enrollment: *54* • Male
Enrollment: *4* • Total Graduates: *22*

FINANCES

Residental Annual Tuition: *$4,368* • Non-Residential
Annual Tuition: *$8,320* • General Institutional Fees: *$132* •
Additional Nursing Fees: *$0*

IDAHO STATE UNIVERSITY

Address: Box 8101 Beackley Building 66 N, Pocatello, ID
            83209-8101
Phone: 208-236-2325
Fax: Not Provided
Contact: Pamela N. Clarke, RN, MPH, PhD, Professor
            and Chair
Email: clarpame@isu.edu

GENERAL INFORMATION

Type of School: *4-Year College or University, Private
(Religious)* • Accreditation: *Northwestern Association of Schools
and Colleges* • Total Enrollment: *4000*

PROGRAM INFORMATION

NLNAC Accreditation: *Not Reported* • CCNE Accreditation:

_____

For specialty program listings, refer to the index.

NURSING STUDENT PROFILE

Total Nursing Enrollments: *44* • Full-Time Enrollment: *13* •
Part-Time Enrollment: *31* • Female Enrollment: *40* • Male
Enrollment: *4* • Total Graduates: *18*

FINANCES

Residental Annual Tuition: *$2,958* • Non-Residential
Annual Tuition: *$6,240* • General Institutional Fees: *$280* •
Additional Nursing Fees: *$50*

BRADLEY UNIVERSITY

Address: Burgess Hall 302, Peoria, IL 61625
Phone: 309-677-2528
Fax: Not Provided
Contact: Francesca A. Armmer, PhD, RN, Chairperson
Email: faa@bradley.edu

GENERAL INFORMATION

Type of School: *4-Year College or University, Private (Independent)* • Accreditation: *North Central Association of Colleges and Schools* • Total Enrollment: *5951*

PROGRAM INFORMATION

NLNAC Accreditation: *Yes* • CCNE Accreditation:

———————

For specialty program listings, refer to the index.

NURSING STUDENT PROFILE

Total Nursing Enrollments: *40* • Full-Time Enrollment: *24* • Part-Time Enrollment: *16* • Female Enrollment: *31* • Male Enrollment: *9* • Total Graduates: *14*

FINANCES

Residental Annual Tuition: *$8,424* • Non-Residential Annual Tuition: *$8,424* • General Institutional Fees: *$25* • Additional Nursing Fees: *$0*

DEPAUL UNIVERSITY

Address: 5504 Krueger Drive, Chicago, IL 60614
Phone: 773-325-7280
Fax: Not Provided
Contact: Susan Poslusny, RN, PhD, Assistant Professor and Chairperson
Email: sposlusn@wppost.depaul.edu

GENERAL INFORMATION

Type of School: *4-Year College or University, Public* • Accreditation: *North Central Association of Colleges and Schools* • Total Enrollment: *1500*

PROGRAM INFORMATION

NLNAC Accreditation: *Yes* • CCNE Accreditation:

———————

For specialty program listings, refer to the index.

NURSING STUDENT PROFILE

Total Nursing Enrollments: *118* • Full-Time Enrollment: *55* • Part-Time Enrollment: *63* • Female Enrollment: *106* • Male Enrollment: *12* • Total Graduates: *28*

FINANCES

Residental Annual Tuition: *$12,640* • Non-Residential Annual Tuition: *$12,640* • General Institutional Fees: *$40* • Additional Nursing Fees: *Not Reported*

ILLINOIS STATE UNIVERSITY

Address: Campus Box 5810, Normal, IL 34981
Phone: 309-438-2203
Fax: 309-438-2620
Contact: Donna Konradi, DNS, RN, Graduate Director,
            Assistant Professor
Email: dbkonra@ilstu.edu

GENERAL INFORMATION

Type of School: *4-Year College or University, Public* •
Accreditation: *North Central Association of Colleges and
Schools* • Total Enrollment: *11740*

PROGRAM INFORMATION

NLNAC Accreditation: *Yes* • CCNE Accreditation:

_____

For specialty program listings, refer to the index.

NURSING STUDENT PROFILE

Total Nursing Enrollments: *37* • Full-Time Enrollment: *7* •
Part-Time Enrollment: *30* • Female Enrollment: *36* • Male
Enrollment: *1* • Total Graduates: *17*

FINANCES

Residental Annual Tuition: *$2,631* • Non-Residential
Annual Tuition: *$7,893* • General Institutional Fees: *$376* •
Additional Nursing Fees: *$0*

LEWIS UNIVERSITY

Address: 5800 Godfrey Rd., Romeoville, IL 62035
Phone: 815-836-5355
Fax: Not Provided
Contact: Lois Stephens, MSN, RN, Acting Director
Email: stephelo@lewisu.edu

GENERAL INFORMATION

Type of School: *4-Year College or University, Private
(Independent)* • Accreditation: *North Central Association of
Colleges and Schools* • Total Enrollment: *1500*

PROGRAM INFORMATION

NLNAC Accreditation: *Yes* • CCNE Accreditation:

_____

For specialty program listings, refer to the index.

NURSING STUDENT PROFILE

Total Nursing Enrollments: *90* • Full-Time Enrollment: *1* •
Part-Time Enrollment: *89* • Female Enrollment: *89* • Male
Enrollment: *1* • Total Graduates: *17*

FINANCES

Residental Annual Tuition: *Not Reported* • Non-Residential
Annual Tuition: *Not Reported* • General Institutional Fees:
Not Reported • Additional Nursing Fees: *Not Reported*

LOYOLA UNIVERSITY— CHICAGO

Address: 750 N Laffoon St., Chicago, IL 60626
Phone: 773-508-3261
Fax: 773-508-3241
Contact: Marcia C. Maurer, RN, Associate Dean/Director
          Graduate Programs in Nursing
Email: mmaurer@luc.edu

GENERAL INFORMATION

Type of School: *4-Year College or University, Private (Religious)* • Accreditation: *North Central Association of Colleges and Schools* • Total Enrollment: *4200*

PROGRAM INFORMATION

NLNAC Accreditation: *Yes* • CCNE Accreditation:

———

For specialty program listings, refer to the index.

NURSING STUDENT PROFILE

Total Nursing Enrollments: *156* • Full-Time Enrollment: *35* • Part-Time Enrollment: *121* • Female Enrollment: *150* • Male Enrollment: *6* • Total Graduates: *33*

FINANCES

Residental Annual Tuition: *$11,208* • Non-Residential Annual Tuition: *$11,208* • General Institutional Fees: *$110* • Additional Nursing Fees: *Not Reported*

NORTH PARK UNIVERSITY

Address: 705 N Grand Ave, Chicago, IL 60625
Phone: 773-244-5698
Fax: Not Provided
Contact: Wendy Burgess, PhD, RN, CS, Interim Director,
          Graduate Programs in Nursing
Email: wburgess@northpark.edu

GENERAL INFORMATION

Type of School: *4-Year College or University, Public* • Accreditation: *North Central Association of Colleges and Schools* • Total Enrollment: *Not Provided*

PROGRAM INFORMATION

NLNAC Accreditation: *Not Reported* • CCNE Accreditation:

———

For specialty program listings, refer to the index.

NURSING STUDENT PROFILE

Total Nursing Enrollments: *104* • Full-Time Enrollment: *14* • Part-Time Enrollment: *90* • Female Enrollment: *94* • Male Enrollment: *10* • Total Graduates: *14*

FINANCES

Residental Annual Tuition: *$6,750* • Non-Residential Annual Tuition: *$6,750* • General Institutional Fees: *Not Reported* • Additional Nursing Fees: *$162*

NORTHERN ILLINOIS UNIVERSITY

Address: 790 Thomas More Parkway, DeKalb, IL 60115
Phone: 815-753-6553
Fax: Not Provided
Contact: Marilyn Frank-Stromborg, RN, EdD, FAAN, Professor and Chair
Email: cancer@niu.edu

GENERAL INFORMATION

Type of School: *4-Year College or University, Public* • Accreditation: *North Central Association of Colleges and Schools* • Total Enrollment: *Not Provided*

PROGRAM INFORMATION

NLNAC Accreditation: *Yes* • CCNE Accreditation:

––––––––

For specialty program listings, refer to the index.

NURSING STUDENT PROFILE

Total Nursing Enrollments: *100* • Full-Time Enrollment: *14* • Part-Time Enrollment: *86* • Female Enrollment: *98* • Male Enrollment: *2* • Total Graduates: *26*

FINANCES

Residental Annual Tuition: *$2,268* • Non-Residential Annual Tuition: *$4,636* • General Institutional Fees: *$465* • Additional Nursing Fees: *$143*

RUSH UNIVERSITY

Address: 600 South Paulina Suite 1080, Chicago, IL 60612
Phone: 312-942-7117
Fax: Not Provided
Contact: Kathleen G. Andreoli, DSN, RN, FAAN, Dean, College of Nursing and Vice President, Nursing Affairs
Email: kandreoli@rushu.rush.edu

GENERAL INFORMATION

Type of School: *4-Year College or University, Public* • Accreditation: *North Central Association of Colleges and Schools* • Total Enrollment: *Not Provided*

PROGRAM INFORMATION

NLNAC Accreditation: *No* • CCNE Accreditation: *Yes*

––––––––

For specialty program listings, refer to the index.

NURSING STUDENT PROFILE

Total Nursing Enrollments: *161* • Full-Time Enrollment: *6* • Part-Time Enrollment: *155* • Female Enrollment: *139* • Male Enrollment: *22* • Total Graduates: *67*

FINANCES

Residental Annual Tuition: *$17,120* • Non-Residential Annual Tuition: *$17,120* • General Institutional Fees: *Not Reported* • Additional Nursing Fees: *Not Reported*

SAINT XAVIER UNIVERSITY

Address: 3700 West 103 Street, Chicago, IL 60655
Phone: 773-298-3700
Fax: 773-298-3704
Contact: Mary M. Lebold, EdD, RN, Dean
Email: lebold@sxu.edu

GENERAL INFORMATION

Type of School: *4-Year College or University, Private (Religious)* • Accreditation: *North Central Association of Colleges and Schools* • Total Enrollment: *4867*

PROGRAM INFORMATION

NLNAC Accreditation: *Yes* • CCNE Accreditation:

_____

For specialty program listings, refer to the index.

NURSING STUDENT PROFILE

Total Nursing Enrollments: *92* • Full-Time Enrollment: *9* • Part-Time Enrollment: *83* • Female Enrollment: *90* • Male Enrollment: *2* • Total Graduates: *15*

FINANCES

Residental Annual Tuition: *$12,000* • Non-Residential Annual Tuition: *$12,000* • General Institutional Fees: *$80* • Additional Nursing Fees: *$150*

SOUTHERN ILLINOIS UNIVERSITY— EDWARDSVILLE

Address: 1701 LaFayette Parkway, Edwadsville, IL 62026
Phone: 618-650-3969
Fax: 618-650-3854
Contact: Felissa R. Lashley, PhD, RN, ACRN, FAAN, Dean
Email: flashle@siue.edu

GENERAL INFORMATION

Type of School: *4-Year College or University, Public* • Accreditation: *North Central Association of Colleges and Schools* • Total Enrollment: *Not Provided*

PROGRAM INFORMATION

NLNAC Accreditation: *Yes* • CCNE Accreditation: *Yes*

_____

For specialty program listings, refer to the index.

NURSING STUDENT PROFILE

Total Nursing Enrollments: *99* • Full-Time Enrollment: *40* • Part-Time Enrollment: *59* • Female Enrollment: *80* • Male Enrollment: *19* • Total Graduates: *78*

FINANCES

Residental Annual Tuition: *$2,712* • Non-Residential Annual Tuition: *$5,424* • General Institutional Fees: *$479* • Additional Nursing Fees: *$180*

UNIVERSITY OF ILLINOIS— CHICAGO

Address:　601 S. Morgan, Chicago, IL 60607
Phone:　312-996-1749
Fax:　312-413-4399
Contact:　Joan Shaver, PhD, RN, FAAN, Dean
Email:　jshaver@uic.edu

GENERAL INFORMATION

Type of School: *4-Year College or University, Public* •
Accreditation: *North Central Association of Colleges and
Schools* • Total Enrollment: *17498*

PROGRAM INFORMATION

NLNAC Accreditation: *No* • CCNE Accreditation: *Yes*

_____

For specialty program listings, refer to the index.

NURSING STUDENT PROFILE

Total Nursing Enrollments: *240* • Full-Time Enrollment:
60 • Part-Time Enrollment: *180* • Female Enrollment: *230* •
Male Enrollment: *10* • Total Graduates: *90*

FINANCES

Residental Annual Tuition: *$3,740* • Non-Residential
Annual Tuition: *$7,368* • General Institutional Fees: *$820* •
Additional Nursing Fees: *$0*

UNIVERSITY OF ST. FRANCIS—JOLIET

Address:　290 N. Springfield Ave., Joliet, IL 60435
Phone:　815-741-7130
Fax:　815-741-7131
Contact:　JoAnn Glotfelty, MS/RN, Interim Dean
Email:　jglotfelty@stfrancis.edu

GENERAL INFORMATION

Type of School: *4-Year College or University, Private
(Independent)* • Accreditation: *North Central Association of
Colleges and Schools* • Total Enrollment: *Not Provided*

PROGRAM INFORMATION

NLNAC Accreditation: *Not Reported* • CCNE Accreditation:

_____

For specialty program listings, refer to the index.

NURSING STUDENT PROFILE

Total Nursing Enrollments: *6* • Full-Time Enrollment: *0* •
Part-Time Enrollment: *6* • Female Enrollment: *6* • Male
Enrollment: *0* • Total Graduates: *Not Provided*

FINANCES

Residental Annual Tuition: *Not Reported* • Non-Residential
Annual Tuition: *Not Reported* • General Institutional Fees:
Not Reported • Additional Nursing Fees: *Not Reported*

BALL STATE UNIVERSITY

Address: 2000 University Blvd, Munice, IN 47306
Phone: 765-285-5764
Fax: 765-285-2169
Contact: Marilyn Ryan, EdD, RN, Associate Director, Graduate Program
Email: mryan@bsu.edu

GENERAL INFORMATION

Type of School: *4-Year College or University, Public* •
Accreditation: *North Central Association of Colleges and Schools* • Total Enrollment: *18000*

PROGRAM INFORMATION

NLNAC Accreditation: *Yes* • CCNE Accreditation:

_____

For specialty program listings, refer to the index.

NURSING STUDENT PROFILE

Total Nursing Enrollments: *233* • Full-Time Enrollment: *0* •
Part-Time Enrollment: *233* • Female Enrollment: *211* • Male Enrollment: *22* • Total Graduates: *28*

FINANCES

Residental Annual Tuition: *$3,722* • Non-Residential Annual Tuition: *$4,944* • General Institutional Fees: *$0* • Additional Nursing Fees: *$400*

INDIANA STATE UNIVERSITY

Address: 2325 Chester Boulevard, Terre Haute, IN 47374
Phone: 812-237-3688
Fax: 812-237-4300
Contact: Suzy Fletcher, RN, DNS, Interim Chair, Baccalaureate and Higher Degree Program
Email: S-Fletcher@indstate.edu

GENERAL INFORMATION

Type of School: *4-Year College or University, Public* •
Accreditation: *North Central Association of Colleges and Schools* • Total Enrollment: *3294*

PROGRAM INFORMATION

NLNAC Accreditation: *Yes* • CCNE Accreditation:

_____

For specialty program listings, refer to the index.

NURSING STUDENT PROFILE

Total Nursing Enrollments: *15* • Full-Time Enrollment: *1* •
Part-Time Enrollment: *14* • Female Enrollment: *13* • Male Enrollment: *2* • Total Graduates: *13*

FINANCES

Residental Annual Tuition: *$1,215* • Non-Residential Annual Tuition: *$2,961* • General Institutional Fees: *$0* • Additional Nursing Fees: *$526*

INDIANA UNIVERSITY—PURDUE UNIVERSITY

Address: 1111 Middle Drive, Indianapolis, IN 46202-
          2896
Phone: 317-274-4413
Fax: 317-274-2996
Contact: Sue Morrissey, RN, DNSc, Acting Associate
          Dean for Graduate Programs
Email: smorriss@iupui.edu

GENERAL INFORMATION

Type of School: *4-Year College or University, Public* •
Accreditation: *North Central Association of Colleges and
Schools* • Total Enrollment: *37963*

PROGRAM INFORMATION

NLNAC Accreditation: *Yes* • CCNE Accreditation: *Yes*

———————

For specialty program listings, refer to the index.

NURSING STUDENT PROFILE

Total Nursing Enrollments: *286* • Full-Time Enrollment:
30 • Part-Time Enrollment: *256* • Female Enrollment: *279* •
Male Enrollment: *7* • Total Graduates: *56*

FINANCES

Residental Annual Tuition: *$5,703* • Non-Residential
Annual Tuition: *$14,886* • General Institutional Fees: *$341* •
Additional Nursing Fees: *$211*

INDIANA UNIVERSITY–PURDUE UNIVERSITY—FORT WAYNE

Address: 3400 Broadway, Indianapolis, IN 46408
Phone: 219-481-6282
Fax: 219-481-5767
Contact: Judith A. Lemise, RN, DNSc, Director of
          Graduate Programs in Nursing and Associate
          Professor
Email: lemisej@ipfw.edu

GENERAL INFORMATION

Type of School: *Not Provided* • Accreditation: *Not Provided* •
Total Enrollment: *2600*

PROGRAM INFORMATION

NLNAC Accreditation: *Not Reported* • CCNE Accreditation:

———————

For specialty program listings, refer to the index.

NURSING STUDENT PROFILE

Total Nursing Enrollments: *7* • Full-Time Enrollment: *0* •
Part-Time Enrollment: *7* • Female Enrollment: *7* • Male
Enrollment: *0* • Total Graduates: *1*

FINANCES

Residental Annual Tuition: *$3,793* • Non-Residential
Annual Tuition: *$8,431* • General Institutional Fees: *$9* •
Additional Nursing Fees: *Not Reported*

INDIANA WESLEYAN UNIVERSITY

Address: 4201 S. Washington Street, Marion, IN 46904
Phone: 765-677-2266
Fax: 765-677-2284
Contact: Susan D. Stranahan, PhD, Chair, Division of Nursing
Email: sstranah@indwes.edu

GENERAL INFORMATION

Type of School: *4-Year College or University, Public* •
Accreditation: *North Central Association of Colleges and Schools* • Total Enrollment: *4649*

PROGRAM INFORMATION

NLNAC Accreditation: *Not Reported* • CCNE Accreditation: *Yes*

_____

For specialty program listings, refer to the index.

NURSING STUDENT PROFILE

Total Nursing Enrollments: *26* • Full-Time Enrollment: *11* • Part-Time Enrollment: *15* • Female Enrollment: *24* • Male Enrollment: *2* • Total Graduates: *14*

FINANCES

Residental Annual Tuition: *$14,420* • Non-Residential Annual Tuition: *$14,420* • General Institutional Fees: *Not Reported* • Additional Nursing Fees: *Not Reported*

PURDUE UNIVERSITY— CALUMET

Address: 3950 Mid-America Boulevard, Hammond, IN 46323
Phone: 219-989-2815
Fax: Not Provided
Contact: Peggy S. Gerard, RN, DNSc, Professor and Coordinator
Email: psgerard@calumet.purdue.edu

GENERAL INFORMATION

Type of School: *4-Year College or University, Public* •
Accreditation: *North Central Association of Colleges and Schools* • Total Enrollment: *37762*

PROGRAM INFORMATION

NLNAC Accreditation: *Yes* • CCNE Accreditation:

_____

For specialty program listings, refer to the index.

NURSING STUDENT PROFILE

Total Nursing Enrollments: *102* • Full-Time Enrollment: *30* • Part-Time Enrollment: *72* • Female Enrollment: *97* • Male Enrollment: *5* • Total Graduates: *28*

FINANCES

Residental Annual Tuition: *$2,282* • Non-Residential Annual Tuition: *$5,184* • General Institutional Fees: *$122* • Additional Nursing Fees: *$160*

UNIVERSITY OF INDIANAPOLIS

Address: 1400 E. Hanna Ave., Indianapolis, IN 46227-3630
Phone: 317-788-3328
Fax: Not Provided
Contact: Anita Siccardi, EdD, RN, Master's Program Coordinator
Email: siccardi@uindy.edu

GENERAL INFORMATION

Type of School: *4-Year College or University, Public* • Accreditation: *North Central Association of Colleges and Schools* • Total Enrollment: *1200*

PROGRAM INFORMATION

NLNAC Accreditation: *Not Reported* • CCNE Accreditation: *Yes*

For specialty program listings, refer to the index.

NURSING STUDENT PROFILE

Total Nursing Enrollments: *25* • Full-Time Enrollment: *5* • Part-Time Enrollment: *20* • Female Enrollment: *24* • Male Enrollment: *1* • Total Graduates: *7*

FINANCES

Residental Annual Tuition: *$16,352* • Non-Residential Annual Tuition: *$16,352* • General Institutional Fees: *$0* • Additional Nursing Fees: *$95*

UNIVERSITY OF SAINT FRANCIS—FORT WAYNE

Address: 2701 Spring Street, Fort Wayne, IN 46808
Phone: 260-434-7687
Fax: 260-434-7404
Contact: Nancy Sweeney, PhD, APRN, BC, Program Director
Email: nsweeney@sf.edu

GENERAL INFORMATION

Type of School: *Not Provided* • Accreditation: *Not Provided* • Total Enrollment: *Not Provided*

PROGRAM INFORMATION

NLNAC Accreditation: *Not Reported* • CCNE Accreditation: *Yes*

For specialty program listings, refer to the index.

NURSING STUDENT PROFILE

Total Nursing Enrollments: *27* • Full-Time Enrollment: *12* • Part-Time Enrollment: *15* • Female Enrollment: *27* • Male Enrollment: *0* • Total Graduates: *10*

FINANCES

Residental Annual Tuition: *$12,690* • Non-Residential Annual Tuition: *$12,690* • General Institutional Fees: *$540* • Additional Nursing Fees: *Not Reported*

UNIVERSITY OF SOUTHERN INDIANA

Address: 8600 University Blvd., Evansville, IN 47712
Phone: 812-465-1171
Fax: 812-465-7092
Contact: Melissa Vandeveer, PHD, C-NP, Director,
            Graduate Nursing
Email: mvandeve@usi.edu

GENERAL INFORMATION

Type of School: *4-Year College or University, Public* •
Accreditation: *North Central Association of Colleges and
Schools* • Total Enrollment: *28766*

PROGRAM INFORMATION

NLNAC Accreditation: *Not Reported* • CCNE Accreditation:
Yes

_____

For specialty program listings, refer to the index.

NURSING STUDENT PROFILE

Total Nursing Enrollments: *112* • Full-Time Enrollment:
25 • Part-Time Enrollment: *87* • Female Enrollment: *100* •
Male Enrollment: *12* • Total Graduates: *15*

FINANCES

Residental Annual Tuition: *$5,928* • Non-Residential
Annual Tuition: *$11,712* • General Institutional Fees: *$60* •
Additional Nursing Fees: *$60*

VALPARAISO UNIVERSITY

Address: PO Box 917, Valparaiso, IN 32593
Phone: 219-464-5289
Fax: Not Provided
Contact: Freda S. Scales, PhD, RN, Dean, College of
            Nursing
Email: Freda.Scales@valpo.edu

GENERAL INFORMATION

Type of School: *4-Year College or University, Public* •
Accreditation: *North Central Association of Colleges and
Schools* • Total Enrollment: *Not Provided*

PROGRAM INFORMATION

NLNAC Accreditation: *No* • CCNE Accreditation:

_____

For specialty program listings, refer to the index.

NURSING STUDENT PROFILE

Total Nursing Enrollments: *63* • Full-Time Enrollment: *12* •
Part-Time Enrollment: *51* • Female Enrollment: *61* • Male
Enrollment: *2* • Total Graduates: *29*

FINANCES

Residental Annual Tuition: *$13,120* • Non-Residential
Annual Tuition: *$13,120* • General Institutional Fees: *$25* •
Additional Nursing Fees: *$20*

ALLEN COLLEGE

Address: 1825 Logan Ave, Waterloo, IA 50703-1999
Phone: 319-226-2047
Fax: 319-226-2070
Contact: Diane Young, PhD, RN, MSN, MSN
Department Chair
Email: YoungDM@ihs.org

GENERAL INFORMATION

Type of School: *4-Year College or University, Private (Independent)* • Accreditation: *North Central Association of Colleges and Schools* • Total Enrollment: *257*

PROGRAM INFORMATION

NLNAC Accreditation: *Yes* • CCNE Accreditation:

For specialty program listings, refer to the index.

NURSING STUDENT PROFILE

Total Nursing Enrollments: *24* • Full-Time Enrollment: *13* • Part-Time Enrollment: *11* • Female Enrollment: *23* • Male Enrollment: *1* • Total Graduates: *7*

FINANCES

Residental Annual Tuition: *$9,320* • Non-Residential Annual Tuition: *$9,320* • General Institutional Fees: *$361* • Additional Nursing Fees: *$0*

CLARKE COLLEGE

Address: 1550 Clarke St, Dubuque, IA 52001
Phone: 319-588-6361
Fax: Not Provided
Contact: Mary Margaret Mooney, DNSc, ARNP, FAAN, Chair
Email: mmooney@clarke.edu

GENERAL INFORMATION

Type of School: *4-Year College or University, Private (Independent)* • Accreditation: *North Central Association of Colleges and Schools* • Total Enrollment: *1249*

PROGRAM INFORMATION

NLNAC Accreditation: *Not Reported* • CCNE Accreditation:

For specialty program listings, refer to the index.

NURSING STUDENT PROFILE

Total Nursing Enrollments: *33* • Full-Time Enrollment: *4* • Part-Time Enrollment: *29* • Female Enrollment: *32* • Male Enrollment: *1* • Total Graduates: *Not Provided*

FINANCES

Residental Annual Tuition: *$6,120* • Non-Residential Annual Tuition: *$6,120* • General Institutional Fees: *$340* • Additional Nursing Fees: *$400*

NLN Official Guide to Undergraduate and Graduate Nursing Programs

DRAKE UNIVERSITY

Address: 2507 University Ave, Des Moines, IA 50311
Phone: 515-271-2830
Fax: 515-271-4569
Contact: Linda H. Brady, PhD, RN, Associate Dean of
          Nursing
Email: linda.brady@drake.edu

GENERAL INFORMATION

Type of School: *4-Year College or University, Private (Independent)* • Accreditation: *North Central Association of Colleges and Schools* • Total Enrollment: *1691*

PROGRAM INFORMATION

NLNAC Accreditation: *Yes* • CCNE Accreditation:

_____

For specialty program listings, refer to the index.

NURSING STUDENT PROFILE

Total Nursing Enrollments: *50* • Full-Time Enrollment: *19* • Part-Time Enrollment: *31* • Female Enrollment: *49* • Male Enrollment: *1* • Total Graduates: *11*

FINANCES

Residental Annual Tuition: *$13,200* • Non-Residential Annual Tuition: *Not Reported* • General Institutional Fees: *Not Reported* • Additional Nursing Fees: *Not Reported*

UNIVERSITY OF IOWA

Address: 101 Nursing Building, Iowa City, IA 52242
Phone: 319-335-8709
Fax: 319-335-7129
Contact: Marion Johnson, PhD, RN, Director - Master's
          Program
Email: marion-johnson@uiowa.edu

GENERAL INFORMATION

Type of School: *4-Year College or University, Private (Religious)* • Accreditation: *North Central Association of Colleges and Schools* • Total Enrollment: *25000*

PROGRAM INFORMATION

NLNAC Accreditation: *Not Reported* • CCNE Accreditation: *Yes*

_____

For specialty program listings, refer to the index.

NURSING STUDENT PROFILE

Total Nursing Enrollments: *142* • Full-Time Enrollment: *48* • Part-Time Enrollment: *94* • Female Enrollment: *126* • Male Enrollment: *16* • Total Graduates: *48*

FINANCES

Residental Annual Tuition: *$3,166* • Non-Residential Annual Tuition: *$10,202* • General Institutional Fees: *$286* • Additional Nursing Fees: *$260*

NEWMAN UNIVERSITY

Address: 3111 Saunders Settlement Rd., Wichita, KS
          67213
Phone: 316-942-4291
Fax: Not Provided
Contact: Jeanette Jeffers, PhD, MN, ARNP-CNS,
          Program Director, MSN Program
Email: jeffersj@newmanu.edu

GENERAL INFORMATION

Type of School: *Other* • Accreditation: *North Central
Association of Colleges and Schools* • Total Enrollment: *Not
Provided*

PROGRAM INFORMATION

NLNAC Accreditation: *Not Reported* • CCNE Accreditation:

_____

For specialty program listings, refer to the index.

NURSING STUDENT PROFILE

Total Nursing Enrollments: *29* • Full-Time Enrollment: *4* •
Part-Time Enrollment: *25* • Female Enrollment: *29* • Male
Enrollment: *0* • Total Graduates: *0*

FINANCES

Residental Annual Tuition: *$15,712* • Non-Residential
Annual Tuition: *$15,712* • General Institutional Fees: *$120* •
Additional Nursing Fees: *Not Reported*

UNIVERSITY OF KANSAS

Address: 3901 Rainbow Blvd., Kansas City, KS 66160-
          7501
Phone: 913-588-1619
Fax: 913-588-1615
Contact: Karen L. Miller, PhD, RN, FAAN, Professor and
          Dean
Email: soninfo@kumc.edu

GENERAL INFORMATION

Type of School: *4-Year College or University, Public* •
Accreditation: *North Central Association of Colleges and
Schools* • Total Enrollment: *2839*

PROGRAM INFORMATION

NLNAC Accreditation: *Yes* • CCNE Accreditation:

_____

For specialty program listings, refer to the index.

NURSING STUDENT PROFILE

Total Nursing Enrollments: *140* • Full-Time Enrollment:
21 • Part-Time Enrollment: *119* • Female Enrollment: *135* •
Male Enrollment: *5* • Total Graduates: *38*

FINANCES

Residental Annual Tuition: *$2,829* • Non-Residential
Annual Tuition: *$8,451* • General Institutional Fees: *$266* •
Additional Nursing Fees: *Not Reported*

Circle 126 on reader card   See in-depth profile for more information

WICHITA STATE UNIVERSITY

Address: 1845 Fairmont, Wichita, KS 67260
Phone: 316-978-5742
Fax: 316-978-3094
Contact: Alicia A. Huckstadt, PhD, ARNP, FNP, |Graduate Program Director
Email: alicia.huckstadt@wichita.edu

GENERAL INFORMATION

Type of School: *Other* • Accreditation: *North Central Association of Colleges and Schools* • Total Enrollment: *12000*

PROGRAM INFORMATION

NLNAC Accreditation: *Yes* • CCNE Accreditation: *Provisional*

_____

For specialty program listings, refer to the index.

NURSING STUDENT PROFILE

Total Nursing Enrollments: *151* • Full-Time Enrollment: *48* • Part-Time Enrollment: *103* • Female Enrollment: *142* • Male Enrollment: *9* • Total Graduates: *36*

FINANCES

Residental Annual Tuition: *$4,284* • Non-Residential Annual Tuition: *$12,207* • General Institutional Fees: *$0* • Additional Nursing Fees: *$755*

BELLARMINE COLLEGE

Address: 2001 Newburg Rd, Miles Hall, Louisville, KY 40205
Phone: 502-452-8414
Fax: Not Provided
Contact: Margaret E. Miller, PhD, RN, MSN Program Director
Email: maggie.miller@bellarmine.edu

GENERAL INFORMATION

Type of School: *Other, Private (Independent)* • Accreditation: *Southern Association of Colleges and Schools* • Total Enrollment: *Not Provided*

PROGRAM INFORMATION

NLNAC Accreditation: *Yes* • CCNE Accreditation:

_____

For specialty program listings, refer to the index.

NURSING STUDENT PROFILE

Total Nursing Enrollments: *89* • Full-Time Enrollment: *0* • Part-Time Enrollment: *89* • Female Enrollment: *Not Provided* • Male Enrollment: *Not Provided* • Total Graduates: *26*

FINANCES

Residental Annual Tuition: *Not Reported* • Non-Residential Annual Tuition: *Not Reported* • General Institutional Fees: *Not Reported* • Additional Nursing Fees: *Not Reported*

EASTERN KENTUCKY UNIVERSITY

Address: Rowlett 203, 521 Lancaster Avenue, Richmond, KY 40475
Phone: 606-622-1956
Fax: Not Provided
Contact: Deborah Whitehouse, RN, DNS, Chair
Email: bsnwhite@acs.eku.edu

GENERAL INFORMATION

Type of School: *Not Provided* • Accreditation: *Not Provided* • Total Enrollment: *1600*

PROGRAM INFORMATION

NLNAC Accreditation: *No* • CCNE Accreditation: *Yes*

_____

For specialty program listings, refer to the index.

NURSING STUDENT PROFILE

Total Nursing Enrollments: *Not Provided* • Full-Time Enrollment: *Not Provided* • Part-Time Enrollment: *Not Provided* • Female Enrollment: *Not Provided* • Male Enrollment: *Not Provided* • Total Graduates: *31*

FINANCES

Residental Annual Tuition: *Not Reported* • Non-Residential Annual Tuition: *Not Reported* • General Institutional Fees: *Not Reported* • Additional Nursing Fees: *Not Reported*

MURRAY STATE UNIVERSITY

Address: 120 Mason Hall, Murray, KY 42071
Phone: 270-762-6671
Fax: Not Provided
Contact: Nancey E.M. France, PhD, RN, Graduate Coordinator
Email: nancey.france@murraystate.edu

GENERAL INFORMATION

Type of School: *4-Year College or University, Public* • Accreditation: *Southern Association of Colleges and Schools* • Total Enrollment: *273*

PROGRAM INFORMATION

NLNAC Accreditation: *Yes* • CCNE Accreditation:

_____

For specialty program listings, refer to the index.

NURSING STUDENT PROFILE

Total Nursing Enrollments: *60* • Full-Time Enrollment: *48* • Part-Time Enrollment: *12* • Female Enrollment: *48* • Male Enrollment: *12* • Total Graduates: *20*

FINANCES

Residental Annual Tuition: *$2,500* • Non-Residential Annual Tuition: *$6,740* • General Institutional Fees: *$0* • Additional Nursing Fees: *$6,500*

NORTHERN KENTUCKY UNIVERSITY

Address: Nunn Drive, AHG 303, Highland Heights, KY 41076
Phone: 606-572-5178
Fax: Not Provided
Contact: Denise L Robinson, PhD, RN, FNP, Director MSN Program
Email: robinson@nku.edu

GENERAL INFORMATION

Type of School: *4-Year College, Public* • Accreditation: *Southern Association of Colleges* • Total Enrollment: *12000*

PROGRAM INFORMATION

NLNAC Accreditation: *Yes* • CCNE Accreditation:

_____

For specialty program listings, refer to the index.

NURSING STUDENT PROFILE

Total Nursing Enrollments: *66* • Full-Time Enrollment: *8* • Part-Time Enrollment: *58* • Female Enrollment: *61* • Male Enrollment: *5* • Total Graduates: *31*

FINANCES

Residental Annual Tuition: *$2,304* • Non-Residential Annual Tuition: *$6,660* • General Institutional Fees: *Not Reported* • Additional Nursing Fees: *$40*

SPALDING UNIVERSITY

Address: Allied Health Building, SUNY Alfred, Louisville, KY 40203
Phone: 502-585-7125
Fax: Not Provided
Contact: Cynthia R. Crabtree, RN, Dean
Email: ccrabtree@spalding.edu

GENERAL INFORMATION

Type of School: *4-Year College or University, Public* • Accreditation: *Southern Association of Colleges and Schools* • Total Enrollment: *4468*

PROGRAM INFORMATION

NLNAC Accreditation: *Yes* • CCNE Accreditation:

_____

For specialty program listings, refer to the index.

NURSING STUDENT PROFILE

Total Nursing Enrollments: *56* • Full-Time Enrollment: *25* • Part-Time Enrollment: *31* • Female Enrollment: *52* • Male Enrollment: *4* • Total Graduates: *16*

FINANCES

Residental Annual Tuition: *$14,720* • Non-Residential Annual Tuition: *$14,720* • General Institutional Fees: *$200* • Additional Nursing Fees: *$500*

UNIVERSITY OF KENTUCKY

Address: 760 Rose Street, Rm 315, Lexington, KY 40536
Phone: 606-323-6685
Fax: Not Provided
Contact: Juliann G. Sebastian, PhD, RN, CS, FAAN,
           Assistant Dean for Advanced Practice Nursing
Email: jgseba00@pop.uky.edu

GENERAL INFORMATION

Type of School: *4-Year College or University, Public* •
Accreditation: *Southern Association of Colleges and Schools* •
Total Enrollment: *28840*

PROGRAM INFORMATION

NLNAC Accreditation: *Yes* • CCNE Accreditation:

_____

For specialty program listings, refer to the index.

NURSING STUDENT PROFILE

Total Nursing Enrollments: *99* • Full-Time Enrollment: *34* •
Part-Time Enrollment: *65* • Female Enrollment: *88* • Male
Enrollment: *11* • Total Graduates: *48*

FINANCES

Residental Annual Tuition: *$3,260* • Non-Residential
Annual Tuition: *$9,780* • General Institutional Fees: *$336* •
Additional Nursing Fees: *$0*

UNIVERSITY OF LOUISVILLE

Address: 555 S. Floyd Street, Louisville, KY 40292
Phone: 502-852-8384
Fax: Not Provided
Contact: Deborah Scott, RN, DSN, Associate Dean for
           Academic Affairs
Email: dlscot02@gwise.louisville.edu

GENERAL INFORMATION

Type of School: *4-Year College or University, Public* •
Accreditation: *Southern Association of Colleges and Schools* •
Total Enrollment: *15740*

PROGRAM INFORMATION

NLNAC Accreditation: *Yes* • CCNE Accreditation:

_____

For specialty program listings, refer to the index.

NURSING STUDENT PROFILE

Total Nursing Enrollments: *110* • Full-Time Enrollment:
14 • Part-Time Enrollment: *96* • Female Enrollment: *103* •
Male Enrollment: *7* • Total Graduates: *21*

FINANCES

Residental Annual Tuition: *$3,546* • Non-Residential
Annual Tuition: *$10,066* • General Institutional Fees: *$30* •
Additional Nursing Fees: *$80*

WESTERN KENTUCKY UNIVERSITY

Address: 1 Big Red Way, Bowling Green, KY 42101
Phone: 270-745-3579
Fax: Not Provided
Contact: Donna Blackburn, PhD, RN, Interim
           Department Head
Email: donna.blackburn@wku.edu

GENERAL INFORMATION

Type of School: *4-Year College or University, Public* •
Accreditation: *Southern Association of Colleges and Schools* •
Total Enrollment: *Public*

PROGRAM INFORMATION

NLNAC Accreditation: *Not Reported* • CCNE Accreditation:

_____

For specialty program listings, refer to the index.

NURSING STUDENT PROFILE

Total Nursing Enrollments: *34* • Full-Time Enrollment: *10* •
Part-Time Enrollment: *24* • Female Enrollment: *32* • Male
Enrollment: *2* • Total Graduates: *9*

FINANCES

Residental Annual Tuition: *$2,220* • Non-Residential
Annual Tuition: *$6,660* • General Institutional Fees: *$370* •
Additional Nursing Fees: *$90*

GRAMBLING STATE UNIVERSITY

Address: Box 4272, Grambling, LA 71245
Phone: 318-274-2897
Fax: 318-274-3491
Contact: Rhonda Hensley, RN, CS, MSN, MSN Program
           Director
Email: hensleyr@alpha.gram.edu

GENERAL INFORMATION

Type of School: *4-Year College or University, Public* •
Accreditation: *Not Provided* • Total Enrollment: *2283*

PROGRAM INFORMATION

NLNAC Accreditation: *Yes* • CCNE Accreditation:

_____

For specialty program listings, refer to the index.

NURSING STUDENT PROFILE

Total Nursing Enrollments: *23* • Full-Time Enrollment: *21* •
Part-Time Enrollment: *2* • Female Enrollment: *18* • Male
Enrollment: *5* • Total Graduates: *10*

FINANCES

Residental Annual Tuition: *$3,000* • Non-Residential
Annual Tuition: *Not Reported* • General Institutional Fees:
$200 • Additional Nursing Fees: *$500*

LOUISIANA STATE UNIVERSITY

Address:　1600 Maple Street, New Orleans, LA 70112
Phone:　504-568-4106
Fax:　504-599-0573
Contact:　Elizabeth A. Humphrey, EdD, RN, Dean and Professor
Email:　ehumph@lsuhsc.edu

GENERAL INFORMATION

Type of School: *Not Provided* • Accreditation: *Not Provided* • Total Enrollment: *1124*

PROGRAM INFORMATION

NLNAC Accreditation: *Not Reported* • CCNE Accreditation: *Yes*

———

For specialty program listings, refer to the index.

NURSING STUDENT PROFILE

Total Nursing Enrollments: *87* • Full-Time Enrollment: *39* • Part-Time Enrollment: *48* • Female Enrollment: *70* • Male Enrollment: *17* • Total Graduates: *12*

FINANCES

Residental Annual Tuition: *$2,522* • Non-Residential Annual Tuition: *$5,022* • General Institutional Fees: *$166* • Additional Nursing Fees: *$0*

LOYOLA UNIVERSITY NEW ORLEANS

Address:　6363 Saint Charles Avenue, New Orleans, LA 70118
Phone:　504-865-3253
Fax:　Not Provided
Contact:　Billie Ann Wilson, PhD, APRN, Director
Email:　bwilson@loyno.edu

GENERAL INFORMATION

Type of School: *4-Year College or University, Public* • Accreditation: *Southern Association of Colleges and Schools* • Total Enrollment: *1300*

PROGRAM INFORMATION

NLNAC Accreditation: *Not Reported* • CCNE Accreditation:

———

For specialty program listings, refer to the index.

NURSING STUDENT PROFILE

Total Nursing Enrollments: *47* • Full-Time Enrollment: *6* • Part-Time Enrollment: *41* • Female Enrollment: *43* • Male Enrollment: *4* • Total Graduates: *Not Provided*

FINANCES

Residental Annual Tuition: *$7,290* • Non-Residential Annual Tuition: *Not Reported* • General Institutional Fees: *$107* • Additional Nursing Fees: *$0*

MCNEESE STATE UNIVERSITY

Address: P.O.Box 90415, Lake Charles, LA 70609
Phone: 337-475-5820
Fax: 337-475-5924
Contact: Peggy L. Wolfe, PhD, RN, Dean, College of Nursing
Email: pwolfe@mail.mcneese.edu

GENERAL INFORMATION

Type of School: *4-Year College or University, Public* •
Accreditation: *Southern Association of Colleges and Schools* •
Total Enrollment: *Not Provided*

PROGRAM INFORMATION

NLNAC Accreditation: *Yes* • CCNE Accreditation:

_____

For specialty program listings, refer to the index.

NURSING STUDENT PROFILE

Total Nursing Enrollments: *53* • Full-Time Enrollment: *9* •
Part-Time Enrollment: *44* • Female Enrollment: *43* • Male
Enrollment: *10* • Total Graduates: *6*

FINANCES

Residental Annual Tuition: *$1,998* • Non-Residential
Annual Tuition: *$6,340* • General Institutional Fees: *$243* •
Additional Nursing Fees: *$100*

NORTHWESTERN STATE UNIVERSITY OF LOUISIANA

Address: H. L. Campus 7350 Cooley Lake Road, Natchitoches, LA 71497
Phone: 318-677-3100
Fax: 318-677-3127
Contact: Norann Y. Panchock, PhD, RN, CS, FNP, Dean
Email: planchockn@nsula.edu

GENERAL INFORMATION

Type of School: *4-Year College or University, Public* •
Accreditation: *Southern Association of Colleges and Schools* •
Total Enrollment: *4173*

PROGRAM INFORMATION

NLNAC Accreditation: *Yes* • CCNE Accreditation:
Provisional

_____

For specialty program listings, refer to the index.

NURSING STUDENT PROFILE

Total Nursing Enrollments: *102* • Full-Time Enrollment: *9* •
Part-Time Enrollment: *93* • Female Enrollment: *93* • Male
Enrollment: *9* • Total Graduates: *26*

FINANCES

Residental Annual Tuition: *$3,223* • Non-Residential
Annual Tuition: *$7,797* • General Institutional Fees: *$83* •
Additional Nursing Fees: *$195*

SOUTHEASTERN LOUISIANA UNIVERSITY

Address: SLU 10781, Hammond, LA 70402
Phone: 225-765-2324
Fax: Not Provided
Contact: Sarah K. Thrornhill, PhD, RN, CNAA, Director, Graduate Nursing Program
Email: sthornhill@selu.edu

GENERAL INFORMATION

Type of School: *Other* • Accreditation: *Not Provided* • Total Enrollment: *1900*

PROGRAM INFORMATION

NLNAC Accreditation: *Yes* • CCNE Accreditation:

_____

For specialty program listings, refer to the index.

NURSING STUDENT PROFILE

Total Nursing Enrollments: *38* • Full-Time Enrollment: *8* • Part-Time Enrollment: *30* • Female Enrollment: *33* • Male Enrollment: *5* • Total Graduates: *10*

FINANCES

Residental Annual Tuition: *$6,654* • Non-Residential Annual Tuition: *Not Reported* • General Institutional Fees: *$15* • Additional Nursing Fees: *$40*

SOUTHERN UNIVERSITY AND A&M COLLEGE

Address: PO BOX 11784, Swan Street building 170, Baton Rouge, LA 70813
Phone: 225-771-2663
Fax: Not Provided
Contact: Sandra C. Brown, DNS, CCRN, FNP-C, Chair, Graduate Programs in Nursing
Email: sandrabrown@suson.subr.edu

GENERAL INFORMATION

Type of School: *4-Year College or University, Public* • Accreditation: *Southern Association of Colleges and Schools* • Total Enrollment: *1847*

PROGRAM INFORMATION

NLNAC Accreditation: *Yes* • CCNE Accreditation:

_____

For specialty program listings, refer to the index.

NURSING STUDENT PROFILE

Total Nursing Enrollments: *38* • Full-Time Enrollment: *12* • Part-Time Enrollment: *26* • Female Enrollment: *35* • Male Enrollment: *3* • Total Graduates: *8*

FINANCES

Residental Annual Tuition: *$2,274* • Non-Residential Annual Tuition: *$7,440* • General Institutional Fees: *$2,274* • Additional Nursing Fees: *$0*

UNIVERSITY OF LOUISIANA—LAFAYETTE

Address: 700 University Avenue, Hammond, LA 71209
Phone: 337-482-5617
Fax: Not Provided
Contact: Carolyn P. Delahoussaye, RN, DNS, MSN
           Program Coordinator
Email: cgp6303@louisiana.edu

GENERAL INFORMATION

Type of School: *4-Year College or University, Public* •
Accreditation: *Southern Association of Colleges and Schools* •
Total Enrollment: *25920*

PROGRAM INFORMATION

NLNAC Accreditation: *Yes* • CCNE Accreditation:

_____

For specialty program listings, refer to the index.

NURSING STUDENT PROFILE

Total Nursing Enrollments: *40* • Full-Time Enrollment: *5* •
Part-Time Enrollment: *35* • Female Enrollment: *30* • Male
Enrollment: *10* • Total Graduates: *7*

FINANCES

Residental Annual Tuition: *$1,985* • Non-Residential
Annual Tuition: *$7,217* • General Institutional Fees: *Not
Reported* • Additional Nursing Fees: *Not Reported*

HUSSON COLLEGE

Address: 1 Circle College, Bangor, ME 04401
Phone: 207-941-7065
Fax: 207-941-7883
Contact: Mary Shea, MSN, Director, Family and
           Community NP Program
Email: sheam@husson.edu

GENERAL INFORMATION

Type of School: *4-Year College or University, Private
(Independent)* • Accreditation: *New England Association of
Schools and Colleges* • Total Enrollment: *1000*

PROGRAM INFORMATION

NLNAC Accreditation: *Yes* • CCNE Accreditation:

_____

For specialty program listings, refer to the index.

NURSING STUDENT PROFILE

Total Nursing Enrollments: *25* • Full-Time Enrollment: *8* •
Part-Time Enrollment: *17* • Female Enrollment: *25* • Male
Enrollment: *0* • Total Graduates: *12*

FINANCES

Residental Annual Tuition: *$7,584* • Non-Residential
Annual Tuition: *$7,584* • General Institutional Fees: *$0* •
Additional Nursing Fees: *$0*

SAINT JOSEPH'S COLLEGE

Address: 5600 Oakland, Standish, ME 04084-5263
Phone: 207-893-7956
Fax: 207-893-7520
Contact: Linda R. Conover, PhD, RN, Chair
Email: LConover@sjcme.edu

GENERAL INFORMATION

Type of School: *4-Year College or University, Private (Independent)* • Accreditation: *New England Association of Schools and Colleges* • Total Enrollment: *Not Provided*

PROGRAM INFORMATION

NLNAC Accreditation: *Not Reported* • CCNE Accreditation: *Yes*

For specialty program listings, refer to the index.

NURSING STUDENT PROFILE

Total Nursing Enrollments: *274* • Full-Time Enrollment: *0* • Part-Time Enrollment: *274* • Female Enrollment: *257* • Male Enrollment: *17* • Total Graduates: *4*

FINANCES

Residental Annual Tuition: *$5,640* • Non-Residential Annual Tuition: *$5,640* • General Institutional Fees: *$0* • Additional Nursing Fees: *$0*

UNIVERSITY OF MAINE

Address: 5724 Dunn Hall, Orono, ME 04469
Phone: 207-581-2605
Fax: 207-581-2585
Contact: Carol Wood, EdD, CNM, Graduate Program
            Coordinator
Email: cwood@maine.edu

GENERAL INFORMATION

Type of School: *4-Year College or University, Public* • Accreditation: *New England Association of Schools and Colleges* • Total Enrollment: *8760*

PROGRAM INFORMATION

NLNAC Accreditation: *Not Reported* • CCNE Accreditation: *Yes*

For specialty program listings, refer to the index.

NURSING STUDENT PROFILE

Total Nursing Enrollments: *33* • Full-Time Enrollment: *23* • Part-Time Enrollment: *10* • Female Enrollment: *30* • Male Enrollment: *3* • Total Graduates: *4*

FINANCES

Residental Annual Tuition: *$3,564* • Non-Residential Annual Tuition: *$10,116* • General Institutional Fees: *$298* • Additional Nursing Fees: *$0*

UNIVERSITY OF SOUTHERN MAINE

Address: PO Box 9300, Portland, ME 04104-9300
Phone: 207-780-4404
Fax: 207-780-4997
Contact: Jane M Kirschling, RN, DNS, Dean and Professor of Nursing
Email: jane.kirschling@usm.maine.edu

GENERAL INFORMATION

Type of School: *4-Year College or University, Public* • Accreditation: *New England Association of Schools and Colleges* • Total Enrollment: *4000*

PROGRAM INFORMATION

NLNAC Accreditation: *Yes* • CCNE Accreditation: *No*

———————

For specialty program listings, refer to the index.

NURSING STUDENT PROFILE

Total Nursing Enrollments: *89* • Full-Time Enrollment: *50* • Part-Time Enrollment: *39* • Female Enrollment: *81* • Male Enrollment: *8* • Total Graduates: *32*

FINANCES

Residental Annual Tuition: *$3,465* • Non-Residential Annual Tuition: *$9,684* • General Institutional Fees: *$400* • Additional Nursing Fees: *$180*

JOHNS HOPKINS UNIVERSITY

Address: 525 North Wolfe Street, Baltimore, MD 21205
Phone: 410-614-4081
Fax: 410-955-7463
Contact: Stella Shiber, PhD, RN, Associate Dean for Professional Education Programs and Practice
Email: sshiber@son.jhmi.edu

GENERAL INFORMATION

Type of School: *Independent, Public* • Accreditation: *Middle States Association of Colleges and Schools* • Total Enrollment: *Not Provided*

PROGRAM INFORMATION

NLNAC Accreditation: *Yes* • CCNE Accreditation: *Provisional*

———————

For specialty program listings, refer to the index.

NURSING STUDENT PROFILE

Total Nursing Enrollments: *178* • Full-Time Enrollment: *45* • Part-Time Enrollment: *133* • Female Enrollment: *164* • Male Enrollment: *14* • Total Graduates: *57*

FINANCES

Residental Annual Tuition: *$21,122* • Non-Residential Annual Tuition: *$21,122* • General Institutional Fees: *$0* • Additional Nursing Fees: *$0*

SALISBURY STATE UNIVERSITY

Address: PO Box 318, Salisbury, MD 21801
Phone: 410-543-6402
Fax: 410-548-3313
Contact: Karen K. Badros, PhD, CFNP, Graduate Program Director
Email: kkbadros@salisbury.edu

GENERAL INFORMATION

Type of School: *4-Year College or University, Public* •
Accreditation: *Not Provided* • Total Enrollment: *Not Provided*

PROGRAM INFORMATION

NLNAC Accreditation: *Yes* • CCNE Accreditation: *No*

For specialty program listings, refer to the index.

NURSING STUDENT PROFILE

Total Nursing Enrollments: *27* • Full-Time Enrollment: *9* •
Part-Time Enrollment: *18* • Female Enrollment: *23* • Male
Enrollment: *4* • Total Graduates: *8*

FINANCES

Residental Annual Tuition: *$3,132* • Non-Residential
Annual Tuition: *$6,390* • General Institutional Fees: *$100* •
Additional Nursing Fees: *$50*

UNIFORMED SERVICES UNIVERSITY

Address: PO Box 21150, Bethesda, MD 20814-4799
Phone: 301-295-9004
Fax: 301-295-9006
Contact: Faye G. Abdellah, EdD, ScD, RN, FAAN, Dean and Professor
Email: fabdellah@usuhs.mil

GENERAL INFORMATION

Type of School: *4-Year College or University, Public* •
Accreditation: *Middle States Association of Colleges and Schools* • Total Enrollment: *2525*

PROGRAM INFORMATION

NLNAC Accreditation: *Yes* • CCNE Accreditation: *No*

For specialty program listings, refer to the index.

NURSING STUDENT PROFILE

Total Nursing Enrollments: *53* • Full-Time Enrollment: *52* •
Part-Time Enrollment: *1* • Female Enrollment: *21* • Male
Enrollment: *32* • Total Graduates: *34*

FINANCES

Residental Annual Tuition: *Not Reported* • Non-Residential
Annual Tuition: *Not Reported* • General Institutional Fees:
Not Reported • Additional Nursing Fees: *Not Reported*

UNIVERSITY OF MARYLAND—BALTIMORE

Address: 655 W. Lombard Street, Baltimore, MD 21210
Phone: 410-706-6741
Fax: 410-706-4231
Contact: Barbara R. Heller, EdD, RN, FAAN, Dean and Professor
Email: heller@son.umaryland.edu

GENERAL INFORMATION

Type of School: *4-Year College or University, Public* • Accreditation: *Middle States Association of Colleges and Schools* • Total Enrollment: *Not Provided*

PROGRAM INFORMATION

NLNAC Accreditation: *Yes* • CCNE Accreditation:

_____

For specialty program listings, refer to the index.

NURSING STUDENT PROFILE

Total Nursing Enrollments: *578* • Full-Time Enrollment: *222* • Part-Time Enrollment: *356* • Female Enrollment: *525* • Male Enrollment: *53* • Total Graduates: *232*

FINANCES

Residental Annual Tuition: *$11,200* • Non-Residential Annual Tuition: *$18,240* • General Institutional Fees: *$276* • Additional Nursing Fees: *$205*

BOSTON COLLEGE

Address: 140 Commonwealth Ave., Chestnut Hill, MA 02467-3812
Phone: 617-552-4279
Fax: 617-552-0931
Contact: Laurel Eisenhauer, PhD, RN, FAAN, Associate Dean for Graduate Programs
Email: laurel.eisenhauer@bc.edu

GENERAL INFORMATION

Type of School: *4-Year College or University, Private (Religious)* • Accreditation: *New England Association of Schools and Colleges* • Total Enrollment: *14000*

PROGRAM INFORMATION

NLNAC Accreditation: *Yes* • CCNE Accreditation:

_____

For specialty program listings, refer to the index.

NURSING STUDENT PROFILE

Total Nursing Enrollments: *102* • Full-Time Enrollment: *72* • Part-Time Enrollment: *30* • Female Enrollment: *98* • Male Enrollment: *4* • Total Graduates: *46*

FINANCES

Residental Annual Tuition: *$17,382* • Non-Residential Annual Tuition: *$17,382* • General Institutional Fees: *$235* • Additional Nursing Fees: *$185*

FITCHBURG STATE COLLEGE

Address: 160 Pearl Street, Fitchburg, MA 01420
Phone: 978-665-3033
Fax: Not Provided
Contact: Andrea Wallen, EdD, RN, Graduate Program
Chairperson
Email: awallen@fsc.edu

GENERAL INFORMATION

Type of School: *4-Year College or University, Public* •
Accreditation: *New England Association of Schools and
Colleges* • Total Enrollment: *Not Provided*

PROGRAM INFORMATION

NLNAC Accreditation: *Not Reported* • CCNE Accreditation:

_____

For specialty program listings, refer to the index.

NURSING STUDENT PROFILE

Total Nursing Enrollments: *22* • Full-Time Enrollment: *0* •
Part-Time Enrollment: *22* • Female Enrollment: *21* • Male
Enrollment: *1* • Total Graduates: *19*

FINANCES

Residental Annual Tuition: *$4,800* • Non-Residential
Annual Tuition: *$4,800* • General Institutional Fees:
$2,304 • Additional Nursing Fees: *$0*

MASSACHUSETTS COLLEGE OF PHARMACY

Address: 1400 College Drive, Boston, MA 02115
Phone: 617-732-2977
Fax: Not Provided
Contact: Gail C. MacDonald, RN, DNSc, Acting
Director
Email: gmacdonald@mcp.edu

GENERAL INFORMATION

Type of School: *4-Year College or University, Public* •
Accreditation: *New England Association of Schools and
Colleges* • Total Enrollment: *2859*

PROGRAM INFORMATION

NLNAC Accreditation: *Not Reported* • CCNE Accreditation:

_____

For specialty program listings, refer to the index.

NURSING STUDENT PROFILE

Total Nursing Enrollments: *33* • Full-Time Enrollment: *29* •
Part-Time Enrollment: *4* • Female Enrollment: *26* • Male
Enrollment: *7* • Total Graduates: *5*

FINANCES

Residental Annual Tuition: *$9,936* • Non-Residential
Annual Tuition: *$9,936* • General Institutional Fees: *$260* •
Additional Nursing Fees: *$0*

NORTHEASTERN UNIVERSITY

Address: 360 Huntington Avenue, Boston, MA 02115
Phone: 617-383-4603
Fax: 617-373-8672
Contact: Margery Chisholm, EdD, Graduate Program
           Director
Email: machisho@lynx.neu.edu

GENERAL INFORMATION

Type of School: *4-Year College or University, Public* •
Accreditation: *New England Association of Schools and
Colleges* • Total Enrollment: *Not Reported*

PROGRAM INFORMATION

NLNAC Accreditation: *Yes* • CCNE Accreditation: *Yes*

———————

For specialty program listings, refer to the index.

NURSING STUDENT PROFILE

Total Nursing Enrollments: *189* • Full-Time Enrollment:
52 • Part-Time Enrollment: *137* • Female Enrollment: *188* •
Male Enrollment: *1* • Total Graduates: *59*

FINANCES

Residental Annual Tuition: *Not Reported* • Non-Residential
Annual Tuition: *Not Reported* • General Institutional Fees:
Not Reported • Additional Nursing Fees: *Not Reported*

REGIS COLLEGE

Address: 235 Wellesley Street, Weston, MA 02493
Phone: 508-768-7090
Fax: 508-768-7089
Contact: Amy Anderson, EdD, RN, Chair, Division of
           Nursing
Email: amy.anderson@regiscollege.edu

GENERAL INFORMATION

Type of School: *4-Year College or University, Public* •
Accreditation: *New England Association of Schools and
Colleges* • Total Enrollment: *3394*

PROGRAM INFORMATION

NLNAC Accreditation: *Yes* • CCNE Accreditation:

———————

For specialty program listings, refer to the index.

NURSING STUDENT PROFILE

Total Nursing Enrollments: *69* • Full-Time Enrollment: *4* •
Part-Time Enrollment: *65* • Female Enrollment: *68* • Male
Enrollment: *1* • Total Graduates: *26*

FINANCES

Residental Annual Tuition: *$17,500* • Non-Residential
Annual Tuition: *$17,500* • General Institutional Fees: *$70* •
Additional Nursing Fees: *$50*

SALEM STATE COLLEGE

Address: 900 West Vest, Salem, MA 01970
Phone: 978-542-6646
Fax: 978-542-6818
Contact: Susan Anderson, EdD, RN, Coordinator
Email: sanderson@shore.net

GENERAL INFORMATION

Type of School: *4-Year College or University, Public* •
Accreditation: *New England Association of Schools and
Colleges* • Total Enrollment: *4867*

PROGRAM INFORMATION

NLNAC Accreditation: *Yes* • CCNE Accreditation: *No*

For specialty program listings, refer to the index.

NURSING STUDENT PROFILE

Total Nursing Enrollments: *40* • Full-Time Enrollment: *0* •
Part-Time Enrollment: *40* • Female Enrollment: *39* • Male
Enrollment: *1* • Total Graduates: *17*

FINANCES

Residental Annual Tuition: *$3,360* • Non-Residential
Annual Tuition: *$5,520* • General Institutional Fees: *$720* •
Additional Nursing Fees: *$20*

SIMMONS COLLEGE

Address: 230 Airport Road, Boston, MA 02115
Phone: 617-521-2139
Fax: 617-521-3045
Contact: Judy A. Beal, RN, DNSc, Professor and Associate
Dean
Email: judy.beal@simmons.edu

GENERAL INFORMATION

Type of School: *4-Year College or University, Private
Independent* • Accreditation: *New England Association of
Schools and Colleges* • Total Enrollment: *4000*

PROGRAM INFORMATION

NLNAC Accreditation: *Yes* • CCNE Accreditation:

For specialty program listings, refer to the index.

NURSING STUDENT PROFILE

Total Nursing Enrollments: *103* • Full-Time Enrollment:
72 • Part-Time Enrollment: *31* • Female Enrollment: *101* •
Male Enrollment: *2* • Total Graduates: *23*

FINANCES

Residental Annual Tuition: *$15,912* • Non-Residential
Annual Tuition: *$15,912* • General Institutional Fees: *$60* •
Additional Nursing Fees: *$0*

UNIVERSITY OF MASSACHUSETTS—AMHERST

Address: 715 North Pleasant, Amherst, MA 01003
Phone: 413-545-5091
Fax: 413-577-2550
Contact: Jeanine Young-Mason, EdD, RN, CS, FAAN,
            Graduate Program Director
Email: youngmason@nursing.umass.edu

GENERAL INFORMATION

Type of School: *Not Provided* • Accreditation: *Not Provided* •
Total Enrollment: *Not Provided*

PROGRAM INFORMATION

NLNAC Accreditation: *Not Reported* • CCNE Accreditation:
No

———————

For specialty program listings, refer to the index.

NURSING STUDENT PROFILE

Total Nursing Enrollments: *55* • Full-Time Enrollment: *25* •
Part-Time Enrollment: *30* • Female Enrollment: *49* • Male
Enrollment: *6* • Total Graduates: *36*

FINANCES

Residental Annual Tuition: *$12,284* • Non-Residential
Annual Tuition: *$26,224* • General Institutional Fees:
$6,004 • Additional Nursing Fees: *Not Reported*

UNIVERSITY OF MASSACHUSETTS—BOSTON

Address: 100 Morrissy Blvd, Boston, MA 02125-3393
Phone: 617-287-7511
Fax: 617-287-7527
Contact: Brenda S. Cherry, PhD, RN, Dean
Email: brenda.cherry@umb.edu

GENERAL INFORMATION

Type of School: *4-Year College or University, Public* •
Accreditation: *New England Association of Schools and
Colleges* • Total Enrollment: *Not Provided*

PROGRAM INFORMATION

NLNAC Accreditation: *Yes* • CCNE Accreditation:
Provisional

———————

For specialty program listings, refer to the index.

NURSING STUDENT PROFILE

Total Nursing Enrollments: *125* • Full-Time Enrollment:
35 • Part-Time Enrollment: *90* • Female Enrollment: *117* •
Male Enrollment: *8* • Total Graduates: *40*

FINANCES

Residental Annual Tuition: *$2,590* • Non-Residential
Annual Tuition: *$9,758* • General Institutional Fees:
$3,230 • Additional Nursing Fees: *$140*

UNIVERSITY OF MASSACHUSETTS— DARTMOUTH

Address: 285 Old Westport Road, Dartmouth, MA 02757
Phone: 508-999-8505
Fax: 508-999-9127
Contact: Nancy Dluhy, PhD, RN, Director, Graduate
           Program
Email: mdluhy@umasse.edu

GENERAL INFORMATION

Type of School: *4-Year College or University, Public* •
Accreditation: *Not Provided* • Total Enrollment: *Not Provided*

PROGRAM INFORMATION

NLNAC Accreditation: *Yes* • CCNE Accreditation: *No*

_____

For specialty program listings, refer to the index.

NURSING STUDENT PROFILE

Total Nursing Enrollments: *74* • Full-Time Enrollment: *8* •
Part-Time Enrollment: *66* • Female Enrollment: *70* • Male
Enrollment: *4* • Total Graduates: *19*

FINANCES

Residental Annual Tuition: *$2,480* • Non-Residential
Annual Tuition: *$7,995* • General Institutional Fees:
$2,888 • Additional Nursing Fees: *$352*

UNIVERSITY OF MASSACHUSETTS—LOWELL

Address: 3 Solomon Way, Suite 2, Lowell, MA 01854-
           5126
Phone: 978-934-4467
Fax: 978-934-3006
Contact: May Futrell, PhD, FAAN, Professor and Chair,
           Department of Nursing
Email: May_Futrell@uml.edu

GENERAL INFORMATION

Type of School: *4-Year College or University, Public* •
Accreditation: *New England Association of Schools and
Colleges* • Total Enrollment: *Not Provided*

PROGRAM INFORMATION

NLNAC Accreditation: *Yes* • CCNE Accreditation: *No*

_____

For specialty program listings, refer to the index.

NURSING STUDENT PROFILE

Total Nursing Enrollments: *60* • Full-Time Enrollment: *21* •
Part-Time Enrollment: *39* • Female Enrollment: *Not
Provided* • Male Enrollment: *Not Provided* • Total Graduates:
17

FINANCES

Residental Annual Tuition: *$1,819* • Non-Residential
Annual Tuition: *$6,559* • General Institutional Fees:
$1,168 • Additional Nursing Fees: *Not Reported*

UNIVERSITY OF MASSACHUSETTS—WORCESTER

Address: 55 Lake Ave North, Worcester, MA 01655
Phone: 508-856-4185
Fax: Not Provided
Contact: Mary K. Alexander, EdD, RNCS, ANP, Associate Dean and Professor
Email: mary.alexander@umassmed.edu

GENERAL INFORMATION

Type of School: *4-Year College or University, Public* • Accreditation: *New England Association of Schools and Colleges* • Total Enrollment: *Not Provided*

PROGRAM INFORMATION

NLNAC Accreditation: *Yes* • CCNE Accreditation:

_____

For specialty program listings, refer to the index.

NURSING STUDENT PROFILE

Total Nursing Enrollments: *49* • Full-Time Enrollment: *28* • Part-Time Enrollment: *21* • Female Enrollment: *44* • Male Enrollment: *5* • Total Graduates: *32*

FINANCES

Residental Annual Tuition: *$1,254* • Non-Residential Annual Tuition: *$4,878* • General Institutional Fees: *Not Reported* • Additional Nursing Fees: *$998*

WORCESTER STATE COLLEGE

Address: 486 Chandler St, Worcester, MA 01602
Phone: 508-929-8129
Fax: 508-929-8168
Contact: Jean Campaniello, EdD, RN, Coordinator
Email: jcampaniello@worcester.edu

GENERAL INFORMATION

Type of School: *4-Year College or University, Public* • Accreditation: *New England Association of Schools and Colleges* • Total Enrollment: *Not Reported*

PROGRAM INFORMATION

NLNAC Accreditation: *Not Reported* • CCNE Accreditation: *No*

_____

For specialty program listings, refer to the index.

NURSING STUDENT PROFILE

Total Nursing Enrollments: *7* • Full-Time Enrollment: *0* • Part-Time Enrollment: *7* • Female Enrollment: *7* • Male Enrollment: *0* • Total Graduates: *Not Provided*

FINANCES

Residental Annual Tuition: *Not Reported* • Non-Residential Annual Tuition: *Not Reported* • General Institutional Fees: *Not Reported* • Additional Nursing Fees: *Not Reported*

ANDREWS UNIVERSITY

Address: Andrews University, Berrien Springs, MI 49104
Phone: 616-471-3578
Fax: Not Provided
Contact: Rilla Taylor, RN, Graduate Program Director
Email: rtaylor@andrews.edu

GENERAL INFORMATION

Type of School: *4-Year College or University, Private (Religious)* • Accreditation: *North Central Association of Colleges and Schools* • Total Enrollment: *3000*

PROGRAM INFORMATION

NLNAC Accreditation: *Yes* • CCNE Accreditation: *No*

For specialty program listings, refer to the index.

NURSING STUDENT PROFILE

Total Nursing Enrollments: *123* • Full-Time Enrollment: *0* • Part-Time Enrollment: *123* • Female Enrollment: *115* • Male Enrollment: *8* • Total Graduates: *37*

FINANCES

Residental Annual Tuition: *$6,000* • Non-Residential Annual Tuition: *$6,000* • General Institutional Fees: *$320* • Additional Nursing Fees: *$0*

EASTERN MICHIGAN UNIVERSITY

Address: 311 Marshall, Ypsilanti, MI 48197
Phone: 734-487-3274
Fax: Not Provided
Contact: Lorraine Wilson, PhD, RN, MSN Program
           Coordinator
Email: nur_wilson@emuvax.emich.edu

GENERAL INFORMATION

Type of School: *4-Year College or University, Private (Religious)* • Accreditation: *North Central Association of Colleges and Schools* • Total Enrollment: *1250*

PROGRAM INFORMATION

NLNAC Accreditation: *Yes* • CCNE Accreditation: *No*

For specialty program listings, refer to the index.

NURSING STUDENT PROFILE

Total Nursing Enrollments: *78* • Full-Time Enrollment: *0* • Part-Time Enrollment: *78* • Female Enrollment: *76* • Male Enrollment: *2* • Total Graduates: *4*

FINANCES

Residental Annual Tuition: *$2,682* • Non-Residential Annual Tuition: *$6,300* • General Institutional Fees: *$0* • Additional Nursing Fees: *$0*

GRAND VALLEY STATE UNIVERSITY

Address: 212 Henry Hall, Allendale, MI 49401
Phone: 616-336-7167
Fax: 616-336-7362
Contact: Jean Martin, RNC, DNSc, PNP, Director, Graduate Programs
Email: martinj@gvsu.edu

GENERAL INFORMATION

Type of School: *4-Year College or University, Public* • Accreditation: *North Central Association of Colleges and Schools* • Total Enrollment: *2000*

PROGRAM INFORMATION

NLNAC Accreditation: *Yes* • CCNE Accreditation: *No*

For specialty program listings, refer to the index.

NURSING STUDENT PROFILE

Total Nursing Enrollments: *133* • Full-Time Enrollment: *21* • Part-Time Enrollment: *112* • Female Enrollment: *126* • Male Enrollment: *7* • Total Graduates: *39*

FINANCES

Residental Annual Tuition: *$3,600* • Non-Residential Annual Tuition: *$7,740* • General Institutional Fees: *$0* • Additional Nursing Fees: *$0*

MADONNA UNIVERSITY

Address: 1467 Mount Vernon Avenue, Livonia, MI 48150
Phone: 731-432-5461
Fax: 734-432-5463
Contact: Mildred S. Braunstein, PhD, RN, Chair, Nursing Graduate Program
Email: mbraunstein@madonna.edu

GENERAL INFORMATION

Type of School: *4-Year College or University, Public* • Accreditation: *North Central Association of Colleges and Schools* • Total Enrollment: *3328*

PROGRAM INFORMATION

NLNAC Accreditation: *Yes* • CCNE Accreditation:

For specialty program listings, refer to the index.

NURSING STUDENT PROFILE

Total Nursing Enrollments: *50* • Full-Time Enrollment: *1* • Part-Time Enrollment: *49* • Female Enrollment: *50* • Male Enrollment: *0* • Total Graduates: *45*

FINANCES

Residental Annual Tuition: *$6,510* • Non-Residential Annual Tuition: *$6,150* • General Institutional Fees: *$100* • Additional Nursing Fees: *$315*

MICHIGAN STATE UNIVERSITY

Address: A230 Life Sciences Building, East Lansing, MI
             48824-1317
Phone: 517-355-6527
Fax: Not Provided
Contact: Marilyn Rothert, RN, Dean and Professor
Email: rothert@msu.edu

GENERAL INFORMATION

Type of School: *4-Year College or University, Public* •
Accreditation: *North Central Association of Colleges and
Schools* • Total Enrollment: *Not Provided*

PROGRAM INFORMATION

NLNAC Accreditation: *Yes* • CCNE Accreditation:

_____

For specialty program listings, refer to the index.

NURSING STUDENT PROFILE

Total Nursing Enrollments: *146* • Full-Time Enrollment:
30 • Part-Time Enrollment: *116* • Female Enrollment: *Not
Provided* • Male Enrollment: *Not Provided* • Total Graduates:
75

FINANCES

Residental Annual Tuition: *Not Reported* • Non-Residential
Annual Tuition: *Not Reported* • General Institutional Fees:
Not Reported • Additional Nursing Fees: *Not Reported*

NORTHERN MICHIGAN UNIVERSITY

Address: 709 Oklahoma Blvd, Marquette, MI 49855
Phone: 906-227-2834
Fax: 906-227-1658
Contact: Kerri D. Schuiling, RM, MSN, CNH, WHNP,
             Associate Director
Email: kschuilli@nmc.edu

GENERAL INFORMATION

Type of School: *4-Year College or University, Public* •
Accreditation: *North Central Association of Colleges and
Schools* • Total Enrollment: *12000*

PROGRAM INFORMATION

NLNAC Accreditation: *Yes* • CCNE Accreditation: *No*

_____

For specialty program listings, refer to the index.

NURSING STUDENT PROFILE

Total Nursing Enrollments: *54* • Full-Time Enrollment: *15* •
Part-Time Enrollment: *39* • Female Enrollment: *51* • Male
Enrollment: *3* • Total Graduates: *Not Provided*

FINANCES

Residental Annual Tuition: *Not Reported* • Non-Residential
Annual Tuition: *Not Reported* • General Institutional Fees:
Not Reported • Additional Nursing Fees: *Not Reported*

OAKLAND UNIVERSITY

Address: 2280 State Road 540, Rochester, MI 48309
Phone: 248-370-4081
Fax: 248-370-4279
Contact: Kathleen Emrich, EdD, RN, Interim Dean
Email: emrich@oakland.edu

GENERAL INFORMATION

Type of School: *4-Year College or University, Public* •
Accreditation: *North Central Association of Colleges and Schools* • Total Enrollment: *Not Provided*

PROGRAM INFORMATION

NLNAC Accreditation: *Yes* • CCNE Accreditation: *Provisional*

For specialty program listings, refer to the index.

NURSING STUDENT PROFILE

Total Nursing Enrollments: *120* • Full-Time Enrollment: *45* • Part-Time Enrollment: *75* • Female Enrollment: *104* • Male Enrollment: *16* • Total Graduates: *23*

FINANCES

Residental Annual Tuition: *$5,448* • Non-Residential Annual Tuition: *$11,738* • General Institutional Fees: *$430* • Additional Nursing Fees: *Not Reported*

SAGINAW VALLEY STATE UNIVERSITY

Address: PO Box 600, University Center, MI 48710
Phone: 517-790-4145
Fax: Not Provided
Contact: Cheryl E. Easley, PhD, RN, Dean
Email: ceasely@svsu.edu

GENERAL INFORMATION

Type of School: *Not Provided* • Accreditation: *Not Provided* • Total Enrollment: *23135*

PROGRAM INFORMATION

NLNAC Accreditation: *Yes* • CCNE Accreditation: *No*

For specialty program listings, refer to the index.

NURSING STUDENT PROFILE

Total Nursing Enrollments: *66* • Full-Time Enrollment: *8* • Part-Time Enrollment: *58* • Female Enrollment: *63* • Male Enrollment: *3* • Total Graduates: *12*

FINANCES

Residental Annual Tuition: *$3,804* • Non-Residential Annual Tuition: *$7,471* • General Institutional Fees: *Not Reported* • Additional Nursing Fees: *Not Reported*

UNIVERSITY OF DETROIT MERCY

Address: 1800 Lincoln Avenue, Detroit, MI 48219
Phone: 313-993-6132
Fax: 313-993-6273
Contact: Suzanne Mellon, PhD, RN, Dean, College of
          Health Professions and McAuley School of
          Nursing
Email: mellonsk@udmercy.edu

GENERAL INFORMATION

Type of School: *4-Year College or University, Private
(Independent)* • Accreditation: *North Central Association of
Colleges and Schools* • Total Enrollment: *16696*

PROGRAM INFORMATION

NLNAC Accreditation: *Yes* • CCNE Accreditation: *No*

———

For specialty program listings, refer to the index.

NURSING STUDENT PROFILE

Total Nursing Enrollments: *13* • Full-Time Enrollment: *3* •
Part-Time Enrollment: *10* • Female Enrollment: *13* • Male
Enrollment: *0* • Total Graduates: *0*

FINANCES

Residental Annual Tuition: *$8,325* • Non-Residential
Annual Tuition: *$8,325* • General Institutional Fees: *$400* •
Additional Nursing Fees: *$100*

UNIVERSITY OF MICHIGAN

Address: 400 N. Ingalls, Ann Arbor, MI 48502-1950
Phone: 734-764-7188
Fax: 734-647-1419
Contact: Carol Loveland-Cherry, PhD,RN, FAAN,
          Executive Associate Dean for Academic Affairs
          and Professor
Email: loveland@umich.edu

GENERAL INFORMATION

Type of School: *4-Year College or University, Public* •
Accreditation: *North Central Association of Colleges and
Schools* • Total Enrollment: *38103*

PROGRAM INFORMATION

NLNAC Accreditation: *Yes* • CCNE Accreditation:

———

For specialty program listings, refer to the index.

NURSING STUDENT PROFILE

Total Nursing Enrollments: *181* • Full-Time Enrollment:
72 • Part-Time Enrollment: *109* • Female Enrollment: *164* •
Male Enrollment: *17* • Total Graduates: *59*

FINANCES

Residental Annual Tuition: *$11,562* • Non-Residential
Annual Tuition: *$23,442* • General Institutional Fees: *$198* •
Additional Nursing Fees: *Not Reported*

BETHEL COLLEGE

Address: 3900 Bethel Drive, Saint Paul, MN 55112
Phone: 651-638-6298
Fax: 651-635-1965
Contact: Marjorie A Schaffer, PhD, RN, Professor and
            Director of Graduate Program
Email: m-schaffer@bethel.edu

GENERAL INFORMATION

Type of School: *4-Year College or University, Private (Religious)* • Accreditation: *North Central Association of Colleges and Schools* • Total Enrollment: *502*

PROGRAM INFORMATION

NLNAC Accreditation: *Not Reported* • CCNE Accreditation:

For specialty program listings, refer to the index.

NURSING STUDENT PROFILE

Total Nursing Enrollments: *38* • Full-Time Enrollment: *38* • Part-Time Enrollment: *0* • Female Enrollment: *37* • Male Enrollment: *1* • Total Graduates: *4*

FINANCES

Residental Annual Tuition: *$6,720* • Non-Residential Annual Tuition: *$6,720* • General Institutional Fees: *$60* • Additional Nursing Fees: *$320*

COLLEGE OF SAINT CATHERINE

Address: 2004 Randolph Avenue, Saint Paul, MN 55105
Phone: 651-690-6575
Fax: 651-690-6941
Contact: Ruth Brink, PhD, RN, MS, CPNP, Director,
            Master's Program
Email: brin0085@tc.umn.edu

GENERAL INFORMATION

Type of School: *4-Year College or University, Private (Religious)* • Accreditation: *North Central Association of Colleges and Schools* • Total Enrollment: *Not Provided*

PROGRAM INFORMATION

NLNAC Accreditation: *Yes* • CCNE Accreditation: *No*

For specialty program listings, refer to the index.

NURSING STUDENT PROFILE

Total Nursing Enrollments: *42* • Full-Time Enrollment: *42* • Part-Time Enrollment: *0* • Female Enrollment: *42* • Male Enrollment: *0* • Total Graduates: *24*

FINANCES

Residental Annual Tuition: *$495* • Non-Residential Annual Tuition: *Not Reported* • General Institutional Fees: *Not Reported* • Additional Nursing Fees: *$90*

COLLEGE OF SAINT SCHOLASTICA

Address: 1901 S. 72nd St., Duluth, MN 55811
Phone: 218-723-6452
Fax: 218-723-6472
Contact: Carleen Maynard, PhD, RN, Director, Graduate Program
Email: cmaynard@css.edu

GENERAL INFORMATION

Type of School: *4-Year College or University, Private (Religious)* • Accreditation: *North Central Association of Colleges and Schools* • Total Enrollment: *930*

PROGRAM INFORMATION

NLNAC Accreditation: *Yes* • CCNE Accreditation: *Provisional*

For specialty program listings, refer to the index.

NURSING STUDENT PROFILE

Total Nursing Enrollments: *49* • Full-Time Enrollment: *14* • Part-Time Enrollment: *35* • Female Enrollment: *45* • Male Enrollment: *4* • Total Graduates: *17*

FINANCES

Residental Annual Tuition: *$13,560* • Non-Residential Annual Tuition: *$13,560* • General Institutional Fees: *$0* • Additional Nursing Fees: *$100*

METROPOLITAN STATE UNIVERSITY

Address: 950 North West 20th Street, St. Paul, MN 55106
Phone: 651-772-7705
Fax: 651-772-6130
Contact: Marilyn Loen, PhD, RN, GNP, Executive Director
Email: marilyn.loen@metrostate.edu

GENERAL INFORMATION

Type of School: *4-Year College or University, Public* • Accreditation: *North Central Association of Colleges and Schools* • Total Enrollment: *5000*

PROGRAM INFORMATION

NLNAC Accreditation: *Not Reported* • CCNE Accreditation: *Yes*

For specialty program listings, refer to the index.

NURSING STUDENT PROFILE

Total Nursing Enrollments: *33* • Full-Time Enrollment: *15* • Part-Time Enrollment: *18* • Female Enrollment: *30* • Male Enrollment: *3* • Total Graduates: *2*

FINANCES

Residental Annual Tuition: *$2,352* • Non-Residential Annual Tuition: *$3,728* • General Institutional Fees: *$101* • Additional Nursing Fees: *$0*

MINNESOTA STATE UNIVERSITY—MANKATO

Address: 360 Wisink Hall, Mankato, MN 56001
Phone: 507-389-1317
Fax: 507-389-6516
Contact: Sharon P. Aadalen, PhD, RN, Graduate Program
            Director
Email: sharon.aadalen@mnsu.edu

GENERAL INFORMATION

Type of School: *4-Year College or University, Public* •
Accreditation: *North Central Association of Colleges and
Schools* • Total Enrollment: *Not Provided*

PROGRAM INFORMATION

NLNAC Accreditation: *Yes* • CCNE Accreditation:

For specialty program listings, refer to the index.

NURSING STUDENT PROFILE

Total Nursing Enrollments: *66* • Full-Time Enrollment: *36* •
Part-Time Enrollment: *30* • Female Enrollment: *63* • Male
Enrollment: *3* • Total Graduates: *11*

FINANCES

Residental Annual Tuition: *$2,364* • Non-Residential
Annual Tuition: *$3,736* • General Institutional Fees: *$480* •
Additional Nursing Fees: *Not Reported*

UNIVERSITY OF MINNESOTA—MINNEAPOLIS

Address: 5-140 WHD, 308 Harvard St SE, Minneapolis,
            MN 55455-0342
Phone: 612-624-5959
Fax: Not Provided
Contact: Sandra Edwardson, PhD, RN, Dean
Email: edwardso@mailbox.mail.umn.edu

GENERAL INFORMATION

Type of School: *4-Year College or University, Public* •
Accreditation: *North Central Association of Colleges and
Schools* • Total Enrollment: *38103*

PROGRAM INFORMATION

NLNAC Accreditation: *No* • CCNE Accreditation: *No*

For specialty program listings, refer to the index.

NURSING STUDENT PROFILE

Total Nursing Enrollments: *246* • Full-Time Enrollment:
142 • Part-Time Enrollment: *104* • Female Enrollment:
227 • Male Enrollment: *19* • Total Graduates: *117*

FINANCES

Residental Annual Tuition: *$5,040* • Non-Residential
Annual Tuition: *$9,900* • General Institutional Fees: *$477* •
Additional Nursing Fees: *Not Reported*

WINONA STATE UNIVERISTY

Address: Stark Hall, 175 West Mark Street, Winona, MN 55987
Phone: 507-285-7489
Fax: 507-292-5127
Contact: William McBreen, PhD, RN, Director, Master's Program in Nursing
Email: wmcbreen@winona.msus.edu

GENERAL INFORMATION

Type of School: *4-Year College or University, Public* • Accreditation: *North Central Association of Colleges and Schools* • Total Enrollment: *7500*

PROGRAM INFORMATION

NLNAC Accreditation: *Yes* • CCNE Accreditation:

_____

For specialty program listings, refer to the index.

NURSING STUDENT PROFILE

Total Nursing Enrollments: *90* • Full-Time Enrollment: *35* • Part-Time Enrollment: *55* • Female Enrollment: *87* • Male Enrollment: *3* • Total Graduates: *31*

FINANCES

Residental Annual Tuition: *$3,254* • Non-Residential Annual Tuition: *$5,140* • General Institutional Fees: *$224* • Additional Nursing Fees: *$85*

ALCORN STATE UNIVERSITY

Address: 15 Campus Drive, Natchez, MS 39096
Phone: 601-304-4303
Fax: 601-304-4398
Contact: Evelyn A. Stiner, PhD, FNP, Chairperson, Department of Graduate Nursing
Email: stiner@lorman.alcorn.edu

GENERAL INFORMATION

Type of School: *4-Year College or University, Public* • Accreditation: *Southern Association of Colleges and Schools* • Total Enrollment: *3109*

PROGRAM INFORMATION

NLNAC Accreditation: *Yes* • CCNE Accreditation: *No*

_____

For specialty program listings, refer to the index.

NURSING STUDENT PROFILE

Total Nursing Enrollments: *33* • Full-Time Enrollment: *11* • Part-Time Enrollment: *22* • Female Enrollment: *31* • Male Enrollment: *2* • Total Graduates: *10*

FINANCES

Residental Annual Tuition: *$3,018* • Non-Residential Annual Tuition: *$9,810* • General Institutional Fees: *$200* • Additional Nursing Fees: *$75*

DELTA STATE UNIVERSITY

Address: DSU Box 3343, Cleveland, MS 38733
Phone: 662-846-4255
Fax: 662-846-4267
Contact: Dana Lamar, EdD, RNC, Coordinator of
             Academic Programs
Email: dlamar@dsu.deltast.edu

GENERAL INFORMATION

Type of School: *4-Year College or University, Public* •
Accreditation: *Southern Association of Colleges and Schools* •
Total Enrollment: *3746*

PROGRAM INFORMATION

NLNAC Accreditation: *Yes* • CCNE Accreditation: *Yes*

For specialty program listings, refer to the index.

NURSING STUDENT PROFILE

Total Nursing Enrollments: *24* • Full-Time Enrollment: *20* •
Part-Time Enrollment: *4* • Female Enrollment: *24* • Male
Enrollment: *0* • Total Graduates: *19*

FINANCES

Residental Annual Tuition: *$3,100* • Non-Residential
Annual Tuition: *$3,100* • General Institutional Fees: *$0* •
Additional Nursing Fees: *$20*

UNIVERSITY OF MISSISSIPPI MEDICAL CENTER

Address: 2500 North State Street, Jackson, MS 39216
Phone: 601-984-6256
Fax: 601-815-5957
Contact: Ola Allen, RN, DNSc, Associate Dean for
             Academics
Email: oallen@son.umsmed.edu

GENERAL INFORMATION

Type of School: *4-Year College or University, Public* •
Accreditation: *Southern Association of Colleges and Schools* •
Total Enrollment: *6320*

PROGRAM INFORMATION

NLNAC Accreditation: *Yes* • CCNE Accreditation: *Yes*

For specialty program listings, refer to the index.

NURSING STUDENT PROFILE

Total Nursing Enrollments: *58* • Full-Time Enrollment: *45* •
Part-Time Enrollment: *13* • Female Enrollment: *53* • Male
Enrollment: *5* • Total Graduates: *34*

FINANCES

Residental Annual Tuition: *$2,378* • Non-Residential
Annual Tuition: *$5,197* • General Institutional Fees:
$1,286 • Additional Nursing Fees: *Not Reported*

UNIVERSITY OF SOUTHERN MISSISSIPPI

Address: PO Box 5095, Hattiesburg, MS 39406
Phone: 601-266-5639
Fax: 601-266-5927
Contact: Bonnie Lee Harbaugh, PhD, RN, Assistant Dean
           for Graduate Program
Email: Bonnie.Harbaugh@usm.edu

GENERAL INFORMATION

Type of School: *4-Year College or University, Public* •
Accreditation: *Southern Association of Colleges and Schools* •
Total Enrollment: *9600*

PROGRAM INFORMATION

NLNAC Accreditation: *Yes* • CCNE Accreditation:

_____

For specialty program listings, refer to the index.

NURSING STUDENT PROFILE

Total Nursing Enrollments: *104* • Full-Time Enrollment:
47 • Part-Time Enrollment: *57* • Female Enrollment: *99* •
Male Enrollment: *5* • Total Graduates: *43*

FINANCES

Residental Annual Tuition: *$2,870* • Non-Residential
Annual Tuition: *$4,239* • General Institutional Fees: *$50* •
Additional Nursing Fees: *$50*

GRACELAND UNIVERSITY

Address: 1401 West Truman Road, Independence, MO
           50140
Phone: 816-833-0524
Fax: 816-833-2990
Contact: Karen Fernengel, PhD, FNP, CS, Associate Dean
           of Nursing
Email: karenf@graceland.edu

GENERAL INFORMATION

Type of School: *4-Year College, Private (Religious)* •
Accreditation: *North Central Association of Colleges and
Schools* • Total Enrollment: *2283*

PROGRAM INFORMATION

NLNAC Accreditation: *Yes* • CCNE Accreditation: *Yes*

_____

For specialty program listings, refer to the index.

NURSING STUDENT PROFILE

Total Nursing Enrollments: *142* • Full-Time Enrollment:
16 • Part-Time Enrollment: *126* • Female Enrollment: *120* •
Male Enrollment: *22* • Total Graduates: *18*

FINANCES

Residental Annual Tuition: *$13,600* • Non-Residential
Annual Tuition: *13,600* • General Institutional Fees: *$0* •
Additional Nursing Fees: *$1,066*

JEWISH HOSPITAL

Address: 306 South Kings Highway Boulevard, St. Louis, MO 63110
Phone: 314-454-8416
Fax: 314-454-5239
Contact: Elizabeth A. Buck, PhD, RN, Academic Dean, Nursing Division
Email: eab1458@bjc.org

GENERAL INFORMATION

Type of School: *4-Year College or University, Public* •
Accreditation: *Not Provided* • Total Enrollment: *6540*

PROGRAM INFORMATION

NLNAC Accreditation: *Yes* • CCNE Accreditation: *Yes*

_____

For specialty program listings, refer to the index.

NURSING STUDENT PROFILE

Total Nursing Enrollments: *53* • Full-Time Enrollment: *18* •
Part-Time Enrollment: *35* • Female Enrollment: *48* • Male
Enrollment: *5* • Total Graduates: *16*

FINANCES

Residental Annual Tuition: *$4,320* • Non-Residential
Annual Tuition: *Not Reported* • General Institutional Fees:
$0 • Additional Nursing Fees: *Not Reported*

SAINT LOUIS UNIVERSITY

Address: 235 Marshall Ave, St Louis, MO 63104
Phone: 314-577-8970
Fax: 314-577-8949
Contact: Patsy L. Ruchala, RN, DNSc, Director, Master's Program
Email: ruchalapl@slv.edu

GENERAL INFORMATION

Type of School: *4-Year College, Private (Religious)* •
Accreditation: *North Central Assoication of Colleges* • Total
Enrollment: *11112*

PROGRAM INFORMATION

NLNAC Accreditation: *Yes* • CCNE Accreditation:
Provisional

_____

For specialty program listings, refer to the index.

NURSING STUDENT PROFILE

Total Nursing Enrollments: *155* • Full-Time Enrollment:
21 • Part-Time Enrollment: *134* • Female Enrollment: *140* •
Male Enrollment: *15* • Total Graduates: *46*

FINANCES

Residental Annual Tuition: *$14,400* • Non-Residential
Annual Tuition: *$14,400* • General Institutional Fees: *Not
Reported* • Additional Nursing Fees: *$480*

SOUTHEAST MISSOURI STATE UNIVERSITY

Address:　3575 College Rd, Cape Girardeau, MO 63701
Phone:　573-651-2871
Fax:　Not Provided
Contact:　Elaine Jackson, PhD, RN, Associate Professor and Director of Graduate Studies
Email:　ejackson@semorm.semo.edu

GENERAL INFORMATION

Type of School: *Not Reported or University, Public (Independent)* • Accreditation: *North Central Association of Colleges and Schools* • Total Enrollment: *7396*

PROGRAM INFORMATION

NLNAC Accreditation: *Yes* • CCNE Accreditation: *No*

For specialty program listings, refer to the index.

NURSING STUDENT PROFILE

Total Nursing Enrollments: *41* • Full-Time Enrollment: *15* • Part-Time Enrollment: *26* • Female Enrollment: *35* • Male Enrollment: *6* • Total Graduates: *17*

FINANCES

Residental Annual Tuition: *$2,003* • Non-Residential Annual Tuition: *$3,749* • General Institutional Fees: *$197* • Additional Nursing Fees: *Not Reported*

SOUTHWEST MISSOURI STATE UNIVERSITY— SPRINGFIELD

Address:　901 S National Ave, Springfield, MO 65804
Phone:　417-836-5310
Fax:　Not Provided
Contact:　Kathryn L. Hope, PhD, RN,CS,FNP, Head, Department of Nursing
Email:　Kathrynhope@mail.smsu.edu

GENERAL INFORMATION

Type of School: *Not Provided* • Accreditation: *Not Provided* • Total Enrollment: *Not Provided*

PROGRAM INFORMATION

NLNAC Accreditation: *Not Reported* • CCNE Accreditation: *No*

For specialty program listings, refer to the index.

NURSING STUDENT PROFILE

Total Nursing Enrollments: *28* • Full-Time Enrollment: *4* • Part-Time Enrollment: *24* • Female Enrollment: *22* • Male Enrollment: *6* • Total Graduates: *6*

FINANCES

Residental Annual Tuition: *$2,070* • Non-Residential Annual Tuition: *$4,140* • General Institutional Fees: *$370* • Additional Nursing Fees: *$0*

UNIVERSITY OF MISSOURI— COLUMBIA

Address: S218 Nursing School Bldg, Columbia, MO 65211
Phone: 573-882-0228
Fax: 573-884-4544
Contact: Roxanne McDaniel, PhD, RN, Director of Graduate Studies
Email: mcdanielr@missouri.edu

GENERAL INFORMATION

Type of School: *Not Provided* • Accreditation: *North Central Association of Colleges and Schools* • Total Enrollment: *1694*

PROGRAM INFORMATION

NLNAC Accreditation: *No* • CCNE Accreditation: *Provisional*

For specialty program listings, refer to the index.

NURSING STUDENT PROFILE

Total Nursing Enrollments: *107* • Full-Time Enrollment: *37* • Part-Time Enrollment: *70* • Female Enrollment: *100* • Male Enrollment: *7* • Total Graduates: *27*

FINANCES

Residental Annual Tuition: *$5,306* • Non-Residential Annual Tuition: *$8,048* • General Institutional Fees: *$460* • Additional Nursing Fees: *Not Reported*

UNIVERSITY OF MISSOURI— KANSAS CITY

Address: 1115 North Roberts Street, Kansas City, MO 64108
Phone: 816-235-5608
Fax: 816-235-1701
Contact: Claudia Beckmann, PhD, RN, Associate Professor
Email: beckmannc@umkc.edu

GENERAL INFORMATION

Type of School: *Not Provided* • Accreditation: *North Central Association of Colleges and Schools* • Total Enrollment: *Not Provided*

PROGRAM INFORMATION

NLNAC Accreditation: *Not Reported* • CCNE Accreditation: *Yes*

For specialty program listings, refer to the index.

NURSING STUDENT PROFILE

Total Nursing Enrollments: *218* • Full-Time Enrollment: *40* • Part-Time Enrollment: *178* • Female Enrollment: *211* • Male Enrollment: *7* • Total Graduates: *61*

FINANCES

Residental Annual Tuition: *$4,157* • Non-Residential Annual Tuition: *$12,504* • General Institutional Fees: *$30* • Additional Nursing Fees: *$113*

UNIVERSITY OF MISSOURI— ST. LOUIS

Address: 8001 Natural Bridge Road, St Louis, MO 63121
Phone: 314-516-6849
Fax: 314-516-6730
Contact: Peggy Ellis, PhD, RN, CS, MSN Program
            Director
Email: pellis@umsl.edu

GENERAL INFORMATION

Type of School: *4-Year College or University, Public* •
Accreditation: *North Central Association of Colleges and
Schools* • Total Enrollment: *Not Provided*

PROGRAM INFORMATION

NLNAC Accreditation: *Not Reported* • CCNE Accreditation:

_____

For specialty program listings, refer to the index.

NURSING STUDENT PROFILE

Total Nursing Enrollments: *221* • Full-Time Enrollment:
19 • Part-Time Enrollment: *202* • Female Enrollment: *213* •
Male Enrollment: *8* • Total Graduates: *69*

FINANCES

Residental Annual Tuition: *$4,152* • Non-Residential
Annual Tuition: *$12,504* • General Institutional Fees:
$2,688 • Additional Nursing Fees: *$0*

WEBSTER UNIVERSITY

Address: 470 E Lockwood, St Louis, MO 63119
Phone: 314-968-7176
Fax: 314-963-6101
Contact: Susan A. Heady, PhD, RN, MSN, Coordinator
Email: headysa@webster.edu

GENERAL INFORMATION

Type of School: *4-Year College or University, Public* •
Accreditation: *North Central Association of Colleges and
Schools* • Total Enrollment: *Not Provided*

PROGRAM INFORMATION

NLNAC Accreditation: *Not Reported* • CCNE Accreditation:

_____

For specialty program listings, refer to the index.

NURSING STUDENT PROFILE

Total Nursing Enrollments: *38* • Full-Time Enrollment: *0* •
Part-Time Enrollment: *38* • Female Enrollment: *37* • Male
Enrollment: *1* • Total Graduates: *10*

FINANCES

Residental Annual Tuition: *$9,192* • Non-Residential
Annual Tuition: *$9,192* • General Institutional Fees: *$0* •
Additional Nursing Fees: *$0*

MONTANA STATE UNIVERSITY—BOZEMAN

Address: MT
Phone: 406-994-3783
Fax: Not Provided
Contact: Gretchen McNeely, RNC, DNSc, Associate
Dean
Email: gmcneely@montana.edu

GENERAL INFORMATION

Type of School: *4-Year College or University, Public* •
Accreditation: *Northwestern Association of Schools and
Colleges* • Total Enrollment: *Not Provided*

PROGRAM INFORMATION

NLNAC Accreditation: *Not Reported* • CCNE Accreditation:
Yes

For specialty program listings, refer to the index.

NURSING STUDENT PROFILE

Total Nursing Enrollments: *28* • Full-Time Enrollment: *18* •
Part-Time Enrollment: *10* • Female Enrollment: *26* • Male
Enrollment: *2* • Total Graduates: *13*

FINANCES

Residental Annual Tuition: *$2,612* • Non-Residential
Annual Tuition: *$8,278* • General Institutional Fees:
$1,637 • Additional Nursing Fees: *$2,461*

CLARKSON COLLEGE

Address: 1550 Clarke St, Omaha, NE 68131
Phone: 402-552-3035
Fax: 402-552-6019
Contact: Mae Timmons, EdD, RN, MSN, Director,
Graduate Program
Email: timmons@clarksoncollege.edu

GENERAL INFORMATION

Type of School: *4-Year College or University, Private
(Independent)* • Accreditation: *North Central Association of
Colleges and Schools* • Total Enrollment: *1249*

PROGRAM INFORMATION

NLNAC Accreditation: *Yes* • CCNE Accreditation: *No*

For specialty program listings, refer to the index.

NURSING STUDENT PROFILE

Total Nursing Enrollments: *116* • Full-Time Enrollment: *6* •
Part-Time Enrollment: *110* • Female Enrollment: *107* • Male
Enrollment: *9* • Total Graduates: *28*

FINANCES

Residental Annual Tuition: *$8,016* • Non-Residential
Annual Tuition: *$8,016* • General Institutional Fees: *$668* •
Additional Nursing Fees: *Not Reported*

CREIGHTON UNIVERSITY

Address: 860 Thurston Road, Omaha, NE 68178
Phone: 402-280-2054
Fax: 402-280-2045
Contact: Eleanor Howell, PhD, RN, Associate Dean for Academic and Clinical Affairs
Email: howell@crreighton.edu

GENERAL INFORMATION

Type of School: *4-Year College or University, Public* • Accreditation: *Not Provided* • Total Enrollment: *Not Provided*

PROGRAM INFORMATION

NLNAC Accreditation: *Yes* • CCNE Accreditation: *No*

———

For specialty program listings, refer to the index.

NURSING STUDENT PROFILE

Total Nursing Enrollments: *74* • Full-Time Enrollment: *28* • Part-Time Enrollment: *46* • Female Enrollment: *71* • Male Enrollment: *3* • Total Graduates: *19*

FINANCES

Residental Annual Tuition: *$10,728* • Non-Residential Annual Tuition: *$10,728* • General Institutional Fees: *$283* • Additional Nursing Fees: *$7*

UNIVERSITY OF NEBRASKA MEDICAL CENTER

Address: 985330 Nebraska Medical Center, Omaha, NE 68198-5330
Phone: 402-559-7457
Fax: 402-559-6379
Contact: Margaret Wilson, PhD, BSN, MN, Associate Professor and Associate Dean
Email: mwilson@unmc.edu

GENERAL INFORMATION

Type of School: *4-Year College or University, Public* • Accreditation: *North Central Association of Colleges and Schools* • Total Enrollment: *Not Provided*

PROGRAM INFORMATION

NLNAC Accreditation: *Not Reported* • CCNE Accreditation: *Yes*

———

For specialty program listings, refer to the index.

NURSING STUDENT PROFILE

Total Nursing Enrollments: *223* • Full-Time Enrollment: *70* • Part-Time Enrollment: *153* • Female Enrollment: *213* • Male Enrollment: *10* • Total Graduates: *44*

FINANCES

Residental Annual Tuition: *$4,672* • Non-Residential Annual Tuition: *$12,288* • General Institutional Fees: *$366* • Additional Nursing Fees: *$200*

UNIVERSITY OF NEVADA—LAS VEGAS

Address: 4505 Maryland Pkwy, Las Vegas, NV 89154
Phone: 702-895-3360
Fax: 702-895-4807
Contact: Margaret Louis, PhD, RN, Coordinator, Graduate Program
Email: Not Provided

GENERAL INFORMATION

Type of School: *4-Year College or University, Public* • Accreditation: *North Central Association of Colleges and Schools* • Total Enrollment: *23000*

PROGRAM INFORMATION

NLNAC Accreditation: *Yes* • CCNE Accreditation:

_____

For specialty program listings, refer to the index.

NURSING STUDENT PROFILE

Total Nursing Enrollments: *36* • Full-Time Enrollment: *16* • Part-Time Enrollment: *20* • Female Enrollment: *33* • Male Enrollment: *3* • Total Graduates: *7*

FINANCES

Residental Annual Tuition: *$2,400* • Non-Residential Annual Tuition: *$2,400* • General Institutional Fees: *$70* • Additional Nursing Fees: *$50*

UNIVERSITY OF NEVADA—RENO

Address: 716 Stevens Avenue, Reno, NV 89507
Phone: 775-784-6841
Fax: 775-784-4262
Contact: Julie E. Johnson, PhD, RN, Director
Email: jej@unr.edu

GENERAL INFORMATION

Type of School: *4-Year College or University, Public* • Accreditation: *Northwestern Association of Schools and Colleges* • Total Enrollment: *2636*

PROGRAM INFORMATION

NLNAC Accreditation: *Yes* • CCNE Accreditation:

_____

For specialty program listings, refer to the index.

NURSING STUDENT PROFILE

Total Nursing Enrollments: *31* • Full-Time Enrollment: *23* • Part-Time Enrollment: *8* • Female Enrollment: *26* • Male Enrollment: *5* • Total Graduates: *9*

FINANCES

Residental Annual Tuition: *$2,400* • Non-Residential Annual Tuition: *$6,980* • General Institutional Fees: *Not Reported* • Additional Nursing Fees: *Not Reported*

RIVIER COLLEGE

Address: 1234 Columbus Avenue, Nashua, NH 03060-
            5086
Phone: 603-897-8529
Fax: Not Provided
Contact: Karen L. Baranowster, RN, DNSc, ANP, Chair,
            Baccalaureate and Master's Programs
Email: kbaranowster@rivier.edu

GENERAL INFORMATION

Type of School: *Other, Private (Independent)* • Accreditation:
Not Provided • Total Enrollment: *27406*

PROGRAM INFORMATION

NLNAC Accreditation: *Yes* • CCNE Accreditation: *No*

For specialty program listings, refer to the index.

NURSING STUDENT PROFILE

Total Nursing Enrollments: *54* • Full-Time Enrollment: *10* •
Part-Time Enrollment: *44* • Female Enrollment: *Not
Provided* • Male Enrollment: *Not Provided* • Total Graduates:
36

FINANCES

Residental Annual Tuition: *Not Reported* • Non-Residential
Annual Tuition: *Not Reported* • General Institutional Fees:
Not Reported • Additional Nursing Fees: *Not Reported*

UNIVERSITY OF NEW HAMPSHIRE

Address: Hewitt Hall, Durham, NH 03824
Phone: 603-862-2285
Fax: Not Provided
Contact: Gene Harkless, DNSc, ARNP, Associate
            Professor
Email: geh@christa.unh.edu

GENERAL INFORMATION

Type of School: *4-Year College or University, Private
(Independent)* • Accreditation: *New England Association of
Schools and Colleges* • Total Enrollment: *12000*

PROGRAM INFORMATION

NLNAC Accreditation: *No* • CCNE Accreditation: *No*

For specialty program listings, refer to the index.

NURSING STUDENT PROFILE

Total Nursing Enrollments: *51* • Full-Time Enrollment: *11* •
Part-Time Enrollment: *40* • Female Enrollment: *48* • Male
Enrollment: *3* • Total Graduates: *22*

FINANCES

Residental Annual Tuition: *$5,750* • Non-Residential
Annual Tuition: *$14,640* • General Institutional Fees: *$897* •
Additional Nursing Fees: *$445*

THE COLLEGE OF NEW JERSEY

Address: Pennington Road, Trenton, NJ 08628-0718
Phone: 609-771-2510
Fax: 609-637-5159
Contact: Claire Lindberg, PhD, RN, APN, C, Family
           Nurse Practitioner Program Coordinator
Email: lindberg@tcnj.edu

GENERAL INFORMATION

Type of School: *4-Year College or University, Public* •
Accreditation: *Middle States Association of Colleges and
Schools* • Total Enrollment: *7828*

PROGRAM INFORMATION

NLNAC Accreditation: *Yes* • CCNE Accreditation: *No*

For specialty program listings, refer to the index.

NURSING STUDENT PROFILE

Total Nursing Enrollments: *21* • Full-Time Enrollment: *0* •
Part-Time Enrollment: *21* • Female Enrollment: *18* • Male
Enrollment: *3* • Total Graduates: *2*

FINANCES

Residental Annual Tuition: *$5,776* • Non-Residential
Annual Tuition: *$8,086* • General Institutional Fees: *Not
Reported* • Additional Nursing Fees: *Not Reported*

FAIRLEIGH DICKINSON UNIVERSITY

Address: 1000 River Hall, Dickinson Hall Room 444,
           Teaneck, NJ 07666
Phone: 203-254-4000
Fax: Not Provided
Contact: Kathleen Wheeler, PhD, APRN, Associate
           Professor Director, Graduate Program
Email: kwheeler@fairl.fairfield.edu

GENERAL INFORMATION

Type of School: *Not Provided* • Accreditation: *Not Provided* •
Total Enrollment: *68*

PROGRAM INFORMATION

NLNAC Accreditation: *No* • CCNE Accreditation: *No*

For specialty program listings, refer to the index.

NURSING STUDENT PROFILE

Total Nursing Enrollments: *52* • Full-Time Enrollment: *16* •
Part-Time Enrollment: *36* • Female Enrollment: *51* • Male
Enrollment: *1* • Total Graduates: *7*

FINANCES

Residental Annual Tuition: *$6,570* • Non-Residential
Annual Tuition: *$6,570* • General Institutional Fees: *$25* •
Additional Nursing Fees: *$360*

FELICIAN COLLEGE

Address: 262 South Main Street, Lodi, NJ 07644
Phone: 201-559-6090
Fax: 201-559-6188
Contact: Margo M. Griffin, EdD, ANPC, Assoc. Prof.,
             Chairperson, Graduate Nursing
Email: griffinm@inet.felician.edu

GENERAL INFORMATION

Type of School: *Not Provided* • Accreditation: *Middle States Association of Colleges and Schools* • Total Enrollment: *1374*

PROGRAM INFORMATION

NLNAC Accreditation: *Not Reported* • CCNE Accreditation: *Provisional*

_____

For specialty program listings, refer to the index.

NURSING STUDENT PROFILE

Total Nursing Enrollments: *23* • Full-Time Enrollment: *17* • Part-Time Enrollment: *6* • Female Enrollment: *22* • Male Enrollment: *1* • Total Graduates: *12*

FINANCES

Residental Annual Tuition: *$9,600* • Non-Residential Annual Tuition: *$9,600* • General Institutional Fees: *$580* • Additional Nursing Fees: *$1,100*

KEAN UNIVERSITY

Address: 3331 Rt. 38 & Hartford Road, Mount Laurel,
             NJ 60621
Phone: 908-527-3147
Fax: Not Provided
Contact: Dula F. Pacquiao, EdD, RN, CTN, Associate
             Professor
Email: dulafp@aol.com

GENERAL INFORMATION

Type of School: *4-Year College or University, Public* • Accreditation: *Not Provided* • Total Enrollment: *2677*

PROGRAM INFORMATION

NLNAC Accreditation: *Yes* • CCNE Accreditation: *No*

_____

For specialty program listings, refer to the index.

NURSING STUDENT PROFILE

Total Nursing Enrollments: *66* • Full-Time Enrollment: *36* • Part-Time Enrollment: *30* • Female Enrollment: *64* • Male Enrollment: *2* • Total Graduates: *30*

FINANCES

Residental Annual Tuition: *Not Reported* • Non-Residential Annual Tuition: *$4,030* • General Institutional Fees: *$236* • Additional Nursing Fees: *Not Reported*

MONMOUTH UNIVERSITY

Address: PO Box 6010, 2100 16th Avenue South, West
             Long Branch, NJ 07764
Phone: 732-263-5271
Fax: 732-263-5131
Contact: Janet Mahoney, PhD, RN, CNS, CEN, CNA,
             Director of MSN Program
Email: jmahoney@monmouth.edu

GENERAL INFORMATION

Type of School: *4-Year College or University, Private
Independent* • Accreditation: *Middle States Association of
Colleges and Schools* • Total Enrollment: *5753*

PROGRAM INFORMATION

NLNAC Accreditation: *No* • CCNE Accreditation: *Yes*

─────────

For specialty program listings, refer to the index.

NURSING STUDENT PROFILE

Total Nursing Enrollments: *105* • Full-Time Enrollment:
13 • Part-Time Enrollment: *92* • Female Enrollment: *101* •
Male Enrollment: *4* • Total Graduates: *Not Provided*

FINANCES

Residental Annual Tuition: *$18,464* • Non-Residential
Annual Tuition: *$18,464* • General Institutional Fees: *$284* •
Additional Nursing Fees: *Not Reported*

NEW JERSEY CITY UNIVERSITY

Address: 5317 Lovington Highway, Jersey City, NJ 07305
Phone: 201-200-3157
Fax: 201-200-3141
Contact: Gloria Boseman, PhD,RN, MS, Associate
             Professor and Chairperson
Email: gboseman@njcu.edu

GENERAL INFORMATION

Type of School: *4-Year College or University, Public* •
Accreditation: *Middle States Association of Colleges and
Schools* • Total Enrollment: *Not Provided*

PROGRAM INFORMATION

NLNAC Accreditation: *Not Reported* • CCNE Accreditation:
No

─────────

For specialty program listings, refer to the index.

NURSING STUDENT PROFILE

Total Nursing Enrollments: *38* • Full-Time Enrollment: *0* •
Part-Time Enrollment: *38* • Female Enrollment: *36* • Male
Enrollment: *2* • Total Graduates: *4*

FINANCES

Residental Annual Tuition: *$5,592* • Non-Residential
Annual Tuition: *$9,744* • General Institutional Fees: *$40* •
Additional Nursing Fees: *Not Reported*

RICHARD STOCKTON COLLEGE OF NEW JERSEY

Address: 500 J Clyde Morris Boulevard, Pomona, NJ
           08240
Phone: 609-652-4496
Fax: 609-652-4858
Contact: Cheryle Fisher Eisele, EdD, RN, NPC,
           Coordinator
Email: ceisele@stockton.edu

GENERAL INFORMATION

Type of School: *4-Year College or University, Public* •
Accreditation: *Middle States Association of Colleges and
Schools* • Total Enrollment: *1100*

PROGRAM INFORMATION

NLNAC Accreditation: *Not Reported* • CCNE Accreditation:
No

————

For specialty program listings, refer to the index.

NURSING STUDENT PROFILE

Total Nursing Enrollments: *26* • Full-Time Enrollment: *0* •
Part-Time Enrollment: *26* • Female Enrollment: *26* • Male
Enrollment: *0* • Total Graduates: *6*

FINANCES

Residental Annual Tuition: *$5,928* • Non-Residential
Annual Tuition: *$8,280* • General Institutional Fees: *$74* •
Additional Nursing Fees: *$0*

RUTGERS—THE STATE UNIVERSITY OF NEW JERSEY

Address: 3835 Freeport Boulevard, Newark, NJ 07102
Phone: 973-353-5293
Fax: Not Provided
Contact: Joanne Stevenson, PhD, RN, Associate Dean for
           Academic Affairs and Research/Graduate
           Program Director
Email: Stevenson@nightingale.rutgers.edu

GENERAL INFORMATION

Type of School: *Not Provided* • Accreditation: *Not Provided* •
Total Enrollment: *1299*

PROGRAM INFORMATION

NLNAC Accreditation: *No* • CCNE Accreditation: *No*

————

For specialty program listings, refer to the index.

NURSING STUDENT PROFILE

Total Nursing Enrollments: *257* • Full-Time Enrollment:
17 • Part-Time Enrollment: *240* • Female Enrollment: *250* •
Male Enrollment: *7* • Total Graduates: *45*

FINANCES

Residental Annual Tuition: *$6,776* • Non-Residential
Annual Tuition: *$9,936* • General Institutional Fees: *$845* •
Additional Nursing Fees: *Not Reported*

SAINT PETER'S COLLEGE

Address: 2800 Main Street, Jersey City, NJ 07306-5997
Phone: 201-568-5208
Fax: 201-569-1254
Contact: Marylou Yam, PhD, RN, CS, Chairperson
Email: Yam_M@spcvxa.spc.edu

GENERAL INFORMATION

Type of School: *4-Year College or University, Private (Religious)* • Accreditation: *Middle States Association of Colleges and Schools* • Total Enrollment: *3300*

PROGRAM INFORMATION

NLNAC Accreditation: *Yes* • CCNE Accreditation: *Yes*

For specialty program listings, refer to the index.

NURSING STUDENT PROFILE

Total Nursing Enrollments: *37* • Full-Time Enrollment: *0* • Part-Time Enrollment: *37* • Female Enrollment: *36* • Male Enrollment: *1* • Total Graduates: *9*

FINANCES

Residental Annual Tuition: *$13,392* • Non-Residential Annual Tuition: *$13,392* • General Institutional Fees: *$225* • Additional Nursing Fees: *$578*

SETON HALL UNIVERSITY

Address: 9500 Old Greensboro Road, South Orange, NJ 07079
Phone: 973-761-9286
Fax: 973-761-9607
Contact: Leona Keinman, EdD, RN, Chairperson, Graduate Nursing Department and Associate Professor
Email: Kleinmle@shu.edu

GENERAL INFORMATION

Type of School: *4-Year College or University, Private (Independent)* • Accreditation: *Not Provided* • Total Enrollment: *1935*

PROGRAM INFORMATION

NLNAC Accreditation: *Yes* • CCNE Accreditation: *Yes*

For specialty program listings, refer to the index.

NURSING STUDENT PROFILE

Total Nursing Enrollments: *133* • Full-Time Enrollment: *48* • Part-Time Enrollment: *85* • Female Enrollment: *128* • Male Enrollment: *5* • Total Graduates: *32*

FINANCES

Residental Annual Tuition: *$20,768* • Non-Residential Annual Tuition: *$20,768* • General Institutional Fees: *$410* • Additional Nursing Fees: *Not Reported*

UNIVERSITY OF MEDICINE & DENTISTRY OF NEW JERSEY

Address: 102 Newport Hall, 610 Goodman Avenue,
           Newark, NJ 07107-3001
Phone: 973-972-7671
Fax: Not Provided
Contact: Anthony Forrester, PhD, RN, Professor and
           Assistant Dean (Acting)
Email: forreste@umdmj.edu

GENERAL INFORMATION

Type of School: *4-Year College or University, Public* •
Accreditation: *Middle States Association of Colleges and
Schools* • Total Enrollment: *Not Provided*

PROGRAM INFORMATION

NLNAC Accreditation: *Yes* • CCNE Accreditation: *No*

_____

For specialty program listings, refer to the index.

NURSING STUDENT PROFILE

Total Nursing Enrollments: *171* • Full-Time Enrollment:
33 • Part-Time Enrollment: *138* • Female Enrollment: *Not
Provided* • Male Enrollment: *Not Provided* • Total Graduates:
38

FINANCES

Residental Annual Tuition: *$4,860* • Non-Residential
Annual Tuition: *$6,876* • General Institutional Fees: *$500* •
Additional Nursing Fees: *$0*

WILLIAM PATERSON UNIVERSITY

Address: 300 Pomton Road, Wayne, NJ 07470-
Phone: 973-720-3495
Fax: 973-720-3517
Contact: Connie G. Bareford, PhD, RN, CS, Graduate
           Program Director
Email: barefordc@wpunj.edu

GENERAL INFORMATION

Type of School: *4-Year College or University, Public* •
Accreditation: *Middle States Association of Colleges and
Schools* • Total Enrollment: *1150*

PROGRAM INFORMATION

NLNAC Accreditation: *Not Reported* • CCNE Accreditation:
Yes

_____

For specialty program listings, refer to the index.

NURSING STUDENT PROFILE

Total Nursing Enrollments: *93* • Full-Time Enrollment: *0* •
Part-Time Enrollment: *93* • Female Enrollment: *90* • Male
Enrollment: *3* • Total Graduates: *15*

FINANCES

Residental Annual Tuition: *$6,672* • Non-Residential
Annual Tuition: *$9,456* • General Institutional Fees: *$30* •
Additional Nursing Fees: *$60*

NEW MEXICO STATE UNIVERSITY

Address: PO Box 30001/MSC 3185, Las Cruces, NM
            88003-8001
Phone: 505-646-3812
Fax: 505-646-2167
Contact: Wendell W. Oderkirk, PhD, RN, Interim
            Academic Department Head
Email: woderkir@nmsu.edu

GENERAL INFORMATION

Type of School: *4-Year College or University, Public* •
Accreditation: *North Central Association of Colleges and
Schools* • Total Enrollment: *9450*

PROGRAM INFORMATION

NLNAC Accreditation: *Yes* • CCNE Accreditation: *No*

For specialty program listings, refer to the index.

NURSING STUDENT PROFILE

Total Nursing Enrollments: *31* • Full-Time Enrollment: *8* •
Part-Time Enrollment: *23* • Female Enrollment: *24* • Male
Enrollment: *7* • Total Graduates: *8*

FINANCES

Residental Annual Tuition: *$2,994* • Non-Residential
Annual Tuition: *$9,402* • General Institutional Fees: *$0* •
Additional Nursing Fees: *$35*

UNIVERSITY OF NEW MEXICO

Address: P. O. Box 5054, Albuquerque, NM 87131
Phone: 505-272-6284
Fax: 505-272-3970
Contact: Sandra L. Ferketich, PhD, RN, FAAN, Dean and
            Professor
Email: sferketich@salud.unm.edu

GENERAL INFORMATION

Type of School: *Not Provided* • Accreditation: *Not Provided* •
Total Enrollment: *3887*

PROGRAM INFORMATION

NLNAC Accreditation: *Yes* • CCNE Accreditation:
Provisional

For specialty program listings, refer to the index.

NURSING STUDENT PROFILE

Total Nursing Enrollments: *85* • Full-Time Enrollment: *41* •
Part-Time Enrollment: *44* • Female Enrollment: *78* • Male
Enrollment: *7* • Total Graduates: *51*

FINANCES

Residental Annual Tuition: *$3,341* • Non-Residential
Annual Tuition: *$11,777* • General Institutional Fees: *$40* •
Additional Nursing Fees: *$150*

ADELPHI UNIVERSITY

Address: 1 South Ave., Garden City, NY 11530
Phone: 516-877-4564
Fax: 516-877-4558
Contact: Veronica Conners, PhD, EdD, RN, Associate
           Dean for Graduate and Research Programs
Email: conners@adelphi.edu

GENERAL INFORMATION

Type of School: *4-Year College or University, Private (Independent)* • Accreditation: *Middle States Association of Colleges and Schools* • Total Enrollment: *6500*

PROGRAM INFORMATION

NLNAC Accreditation: *Yes* • CCNE Accreditation:

―――――――

For specialty program listings, refer to the index.

NURSING STUDENT PROFILE

Total Nursing Enrollments: *123* • Full-Time Enrollment: *0* • Part-Time Enrollment: *123* • Female Enrollment: *116* • Male Enrollment: *7* • Total Graduates: *21*

FINANCES

Residental Annual Tuition: *$18,000* • Non-Residential Annual Tuition: *$18,000* • General Institutional Fees: *$0* • Additional Nursing Fees: *$7*

COLLEGE OF MOUNT ST. VINCENT

Address: 6301 Riverdale Avenue, Bronx, NY 10471-1093
Phone: 718-405-3355
Fax: Not Provided
Contact: Kem Louie, PhD, RN, CS, FAAN, Chairperson
Email: klouie@cmsv.edu

GENERAL INFORMATION

Type of School: *4-Year College or University, Private (Religious)* • Accreditation: *Middle States Association of Colleges and Schools* • Total Enrollment: *2300*

PROGRAM INFORMATION

NLNAC Accreditation: *Not Reported* • CCNE Accreditation: *Yes*

―――――――

For specialty program listings, refer to the index.

NURSING STUDENT PROFILE

Total Nursing Enrollments: *112* • Full-Time Enrollment: *6* • Part-Time Enrollment: *106* • Female Enrollment: *106* • Male Enrollment: *6* • Total Graduates: *16*

FINANCES

Residental Annual Tuition: *$11,520* • Non-Residential Annual Tuition: *$11,520* • General Institutional Fees: *Not Reported* • Additional Nursing Fees: *Not Reported*

COLLEGE OF NEW ROCHELLE

Address: P.O. Box 7718, New Rochelle, NY 10805
Phone: 914-654-5813
Fax: Not Provided
Contact: Barbara Joyce, PhD, RN, Chairperson, Graduate Nursing Program
Email: bjoyce@cnr.edu

GENERAL INFORMATION

Type of School: *4-Year College or University, Public* • Accreditation: *Middle States Association of Colleges and Schools* • Total Enrollment: *6500*

PROGRAM INFORMATION

NLNAC Accreditation: *Not Reported* • CCNE Accreditation: *No*

_____

For specialty program listings, refer to the index.

NURSING STUDENT PROFILE

Total Nursing Enrollments: *66* • Full-Time Enrollment: *1* • Part-Time Enrollment: *65* • Female Enrollment: *Not Provided* • Male Enrollment: *Not Provided* • Total Graduates: *25*

FINANCES

Residental Annual Tuition: *Not Reported* • Non-Residential Annual Tuition: *Not Reported* • General Institutional Fees: *Not Reported* • Additional Nursing Fees: *Not Reported*

COLUMBIA UNIVERSITY

Address: 617 West 168th Street, New York, NY 10032
Phone: 212-305-3582
Fax: 212-305-1116
Contact: Sarah Sheets Cook, MEd, Vice Dean
Email: ssc3@columbia.edu

GENERAL INFORMATION

Type of School: *4-Year College or University, Private (Religious)* • Accreditation: *None* • Total Enrollment: *19000*

PROGRAM INFORMATION

NLNAC Accreditation: *Yes* • CCNE Accreditation:

_____

For specialty program listings, refer to the index.

NURSING STUDENT PROFILE

Total Nursing Enrollments: *323* • Full-Time Enrollment: *120* • Part-Time Enrollment: *203* • Female Enrollment: *288* • Male Enrollment: *35* • Total Graduates: *136*

FINANCES

Residental Annual Tuition: *$18,384* • Non-Residential Annual Tuition: *$18,384* • General Institutional Fees: *$1,478* • Additional Nursing Fees: *$100*

DAEMEN COLLEGE

Address: 4380 Main Street, Amherst, NY 14226
Phone: 716-839-8387
Fax: 716-839-8516
Contact: Mary Lou Rusin, EdD, RN, Professor and Chair
Email: mrusin@daemen.edu

GENERAL INFORMATION

Type of School: *4-Year College or University, Private Independent* • Accreditation: *Middle States Association of Colleges and Schools* • Total Enrollment: *2000*

PROGRAM INFORMATION

NLNAC Accreditation: *Yes* • CCNE Accreditation: *No*

For specialty program listings, refer to the index.

NURSING STUDENT PROFILE

Total Nursing Enrollments: *39* • Full-Time Enrollment: *6* • Part-Time Enrollment: *33* • Female Enrollment: *38* • Male Enrollment: *1* • Total Graduates: *10*

FINANCES

Residental Annual Tuition: *$11,520* • Non-Residential Annual Tuition: *$11,520* • General Institutional Fees: *$336* • Additional Nursing Fees: *$50*

D'YOUVILLE COLLEGE

Address: 320 Porter Ave., Buffalo, NY 14201
Phone: 716-881-3200
Fax: 716-881-8159
Contact: Verna Kieffer, RN, DNS, Chair
Email: kiefferv@dyc.edu

GENERAL INFORMATION

Type of School: *4-Year College or University, Private Independent* • Accreditation: *Middle States Association of Colleges and Schools* • Total Enrollment: *15000*

PROGRAM INFORMATION

NLNAC Accreditation: *Yes* • CCNE Accreditation:

For specialty program listings, refer to the index.

NURSING STUDENT PROFILE

Total Nursing Enrollments: *174* • Full-Time Enrollment: *32* • Part-Time Enrollment: *142* • Female Enrollment: *160* • Male Enrollment: *14* • Total Graduates: *33*

FINANCES

Residental Annual Tuition: *$7,749* • Non-Residential Annual Tuition: *$7,749* • General Institutional Fees: *$200* • Additional Nursing Fees: *$60*

Circle 41 on reader card   See in-depth profile for more information

EXCELSIOR COLLEGE

Address: 7 Columbia Circle, Albany, NY 12203
Phone: 518-464-8728
Fax: 518-464-8777
Contact: Deborah Sopczyk, RN, MS, Director of MSN
Program
Email: dsopczyk@excelsior.edu

GENERAL INFORMATION

Type of School: *4-Year College or University, Private Independent* • Accreditation: *Middle States Association of Colleges and Schools* • Total Enrollment: *17250*

PROGRAM INFORMATION

NLNAC Accreditation: *No* • CCNE Accreditation: *No*

For specialty program listings, refer to the index.

NURSING STUDENT PROFILE

Total Nursing Enrollments: *88* • Full-Time Enrollment: *7* • Part-Time Enrollment: *81* • Female Enrollment: *81* • Male Enrollment: *7* • Total Graduates: *0*

FINANCES

Residental Annual Tuition: *$7,200* • Non-Residential Annual Tuition: *$7,200* • General Institutional Fees: *$150* • Additional Nursing Fees: *Not Reported*

HERBERT H. LEHMAN COLLEGE

Address: 250 Bedford Park Blvd. West, Bronx, NY 38901
Phone: 718-960-8794
Fax: Not Provided
Contact: Ngozi Nkonglo, RN, Chairperson
Email: Not Provided

GENERAL INFORMATION

Type of School: *4-Year College or University, Public* • Accreditation: *Middle States Association of Colleges and Schools* • Total Enrollment: *Not Provided*

PROGRAM INFORMATION

NLNAC Accreditation: *Yes* • CCNE Accreditation: *No*

For specialty program listings, refer to the index.

NURSING STUDENT PROFILE

Total Nursing Enrollments: *Not Provided* • Full-Time Enrollment: *Not Provided* • Part-Time Enrollment: *Not Provided* • Female Enrollment: *Not Provided* • Male Enrollment: *Not Provided* • Total Graduates: *Not Provided*

FINANCES

Residental Annual Tuition: *Not Reported* • Non-Residential Annual Tuition: *Not Reported* • General Institutional Fees: *Not Reported* • Additional Nursing Fees: *Not Reported*

LONG ISLAND UNIVERSITY

Address: CW Post Campus of LIU, Brookville, NY 11548
Phone: 516-299-4158
Fax: 516-299-2352
Contact: Loretta Knapp, PhD, RN, Chairperson
Email: lknapp@lui.edu

GENERAL INFORMATION

Type of School: *4-Year College or University, Private (Independent)* • Accreditation: *Not Provided* • Total Enrollment: *27000*

PROGRAM INFORMATION

NLNAC Accreditation: *Yes* • CCNE Accreditation: *No*

_____

For specialty program listings, refer to the index.

NURSING STUDENT PROFILE

Total Nursing Enrollments: *80* • Full-Time Enrollment: *0* • Part-Time Enrollment: *80* • Female Enrollment: *68* • Male Enrollment: *12* • Total Graduates: *9*

FINANCES

Residental Annual Tuition: *$11,520* • Non-Residential Annual Tuition: *$11,520* • General Institutional Fees: *Not Reported* • Additional Nursing Fees: *Not Reported*

LONG ISLAND UNIVERSITY—BROOKLYN

Address: PO Box 878, Brooklyn, NY 11201
Phone: 718-624-2285
Fax: Not Provided
Contact: Dawn F. Kits, MA, CEN, CANP, Director
Email: cpk1217@aol.com

GENERAL INFORMATION

Type of School: *4-Year College or University, Private (Independent)* • Accreditation: *Middle States Association of Colleges and Schools* • Total Enrollment: *29774*

PROGRAM INFORMATION

NLNAC Accreditation: *Not Reported* • CCNE Accreditation: *No*

_____

For specialty program listings, refer to the index.

NURSING STUDENT PROFILE

Total Nursing Enrollments: *90* • Full-Time Enrollment: *6* • Part-Time Enrollment: *84* • Female Enrollment: *85* • Male Enrollment: *5* • Total Graduates: *14*

FINANCES

Residental Annual Tuition: *$9,090* • Non-Residential Annual Tuition: *$9,090* • General Institutional Fees: *$400* • Additional Nursing Fees: *Not Reported*

MOUNT SAINT MARY COLLEGE

Address: 330 Powell Ave., Newburgh, NY 12550
Phone: 845-569-3138
Fax: Not Provided
Contact: Leona Deboer, PhD, RN, Graduate Program Coordinator and Professor
Email: deboer@msmc.edu

GENERAL INFORMATION

Type of School: *Independent, Private Independent* • Accreditation: *Middle States Association of Colleges and Schools* • Total Enrollment: *2221*

PROGRAM INFORMATION

NLNAC Accreditation: *No* • CCNE Accreditation: *Yes*

_____

For specialty program listings, refer to the index.

NURSING STUDENT PROFILE

Total Nursing Enrollments: *25* • Full-Time Enrollment: *3* • Part-Time Enrollment: *22* • Female Enrollment: *23* • Male Enrollment: *2* • Total Graduates: *1*

FINANCES

Residental Annual Tuition: *$7,002* • Non-Residential Annual Tuition: *$7,002* • General Institutional Fees: *$40* • Additional Nursing Fees: *$25*

NEW YORK UNIVERSITY

Address: PO Box 799, New York, NY 10003-6677
Phone: 212-998-9020
Fax: 212-995-4679
Contact: Judith Haber, PhD, APRN, CS, FAAN, Professor and Director, MA and Post-MA Program
Email: jh33@nyu.edu

GENERAL INFORMATION

Type of School: *4-Year College, Private (Independent)* • Accreditation: *Middle State Association of Colleges* • Total Enrollment: *Not Reported*

PROGRAM INFORMATION

NLNAC Accreditation: *Yes* • CCNE Accreditation:

_____

For specialty program listings, refer to the index.

NURSING STUDENT PROFILE

Total Nursing Enrollments: *500* • Full-Time Enrollment: *23* • Part-Time Enrollment: *477* • Female Enrollment: *468* • Male Enrollment: *32* • Total Graduates: *74*

FINANCES

Residental Annual Tuition: *$17,640* • Non-Residential Annual Tuition: *$17,640* • General Institutional Fees: *$1,224* • Additional Nursing Fees: *$0*

NIAGARA UNIVERSITY

Address: 1617 East Ball Road, Niagara, NY 14109-2203
Phone: 716-286-8310
Fax: 716-586-8308
Contact: Joan Dulce Dunn, RN, DNS, SNP, Director, Graduate Nursing
Email: joandd@niagara.edu

GENERAL INFORMATION

Type of School: *4-Year College or University, Private (Religious)* • Accreditation: *Middle States Association of Colleges and Schools* • Total Enrollment: *3000*

PROGRAM INFORMATION

NLNAC Accreditation: *Yes* • CCNE Accreditation:

For specialty program listings, refer to the index.

NURSING STUDENT PROFILE

Total Nursing Enrollments: *14* • Full-Time Enrollment: *12* • Part-Time Enrollment: *2* • Female Enrollment: *12* • Male Enrollment: *2* • Total Graduates: *8*

FINANCES

Residental Annual Tuition: *$14,820* • Non-Residential Annual Tuition: *Not Reported* • General Institutional Fees: *$35* • Additional Nursing Fees: *$50*

PACE UNIVERSITY

Address: 3160 Redhill Avenue, Pleasantville, NY 10570
Phone: 914-773-3553
Fax: 914-773-3345
Contact: Karen Anderson Keith, PhD, RN, FNP, Chairperson, Department of Graduate Studies
Email: kkeith@pace.edu

GENERAL INFORMATION

Type of School: *4-Year College or University, Private Independent* • Accreditation: *Middle States Association of Colleges and Schools* • Total Enrollment: *13000*

PROGRAM INFORMATION

NLNAC Accreditation: *Not Reported* • CCNE Accreditation: *Yes*

For specialty program listings, refer to the index.

NURSING STUDENT PROFILE

Total Nursing Enrollments: *181* • Full-Time Enrollment: *45* • Part-Time Enrollment: *136* • Female Enrollment: *170* • Male Enrollment: *11* • Total Graduates: *65*

FINANCES

Residental Annual Tuition: *Not Reported* • Non-Residential Annual Tuition: *Not Reported* • General Institutional Fees: *Not Reported* • Additional Nursing Fees: *Not Reported*

SAINT JOHN FISHER COLLEGE

Address: 245 Clinton Ave., Rochester, NY 11205
Phone: 716-385-8472
Fax: Not Provided
Contact: Patricia Lindley, PhD, RN, FNP, Chairperson
Email: lindley@sjfc.edu

GENERAL INFORMATION

Type of School: *4-Year College or University, Private (Independent)* • Accreditation: *Middle States Association of Colleges and Schools* • Total Enrollment: *2175*

PROGRAM INFORMATION

NLNAC Accreditation: *Yes* • CCNE Accreditation: *No*

_____

For specialty program listings, refer to the index.

NURSING STUDENT PROFILE

Total Nursing Enrollments: *84* • Full-Time Enrollment: *83* • Part-Time Enrollment: *1* • Female Enrollment: *78* • Male Enrollment: *6* • Total Graduates: *33*

FINANCES

Residental Annual Tuition: *$7,560* • Non-Residential Annual Tuition: *Not Reported* • General Institutional Fees: *$610* • Additional Nursing Fees: *$0*

STATE UNIVERSITY OF NEW YORK—BUFFALO

Address: 1040 Kimball Tower, 3435 Man Street, Buffalo, NY 12901
Phone: 716-829-2533
Fax: 716-829-2566
Contact: Karen J. Radke, PhD, RN, Associate Dean for Academic Affairs
Email: radke@buffalo.edu

GENERAL INFORMATION

Type of School: *Other* • Accreditation: *Middle States Association of Colleges and Schools* • Total Enrollment: *1483*

PROGRAM INFORMATION

NLNAC Accreditation: *Not Reported* • CCNE Accreditation: *Yes*

_____

For specialty program listings, refer to the index.

NURSING STUDENT PROFILE

Total Nursing Enrollments: *125* • Full-Time Enrollment: *72* • Part-Time Enrollment: *53* • Female Enrollment: *115* • Male Enrollment: *10* • Total Graduates: *66*

FINANCES

Residental Annual Tuition: *$5,100* • Non-Residential Annual Tuition: *$8,416* • General Institutional Fees: *$870* • Additional Nursing Fees: *Not Reported*

STATE UNIVERSITY OF NEW YORK—STONY BROOK

Address: Health Care Center, Level 2, Rm 235, Stony Brook, NY 11794
Phone: 631-444-3260
Fax: 631-444-3136
Contact: Lenora J. McClean, EdD, RN, Dean and Chief Nursing Officer
Email: Lenora.McClean@sunysb.edu

GENERAL INFORMATION

Type of School: *4-Year College or University, Public* • Accreditation: *Middle States Association of Colleges and Schools* • Total Enrollment: *5000*

PROGRAM INFORMATION

NLNAC Accreditation: *Yes* • CCNE Accreditation: *No*

—————
For specialty program listings, refer to the index.

NURSING STUDENT PROFILE

Total Nursing Enrollments: *528* • Full-Time Enrollment: *58* • Part-Time Enrollment: *470* • Female Enrollment: *486* • Male Enrollment: *42* • Total Graduates: *185*

FINANCES

Residental Annual Tuition: *$5,100* • Non-Residential Annual Tuition: *$8,416* • General Institutional Fees: *$240* • Additional Nursing Fees: *$236*

STATE UNIVERSITY OF NEW YORK—SYRACUSE

Address: 750 East Adams St., Syracuse, NY 12540
Phone: 315-464-4277
Fax: Not Provided
Contact: Elvira Szigeti, PhD, RN, Dean and Chair, Graduate Nursing
Email: szigetie@mail.upstate.edu

GENERAL INFORMATION

Type of School: *4-Year College or University, Public* • Accreditation: *Middle States Association of Colleges and Schools* • Total Enrollment: *6000*

PROGRAM INFORMATION

NLNAC Accreditation: *Yes* • CCNE Accreditation: *No*

—————
For specialty program listings, refer to the index.

NURSING STUDENT PROFILE

Total Nursing Enrollments: *79* • Full-Time Enrollment: *20* • Part-Time Enrollment: *59* • Female Enrollment: *77* • Male Enrollment: *2* • Total Graduates: *38*

FINANCES

Residental Annual Tuition: *$5,100* • Non-Residential Annual Tuition: *$8,416* • General Institutional Fees: *$210* • Additional Nursing Fees: *Not Reported*

STATE UNIVERSITY OF NEW YORK—UTICA/ROME

Address: 1250 East Cooley Drive, Utica, NY 13504-3050
Phone: 315-792-7295
Fax: 315-792-7555
Contact: Jeannine D. Muldoon, PhD, RN, Dean and Professor
Email: muldooj@sunyit.edu

GENERAL INFORMATION

Type of School: *Other* • Accreditation: *Not Provided* • Total Enrollment: *19929*

PROGRAM INFORMATION

NLNAC Accreditation: *Yes* • CCNE Accreditation: *Provisional*

For specialty program listings, refer to the index.

NURSING STUDENT PROFILE

Total Nursing Enrollments: *48* • Full-Time Enrollment: *9* • Part-Time Enrollment: *39* • Female Enrollment: *46* • Male Enrollment: *2* • Total Graduates: *15*

FINANCES

Residental Annual Tuition: *$5,100* • Non-Residential Annual Tuition: *$8,416* • General Institutional Fees: *$515* • Additional Nursing Fees: *Not Reported*

SUNY HEALTH SCIENCE CENTER—BROOKLYN

Address: 450 Clarkson Ave., Box 22, Brooklyn, NY 13202
Phone: 718-270-7605
Fax: Not Provided
Contact: Laila N. Sedhom, PhD, RN, Professor and Associate Dean
Email: LSedhom@netmail.hscbklyn.edu

GENERAL INFORMATION

Type of School: *Not Provided* • Accreditation: *Not Provided* • Total Enrollment: *22*

PROGRAM INFORMATION

NLNAC Accreditation: *Yes* • CCNE Accreditation: *Yes*

For specialty program listings, refer to the index.

NURSING STUDENT PROFILE

Total Nursing Enrollments: *186* • Full-Time Enrollment: *63* • Part-Time Enrollment: *123* • Female Enrollment: *157* • Male Enrollment: *29* • Total Graduates: *37*

FINANCES

Residental Annual Tuition: *$6,618* • Non-Residential Annual Tuition: *$8,461* • General Institutional Fees: *$108* • Additional Nursing Fees: *$685*

SYRACUSE UNIVERSITY

Address: 426 Ostrom Avenue, Syracuse, NY 13210
Phone: 315-443-2141
Fax: 315-443-2164
Contact: Cecilia F. Mulvey, PhD, RN, Interim Dean
Email: cfmulvey@nursing.syr.edu

GENERAL INFORMATION

Type of School: *4-Year College or University, Public* •
Accreditation: *Middle States Association of Colleges and Schools* • Total Enrollment: *Not Provided*

PROGRAM INFORMATION

NLNAC Accreditation: *Yes* • CCNE Accreditation: *No*

For specialty program listings, refer to the index.

NURSING STUDENT PROFILE

Total Nursing Enrollments: *81* • Full-Time Enrollment: *27* • Part-Time Enrollment: *54* • Female Enrollment: *78* • Male Enrollment: *3* • Total Graduates: *42*

FINANCES

Residental Annual Tuition: *$12,992* • Non-Residential Annual Tuition: *$13,992* • General Institutional Fees: *$390* • Additional Nursing Fees: *$110*

UNIVERSITY OF ROCHESTER

Address: 601 Elmwood Ave., Box SON, Rochester, NY 14642
Phone: 585-275-5713
Fax: 585-756-8299
Contact: Charlotte Torres, EdD, RN, CS, Director, Master's Program
Email: Charlotte_Torres@urmc.rochester.edu

GENERAL INFORMATION

Type of School: *4-Year University, Private Independent* •
Accreditation: *Middle State* • Total Enrollment: *8201*

PROGRAM INFORMATION

NLNAC Accreditation: *Yes* • CCNE Accreditation: *No*

For specialty program listings, refer to the index.

NURSING STUDENT PROFILE

Total Nursing Enrollments: *102* • Full-Time Enrollment: *26* • Part-Time Enrollment: *76* • Female Enrollment: *92* • Male Enrollment: *10* • Total Graduates: *49*

FINANCES

Residental Annual Tuition: *$18,120* • Non-Residential Annual Tuition: *$18,120* • General Institutional Fees: *$429* • Additional Nursing Fees: *$75*

DUKE UNIVERSITY

Address: 2507 University Ave, Durham, NC 27710
Phone: 919-684-3786
Fax: Not Provided
Contact: Mary T. Champagne, PhD, Dean
Email: Champ001@mc.duke.edu

GENERAL INFORMATION

Type of School: *4-Year College or University, Private (Independent)* • Accreditation: *Southern Association of Colleges and Schools* • Total Enrollment: *11535*

PROGRAM INFORMATION

NLNAC Accreditation: *Yes* • CCNE Accreditation: *Yes*

_____

For specialty program listings, refer to the index.

NURSING STUDENT PROFILE

Total Nursing Enrollments: *246* • Full-Time Enrollment: *63* • Part-Time Enrollment: *183* • Female Enrollment: *230* • Male Enrollment: *16* • Total Graduates: *80*

FINANCES

Residental Annual Tuition: *$20,664* • Non-Residential Annual Tuition: *$20,664* • General Institutional Fees: *$134* • Additional Nursing Fees: *$173*

EAST CAROLINA UNIVERSITY

Address: East 5th Street, Greenville, NC 27858
Phone: 252-328-4302
Fax: 252-328-4300
Contact: Judy Hayes Bernhardt, PhD, RN, Interim Associate Dean for Graduate Programs
Email: bernhardtj@mail.ecu.edu

GENERAL INFORMATION

Type of School: *4-Year College or University, Public* • Accreditation: *Southern Association of Colleges and Schools* • Total Enrollment: *2284*

PROGRAM INFORMATION

NLNAC Accreditation: *Yes* • CCNE Accreditation: *No*

_____

For specialty program listings, refer to the index.

NURSING STUDENT PROFILE

Total Nursing Enrollments: *88* • Full-Time Enrollment: *42* • Part-Time Enrollment: *46* • Female Enrollment: *84* • Male Enrollment: *4* • Total Graduates: *37*

FINANCES

Residental Annual Tuition: *$1,524* • Non-Residential Annual Tuition: *$10,252* • General Institutional Fees: *$557* • Additional Nursing Fees: *$162*

QUEENS COLLEGE

Address: 1900 Selwyn Ave., Charlotte, NC 28274
Phone: 704-337-2295
Fax: 704-337-2477
Contact: Joan S. McGill, RN, BSN, MSN, DSN,
         Professor and Chair
Email: mcgillj@queens.edu

GENERAL INFORMATION

Type of School: *Not Provided* • Accreditation: *Not Provided* •
Total Enrollment: *9100*

PROGRAM INFORMATION

NLNAC Accreditation: *Not Reported* • CCNE Accreditation:
Yes

_____

For specialty program listings, refer to the index.

NURSING STUDENT PROFILE

Total Nursing Enrollments: *31* • Full-Time Enrollment: *0* •
Part-Time Enrollment: *31* • Female Enrollment: *30* • Male
Enrollment: *1* • Total Graduates: *6*

FINANCES

Residental Annual Tuition: *$235* • Non-Residential Annual
Tuition: *$235* • General Institutional Fees: *$0* • Additional
Nursing Fees: *$0*

UNIVERSITY OF NORTH CAROLINA—CHAPEL HILL

Address: Carrington Hall, Campus Box 7460, Chapel
         Hill, NC 27599
Phone: 919-966-3586
Fax: 919-843-6212
Contact: Jennifer D'Auria, PhD, RN, Associate Professor
         and Director, Master's Program
Email: jdauria@email.unc.edu

GENERAL INFORMATION

Type of School: *4-Year College or University, Public* •
Accreditation: *Southern Association of Colleges and Schools* •
Total Enrollment: *23659*

PROGRAM INFORMATION

NLNAC Accreditation: *Yes* • CCNE Accreditation: *Yes*

_____

For specialty program listings, refer to the index.

NURSING STUDENT PROFILE

Total Nursing Enrollments: *167* • Full-Time Enrollment:
110 • Part-Time Enrollment: *57* • Female Enrollment: *153* •
Male Enrollment: *14* • Total Graduates: *45*

FINANCES

Residental Annual Tuition: *$1,256* • Non-Residential
Annual Tuition: *$6,411* • General Institutional Fees: *$446* •
Additional Nursing Fees: *$150*

UNIVERSITY OF NORTH CAROLINA—CHARLOTTE

Address: 9201 University City Blvd, Charlotte, NC 28223
Phone: 704-687-4687
Fax: 704-687-3180
Contact: Sue Marquis Bishop, PhD, RN, FAAN, Dean
Email: isbishop@email.uncc.edu

GENERAL INFORMATION

Type of School: *4-Year College or University, Public* •
Accreditation: *Southern Association of Colleges and Schools* •
Total Enrollment: *5601*

PROGRAM INFORMATION

NLNAC Accreditation: *Yes* • CCNE Accreditation: *No*

For specialty program listings, refer to the index.

NURSING STUDENT PROFILE

Total Nursing Enrollments: *166* • Full-Time Enrollment:
58 • Part-Time Enrollment: *108* • Female Enrollment: *135* •
Male Enrollment: *31* • Total Graduates: *62*

FINANCES

Residental Annual Tuition: *$1,940* • Non-Residential
Annual Tuition: *$9,210* • General Institutional Fees: *Not
Reported* • Additional Nursing Fees: *Not Reported*

UNIVERSITY OF NORTH CAROLINA—GREENSBORO

Address: PO Box 26172, Greensboro, NC 27402
Phone: 336-334-5010
Fax: 336-334-3628
Contact: Lynne G. Pearcey, RN, Dean
Email: l-pearce@uncg.edu

GENERAL INFORMATION

Type of School: *4-Year College or University, Public* •
Accreditation: *Southern Association of Colleges and Schools* •
Total Enrollment: *24180*

PROGRAM INFORMATION

NLNAC Accreditation: *Yes* • CCNE Accreditation: *No*

For specialty program listings, refer to the index.

NURSING STUDENT PROFILE

Total Nursing Enrollments: *244* • Full-Time Enrollment:
149 • Part-Time Enrollment: *95* • Female Enrollment: *220* •
Male Enrollment: *24* • Total Graduates: *59*

FINANCES

Residental Annual Tuition: *$1,555* • Non-Residential
Annual Tuition: *$4,744* • General Institutional Fees: *$215* •
Additional Nursing Fees: *Not Reported*

UNIVERSITY OF NORTH CAROLINA—WILMINGTON

Address: 601 S. College Road, Wilmington, NC 28403
Phone: 910-962-3784
Fax: 910-962-3723
Contact: Bettie J. Glenn, EdD, MSN, BS, Associate Dean for Academic Affairs
Email: glennb@uncw.edu

GENERAL INFORMATION

Type of School: *4-Year College or University, Public* •
Accreditation: *Southern Association of Colleges and Schools* •
Total Enrollment: *17000*

PROGRAM INFORMATION

NLNAC Accreditation: *Yes* • CCNE Accreditation: *No*

_____

For specialty program listings, refer to the index.

NURSING STUDENT PROFILE

Total Nursing Enrollments: *24* • Full-Time Enrollment: *8* •
Part-Time Enrollment: *16* • Female Enrollment: *21* • Male
Enrollment: *3* • Total Graduates: *12*

FINANCES

Residental Annual Tuition: *$1,200* • Non-Residential
Annual Tuition: *$4,875* • General Institutional Fees: *$0* •
Additional Nursing Fees: *$18*

TRI-COLLEGE UNIVERSITY NURSING CONSORTIUM

Address: 360 Choate Ave., Fargo, ND 58105
Phone: 218-236-4699
Fax: 218-299-5990
Contact: Jane F. Giedt, PhD, RN, Chair, Graduate Nursing Program
Email: giedt@mnstate.edu

GENERAL INFORMATION

Type of School: *4-Year College or University, Other* •
Accreditation: *North Central Association of Colleges and Schools* • Total Enrollment: *365*

PROGRAM INFORMATION

NLNAC Accreditation: *Not Reported* • CCNE Accreditation: *No*

_____

For specialty program listings, refer to the index.

NURSING STUDENT PROFILE

Total Nursing Enrollments: *23* • Full-Time Enrollment: *3* •
Part-Time Enrollment: *20* • Female Enrollment: *22* • Male
Enrollment: *1* • Total Graduates: *0*

FINANCES

Residental Annual Tuition: *$5,500* • Non-Residential
Annual Tuition: *$5,500* • General Institutional Fees: *$0* •
Additional Nursing Fees: *$300*

UNIVERSITY OF MARY

Address: 900 College Street, Bismarck, ND 58501
Phone: 701-255-7500
Fax: Not Provided
Contact: Betty Rambur, RN, DNSc, Chairperson
Email: barambur@umary.edu

GENERAL INFORMATION

Type of School: *4-Year College or University, Public* •
Accreditation: *North Central Association of Colleges and
Schools* • Total Enrollment: *5617*

PROGRAM INFORMATION

NLNAC Accreditation: *Yes* • CCNE Accreditation: *No*

———

For specialty program listings, refer to the index.

NURSING STUDENT PROFILE

Total Nursing Enrollments: *48* • Full-Time Enrollment: *33* •
Part-Time Enrollment: *15* • Female Enrollment: *42* • Male
Enrollment: *6* • Total Graduates: *15*

FINANCES

Residental Annual Tuition: *Not Reported* • Non-Residential
Annual Tuition: *Not Reported* • General Institutional Fees:
Not Reported • Additional Nursing Fees: *Not Reported*

UNIVERSITY OF NORTH DAKOTA

Address: Box 9025 University Station, Grand Forks, ND
58202
Phone: Not Provided
Fax: Not Provided
Contact: Not Provided
Email: Not Provided

GENERAL INFORMATION

Type of School: *Not Provided* • Accreditation: *North Central
Association of Colleges and Schools* • Total Enrollment: *Not
Provided*

PROGRAM INFORMATION

NLNAC Accreditation: *Yes* • CCNE Accreditation: *No*

———

For specialty program listings, refer to the index.

NURSING STUDENT PROFILE

Total Nursing Enrollments: *Not Provided* • Full-Time
Enrollment: *Not Provided* • Part-Time Enrollment: *Not
Provided* • Female Enrollment: *Not Provided* • Male
Enrollment: *Not Provided* • Total Graduates: *Not Provided*

FINANCES

Residental Annual Tuition: *Not Reported* • Non-Residential
Annual Tuition: *Not Reported* • General Institutional Fees:
Not Reported • Additional Nursing Fees: *Not Reported*

CAPITAL UNIVERSITY

Address: 2199 E. Main St., Columbus, OH 43209-2394
Phone: 614-236-6703
Fax: Not Provided
Contact: Doris S. Edwards, EdD, RN, Dean and Professor
Email: dedwards@capital.edu

GENERAL INFORMATION

Type of School: *4-Year College or University, Private (Religious)* • Accreditation: *North Central Association of Colleges and Schools* • Total Enrollment: *4000*

PROGRAM INFORMATION

NLNAC Accreditation: *Not Reported* • CCNE Accreditation: *Yes*

_____

For specialty program listings, refer to the index.

NURSING STUDENT PROFILE

Total Nursing Enrollments: *46* • Full-Time Enrollment: *6* • Part-Time Enrollment: *40* • Female Enrollment: *46* • Male Enrollment: *0* • Total Graduates: *8*

FINANCES

Residental Annual Tuition: *$4,860* • Non-Residential Annual Tuition: *Not Reported* • General Institutional Fees: *$0* • Additional Nursing Fees: *$0*

CASE WESTERN RESERVE UNIVERSITY

Address: 10900 Euclid Avenue, Cleveland, OH 44106-4904
Phone: 216-368-6304
Fax: 216-368-3542
Contact: Georgia L. Narsavage, PhD, RN, CS, Associate Professor and Director MSN Program
Email: gln2@po.cwru.edu

GENERAL INFORMATION

Type of School: *4-Year College or University, Private (Independent)* • Accreditation: *North Central Association of Colleges and Schools* • Total Enrollment: *Not Provided*

PROGRAM INFORMATION

NLNAC Accreditation: *Yes* • CCNE Accreditation:

_____

For specialty program listings, refer to the index.

NURSING STUDENT PROFILE

Total Nursing Enrollments: *218* • Full-Time Enrollment: *76* • Part-Time Enrollment: *142* • Female Enrollment: *190* • Male Enrollment: *28* • Total Graduates: *135*

FINANCES

Residental Annual Tuition: *$21,000* • Non-Residential Annual Tuition: *$21,000* • General Institutional Fees: *$0* • Additional Nursing Fees: *$15*

CLEVELAND STATE UNIVERSITY

Address: 1860 East 22 Street, Cleveland, OH 44115
Phone: 216-687-3548
Fax: 216-687-3556
Contact: June Romeo, PhD, MSN, MEd, NP-C, Program
           Director
Email: j.romeo@csuohio.edu

GENERAL INFORMATION

Type of School: *Other, Public* • Accreditation: *North Central Association of Colleges and Schools* • Total Enrollment: *3006*

PROGRAM INFORMATION

NLNAC Accreditation: *Not Reported* • CCNE Accreditation: *No*

For specialty program listings, refer to the index.

NURSING STUDENT PROFILE

Total Nursing Enrollments: *12* • Full-Time Enrollment: *5* • Part-Time Enrollment: *7* • Female Enrollment: *10* • Male Enrollment: *2* • Total Graduates: *14*

FINANCES

Residental Annual Tuition: *Not Reported* • Non-Residential Annual Tuition: *Not Reported* • General Institutional Fees: *Not Reported* • Additional Nursing Fees: *Not Reported*

FRANCISCAN UNIVERSITY—STEUBENVILLE

Address: 1235 University Boulevard, Steubenville, OH
           43952
Phone: 740-284-7245
Fax: Not Provided
Contact: Joan A. Davis, PhD, CRNP, Director of
           Graduate Nursing
Email: jdavis@franuniv.edu

GENERAL INFORMATION

Type of School: *4-Year College or University, Private (Religious)* • Accreditation: *Not Provided* • Total Enrollment: *Not Provided*

PROGRAM INFORMATION

NLNAC Accreditation: *Not Reported* • CCNE Accreditation: *No*

For specialty program listings, refer to the index.

NURSING STUDENT PROFILE

Total Nursing Enrollments: *17* • Full-Time Enrollment: *11* • Part-Time Enrollment: *6* • Female Enrollment: *17* • Male Enrollment: *0* • Total Graduates: *Not Provided*

FINANCES

Residental Annual Tuition: *$7,590* • Non-Residential Annual Tuition: *$7,590* • General Institutional Fees: *$120* • Additional Nursing Fees: *$230*

MEDICAL COLLEGE OF OHIO

Address: 3015 Arlington Avenue, Toledo, OH 43614-
            5803
Phone: 419-383-5892
Fax: 419-383-5894
Contact: Janet H. Robinson, PhD, RN, Associate Dean,
            Graduate Nursing Program
Email: jrobinson@mco.edu

GENERAL INFORMATION

Type of School: *4-Year College or University, Public* •
Accreditation: *North Central Association of Colleges and
Schools* • Total Enrollment: *Not Provided*

PROGRAM INFORMATION

NLNAC Accreditation: *Not Reported* • CCNE Accreditation:
Yes

_____

For specialty program listings, refer to the index.

NURSING STUDENT PROFILE

Total Nursing Enrollments: *89* • Full-Time Enrollment: *11* •
Part-Time Enrollment: *78* • Female Enrollment: *87* • Male
Enrollment: *2* • Total Graduates: *32*

FINANCES

Residental Annual Tuition: *$5,298* • Non-Residential
Annual Tuition: *$12,178* • General Institutional Fees: *$678* •
Additional Nursing Fees: *$70*

THE OHIO STATE UNIVERSITY

Address: Newton Hall, 1585 Neil Avenue, Columbus,
            OH 43210
Phone: 614-292-8900
Fax: 614-292-4535
Contact: Ursulay A. Anderson, PhD, RN, FAAN, Dean,
            Professor and Assistant Vice President for Health
            Sciences
Email: anderson.328@osu.edu

GENERAL INFORMATION

Type of School: *4-Year College or University, Public* •
Accreditation: *North Central Association of Colleges and
Schools* • Total Enrollment: *55233*

PROGRAM INFORMATION

NLNAC Accreditation: *Not Reported* • CCNE Accreditation:
Yes

_____

For specialty program listings, refer to the index.

NURSING STUDENT PROFILE

Total Nursing Enrollments: *128* • Full-Time Enrollment:
63 • Part-Time Enrollment: *65* • Female Enrollment: *122* •
Male Enrollment: *6* • Total Graduates: *44*

FINANCES

Residental Annual Tuition: *$5,757* • Non-Residential
Annual Tuition: *$14,892* • General Institutional Fees: *Not
Reported* • Additional Nursing Fees: *Not Reported*

OTTERBEIN COLLEGE

Address: One Otterbein College, Westerville, OH 43081
Phone: 614-823-1614
Fax: Not Provided
Contact: Eda L. Mikolai, PhD, RN, CNAA, Director of Graduate Studies
Email: EMikolai@otterbein.edu

GENERAL INFORMATION

Type of School: *4-Year College or University, Public* • Accreditation: *North Central Association of Colleges and Schools* • Total Enrollment: *3000*

PROGRAM INFORMATION

NLNAC Accreditation: *Yes* • CCNE Accreditation: *No*

For specialty program listings, refer to the index.

NURSING STUDENT PROFILE

Total Nursing Enrollments: *109* • Full-Time Enrollment: *18* • Part-Time Enrollment: *91* • Female Enrollment: *Not Provided* • Male Enrollment: *Not Provided* • Total Graduates: *18*

FINANCES

Residental Annual Tuition: *Not Reported* • Non-Residential Annual Tuition: *Not Reported* • General Institutional Fees: *Not Reported* • Additional Nursing Fees: *Not Reported*

THE UNIVERSITY OF AKRON

Address: 209 Carroll Street, Akron, OH 44325-3701
Phone: 330-972-5936
Fax: 330-972-5737
Contact: Kathleen Ross-Alaolmolki, PhD, RN, Coordinator, Master's Program
Email: krl@uakron.edu

GENERAL INFORMATION

Type of School: *4-Year College or University, Private (Independent)* • Accreditation: *North Central Association of Colleges and Schools* • Total Enrollment: *Not Provided*

PROGRAM INFORMATION

NLNAC Accreditation: *Yes* • CCNE Accreditation: *No*

For specialty program listings, refer to the index.

NURSING STUDENT PROFILE

Total Nursing Enrollments: *193* • Full-Time Enrollment: *58* • Part-Time Enrollment: *135* • Female Enrollment: *145* • Male Enrollment: *48* • Total Graduates: *53*

FINANCES

Residental Annual Tuition: *$4,986* • Non-Residential Annual Tuition: *$8,929* • General Institutional Fees: *$92* • Additional Nursing Fees: *$300*

UNIVERSITY OF CINCINNATI

Address: 9555 Plainfield Road, Cincinnati, OH 45236
Phone: 513-558-0310
Fax: 513-558-5054
Contact: Susan Kennerly, PhD, RN, Associate Dean for
           Academic Affairs
Email: Susan.Kennerly@uc.edu

GENERAL INFORMATION

Type of School: *4-Year College or University, Private
(Independent)* • Accreditation: *North Central Association of
Colleges and Schools* • Total Enrollment: *14195*

PROGRAM INFORMATION

NLNAC Accreditation: *Yes* • CCNE Accreditation: *No*

_____

For specialty program listings, refer to the index.

NURSING STUDENT PROFILE

Total Nursing Enrollments: *201* • Full-Time Enrollment:
115 • Part-Time Enrollment: *86* • Female Enrollment: *172* •
Male Enrollment: *29* • Total Graduates: *81*

FINANCES

Residental Annual Tuition: *$5,394* • Non-Residential
Annual Tuition: *$10,839* • General Institutional Fees: *$870* •
Additional Nursing Fees: *$0*

URSULINE COLLEGE

Address: 2550 Lander Road, Pepper Pike, OH 44124
Phone: 440-449-3425
Fax: 440-449-4267
Contact: Carol H. Waggoner, PhD, RN, Professor and
           Director
Email: cwaggone@ursuline.edu

GENERAL INFORMATION

Type of School: *Not Provided* • Accreditation: *Not Provided* •
Total Enrollment: *Not Provided*

PROGRAM INFORMATION

NLNAC Accreditation: *Not Reported* • CCNE Accreditation:
Yes

_____

For specialty program listings, refer to the index.

NURSING STUDENT PROFILE

Total Nursing Enrollments: *53* • Full-Time Enrollment: *0* •
Part-Time Enrollment: *53* • Female Enrollment: *51* • Male
Enrollment: *2* • Total Graduates: *8*

FINANCES

Residental Annual Tuition: *Not Reported* • Non-Residential
Annual Tuition: *Not Reported* • General Institutional Fees:
Not Reported • Additional Nursing Fees: *Not Reported*

WRIGHT STATE UNIVERSITY

Address: 3640 Colonel, Dayton, OH 45435
Phone: 937-775-3133
Fax: 937-775-4571
Contact: Patricia A. Martin, PhD, RN, Dean
Email: patricia.martin@wright.edu

GENERAL INFORMATION

Type of School: *4-Year College or University, Public* •
Accreditation: *North Central Association of Colleges and
Schools* • Total Enrollment: *Not Provided*

PROGRAM INFORMATION

NLNAC Accreditation: *Yes* • CCNE Accreditation:

For specialty program listings, refer to the index.

NURSING STUDENT PROFILE

Total Nursing Enrollments: *156* • Full-Time Enrollment:
48 • Part-Time Enrollment: *108* • Female Enrollment: *144* •
Male Enrollment: *12* • Total Graduates: *39*

FINANCES

Residental Annual Tuition: *$5,594* • Non-Residential
Annual Tuition: *$10,938* • General Institutional Fees: *$687* •
Additional Nursing Fees: *$0*

XAVIER UNIVERSITY

Address: 3800 Victoria, Cincinnati, OH 45007
Phone: 513-745-3815
Fax: 513-745-1087
Contact: Susan M. Schmidt, PhD, RN, COHM-S, CNS,
           Chair
Email: Schmidts@xu.edu

GENERAL INFORMATION

Type of School: *4-Year College or University, Private
(Religious)* • Accreditation: *North Central Association of
Colleges and Schools* • Total Enrollment: *6523*

PROGRAM INFORMATION

NLNAC Accreditation: *Yes* • CCNE Accreditation: *No*

For specialty program listings, refer to the index.

NURSING STUDENT PROFILE

Total Nursing Enrollments: *43* • Full-Time Enrollment: *1* •
Part-Time Enrollment: *42* • Female Enrollment: *41* • Male
Enrollment: *2* • Total Graduates: *9*

FINANCES

Residental Annual Tuition: *$9,840* • Non-Residential
Annual Tuition: *Not Reported* • General Institutional Fees:
Not Reported • Additional Nursing Fees: *$70*

Circle 151 on reader card   See in-depth profile for more information

YOUNGSTOWN STATE UNIVERSITY

Address: One University Plaza, Youngstown, OH 44555-0002
Phone: 330-742-1792
Fax: Not Provided
Contact: Sharon P. Shipton, PhD, MSN Program Director
Email: micah12@pathway.net

GENERAL INFORMATION

Type of School: *4-Year College or University, Public* • Accreditation: *North Central Association of Colleges and Schools* • Total Enrollment: *Not Provided*

PROGRAM INFORMATION

NLNAC Accreditation: *Not Reported* • CCNE Accreditation: *No*

_____

For specialty program listings, refer to the index.

NURSING STUDENT PROFILE

Total Nursing Enrollments: *16* • Full-Time Enrollment: *0* • Part-Time Enrollment: *16* • Female Enrollment: *16* • Male Enrollment: *0* • Total Graduates: *10*

FINANCES

Residental Annual Tuition: *$3,768* • Non-Residential Annual Tuition: *$6,096* • General Institutional Fees: *$768* • Additional Nursing Fees: *$420*

UNIVERSITY OF OKLAHOMA

Address: PO Box 26901, Oklahoma City, OK 73190-0001
Phone: 405-271-2420
Fax: 405-271-3443
Contact: Patricia R. Forni, PhD, RN, FAAN, Dean and Professor
Email: Patricia-Forni@ouhsc.edu

GENERAL INFORMATION

Type of School: *4-Year College or University, Public* • Accreditation: *North Central Association of Colleges and Schools* • Total Enrollment: *12687*

PROGRAM INFORMATION

NLNAC Accreditation: *Yes* • CCNE Accreditation: *No*

_____

For specialty program listings, refer to the index.

NURSING STUDENT PROFILE

Total Nursing Enrollments: *205* • Full-Time Enrollment: *51* • Part-Time Enrollment: *154* • Female Enrollment: *189* • Male Enrollment: *16* • Total Graduates: *63*

FINANCES

Residental Annual Tuition: *$2,580* • Non-Residential Annual Tuition: *$8,250* • General Institutional Fees: *$390* • Additional Nursing Fees: *$339*

OREGON HEALTH SCIENCES UNIVERSITY

Address: 18th and Colorado, Portland, OR 97201
Phone: 503-494-3894
Fax: 503-494-4350
Contact: Beverly Hoeffer, RN, DNSc, FAAN, Associate Dean for Academic Affairs
Email: hoefferb@ohsu.edu

GENERAL INFORMATION

Type of School: *4-Year College or University, Public* • Accreditation: *Northwestern Association of Schools and Colleges* • Total Enrollment: *Not Provided*

PROGRAM INFORMATION

NLNAC Accreditation: *Yes* • CCNE Accreditation: *No*

———

For specialty program listings, refer to the index.

NURSING STUDENT PROFILE

Total Nursing Enrollments: *138* • Full-Time Enrollment: *83* • Part-Time Enrollment: *55* • Female Enrollment: *122* • Male Enrollment: *16* • Total Graduates: *47*

FINANCES

Residental Annual Tuition: *$6,192* • Non-Residential Annual Tuition: *$10,296* • General Institutional Fees: *$514* • Additional Nursing Fees: *$600*

UNIVERSITY OF PORTLAND

Address: 5000 North Willamette Boulevard, Portland, OR 97203
Phone: 503-943-7211
Fax: 503-943-7729
Contact: Terry R. Misener, PhD, RN, FAAN, Dean and Professor
Email: misener@up.edu

GENERAL INFORMATION

Type of School: *4-Year College or University, Other* • Accreditation: *Northwestern Association of Schools and Colleges* • Total Enrollment: *25461*

PROGRAM INFORMATION

NLNAC Accreditation: *Yes* • CCNE Accreditation: *Yes*

———

For specialty program listings, refer to the index.

NURSING STUDENT PROFILE

Total Nursing Enrollments: *40* • Full-Time Enrollment: *36* • Part-Time Enrollment: *4* • Female Enrollment: *38* • Male Enrollment: *2* • Total Graduates: *5*

FINANCES

Residental Annual Tuition: *$12,912* • Non-Residential Annual Tuition: *$12,912* • General Institutional Fees: *Not Reported* • Additional Nursing Fees: *$25*

BLOOMSBURG UNIVERSITY

Address: 400 E. 2nd Street, RM 3109, MCHS, Lakes County, PA 17815
Phone: 570-389-3121
Fax: 570-389-5008
Contact: Sharon Haymaker, PhD, Graduate Coordinator
Email: haymaker@husky.bloomu.edu

GENERAL INFORMATION

Type of School: *4-Year College or University, Public* • Accreditation: *Middle States Association of Colleges and Schools* • Total Enrollment: *7916*

PROGRAM INFORMATION

NLNAC Accreditation: *Yes* • CCNE Accreditation: *No*

For specialty program listings, refer to the index.

NURSING STUDENT PROFILE

Total Nursing Enrollments: *34* • Full-Time Enrollment: *1* • Part-Time Enrollment: *33* • Female Enrollment: *31* • Male Enrollment: *3* • Total Graduates: *6*

FINANCES

Residental Annual Tuition: *$4,600* • Non-Residential Annual Tuition: *$7,554* • General Institutional Fees: *$834* • Additional Nursing Fees: *$0*

CARLOW COLLEGE

Address: 3333 5th Avenue, Pittsburgh, PA 15213
Phone: 412-578-6596
Fax: 412-578-6114
Contact: Susan Sterrett, RN, MSN, MBA, Master's Program Director
Email: ssterret@carlow.edu

GENERAL INFORMATION

Type of School: *4-Year College or University, Private (Religious)* • Accreditation: *Middle States Association of Colleges and Schools* • Total Enrollment: *1933*

PROGRAM INFORMATION

NLNAC Accreditation: *Not Reported* • CCNE Accreditation: *Yes*

For specialty program listings, refer to the index.

NURSING STUDENT PROFILE

Total Nursing Enrollments: *51* • Full-Time Enrollment: *30* • Part-Time Enrollment: *21* • Female Enrollment: *49* • Male Enrollment: *2* • Total Graduates: *37*

FINANCES

Residental Annual Tuition: *$10,248* • Non-Residential Annual Tuition: *$10,248* • General Institutional Fees: *$600* • Additional Nursing Fees: *Not Reported*

CLARION UNIVERSITY

Address: 1801 West 1st Street, Santa Rosa, PA 16301
Phone: 724-738-2323
Fax: 724-738-2881
Contact: Joyce Denrose-White, RN, CRNP, BC, MPH,
            Coordinator
Email: joyce.white@clarion.edu

GENERAL INFORMATION

Type of School: *4-Year College or University, Public •*
Accreditation: *Middle States Association of Colleges and
Schools •* Total Enrollment: *6192*

PROGRAM INFORMATION

NLNAC Accreditation: *Yes •* CCNE Accreditation: *No*

_____

For specialty program listings, refer to the index.

NURSING STUDENT PROFILE

Total Nursing Enrollments: *35 •* Full-Time Enrollment: *2 •*
Part-Time Enrollment: *33 •* Female Enrollment: *31 •* Male
Enrollment: *4 •* Total Graduates: *12*

FINANCES

Residental Annual Tuition: *$5,400 •* Non-Residential
Annual Tuition: *$9,000 •* General Institutional Fees: *Not
Reported •* Additional Nursing Fees: *$320*

COLLEGE MISERICORDIA

Address: 100 Main Street, Dallas, PA 18612
Phone: 570-674-6440
Fax: 570-674-8902
Contact: Jean R. Bohlander, RN, Coordinator, Graduate
            Nursing Programs
Email: jbohland@miseri.edu

GENERAL INFORMATION

Type of School: *4-Year College or University, Private
(Independent) •* Accreditation: *Middle States Association of
Colleges and Schools •* Total Enrollment: *Not Provided*

PROGRAM INFORMATION

NLNAC Accreditation: *Yes •* CCNE Accreditation: *No*

_____

For specialty program listings, refer to the index.

NURSING STUDENT PROFILE

Total Nursing Enrollments: *79 •* Full-Time Enrollment: *16 •*
Part-Time Enrollment: *63 •* Female Enrollment: *Not
Provided •* Male Enrollment: *Not Provided •* Total Graduates:
25

FINANCES

Residental Annual Tuition: *Not Reported •* Non-Residential
Annual Tuition: *Not Reported •* General Institutional Fees:
Not Reported • Additional Nursing Fees: *Not Reported*

DUQUESNE UNIVERSITY

Address: 600 Forbes Avenue, Pittsburgh, PA 15282
Phone: 412-396-6537
Fax: 412-396-4180
Contact: Ellen Olshansky, RNC, DNCs, Associate Dean, Graduate Programs and Professor
Email: olshansky@duq.edu

GENERAL INFORMATION

Type of School: *4-Year College, Private (Religious)* • Accreditation: *Middle States Association of Colleges and Schools* • Total Enrollment: *9555*

PROGRAM INFORMATION

NLNAC Accreditation: *Yes* • CCNE Accreditation: *No*

For specialty program listings, refer to the index.

NURSING STUDENT PROFILE

Total Nursing Enrollments: *53* • Full-Time Enrollment: *1* • Part-Time Enrollment: *52* • Female Enrollment: *53* • Male Enrollment: *0* • Total Graduates: *9*

FINANCES

Residental Annual Tuition: *$622* • Non-Residential Annual Tuition: *$622* • General Institutional Fees: *$56* • Additional Nursing Fees: *$0*

EDINBORO UNIVERSITY OF PENNSYLVANIA

Address: 125 Centennial Hall, Edinboro, PA 16444
Phone: 814-732-2900
Fax: 814-732-2536
Contact: Patricia L. Nosel, RN, MN, Chairperson
Email: nosel@edinboro.edu

GENERAL INFORMATION

Type of School: *4-Year College or University, Private (Religious)* • Accreditation: *Middle States Association of Colleges and Schools* • Total Enrollment: *Not Provided*

PROGRAM INFORMATION

NLNAC Accreditation: *Not Reported* • CCNE Accreditation: *No*

For specialty program listings, refer to the index.

NURSING STUDENT PROFILE

Total Nursing Enrollments: *7* • Full-Time Enrollment: *7* • Part-Time Enrollment: *0* • Female Enrollment: *6* • Male Enrollment: *1* • Total Graduates: *13*

FINANCES

Residental Annual Tuition: *$4,138* • Non-Residential Annual Tuition: *$7,008* • General Institutional Fees: *$526* • Additional Nursing Fees: *$0*

GANNON UNIVERSITY

Address:	109 University Square, Erie, PA 16541
Phone:	814-871-5363
Fax:	814-871-5662
Contact:	Ruth Shoemaker, RN, MBA, MSN, Assistant Professor
Email:	shoemake001@gannon.edu

GENERAL INFORMATION

Type of School: *4-Year College or University, Public* • Accreditation: *Middle States Association of Colleges and Schools* • Total Enrollment: *Not Provided*

PROGRAM INFORMATION

NLNAC Accreditation: *Yes* • CCNE Accreditation: *No*

For specialty program listings, refer to the index.

NURSING STUDENT PROFILE

Total Nursing Enrollments: *73* • Full-Time Enrollment: *36* • Part-Time Enrollment: *37* • Female Enrollment: *48* • Male Enrollment: *25* • Total Graduates: *17*

FINANCES

Residental Annual Tuition: *$11,520* • Non-Residential Annual Tuition: *$11,520* • General Institutional Fees: *$350* • Additional Nursing Fees: *Not Reported*

GWYNEDD-MERCY COLLEGE

Address:	P.O. Box 901, 1301 Sumneytown Pike, Gwynedd Valley, PA 19437
Phone:	215-646-7300
Fax:	Not Provided
Contact:	Barbara A. Jones, DNSc, Program Director
Email:	Not Provided

GENERAL INFORMATION

Type of School: *Not Provided* • Accreditation: *Middle States Association of Colleges and Schools* • Total Enrollment: *5930*

PROGRAM INFORMATION

NLNAC Accreditation: *Yes* • CCNE Accreditation: *No*

For specialty program listings, refer to the index.

NURSING STUDENT PROFILE

Total Nursing Enrollments: *67* • Full-Time Enrollment: *10* • Part-Time Enrollment: *57* • Female Enrollment: *63* • Male Enrollment: *4* • Total Graduates: *24*

FINANCES

Residental Annual Tuition: *$9,600* • Non-Residential Annual Tuition: *$9,600* • General Institutional Fees: *$70* • Additional Nursing Fees: *$180*

HOLY FAMILY COLLEGE

Address: Grand Frankford, Philadelphia, PA 19114
Phone: 215-637-7700
Fax: Not Provided
Contact: Sara Wuthnow, EdD, RN, Interim MSN Chair
Email: swuthnow@hfc.edu

GENERAL INFORMATION

Type of School: *4-Year College or University, Private (Religious)* • Accreditation: *Middle States Association of Colleges and Schools* • Total Enrollment: *2800*

PROGRAM INFORMATION

NLNAC Accreditation: *Yes* • CCNE Accreditation: *No*

For specialty program listings, refer to the index.

NURSING STUDENT PROFILE

Total Nursing Enrollments: *13* • Full-Time Enrollment: *0* • Part-Time Enrollment: *13* • Female Enrollment: *12* • Male Enrollment: *1* • Total Graduates: *0*

FINANCES

Residental Annual Tuition: *$5,940* • Non-Residential Annual Tuition: *$5,940* • General Institutional Fees: *$85* • Additional Nursing Fees: *$40*

INDIANA UNIVERSITY OF PENNSYLVANIA

Address: 1010 Oakland Avenue, Indiana, PA 45623
Phone: 724-357-2557
Fax: Not Provided
Contact: Jodell Kuzneski, RN, MNEd, Chairperson, Department of Nursing/Allied Health Professions
Email: kuzneski@grove.iup.edu

GENERAL INFORMATION

Type of School: *4-Year College or University, Public* • Accreditation: *Middle States Association of Colleges and Schools* • Total Enrollment: *11321*

PROGRAM INFORMATION

NLNAC Accreditation: *Not Reported* • CCNE Accreditation: *No*

For specialty program listings, refer to the index.

NURSING STUDENT PROFILE

Total Nursing Enrollments: *27* • Full-Time Enrollment: *4* • Part-Time Enrollment: *23* • Female Enrollment: *Not Provided* • Male Enrollment: *Not Provided* • Total Graduates: *14*

FINANCES

Residental Annual Tuition: *Not Reported* • Non-Residential Annual Tuition: *Not Reported* • General Institutional Fees: *Not Reported* • Additional Nursing Fees: *Not Reported*

LA ROCHE COLLEGE

Address: 9000 Babcock Blvd., Pittsburgh, PA 15327
Phone: 412-536-1173
Fax: 412-536-1175
Contact: Rosemary McCarthy, RN, MSN, Graduate
            Program Director
Email: mccartr1@laroche.edu

GENERAL INFORMATION

Type of School: *4-Year College or University, Private (Religious)* • Accreditation: *Middle States Association of Colleges and Schools* • Total Enrollment: *7700*

PROGRAM INFORMATION

NLNAC Accreditation: *Yes* • CCNE Accreditation:

_____

For specialty program listings, refer to the index.

NURSING STUDENT PROFILE

Total Nursing Enrollments: *48* • Full-Time Enrollment: *0* • Part-Time Enrollment: *48* • Female Enrollment: *48* • Male Enrollment: *0* • Total Graduates: *15*

FINANCES

Residental Annual Tuition: *$10,560* • Non-Residential Annual Tuition: *Not Reported* • General Institutional Fees: *$14* • Additional Nursing Fees: *$0*

LA SALLE UNIVERSITY

Address: 1900 W. Olney Avenue, Philadelphia, PA 19141
Phone: 215-951-1322
Fax: 215-951-1896
Contact: Janice M. Beitz, PhD, RN, CS, CNOR,
            CWOCN, Associate Professor
Email: beitz@lasalle.edu

GENERAL INFORMATION

Type of School: *4-Year College or University, Private (Religious)* • Accreditation: *Middle States Association of Colleges and Schools* • Total Enrollment: *Not Reported*

PROGRAM INFORMATION

NLNAC Accreditation: *Yes* • CCNE Accreditation: *Provisional*

_____

For specialty program listings, refer to the index.

NURSING STUDENT PROFILE

Total Nursing Enrollments: *136* • Full-Time Enrollment: *86* • Part-Time Enrollment: *50* • Female Enrollment: *122* • Male Enrollment: *14* • Total Graduates: *36*

FINANCES

Residental Annual Tuition: *$550* • Non-Residential Annual Tuition: *$0* • General Institutional Fees: *$75* • Additional Nursing Fees: *$100*

MCP HAHNEMANN UNIVERSITY

Address: 245 North 15th St., Mail Stop 501, Philadelphia, PA 19102
Phone: 215-762-1644
Fax: 215-762-1259
Contact: Elizabeth Blunt, MSN, CEN, CRNP, Program Director
Email: elizabeth.blunt@drexel.edu

MILLERSVILLE UNIVERSITY

Address: 110 Galewski Drive, Millersville, PA 17551
Phone: 717-871-5276
Fax: 717-871-4877
Contact: Barbara F. Haus, EdD, CRNP, APRN-BC, CPNP, Graduate Program Coordinator
Email: Barbara.Haus@millersville.edu

GENERAL INFORMATION

Type of School: *4-Year College or University, Private Independent* • Accreditation: *Middle States Association of Colleges and Schools* • Total Enrollment: *3000*

GENERAL INFORMATION

Type of School: *4-Year College or University, Public* • Accreditation: *Middle States Association of Colleges and Schools* • Total Enrollment: *5800*

PROGRAM INFORMATION

NLNAC Accreditation: *Yes* • CCNE Accreditation: *No*

For specialty program listings, refer to the index.

PROGRAM INFORMATION

NLNAC Accreditation: *Yes* • CCNE Accreditation: *No*

For specialty program listings, refer to the index.

NURSING STUDENT PROFILE

Total Nursing Enrollments: *184* • Full-Time Enrollment: *52* • Part-Time Enrollment: *132* • Female Enrollment: *150* • Male Enrollment: *34* • Total Graduates: *79*

NURSING STUDENT PROFILE

Total Nursing Enrollments: *27* • Full-Time Enrollment: *0* • Part-Time Enrollment: *27* • Female Enrollment: *25* • Male Enrollment: *2* • Total Graduates: *9*

FINANCES

Residental Annual Tuition: *$6,440* • Non-Residential Annual Tuition: *Not Provided* • General Institutional Fees: *$600* • Additional Nursing Fees: *$100*

FINANCES

Residental Annual Tuition: *$4,600* • Non-Residential Annual Tuition: *$7,554* • General Institutional Fees: *$783* • Additional Nursing Fees: *$0*

NEUMANN COLLEGE

Address: 1 Neuman Road, Aston, PA 19014
Phone: 610-558-5561
Fax: 610-361-5265
Contact: Gregg E. Newschwander, PhD, RN, Professor
      and Chair Division of Nursing and Health
      Sciences
Email: newschwg@neumann.edu

GENERAL INFORMATION

Type of School: *4-Year College or University, Private (Religious)* • Accreditation: *Middle States Association of Colleges and Schools* • Total Enrollment: *Not Provided*

PROGRAM INFORMATION

NLNAC Accreditation: *Not Reported* • CCNE Accreditation: *No*

_____

For specialty program listings, refer to the index.

NURSING STUDENT PROFILE

Total Nursing Enrollments: *3* • Full-Time Enrollment: *0* • Part-Time Enrollment: *3* • Female Enrollment: *3* • Male Enrollment: *0* • Total Graduates: *1*

FINANCES

Residental Annual Tuition: *$10,080* • Non-Residential Annual Tuition: *$10,080* • General Institutional Fees: *$0* • Additional Nursing Fees: *$0*

PENNSYLVANIA STATE UNIVERSITY

Address: 203 Hlth and Human Development E,
      University Park, PA 16802
Phone: 814-863-7755
Fax: 814-865-3779
Contact: Karen H. Morin, RN, DSN, Professor-in-Charge
      of Graduate Programs
Email: khm10@psu.edu

GENERAL INFORMATION

Type of School: *4-Year College or University, Public* • Accreditation: *Middle States Association of Colleges and Schools* • Total Enrollment: *3154*

PROGRAM INFORMATION

NLNAC Accreditation: *Yes* • CCNE Accreditation:

_____

For specialty program listings, refer to the index.

NURSING STUDENT PROFILE

Total Nursing Enrollments: *55* • Full-Time Enrollment: *24* • Part-Time Enrollment: *31* • Female Enrollment: *53* • Male Enrollment: *2* • Total Graduates: *23*

FINANCES

Residental Annual Tuition: *$7,314* • Non-Residential Annual Tuition: *$14,980* • General Institutional Fees: *$306* • Additional Nursing Fees: *$0*

TEMPLE UNIVERSITY

Address: Jones Hall, 3307 North Broad Street,
           Philadelphia, PA 19140
Phone: 215-707-4617
Fax: 215-707-1599
Contact: Margaret Shepard, PhD, RN, Director, Graduate
           Studies
Email: mshepard@unix.temple.edu

GENERAL INFORMATION

Type of School: *4-Year College or University, Public* •
Accreditation: *Middle States Association of Colleges and
Schools* • Total Enrollment: *3405*

PROGRAM INFORMATION

NLNAC Accreditation: *Yes* • CCNE Accreditation:

_____

For specialty program listings, refer to the index.

NURSING STUDENT PROFILE

Total Nursing Enrollments: *63* • Full-Time Enrollment: *33* •
Part-Time Enrollment: *30* • Female Enrollment: *52* • Male
Enrollment: *11* • Total Graduates: *32*

FINANCES

Residental Annual Tuition: *$8,448* • Non-Residential
Annual Tuition: *$11,616* • General Institutional Fees: *Not
Reported* • Additional Nursing Fees: *Not Reported*

THOMAS JEFFERSON UNIVERSITY

Address: PO Box 587, Philadelphia, PA 19107
Phone: 215-503-7937
Fax: 215-503-0376
Contact: Mary G. Schaal, EdD, RN, Vice Chair and
           Director of Graduate Programs
Email: mary.schaal@mail.tju.edu

GENERAL INFORMATION

Type of School: *4-Year College or University, Public* •
Accreditation: *Middle States Association of Colleges and
Schools* • Total Enrollment: *1000*

PROGRAM INFORMATION

NLNAC Accreditation: *Yes* • CCNE Accreditation: *No*

_____

For specialty program listings, refer to the index.

NURSING STUDENT PROFILE

Total Nursing Enrollments: *138* • Full-Time Enrollment:
65 • Part-Time Enrollment: *73* • Female Enrollment: *125* •
Male Enrollment: *13* • Total Graduates: *17*

FINANCES

Residental Annual Tuition: *$19,500* • Non-Residential
Annual Tuition: *$19,500* • General Institutional Fees: *$0* •
Additional Nursing Fees: *$0*

UNIVERSITY OF PENNSYLVANIA

Address: 420 Guardian Drive, Philadelphia, PA 19104
Phone: 215-898-8286
Fax: 215-573-8857
Contact: Anne Keane, EdD, RN, FAAN, Interim Associate Dean for Graduate Studies and Professional Development
Email: Not Provided

GENERAL INFORMATION

Type of School: *4-Year College or University, Private Independent* • Accreditation: *Middle States Association of Colleges and Schools* • Total Enrollment: *21800*

PROGRAM INFORMATION

NLNAC Accreditation: *Yes* • CCNE Accreditation: *Yes*

For specialty program listings, refer to the index.

NURSING STUDENT PROFILE

Total Nursing Enrollments: *263* • Full-Time Enrollment: *127* • Part-Time Enrollment: *136* • Female Enrollment: *256* • Male Enrollment: *7* • Total Graduates: *147*

FINANCES

Residental Annual Tuition: *$23,636* • Non-Residential Annual Tuition: *$23,636* • General Institutional Fees: *$1,272* • Additional Nursing Fees: *$488*

UNIVERSITY OF PITTSBURGH

Address: 3500 Victoria St Building 350, Pittsburgh, PA 16701
Phone: 412-624-6910
Fax: Not Provided
Contact: Kathleen T. Lucke, PhD, RN, CNRN, Assistant Dean for Student Services
Email: luck01+@pitt.edu

GENERAL INFORMATION

Type of School: *4-Year College or University, Private (Independent)* • Accreditation: *Middle States Association of Colleges and Schools* • Total Enrollment: *21800*

PROGRAM INFORMATION

NLNAC Accreditation: *Not Reported* • CCNE Accreditation: *Yes*

For specialty program listings, refer to the index.

NURSING STUDENT PROFILE

Total Nursing Enrollments: *237* • Full-Time Enrollment: *96* • Part-Time Enrollment: *141* • Female Enrollment: *193* • Male Enrollment: *44* • Total Graduates: *88*

FINANCES

Residental Annual Tuition: *$9,778* • Non-Residential Annual Tuition: *$20,146* • General Institutional Fees: *$251* • Additional Nursing Fees: *$11*

UNIVERSITY OF SCRANTON

Address: 800 Linden Street, Scranton, PA 18510
Phone: 570-941-7673
Fax: 570-941-7903
Contact: Mary Jane S. Hanson, PhD, RN, CRNP, CS, Associate Professor
Email: hansonm2@scranton.edu

GENERAL INFORMATION

Type of School: *4-Year College or University, Private (Independent)* • Accreditation: *Middle States Association of Colleges and Schools* • Total Enrollment: *1650*

PROGRAM INFORMATION

NLNAC Accreditation: *Yes* • CCNE Accreditation:

_____

For specialty program listings, refer to the index.

NURSING STUDENT PROFILE

Total Nursing Enrollments: *60* • Full-Time Enrollment: *13* • Part-Time Enrollment: *47* • Female Enrollment: *58* • Male Enrollment: *2* • Total Graduates: *0*

FINANCES

Residental Annual Tuition: *$12,120* • Non-Residential Annual Tuition: *$12,120* • General Institutional Fees: *$100* • Additional Nursing Fees: *$220*

VILLANOVA UNIVERSITY

Address: 2925 North Landing Road, Villanova, PA 19085
Phone: 610-519-4907
Fax: 610-519-7650
Contact: Claire Manfredi, EdD, RN, MSN, MA, Professor and Director, Graduate Nursing Programs
Email: claire.manfredi@villanova.edu

GENERAL INFORMATION

Type of School: *Not Reported, Other* • Accreditation: *Middle States Association of Colleges and Schools* • Total Enrollment: *Not Provided*

PROGRAM INFORMATION

NLNAC Accreditation: *Yes* • CCNE Accreditation: *Yes*

_____

For specialty program listings, refer to the index.

NURSING STUDENT PROFILE

Total Nursing Enrollments: *148* • Full-Time Enrollment: *44* • Part-Time Enrollment: *104* • Female Enrollment: *133* • Male Enrollment: *15* • Total Graduates: *41*

FINANCES

Residental Annual Tuition: *$12,000* • Non-Residential Annual Tuition: *$12,000* • General Institutional Fees: *$30* • Additional Nursing Fees: *$0*

Circle 142 on reader card   **See in-depth profile for more information**

WEST CHESTER UNIVERSITY

Address: PO Box 277, West Chester, PA 19383
Phone: 610-436-2258
Fax: 610-436-3083
Contact: Janet S. Hickman, EdD, RN, Graduate Program
            Coordinator
Email: jhickman@wcupa.edu

GENERAL INFORMATION

Type of School: *4-Year College or University, Public* •
Accreditation: *Middle States Association of Colleges and
Schools* • Total Enrollment: *2150*

PROGRAM INFORMATION

NLNAC Accreditation: *Yes* • CCNE Accreditation: *No*

For specialty program listings, refer to the index.

NURSING STUDENT PROFILE

Total Nursing Enrollments: *20* • Full-Time Enrollment: *2* •
Part-Time Enrollment: *18* • Female Enrollment: *20* • Male
Enrollment: *0* • Total Graduates: *6*

FINANCES

Residental Annual Tuition: *$5,520* • Non-Residential
Annual Tuition: *$9,336* • General Institutional Fees: *$768* •
Additional Nursing Fees: *Not Reported*

WIDENER UNIVERSITY

Address: One University Place, Chester, PA 19013
Phone: 610-499-4208
Fax: 610-499-4216
Contact: Mary B. Walker, EdD, RN, Assistant Dean for
            Graduate Studies
Email: mary.b.walker@widener.edu

GENERAL INFORMATION

Type of School: *4-Year College or University, Public* •
Accreditation: *Middle States Association of Colleges and
Schools* • Total Enrollment: *500*

PROGRAM INFORMATION

NLNAC Accreditation: *Yes* • CCNE Accreditation: *No*

For specialty program listings, refer to the index.

NURSING STUDENT PROFILE

Total Nursing Enrollments: *104* • Full-Time Enrollment:
15 • Part-Time Enrollment: *89* • Female Enrollment: *93* •
Male Enrollment: *11* • Total Graduates: *42*

FINANCES

Residental Annual Tuition: *$525* • Non-Residential Annual
Tuition: *$525* • General Institutional Fees: *$100* • Additional
Nursing Fees: *$140*

WILKES UNIVERSITY

Address: 109 S Franklin St, Wilkes-Barre, PA 18766
Phone: 570-408-4074
Fax: 570-408-9807
Contact: Mary Ann Merrigan, PhD, RN, Chairperson
Email: merrigan@wilkes.edu

GENERAL INFORMATION

Type of School: *Not Provided* • Accreditation: *Middle States Association of Colleges and Schools* • Total Enrollment: *4000*

PROGRAM INFORMATION

NLNAC Accreditation: *Not Reported* • CCNE Accreditation: *Yes*

―――――――

For specialty program listings, refer to the index.

NURSING STUDENT PROFILE

Total Nursing Enrollments: *20* • Full-Time Enrollment: *7* • Part-Time Enrollment: *13* • Female Enrollment: *17* • Male Enrollment: *3* • Total Graduates: *9*

FINANCES

Residental Annual Tuition: *$13,008* • Non-Residential Annual Tuition: *$13,008* • General Institutional Fees: *$200* • Additional Nursing Fees: *Not Reported*

PONTIFICAL CATHOLIC UNIVERSITY—PUERTO RICO

Address: 1401 S. US 421, Ponce, PR 00717-0777
Phone: 787-841-2000
Fax: Not Provided
Contact: Mildred Lespier, MSN, Master of Nursing
          Coordinator
Email: mlespier@pucpr.edu

GENERAL INFORMATION

Type of School: *Not Provided* • Accreditation: *Not Provided* • Total Enrollment: *2300*

PROGRAM INFORMATION

NLNAC Accreditation: *Yes* • CCNE Accreditation: *No*

―――――――

For specialty program listings, refer to the index.

NURSING STUDENT PROFILE

Total Nursing Enrollments: *53* • Full-Time Enrollment: *21* • Part-Time Enrollment: *32* • Female Enrollment: *49* • Male Enrollment: *4* • Total Graduates: *17*

FINANCES

Residental Annual Tuition: *$3,600* • Non-Residential Annual Tuition: *$3,600* • General Institutional Fees: *$470* • Additional Nursing Fees: *$1,800*

UNIVERSITY OF PUERTO RICO—MAYAGUEZ

Address: PO Box 9015, San Juan, PR 00681-9015
Phone: 787-758-2525
Fax: 787-281-0721
Contact: Rebecca Alberti, ND, MS, FNP, Director
Email: ralberti@rcm.upr.edu

GENERAL INFORMATION

Type of School: *Governmental Agency, Public (Religious)* •
Accreditation: *Middle States Association* • Total Enrollment:
12000

PROGRAM INFORMATION

NLNAC Accreditation: *No* • CCNE Accreditation: *No*

For specialty program listings, refer to the index.

NURSING STUDENT PROFILE

Total Nursing Enrollments: *162* • Full-Time Enrollment:
162 • Part-Time Enrollment: *0* • Female Enrollment: *134* •
Male Enrollment: *28* • Total Graduates: *59*

FINANCES

Residental Annual Tuition: *Not Provided* • Non-Residential
Annual Tuition: *Not Provided* • General Institutional Fees:
Not Provided • Additional Nursing Fees: *Not Provided*

UNIVERSITY OF RHODE ISLAND

Address: White Hall, 2 Heathman Road, Kingston, RI
02881
Phone: 401-874-5337
Fax: Not Provided
Contact: Donna Schwartz-Barcott, PhD, RN, Professor
and Director of Graduate Studies in Nursing
Email: dsb@uri.edu

GENERAL INFORMATION

Type of School: *4-Year College or University, Public* •
Accreditation: *New England Association of Schools and
Colleges* • Total Enrollment: *Not Provided*

PROGRAM INFORMATION

NLNAC Accreditation: *Yes* • CCNE Accreditation: *No*

For specialty program listings, refer to the index.

NURSING STUDENT PROFILE

Total Nursing Enrollments: *102* • Full-Time Enrollment:
42 • Part-Time Enrollment: *60* • Female Enrollment: *96* •
Male Enrollment: *6* • Total Graduates: *32*

FINANCES

Residental Annual Tuition: *$3,540* • Non-Residential
Annual Tuition: *$10,116* • General Institutional Fees: *$626* •
Additional Nursing Fees: *$75*

CLEMSON UNIVERSITY

Address: 510 Edwards Hall, Clemson, SC 29634
Phone: 864-656-5528
Fax: 864-656-5488
Contact: Rosanne H. Pruitt, PhD, RNC, FNP, Professor
Email: prosan@clemson.edu

MEDICAL UNIVERSITY OF SOUTH CAROLINA

Address: P. O. Box 173362, Charleston, SC 29425
Phone: 843-792-0686
Fax: 843-792-9258
Contact: Jean D'Meza Leuner, PhD, RN, Associate Dean
           for Academics and Evaluation
Email: leunerj@musc.edu

GENERAL INFORMATION

Type of School: *4-Year College or University, Public* •
Accreditation: *Southern Association of Colleges and Schools* •
Total Enrollment: *Not Provided*

GENERAL INFORMATION

Type of School: *Other* • Accreditation: *Southern Association of Colleges and Schools* • Total Enrollment: *1939*

PROGRAM INFORMATION

NLNAC Accreditation: *Yes* • CCNE Accreditation: *No*

For specialty program listings, refer to the index.

PROGRAM INFORMATION

NLNAC Accreditation: *Yes* • CCNE Accreditation: *No*

For specialty program listings, refer to the index.

NURSING STUDENT PROFILE

Total Nursing Enrollments: 55 • Full-Time Enrollment: *16* •
Part-Time Enrollment: *39* • Female Enrollment: *50* • Male
Enrollment: *5* • Total Graduates: *15*

NURSING STUDENT PROFILE

Total Nursing Enrollments: *122* • Full-Time Enrollment:
51 • Part-Time Enrollment: *71* • Female Enrollment: *114* •
Male Enrollment: *8* • Total Graduates: *67*

FINANCES

Residental Annual Tuition: *$3,810* • Non-Residential
Annual Tuition: *$9,784* • General Institutional Fees: *$240* •
Additional Nursing Fees: *$80*

FINANCES

Residental Annual Tuition: *$4,578* • Non-Residential
Annual Tuition: *$6,872* • General Institutional Fees: *$176* •
Additional Nursing Fees: *$600*

UNIVERSITY OF SOUTH CAROLINA—COLUMBIA

Address: 414 East Clark, Julian Hall 212, Columbia, SC 29208
Phone: 803-777-3862
Fax: 803-777-2027
Contact: Mary Ann Parsons, PhD, Dean
Email: maryann.parsons@sc.edu

GENERAL INFORMATION

Type of School: *4-Year College or University, Public* • Accreditation: *Southern Association of Colleges and Schools* • Total Enrollment: *11792*

PROGRAM INFORMATION

NLNAC Accreditation: *Yes* • CCNE Accreditation: *Yes*

For specialty program listings, refer to the index.

NURSING STUDENT PROFILE

Total Nursing Enrollments: *89* • Full-Time Enrollment: *28* • Part-Time Enrollment: *61* • Female Enrollment: *87* • Male Enrollment: *2* • Total Graduates: *41*

FINANCES

Residental Annual Tuition: *$5,410* • Non-Residential Annual Tuition: *$11,236* • General Institutional Fees: *$100* • Additional Nursing Fees: *$22*

AUGUSTANA COLLEGE

Address: 2001 South Summit Avenue, Sioux Falls, SD 57197
Phone: 605-274-4729
Fax: 605-274-4723
Contact: Margot Nelson, PhD, RN, Assoc. Professor and Master's Program Coordinator
Email: mnelson@inst.augie.edu

GENERAL INFORMATION

Type of School: *4-Year College or University, Private (Religious)* • Accreditation: *North Central Association of Colleges and Schools* • Total Enrollment: *1783*

PROGRAM INFORMATION

NLNAC Accreditation: *No* • CCNE Accreditation: *Yes*

For specialty program listings, refer to the index.

NURSING STUDENT PROFILE

Total Nursing Enrollments: *33* • Full-Time Enrollment: *0* • Part-Time Enrollment: *33* • Female Enrollment: *32* • Male Enrollment: *1* • Total Graduates: *9*

FINANCES

Residental Annual Tuition: *$6,420* • Non-Residential Annual Tuition: *$6,420* • General Institutional Fees: *$0* • Additional Nursing Fees: *$15*

SOUTH DAKOTA STATE UNIVERSITY

Address: 1819 Broadway, Brookings, SD 57007
Phone: 605-688-4114
Fax: 605-688-6119
Contact: Penny Powers, PhD, RN, Department Head,
             Graduate Nursing
Email: Penny_Powers@sdstate.edu

GENERAL INFORMATION

Type of School: *4-Year College or University, Public* •
Accreditation: *North Central Association of Colleges and
Schools* • Total Enrollment: *Not Provided*

PROGRAM INFORMATION

NLNAC Accreditation: *Yes* • CCNE Accreditation: *No*

_____

For specialty program listings, refer to the index.

NURSING STUDENT PROFILE

Total Nursing Enrollments: *85* • Full-Time Enrollment: *11* •
Part-Time Enrollment: *74* • Female Enrollment: *78* • Male
Enrollment: *7* • Total Graduates: *23*

FINANCES

Residental Annual Tuition: *$2,017* • Non-Residential
Annual Tuition: *$5,949* • General Institutional Fees: *$104* •
Additional Nursing Fees: *$288*

BELMONT UNIVERSITY

Address: 1900 Belmont Boulevard, Nashville, TN 37212
Phone: 615-460-6142
Fax: Not Provided
Contact: Leslie J. Higgins, PhD, RN, CFNP, Director,
             Graduate Studies in Nursing
Email: higginsl@mail.belmont.edu

GENERAL INFORMATION

Type of School: *4-Year College or University, Private
(Religious)* • Accreditation: *Southern Association of Colleges
and Schools* • Total Enrollment: *3026*

PROGRAM INFORMATION

NLNAC Accreditation: *Yes* • CCNE Accreditation:

_____

For specialty program listings, refer to the index.

NURSING STUDENT PROFILE

Total Nursing Enrollments: *15* • Full-Time Enrollment: *5* •
Part-Time Enrollment: *10* • Female Enrollment: *15* • Male
Enrollment: *0* • Total Graduates: *15*

FINANCES

Residental Annual Tuition: *$10,530* • Non-Residential
Annual Tuition: *$10,530* • General Institutional Fees: *$0* •
Additional Nursing Fees: *$0*

CARSON NEWMAN COLLEGE

Address: 1646 Russell Avenue, Hammond, TN 37760
Phone: 865-471-3426
Fax: Not Provided
Contact: Ann Harley, PhD, Dean and Chair, Graduate
           Studies in Nursing
Email: harley@cncacc.cn.edu

GENERAL INFORMATION

Type of School: _4-Year College or University, Private
(Religious)_ • Accreditation: _Southern Association of Colleges
and Schools_ • Total Enrollment: _2230_

PROGRAM INFORMATION

NLNAC Accreditation: _Yes_ • CCNE Accreditation: _No_

For specialty program listings, refer to the index.

NURSING STUDENT PROFILE

Total Nursing Enrollments: _23_ • Full-Time Enrollment: _17_ •
Part-Time Enrollment: _6_ • Female Enrollment: _21_ • Male
Enrollment: _2_ • Total Graduates: _5_

FINANCES

Residental Annual Tuition: _$8,100_ • Non-Residential
Annual Tuition: _$8,100_ • General Institutional Fees: _$250_ •
Additional Nursing Fees: _$80_

EAST TENNESSEE STATE UNIVERSITY

Address: P.O. Box 70617, Johnson City, TN 37614
Phone: 423-439-4624
Fax: 423-439-4522
Contact: Patricia Smith, EdD, RN, Associate Dean,
           Academic Programs
Email: smithp@etsu.edu

GENERAL INFORMATION

Type of School: _Other_ • Accreditation: _Southern Association of
Colleges and Schools_ • Total Enrollment: _Not Provided_

PROGRAM INFORMATION

NLNAC Accreditation: _Yes_ • CCNE Accreditation: _No_

For specialty program listings, refer to the index.

NURSING STUDENT PROFILE

Total Nursing Enrollments: _91_ • Full-Time Enrollment: _43_ •
Part-Time Enrollment: _48_ • Female Enrollment: _74_ • Male
Enrollment: _17_ • Total Graduates: _36_

FINANCES

Residental Annual Tuition: _$3,592_ • Non-Residential
Annual Tuition: _$10,064_ • General Institutional Fees: _$203_ •
Additional Nursing Fees: _$0_

SOUTHERN ADVENTIST UNIVERSITY

Address: P.O. Box 370, Collegedale, TN 37315
Phone: 423-238-2942
Fax: 423-238-3004
Contact: L. Phil Hunt, EdD, MEd, RN, Dean and
           Professor
Email: phunt@southern.edu

GENERAL INFORMATION

Type of School: *4-Year College or University, Private (Religious)* • Accreditation: *Southern Association of Colleges and Schools* • Total Enrollment: *1800*

PROGRAM INFORMATION

NLNAC Accreditation: *Not Reported* • CCNE Accreditation: *No*

For specialty program listings, refer to the index.

NURSING STUDENT PROFILE

Total Nursing Enrollments: *17* • Full-Time Enrollment: *0* • Part-Time Enrollment: *17* • Female Enrollment: *16* • Male Enrollment: *1* • Total Graduates: *Not Provided*

FINANCES

Residental Annual Tuition: *$5,580* • Non-Residential Annual Tuition: *$5,580* • General Institutional Fees: *Not Reported* • Additional Nursing Fees: *Not Reported*

TENNESSEE STATE UNIVERSITY

Address: 5201 University Boulevard, Nashville, TN
          37209-1561
Phone: 615-963-5261
Fax: 615-963-7614
Contact: Barbara E. Brown, EdD, MSN, BSN, MSN
          Director
Email: bbrown@tnstate.edu

GENERAL INFORMATION

Type of School: *4-Year College or University, Public* • Accreditation: *Southern Association of Colleges and Schools* • Total Enrollment: *3405*

PROGRAM INFORMATION

NLNAC Accreditation: *Yes* • CCNE Accreditation: *No*

For specialty program listings, refer to the index.

NURSING STUDENT PROFILE

Total Nursing Enrollments: *16* • Full-Time Enrollment: *7* • Part-Time Enrollment: *9* • Female Enrollment: *16* • Male Enrollment: *0* • Total Graduates: *13*

FINANCES

Residental Annual Tuition: *$2,962* • Non-Residential Annual Tuition: *$7,788* • General Institutional Fees: *Not Reported* • Additional Nursing Fees: *Not Reported*

UNIVERSITY OF TENNESSEE— CHATTANOOGA

Address: 615 McCallie Avenue, Chattanooga, TN 37403
Phone: 423-755-4724
Fax: 423-755-4668
Contact: Dana Hames Wertenberger, PhD, RN, Director and Professor
Email: Dana-Wertenberger@utc.edu

GENERAL INFORMATION

Type of School: *4-Year College or University, Public* •
Accreditation: *Southern Association of Colleges and Schools* •
Total Enrollment: *5877*

PROGRAM INFORMATION

NLNAC Accreditation: *Not Reported* • CCNE Accreditation: *Yes*

_____

For specialty program listings, refer to the index.

NURSING STUDENT PROFILE

Total Nursing Enrollments: *64* • Full-Time Enrollment: *55* •
Part-Time Enrollment: *9* • Female Enrollment: *43* • Male
Enrollment: *21* • Total Graduates: *23*

FINANCES

Residental Annual Tuition: *$3,214* • Non-Residential
Annual Tuition: *$9,744* • General Institutional Fees: *$538* •
Additional Nursing Fees: *$42*

THE UNIVERSITY OF TENNESSEE—KNOXVILLE

Address: 1200 Volunteer Boulevard, Knoxville, TN 37996
Phone: 865-974-6804
Fax: 865-974-3569
Contact: Martha R. Alligood, PhD, RN, Chair
Email: malligoo@utk.edu

GENERAL INFORMATION

Type of School: *4-Year College or University, Public* •
Accreditation: *Southern Association of Colleges and Schools* •
Total Enrollment: *26000*

PROGRAM INFORMATION

NLNAC Accreditation: *Yes* • CCNE Accreditation: *No*

_____

For specialty program listings, refer to the index.

NURSING STUDENT PROFILE

Total Nursing Enrollments: *40* • Full-Time Enrollment: *25* •
Part-Time Enrollment: *15* • Female Enrollment: *38* • Male
Enrollment: *2* • Total Graduates: *22*

FINANCES

Residental Annual Tuition: *$4,004* • Non-Residential
Annual Tuition: *$10,596* • General Institutional Fees: *$550* •
Additional Nursing Fees: *$19*

UNIVERSITY OF TENNESSEE— MEMPHIS

Address: 877 Madison Ave, Memphis, TN 38163
Phone: 901-448-6128
Fax: Not Provided
Contact: Michael A. Carter, DNSc, Professor and Dean
Email: mcarter@utmem.edu

GENERAL INFORMATION

Type of School: *4-Year College or University, Public* •
Accreditation: *Southern Association of Colleges and Schools* •
Total Enrollment: *3474*

PROGRAM INFORMATION

NLNAC Accreditation: *No* • CCNE Accreditation: *Yes*

For specialty program listings, refer to the index.

NURSING STUDENT PROFILE

Total Nursing Enrollments: *95* • Full-Time Enrollment: *91* •
Part-Time Enrollment: *4* • Female Enrollment: *71* • Male
Enrollment: *24* • Total Graduates: *47*

FINANCES

Residental Annual Tuition: *$5,184* • Non-Residential
Annual Tuition: *$11,948* • General Institutional Fees: *$60* •
Additional Nursing Fees: *$32*

VANDERBILT UNIVERSITY

Address: 1525 Green Spring Valley Rd, Nashville, TN 37240
Phone: 615-322-3804
Fax: 615-322-1708
Contact: Linda Norman, RN, Chairperson
Email: linda.norman@mcmail.vanderbilt.edu

GENERAL INFORMATION

Type of School: *4-Year College, Private Independent* •
Accreditation: *Southern Association of Colleges and Schools* •
Total Enrollment: *3650*

PROGRAM INFORMATION

NLNAC Accreditation: *Yes* • CCNE Accreditation: *No*

For specialty program listings, refer to the index.

NURSING STUDENT PROFILE

Total Nursing Enrollments: *383* • Full-Time Enrollment:
316 • Part-Time Enrollment: *67* • Female Enrollment: *339* •
Male Enrollment: *44* • Total Graduates: *219*

FINANCES

Residental Annual Tuition: *$24,900* • Non-Residential
Annual Tuition: *$24,900* • General Institutional Fees: *$961* •
Additional Nursing Fees: *$263*

ACU-HSU-MCM CONSORTIUM

Address: 2149 Hickory, Abilene, TX 79601
Phone: 915-672-2441
Fax: 915-672-5023
Contact: Cecilia Tiller, RNC, DSN, WHNP, Dean and Professor
Email: ctiller.aisn@hsutx.edu

GENERAL INFORMATION

Type of School: *Not Provided* • Accreditation: *Southern Association of Colleges and Schools* • Total Enrollment: *Not Provided*

PROGRAM INFORMATION

NLNAC Accreditation: *Not Reported* • CCNE Accreditation: *Yes*

_____

For specialty program listings, refer to the index.

NURSING STUDENT PROFILE

Total Nursing Enrollments: *21* • Full-Time Enrollment: *16* • Part-Time Enrollment: *5* • Female Enrollment: *17* • Male Enrollment: *4* • Total Graduates: *3*

FINANCES

Residental Annual Tuition: *$8,040* • Non-Residential Annual Tuition: *$8,040* • General Institutional Fees: *$300* • Additional Nursing Fees: *$100*

ANGELO STATE UNIVERSITY

Address: 2601 W. Ave. N, San Angelo, TX 76909
Phone: 915-942-2224
Fax: 915-942-2236
Contact: Leslie M. Mayrand, PhD, RN, CNS, Graduate Advisor and Program Director
Email: leslie.mayrand@angelo.edu

GENERAL INFORMATION

Type of School: *4-Year College or University, Public* • Accreditation: *Southern Association of Colleges and Schools* • Total Enrollment: *6000*

PROGRAM INFORMATION

NLNAC Accreditation: *Yes* • CCNE Accreditation: *No*

_____

For specialty program listings, refer to the index.

NURSING STUDENT PROFILE

Total Nursing Enrollments: *16* • Full-Time Enrollment: *0* • Part-Time Enrollment: *16* • Female Enrollment: *13* • Male Enrollment: *3* • Total Graduates: *3*

FINANCES

Residental Annual Tuition: *$1,043* • Non-Residential Annual Tuition: *$3,623* • General Institutional Fees: *$563* • Additional Nursing Fees: *$0*

BAYLOR UNIVERSITY

Address: 3700 Worth Street, Dallas, TX 75246
Phone: 214-820-4191
Fax: 214-818-8692
Contact: Pauline T. Johnson, PhD, RN, Professor and Director of the Graduate Program
Email: Pauline_Johnson@baylor.edu

GENERAL INFORMATION

Type of School: *4-Year College or University, Private (Religious)* • Accreditation: *Southern Association of Colleges and Schools* • Total Enrollment: *13000*

PROGRAM INFORMATION

NLNAC Accreditation: *Not Reported* • CCNE Accreditation: *Yes*

_____

For specialty program listings, refer to the index.

NURSING STUDENT PROFILE

Total Nursing Enrollments: *43* • Full-Time Enrollment: *16* • Part-Time Enrollment: *27* • Female Enrollment: *40* • Male Enrollment: *3* • Total Graduates: *8*

FINANCES

Residental Annual Tuition: *$379* • Non-Residential Annual Tuition: *$379* • General Institutional Fees: *$1,180* • Additional Nursing Fees: *$300*

HOUSTON BAPTIST UNIVERSITY

Address: 7502 Fondren Rd, Houston, TX 21044
Phone: 281-649-3300
Fax: 281-649-3340
Contact: Nancy Yuill, PhD, RN, Dean, College of Nursing
Email: nyuill@hbu.edu

GENERAL INFORMATION

Type of School: *4-Year College or University, Private Independent* • Accreditation: *Southern Association of Colleges and Schools* • Total Enrollment: *2300*

PROGRAM INFORMATION

NLNAC Accreditation: *No* • CCNE Accreditation:

_____

For specialty program listings, refer to the index.

NURSING STUDENT PROFILE

Total Nursing Enrollments: *30* • Full-Time Enrollment: *5* • Part-Time Enrollment: *25* • Female Enrollment: *29* • Male Enrollment: *1* • Total Graduates: *5*

FINANCES

Residental Annual Tuition: *$8,750* • Non-Residential Annual Tuition: *$8,750* • General Institutional Fees: *$940* • Additional Nursing Fees: *$128*

MIDWESTERN STATE UNIVERSITY

Address: 2715 Dickinson Street, Wichita Falls, TX 76308
Phone: 940-397-4594
Fax: Not Provided
Contact: Susan Sportsman, PhD, RN, Dean
Email: fsprtsms@nexos.mwsu.edu

GENERAL INFORMATION

Type of School: *4-Year College or University, Private (Religious)* • Accreditation: *Southern Association of Colleges and Schools* • Total Enrollment: *Not Provided*

PROGRAM INFORMATION

NLNAC Accreditation: *Yes* • CCNE Accreditation:

_____

For specialty program listings, refer to the index.

NURSING STUDENT PROFILE

Total Nursing Enrollments: *15* • Full-Time Enrollment: *2* • Part-Time Enrollment: *13* • Female Enrollment: *13* • Male Enrollment: *2* • Total Graduates: *2*

FINANCES

Residental Annual Tuition: *$864* • Non-Residential Annual Tuition: *$4,752* • General Institutional Fees: *$600* • Additional Nursing Fees: *$164*

TEXAS A&M UNIVERSITY— CORPUS CRISTI

Address: 6300 Ocean Drive, Corpus Christi, TX 78412
Phone: 361-825-3323
Fax: 361-825-2484
Contact: Joyce Esperanza, EdD, RN, Outreach Coordinator and Professor
Email: ejoyce@falcon.tamucc.edu

GENERAL INFORMATION

Type of School: *4-Year College or University, Public* • Accreditation: *Southern Association of Colleges and Schools* • Total Enrollment: *3735*

PROGRAM INFORMATION

NLNAC Accreditation: *No* • CCNE Accreditation: *No*

_____

For specialty program listings, refer to the index.

NURSING STUDENT PROFILE

Total Nursing Enrollments: *80* • Full-Time Enrollment: *9* • Part-Time Enrollment: *71* • Female Enrollment: *60* • Male Enrollment: *20* • Total Graduates: *26*

FINANCES

Residental Annual Tuition: *$2,880* • Non-Residential Annual Tuition: *$6,120* • General Institutional Fees: *Not Reported* • Additional Nursing Fees: *Not Reported*

TEXAS TECH UNIVERSITY HEALTH SCIENCES CENTER

Address: 1241 Hawthorne Suite 228, Lubbock, TX 79430
Phone: 806-743-3055
Fax: 806-743-1622
Contact: Barbara Johnston, PhD, RN, Associate Dean, Graduate Program
Email: barbara.johnston@ttmc.ttuhsc.edu

GENERAL INFORMATION

Type of School: *Not Provided, Public* • Accreditation: *SACS* • Total Enrollment: *1788*

PROGRAM INFORMATION

NLNAC Accreditation: *Yes* • CCNE Accreditation: *Yes*

For specialty program listings, refer to the index.

NURSING STUDENT PROFILE

Total Nursing Enrollments: *64* • Full-Time Enrollment: *3* • Part-Time Enrollment: *61* • Female Enrollment: *56* • Male Enrollment: *8* • Total Graduates: *10*

FINANCES

Residental Annual Tuition: *$1,566* • Non-Residential Annual Tuition: *$7,398* • General Institutional Fees: *$116* • Additional Nursing Fees: *$83*

TEXAS WOMAN'S UNIVERSITY

Address: 101 West State Street, Denton, TX 76201
Phone: 940-898-2401
Fax: 940-898-2437
Contact: Carolyn S. Gunning, PhD, RN, Dean
Email: cgunning@twu.edu

GENERAL INFORMATION

Type of School: *4-Year College or University, Private (Independent)* • Accreditation: *Not Provided* • Total Enrollment: *1788*

PROGRAM INFORMATION

NLNAC Accreditation: *Yes* • CCNE Accreditation: *No*

For specialty program listings, refer to the index.

NURSING STUDENT PROFILE

Total Nursing Enrollments: *283* • Full-Time Enrollment: *47* • Part-Time Enrollment: *236* • Female Enrollment: *267* • Male Enrollment: *16* • Total Graduates: *57*

FINANCES

Residental Annual Tuition: *Not Reported* • Non-Residential Annual Tuition: *Not Reported* • General Institutional Fees: *Not Reported* • Additional Nursing Fees: *Not Reported*

UNIVERSITY OF TEXAS— ARLINGTON

Address: 411 S Nedderman Drive, Arlington, TX 76019
Phone: 817-272-2776
Fax: 817-272-5006
Contact: Susan K. Grove, PhD, RN, Assistant Dean
Email: grove@uta.edu

GENERAL INFORMATION

Type of School: *4-Year College or University, Public* •
Accreditation: *Southern Association of Colleges and Schools* •
Total Enrollment: *Not Provided*

PROGRAM INFORMATION

NLNAC Accreditation: *Yes* • CCNE Accreditation:

_____

For specialty program listings, refer to the index.

NURSING STUDENT PROFILE

Total Nursing Enrollments: *Not Provided* • Full-Time
Enrollment: *Not Provided* • Part-Time Enrollment: *Not
Provided* • Female Enrollment: *Not Provided* • Male
Enrollment: *Not Provided* • Total Graduates: *Not Provided*

FINANCES

Residental Annual Tuition: *Not Reported* • Non-Residential
Annual Tuition: *Not Reported* • General Institutional Fees:
Not Reported • Additional Nursing Fees: *Not Reported*

UNIVERSITY OF TEXAS— AUSTIN

Address: 1700 Red River, Austin, TX 78701
Phone: 512-232-4751
Fax: Not Provided
Contact: Lorraine O. Walker, EdD, RN, FAAN, Assistant Dean
Email: walkerl@mail.utexas.edu

GENERAL INFORMATION

Type of School: *4-Year College, Public* • Accreditation: *Data
Not Provided* • Total Enrollment: 2874

PROGRAM INFORMATION

NLNAC Accreditation: *No* • CCNE Accreditation: *No*

_____

For specialty program listings, refer to the index.

NURSING STUDENT PROFILE

Total Nursing Enrollments: *149* • Full-Time Enrollment:
107 • Part-Time Enrollment: *42* • Female Enrollment: *136* •
Male Enrollment: *13* • Total Graduates: *47*

FINANCES

Residental Annual Tuition: *$2,052* • Non-Residential
Annual Tuition: *$5,940* • General Institutional Fees: *$650* •
Additional Nursing Fees: *$430*

UNIVERSITY OF TEXAS— BROWNSVILLE AND TEXAS SOUTHMOST COLLEGE

Address: 80 Fort Brown, Brownsville, TX 78520
Phone: 956-574-6690
Fax: 956-574-6778
Contact: Ella Herriage, PhD, RN, MPH, Director, Graduate Program
Email: eherriage@utbl.utb.edu

GENERAL INFORMATION

Type of School: *4-Year College or University, Public* •
Accreditation: *Southern Association of Colleges and Schools* •
Total Enrollment: *1927*

PROGRAM INFORMATION

NLNAC Accreditation: *Not Reported* • CCNE Accreditation:

_____

For specialty program listings, refer to the index.

NURSING STUDENT PROFILE

Total Nursing Enrollments: *15* • Full-Time Enrollment: *15* •
Part-Time Enrollment: *0* • Female Enrollment: *14* • Male
Enrollment: *1* • Total Graduates: *Not Provided*

FINANCES

Residental Annual Tuition: *$864* • Non-Residential Annual
Tuition: *$4,770* • General Institutional Fees: *$864* •
Additional Nursing Fees: *$0*

UNIVERSITY OF TEXAS— EL PASO

Address: 1101 N. Campbell, El Paso, TX 79902
Phone: 915-747-7230
Fax: Not Provided
Contact: Dorothy Stuppy, PhD, RN, Graduate Program Coordinator
Email: dstuppy@utep.edu

GENERAL INFORMATION

Type of School: *4-Year College or University, Public* •
Accreditation: *Southern Association of Colleges and Schools* •
Total Enrollment: *8485*

PROGRAM INFORMATION

NLNAC Accreditation: *Not Reported* • CCNE Accreditation:

_____

For specialty program listings, refer to the index.

NURSING STUDENT PROFILE

Total Nursing Enrollments: *90* • Full-Time Enrollment: *20* •
Part-Time Enrollment: *70* • Female Enrollment: *Not
Provided* • Male Enrollment: *Not Provided* • Total Graduates:
30

FINANCES

Residental Annual Tuition: *Not Reported* • Non-Residential
Annual Tuition: *Not Reported* • General Institutional Fees:
Not Reported • Additional Nursing Fees: *Not Reported*

UNIVERSITY OF TEXAS— PAN AMERICAN

Address: 1201 W. University Drive, Edinburg, TX 78539
Phone: 956-316-7082
Fax: 956-381-2384
Contact: Barbara Tucker, PhD, RNSC, FNP, MSN
Program Coordinator
Email: msnprogram@panam.edu

GENERAL INFORMATION

Type of School: *4-Year College or University, Public* •
Accreditation: *Southern Association of Colleges and Schools* •
Total Enrollment: *20424*

PROGRAM INFORMATION

NLNAC Accreditation: *Yes* • CCNE Accreditation:
Provisional

For specialty program listings, refer to the index.

NURSING STUDENT PROFILE

Total Nursing Enrollments: *55* • Full-Time Enrollment: *15* •
Part-Time Enrollment: *40* • Female Enrollment: *41* • Male
Enrollment: *14* • Total Graduates: *8*

FINANCES

Residental Annual Tuition: *$1,877* • Non-Residential
Annual Tuition: *$5,747* • General Institutional Fees: *$450* •
Additional Nursing Fees: *$61*

UNIVERSITY OF TEXAS— TYLER

Address: 3900 University Blvd, Tyler, TX 75799
Phone: 903-566-7220
Fax: 903-565-5533
Contact: Susan Yarbrough, PhD, RN, Assistant Dean for
Graduate Nursing Programs
Email: syarbrough@mail.uttly.edu

GENERAL INFORMATION

Type of School: *4-Year College or University, Public* •
Accreditation: *Southern Association of Colleges and Schools* •
Total Enrollment: *Not Provided*

PROGRAM INFORMATION

NLNAC Accreditation: *Yes* • CCNE Accreditation:
Provisional

For specialty program listings, refer to the index.

NURSING STUDENT PROFILE

Total Nursing Enrollments: *60* • Full-Time Enrollment: *8* •
Part-Time Enrollment: *52* • Female Enrollment: *52* • Male
Enrollment: *8* • Total Graduates: *4*

FINANCES

Residental Annual Tuition: *$1,008* • Non-Residential
Annual Tuition: *$6,072* • General Institutional Fees:
$1,572 • Additional Nursing Fees: *$125*

UNIVERSITY OF TEXAS HEALTH SCIENCE CENTER— HOUSTON

Address: 1100 Holcombe Blvd, Houston, TX 77030
Phone: 713-500-2002
Fax: Not Provided
Contact: Patricia L. Starck, RN, DSN, FAAN, Dean and
           John P. McGovern Professor
Email: pstarck@sonl.nur.uth.tmc.edu

GENERAL INFORMATION

Type of School: *4-Year College or University, Public* •
Accreditation: *Southern Association of Colleges and Schools* •
Total Enrollment: *Not Provided*

PROGRAM INFORMATION

NLNAC Accreditation: *Yes* • CCNE Accreditation: *No*

For specialty program listings, refer to the index.

NURSING STUDENT PROFILE

Total Nursing Enrollments: *336* • Full-Time Enrollment:
211 • Part-Time Enrollment: *125* • Female Enrollment:
241 • Male Enrollment: *95* • Total Graduates: *110*

FINANCES

Residental Annual Tuition: *$1,566* • Non-Residential
Annual Tuition: *$7,398* • General Institutional Fees: *$116* •
Additional Nursing Fees: *$83*

UNIVERSITY OF TEXAS HEALTH SCIENCE CENTER— SAN ANTONIO

Address: 7703 Floyd Curl Drive - MSC 7942, San
           Antonio, TX 78229-3900
Phone: 210-567-5815
Fax: 210-567-3813
Contact: Beverly H. Robinson, PhD, RN, C, FAAN,
           Professor and Associate Dean for Graduate
           Nursing Program
Email: robinsonb@uthscsa.edu

GENERAL INFORMATION

Type of School: *Other* • Accreditation: *Not Provided* • Total
Enrollment: *2544*

PROGRAM INFORMATION

NLNAC Accreditation: *Yes* • CCNE Accreditation: *No*

For specialty program listings, refer to the index.

NURSING STUDENT PROFILE

Total Nursing Enrollments: *121* • Full-Time Enrollment:
32 • Part-Time Enrollment: *89* • Female Enrollment: *103* •
Male Enrollment: *18* • Total Graduates: *46*

FINANCES

Residental Annual Tuition: *$1,008* • Non-Residential
Annual Tuition: *$6,124* • General Institutional Fees: *$986* •
Additional Nursing Fees: *$60*

UNIVERSITY OF TEXAS MEDICAL BRANCH— GALVESTON

Address: 301 University Blvd, Galveston, TX 77555
Phone: 409-772-7311
Fax: 409-747-1519
Contact: Jeanette C. Hartshorn, PhD, RN, FAAN, Associate Dean for Academic Administration and Director, Master's Program
Email: jhartsho@utmb.edu

GENERAL INFORMATION

Type of School: *Not Provided* • Accreditation: *Not Provided* • Total Enrollment: *2544*

PROGRAM INFORMATION

NLNAC Accreditation: *Yes* • CCNE Accreditation: *Yes*

For specialty program listings, refer to the index.

NURSING STUDENT PROFILE

Total Nursing Enrollments: *83* • Full-Time Enrollment: *48* • Part-Time Enrollment: *35* • Female Enrollment: *77* • Male Enrollment: *6* • Total Graduates: *31*

FINANCES

Residental Annual Tuition: *$960* • Non-Residential Annual Tuition: *$6,120* • General Institutional Fees: *$1,745* • Additional Nursing Fees: *$60*

UNIVERSITY OF THE INCARNATE WORD

Address: 600 S College Ave, San Antonio, TX 78209-6397
Phone: 210-829-3988
Fax: 210-829-3174
Contact: Sandra Strickland, PhD, RN, Associate Professor and Chair, MSN Program
Email: strickla@universe.uiwtx.edu

GENERAL INFORMATION

Type of School: *Not Provided* • Accreditation: *Not Provided* • Total Enrollment: *3742*

PROGRAM INFORMATION

NLNAC Accreditation: *Yes* • CCNE Accreditation: *Yes*

For specialty program listings, refer to the index.

NURSING STUDENT PROFILE

Total Nursing Enrollments: *33* • Full-Time Enrollment: *4* • Part-Time Enrollment: *29* • Female Enrollment: *29* • Male Enrollment: *4* • Total Graduates: *13*

FINANCES

Residental Annual Tuition: *$445* • Non-Residential Annual Tuition: *$445* • General Institutional Fees: *Not Reported* • Additional Nursing Fees: *Not Reported*

WEST TEXAS A&M UNIVERSITY

Address: 2501 Fourth Avenue, Canyon, TX 79016
Phone: 806-651-2641
Fax: 806-651-2632
Contact: Barbara Biehler, EdD, RN, PNP, Graduate
           Program Coordinator
Email: bbiehler@mail.wtamu.edu

GENERAL INFORMATION

Type of School: *4-Year College or University, Public* •
Accreditation: *Southern Association of Colleges and Schools* •
Total Enrollment: *2450*

PROGRAM INFORMATION

NLNAC Accreditation: *Not Reported* • CCNE Accreditation:
Yes

———

For specialty program listings, refer to the index.

NURSING STUDENT PROFILE

Total Nursing Enrollments: *40* • Full-Time Enrollment: *34* •
Part-Time Enrollment: *6* • Female Enrollment: *37* • Male
Enrollment: *3* • Total Graduates: *15*

FINANCES

Residental Annual Tuition: *$1,431* • Non-Residential
Annual Tuition: *$229* • General Institutional Fees: *$540* •
Additional Nursing Fees: *$200*

BRIGHAM YOUNG UNIVERSITY

Address: B-130 ASB, Provo, UT 84602
Phone: 801-378-5626
Fax: 801-422-0536
Contact: Mary Williams, PhD, RN, MS, Associate Dean
Email: mary_williams@byu.edu

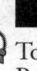

GENERAL INFORMATION

Type of School: *4-Year College or University, Private
(Religious)* • Accreditation: *Northwestern Association of Schools
and Colleges* • Total Enrollment: *32771*

PROGRAM INFORMATION

NLNAC Accreditation: *Yes* • CCNE Accreditation: *Yes*

———

For specialty program listings, refer to the index.

NURSING STUDENT PROFILE

Total Nursing Enrollments: *21* • Full-Time Enrollment: *13* •
Part-Time Enrollment: *8* • Female Enrollment: *15* • Male
Enrollment: *6* • Total Graduates: *11*

FINANCES

Residental Annual Tuition: *$1,930* • Non-Residential
Annual Tuition: *$2,895* • General Institutional Fees: *$400* •
Additional Nursing Fees: *$0*

UNIVERSITY OF UTAH

Address: 10 S. 2000 E. Front, Salt Lake City, UT 84112
Phone: 801-581-8480
Fax: Not Provided
Contact: B. Lee Walker, PhD, RN, Interim Associate Dean
           for Academic Affairs
Email: lee.walker@nurs.utah.edu

GENERAL INFORMATION

Type of School: *Not Provided* • Accreditation: *Northwestern Association of Schools and Colleges* • Total Enrollment: *Not Provided*

PROGRAM INFORMATION

NLNAC Accreditation: *Yes* • CCNE Accreditation: *No*

———

For specialty program listings, refer to the index.

NURSING STUDENT PROFILE

Total Nursing Enrollments: *205* • Full-Time Enrollment: *75* • Part-Time Enrollment: *130* • Female Enrollment: *170* • Male Enrollment: *35* • Total Graduates: *66*

FINANCES

Residental Annual Tuition: *$2,104* • Non-Residential Annual Tuition: *$6,310* • General Institutional Fees: *Not Reported* • Additional Nursing Fees: *$50*

THE UNIVERSITY OF VERMONT

Address: 194 Prospect St, Burlington, VT 05405
Phone: 802-656-3051
Fax: 802-656-8306
Contact: Gail Ann Deluca Havens, PhD, APRN, BC,
           Associate Professor and Chair of Nursing
Email: Gail.Havens@uvm.edu

GENERAL INFORMATION

Type of School: *4-Year College or University, Public* • Accreditation: *New England Association of Schools and Colleges* • Total Enrollment: *Not Provided*

PROGRAM INFORMATION

NLNAC Accreditation: *Yes* • CCNE Accreditation: *No*

———

For specialty program listings, refer to the index.

NURSING STUDENT PROFILE

Total Nursing Enrollments: *56* • Full-Time Enrollment: *24* • Part-Time Enrollment: *32* • Female Enrollment: *55* • Male Enrollment: *1* • Total Graduates: *7*

FINANCES

Residental Annual Tuition: *$8,040* • Non-Residential Annual Tuition: *$20,100* • General Institutional Fees: *$605* • Additional Nursing Fees: *$39*

GEORGE MASON UNIVERSITY

Address: 4400 University Drive, Fairfax, VA 22030-4444
Phone: 703-993-1731
Fax: 703-993-1949
Contact: Ellen Dawson, PhD, RN, ANP, Assistant Dean, Graduate Nursing Program
Email: edawson@gmu.edu

GENERAL INFORMATION

Type of School: *4-Year College or University, Private (Independent)* • Accreditation: *Not Provided* • Total Enrollment: *Not Provided*

PROGRAM INFORMATION

NLNAC Accreditation: *Yes* • CCNE Accreditation: *Yes*

For specialty program listings, refer to the index.

NURSING STUDENT PROFILE

Total Nursing Enrollments: *284* • Full-Time Enrollment: *101* • Part-Time Enrollment: *183* • Female Enrollment: *267* • Male Enrollment: *17* • Total Graduates: *84*

FINANCES

Residental Annual Tuition: *$191* • Non-Residential Annual Tuition: *$525* • General Institutional Fees: *$0* • Additional Nursing Fees: *$10*

HAMPTON UNIVERSITY

Address: Tyler and Emancipation Drive, Hampton, VA 23668
Phone: 757-727-5672
Fax: 757-727-5423
Contact: Shirley V. Gore, PhD, RN, CS/FNP, Chairperson, Department of Graduate Nursing Education
Email: shirley.gore@hamptonu.edu

GENERAL INFORMATION

Type of School: *4-Year College or University, Private Independent* • Accreditation: *Southern Association of Colleges and Schools* • Total Enrollment: *5743*

PROGRAM INFORMATION

NLNAC Accreditation: *Yes* • CCNE Accreditation: *No*

For specialty program listings, refer to the index.

NURSING STUDENT PROFILE

Total Nursing Enrollments: *65* • Full-Time Enrollment: *49* • Part-Time Enrollment: *16* • Female Enrollment: *59* • Male Enrollment: *6* • Total Graduates: *14*

FINANCES

Residental Annual Tuition: *$9,966* • Non-Residential Annual Tuition: *$9,966* • General Institutional Fees: *$70* • Additional Nursing Fees: *Not Reported*

MARYMOUNT UNIVERSITY

Address: 2807 North Glebe Road, Arlington, VA 22707
Phone: 703-526-6836
Fax: 703-284-3819
Contact: Christine M. Galante, PhD, RN, CHE, Chair, Graduate Nursing Program
Email: cgala77767@aol.com

GENERAL INFORMATION

Type of School: _4-Year College or University, Private (Religious)_ • Accreditation: _Southern Association of Colleges and Schools_ • Total Enrollment: _3600_

PROGRAM INFORMATION

NLNAC Accreditation: _Yes_ • CCNE Accreditation: _No_

———

For specialty program listings, refer to the index.

NURSING STUDENT PROFILE

Total Nursing Enrollments: _47_ • Full-Time Enrollment: _7_ • Part-Time Enrollment: _40_ • Female Enrollment: _42_ • Male Enrollment: _5_ • Total Graduates: _7_

FINANCES

Residental Annual Tuition: _$10,000_ • Non-Residential Annual Tuition: _Not Provided_ • General Institutional Fees: _$300_ • Additional Nursing Fees: _$115_

OLD DOMINION UNIVERSITY

Address: 4601 Hampton Blvd, Norfolk, VA 23529-0500
Phone: 757-683-4298
Fax: Not Provided
Contact: Laurel S. Garzon, DNSc, Graduate Program Director
Email: lgarzon@odu.edu

GENERAL INFORMATION

Type of School: _4-Year College or University, Public_ • Accreditation: _Southern_ • Total Enrollment: _18500_

PROGRAM INFORMATION

NLNAC Accreditation: _Yes_ • CCNE Accreditation:

———

For specialty program listings, refer to the index.

NURSING STUDENT PROFILE

Total Nursing Enrollments: _139_ • Full-Time Enrollment: _80_ • Part-Time Enrollment: _59_ • Female Enrollment: _Not Provided_ • Male Enrollment: _Not Provided_ • Total Graduates: _71_

FINANCES

Residental Annual Tuition: _Not Reported_ • Non-Residential Annual Tuition: _Not Reported_ • General Institutional Fees: _Not Reported_ • Additional Nursing Fees: _Not Reported_

RADFORD UNIVERSITY

Address: Freelander Drive, Radford, VA 24142
Phone: 540-831-7700
Fax: 540-831-7716
Contact: Karolyn Givens, EdD, RN, Coordinator, Graduate Program
Email: kgivens@radford.edu

GENERAL INFORMATION

Type of School: *4-Year College or University, Public* • Accreditation: *Southern Association of Colleges and Schools* • Total Enrollment: *Not Provided*

PROGRAM INFORMATION

NLNAC Accreditation: *Yes* • CCNE Accreditation:

For specialty program listings, refer to the index.

NURSING STUDENT PROFILE

Total Nursing Enrollments: *38* • Full-Time Enrollment: *14* • Part-Time Enrollment: *24* • Female Enrollment: *36* • Male Enrollment: *2* • Total Graduates: *6*

FINANCES

Residental Annual Tuition: *$3,696* • Non-Residential Annual Tuition: *$7,260* • General Institutional Fees: *Not Reported* • Additional Nursing Fees: *$100*

SHENANDOAH UNIVERSITY

Address: 3192 Los Angeles Avenue, Winchester, VA 22601
Phone: 540-678-4381
Fax: 540-665-5519
Contact: Sheila M. Sparks, RN, DNSc, CS, Interim Director
Email: ssparks@su.edu

GENERAL INFORMATION

Type of School: *4-Year College or University, Private Independent* • Accreditation: *Southern Association of Colleges and Schools* • Total Enrollment: *Not Provided*

PROGRAM INFORMATION

NLNAC Accreditation: *Yes* • CCNE Accreditation: *No*

For specialty program listings, refer to the index.

NURSING STUDENT PROFILE

Total Nursing Enrollments: *32* • Full-Time Enrollment: *8* • Part-Time Enrollment: *24* • Female Enrollment: *27* • Male Enrollment: *5* • Total Graduates: *9*

FINANCES

Residental Annual Tuition: *$12,000* • Non-Residential Annual Tuition: *$12,000* • General Institutional Fees: *$0* • Additional Nursing Fees: *$195*

UNIVERSITY OF VIRGINIA

Address: 1 College Ave., Charlottesville, VA 24293
Phone: 434-924-0112
Fax: 434-982-1809
Contact: Anne Hamric, PhD, Associate Professor
Email: abh4f@virginia.edu

GENERAL INFORMATION

Type of School: *4-Year College or University, Public* •
Accreditation: *Southern Association of Colleges and Schools* •
Total Enrollment: *1494*

PROGRAM INFORMATION

NLNAC Accreditation: *Yes* • CCNE Accreditation:
Provisional

_____

For specialty program listings, refer to the index.

NURSING STUDENT PROFILE

Total Nursing Enrollments: *106* • Full-Time Enrollment:
65 • Part-Time Enrollment: *41* • Female Enrollment: *98* •
Male Enrollment: *8* • Total Graduates: *46*

FINANCES

Residental Annual Tuition: *$3,988* • Non-Residential
Annual Tuition: *$17,078* • General Institutional Fees:
$1,245 • Additional Nursing Fees: *Not Reported*

VIRGINIA COMMONWEALTH UNIVERSITY

Address: 3097 Colonial Avenue, SW, PO Box 14007,
            Richmond, VA 24038
Phone: 804-828-0521
Fax: 804-828-7743
Contact: Janet B. Younger, PhD, RN, CPNP, Asst. Dean
            & Professor
Email: younger@hsc.vcu.edu

GENERAL INFORMATION

Type of School: *4-Year College or University, Public* •
Accreditation: *Southern Association of Colleges and Schools* •
Total Enrollment: *25000*

PROGRAM INFORMATION

NLNAC Accreditation: *Yes* • CCNE Accreditation: *No*

_____

For specialty program listings, refer to the index.

NURSING STUDENT PROFILE

Total Nursing Enrollments: *186* • Full-Time Enrollment:
101 • Part-Time Enrollment: *85* • Female Enrollment: *177* •
Male Enrollment: *9* • Total Graduates: *57*

FINANCES

Residental Annual Tuition: *$4,276* • Non-Residential
Annual Tuition: *$12,672* • General Institutional Fees: *$967* •
Additional Nursing Fees: *$0*

GONZAGA UNIVERSITY

Address: 502 East Brooke Avenue, Spokane, WA 99258
Phone: 509-323-6646
Fax: 509-328-5827
Contact: Susan Norwood, EdD, ARNP, Chairperson
Email: norwood@gu.gonzaga.edu

GENERAL INFORMATION

Type of School: *4-Year College or University, Private (Religious)* • Accreditation: *Northwestern Association of Schools and Colleges* • Total Enrollment: *1121*

PROGRAM INFORMATION

NLNAC Accreditation: *Yes* • CCNE Accreditation: *Yes*

For specialty program listings, refer to the index.

NURSING STUDENT PROFILE

Total Nursing Enrollments: *232* • Full-Time Enrollment: *200* • Part-Time Enrollment: *32* • Female Enrollment: *222* • Male Enrollment: *10* • Total Graduates: *39*

FINANCES

Residental Annual Tuition: *$10,800* • Non-Residential Annual Tuition: *$10,800* • General Institutional Fees: *$200* • Additional Nursing Fees: *$50*

PACIFIC LUTHERAN UNIVERSITY

Address: One College Avenue, Tacoma, WA 98447
Phone: 253-535-7674
Fax: 253-535-7590
Contact: Terry W. Miller, PhD, RN, Dean and Professor
Email: millertw@plu.edu

GENERAL INFORMATION

Type of School: *4-Year College or University, Private (Independent)* • Accreditation: *Not Provided* • Total Enrollment: *13000*

PROGRAM INFORMATION

NLNAC Accreditation: *Yes* • CCNE Accreditation: *No*

For specialty program listings, refer to the index.

NURSING STUDENT PROFILE

Total Nursing Enrollments: *33* • Full-Time Enrollment: *11* • Part-Time Enrollment: *22* • Female Enrollment: *30* • Male Enrollment: *3* • Total Graduates: *21*

FINANCES

Residental Annual Tuition: *$9,126* • Non-Residential Annual Tuition: *$9,126* • General Institutional Fees: *$0* • Additional Nursing Fees: *$55*

SEATTLE UNIVERSITY

Address: 900 Broadway, Seattle, WA 98122
Phone: 206-296-5663
Fax: 206-296-5544
Contact: Marilyn Whitley, PhD, RN, Director
Email: mpwhitley@seattleu.edu

GENERAL INFORMATION

Type of School: *4-Year College or University, Private (Religious)* • Accreditation: *WASC* • Total Enrollment: *6000*

PROGRAM INFORMATION

NLNAC Accreditation: *Yes* • CCNE Accreditation: *No*

For specialty program listings, refer to the index.

NURSING STUDENT PROFILE

Total Nursing Enrollments: *17* • Full-Time Enrollment: *8* • Part-Time Enrollment: *9* • Female Enrollment: *13* • Male Enrollment: *4* • Total Graduates: *9*

FINANCES

Residental Annual Tuition: *$11,370* • Non-Residential Annual Tuition: *$11,370* • General Institutional Fees: *$75* • Additional Nursing Fees: *$0*

UNIVERSITY OF WASHINGTON

Address: 2420 Nicolet Drive, Seattle, WA 98195
Phone: 206-616-8407
Fax: Not Provided
Contact: Susan L. Woods, PhD, Associate Dean for Academic Programs
Email: slwoods@u.washington.edu

GENERAL INFORMATION

Type of School: *Other* • Accreditation: *Not Provided* • Total Enrollment: *23717*

PROGRAM INFORMATION

NLNAC Accreditation: *Yes* • CCNE Accreditation: *No*

For specialty program listings, refer to the index.

NURSING STUDENT PROFILE

Total Nursing Enrollments: *286* • Full-Time Enrollment: *138* • Part-Time Enrollment: *148* • Female Enrollment: *265* • Male Enrollment: *21* • Total Graduates: *102*

FINANCES

Residental Annual Tuition: *$5,463* • Non-Residential Annual Tuition: *$13,752* • General Institutional Fees: *$160* • Additional Nursing Fees: *$0*

WASHINGTON STATE UNIVERSITY

Address: 3903 University Circle, Pullman, WA 99163
Phone: 509-324-7335
Fax: 509-324-7336
Contact: Anne M. Hirsch, DNS, ARNP, Associate Dean for Academic Affairs
Email: hirsch@wsu.edu

GENERAL INFORMATION

Type of School: *Not Provided* • Accreditation: *Not Provided* • Total Enrollment: *17000*

PROGRAM INFORMATION

NLNAC Accreditation: *Yes* • CCNE Accreditation: *Provisional*

_____

For specialty program listings, refer to the index.

NURSING STUDENT PROFILE

Total Nursing Enrollments: *132* • Full-Time Enrollment: *35* • Part-Time Enrollment: *97* • Female Enrollment: *109* • Male Enrollment: *23* • Total Graduates: *38*

FINANCES

Residental Annual Tuition: *$5,886* • Non-Residential Annual Tuition: *$14,426* • General Institutional Fees: *$0* • Additional Nursing Fees: *$40*

MARSHALL UNIVERSITY

Address: 12300 McCracken Road, Huntington, WV 25755-9500
Phone: 304-696-2366
Fax: 304-696-6739
Contact: Linda M. Scott, PhD, RN, C-FNP, Associate Dean
Email: scott@marshall.edu

GENERAL INFORMATION

Type of School: *4-Year College or University, Private (Religious)* • Accreditation: *North Central Association of Colleges and Schools* • Total Enrollment: *1595*

PROGRAM INFORMATION

NLNAC Accreditation: *Yes* • CCNE Accreditation: *No*

_____

For specialty program listings, refer to the index.

NURSING STUDENT PROFILE

Total Nursing Enrollments: *64* • Full-Time Enrollment: *17* • Part-Time Enrollment: *47* • Female Enrollment: *57* • Male Enrollment: *7* • Total Graduates: *21*

FINANCES

Residential Annual Tuition: *$2,238* • Non-Residential Annual Tuition: *$6,810* • General Institutional Fees: *$488* • Additional Nursing Fees: *$250*

WEST VIRGINIA UNIVERSITY

Address: 6700 Hlth Sciences S Box 9600, Morgantown, WV 26506-9600
Phone: 304-293-4298
Fax: 304-293-2546
Contact: Mary Jane Smith, PhD, RN, Associate Dean Graduate Academic Affairs
Email: mjsmith@hsc.wvu.edu

GENERAL INFORMATION

Type of School: *4-Year College or University, Public* • Accreditation: *North Central Association of Colleges and Schools* • Total Enrollment: *6678*

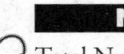

PROGRAM INFORMATION

NLNAC Accreditation: *No* • CCNE Accreditation: *Yes*

_____

For specialty program listings, refer to the index.

NURSING STUDENT PROFILE

Total Nursing Enrollments: *71* • Full-Time Enrollment: *37* • Part-Time Enrollment: *34* • Female Enrollment: *64* • Male Enrollment: *7* • Total Graduates: *40*

FINANCES

Residental Annual Tuition: *$1,270* • Non-Residential Annual Tuition: *$3,910* • General Institutional Fees: *$749* • Additional Nursing Fees: *$366*

WHEELING JESUIT UNIVERSITY

Address: 316 Washington Ave, Wheeling, WV 26003
Phone: 304-243-2227
Fax: 304-243-4441
Contact: Rose Kutlenios, PhD, RN, CS, Chair and Professor, Department of Nursing
Email: rosekut@wju.edu

GENERAL INFORMATION

Type of School: *4-Year College or University, Private (Religious)* • Accreditation: *North Central Association of Colleges and Schools* • Total Enrollment: *1280*

PROGRAM INFORMATION

NLNAC Accreditation: *Yes* • CCNE Accreditation:

_____

For specialty program listings, refer to the index.

NURSING STUDENT PROFILE

Total Nursing Enrollments: *36* • Full-Time Enrollment: *2* • Part-Time Enrollment: *34* • Female Enrollment: *Not Provided* • Male Enrollment: *Not Provided* • Total Graduates: *3*

FINANCES

Residental Annual Tuition: *$9,840* • Non-Residential Annual Tuition: *$9,840* • General Institutional Fees: *Not Reported* • Additional Nursing Fees: *$60*

CARDINAL STRITCH UNIVERSITY

Address: 6801 North Yates Road, Benton Harbor, WI
          53217
Phone: 414-410-4388
Fax: 414-410-4385
Contact: Ruth M. Waite, PhD, RN, MSN Program Chair
Email: rwaite@stritch.edu

GENERAL INFORMATION

Type of School: *4-Year College or University, Private (Religious)* • Accreditation: *North Central Association of Colleges and Schools* • Total Enrollment: *5700*

PROGRAM INFORMATION

NLNAC Accreditation: *Yes* • CCNE Accreditation:

_____

For specialty program listings, refer to the index.

NURSING STUDENT PROFILE

Total Nursing Enrollments: *26* • Full-Time Enrollment: *2* • Part-Time Enrollment: *24* • Female Enrollment: *26* • Male Enrollment: *0* • Total Graduates: *0*

FINANCES

Residental Annual Tuition: *$5,925* • Non-Residential Annual Tuition: *$5,925* • General Institutional Fees: *$75* • Additional Nursing Fees: *$15*

CONCORDIA UNIVERSITY WISCONSIN (LCMS)

Address: 12800 North Lake Shore Dirve, Mequon, WI
          53097
Phone: 262-243-4452
Fax: 262-243-4466
Contact: Ruth Gresley, PhD, RN, MSN, Director of
          Master's in Nursing Program and Dean of
          Human Services
Email: ruth.gresley@cuw.edu

GENERAL INFORMATION

Type of School: *4-Year College or University, Private (Independent)* • Accreditation: *North Central Association of Colleges and Schools* • Total Enrollment: *4600*

PROGRAM INFORMATION

NLNAC Accreditation: *Yes* • CCNE Accreditation: *Yes*

_____

For specialty program listings, refer to the index.

NURSING STUDENT PROFILE

Total Nursing Enrollments: *84* • Full-Time Enrollment: *26* • Part-Time Enrollment: *58* • Female Enrollment: *79* • Male Enrollment: *5* • Total Graduates: *12*

FINANCES

Residental Annual Tuition: *$7,200* • Non-Residential Annual Tuition: *$7,200* • General Institutional Fees: *$0* • Additional Nursing Fees: *$0*

EDGEWOOD COLLEGE

Address: 1000 Edgewood College Drive, Madison, WI 53711
Phone: 608-663-2292
Fax: Not Provided
Contact: Mary Kelly-Powell, PhD, RN, Interim Chair and Associate Professor
Email: mkellypowell@edgewood.edu

GENERAL INFORMATION

Type of School: *Not Provided* • Accreditation: *North Central Association of Colleges and Schools* • Total Enrollment: *Not Provided*

PROGRAM INFORMATION

NLNAC Accreditation: *Not Reported* • CCNE Accreditation: *Yes*

For specialty program listings, refer to the index.

NURSING STUDENT PROFILE

Total Nursing Enrollments: *21* • Full-Time Enrollment: *0* • Part-Time Enrollment: *21* • Female Enrollment: *21* • Male Enrollment: *0* • Total Graduates: *10*

FINANCES

Residental Annual Tuition: *$6,480* • Non-Residential Annual Tuition: *$6,480* • General Institutional Fees: *Not Reported* • Additional Nursing Fees: *Not Reported*

MARQUETTE UNIVERSITY

Address: PO Box 1881, Milwaukee, WI 53201-1881
Phone: 414-288-3812
Fax: 414-288-1597
Contact: Madeline Wake, PhD, RN, FAAN, Dean and Professor
Email: madeline.wake@marquette.edu

GENERAL INFORMATION

Type of School: *4-Year College or University, Public* • Accreditation: *North Central Association of Colleges and Schools* • Total Enrollment: *Not Provided*

PROGRAM INFORMATION

NLNAC Accreditation: *Yes* • CCNE Accreditation: *Yes*

For specialty program listings, refer to the index.

NURSING STUDENT PROFILE

Total Nursing Enrollments: *140* • Full-Time Enrollment: *56* • Part-Time Enrollment: *84* • Female Enrollment: *133* • Male Enrollment: *7* • Total Graduates: *37*

FINANCES

Residental Annual Tuition: *$565* • Non-Residential Annual Tuition: *$565* • General Institutional Fees: *Not Reported* • Additional Nursing Fees: *Not Reported*

UNIVERSITY OF WISCONSIN—EAU CLAIRE

Address: 600 Highland Avenue, H6/150, Eau Claire, WI 53792-2455
Phone: 715-836-5287
Fax: 715-836-5925
Contact: Rita Kisting Sparks, PhD, RN, Interim Associate Dean and Educational Administrator
Email: sparksrk@vwec.edu

GENERAL INFORMATION

Type of School: *4-Year College or University, Public* • Accreditation: *North Central Association of Colleges and Schools* • Total Enrollment: *9500*

PROGRAM INFORMATION

NLNAC Accreditation: *Not Reported* • CCNE Accreditation: *Yes*

_____

For specialty program listings, refer to the index.

NURSING STUDENT PROFILE

Total Nursing Enrollments: *62* • Full-Time Enrollment: *12* • Part-Time Enrollment: *50* • Female Enrollment: *57* • Male Enrollment: *5* • Total Graduates: *28*

FINANCES

Residental Annual Tuition: *$4,505* • Non-Residential Annual Tuition: *$14,247* • General Institutional Fees: *$461* • Additional Nursing Fees: *$25*

UNIVERSITY OF WISCONSIN—MILWAUKEE

Address: PO Box 413, Milwaukee, WI 53201
Phone: 414-229-5468
Fax: Not Provided
Contact: Susan Dean-Baar, PhD, RN, FAAN, Associate Dean for Academic Affairs
Email: deanbaar@uwm.edu

GENERAL INFORMATION

Type of School: *4-Year College or University, Public* • Accreditation: *North Central Association of Colleges and Schools* • Total Enrollment: *24223*

PROGRAM INFORMATION

NLNAC Accreditation: *No* • CCNE Accreditation:

_____

For specialty program listings, refer to the index.

NURSING STUDENT PROFILE

Total Nursing Enrollments: *108* • Full-Time Enrollment: *47* • Part-Time Enrollment: *61* • Female Enrollment: *99* • Male Enrollment: *9* • Total Graduates: *43*

FINANCES

Residental Annual Tuition: *$5,057* • Non-Residential Annual Tuition: *$16,231* • General Institutional Fees: *$306* • Additional Nursing Fees: *$0*

Circle 139 on reader card   See in-depth profile for more information

UNIVERSITY OF WISCONSIN—OSHKOSH

Address: 800 Algoma Blvd, Oshkosh, WI 54901
Phone: 920-424-2121
Fax: 920-424-0123
Contact: Rosemary Smith, PhD, RN, Graduate Program
            Director
Email: smithr@uwosh.edu

GENERAL INFORMATION

Type of School: *4-Year College or University, Public* •
Accreditation: *North Central Association of Colleges and
Schools* • Total Enrollment: *Not Provided*

PROGRAM INFORMATION

NLNAC Accreditation: *Not Reported* • CCNE Accreditation:
Yes

_____

For specialty program listings, refer to the index.

NURSING STUDENT PROFILE

Total Nursing Enrollments: *58* • Full-Time Enrollment: *27* •
Part-Time Enrollment: *31* • Female Enrollment: *53* • Male
Enrollment: *5* • Total Graduates: *15*

FINANCES

Residental Annual Tuition: *$3,972* • Non-Residential
Annual Tuition: *$12,330* • General Institutional Fees: *Not
Reported* • Additional Nursing Fees: *$0*

VITERBO COLLEGE

Address: 815 South 9th Street, La Crosse, WI 54601
Phone: 608-796-3688
Fax: 608-796-3050
Contact: Bonnie Nesbitt, PhD, RN, CS, Professor
Email: bjnesbitt@viterbo.edu

GENERAL INFORMATION

Type of School: *4-Year College or University, Private
Independent* • Accreditation: *North Central Association of
Colleges and Schools* • Total Enrollment: *1750*

PROGRAM INFORMATION

NLNAC Accreditation: *Not Reported* • CCNE Accreditation:
No

_____

For specialty program listings, refer to the index.

NURSING STUDENT PROFILE

Total Nursing Enrollments: *31* • Full-Time Enrollment: *30* •
Part-Time Enrollment: *1* • Female Enrollment: *31* • Male
Enrollment: *0* • Total Graduates: *0*

FINANCES

Residental Annual Tuition: *$9,360* • Non-Residential
Annual Tuition: *$9,360* • General Institutional Fees: *$0* •
Additional Nursing Fees: *$0*

UNIVERSITY OF WYOMING

Address: PO Box 3065, Laramie, WY 82071
Phone: 307-766-6569
Fax: 307-766-4294
Contact: Marcia L. Dale, EdD, RN, FAAN, Dean, School
           of Nursing
Email: marcia@uwyo.edu

GENERAL INFORMATION

Type of School: *4-Year College, Public* • Accreditation: *Northwestern Association of Schools and Colleges* • Total Enrollment: *11057*

PROGRAM INFORMATION

NLNAC Accreditation: *Yes* • CCNE Accreditation: *Yes*

_____

For specialty program listings, refer to the index.

NURSING STUDENT PROFILE

Total Nursing Enrollments: *67* • Full-Time Enrollment: *20* • Part-Time Enrollment: *47* • Female Enrollment: *60* • Male Enrollment: *7* • Total Graduates: *9*

FINANCES

Residental Annual Tuition: *$2,895* • Non-Residential Annual Tuition: *$8,367* • General Institutional Fees: *$491* • Additional Nursing Fees: *$200*

DOCTORAL PROGRAMS

UNIVERSITY OF ARIZONA

Address: 1305 North Martin, PO Box 210203, Tucson, AZ 85721-0203
Phone: 520-626-6151
Fax: Not Provided
Contact: Pamela G. Reed, PhD, RN, FAAN, Professor and Associate Dean for Academic Affairs
Email: preed@nursing.arizona.edu

GENERAL INFORMATION

Type of School: *4-Year College or University, Public* • Accreditation: *North Central Association of Colleges and Schools* • Total Enrollment: *34300*

PROGRAM INFORMATION

Degree Awarded: *Ph.D* • Specialty Focuses: *Research*

NURSING STUDENT PROFILE

Total Nursing Enrollment: *48* • Full-Time Enrollment: *17* • Part-Time Enrollment: *31* • Female Enrollment: *44* • Male Enrollment: *4* • Total Graduates: *5*

FINANCES

Residential Annual Tuition: *$2,272* • Non-Residential Annual Tuition: *$7,290* • General Institutional Fees: *$38* • Additional Nursing Fees: *$0*

UNIVERSITY OF ARKANSAS FOR MEDICAL SCIENCES

Address: 4301 West Markham, Slot 529, Little Rock, AR 72205
Phone: 501-686-7967
Fax: Not Provided
Contact: Janet E. Lord, PhD, RN, Interim Associate Dean for Doctoral Program
Email: lordjanete@uams.edu

GENERAL INFORMATION

Type of School: *4-Year College or University, Public* • Accreditation: *North Central Association of Colleges and Schools* • Total Enrollment: *5000*

PROGRAM INFORMATION

Degree Awarded: *PhD* • Specialty Focuses: *Research, Clinical Practice, Educational/Professorial Role, and Administration/Executive Role*

NURSING STUDENT PROFILE

Total Nursing Enrollment: *12* • Full-Time Enrollment: *6* • Part-Time Enrollment: *6* • Female Enrollment: *12* • Male Enrollment: *0* • Total Graduates: *1*

FINANCES

Residential Annual Tuition: *$3,540* • Non-Residential Annual Tuition: *$7,600* • General Institutional Fees: *$50* • Additional Nursing Fees: *$150*

UNIVERSITY OF CALIFORNIA—LOS ANGELES

Address: Box 951702, Los Angeles, CA 90095-1702
Phone: 310-825-9621
Fax: Not Provided
Contact: Marie J. Cowan, PhD, RN, FAAN, Dean and Professor
Email: mcowan@sonnet.ucla.edu

GENERAL INFORMATION

Type of School: *4-Year College or University, Public* •
Accreditation: *Western Association of Schools and Colleges* •
Total Enrollment: *34000*

PROGRAM INFORMATION

Degree Awarded: *Other* • Specialty Focuses: *Other*

NURSING STUDENT PROFILE

Total Nursing Enrollment: *Not Provided* • Full-Time Enrollment: *Not Provided* • Part-Time Enrollment: *Not Provided* • Female Enrollment: *Not Provided* • Male Enrollment: *Not Provided* • Total Graduates: *Not Provided*

FINANCES

Residential Annual Tuition: *Not Provided* • Non-Residential Annual Tuition: *Not Provided* • General Institutional Fees: *Not Provided* • Additional Nursing Fees: *Not Provided*

UNIVERSITY OF CALIFORNIA— SAN FRANCISCO

Address: 500 Parnassus Avenue, San Francisco, CA 94143
Phone: 415-476-9710
Fax: 415-476-9707
Contact: Dorrie Fontaine, DNSc, RN, FAAN, Associate Dean, Academic Programs
Email: dorrie.fontaine@nursing.ucsf.edu

GENERAL INFORMATION

Type of School: *4-Year College or University, Public* •
Accreditation: *Western Association of Schools and Colleges* •
Total Enrollment: *2500*

PROGRAM INFORMATION

Degree Awarded: *PhD and DNS/DNSc* • Specialty Focuses: *Research*

NURSING STUDENT PROFILE

Total Nursing Enrollment: *103* • Full-Time Enrollment: *103* • Part-Time Enrollment: *0* • Female Enrollment: *92* • Male Enrollment: *11* • Total Graduates: *11*

FINANCES

Residential Annual Tuition: *$3,086* • Non-Residential Annual Tuition: *$14,931* • General Institutional Fees: *$1,219* • Additional Nursing Fees: *$0*

UNIVERSITY OF COLORADO—DENVER

Address: 4200 East Ninth Avenue, Denver, CO 80262
Phone: 303-315-4246
Fax: Not Provided
Contact: Kathy Magilvy, PhD, RN, Director
Email: kathy.magilvy@uchsc.edu

GENERAL INFORMATION

Type of School: *Not Provided* • Accreditation: *Not Provided* • Total Enrollment: *Not Provided*

PROGRAM INFORMATION

Degree Awarded: *Other* • Specialty Focuses: *Other*

NURSING STUDENT PROFILE

Total Nursing Enrollment: *Not Provided* • Full-Time Enrollment: *Not Provided* • Part-Time Enrollment: *Not Provided* • Female Enrollment: *Not Provided* • Male Enrollment: *Not Provided* • Total Graduates: *Not Provided*

FINANCES

Residential Annual Tuition: *Not Provided* • Non-Residential Annual Tuition: *Not Provided* • General Institutional Fees: *Not Provided* • Additional Nursing Fees: *Not Provided*

UNIVERSITY OF SOUTHERN COLORADO

Address: 2200 Bonforte Boulevard, Pueblo, CO 81001
Phone: 803-777-3862
Fax: 803-777-2027
Contact: Mary Ann Parsons, PhD, RN, Dean
Email: maryann.parsons@sc.edu

GENERAL INFORMATION

Type of School: *4-Year College or University, Public* • Accreditation: *North Central Association of Colleges and Schools* • Total Enrollment: *4000*

PROGRAM INFORMATION

Degree Awarded: *Other* • Specialty Focuses: *Research and Clinical Practice*

NURSING STUDENT PROFILE

Total Nursing Enrollment: *14* • Full-Time Enrollment: *9* • Part-Time Enrollment: *5* • Female Enrollment: *13* • Male Enrollment: *1* • Total Graduates: *1*

FINANCES

Residential Annual Tuition: *$5,410* • Non-Residential Annual Tuition: *$11,236* • General Institutional Fees: *$100* • Additional Nursing Fees: *$750*

UNIVERSITY OF CONNECTICUT

Address: 231 Glenbrook Road, Storrs Mansfield, CT
             06269
Phone: 860-486-3716
Fax: Not Provided
Contact: Kathleen Bruttomesso, PhD, RN, Interim Dean
Email: bruttome@uconnvm.uconn.edu

GENERAL INFORMATION

Type of School: *4-Year College or University, Public* •
Accreditation: *New England Association of Schools and
Colleges* • Total Enrollment: *16696*

PROGRAM INFORMATION

Degree Awarded: *PhD* • Specialty Focuses: *Research*

NURSING STUDENT PROFILE

Total Nursing Enrollment: *33* • Full-Time Enrollment: *12* •
Part-Time Enrollment: *21* • Female Enrollment: *30* • Male
Enrollment: *3* • Total Graduates: *1*

FINANCES

Residential Annual Tuition: *$5,272* • Non-Residential
Annual Tuition: *$13,696* • General Institutional Fees: *$506* •
Additional Nursing Fees: *$0*

YALE UNIVERSITY

Address: 100 Church Street South, New Haven, CT
             06537
Phone: 203-737-5501
Fax: Not Provided
Contact: Ruth McCorkle, PhD, FAAN, Chairperson
Email: ruth.mccorkle@yale.edu

GENERAL INFORMATION

Type of School: *4-Year College or University, Private
(Independent)* • Accreditation: *New England Association of
Schools and Colleges* • Total Enrollment: *11017*

PROGRAM INFORMATION

Degree Awarded: *Other* • Specialty Focuses: *Other*

NURSING STUDENT PROFILE

Total Nursing Enrollment: *Not Provided* • Full-Time
Enrollment: *Not Provided* • Part-Time Enrollment: *Not
Provided* • Female Enrollment: *Not Provided* • Male
Enrollment: *Not Provided* • Total Graduates: *Not Provided*

FINANCES

Residential Annual Tuition: *Not Provided* • Non-Residential
Annual Tuition: *Not Provided* • General Institutional Fees:
Not Provided • Additional Nursing Fees: *Not Provided*

THE CATHOLIC UNIVERSITY OF AMERICA

Address: 620 Michigan Avenue, North East, Washington, DC 20064
Phone: 202-319-5405
Fax: Not Provided
Contact: Ann Marie Brooks, DNSc, RN, FAAN, FACHE, Dean
Email: brooks@cua.edu

GENERAL INFORMATION

Type of School: *4-Year College or University, Private (Independent)* • Accreditation: *Middle States Association of Colleges and Schools* • Total Enrollment: *5500*

PROGRAM INFORMATION

Degree Awarded: *Other* • Specialty Focuses: *Other*

NURSING STUDENT PROFILE

Total Nursing Enrollment: *Not Provided* • Full-Time Enrollment: *Not Provided* • Part-Time Enrollment: *Not Provided* • Female Enrollment: *Not Provided* • Male Enrollment: *Not Provided* • Total Graduates: *Not Provided*

FINANCES

Residential Annual Tuition: *Not Provided* • Non-Residential Annual Tuition: *Not Provided* • General Institutional Fees: *Not Provided* • Additional Nursing Fees: *Not Provided*

BARRY UNIVERSITY

Address: 11300 North East Second Avenue, Miami Shores, FL 33161-6695
Phone: 305-899-3800
Fax: 305-899-3831
Contact: Janyce Dyer, DNSc, CS, FNP, C, Associate Dean Graduate Program
Email: jdyer@mail.barry.edu

GENERAL INFORMATION

Type of School: *4-Year College or University, Private (Religious)* • Accreditation: *Southern Association of Colleges and Schools* • Total Enrollment: *8700*

PROGRAM INFORMATION

Degree Awarded: *PhD* • Specialty Focuses: *Research*

NURSING STUDENT PROFILE

Total Nursing Enrollment: *26* • Full-Time Enrollment: *0* • Part-Time Enrollment: *26* • Female Enrollment: *23* • Male Enrollment: *3* • Total Graduates: *3*

FINANCES

Residential Annual Tuition: *Not Provided* • Non-Residential Annual Tuition: *Not Provided* • General Institutional Fees: *Not Provided* • Additional Nursing Fees: *Not Provided*

UNIVERSITY OF FLORIDA

Address: P.O. Box 100197, Gainesville, FL 32610
Phone: 352-392-3752
Fax: Not Provided
Contact: Kathleen Ann Long, PhD, RNCS, FAAN, Dean and Professor
Email: longka@nursing.ufl.edu

UNIVERSITY OF MIAMI

Address: 58010 Red Road, Miami, FL 33143
Phone: 305-284-1554
Fax: Not Provided
Contact: Ellen Baer, PhD, RN, Coordinator
Email: ebaer@miami.edu

GENERAL INFORMATION

Type of School: *4-Year College or University, Public* •
Accreditation: *Southern Association of Colleges and Schools* •
Total Enrollment: *43000*

GENERAL INFORMATION

Type of School: *Independent, Private (Independent)* •
Accreditation: *Southern Association of Colleges and Schools* •
Total Enrollment: *13963*

PROGRAM INFORMATION

Degree Awarded: *PhD* • Specialty Focuses: *Research*

PROGRAM INFORMATION

Degree Awarded: *Other* • Specialty Focuses: *Other*

NURSING STUDENT PROFILE

Total Nursing Enrollment: *34* • Full-Time Enrollment: *9* •
Part-Time Enrollment: *25* • Female Enrollment: *31* • Male
Enrollment: *3* • Total Graduates: *5*

NURSING STUDENT PROFILE

Total Nursing Enrollment: *Not Provided* • Full-Time
Enrollment: *Not Provided* • Part-Time Enrollment: *Not
Provided* • Female Enrollment: *Not Provided* • Male
Enrollment: *Not Provided* • Total Graduates: *Not Provided*

FINANCES

Residential Annual Tuition: *Not Provided* • Non-Residential
Annual Tuition: *Not Provided* • General Institutional Fees:
Not Provided • Additional Nursing Fees: *Not Provided*

FINANCES

Residential Annual Tuition: *Not Provided* • Non-Residential
Annual Tuition: *Not Provided* • General Institutional Fees:
Not Provided • Additional Nursing Fees: *Not Provided*

UNIVERSITY OF SOUTH FLORIDA

Address: 4202 East Fowler Avenue, Tampa, FL 33620
Phone: 813-974-9091
Fax: 813-974-5418
Contact: Patricia A Burns, PhD, RN, FAAN, Dean and Professor
Email: pburns@hsc.usf.edu

GENERAL INFORMATION

Type of School: *4-Year College or University, Public* • Accreditation: *Southern Association of Colleges and Schools* • Total Enrollment: *37814*

PROGRAM INFORMATION

Degree Awarded: *PhD* • Specialty Focuses: *None*

NURSING STUDENT PROFILE

Total Nursing Enrollment: *27* • Full-Time Enrollment: *10* • Part-Time Enrollment: *17* • Female Enrollment: *26* • Male Enrollment: *1* • Total Graduates: *6*

FINANCES

Residential Annual Tuition: *$3,824* • Non-Residential Annual Tuition: *$13,188* • General Institutional Fees: *Not Provided* • Additional Nursing Fees: *Not Provided*

EMORY UNIVERSITY

Address: 1520 Clifton Rd. NE, Ste. 402, Atlanta, GA 30322
Phone: 404-727-6939
Fax: 404-727-8514
Contact: Sandra B. Bunbar, DSN, RN, FAAN, Professor and Director of the Doctoral Program
Email: sbdunba@emory.edu

GENERAL INFORMATION

Type of School: *4-Year College or University, Private (Religious)* • Accreditation: *Southern Association of Colleges and Schools* • Total Enrollment: *11400*

PROGRAM INFORMATION

Degree Awarded: *PhD* • Specialty Focuses: *Research*

NURSING STUDENT PROFILE

Total Nursing Enrollment: *12* • Full-Time Enrollment: *12* • Part-Time Enrollment: *0* • Female Enrollment: *12* • Male Enrollment: *0* • Total Graduates: *0*

FINANCES

Residential Annual Tuition: *$24,770* • Non-Residential Annual Tuition: *$24,770* • General Institutional Fees: *$176* • Additional Nursing Fees: *$0*

GEORGIA STATE UNIVERSITY

Address: University Plaza, Atlanta, GA 30303
Phone: 404-463-9284
Fax: Not Provided
Contact: Sherry Gaines, PhD, RN, Interim Associate
Director, Graduate
Email: Not Provided

GENERAL INFORMATION

Type of School: *4-Year College or University, Public* •
Accreditation: *Southern Association of Colleges and Schools* •
Total Enrollment: *24000*

PROGRAM INFORMATION

Degree Awarded: *PhD* • Specialty Focuses: *Research*

NURSING STUDENT PROFILE

Total Nursing Enrollment: *31* • Full-Time Enrollment: *3* •
Part-Time Enrollment: *28* • Female Enrollment: *Not
Provided* • Male Enrollment: *Not Provided* • Total Graduates:
7

FINANCES

Residential Annual Tuition: *Not Provided* • Non-Residential
Annual Tuition: *Not Provided* • General Institutional Fees:
Not Provided • Additional Nursing Fees: *Not Provided*

MEDICAL COLLEGE OF GEORGIA

Address: 997 St. Sebastian Way, Augusta, GA 30912
Phone: 706-721-2787
Fax: 706-721-7390
Contact: Katherine E. Nugent, PhD, RN, Professor and
Associate Dean for Academic Programs
Email: knugent@mail.mcg.edu

GENERAL INFORMATION

Type of School: *4-Year College or University, Public* •
Accreditation: *Southern Association of Colleges and Schools* •
Total Enrollment: *1939*

PROGRAM INFORMATION

Degree Awarded: *PhD* • Specialty Focuses: *Research and
Other*

NURSING STUDENT PROFILE

Total Nursing Enrollment: *14* • Full-Time Enrollment: *0* •
Part-Time Enrollment: *14* • Female Enrollment: *13* • Male
Enrollment: *1* • Total Graduates: *4*

FINANCES

Residential Annual Tuition: *$1,578* • Non-Residential
Annual Tuition: *$6,312* • General Institutional Fees: *$218* •
Additional Nursing Fees: *$0*

| Circle 79 on reader card | See in-depth profile for more information |

UNIVERSITY OF HAWAII AT MANOA

Address: 2528 McCarthy Mall, Webster 330, Honolulu, HI 96822
Phone: 808-956-8522
Fax: 808-856-3257
Contact: Rosanne C. Harrigan, EdD, APRNRx, FAAN, Dean
Email: harrigan@hawaii.edu

GENERAL INFORMATION

Type of School: *4-Year College or University, Public* • Accreditation: *Western Association of Schools and Colleges* • Total Enrollment: *17498*

PROGRAM INFORMATION

Degree Awarded: *PhD* • Specialty Focuses: *Research*

NURSING STUDENT PROFILE

Total Nursing Enrollment: *22* • Full-Time Enrollment: *3* • Part-Time Enrollment: *19* • Female Enrollment: *17* • Male Enrollment: *5* • Total Graduates: *0*

FINANCES

Residential Annual Tuition: *$4,368* • Non-Residential Annual Tuition: *$8,320* • General Institutional Fees: *$132* • Additional Nursing Fees: *$0*

LOYOLA UNIVERSITY— CHICAGO

Address: 6525 North Sheridan Rd., Chicago, IL 60625
Phone: 773-508-3261
Fax: Not Provided
Contact: Marica C. Maurer, PhD, RN, Associate Dean and Director
Email: mmaurer@luc.edu

GENERAL INFORMATION

Type of School: *4-Year College or University, Private (Religious)* • Accreditation: *North Central Association of Colleges and Schools* • Total Enrollment: *13358*

PROGRAM INFORMATION

Degree Awarded: *PhD* • Specialty Focuses: *None*

NURSING STUDENT PROFILE

Total Nursing Enrollment: *53* • Full-Time Enrollment: *20* • Part-Time Enrollment: *33* • Female Enrollment: *47* • Male Enrollment: *6* • Total Graduates: *1*

FINANCES

Residential Annual Tuition: *Not Provided* • Non-Residential Annual Tuition: *Not Provided* • General Institutional Fees: *$118* • Additional Nursing Fees: *$1,550*

RUSH UNIVERSITY

Address: 600 S. Paulina, Chicago, IL 60612
Phone: 312-942-7117
Fax: Not Provided
Contact: Kathleen Andreoli, DSN, RN, FAAN, Dean and Vice President
Email: kandreoli@rushu.rush.edu

UNIVERSITY OF ILLINOIS—CHICAGO

Address: 601 S. Morgan, Chicago, IL 60607
Phone: 312-996-1749
Fax: 312-413-4399
Contact: Joan Shaver, PhD, RN, FAAN, Dean
Email: jshaver@uic.edu

GENERAL INFORMATION

Type of School: *Hospital, Private (Independent)* • Accreditation: *North Central Association of Colleges and Schools* • Total Enrollment: *1299*

GENERAL INFORMATION

Type of School: *4-Year College or University, Public* • Accreditation: *North Central Association of Colleges and Schools* • Total Enrollment: *25000*

PROGRAM INFORMATION

Degree Awarded: *DNS/DNSc* • Specialty Focuses: *Research Clinical Practice*

PROGRAM INFORMATION

Degree Awarded: *PhD* • Specialty Focuses: *Research*

NURSING STUDENT PROFILE

Total Nursing Enrollment: *154* • Full-Time Enrollment: *0* • Part-Time Enrollment: *154* • Female Enrollment: *142* • Male Enrollment: *12* • Total Graduates: *31*

NURSING STUDENT PROFILE

Total Nursing Enrollment: *64* • Full-Time Enrollment: *24* • Part-Time Enrollment: *40* • Female Enrollment: *64* • Male Enrollment: *0* • Total Graduates: *5*

FINANCES

Residential Annual Tuition: *$14,565* • Non-Residential Annual Tuition: *Not Provided* • General Institutional Fees: *Not Provided* • Additional Nursing Fees: *Not Provided*

FINANCES

Residential Annual Tuition: *$3,740* • Non-Residential Annual Tuition: *$7,380* • General Institutional Fees: *Not Provided* • Additional Nursing Fees: *$820*

Circle 124 on reader card   See in-depth profile for more information

INDIANA UNIVERSITY—PURDUE UNIVERSITY

Address: 355 Lansing Street, Indianapolis, IN 46202-2896
Phone: 317-274-3670
Fax: 317-274-2996
Contact: Sharon Farley, PhD, RN, FAAN, Acting Director, PhD Program and Executive Associate Dean
Email: Sfarley@iupui.edu

GENERAL INFORMATION

Type of School: *4-Year College or University, Public* • Accreditation: *North Central Association of Colleges and Schools* • Total Enrollment: *27500*

PROGRAM INFORMATION

Degree Awarded: *PhD and DNS/DNSc* • Specialty Focuses: *Research*

NURSING STUDENT PROFILE

Total Nursing Enrollment: *29* • Full-Time Enrollment: *10* • Part-Time Enrollment: *19* • Female Enrollment: *28* • Male Enrollment: *1* • Total Graduates: *7*

FINANCES

Residential Annual Tuition: *$171* • Non-Residential Annual Tuition: *$494* • General Institutional Fees: *$431* • Additional Nursing Fees: *$211*

UNIVERSITY OF IOWA

Address: 101 Nursing Building, Iowa City, IA 52242
Phone: 319-335-7021
Fax: Not Provided
Contact: Meridean Mass, PhD, RN, FAAN, Professor and Director
Email: meridean-maas@uiowa.edu

GENERAL INFORMATION

Type of School: *4-Year College or University, Public* • Accreditation: *North Central Association of Colleges and Schools* • Total Enrollment: *28840*

PROGRAM INFORMATION

Degree Awarded: *PhD* • Specialty Focuses: *Administration/Executive Role and Other*

NURSING STUDENT PROFILE

Total Nursing Enrollment: *37* • Full-Time Enrollment: *25* • Part-Time Enrollment: *12* • Female Enrollment: *34* • Male Enrollment: *3* • Total Graduates: *4*

FINANCES

Residential Annual Tuition: *Not Provided* • Non-Residential Annual Tuition: *Not Provided* • General Institutional Fees: *Not Provided* • Additional Nursing Fees: *Not Provided*

UNIVERSITY OF KANSAS

Address: 3901 Rainbow Blvd., Kansas City, KS 66160-
            7501
Phone: 913-588-1619
Fax: Not Provided
Contact: Karen L. Miller, PhD, RN, FAAN, Professor and
            Dean
Email: soninfo@kumc.edu

GENERAL INFORMATION

Type of School: *4-Year College or University, Public* •
Accreditation: *North Central Association of Colleges and
Schools* • Total Enrollment: *25920*

PROGRAM INFORMATION

Degree Awarded: *PhD* • Specialty Focuses: *Research*

NURSING STUDENT PROFILE

Total Nursing Enrollment: *42* • Full-Time Enrollment: *9* •
Part-Time Enrollment: *33* • Female Enrollment: *41* • Male
Enrollment: *1* • Total Graduates: *5*

FINANCES

Residential Annual Tuition: *Not Provided* • Non-Residential
Annual Tuition: *Not Provided* • General Institutional Fees:
$266 • Additional Nursing Fees: *Not Provided*

LOUISIANA STATE UNIVERSITY

Address: 433 Bolivar Street, New Orleans, LA 70112
Phone: 504-568-4106
Fax: 504-599-0573
Contact: Elizabeth A. Humphrey, EdD, RN, Professor and
            Dean
Email: ehumph@lsuhsc.edu

GENERAL INFORMATION

Type of School: *Other , Public* • Accreditation: *Southern
Association of Colleges and Schools* • Total Enrollment: *2755*

PROGRAM INFORMATION

Degree Awarded: *DNS./DNSc.* • Specialty Focuses: *Clinical
Practice and Administration/Executive Role*

NURSING STUDENT PROFILE

Total Nursing Enrollment: *62* • Full-Time Enrollment: *6* •
Part-Time Enrollment: *56* • Female Enrollment: *57* • Male
Enrollment: *5* • Total Graduates: *6*

FINANCES

Residential Annual Tuition: *$2,522* • Non-Residential
Annual Tuition: *$5,022* • General Institutional Fees: *$166* •
Additional Nursing Fees: *$0*

JOHNS HOPKINS UNIVERSITY

Address: 525 N. Wolfe St., Room 501, Baltimore, MD 21205
Phone: 410-614-5322
Fax: Not Provided
Contact: Jacquelyn Campbell, PhD, RN, Associate Dean of PdD Programs and Research
Email: jcampbel@son.jhmi.edu

GENERAL INFORMATION

Type of School: *Independent, Private (Independent)* • Accreditation: *Middle States Association of Colleges and Schools* • Total Enrollment: *Not Provided*

PROGRAM INFORMATION

Degree Awarded: *PhD* • Specialty Focuses: *Research*

NURSING STUDENT PROFILE

Total Nursing Enrollment: *24* • Full-Time Enrollment: *10* • Part-Time Enrollment: *14* • Female Enrollment: *22* • Male Enrollment: *2* • Total Graduates: *4*

FINANCES

Residential Annual Tuition: *$25,880* • Non-Residential Annual Tuition: *$25,880* • General Institutional Fees: *$500* • Additional Nursing Fees: *Not Provided*

UNIVERSITY OF MARYLAND—BALTIMORE

Address: 655 W Lombard St, Baltimore, MD 21210
Phone: 410-706-6741
Fax: 410-706-4231
Contact: Barbara R Heller, EdD, RN, FAAN, Dean and Professor
Email: heller@son.umaryland.edu

GENERAL INFORMATION

Type of School: *4-Year College or University, Public* • Accreditation: *Middle States Association of Colleges and Schools* • Total Enrollment: *Not Provided*

PROGRAM INFORMATION

Degree Awarded: *PhD* • Specialty Focuses: *Research*

NURSING STUDENT PROFILE

Total Nursing Enrollment: *71* • Full-Time Enrollment: *38* • Part-Time Enrollment: *33* • Female Enrollment: *65* • Male Enrollment: *6* • Total Graduates: *10*

FINANCES

Residential Annual Tuition: *$5,058* • Non-Residential Annual Tuition: *$9,054* • General Institutional Fees: *$276* • Additional Nursing Fees: *$205*

BOSTON COLLEGE

Address: 140 Commonwealth Ave., Chestnut Hill, MA
          02467-3812
Phone: 617-552-4279
Fax: 617-552-0745
Contact: Laurel Eisenhauer, PhD, RN, FAAN, Associate
          Dean
Email: laurel_eisenhauer@bc.edu

GENERAL INFORMATION

Type of School: *4-Year College or University, Private
(Religious)* • Accreditation: *New England Association of Schools
and Colleges* • Total Enrollment: *14000*

PROGRAM INFORMATION

Degree Awarded: *PhD and DNS/DNSc* • Specialty Focuses:
Other

NURSING STUDENT PROFILE

Total Nursing Enrollment: *40* • Full-Time Enrollment: *24* •
Part-Time Enrollment: *16* • Female Enrollment: *38* • Male
Enrollment: *2* • Total Graduates: *7*

FINANCES

Residential Annual Tuition: *$12,996* • Non-Residential
Annual Tuition: *$12,996* • General Institutional Fees: *$65* •
Additional Nursing Fees: *$722*

UNIVERSITY OF MASSACHUSETTS—AMHERST

Address: 715 North Pleasant, Amherst, MA 01003
Phone: 508-856-5661
Fax: Not Provided
Contact: James Fain, PhD, RN, Director, Collaborative
          PhD Program
Email: james.fain@umassmed.edu

GENERAL INFORMATION

Type of School: *4-Year College or University, Public* •
Accreditation: *Not Provided* • Total Enrollment: *Not Provided*

PROGRAM INFORMATION

Degree Awarded: *PhD* • Specialty Focuses: *Research and
Educational/Professorial Role*

NURSING STUDENT PROFILE

Total Nursing Enrollment: *30* • Full-Time Enrollment: *Not
Provided* • Part-Time Enrollment: *Not Provided* • Female
Enrollment: *29* • Male Enrollment: *1* • Total Graduates: *7*

FINANCES

Residential Annual Tuition: *$2,640* • Non-Residential
Annual Tuition: *$9,856* • General Institutional Fees:
$1,501 • Additional Nursing Fees: *$1,109*

UNIVERSITY OF MASSACHUSETTS—BOSTON

Address: 100 Morrissy Blvd, Boston, MA 02125-3393
Phone: 617-287-7548
Fax: 617-287-7527
Contact: Gail Russell, EdD, RN, Director
Email: gail.russell@umb.edu

GENERAL INFORMATION

Type of School: *4-Year College or University, Public* • Accreditation: *New England Association of Schools and Colleges* • Total Enrollment: *Not Provided*

PROGRAM INFORMATION

Degree Awarded: *PhD* • Specialty Focuses: *Research|Other*

NURSING STUDENT PROFILE

Total Nursing Enrollment: *23* • Full-Time Enrollment: *9* • Part-Time Enrollment: *14* • Female Enrollment: *23* • Male Enrollment: *0* • Total Graduates: *1*

FINANCES

Residential Annual Tuition: *$2,590* • Non-Residential Annual Tuition: *$9,758* • General Institutional Fees: *$3,230* • Additional Nursing Fees: *Not Provided*

UNIVERSITY OF MASSACHUSETTS—LOWELL

Address: 3 Solomont Way, Suite 2, Lowell, MA 01854-5126
Phone: 978-934-4537
Fax: Not Provided
Contact: Cheryl Cox, PhD, RN, Director
Email: cheryl_cox@uml.edu

GENERAL INFORMATION

Type of School: *4-Year College or University, Public* • Accreditation: *New England Association of Schools and Colleges* • Total Enrollment: *Not Provided*

PROGRAM INFORMATION

Degree Awarded: *PhD* • Specialty Focuses: *Research, Clinical Practice, Educational/Professorial Role, and Other*

NURSING STUDENT PROFILE

Total Nursing Enrollment: *12* • Full-Time Enrollment: *6* • Part-Time Enrollment: *6* • Female Enrollment: *11* • Male Enrollment: *1* • Total Graduates: *1*

FINANCES

Residential Annual Tuition: *$2,336* • Non-Residential Annual Tuition: *$6,559* • General Institutional Fees: *$1819* • Additional Nursing Fees: *$0*

MICHIGAN STATE UNIVERSITY

Address: A219 Life Sciences, East Lansing, MI 48824-1317
Phone: 517-432-6220
Fax: Not Provided
Contact: Audrey G Gift, PhD, RN, FAAN, Associate Dean
Email: agift@msu.edu

GENERAL INFORMATION

Type of School: *4-Year College or University, Public* • Accreditation: *North Central Association of Colleges and Schools* • Total Enrollment: *43366*

PROGRAM INFORMATION

Degree Awarded: *PhD* • Specialty Focuses: *Research*

NURSING STUDENT PROFILE

Total Nursing Enrollment: *6* • Full-Time Enrollment: *6* • Part-Time Enrollment: *0* • Female Enrollment: *6* • Male Enrollment: *0* • Total Graduates: *Not Provided*

FINANCES

Residential Annual Tuition: *$4,266* • Non-Residential Annual Tuition: *$8,631* • General Institutional Fees: *Not Provided* • Additional Nursing Fees: *Not Provided*

UNIVERSITY OF MICHIGAN

Address: 400 N. Ingalls, Ann Arbor, MI 48109
Phone: 734-764-9454
Fax: 734-763-6668
Contact: Carol Loveland-Cherry, PhD, RN, FAAN, Interim Director
Email: loveland@umich.edu

GENERAL INFORMATION

Type of School: *4-Year College or University, Public* • Accreditation: *North Central Association of Colleges and Schools* • Total Enrollment: *38103*

PROGRAM INFORMATION

Degree Awarded: *PhD* • Specialty Focuses: *Research and Administration/Executive Role*

NURSING STUDENT PROFILE

Total Nursing Enrollment: *72* • Full-Time Enrollment: *34* • Part-Time Enrollment: *38* • Female Enrollment: *70* • Male Enrollment: *2* • Total Graduates: *10*

FINANCES

Residential Annual Tuition: *$11,562* • Non-Residential Annual Tuition: *$23,442* • General Institutional Fees: *$198* • Additional Nursing Fees: *Not Provided*

UNIVERSITY OF MISSISSIPPI MEDICAL CENTER

Address: 2500 North State Street, Jackson, MS 39216
Phone: 601-815-3925
Fax: Not Provided
Contact: Peggy O Hewlett, PhD, RN, Director of
           Doctorate Program
Email: phewlett@son.umsmed.edu

GENERAL INFORMATION

Type of School: *Technical/Specialized Institution, Public* •
Accreditation: *Southern Association of Colleges and Schools* •
Total Enrollment: *1694*

PROGRAM INFORMATION

Degree Awarded: *PhD* • Specialty Focuses: *Research and Other*

NURSING STUDENT PROFILE

Total Nursing Enrollment: *17* • Full-Time Enrollment: *1* •
Part-Time Enrollment: *16* • Female Enrollment: *17* • Male
Enrollment: *0* • Total Graduates: *0*

FINANCES

Residential Annual Tuition: *$2,378* • Non-Residential
Annual Tuition: *$4,691* • General Institutional Fees: *Not
Provided* • Additional Nursing Fees: *Not Provided*

THE UNIVERSITY OF SOUTHERN MISSISSIPPI

Address: PO Box 5095, Hattiesburg, MS 39406
Phone: 601-266-5471
Fax: Not Provided
Contact: Bonnie Lee Harbaugh, PhD, RN, Assistant Dean
Email: Bonnie.Harbaugh@usm.edu

GENERAL INFORMATION

Type of School: *4-Year College or University, Public* •
Accreditation: *Southern Association of Colleges and Schools* •
Total Enrollment: *14510*

PROGRAM INFORMATION

Degree Awarded: *PhD* • Specialty Focuses:
*Educational/Professorial Role, Administration/Executive Role,
and Other*

NURSING STUDENT PROFILE

Total Nursing Enrollment: *8* • Full-Time Enrollment: *5* •
Part-Time Enrollment: *3* • Female Enrollment: *6* • Male
Enrollment: *2* • Total Graduates: *0*

FINANCES

Residential Annual Tuition: *$3,868* • Non-Residential
Annual Tuition: *$8,846* • General Institutional Fees: *$0* •
Additional Nursing Fees: *$0*

SAINT LOUIS UNIVERSITY

Address: 3525 Caroline Mall, Saint Louis, MO 63104
Phone: 314-577-8971
Fax: Not Provided
Contact: Irene I Riddle, PhD, RN, Director and Professor
Email: riddleii@slu.edu

GENERAL INFORMATION

Type of School: *4-Year College or University, Private (Religious)* • Accreditation: *North Central Association of Colleges and Schools* • Total Enrollment: *11112*

PROGRAM INFORMATION

Degree Awarded: *PhD* • Specialty Focuses: *Research*

NURSING STUDENT PROFILE

Total Nursing Enrollment: *37* • Full-Time Enrollment: *7* • Part-Time Enrollment: *30* • Female Enrollment: *35* • Male Enrollment: *2* • Total Graduates: *4*

FINANCES

Residential Annual Tuition: *$10,800* • Non-Residential Annual Tuition: *$10,800* • General Institutional Fees: *Not Provided* • Additional Nursing Fees: *$20*

UNIVERSITY OF MISSOURI— COLUMBIA

Address: S218 Nursing School Bldg, Columbia, MO 65211
Phone: 573-884-7268
Fax: Not Provided
Contact: Eileen Porter, PhD, RN, Co-Director
Email: PorterE@health.missouri.edu

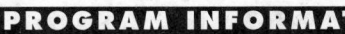

GENERAL INFORMATION

Type of School: *Not Provided* • Accreditation: *North Central Association of Colleges and Schools* • Total Enrollment: *Not Provided*

PROGRAM INFORMATION

Degree Awarded: *PhD* • Specialty Focuses: *Research and Other*

NURSING STUDENT PROFILE

Total Nursing Enrollment: *31* • Full-Time Enrollment: *21* • Part-Time Enrollment: *10* • Female Enrollment: *29* • Male Enrollment: *2* • Total Graduates: *2*

FINANCES

Residential Annual Tuition: *Not Provided* • Non-Residential Annual Tuition: *Not Provided* • General Institutional Fees: *Not Provided* • Additional Nursing Fees: *Not Provided*

UNIVERSITY OF MISSOURI—KANSAS CITY

Address: 2220 Holmes Street, Kansas City, MO 64108
Phone: 816-235-1724
Fax: Not Provided
Contact: Katharine Smith, PhD, RN, Associate Professor
Email: smithkv@umkc.edu

GENERAL INFORMATION

Type of School: *Not Provided* • Accreditation: *North Central Association of Colleges and Schools* • Total Enrollment: *Not Provided*

PROGRAM INFORMATION

Degree Awarded: *PhD* • Specialty Focuses: *Other*

NURSING STUDENT PROFILE

Total Nursing Enrollment: *18* • Full-Time Enrollment: *1* • Part-Time Enrollment: *17* • Female Enrollment: *18* • Male Enrollment: *0* • Total Graduates: *Not Provided*

FINANCES

Residential Annual Tuition: *$3,118* • Non-Residential Annual Tuition: *$9,378* • General Institutional Fees: *$60* • Additional Nursing Fees: *Not Provided*

UNIVERSITY OF MISSOURI—ST. LOUIS

Address: 8001 Natural Bridge Road, Saint Louis, MO 63121
Phone: 314-516-6849
Fax: Not Provided
Contact: Sally Hardin, PhD, RN, FAAN, Program Director
Email: hardins@msx.umsl.edu

GENERAL INFORMATION

Type of School: *Not Provided* • Accreditation: *North Central Association of Colleges and Schools* • Total Enrollment: *Not Provided*

PROGRAM INFORMATION

Degree Awarded: *PhD* • Specialty Focuses: *Research*

NURSING STUDENT PROFILE

Total Nursing Enrollment: *30* • Full-Time Enrollment: *10* • Part-Time Enrollment: *20* • Female Enrollment: *29* • Male Enrollment: *1* • Total Graduates: *4*

FINANCES

Residential Annual Tuition: *$4,000* • Non-Residential Annual Tuition: *$9,000* • General Institutional Fees: *Not Provided* • Additional Nursing Fees: *Not Provided*

UNIVERSITY OF NEBRASKA MEDICAL CENTER

Address: 985330 Nebraska Medical Center, Omaha, NE 68198-5330
Phone: 402-559-7457
Fax: 402-559-6379
Contact: Margaret Wilson, PhD, RN, Associate Professor and Associate Dean
Email: mwilson@unmc.edu

GENERAL INFORMATION

Type of School: *4-Year College or University, Public* • Accreditation: *North Central Association of Colleges and Schools* • Total Enrollment: *2636*

PROGRAM INFORMATION

Degree Awarded: *PhD* • Specialty Focuses: *Research*

NURSING STUDENT PROFILE

Total Nursing Enrollment: *36* • Full-Time Enrollment: *4* • Part-Time Enrollment: *32* • Female Enrollment: *35* • Male Enrollment: *1* • Total Graduates: *1*

FINANCES

Residential Annual Tuition: *$2,623* • Non-Residential Annual Tuition: *$6,993* • General Institutional Fees: *$356* • Additional Nursing Fees: *$200*

UNIVERSITY OF MEDICAL DENTISTRY OF NEW JERSEY/NJIT JOINT BSN PROGRAM

Address: 65 Bergen Street, Rm. 1141, Newark, NJ 07107-3001
Phone: 973-972-8564
Fax: Not Provided
Contact: Joseph Holtzman, PhD, RN, Program Director
Email: holtzman@umdnj.edu

GENERAL INFORMATION

Type of School: *Other, Public* • Accreditation: *Middle States Association of Colleges and Schools* • Total Enrollment: *600*

PROGRAM INFORMATION

Degree Awarded: *PhD* • Specialty Focuses: *Research*

NURSING STUDENT PROFILE

Total Nursing Enrollment: *15* • Full-Time Enrollment: *Not Provided* • Part-Time Enrollment: *Not Provided* • Female Enrollment: *Not Provided* • Male Enrollment: *Not Provided* • Total Graduates: *Not Provided*

FINANCES

Residential Annual Tuition: *$5,058* • Non-Residential Annual Tuition: *$7,146* • General Institutional Fees: *$250* • Additional Nursing Fees: *Not Provided*

ADELPHI UNIVERSITY

Address: 1 South Ave., Garden City, NY 11530
Phone: 516-877-4564
Fax: 516-877-4558
Contact: Veronica Conners, PhD, EdD, RN, Associate
            Dean
Email: conners@adelphi.edu

GENERAL INFORMATION

Type of School: *4-Year College or University, Private
(Independent)* • Accreditation: *Middle States Association of
Colleges and Schools* • Total Enrollment: *6500*

PROGRAM INFORMATION

Degree Awarded: *PhD* • Specialty Focuses: *Research and
Educational/Professorial Role*

NURSING STUDENT PROFILE

Total Nursing Enrollment: *10* • Full-Time Enrollment: *0* •
Part-Time Enrollment: *10* • Female Enrollment: *10* • Male
Enrollment: *0* • Total Graduates: *5*

FINANCES

Residential Annual Tuition: *$9,720* • Non-Residential
Annual Tuition: *$9,720* • General Institutional Fees: *$300* •
Additional Nursing Fees: *Not Provided*

COLUMBIA UNIVERSITY

Address: 630 West 168th St. Box 6, New York, NY 10032
Phone: 212-305-5538
Fax: 212-305-6937
Contact: Elizabeth R Lenz, PhD, Associate Dean for
            Research and Doctoral Studies
Email: er113@columbia.edu

GENERAL INFORMATION

Type of School: *4-Year College or University, Private
(Independent)* • Accreditation: *None* • Total Enrollment:
19000

PROGRAM INFORMATION

Degree Awarded: *DNS/DNSc* • Specialty Focuses: *Research*

NURSING STUDENT PROFILE

Total Nursing Enrollment: *34* • Full-Time Enrollment: *15* •
Part-Time Enrollment: *19* • Female Enrollment: *32* • Male
Enrollment: *2* • Total Graduates: *1*

FINANCES

Residential Annual Tuition: *$18,720* • Non-Residential
Annual Tuition: *$18,720* • General Institutional Fees:
$3,156 • Additional Nursing Fees: *$4,040*

NEW YORK UNIVERSITY

Address: 246 Greene St., New York, NY 10003
Phone: 212-998-5412
Fax: Not Provided
Contact: Elizabeth Norman, PhD, RN, FAAN, Director
Email: elizabeth.norman@nyu.edu

GENERAL INFORMATION

Type of School: *4-Year College or University, Private (Independent)* • Accreditation: *Middle States Association of Colleges and Schools* • Total Enrollment: *Not Provided*

PROGRAM INFORMATION

Degree Awarded: *PhD* • Specialty Focuses: *Research*

NURSING STUDENT PROFILE

Total Nursing Enrollment: *80* • Full-Time Enrollment: *10* • Part-Time Enrollment: *70* • Female Enrollment: *75* • Male Enrollment: *5* • Total Graduates: *4*

FINANCES

Residential Annual Tuition: *$2,447* • Non-Residential Annual Tuition: *Not Provided* • General Institutional Fees: *Not Provided* • Additional Nursing Fees: *Not Provided*

STATE UNIVERSITY OF NEW YORK—BUFFALO

Address: 3435 Main St., 1030 Kimball Tower, Buffalo, NY 14214
Phone: 716-829-2533
Fax: Not Provided
Contact: Karen J Radke, PhD, RN, Associate Dean
Email: radke@buffalo.edu

GENERAL INFORMATION

Type of School: *4-Year College or University, Public* • Accreditation: *Middle States Association of Colleges and Schools* • Total Enrollment: *24830*

PROGRAM INFORMATION

Degree Awarded: *DNS/DNSc* • Specialty Focuses: *Research, Clinical Practice, Educational/Professorial Role and Administration/Executive Role*

NURSING STUDENT PROFILE

Total Nursing Enrollment: *25* • Full-Time Enrollment: *16* • Part-Time Enrollment: *9* • Female Enrollment: *23* • Male Enrollment: *2* • Total Graduates: *7*

FINANCES

Residential Annual Tuition: *$5,100* • Non-Residential Annual Tuition: *$8,416* • General Institutional Fees: *$870* • Additional Nursing Fees: *Not Provided*

TEACHERS COLLEGE, COLUMBIA UNIVERSITY

Address: 525 West 120th St. Box 35, New York, NY
           10027
Phone: 212-678-3120
Fax: Not Provided
Contact: Kathleen O'Connell, PhD, RN, FAAN,
           Professor
Email: oconnell@exchange.tc.columbia.edu

GENERAL INFORMATION

Type of School: *Not Provided, Private (Independent)* •
Accreditation: *Not Provided* • Total Enrollment: *Not Provided*

PROGRAM INFORMATION

Degree Awarded: *EdD* • Specialty Focuses: *Research and
Educational/Professorial Role*

NURSING STUDENT PROFILE

Total Nursing Enrollment: *12* • Full-Time Enrollment: *0* •
Part-Time Enrollment: *12* • Female Enrollment: *12* • Male
Enrollment: *0* • Total Graduates: *3*

FINANCES

Residential Annual Tuition: *$12,690* • Non-Residential
Annual Tuition: *$12,690* • General Institutional Fees: *$170* •
Additional Nursing Fees: *Not Provided*

UNIVERSITY OF ROCHESTER

Address: 601 Elmwood Ave., Box SON, Rochester, NY
           14642
Phone: 585-275-8889
Fax: 585-756-8299
Contact: Madeline Schmitt, PhD, RN, FAAN,
           Coordinator for Doctoral Program
Email: Madeline_Schmitt@urmc.rochester.edu

GENERAL INFORMATION

Type of School: *4-Year College or University, Private
(Independent)* • Accreditation: *Middle States Association of
Colleges and Schools* • Total Enrollment: *8201*

PROGRAM INFORMATION

Degree Awarded: *PhD* • Specialty Focuses: *Research*

NURSING STUDENT PROFILE

Total Nursing Enrollment: *38* • Full-Time Enrollment: *15* •
Part-Time Enrollment: *23* • Female Enrollment: *35* • Male
Enrollment: *3* • Total Graduates: *4*

FINANCES

Residential Annual Tuition: *$13,590* • Non-Residential
Annual Tuition: *$13,590* • General Institutional Fees: *$429* •
Additional Nursing Fees: *Not Provided*

Circle 134 on reader card   **See in-depth profile for more information**

UNIVERSITY OF NORTH CAROLINA—CHAPEL HILL

Address: Carrington Hall, Campus Box 7460, Chapel
            Hill, NC 27599
Phone: 919-966-4274
Fax: 919-843-6212
Contact: Diane Davis, PhD, RN, Professor and Director
Email: holditch@email.unc.edu

CASE WESTERN RESERVE UNIVERSITY

Address: 10900 Euclid Avenue, Cleveland, OH 44106-
            4904
Phone: 216-368-3612
Fax: 216-368-3542
Contact: Jaclene Zauszniewski, PhD, RNC, Program
            Director and Associate Professor
Email: jaz@po.cwru.edu

GENERAL INFORMATION

Type of School: *4-Year College or University, Public* •
Accreditation: *Southern Association of Colleges and Schools* •
Total Enrollment: *24180*

GENERAL INFORMATION

Type of School: *4-Year College or University, Private
(Independent)* • Accreditation: *North Central Association of
Colleges and Schools* • Total Enrollment: *Not Provided*

PROGRAM INFORMATION

Degree Awarded: *PhD* • Specialty Focuses: *Research*

PROGRAM INFORMATION

Degree Awarded: *PhD* • Specialty Focuses: *Research and
Clinical Practice*

NURSING STUDENT PROFILE

Total Nursing Enrollment: *50* • Full-Time Enrollment: *24* •
Part-Time Enrollment: *26* • Female Enrollment: *47* • Male
Enrollment: *3* • Total Graduates: *3*

NURSING STUDENT PROFILE

Total Nursing Enrollment: *73* • Full-Time Enrollment: *15* •
Part-Time Enrollment: *58* • Female Enrollment: *67* • Male
Enrollment: *6* • Total Graduates: *18*

FINANCES

Residential Annual Tuition: *$1,255* • Non-Residential
Annual Tuition: *$6,411* • General Institutional Fees: *$466* •
Additional Nursing Fees: *Not Provided*

FINANCES

Residential Annual Tuition: *$7,875* • Non-Residential
Annual Tuition: *$7,875* • General Institutional Fees: *$15* •
Additional Nursing Fees: *$5*

THE UNIVERSITY OF AKRON

Address: 302 East Buthcel Mall, Akron, OH 44325-3701
Phone: Not Provided
Fax: Not Provided
Contact: Carol Deets, EdD, RN, Associate Dean and
           Director
Email: Carol.Deets@uc.edu

GENERAL INFORMATION

Type of School: *Not Provided* • Accreditation: *Not Provided* •
Total Enrollment: *Not Provided*

PROGRAM INFORMATION

Degree Awarded: *Other* • Specialty Focuses: *Other*

NURSING STUDENT PROFILE

Total Nursing Enrollment: *Not Provided* • Full-Time
Enrollment: *Not Provided* • Part-Time Enrollment: *Not
Provided* • Female Enrollment: *Not Provided* • Male
Enrollment: *Not Provided* • Total Graduates: *Not Provided*

FINANCES

Residential Annual Tuition: *Not Provided* • Non-Residential
Annual Tuition: *Not Provided* • General Institutional Fees:
Not Provided • Additional Nursing Fees: *Not Provided*

UNIVERSITY OF CINCINNATI

Address: 9555 Plainfield Road, Cincinnati, OH 45236
Phone: 513-558-5218
Fax: 513-558-5054
Contact: Carol Deets, EdD, RN, Associate Dean and
           Director of Doctoral Program
Email: carol.deets@uc.edu

GENERAL INFORMATION

Type of School: *2-Year College or University, Public* •
Accreditation: *North Central Association of Colleges and
Schools* • Total Enrollment: *3500*

PROGRAM INFORMATION

Degree Awarded: *PhD* • Specialty Focuses: *Research*

NURSING STUDENT PROFILE

Total Nursing Enrollment: *26* • Full-Time Enrollment: *14* •
Part-Time Enrollment: *12* • Female Enrollment: *11* • Male
Enrollment: *15* • Total Graduates: *9*

FINANCES

Residential Annual Tuition: *$5,394* • Non-Residential
Annual Tuition: *$10,839* • General Institutional Fees: *$870* •
Additional Nursing Fees: *Not Provided*

OREGON HEALTH SCIENCES UNIVERSITY

Address: 3181 South West Sam Jackson Park Road,
           Portland, OR 97201
Phone: 503-494-7725
Fax: Not Provided
Contact: Beverly Hoeffer, DNSc, RN, FAAN, Associate
           Dean for Academic Affairs
Email: proginfo@ohsu.edu

GENERAL INFORMATION

Type of School: *Other , Public* • Accreditation: *Northwestern Association of Schools and Colleges* • Total Enrollment: *2679*

PROGRAM INFORMATION

Degree Awarded: *PhD* • Specialty Focuses: *Research*

NURSING STUDENT PROFILE

Total Nursing Enrollment: *39* • Full-Time Enrollment: *16* • Part-Time Enrollment: *23* • Female Enrollment: *39* • Male Enrollment: *0* • Total Graduates: *7*

FINANCES

Residential Annual Tuition: *$6,780* • Non-Residential Annual Tuition: *$11,256* • General Institutional Fees: *$680* • Additional Nursing Fees: *$40*

DUQUESNE UNIVERSITY

Address: 600 Forbes Ave., Pittsburgh, PA 15282
Phone: 412-396-6537
Fax: 412-396-4180
Contact: Ellen Olshansky, DNSc, RNC, Associate Dean
           of Graduate Programs
Email: olshansky@duq.edu

GENERAL INFORMATION

Type of School: *4-Year College or University, Private (Religious)* • Accreditation: *Middle States Association of Colleges and Schools* • Total Enrollment: *9555*

PROGRAM INFORMATION

Degree Awarded: *PhD* • Specialty Focuses: *Research*

NURSING STUDENT PROFILE

Total Nursing Enrollment: *50* • Full-Time Enrollment: *2* • Part-Time Enrollment: *48* • Female Enrollment: *50* • Male Enrollment: *0* • Total Graduates: *7*

FINANCES

Residential Annual Tuition: *$11,196* • Non-Residential Annual Tuition: *$11,196* • General Institutional Fees: *$56* • Additional Nursing Fees: *Not Provided*

PENNSYLVANIA STATE UNIVERSITY

Address: 203 Health and Human Development,
            University Park, PA 16802-6508
Phone: 814-863-7755
Fax: Not Provided
Contact: Karen H Morin, DSN, RN, Professor
Email: khm10@psu.edu

GENERAL INFORMATION

Type of School: *4-Year College or University, Public* •
Accreditation: *Middle States Association of Colleges and Schools* • Total Enrollment: *15582*

PROGRAM INFORMATION

Degree Awarded: *PhD* • Specialty Focuses: *Research, Clinical Practice, Educational/Professorial Role, Other*

NURSING STUDENT PROFILE

Total Nursing Enrollment: *17* • Full-Time Enrollment: *7* • Part-Time Enrollment: *10* • Female Enrollment: *17* • Male Enrollment: *0* • Total Graduates: *0*

FINANCES

Residential Annual Tuition: *$7,314* • Non-Residential Annual Tuition: *$14,980* • General Institutional Fees: *$306* • Additional Nursing Fees: *Not Provided*

UNIVERSITY OF PENNSYLVANIA

Address: 420 Guardian Drive, Philadelphia, PA 1910
Phone: 215-898-1844
Fax: Not Provided
Contact: Susan Gennaro, DSN, RN, FAAN, Director of
            Doctoral and Post-Doctoral Studies
Email: gennaro@nursing.upenn.edu

GENERAL INFORMATION

Type of School: *4-Year College or University, Private (Independent)* • Accreditation: *Middle States Association of Colleges and Schools* • Total Enrollment: *21800*

PROGRAM INFORMATION

Degree Awarded: *PhD* • Specialty Focuses: *Research*

NURSING STUDENT PROFILE

Total Nursing Enrollment: *59* • Full-Time Enrollment: *21* • Part-Time Enrollment: *38* • Female Enrollment: *57* • Male Enrollment: *2* • Total Graduates: *15*

FINANCES

Residential Annual Tuition: *$27,850* • Non-Residential Annual Tuition: *$27,850* • General Institutional Fees: *$1,612* • Additional Nursing Fees: *$488*

UNIVERSITY OF PITTSBURGH

Address: 3500 Victoria Street, Room 350, Pittsburgh, PA 15261
Phone: 412-624-1905
Fax: Not Provided
Contact: Judith A Erlen, PhD, RN, FAAN, Professor
Email: jae001@pitt.edu

GENERAL INFORMATION

Type of School: *4-Year College or University, Public* • Accreditation: *Middle States Association of Colleges and Schools* • Total Enrollment: *25461*

PROGRAM INFORMATION

Degree Awarded: *PhD* • Specialty Focuses: *Research*

NURSING STUDENT PROFILE

Total Nursing Enrollment: *41* • Full-Time Enrollment: *16* • Part-Time Enrollment: *25* • Female Enrollment: *39* • Male Enrollment: *2* • Total Graduates: *9*

FINANCES

Residential Annual Tuition: *$13,772* • Non-Residential Annual Tuition: *$26,884* • General Institutional Fees: *$240* • Additional Nursing Fees: *$11*

WIDENER UNIVERSITY

Address: One University Place, Chester, PA 19013
Phone: 610-499-4208
Fax: 610-499-4216
Contact: Mary B Walker, EdD, RN, Assistant Dean for Graduate Studies
Email: mary.b.walker@widener.edu

GENERAL INFORMATION

Type of School: *Not Provided* • Accreditation: *Middle States Association of Colleges and Schools* • Total Enrollment: *Not Provided*

PROGRAM INFORMATION

Degree Awarded: *DNS/DNSc* • Specialty Focuses: *Educational/Professorial Role*

NURSING STUDENT PROFILE

Total Nursing Enrollment: *72* • Full-Time Enrollment: *49* • Part-Time Enrollment: *23* • Female Enrollment: *69* • Male Enrollment: *3* • Total Graduates: *9*

FINANCES

Residential Annual Tuition: *$10,080* • Non-Residential Annual Tuition: *$10,080* • General Institutional Fees: *$115* • Additional Nursing Fees: *Not Provided*

UNIVERSITY OF RHODE ISLAND

Address: White Hall, 2 Heathman Road, Kingston, RI 02881
Phone: 401-874-5337
Fax: Not Provided
Contact: Donna Schwartz-Barcott, PhD, RN, Director
Email: dsb@uri.edu

GENERAL INFORMATION

Type of School: *4-Year College or University, Public* •
Accreditation: *New England Association of Schools and Colleges* • Total Enrollment: *14362*

PROGRAM INFORMATION

Degree Awarded: *PhD* • Specialty Focuses: *Research and Educational/Professorial Role*

NURSING STUDENT PROFILE

Total Nursing Enrollment: *52* • Full-Time Enrollment: *8* •
Part-Time Enrollment: *44* • Female Enrollment: *49* • Male
Enrollment: *3* • Total Graduates: *5*

FINANCES

Residential Annual Tuition: *$3,636* • Non-Residential
Annual Tuition: *$10,400* • General Institutional Fees:
$1,428 • Additional Nursing Fees: *$240*

MEDICAL UNIVERSITY OF SOUTH CAROLINA

Address: 99 Johnathan Lucas St, Charleston, SC 29425
Phone: 843-792-4627
Fax: Not Provided
Contact: Gail Stuart, PhD, RN, FAAN, Professor and Director of the Doctoral Program
Email: stuartg@musc.edu

GENERAL INFORMATION

Type of School: *4-Year College or University, Public* •
Accreditation: *Southern Association of Colleges and Schools* •
Total Enrollment: *Not Provided*

PROGRAM INFORMATION

Degree Awarded: *PhD* • Specialty Focuses: *Other*

NURSING STUDENT PROFILE

Total Nursing Enrollment: *Not Provided* • Full-Time
Enrollment: *Not Provided* • Part-Time Enrollment: *Not
Provided* • Female Enrollment: *Not Provided* • Male
Enrollment: *Not Provided* • Total Graduates: *Not Provided*

FINANCES

Residential Annual Tuition: *$2,729* • Non-Residential
Annual Tuition: *$4,361* • General Institutional Fees: *$60* •
Additional Nursing Fees: *$242*

UNIVERSITY OF TENNESSEE—MEMPHIS

Address: 877 Madison Avenue, Memphis, TN 38163
Phone: 901-448-6135
Fax: Not Provided
Contact: Donna Hathaway, PhD, RN, Professor and Dean
Email: DHathaway@utmem.edu

GENERAL INFORMATION

Type of School: *Not Provided* • Accreditation: *Not Provided* • Total Enrollment: *Not Provided*

PROGRAM INFORMATION

Degree Awarded: *PhD and DNS/DNSc* • Specialty Focuses: *Research and Clinical Practice*

NURSING STUDENT PROFILE

Total Nursing Enrollment: *56* • Full-Time Enrollment: *53* • Part-Time Enrollment: *3* • Female Enrollment: *46* • Male Enrollment: *10* • Total Graduates: *2*

FINANCES

Residential Annual Tuition: *$2,959* • Non-Residential Annual Tuition: *$6,977* • General Institutional Fees: *Not Provided* • Additional Nursing Fees: *Not Provided*

UNIVERSITY OF TENNESSEE—KNOXVILLE

Address: 1200 Volunteer Blvd, Knoxville, TN 37996
Phone: 865-974-7581
Fax: Not Provided
Contact: Sandra Thomas, PhD, RN, Director
Email: sthomas@utk.edu

GENERAL INFORMATION

Type of School: *Not Provided* • Accreditation: *Not Provided* • Total Enrollment: *Not Provided*

PROGRAM INFORMATION

Degree Awarded: *PhD* • Specialty Focuses: *Research, Educational/Professorial Role, Administration/Executive Role*

NURSING STUDENT PROFILE

Total Nursing Enrollment: *22* • Full-Time Enrollment: *5* • Part-Time Enrollment: *17* • Female Enrollment: *20* • Male Enrollment: *2* • Total Graduates: *7*

FINANCES

Residential Annual Tuition: *Not Provided* • Non-Residential Annual Tuition: *Not Provided* • General Institutional Fees: *Not Provided* • Additional Nursing Fees: *Not Provided*

UNIVERSITY OF TEXAS MEDICAL BRANCH— GALVESTON

Address: 301 University Blvd, Galveston, TX 77555
Phone: 409-772-1510
Fax: Not Provided
Contact: Mary V Fenton, PhD, RN, Dean and Interim Director
Email: mfenton@utmb.edu

GENERAL INFORMATION

Type of School: *4-Year College or University, Public* •
Accreditation: *Southern Association of Colleges and Schools* •
Total Enrollment: *1927*

PROGRAM INFORMATION

Degree Awarded: *PhD* • Specialty Focuses: *None*

NURSING STUDENT PROFILE

Total Nursing Enrollment: *20* • Full-Time Enrollment: *20* •
Part-Time Enrollment: *0* • Female Enrollment: *17* • Male
Enrollment: *3* • Total Graduates: *0*

FINANCES

Residential Annual Tuition: *$1,080* • Non-Residential
Annual Tuition: *$6,885* • General Institutional Fees: *$136* •
Additional Nursing Fees: *Not Provided*

GEORGE MASON UNIVERSITY

Address: 4400 University Drive/3C4, Fairfax, VA 22030-4444
Phone: 703-993-1920
Fax: 703-993-1942
Contact: Stephanie Ferguson, PhD, RN, FAAN, Coordinator of PhD Program
Email: sfergusl@gmu.edu

GENERAL INFORMATION

Type of School: *4-Year College or University, Public* •
Accreditation: *Southern Association of Colleges and Schools* •
Total Enrollment: *24897*

PROGRAM INFORMATION

Degree Awarded: *PhD* • Specialty Focuses:
Administration/Executive Role and Other

NURSING STUDENT PROFILE

Total Nursing Enrollment: *78* • Full-Time Enrollment: *31* •
Part-Time Enrollment: *47* • Female Enrollment: *69* • Male
Enrollment: *9* • Total Graduates: *10*

FINANCES

Residential Annual Tuition: *$2,292* • Non-Residential
Annual Tuition: *$6,348* • General Institutional Fees: *$150* •
Additional Nursing Fees: *$0*

HAMPTON UNIVERSITY

Address: W. Adrian Freeman Hall, Hampton, VA 23668
Phone: 757-727-5252
Fax: Not Provided
Contact: Pamela V Hammond, PhD, RN, FAAN, Dean
Email: pamela.hammond@hamptonu.edu

UNIVERSITY OF VIRGINIA

Address: PO Box 800782, Charlottesville, VA 22908-0782
Phone: 434-982-1976
Fax: Not Provided
Contact: Barbara Parker, PhD, RN, Professor
Email: bjp8c@virgina.edu

GENERAL INFORMATION

Type of School: *4-Year College or University, Private (Independent)* • Accreditation: *Southern Association of Colleges and Schools* • Total Enrollment: *5743*

GENERAL INFORMATION

Type of School: *4-Year College or University, Public* • Accreditation: *Southern Association of Colleges and Schools* • Total Enrollment: *23717*

PROGRAM INFORMATION

Degree Awarded: *PhD* • Specialty Focuses: *Other*

PROGRAM INFORMATION

Degree Awarded: *PhD* • Specialty Focuses: *Research and Clinical Practice and Educational/Professorial Role and Administration/Executive Role*

NURSING STUDENT PROFILE

Total Nursing Enrollment: *8* • Full-Time Enrollment: *6* • Part-Time Enrollment: *2* • Female Enrollment: *8* • Male Enrollment: *0* • Total Graduates: *Not Provided*

NURSING STUDENT PROFILE

Total Nursing Enrollment: *34* • Full-Time Enrollment: *27* • Part-Time Enrollment: *7* • Female Enrollment: *30* • Male Enrollment: *4* • Total Graduates: *7*

FINANCES

Residential Annual Tuition: *$6,615* • Non-Residential Annual Tuition: *$6,615* • General Institutional Fees: *$245* • Additional Nursing Fees: *$35*

FINANCES

Residential Annual Tuition: *$3,988* • Non-Residential Annual Tuition: *$17,078* • General Institutional Fees: *$1,245* • Additional Nursing Fees: *Not Provided*

VIRGINIA COMMONWEALTH UNIVERSITY

Address: 910 W. Franklin, Richmond, VA 23284
Phone: 804-828-3474
Fax: 804-828-7743
Contact: Inez Tuck, PhD, RN, Associate Dean and
           Professor
Email: ituck@hsc.vcu.edu

GENERAL INFORMATION

Type of School: *4-Year College or University, Public* •
Accreditation: *Southern Association of Colleges and Schools* •
Total Enrollment: *25000*

PROGRAM INFORMATION

Degree Awarded: *PhD* • Specialty Focuses: *Research*

NURSING STUDENT PROFILE

Total Nursing Enrollment: *28* • Full-Time Enrollment: *16* •
Part-Time Enrollment: *12* • Female Enrollment: *25* • Male
Enrollment: *3* • Total Graduates: *6*

FINANCES

Residential Annual Tuition: *$4,276* • Non-Residential
Annual Tuition: *$12,672* • General Institutional Fees: *$967* •
Additional Nursing Fees: *$0*

WEST VIRGINIA UNIVERSITY

Address: PO Box 9600, Morgantown, WV 26506
Phone: 304-293-4298
Fax: Not Provided
Contact: Mary Jane Smith, PhD, RN, Professor and
           Associate Dean
Email: mjsmith@hsc.wvu.edu

GENERAL INFORMATION

Type of School: *4-Year College or University, Public* •
Accreditation: *North Central Association of Colleges and
Schools* • Total Enrollment: *22150*

PROGRAM INFORMATION

Degree Awarded: *Other* • Specialty Focuses: *Other*

NURSING STUDENT PROFILE

Total Nursing Enrollment: *Not Provided* • Full-Time
Enrollment: *Not Provided* • Part-Time Enrollment: *Not
Provided* • Female Enrollment: *Not Provided* • Male
Enrollment: *Not Provided* • Total Graduates: *Not Provided*

FINANCES

Residential Annual Tuition: *Not Provided* • Non-Residential
Annual Tuition: *Not Provided* • General Institutional Fees:
Not Provided • Additional Nursing Fees: *Not Provided*

Circle 143 on reader card   See in-depth profile for more information

UNIVERSITY OF WISCONSIN—MILWAUKEE

Address: PO Box 413, Milwaukee, WI 53201
Phone: 414-229-5468
Fax: Not Provided
Contact: Susan Dean-Baar, PhD, RN, FAAN, Associate
            Dean
Email: deanbaar@uwm.edu

GENERAL INFORMATION

Type of School: *4-Year College or University, Public* •
Accreditation: *North Central Association of Colleges and
Schools* • Total Enrollment: *24223*

PROGRAM INFORMATION

Degree Awarded: *PhD* • Specialty Focuses: *Research*

NURSING STUDENT PROFILE

Total Nursing Enrollment: *42* • Full-Time Enrollment: *8* •
Part-Time Enrollment: *34* • Female Enrollment: *38* • Male
Enrollment: *4* • Total Graduates: *2*

FINANCES

Residential Annual Tuition: *$5,720* • Non-Residential
Annual Tuition: *$17,678* • General Institutional Fees: *$318* •
Additional Nursing Fees: *Not Provided*

Section 4

IN-DEPTH SCHOOL PROFILES

ABINGTON MEMORIAL HOSPITAL
Dixon School of Nursing
Willow Grove, Pennsylvania

THE HOSPITAL
Abington Memorial Hospital (AMH), located at 1200 Old York Road in Abington, PA, is a 508-bed comprehensive regional teaching hospital and comprehensive health center, serving people in Montgomery, Bucks, and Philadelphia counties. AMH has a strong educational mission and provides clinical experiences and educational programs for students in nursing, medicine, dentistry, and medical and radiologic technology. It is designated as the only Level II accredited Trauma Center in Montgomery County and has facilities for helicopter transport of critically ill patients. Comprehensive services include inpatient and outpatient surgery (including open heart surgery), obstetrics/gynecology, pediatrics, geriatrics, oncology, cardiology, rehabilitation, and psychiatry. AMH also provides highly specialized high-risk obstetrics, Level III neonatal intensive care, and home healthcare. AMH is affiliated with The Children's Hospital of Philadelphia through the CHOP Connection.

THE SCHOOL OF NURSING
The School of Nursing is located in Willow Grove, Pennsylvania just north of historic Center City Philadelphia in a suburban teaching hospital setting, where student nurses work with outstanding healthcare professionals. Abington's hospital-based, student-oriented educational program combines academic excellence with strong clinical experience. Our students are prepared to confidently meet the needs of today's healthcare field where nurses are expected to be both clinically competent and theoretically strong. We are especially proud of our outstanding success rate on the RN licensing examination.

PROGRAM OF STUDY
The School of Nursing offers a strong clinically-based course of study in preparation for an exciting career as a professional nurse. The program is planned over three academic years. After one year of college course work in related science and liberal arts, there are two years of nursing education, preparing the graduate for a rewarding career in a variety of healthcare settings.

Graduates are eligible to take the National Council Licensure Examination-Registered Nurse, and with successful completion can use the title, Registered Nurse.

AFFILIATIONS WITH HEALTH CARE FACILITIES
The School of Nursing uses various clinical facilities to provide students with diverse experiences in clinical practice. Abington Memorial Hospital offers experiences in medical-surgical, operating room, obstetrical, and critical care nursing. Clinical facilities at affiliating agencies provide additional experiences in specialized nursing practice, including psychiatric, pediatric, community, and oncologic nursing.

ACADEMIC RESOURCES
The School of Nursing's resources are housed in Abington Memorial Health Center (home of the School of Nursing) and the Abington Memorial Hospital Dixon Building (location of the Wilmer Memorial Medical Library).

Students benefit from state-of-the art skills laboratories, library/media center, and extensive clinical opportunities both on the hospital campus and in the community.

COSTS
Tuition for years two and three at Abington (nursing theory and practice) is $6,000 per year. Tuition for year one at the college of the student's choice (related liberal arts and sciences) varies depending upon the institution selected.

FINANCIAL AID
The School of Nursing participates in the Federal Pell Grant Program, the Pennsylvania Higher Education Assistance Agency Grant Program, The Abington Memorial Hospital Scholarship program, Federal Stafford Loan Program, the Federal PLUS Loan Program, and other community, state, and national scholarship programs.

APPLYING
For acceptance into Abington's hospital-based (one year of college and two years of nursing) program the following is required: a high school diploma or a GED (General Education Diploma); an official transcript from each secondary and postsecondary school attended; acceptable standardized test scores, class rank, and grade point average; and participation in an interview with a member(s) of the Admission Committee. Application deadlines are: early decision, November 15; regular decision, February 15.

CORRESPONDENCE AND INFORMATION
Coordinator of Admission
Abington Memorial Hospital
School of Nursing
2500 Maryland Road
Pennwood Building, Suite 200
Willow Grove, PA 19090-1284
(215) 481-5500
Fax: (215) 481-5597

ADELPHI UNIVERSITY
School of Nursing
Garden City, New York

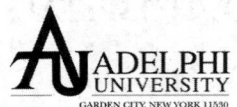

THE UNIVERSITY
Adelphi University, the oldest institution of higher education on Long Island, is located in historic Garden City — 45 minutes from Manhattan. Today, a faculty of more than 500 full and part-time professors serve a student body of 6,000. Adelphi offers over 100 undergraduate and graduate degree and certificate programs, small classes, a committed expert and approachable faculty, accelerated programs, and lifelong career development.

THE SCHOOL OF NURSING
Founded in 1943, the School of Nursing was the first collegiate program on Long Island. In 1949, Adelphi became one of the few schools to offer a master's degree in nursing. The School remains on the cutting edge as it moves into a new era of health care. Its revised curricula emphasizes self-directed learning, concentrates on case studies, and promotes clinical nursing competence using a wide array of learning resources.

PROGRAMS OF STUDY
On the undergraduate level, the School offers a Bachelor of Science in Nursing for students seeking to obtain the degree and become eligible to take the licensing examination for Registered Professional Nurse. The School also offers programs for registered nurses from associate degree or diploma nursing programs, and an accelerated BS/MS for qualified RN students.

The graduate Master of Science program in Nursing prepares advanced practice nurses for the roles of nursing administrator and nurse practitioner in adult-health nursing. The Post-Master's Certificate programs in nursing administration and advanced practice nurse practitioner are designed for students who already hold a master's degree in nursing.

AFFILIATIONS WITH HEALTH CARE FACILITIES
The school's clinical resources include a wide array of community hospitals and clinics, home health care agencies, and specialized geriatric and children's facilities. Numerous community agencies, such as HMOs, school clinics, and senior centers, are also used throughout the course of study.

ACADEMIC FACILITIES
The school's Nursing Resource Center features learning and computer laboratories. The learning laboratories simulate the hospital and home settings with all appropriate and supportive models and supplies. The Swirbul Library is fully computerized and houses over 1.2 million bound volumes, microfilms, and documents.

COSTS
For 2002-2003, undergraduate tuition is $525 per credit or $16,980 for full-time study. Graduate tuition is $500 per credit. University fees range from $200 to $400 per semester. Other fees and housing costs are determined on an individual basis.

FINANCIAL AID
Adelphi University offers a wide variety of financial assistance programs in addition to the various federal and state programs that exist. The amount and types of financial assistance that a student receives are determined by the eligibility of the applicant for each program.

APPLYING
Applicants for the bachelor's program must meet the general conditions for admission to the University. Transfer applicants must interview, and have a minimum GPA of 2.8. RN applicants must hold a current RN license; meet general admission requirements; must have graduated from a professionally accredited program or, if a graduate of a non-accredited or diploma program, must have completed the Regents Examinations; and must have a minimum GPA of 2.5. Applicants to the master's and post-master's programs are required to have a current RN license, hold a BSN or MSN degree from a professionally accredited school, have a minimum GPA of 3.0, and provide letters of reference.

CORRESPONDENCE AND INFORMATION
Adelphi University
Office of University Admissions
One South Avenue
Garden City, New York 11530
(516) 877-3050
Fax: (516) 877-3039
Web: www.adelphi.edu

ANDREWS UNIVERSITY
Department of Nursing
Berrien Springs, MI

Andrews ☙ University

THE UNIVERSITY
Andrews University was founded in 1874 and is now located in Berrien Springs, Michigan near the banks of the St Joseph River. The AU campus is a 1,600-acre arboretum of beautiful landscaping and trees.

MISSION STATEMENT
Based on a framework of Seventh-day Adventist precepts, the Andrews University Department of Nursing prepares nurses at the baccalaureate and master's degree levels for lifelong Christian service in practice, education, leadership, and research to the local, national, and international communities.

Within a culturally diverse context, the faculty create a learning environment that develops and enhances critical thinking, communication, therapeutic nursing skills, and professional development.

THE DEPARTMENT OF NURSING
The Department of Nursing is located in Marsh Hall and is continually being updated to meet the needs of today's nursing student. It offers both a supervised skills lab and computer lab with tutorials.

PROGRAMS OF STUDY
The Department of Nursing offers courses toward two undergraduate degrees: (1) a generic baccalaureate and (2) a BS completion program for RNs. The Department of Nursing also offers courses leading to the Master of Science degree in nursing with a specialty in either adult nurse practitioner or nursing administration/ leadership. The graduate program also offers a post-master's certificate program that will allow advance practice nursing as a family or adult nurse practitioner.

AFFILIATIONS WITH HEALTH CARE FACILITIES
The AU Department of Nursing has various contracts with local health-care agencies. The school's clinical resources include community teaching and specialty hospitals and clinics, a specialized outpatient dialysis unit, a psychiatric and mental health facility, community-based outpatient settings, and acute care inpatient facilities.

ACADEMIC RESOURCES
The school's best and most noted resource is its student/teacher ratio. The campus offers 3 public-access labs containing PC-compatible computers and a variety of software. The AU Writing Center offers computer-assisted tutorials and drop-in help. The James White Library houses collections totaling more than one million volumes, as well as study and research facilities. The library's computerized catalog is accessible through the campus electronic network, as well as globally via the Internet.

COSTS
The undergraduate program offers a per-quarter package for students taking 14-16 credit hours at the cost of $4,010. Charges per quarter hour credit are $285 for 17 or more credits (per credit) and $305 for 13 or fewer credits (per credit).

FINANCIAL AID
AU offers RNs working in hospitals affiliated with the university or located in Berrien County and the South Bend/Mishawaka area a 33% tuition discount. AU also offers Federal Perkins Loans, Federal Supplemental Educational Grants, Federal/State Work-Study, AU Grants and Scholarships, Federal Pell Grants, Michigan Grants and Scholarships, Ford Federal Direct Loan Program subsidized and unsubsidized, Federal Direct Plus, and various other scholarships.

APPLYING
For the Generic BS program, the minimum GPA required is 2.50, with a minimum of 2.50 in cognate subjects. The Nelson Denny Reading test is required for all applicants whose native language is English. The MELAB or the TOEFL exam is required for nonnative speakers of English. An acceptable report on the COPS is required.

For the BS Completion program for RNs, U.S.-educated nurses must pass the NCLEX-RN examination. Nurses registered or licensed outside the U.S. must pass the examination within 6 months.

For the MS Nursing program, students must have a current licensure as an RN in the state in which the course is offered, a baccalaureate degree in nursing from an accredited school, a GPA of 2.75 in nursing courses, positive recommendations by their present employer, one year of nursing experience after graduation, and an undergraduate course in statistics. Nurses preparing to write examinations as Adult Nurse Practitioners must have a GPA of 3.25 or higher.

CORRESPONDENCE AND INFORMATION:
Andrews University
Department of Nursing
Marsh Hall
Berrien Springs, MI 49104-0200
(616) 471-3311
Fax: (616) 417-3454

ARNOT OGDEN MEDICAL CENTER
SCHOOL OF NURSING
Elmira, New York

THE SCHOOL OF NURSING

The Arnot Ogden Medical Center School of Nursing, founded in 1889, is located in the heart of upstate New York's scenic Finger Lakes region. Since opening, the School of Nursing has educated more than 2,000 professional nurses whose skills, talents, and expertise Arnot Ogden Medical Center acknowledges by seeking to employ graduates on completion of training. Graduates are highly employable in other states and settings due to the strong clinical component of the nursing school curriculum.

Arnot Ogden Medical Center, a regional center for tertiary care, primarily serves southern New York and northern Pennsylvania, offering a range of specialty services and technologies normally associated with major urban medical centers. The School of Nursing is accredited by the National League for Nursing Accrediting Commission and registered by the New York State Education Department. The School is a member of the National League for Nursing, the New York State Council of Hospital Schools of Professional Nursing, and the American Hospital Association Assembly of Hospital Schools.

PROGRAM OF STUDY

The School of Nursing offers a diploma in nursing. The program prepares graduates to function competently as beginning practitioners in a variety of health care settings, using the nursing process based on scientific principles and therapeutic communication skills in meeting the holistic needs of the individual and family. Coursework prepares new practitioners to participate in educational and professional activities with the goal of being self-directed, contributing members of the nursing profession and society. Graduates accept professional accountability for nursing practice within the framework of legal and ethical guidelines.

STUDENT POPULATION

The School of Nursing is coeducational and comprised of students representing diverse cultural and educational backgrounds. The student body includes recent high school graduates, college graduates, persons seeking new career goals, students with some college credit seeking a career in nursing, individuals preparing to reenter the workforce, and licensed practical nurses seeking further professional education.

EDUCATIONAL FACILITIES

The School of Nursing's main teaching center is located within the L.D. Clute Education Building on the Arnot Ogden Medical Center campus. The teaching center includes a computer laboratory and a nursing demonstration laboratory, as well as lecture and conference rooms and faculty offices.

ASSOCIATE AGENCIES AND INSTITUTIONS

Elmira College faculty members teach first- and second-year foundation courses in physical, biological, and social sciences and a course in English for School of Nursing students on the Elmira College campus. Elmira College is fully accredited by the Middle States Association of Colleges and Secondary Schools. The Elmira Psychiatric Center, located in downtown Elmira, provides clinical facilities for psychiatric nursing.

CURRICULUM OPTIONS

The School of Nursing offers curriculum options:

Track I: Six 13-week and three 9-week terms within three academic years lead to a diploma in nursing.

Alternate Track: Same as Track I plus summer sessions to permit January graduation for seniors.

LPN to RN: Developed for the licensed practical nurse desiring career advancement to an RN level.

APPLICATION AND ACCEPTANCE

Office of the Director, School of Nursing
Arnot Ogden Medical Center
600 Roe Avenue
Elmira, New York 14905
(607) 737-4153
Fax: (607) 737-4116
E-Mail: schoolofnursing@aomc.org

ATLANTIC UNION COLLEGE
Department of Nursing
South Lancaster, MA

THE COLLEGE
Atlantic Union College is a four-year accredited, coeducational, liberal arts institution with a number of professional and pre-professional programs, several alternative education programs, and a master's degree program in education. Established by the Seventh-day Adventist Church, it welcomes applications from Adventist students all over the world and non-Adventist students who desire a campus atmosphere consciously structured on Christian principles. The college is located in South Lancaster, Massachusetts on a 324-acre campus spread over quiet tree-lined streets and rolling New England countryside. The Department of Nursing is located in Haskell Hall.

PROGRAMS OF STUDY
The Department of Nursing offers Associate Degree in Nursing, LPN to Associate Degree, and RN to BSN opportunities. The Associate degree (A.S.) provides the student with basic preparation in nursing and eligibility to write the NCLEX-RN licensing examination. Successful passing of the NCLEX-RN qualifies the individual for the title, Registered Nurse (RN) and for practice in entry-level staff positions in various health care agencies.

The RN/BSN completion program is open to RNs who have graduated from an NLNAC-accredited diploma or associate degree program. The program may be taken on either full-time or a part-time basis. Part-time students take classes through the Center for Continuing Education at a reduced tuition rate. All nursing classes in the RN/BSN program are taught after 4:00 p.m. and are designed for the working RN. A satellite campus is located in Stoneham, MA where RN to BSN classes are offered. The baccalaureate curriculum is designed for registered nurses who wish to continue their education toward advanced practice. In addition to liberal arts requirements, nursing education includes theoretical and practical components that prepare the professional nurse to fulfill an active and unique role in the delivery of health care for individuals, families, and groups.

ADMISSION
Associate Degree: There are two tracks for acceptance as a nursing major at Atlantic Union College—Track One (pre-nursing) and Track Two (direct acceptance to the nursing program). Track I is a pre-nursing year, followed by Track II. Track II is direct acceptance into the nursing program without one year of pre-nursing. Applicants with previous nursing education (LPNs and transfer students) may apply for advanced placement. Requests will be evaluated on an individual basis.

RN/BSN Completion Program: To be admitted to the RN/BSN completion program, the student must have an associate degree or diploma from an NLNAC-accredited program and a current Massachusetts RN license. Graduates may qualify for direct articulation or may require validation testing.

Acceptance into the AS or BS Nursing Program requires application and acceptance to both the college and nursing program. Applications may be obtained from the College Admissions Office or the Nursing Program.

FURTHER INFORMATION
Chairperson
Department of Nursing
Atlantic Union College
338 Main St.
P.O. Box 1000
South Lancaster, MA 01561-1000
(978) 368-2400
Fax: (978) 368-2518
Web: www.atlanticuc.edu

AUGUSTANA COLLEGE
Department of Nursing
Sioux Falls, South Dakota

THE COLLEGE
Augustana College, founded in 1860, is a fully accredited liberal arts college of the Evangelical Lutheran Church in America. With 1700 students, Augustana is the largest private college in South Dakota and consists of 20 academic departments, a 13-to-1 student-teacher ratio, and a curriculum designed to provide an education of enduring worth by blending the broad learning experiences of the liberal arts with the student's professional goals.

DEPARTMENT OF NURSING
Augustana has offered a program of study in nursing since 1941. Both the Baccalaureate and Master's programs in nursing are recognized for their excellence and contributions to the greater South Dakota community.

MASTER'S PROGRAM IN NURSING
The program of study for Advanced Nursing Practice in Emerging Health Systems is designed to prepare nurses for population and community-focused practice in changing health care systems. Graduates are equipped to address a broad spectrum of health care needs across settings and populations in communities. Health care needs of aggregate populations, which include the underserved, are a special emphasis of the program. The curriculum builds on basic community health nursing preparation and includes health care economics and the dynamics of health care policy-making as well as a nursing core of theoretical, ethical, and research foundations for advanced nursing practice. The track courses provide an advanced clinical component with opportunities for application to practice in a variety of health care settings.

Graduates of the program possess skills in planning and providing care across a broad spectrum of established and emerging health care settings, participating effectively in interdisciplinary models of health care, and providing leadership to develop new approaches to health promotion and illness prevention. Completion of the program of study qualifies graduates for certification.

The curriculum is designed to prepare nurses for health service provision to individuals, families, groups, and communities, with particular emphasis upon populations who have limited access to health care by virtue of age, ethnicity, health status, geographic location, or economic resources.

ADMISSION
Students are admitted to the graduate program in nursing each semester, following their admission to the Graduate Program of the college. Basic requirements for admission are:

- Baccalaureate degree in nursing from an NLNAC-accredited program
- Cumulative grade point average of 3.0 (4.0 scale) for undergraduate preparation
- Current licensure or eligibility for licensure to practice nursing in South Dakota
- Evidence of a completed course in descriptive and inferential statistics
- A two- to three-page typed essay describing professional and educational goals and plans for graduate study
- Two letters of reference supporting the applicant's character and ability for graduate study
- One year of clinical practice experience as an RN is preferred
- Official transcripts from each college and university attended

COSTS
Graduate tuition is $250 per semester credit. Most courses are 3 credits. Students may take up to 6 credits per semester.

CORRESPONDENCE AND INFORMATION
Margot Nelson, RN, PhD
Coordinator of Master's in Nursing Program
Augustana College
Department of Nursing
2001 South Summit Avenue
Sioux Falls, SD, 57197
(605) 336-4721
Fax: (605) 336-4723
E-Mail: mnelson@inst.augie.edu
Web: http://www.augie.edu/dept/nurs/nsgweb1.htm

AUSTIN COMMUNITY COLLEGE
Nursing Programs
Austin, Texas

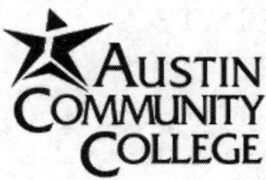

AUSTIN
COMMUNITY
COLLEGE

THE COLLEGE
Located in Austin, Texas, Austin Community College is a comprehensive community college, fully accredited by the Southern Association of Colleges and Schools. ACC opened its doors to 1,793 students in September 1973, and now has more than 29,156 students (Fall 2002). Full-time enrollment is approximately 7,077 (Fall 2002), while part-time enrollment is 22,079. An additional 10,301 students are enrolled throughout the year in continuing education programs.

THE ASSOCIATE DEGREE NURSING PROGRAM
Austin Community College has been providing quality nursing education in central Texas since 1982.
The Associate Degree Nursing (ADN) Program offers two educational tracks:

- The ADN Program—Traditional Track offers basic nursing education to the unlicensed individual. The degree plan consists of 33 semester credit hours of non-nursing course work and 37 semester credit hours of nursing course work that includes classroom, laboratory, and clinical learning experiences.

- The ADN Program—Mobility Track is an accelerated program of study for selected experienced licensed vocational nurses and paramedics. The degree plan consists of 33 semester credit hours of non-nursing course work and 24 semester credit hours of nursing course work that includes classroom, laboratory, and clinical learning experiences.

Graduates of the ADN Program receive an Associate of Applied Science degree and are eligible to apply for the registered nurse (RN) licensure examination.
The pass rate on the NCLEX-RN for the past 5 years has ranged from 96% to 99%.

THE VOCATIONAL NURSING PROGRAM
The fifteen month, part time, Vocational Nursing Program, established in 1973, prepares graduates to care for patients with commonly occurring health needs in a variety of health care settings. The innovative curriculum includes several prerequisite courses that also meet the requirements for admission to the Associated Degree Program.
Graduates of the Vocational Nursing Program receive a certificate of completion and are eligible to apply for the licensed vocational nurse (LVN) licensure examination.
The pass rate on the NCLEX-PN for the past 5 years has ranged from 95% to 100%.

DISTANCE EDUCATION INITIATIVES
The Vocational Nursing Program is offered via interactive video conferencing at the Teaching Center 86 miles southwest of Austin in Fredericksburg, Texas.

The ADN Program—Mobility Track has been offered at the Fredericksburg Teaching Center since Fall 2001.

ACADEMIC RESOURCES
Educational resources include the Health Sciences Library, Nursing Computer Lab, Nursing Skills Lab, and Nursing Tutoring Services.

TUITION & FEES
In-District $32/semester hour
In-State $84/semester hour
Out-of-State $171/semester hour

FINANCIAL AID
The Office of Student Financial Aid provides grants, loans, and work-study to those students who may otherwise be unable to attend college. The amount and type of aid a student may receive depends on the availability of funds and the student's established financial need.

CORRESPONDENCE AND INFORMATION
Jere Hammer, RN, MSN, Coordinator
Associate Degree Nursing Program
Austin Community College
1020 Grove Blvd.
Austin, Texas 78741
(512) 223-6105
E-Mail: adn@austin.cc.tx.us
Web: http://www2.austin.cc.tx.us/adn

Yvonne Van Dyke, RN, MSN, Coordinator
Vocational Nursing Program
Austin Community College
1020 Grove Blvd.
Austin, Texas 78741
(512) 223-6105
E-Mail: hlth_sci@austin.cc.tx.us
Web: http://www2.austin.cc.tx.us/hltsci/lvn

AZUSA PACIFIC UNIVERSITY
Azusa, California

Azusa Pacific University (APU) is a comprehensive, Christian university accredited by the Western Association of Schools and Colleges, that offers more than 40 areas of undergraduate study in the liberal arts and professional programs, 20 master's degree programs, and 4 doctoral programs. Founded on the motto of *God First*, APU has been developing disciples and scholars since 1899. Azusa is located 26 miles northeast of downtown Los Angeles at the base of the San Gabriel Mountains and has a student body of 3,654 undergraduates and 3,181 graduate students.

THE SCHOOL OF NURSING
Azusa Pacific University's School of Nursing celebrates 28 years of excellence in the preparation of generalist and advanced practice nurses who demonstrate subject-matter expertise, clinical competence, and dedication to the treatment of the whole person. In 1975, four nurses came together to create a different caliber of nursing school, now the only Christian university providing nursing education in the San Gabriel Valley and the largest in the Council for Christian Colleges and Universities. The School of Nursing is accredited by the National League for Nursing Accrediting Commission and the California State Board of Registered Nursing.

PROGRAMS OF STUDY
Current graduate offerings include pathways to the Master of Science in Nursing degree and post-master's credential programs in several areas: Articulated RN to Master of Science in Nursing Program (for those with an A.A. degree or diploma in nursing who have a baccalaureate degree in a field other than nursing); BSN to Master of Science in Nursing Program (for those who have completed a bachelor's degree in nursing); School Nurse Services Credential Program plus a Master of Science in Nursing; Post-Master's Nursing Credential Programs in Adult, High Risk Home Health, Nursing Administration, Nursing Education, Parent-Child, or Parish Nursing, and Family Nurse Practitioner (for nurses who have already completed a master's degree). Since its inception, there have been 210 graduates. Plans also call for the debut of a doctorate in nursing within five years.

COSTS
Graduate tuition for most programs is $395 per unit.

FINANCIAL AID
Three types of financial aid are available to students attending Azusa Pacific University—scholarships and grants, educational loans, and student employment (on and off campus). Scholarships and grants do not have to be repaid and may be used to pay for educational expenses. Educational loans may be applied for and require repayment. The federal government provides low interest loans to students. Private lenders provide educational loans to students who are either credit worthy or credit ready. APU provides numerous job opportunities for students needing additional resources to pay for their education.

APPLYING
Apply online at www.apu.edu.

CORRESPONDENCE AND INFORMATION
Azusa Pacific University
901 E. Alosta Ave.
PO Box 7000
Azusa, CA 92821-7000
(800) 825-5278
Web: www.apu.edu

Graduate Center
(626) 815-4570

Office of International Student Services
(626) 812-3055

BALL STATE UNIVERSITY
School of Nursing
Muncie, Indiana

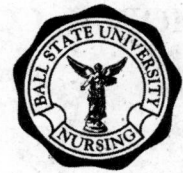

THE UNIVERSITY
Ball State University, founded in 1918, is a comprehensive, publicly assisted institution of higher education whose mission is to provide excellent education. Located in East Central Indiana, Ball State University offers more varied academic programs than a small liberal arts college while providing a more personalized educational experience that may be found at a large research institution.

THE SCHOOL OF NURSING
The School of Nursing, located in the Cooper Science Complex, was founded in 1963. The School of Nursing is a leader in using technology in nursing education, and is accredited by the National League for Nursing Accrediting Commission, 61 Broadway, New York, NY 10006 (212-363-555 or 1-800-669-9656 x 153).

PROGRAMS OF STUDY
The School of Nursing offers the basic baccalaureate, RN-to-baccalaureate, and master's degrees. The master's program offers tracks in education, leadership, and adult/family nurse practitioner. Post-master's educator and NP certificates are available. The RN-to-baccalaureate and the master's programs are available through distance education.

AFFILIATIONS WITH HEALTH CARE FACILITIES
The School of Nursing maintains contractual agreements with many health care facilities, clinics, public health departments, and other resources.

ACADEMIC RESOURCES
Ball State University, whose motto is "everything you need," has a multitude of resources to help students, such as a counseling center, learning and writing centers, computer laboratories, and library system. The School of Nursing has its own learning resource center, which includes simulated hospital, clinic, and community learning experiences. The School of Nursing is connected electronically to Ball Memorial Hospital via the training portion of the hospital information system. The School and the University resources support distance learning.

COSTS
State resident full-time undergraduate tuition is $2,266 per semester. Nonresident full-time tuition per semester is $6,475 (an additional $8 per credit hour is added for on-campus graduate students). Fees for distance education courses are $174 per semester hour of undergraduate credit and $184 per semester hour of graduate credit for residents, and $300 per semester hour of undergraduate credit and $325 per semester hour of graduate credit for nonresidents. Clinical fees are applied to select graduate courses. Room and board is approximately $5,880 per year for undergraduates. These fees, current for 2003-2004, may change.

FINANCIAL AID
Ball State University offers institutionally sponsored non-need scholarships, Federal Nursing Student Loans, Federal Pell Grants, Federal Perkins Loans, Federal Supplemental Educational Opportunity Grants, Federal Work-Study, Federal PLUS Loans, Federal Stafford Loans, and state aid.

APPLYING
Applicants for the basic baccalaureate program apply during the sophomore year. RN to baccalaureate students apply the summer before the fall Nursing progression. The application deadline for the master's program is four months prior to a given semester and can be done via the Internet. Contact the School of Nursing for specific criteria for admission.

CORRESPONDENCE AND INFORMATION
Director, School of Nursing
Ball State University
Muncie IN 47306-0219
(765) 285-5571
Fax: (765) 285-2169
Web: www.bsu.edu/nursing

BAPTIST MEMORIAL COLLEGE OF HEALTH SCIENCES
Memphis, Tennessee

THE COLLEGE

Baptist College of Health Sciences is a private, coeducational, urban, specialized institution. The College focuses on the preparation of healthcare practitioners for the Southern region. Grounded in Christian principles, the College seeks to attract diverse students who demonstrate a commitment to spiritual values and ethics, academic excellence, and lifelong professional development. The educational programs of the College emphasize the importance of collaboration, teamwork, and service in promoting the health and wellness of the communities served.

Baptist College of Health Sciences provides quality post-secondary, baccalaureate, and continuing education in a Christian atmosphere in order to prepare healthcare professionals for the community-focused health care environment of the twenty-first century. The College was chartered in December 1994 as a specialized college offering baccalaureate degrees in nursing (BSN) and health sciences (BHS). The College is accredited by the Commission on Colleges of the Southern Association of Colleges and Schools (1866 Southern Lane, Decatur, Georgia 30033-4097, Telephone: 404-679-4501). The nursing division is accredited by the Commission on Collegiate Nursing Education.

PROGRAMS OF STUDY

Baptist College offers professional nursing education through the baccalaureate program. There are various tracks available to attain the BSN degree including a generic program, an RN to BSN program and an LPN to BSN program. Night and weekend courses are available for students who must work full-time while earning the BSN degree. The College also offers a post-secondary program of one year in Practical Nursing. The goal of this certificate education program is the development of a beginning practitioner who is an integral part of the health care team.

In addition to nursing education, the College offers the majors leading to a Bachelor of Health Sciences degree. They are Diagnostic Medical Sonography, Health Care Management, Medical Radiography, Nuclear Medicine, Radiation Therapy Technology, and Respiratory Care.

AFFILIATIONS WITH HEALTH CARE FACILITIES

Baptist College is the educational arm of a comprehensive healthcare system that offers a wealth of clinical experiences within a three-state region. Extremely competent clinical practitioners are the hallmark of a Baptist education. Clinical facilities available within the nationally-known Memphis medical community enrich the learning environment for students. Experiences include acute care, ambulatory care, home health, rehabilitation, and other diverse community-based clinical sites.

Facilities available in the Memphis community include Baptist Memorial Health Care Corporation Hospitals, the Memphis and Shelby County Public Health Department, St. Jude Children's Research Hospital, The Regional Medical Center at Memphis, and the Women's Health Center. A myriad of other agencies and support groups meet the unique learning needs associated with particular courses and provide additional alternatives for learning experiences.

ACADEMIC RESOURCES

The primary physical facility for Baptist Memorial College of Health Sciences is located at 1003 Monroe Avenue, Memphis, Tennessee, and contains 110,000 square feet with an atrium design. This building includes both educational facilities and residence quarters. The facility contains numerous classroom/conference rooms and an auditorium with a seating capacity of 250. The Health Sciences Library offers online indexes, an online catalog, journals, books, and various multi-media resources. A laboratory with individual work areas is present for client simulation. A computer classroom is equipped with computers and laser printers. The dormitory facility provides both single- and double-occupancy rooms for residency. Science laboratories are located approximately one block from the main facility. Energized radiological sciences laboratories are located adjacent to the campus. These laboratories allow students to perfect their skills in simulated environments prior to performing patient care.

COSTS

Tuition is $150.00 per academic hour. All hours taken are charged at a per hour rate. The total cost of the practical nursing program is $3,800.00. Housing is available on campus at the rate of $630.00 for the fall or spring term for a double occupancy room, or $1,260.00 for a single occupancy room. Summer housing rates are pro-rated. Other costs include books, supplies, uniforms, transportation, immunization fees, and payment of professional liability insurance premiums. Health insurance is required.

FINANCIAL AID

In support of our mission of preparing health care professionals for the twenty-first century, Baptist College of Health Sciences is committed to assisting students in securing financial resources needed to pursue their education. To that end, very generous scholarships are available for first time freshmen. There are four Joseph Powell scholarships each with a four year total award of $20,000. There are ten Health Care Foundation Scholarships of $3,000 each renewable yearly. The Ruby Turrell Scholarship is awarded to a first time freshmen majoring in nursing with a total award over four years of $20,000. There are several other scholarships of varying amounts for incumbent students.

The College participates in Federal Financial Aid programs. Our Federal Financial Aid identification number is 034403 and is available for use on applications for Federal Student Assistance and for deferments. Federal programs that are available include Federal Pell Grants, Subsidized Federal Stafford Loans, Unsubsidized Federal Stafford Loans, Federal PLUS Loans, and Federal Supplemental Opportunity Grants.

CORRESPONDENCE AND INFORMATION

Admissions Office
Baptist College of Health Sciences
1003 Monroe Avenue
Memphis, TN 38104
(901) 575-2247 or (866) 575-2247
Fax: (901) 572-2461
Web: www.bchs.edu

BAPTIST SCHOOLS OF NURSING AND ALLIED HEALTH
Little Rock, Arkansas

THE SPONSOR
Baptist Health sponsors nine health professions schools. It is the largest not-for-profit multi-unit healthcare system in Arkansas and includes: Baptist Medical Center and Baptist Rehabilitation Institute in Little Rock, Baptist Memorial Medical Center in North Little Rock, Baptist Medical Center Arkadelphia in Arkadelphia, Baptist Medical Center Heber Springs in Heber Springs, and Practice Plus in Little Rock.

THE SCHOOLS
The nine schools include seven allied health and two nursing programs. The Baptist School of Coding Technology opened in 1985, the first school established in Arkansas exclusively for coding training. The Baptist School of Histo-technology, founded in 1978, is one of only 50 fully accredited programs of its kind in the United States. The Baptist School of Medical Technology was founded in 1966. The Baptist School of Medical Transcription opened in 1987. The Baptist School of Nuclear Medicine Technology opened in 1979 and came under the sponsorship of Baptist Health in 1987. The Baptist School of Radiography opened in 1953. The Baptist School of Nursing opened in 1921 and, following closure for a ten year period, was reestablished in 1976. In 1987, the school added an accelerated LPN / LPTN to RN track. The Baptist School of Practical Nursing opened in 1964. The Baptist School of Surgical Technology opened in 1999.

PROGRAMS OF STUDY
Graduates of each school are awarded a diploma and are prepared to function as a beginning practitioner in the field of each respective program. Graduates are eligible to apply for a national certification or licensure examination appropriate to the school. Successful candidates become one of the following: Certified Coding Specialist, Registered Histologic Technician, Registered Medical Technologist, Certified Medical Transcriptionist, Registered Nuclear Medicine Technologist, Registered Radiologic Technologist, Certified Surgical Technologist, Registered Nurse, or Licensed Practical Nurse.

AFFILIATIONS WITH HEALTH CARE FACILITIES, COLLEGES, UNIVERSITIES
The Baptist Schools of Nursing and Allied Health maintain contractual agreements with more than sixty healthcare agencies. Clinical resources include acute care hospitals, physician clinics, a specialized children's hospital, psychiatric/mental health facilities, and other outpatient settings. The schools affiliate with five colleges and universities in the state.

ACADEMIC RESOURCES
The schools' resources are located primarily at the Baptist Health Support Center. Students have access to well-equipped classrooms, laboratories, and a learning resource center for audiovisuals. The main library holdings, over 5000, are in the Margaret Clark Gilbreath Memorial Library located at Baptist Medical Center.

COSTS / FINANCIAL AID
Resident full-time student tuition ranges from $2,800 to $9,800 according to the respective school. Nonresidents pay additional tuition. Baptist Health Foundation provides scholarships for qualifying students. The Baptist Health Student Work-Contract Loan Program is available in selected programs. Federal Pell Grants are available.

APPLYING
All schools require high school diploma or GED. ACT or SAT is a requirement for selected schools. Application deadline is March 15 for all allied health schools except surgical technology, which is November 15. Applications are accepted continually for nursing schools. For LPN / LPTN-to-RN applicants, an unencumbered LPN or LPTN license is required. Information for additional requirements is available from each specific school.

CORRESPONDENCE AND INFORMATION
Baptist Schools of Nursing and Allied Health
11900 Colonel Glenn Road, Suite 1000
Little Rock, AR 72210-2820
(501) 202-7415 / (800) 345-3046
Fax: (501) 202-7406
Web: www.baptist-health.com

BARRY UNIVERSITY
School of Nursing
Miami Shores, Florida

THE UNIVERSITY

Barry University, founded in 1940, is an independent, coeducational Catholic institution that fosters academic distinction in the liberal arts and professional studies within the Judeo-Christian and Dominican traditions. We are a values-based institution that seeks to deliver quality education within a caring environment. The University enrolls over 7,000 students drawn from 49 states and 80 countries.

PROGRAMS OF STUDY

The BSN program prepares students for professional nursing practice. The MSN program prepares leaders in nursing administration, nursing education, and nurse practitioner. At the bachelor's and master's level, Barry offers several options for study designed to meet the needs of students. The Ph.D. in Nursing program prepares nurses to be researchers, professors, and executives.

UNDERGRADUATE PROGRAM

The BSN may be earned in several ways. The Basic Option is designed for high school graduates or students with some university/college credit, including LPNs. The Accelerated Option is for students with a bachelor's degree in another field or who have a 3.0 GPA and meet other criteria. RNs have options designed for them. Visit our website at www.barry.edu/nursing.

OPPORTUNITIES

The Nursing Student Association offers financial aid opportunities and activities for community service, student recognition, and socialization. Faculty and students in several academic disciplines come together to respond to societal needs and health care reform through the Barry University Primary Care Nursing Center. The PCNC provides primary care and health education to children and families in selected elementary schools in Miami's under-served areas and to women and children at a domestic abuse shelter. The Center for Nursing Research provides consultation, disseminates research findings, and creates an environment that perpetuates scholarship.

COSTS

Full-time undergraduate tuition is $9,450 per semester; part-time tuition is $545 per credit. Room and board ranges from $2,880 to $3,370 per semester. Working RNs returning for a BSN or MSN receive a 30% tuition discount. A variety of financial aid programs are available.

ADMISSION REQUIREMENTS

Contact the school for details. The application deadline is rolling. University and school admissions requirements must be met.

Basic Option: High school graduates or applicants with fewer than 15 college credits must have C in high school or college biology and chemistry; C in Algebra II or equivalent; 970 total SAT I score or 20 on the ACT, and 2.70 high school or college GPA, with fewer than 5 Ws, Ds, or Fs. Transfer students with 15 or more college credits must have a 2.70 college GPA, with fewer than 5 Ws, Ds, or Fs. LPNs must average 80% in practical nursing coursework and hold a current Florida LPN license or eligibility for NCLEX-PN.

The *Accelerated Option* requires either a bachelor's degree from an accredited college/university or completion of all liberal arts; 2.70 GPA for the most recent 60 credits for those with a bachelor's degree, or 3.00 GPA for those working on their first bachelor's degree; C in 4 required sciences. RN graduates of diploma and ADN programs apply to the *RN-to-BSN Option* or *RN-to-MSN Seamless Option.* The length of these programs depends upon the amount of acceptable transfer credit; success in completion of CLEP, proficiency, and nursing examinations; and part-time or full-time status. The *RN-to-BSN Option* requires 2.70 GPA and current Florida RN licensure. In the *RN-to-MSN Seamless Option,* students earn the BS and the MSN.

INFORMATION

Barry University School of Nursing
11300 N.E. Second Avenue
Miami Shores, Florida 33161-6695
(305) 899-3800
E-Mail: dnogueras@mail.barry.edu
Web: www.barry.edu/nursing

BAYLOR UNIVERSITY
School of Nursing
Dallas, Texas

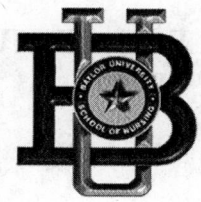

THE UNIVERSITY
Baylor University is the largest Baptist university in the world, and the oldest university in Texas. The main campus is in Waco, Texas, but the School of Nursing is in Dallas. The mission of Baylor University is to educate men and women for worldwide Christian leadership and service by integrating academic excellence and Christian commitment within a caring community.

HISTORY OF THE SCHOOL OF NURSING
The School of Nursing is located in the heart of the Baylor University Medical Center campus, two miles east of downtown Dallas. The Bachelor of Science degree in Nursing was first awarded in 1954. The graduate program began in 1990 and was ranked 59th in the nation by U.S. News and World Report in their 2001 rankings. Baylor continues to educate baccalaureate and graduate prepared nurses for various positions of leadership and service throughout the United States and the world.

PROGRAMS OF STUDY
Both undergraduate and graduate programs are offered on the Baylor campus in Dallas, Texas. The prenursing prerequisites may be completed on the Baylor-Waco campus or at another approved college or university. All students spend the last two years of the upper-division major at the School of Nursing in Dallas. The graduate program offers four tracks: Nursing Administration and Management, Family Nurse Practitioner, Advanced Neonatal Nursing (NNP/CNS), and RN to Masters (Joint BSN/MSN).

All programs are fully accredited by CCNE through 2010.

FACULTY
All faculty members in the School of Nursing hold advanced degrees and teach in their areas of specialization. Nursing faculty members serve on a variety of councils and organizations related to their areas of clinical and professional interests.

STUDENTS AND STUDENT LIFE
Students come from all over the world to attend Baylor University Louise Herrington School of Nursing. The Student Services Department on the Dallas campus provides a wide array of services that promote and provide opportunity for social, cultural, spiritual, intellectual, and physical development.

FACILITIES
Classrooms, laboratories, faculty and administrative offices, and library facilities are all located in the School of Nursing building on the Baylor-Dallas campus. State of the art computers and technologically equipped classrooms and laboratories demonstrate the school's commitment to academic excellence in all areas. A residence hall for students is provided by Baylor University Medical Center and physically adjoins the School of Nursing building.

FINANCIAL AID
The School of Nursing is committed to helping students with financial need achieve a degree from Baylor University. The Financial Aid Office on the Baylor-Waco campus processes all applications for financial aid. To be eligible for any merit- or need-based scholarships through Baylor, you must complete the Federal FAFSA form each year.

To obtain an application for financial aid, contact
Office of Academic Scholarships and Financial Aid Baylor University
PO Box 97028
Waco, Texas 76798-7028
(254) 710-2611
E-Mail: FinancialAid_Office@baylor.edu

Also, please visit Financial Aid Web site at
http://www.baylor.edu/finaid/

ADMISSION
Undergraduate admission information may be obtained by contacting:
Baylor University
Louise Herrington School of Nursing
Pre-Nursing Office
PO Box 97333
Waco, Texas 76798-7333
(254) 710-1821
E-Mail: BU_Nursing@baylor.edu

To obtain information about the graduate program, contact:
Director of Graduate Studies
Baylor University
Louise Herrington School of Nursing
3700 Worth Street
Dallas, Texas 75246
(214) 820-4111
E-Mail: Graduate_Nursing@baylor.edu

Also, please visit our Web site at:
http://www.baylor.edu/Nursing/

BELLIN COLLEGE OF NURSING
Green Bay, Wisconsin

THE COLLEGE OF NURSING

Bellin College of Nursing (BCON) is an independent, coeducational institution located in the heart of Green Bay, Wisconsin within the medical corridor of Bellin and St. Vincent Hospitals. BCON offers a Bachelor of Science in Nursing (BSN) degree only. Bellin's primary mission is "to provide nursing professionals for this region who have a broad theory base, are clinically competent and values-oriented in their practice of nursing, and contributing members of society." Bellin College of Nursing has a consortium agreement with the University of Wisconsin-Green Bay (UWGB). Students normally take the Bellin required general education courses at UWGB. All nursing courses are taught by Bellin College of Nursing faculty, and apart from two introductory freshman nursing courses that are taught on the UWGB campus, the remainder are held on the Bellin College of Nursing campus. In addition to the consortium agreement with UWGB, Bellin also has articulation agreements established with Lakeland College, Silver Lake College, and the College of the Menominee Nation. For those students who are transferring from other accredited institutions, general education courses completed will be assessed by the registrar at Bellin College of Nursing. BCON is accredited by North Central Association of Colleges and Schools and the National League for Nursing Accrediting Commission.

PROGRAMS OF STUDY

Bellin College of Nursing offers a Bachelor of Science in Nursing (BSN) degree. Bellin College of Nursing offers a four-year traditional track program for those students coming into Bellin directly from high school or for students who do not meet the criteria for either the Accelerated Transfer Option or the Sophomore Transfer Option.

Accelerated Transfer Option: Students with prior general education credits may be eligible for this fast-track program. Students with 62 of Bellin's required general education credits are able to complete the program in approximately 21 months or four semesters plus a summer session. Students with 46 of the Bellin required credits are eligible for an accelerated option and will require an individual academic plan. Students need to have at least a 2.7 GPA in the required general education courses.

Sophomore Transfer Option: Students who have completed all of the freshman required general education courses (29 credits) and have a 2.7 GPA are eligible for the sophomore option. Students are able to complete the program in three years and a summer school.

AFFILIATIONS WITH HEALTH CARE FACILITIES

Within the Green Bay area, Bellin College of Nursing has clinical affiliations with Bellin Hospital, Bellin Psychiatric Center, St. Mary's Hospital, St. Vincent Hospital, Odd Fellows Home, Rebekah Home, and Parkview Manor Nursing Home. Other affiliations include 30 public health, community, and home care agencies as well as clinics, childcare centers, older adult independent living centers, and industrial health programs within a four-county region.

ACADEMIC RESOURCES

The Rose Health Sciences Library and the Fuld Learning Resource Center are located on the first floor of the College. The library includes 4000 volumes, books, journals, newspapers and 350 videos.

The Fuld Resource Center includes a skills practice laboratory, a computer room, an assessment room, and a viewing room. Students also have access to the UWGB Library Learning Center. This library has over 280,000 books and bound periodicals and maintains current subscriptions to 1400 scholarly journals, magazines, and newspapers.

COSTS

Tuition costs for the four-year nursing program for the 2002-2003 academic year are approximately $11,000.00; this includes the projected tuition costs for general education courses taken at UWGB (Wisconsin residents). Non-Wisconsin residents enrolled at UWGB are subject to out-of-state tuition charges. Tuition for the accelerated program is based upon a per-credit charge for enrolled nursing courses. Actual tuition costs are determined annually, therefore the above information is subject to change.

FINANCIAL AID

BCON offers need-based scholarships, academic merit scholarships, Federal Pell Grants, Federal Supplemental Educational Opportunity Grants, Federal Work-Study, Federal PLUS Loans, Federal Stafford Loans, and state aid. Under the consortium agreement with UWGB, concurrently enrolled freshman and sophomore students receive financial aid awarded through UWGB.

ADMISSION

High School course requirements required by BCON are:

- 4 years of English
- 3 years of social science
- 3 years of mathematics (one year of algebra and two advanced math courses)
- 1 year of biology
- 1 year of chemistry
- 1 year of advanced science

Students are required to submit an official high school transcript, ACT results, one official copy of any post-high school transcripts, and three references. High School ranking should be in the 66th percentile or higher with at least a 2.9 grade point average on a 4.0 scale. A composite score of 21 or above on the ACT is recognized as competitive.

Students in the four-year program and those in the accelerated option who have general education requirements to fulfill need to apply to and be accepted by UWGB to complete the necessary courses.

CORRESPONDENCE AND INFORMATION

Bellin College of Nursing
Admissions Department
725 S. Webster Avenue
P.O. Box 23400
Green Bay, WI 54305-3400
(920) 433-5803 (Admissions Office)
(920) 433-5801 (Financial Aid Office)
(800) 236-8707 (in Wisconsin only)
Fax: (920) 433-7416
E-Mail: admissio@bcon.edu
Web: www.bcon.edu

BLOOMFIELD COLLEGE
Presbyterian Division of Nursing
Bloomfield, New Jersey

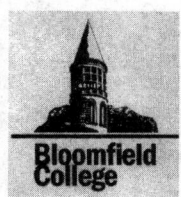

THE COLLEGE
Bloomfield College, founded in 1868, is an independent college historically related to the Presbyterian Church (U.S.A.). Located in the New York metropolitan area, the College awards Bachelor of Arts and Bachelor of Science degrees. The curriculum is designed to provide students with a liberal arts education as well as specialized career preparation. More than 55 nationalities are represented on campus, reflecting the College's commitment to its distinctive mission: to prepare students to attain academic, personal, and professional excellence in a multicultural and global society.

THE PRESBYTERIAN DIVISION OF NURSING
The Presbyterian Division of Nursing revised its curriculum in 1997 to reflect the realities of today's health care system and to prepare graduates to function in the evolving health care market. The new curriculum places emphasis on health promotion, illness prevention, and the delivery of health care in the community. The nursing program is accredited by the New Jersey Board of Nursing and the Commission on Collegiate Nursing Education. The Division is a member of the National League for Nursing.

PROGRAMS OF STUDY
Bloomfield College accepts freshman applicants, transfer students, and RNs who are graduates of associate degree and diploma programs.

AFFILIATIONS WITH HEALTH CARE FACILITIES
The Presbyterian Division of Nursing maintains contractual agreements with more than 25 health care agencies. Clinical settings provide a variety of direct practice sites such as hospitals, extended care, clinics, schools, homes, and other community venues.

ACADEMIC RESOURCES
Resources include the Bloomfield College Library, as well as the Nursing Learning Resource Center. The new library opened in 2000 and provides material in both print and digital formats. The Center for Academic Development offers workshops and tutoring.

COSTS
Full-time students (3-4.5 course units) $6,450 per semester. Part-time students (less than 3 course units) $1,300 per course. Additional fees including comprehensive fee, registration fees, student medical insurance, orientation fee, nursing malpractice insurance, and laboratory fees apply.

FINANCIAL AID
Bloomfield College recognizes that many families need assistance in meeting the costs of their education. Students are encouraged to seek advice and assistance through the Financial Aid Office, whose staff provides detailed information regarding federal, state, and college financial aid. The office can be reached at (973) 748-9000, ext. 212 or 383. Additional financial aid programs, as well as scholarships designated for nursing students, are available at Bloomfield College.

APPLYING
The Bloomfield College catalog provides full details of admission requirements. Note the following:

Admission to the nursing major:

Students entering directly from high school must enter with the following: completion of high school biology, chemistry, and two years of college preparatory mathematics, all with a minimum grade of C; high school GPA of B, with 80% in college prep curriculum; high school rank in the top 1/3 of the class; two references from high school faculty.

College Transfer Students must have a minimum GPA of 2.5. The transfer of nursing courses is subject to evaluation by the Division of Nursing. For generic transfer students, nursing courses six years or older may not be transferred.

Admission for RN students:

Graduates of diploma and associate degree programs in nursing may apply as matriculated candidates for the BS degree with a major in nursing. Registered nurses who have college credits should apply as transfer students.

RN students seeking admission to Bloomfield College pursuant to a BS degree should:

1. Complete general admissions applications for registered nurses.
2. Forward official transcripts of academic work pursued at other institutions.
3. Forward two letters of recommendation.
4. Show proof of RN licensure in the State of New Jersey. RNs licensed in other states must obtain New Jersey licensure.
5. Forward copies of liability/malpractice insurance (min. coverage of $1,000,000/$3,000,000).

CORRESPONDENCE AND INFORMATION
Presbyterian Division of Nursing
Bloomfield College
467 Franklin Street
Bloomfield, NJ 07003
(973) 748-9000, ext. 230
E-Mail: admission@bloomfield.edu
Web: www.bloomfield.edu

BON SECOURS MEMORIAL SCHOOL OF NURSING
Richmond, VA

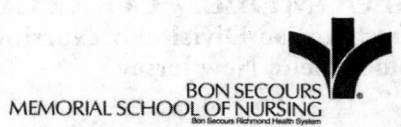

HISTORY OF THE SCHOOL

Bon Secours Memorial School of Nursing is sponsored and supported by Bon Secours Memorial Regional Medical Center. The mission of the school is to benefit the students, the hospital, and the community, and to improve the quality of nursing care. The program focuses on strong clinical practice application and nursing theory beginning early in the first year.

The first class entered the school in September 1961, and over 900 nurses have completed the program since that time.

ADMISSION REQUIREMENTS

Qualified applicants are considered for admission regardless of age, gender, race, color, religion, national origin, marital or veteran status, or physical ability to perform the essential functions of a nursing student with or without reasonable accomodation. Admission into the School of Nursing is competitive. The admissions process for all applicants involves two stages: conditional acceptance and full acceptance.

Basic admission requirements include the following:

- Graduation from an accredited high school or GED certificate in lieu of high school diploma.
- Achievement of a cumulative grade point average of 2.0 or above from high school courses and a minimum grade of C in Algebra, Biology, and college-prep Chemistry. Courses taken after high school may satisfy these requirements.
- Achievement of a cumulative grade point average of 2.0 or above for any college courses taken. Transfer credit is given for a grade of C or above in comparable college non-nursing courses. Science courses must have been completed within the previous 10 years. There is no time limitation on other non-nursing courses.
- Three professional references must be submitted with application.

ADVANCED PLACEMENT FOR LPNs

- Meet all basic admission requirements including high school Algebra, Biology, and college prep Chemistry.
- Submit evidence of current LPN license.
- Submit reference from most recent employer.
- Provide nursing school catalog, course outline/syllabus, and unit outlines as required.
- Take and pay for any necessary placement tests.
- Demonstrate clinical proficiency as required.

FINANCIAL INFORMATION

Loans and scholarships are available to qualifying students after full acceptance into the School of Nursing. Amounts awarded depend on verified need, academic standing, credit ratings, and number of credit hours to be taken.

The School of Nursing participates in the Pell Grant Program, Federal Family Education Loan Program, Veteran's Educational Benefits, and various other scholarship programs. Additionally, Bon Secours also provides a work cancellation loan program for eligible students. The Bon Secours Memorial student loans are made based on academic standing and financial need. These loans are repaid either through cash repayment or work cancellation through employment within the Bon Secours Richmond Health System. The Work Cancellation Program requires that the graduate be licensed and employed as a registered nurse. Loan applications are made prior to the beginning of each school year.

CORRESPONDENCE AND INFORMATION

Bon Secours Memorial School of Nursing
8550 Magellan Pkwy., Suite 1100
Richmond, VA 23227
(804) 627-5380
Web: www.bonsecours.com/son/index.htm

BRIAR CLIFF UNIVERSITY
Sioux City, Iowa

THE PROGRAM
Briar Cliff University Department of Nursing offers three options to attain the Bachelor of Science in Nursing (BSN) degree:

- BASIC BSN OPTION: Students who are not already registered nurses may elect to enroll at Briar Cliff for the entire four-year basic BSN program leading to eligibility to take the registered nursing licensure exam.
- LPN-BSN OPTION: Licensed Practical Nurses may pursue a program of studies leading to a BSN
- RN-BSN OPTION: Registered nurses may pursue a program of studies leading to a BSN

With each option the nursing major is directed toward:

- Providing a foundation for continued learning, for integration of new knowledge into practice, and for graduate education in nursing
- Preparing nurses who will independently and interdependently promote, restore, and maintain the health of client systems in a variety of health care settings
- Developing nurses who will participate in decision making designed to improve health care delivery in a rapidly changing society and complex health care system
- Fostering wholistic personal and professional development

Briar Cliff provides a range of real-world experiences that begin as early as your freshman year. As a senior, you will complete clinical preceptorships (internships) in local, regional, and national hospital and community-based settings. Throughout your college career, you'll be encouraged to participate in service learning opportunities that provide practical experience and better the world in which you live.

ACADEMIC RESOURCES
The Nursing Department's recently remodeled lab, along with its on-site and mobile classrooms, prepare you to meet the complex needs of client as future health professionals.

THE FACULTY
The nursing profession relies upon one-on-one client care, and the advantages of learning within that same close-knit environment are undeniable. Briar Cliff nursing faculty members provide the personal attention you need to excel in classroom and clinical experiences. Working side-by-side with your professors, you'll benefit from their insight and expertise, as they become your role models and mentors. These talented and dedicated professionals are also highly qualified nurse practitioners who connect nursing theories with real-world examples.

OUR FACULTY BELIEVES THAT

- Health is a process in which all dimensions of the person are in harmony with the whole.
- Nursing is a discipline with a unique body of knowledge that facilitates clients' optimal holistic health.
- Baccalaureate nursing education offers students the opportunity to obtain a liberating education, elect areas of study, and develop competencies in their chosen discipline.
- As a Catholic and Franciscan College, inspired by our dedication to God as Creator, Redeemer, and Sanctifier, we value the sanctity of human life, human community, service, openness to all, and hold a reverence for all of creation.

Briar Cliff offers exceptional nursing education with important strengths.

- Accreditation by the National League for Nursing Accrediting Commission
- Approval by the Iowa Board of Nursing
- Graduates who score well above the national average on the NCLEX licensure exam
- Clinical experiences (no other college nursing program in Iowa offers more)
- Graduates who enjoy a 100 percent employment and graduate school acceptance and accept positions of leadership and challenge throughout the country
- Small classes, individual attention, and caring faculty mentors who are master teachers and active professionals
- Flexible acceptance of transfer credit
- Individualized study options and generous financial aid packages
- Networking connections through the Iowa Association of Nursing Students and Theta Gamma chapter of Sigma Theta Tau (International Honor Society of Nursing)
- Basic BSN can be completed in 4 years

Briar Cliff's nursing program prepares you for many professional roles

RECENT GRADUATES HOLD POSITIONS AS

Community health nurse	Nurse practitioner/midwife
Emergency care nurse	Nursing home administrator
Health & wellness educator	Occupational health nurse
Hospital clinical specialist	Private duty nurse
Intensive care nurse	School nurse
Nurse anesthetist	Nursing faculty

Many of our over 700 graduates earn their master's degrees in nursing, thereby improving the health of their communities as nurse practitioners, clinical nurse specialists, nursing leaders, and health care entrepreneurs.

CONTACT INFORMATION
BRIAR CLIFF UNIVERSITY
3303 Rebecca Street
P.O. Box 2100
Sioux City, Iowa 51104-0100
(712) 279-5200 or (800) 662-3303, ext. 5200
E-Mail: admission@briarcliff.edu
or contact
Ruth Dankanich Daumer, EdD, MSN, ARNP, BC
Associate Professor and Chairperson
Department of Nursing
(712) 279-5458 or (800) 662-3303 ext. 5458
E-Mail daumer@briarcliff.edu
Web: http:www.briarcliff.edu/nursing

The Catholic Franciscan Learning Place

BRIDGEPORT HOSPITAL SCHOOL OF NURSING
Bridgeport, Connecticut

HISTORY
Bridgeport Hospital School of Nursing offers an intensive course of study in preparation for nursing in the 21st century within the dynamic setting of a full-service medical center. Established in 1878, Bridgeport Hospital is a licensed 425-bed state-of-the-art facility with specialized services including obstetric, pediatric, cardiovascular care, psychiatry, rehabilitation, critical care, and community health centers. Bridgeport Hospital is part of the Yale-New Haven Health Network and is a teaching affiliate of Yale University.

The School of Nursing, established in 1884, is the oldest school for nursing in Connecticut. Over the last century, the school's graduates have been noted for their clinical excellence and commitment to caring.

The student body is drawn from a diverse pool of applicants. Over 75% of students who began the program in recent years went on to graduate. Of those who graduated, over 95% passed the registered nurse licensure examination (NCLEX). The School boasts an award-winning Student Nurse Association.

PROGRAMS OF STUDY
The school offers three unique programs of study:

A Diploma Nursing program consisting of 4 academic semesters plus a summer course between the first and second year. Graduates are eligible to take the registered nurse licensure exam. Accelerated LPN-to-RN opportunities are available. An Associate in Science Degree in Nursing can be earned through a collaborative effort between Bridgeport Hospital School of Nursing and Housatonic College.

A 20-week Certificate Perioperative Nursing Program prepares registered nurses to function in the operating room.

A 10-month CAAHEP accredited Certificate Program of Surgical Technology prepares graduates to function in a variety of surgical settings. Graduates are eligible to sit for the National Certifying Examination for Surgical Technologists.

All programs incorporate extensive clinical experience where critical thinking is encouraged and fostered. The nursing curriculum is based on a philosophy of holism. The faculty designs learning experiences that complement, respect, and nurture each learner's uniqueness.

CLINICAL SITES
In addition to Bridgeport Hospital, the School utilizes a variety of other acute care settings as well as community health and extended care facilities. Alternate practice sites are selected that maintain the School's strong clinical orientation while exposing students to settings where nurses will be practicing in the new millennium.

ADMISSIONS
Students are admitted to all three programs once a year in September.

Requirements for the RN and Surgical Technologist Programs: 4 years of high school English and 2 years of Mathematics and Science. The TOEFL may be required for non-native speakers of English. Applicants possessing a GED must submit other documented evidence of scholastic aptitude. All Surgical Technology applicants are required to complete a pre-admission test of basic adult education.

Requirements for Perioperative Program: Connecticut RN License.

TUITION & FINANCIAL AID
RN Program: $10,400 for 40 Nursing credits and $2,300 for 30 Non-Nursing credits.
Perioperative Nursing: $2,500
Surgical Technology: $3,500

Scholarships, Federal Pell Grants, Supplemental Educational Opportunity Grants, PLUS Loans, and Stafford Loans are available.

CORRESPONDENCE
Admissions Office
Bridgeport Hospital School of Nursing
200 Mill Hill Avenue
Bridgeport, CT 06610
(203) 384-3022
Fax: (203) 384-3046
Web: http://BHSN.BPTHOSP.ORG

BRIGHAM YOUNG UNIVERSITY
College of Nursing
Provo, Utah

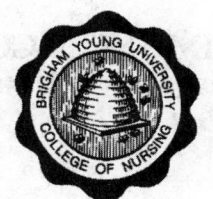

THE UNIVERSITY
Brigham Young University, founded in 1875, is sponsored and operated by The Church of Jesus Christ of Latter-day Saints. It is currently the largest privately owned, church-sponsored university in the United States with approximately 1,500 faculty and 30,000 students, and is nestled at the foot of the beautifully rugged Wasatch Range of the Rocky Mountains on 600 acres. Inscribed at the entrance of the campus is, "The World is Our Campus," reflecting the many local and international learning experiences. Facilities and programs include a 793-acre research farm, a PBS television station, and a three-million-volume library.

THE COLLEGE OF NURSING
The college was established in 1952. Following in the footsteps of pioneer nurses and midwives, college alumni have established a legacy of service as clinicians, nurse practitioners, administrators, educators, and scholars. Today, the nationally accredited program offers a baccalaureate and two masters degrees.

PROGRAMS OF STUDY
The College of Nursing offers a generic baccalaureate degree. Two Masters of Science specializations are offered as a Family Nurse Practitioner and in Adult Med/Surg Clinical Nurse Specialist. Graduates are eligible to apply for certification.

AFFILIATIONS WITH HEALTH CARE FACILITIES
BYU College of Nursing maintains contractual agreements with more than one hundred and twenty-five health-care agencies. Excellent learning experiences are found in a number of urban and rural hospitals as well as home and community settings. Students also have opportunities for clinical experiences among cultures of Native America, Guatemala, and Jordan.

ACADEMIC RESOURCES
College of Nursing facilities include a learning resource center, clinical simulations laboratory, research center, student computer lab, and media development areas. These resources enrich student learning experiences and foster research opportunities for students and faculty.

COSTS
Undergraduate full-time tuition for members of the Church is $1,530 per semester. Non-members full-time tuition is $2,300 per semester. Graduate full-time tuition for members is $1,930 per semester and is $2,895 for non-members.

FINANCIAL AID
BYU offers institutionally-sponsored scholarships, Federal Pell Grants, Federal Subsidized Stafford Loans, Federal Unsubsidized Stafford Loans, and Federal Parent Loan for Undergraduate Students.

APPLYING
For the BSN Program, students must be fully matriculated at BYU, receive a minimum of a C grade in prerequisite courses, and not less than an overall GPA of 3.0 in prerequisite courses. Students with English as a second language, in addition, take the English Proficiency Examination and complete courses recommended by the examination outcome, and complete TOEFL with at least a 580 score.

For the MS program, a baccalaureate degree, eligibility for RN licensure in Utah, satisfactory GRE scores, a minimum GPA on last 60 hours of 3.0, evidence of a statistics course and clinical experience, are recommended. An interview is required.

CORRESPONDENCE AND INFORMATION
Undergraduate:
Linda T. Stevens
Nursing Advisement Center
551 SWKT
Brigham Young University
Provo, UT 84602

Graduate:
Denise Gibbons Davis
Graduate Program
500 SWKT
Brigham Young University
Provo, UT 84602

BRONX COMMUNITY COLLEGE
Department of Nursing and Allied Health Sciences
Bronx, New York

THE COLLEGE
Bronx Community College is a beautiful place to learn. The magnificent 50-acre campus—with trees, spacious lawns and columned buildings—is one of the most inspiring settings in the city. An ethnically diverse student body studies in our modern, state-of-the-art multimedia facilities and library and relaxes in our Olympic-size pool or by attending concerts, theatrical performances, and other special campus events.

THE DEPARTMENT
The Department of Nursing and Allied Health Sciences offers courses designed to make you competitive in today's job market and to make it easy to transfer to baccalaureate programs. Classes are taught in the Nursing Computer Laboratory/College Practice Laboratory, lecture rooms, and clinical facilities.

PROGRAMS OF STUDY
Three programs of study lead to an Associate in Applied Sciences (A.A.S.) degree and eligibility to sit for the Licensure Examination (NCLEX-RN) to practice as a Registered Professional Nurse. The generic two-year program is open to all Bronx Community College and transfer students who meet Nursing program criteria. Qualified LPNs may progress rapidly through the Fast Track RN or the RN Pathway sequence.

ACADEMIC/CLINICAL RESOURCES
The Library and Learning Resources Center at Bronx Community College offer electronic access to information held at all 22 colleges in the City University of New York library system, in addition to its own large print collection. The Nursing program maintains contracts with numerous clinical facilities located in the Bronx and metropolitan area. These include acute care hospitals, psychiatric and mental health settings, children's day care agencies, and long-term care facilities.

COST
Tuition for full-time students is $1,250 to $1,538/semester or $105 to $130/credit for part-time students.

FINANCIAL AID
BCC offers Lincoln/Rudin Fund grants to Nursing students; Federal Pell Grants, Federal Supplemental Educational Opportunity Grants, Perkins Loans, the College Work Study Program, Veterans Administration Education Benefits, the William D. Ford Subsidized Direct Loan Program, the New York State Tuition Assistance Program, the College Discovery Program, the CUNY Assistance Program, and Emergency Loan Funds are also available.

APPLYING
All College applicants must have a diploma from an accredited high school or a New York State Equivalency Diploma.

Generic RN program applicants must meet acceptable standards in reading, writing, mathematics, and chemistry; complete a pre-clinical sequence of courses (Communication, English, Psychology, Pharmacology Computation, and Anatomy and Physiology) with a minimum C+ average; and pass the National League for Nursing Pre-admission Examination-RN Test at an acceptable level.

Fast Track RN and RN Pathway applicants must meet the above requirements and be a qualified Licensed Practical Nurse.

CORRESPONDENCE AND INFORMATION
Nursing Program Director—GT 413
Department of Nursing & Allied Health Sciences
Bronx Community College
West 181st Street & University Avenue
Bronx, NY 10453
(718) 289-5425
Web: www.bcc.cuny.edu

CALIFORNIA STATE UNIVERSITY, DOMINGUEZ HILLS
School of Health – Division of Nursing
Carson, California

THE UNIVERSITY

California State University, Dominguez Hills (CSUDH) is a public institution in the California State University system. CSUDH is accredited by the Western Association of Schools and Colleges. Founded in 1960, CSUDH is a multi-cultural, multi-ethnic teaching and learning community dedicated to excellence. Within CSUDH, the School of Health comprises the Division of Nursing and the Division of Health Sciences. The School of Health offers many diverse programs and options at both the undergraduate and graduate levels. CSUDH is located just minutes from downtown Los Angeles and L.A. airport.

DIVISION OF NURSING

The Division of Nursing's mission is to provide adult learners with the knowledge, skills, and values to improve nursing and health care for populations of unprecedented diversity in the community. Guiding principles are respect for each learner's uniqueness, the ethic of caring, collaborative partnerships with the community, and health as a fundamental right for all. Originating in 1981 to offer nursing programs throughout the state of California, the Division of Nursing has expanded its programs both nationally and internationally. The nursing programs are accessible, current, innovative, and culturally sensitive. Supportive of the working professional, the Division of Nursing's non-traditional curriculum is offered on the Internet using distance education instructional technology. Classes are also available in the evenings and weekends, in a variety of community settings in California. The curricula are updated continually to provide the necessary clinical skills and expertise that are in high demand.

In addition to program-specific content and skills, the SOH programs are designed to emphasize the development of critical thinking and strategies needed for successful adaptation to a rapidly evolving and complex health care environment. Nursing graduates from CSUDH are prepared for a variety of career opportunities in many settings as competent providers of nursing care and leaders in the profession.

CSUDH Division of Nursing provides students with personal attention from some of the finest faculty in the nation. The faculty has extensive knowledge and hands-on experience in teaching, management, clinical practice, and community-based research.

The Division of Nursing offers programs leading to the BSN and MSN degrees. The programs are designed for registered nurses (RNs) whose time, lifestyles, or work schedules make it difficult to complete a traditional course of study. These programs are fully accredited by the National League for Nursing Accreditation Commission (NLNAC), and the Family Nurse Practitioner program is approved by the California Board of Registered Nursing. The Division of Nursing also offers programs leading to the Public Health Certificate, the FNP Post-Master's Certificate, and the Quality Improvement Certificate.

BSN PROGRAM

The BSN program prepares registered nurses as generalists in professional nursing practice. Graduates function as clinicians, leaders, managers, and resource persons in a variety of health care settings.

ADMISSIONS REQUIREMENTS

1. Minimum of 56 semester units of transferable college credit with a cumulative grade point average of at least 2.0 (C) or better (non-residents, 2.4), all grades of C- (70%) or better in all transferable course work. English composition, Speech, general education Math and Logic/Critical Thinking must be completed prior to admission for new applicants.
2. Current RN licensure in the United States or an RN interim permit.

BSN CURRICULUM

A minimum total of 120 semester units are required for the degree. In addition to the major, students must complete general education requirements. Students transferring from a community college can transfer a maximum of 70 units and students from a four-year institution may transfer a maximum of 96 units.

The baccalaureate program comprises classes and/or examinations that include content essential for professional nursing practice. Three options are open to the student:

1. A series of classes. Classes may require onsite attendance, Web-based interaction, or a combination of both.
2. Written assessments which may be taken in lieu of selected courses. The student receives a study packet and takes the examination. Students MUST enroll in the corresponding nursing course before credit can be given.
3. A combination of classes and assessments.

The BSN curriculum features coursework in community-based nursing, leadership and management, informatics, cultural diversity, health promotion, and other content areas that support professional nursing practice.

CERTIFICATE IN PUBLIC HEALTH NURSE (POSTBACCALAUREATE)

This program satisfies the State of California Department of Health academic requirements to be eligible for the state Public Health Nurse (PHN) Certificate. For more information about eligibility requirements and workshops see www.csudh.edu/soh/don.

MSN PROGRAM

The graduate program prepares professional nurses for advanced and specialized practice. The curriculum is organized around the role of the nurse with emphasis on the application of theory through excellence in professional practice, and the advancement of the profession through research, leadership, and scholarship benefit health care needs in society.

ADMISSION REQUIREMENTS

1. Completion of a baccalaureate degree program with a NLNAC or CCNE accredited upper division major in nursing (BSN) from a regionally accredited institution or equivalent as determined by the DON Student Affairs Committee.
2. Overall grade point average of 3.0 (on a four-point scale) or higher in the last 60 semester (90 quarter) units attempted.
3. Current RN licensure in the United States.
4. Satisfaction of the Graduation Writing Assessment Requirement (GWAR).
5. Completion of statistics course that includes both inferential and descriptive components.
6. Completion of introductory research course or equivalent.

7. Part B of CSU Graduate Application including a 100-200 word statement describing the congruence of the applicant's educational goals with the CSUDH Division of Nursing MSN Program.
8. Submission of a professional resume.
9. An interview may be required by the faculty or requested by the applicant.

NURSES WITH NON-NURSING BACHELOR'S DEGREES

Registered nurses who have earned a bachelor's degree in another field may be eligible for the Pathway program to MSN degree upon completion of designated courses. Contact the Pathway advisor for further information. Registered nurse applicants who have earned a master's degree in a major other than nursing should contact the graduate program coordinator to arrange for preadmission advisement.

The program consists of 33-53 semester units of approved graduate study. The curriculum includes core courses, role option courses, role performance courses, and a comprehensive examination. Elective units round out the graduate program requirements. Up to nine approved units may be accepted for transfer credit.

MSN CURRICULUM

Core Courses (20 units)

Role Options (13-33 units)
Parent-Child Clinical Nurse Specialist Option (23 units)
Gerontology Clinical Nurse Specialist Option (23 units)
Nurse Education Option (10 units + 3 units electives)
Nurse Administrator Option (10 units + 3 units electives)
Family Nurse Practitioner (33 units)

AFFILIATION WITH HEALTH CARE FACILITIES

The Division of Nursing maintains affiliations with a broad range of clinical facilities including major medical centers, community health centers, clinics, HMOs, private group practices, schools, and other community-based institutions. Students in clinical role performance courses work on a 1:1 basis with preceptors to achieve the course objectives and the goals of their individual learning contracts.

ACADEMIC FACILITIES

The School of Health has a dedicated unit to support the extensive online educational programs offered to students. The Academic Technology professionals work with the faculty and students to assist in providing a rich online learning environment using advanced Web-based technology. The CSUDH Library is fully equipped and staffed to support online learning with comprehensive online databases that are accessible on and off campus.

STUDENT SERVICES

Careful and comprehensive advisement is a key to student success at CSUDH. To assist in reaching this goal, the School of Health Student Services Center offers students general advising with a Student Services Advisor. Students who need specific program guidance and professional mentoring are referred to their Faculty Advisor. All students must seek faculty advisement to discuss clinical placements and progress in their majors.

NURSING STUDENT GROUP

One of the largest nursing programs in California, CSUDH has a nursing student body of approximately 725 BSN and 275 MSN students. The CSUDH nursing students are working RNs who reflect a very culturally and ethnically diverse population. The more than 5,000 nursing alumni are employed in all areas of nursing as clinicians, educators, and administrators throughout the state and nationally.

COSTS

For California Residents:
Undergraduate fees – 0-6 units is $530.00 and 6.1+ units is $830.00 per semester

Graduate fees – 0-6 units is $549.00 and 6.1+ units is $864.00 per semester

National Students (Graduate and Undergraduate): $225 per unit

FINANCIAL AID

Financial Aid and Scholarships are available. MSN students may be eligible for Professional Nurse Traineeship awards.

APPLYING

Contact the Student Services Center at (800) 344-5484 to request a CSU application packet and for further information or apply online at www.csumentor.edu. Visit the Division of Nursing website, www.csudh.edu/soh/don, to learn more.

The application deadline for the Spring semester is November 1, for the Summer semester is April 1, and for the Fall semester is June 1.

CORRESPONDENCE AND INFORMATION

To obtain additional information, call a School of Health Student Services Center Advisor at (800) 344-5484 (option 1), contact by email at sohadvising@soh.csudh.edu or visit us at www.csudh.edu/soh.

THE FACULTY

The faculty consists of 25 full-time professors and about 40 part-time instructors. Their research interests include distance education, women's health, HIV/AIDS care, health beliefs and practices of underserved populations, and pain management.

CAPITAL HEALTH SYSTEMS SCHOOL OF NURSING
Trenton, New Jersey

THE SETTING
Capital Health System School of Nursing (CHSSON), founded in 1890, is located in Trenton, NJ, an urban area rich in history. CHSSON is within easy reach of Princeton, Philadelphia, New York, the Jersey shore, and Bucks County. College courses are offered at Mercer County Community College, located approximately 10 miles from the school in beautiful, suburban West Windsor Township.

PROGRAMS OF STUDY
The hospital-based school with over a century of excellence offers a three-year, cooperative nursing program with Mercer County Community College. This co-educational program offers opportunities for part- or full-time study. Graduates of the program are eligible to apply for licensure as a Registered Nurse (RN). They are also eligible to continue their education towards a bachelor's degree in nursing at various institutions of higher learning.

AFFILIATIONS
The School of Nursing maintains contractual agreements with more than 20 healthcare agencies. The school's clinical resources include community hospitals and clinics (Mercer and Fuld Campuses), psychiatric and mental health facilities, community-based outpatient settings, visiting nurses agencies, extended care facilities, schools, and hospices.

ACADEMIC RESOURCES
Academic resources at the Fuld Campus include state-of-the-art laboratory and computer centers, and modern classroom facilities with multimedia resources. Mercer County Community College resources include a student writing center, physical education facilities with an Olympic-sized pool, and a library with more than 325,000 print and non-print resources.

TUITION/FINANCIAL AID
Every candidate who is accepted is a recipient of the Helene Fuld Trust Fund Scholarship, which provides tuition for all nursing courses taught at Capital Health System School of Nursing. There are fees for nursing courses as well as tuition and fees for college courses, which are the student's responsibilities. Financial aid is available through MCCC for qualified students. The cost for tuition and fees is approximately $3,000 annually.

ADMISSIONS
Applicants to the School of Nursing are evaluated on an individual basis. The school does not discriminate against applicants or students because of race, color, religious creed, national origin, ancestry, sex, age, marital status, sexual orientation, atypical hereditary cellular or blood trait, medical condition or physical disability, or liability for services in the Armed Forces of the United States. Admission requirements include a completed application form (which can now be completed online at www.capitalhealth.org) with the required application fee; high school diploma or GED equivalency; RN entrance exam, if required; and three recommendations.

CORRESPONDENCE AND INFORMATION:
Registrar
CHSSON
832 Brunswick Avenue
Trenton, NJ 08638
(609) 394-3174 extension 3146
Fax: (609) 695-9247
Web: www.capitalhealth.org

Contact: Casey A. Cruser
(609) 394-6091
ccruser@chsnj.org

CARDINAL STRITCH UNIVERSITY
College of Nursing
Milwaukee, Wisconsin

THE UNIVERSITY
Cardinal Stritch University is a coeducational university, rooted in the liberal arts and established in the Franciscan Catholic tradition. Since its founding in 1937 by the Sisters of St. Francis of Assisi, Stritch has emerged as the largest Franciscan institution of higher education in North America and the second-largest university in Wisconsin.

PROGRAMS OF STUDY
Stritch is the only school in Wisconsin to offer the full range of nursing programs, from ADN through MSN degrees. Each of these programs is accredited by the National League for Nursing Accrediting Commisssion.

The associate's degree prepares students for entry into nursing practice. Upon completion of the ADN, the graduate is eligible to take the National Council Licensure Examinations - Registered Nurse (NCLEX-RN) to become a registered nurse. To complete the degree, 70 credit hours are required—38 in nursing and 32 in liberal arts core courses.

The five-semester ADN includes a full range of studies encompassing the entire life cycle. The program also features community contact and substantial clinical experience. Faculty emphasize theory, problem-solving, critical thinking, and a broad perspective of the nursing field. The ADN naturally feeds into the BSN completion program for those who choose to continue their education.

In addition to the traditional ADN program, Stritch offers an LPN to ADN progression option for licensed practical nurses who want to further develop their abilities to practice nursing and to become licensed as registered nurses. This program allows the LPN to complete requirements for the degree in three semesters following the completion of prerequisite courses and offers all of the benefits of the traditional ADN program.

The BSN completion program prepares the ADN or diploma graduate to practice professional nursing with a broadened knowledge base. Nurses will find this two-year, accelerated program to be a flexible complement to their full-time work schedule. With classes meeting just one night per week, nurses can gain valuable experience in the field while earning the BSN.

Stritch offers a semi-accelerated MSN with an educational focus for working nurses who want to function as "nurse educator" in a variety of client communities. Course theory is carefully merged with practical applications, allowing students to identify their individual needs of study and to create final projects that they can present to employers. Coursework and study provide a foundation for doctoral or advanced study. Students in this 30-month program attend classes one to two nights a week for six semesters to complete the requirements for the MSN. To complete the degree, 36 credit hours are required.

LOCATION
Stritch's 40-acre, park-like main campus is situated in a quiet suburban neighborhood just 15 minutes north of downtown Milwaukee. Access to Lake Michigan is available within several blocks.

COSTS
Full-time ADN tuition for 2002-2003 is $14,240/year. Room and board are $5,060. BSN Completion tuition is $385/credit. Graduate tuition is $445/credit.

FINANCIAL AID
Many financial aid options are available. Eligibility for need-based grant and loan programs is determined after the Free Application for Federal Student Aid (FAFSA) is filed. Candidates for financial aid are encouraged to complete and mail the FAFSA by March 1.

APPLYING
The University accepts applications on a rolling admission basis. Each nursing program adheres to the general admission requirements of the University with the addition of some requirements specific to the ADN, BSN Completion, or MSN program. Both general and specific admission requirements are listed in detail in the University's undergraduate and graduate catalogs.

CORRESPONDENCE AND INFORMATION
To learn more about the ADN or BSN programs:
Janet Beitz, College of Nursing
(414) 410-4391 or 800-347-8822, Ext. 4391
E-Mail: jbeitz@stritch.edu
or
Office of Undergraduate Admissions
Cardinal Stritch University
6801 North Yates Road
Milwaukee, WI 53217-3985
(414) 410-4040 or 800-347-8822, Ext. 4040
E-Mail: admityou@stritch.edu
Web: www.stritch.edu

For the MSN program:
Linda M. Steiner
(414) 410-4062 or 800-347-8822, Ext. 4062
E-Mail: lmsteiner@stritch.edu
or
Office of Graduate Admissions
Cardinal Stritch University
6801 North Yates Road
Milwaukee, WI 53217-3985
(414) 410-4042 or 800-347-8822 Ext. 4042
E-Mail: gradadm@stritch.edu
Web: www.stritch.edu

CASE WESTERN RESERVE UNIVERSITY
The Frances Payne Bolton School of Nursing
Cleveland, Ohio

THE UNIVERSITY

Case Western Reserve University was formed in 1967 by the federation of Case Institute of Technology and Western Reserve University. With almost 10,000 undergraduate and graduate students, it is recognized as one of the major independent universities in the United States.

THE SCHOOL OF NURSING

The Frances Payne Bolton School of Nursing traces its heritage to the Lakeside Hospital Training School for Nurses, which was established in 1898. Largely as a result of a generous endowment from Frances Payne Bolton, the School of Nursing as it now exists was established in 1923.

PROGRAMS OF STUDY

In addition to the Bachelor of Science in Nursing (BSN), the School of Nursing offers the Master of Science in Nursing (MSN), the Doctor of Nursing (ND), and the Doctor of Philosophy (PhD) in nursing.

The Bolton school offers a traditional BSN and a BSN for registered nurses (RN-to-BSN). The RN-to-BSN program may be completed on a full-time or a part-time basis. The BSN program allows for direct entry into nursing with clinical experience beginning the first semester of the freshman year.

The MSN degree is designed for nurses seeking preparation for advanced practice nursing. Nurses from all basic nursing programs accredited by the NLNAC are eligible to apply. Associate or diploma nurses may also qualify for admission to the program. The MSN requires approximately 40 semester hours of study. Specialization is offered in nurse midwifery; nurse anesthesia; medical-surgical, community health, critical-care, and oncology nursing; and acute care, neonatal, adult, family, gerontological, pediatric, psychiatric-mental health, and women's health nurse practitioner studies. Baccalaureate-prepared, certified advanced practice nurses may qualify to complete the MSN in 18-19 semester hours in the intensive summer format.

The Doctor of Nursing (ND) degree is a four-year, entry-level graduate program designed for college graduates with a baccalaureate degree in a discipline other than nursing. The first two years (levels) of the program consist of the prelicensure nursing curriculum and include all course work required to sit for the professional nursing licensing examination (NCLEX-RN). The goal of the postlicensure component of the program is to prepare students for advanced practice and clinical research in nursing. Clinical specialties offered at this level are nurse midwifery and adult, family, gerontological, pediatric, psychiatric-mental health, and women's health nurse practitioner studies. Entry into level III of the program requires a license to practice nursing and is available to graduates of baccalaureate nursing programs. Master's-prepared, nationally certified, advanced practice nurses may qualify for entry to level IV of the ND program.

The Doctor of Philosophy in nursing (PhD) degree program is designed for individuals who seek preparation in research and who have completed either an MSN degree with a clinical nursing major or at least 24 semester hours of graduate study beyond the BSN, including 12 semester hours of supervised clinical practice. The PhD student concentrates on the organization and development of knowledge requisite to nursing practice. Research, which focuses on acute care, pediatric nursing, gerontological nursing, and health systems, is conducted by an internationally known faculty. Opportunities for postdoctoral study and combined-degree programs are also available.

ACADEMIC RESOURCES

The Bolton School of Nursing is in the University Health Science Center, adjacent to the University Hospitals of Cleveland. The facility offers library resources, computer space, audiovisual capabilities, and laboratory and research space.

THE NURSING STUDENTS

More than half of The Bolton School's nursing students are registered nurses who work in hospitals and academic settings. They come from twelve different countries and thirty-five states, totaling over 800 students.

COSTS

For the 2002–2003 academic year, tuition was $1,004 per credit hour for students taking 1 to 11 credit hours and $24,100 for students taking 12 or more credit hours. Nonlocal undergraduate students are required to live on campus. Housing costs ranged from $4,200 to $6,320. For graduate students, there are a variety of options available off campus. University meal plans ranged in cost from $2,676 to $2,890. The University requires students to have health insurance and offers a policy for $874 per year. This fee may be waived if the student has other coverage.

FINANCIAL AID

Each year, undergraduate students identified as Bolton Scholars receive paid awards ranging from 40 to 50 percent of tuition. Additional financial assistance is available through grants, loans, and work-study. Additional information is available from the Registrar's Office at Case Western Reserve University.

At the graduate level, financial assistance is awarded through grants, scholarships, loans, and work agreements. Information may be obtained from the Registrar's Office at The Bolton School.

ADMISSIONS

The programs of study for the BSN, the MSN in nurse anesthesia, and the ND prelicensure curriculum begin in the fall term each year. Students in all other programs may begin in the fall, spring, or summer term. The application deadline for the BSN and the MSN in nurse anesthesia is January 15. Applications for all other programs are processed on a rolling basis and must be completed two months before the term begins. It is recommended that students apply at least six months prior to the term in which they intend to enroll.

CONTACT INFORMATION

Office of Student Services
Frances Payne Bolton School of Nursing
Case Western Reserve University
10900 Euclid Avenue
Cleveland, OH 44106-4904
(800) 825-2540 x2529
E-Mail: admissions@fpb.cwru.edu
Web: http://fpb.cwru.edu

CAYUGA COMMUNITY COLLEGE
Auburn, New York

Cayuga Community College is a public, two-year college sponsored by Cayuga County and a unit of The State University of New York. Located in rural upstate New York, the college offers over 20 degree programs with over 50% of students transferring to four-year colleges and the remainder seeking employment or military service upon completion of degree requirements. The College was one of the first community colleges to open its doors in 1953. Currently the College serves over 2,500 full and part-time students on 2 campuses—the main campus in Auburn, and the extension center in Fulton. Cayuga is accredited by the National League for Nursing Accrediting Commission as well as Middle States Association of Colleges and Universities. Our award-winning, state recognized faculty members are committed to student learning.

NURSING PROGRAM HISTORY
The nursing program was founded in 1972 to meet the needs of the community for skilled, caring registered nurses. In 1974 the College graduated its first nursing class and since then has awarded over 1,000 degrees in nursing. Our current first time NCLEX-RN pass rate of 94% is higher than most in New York State. Our graduates are highly regarded by local hospitals and 100% of our graduates obtain employment.

PROGRAM OF STUDY
The Associate of Applied Science (AAS) degree in Nursing prepares students for entry level nursing positions in acute and long term care as well as community settings. The program is among the first to include 4 credits of Health Assessment along with a semester of community/family-focused nursing care. Students receive their clinical experience at SUNY Upstate Medical Center and Syracuse Community General Hospital, along with Auburn Memorial Hospital and other local health care facilities. The Cayuga County Health Department provides the clinical practice setting for community health and home care visits.

Upon successful completion of the curriculum, students are eligible to sit for the state licensure examination to become registered nurses (NCLEX-RN).

Licensed Practical Nurses may qualify for advance standing in the program.

Students who choose to move on to a baccalaureate degree program may do so through articulations with:

Syracuse University
SUNY Health Science Center at Syracuse
SUNY College of Technology at Utica/Rome
SUNY Plattsburgh (offered distance learning on the Cayuga campus)
Keuka College

COSTS
Tuition for 2001–2002 was the following:

Full-time (12–19 credit hours): $1,260/semester (New York State residents)

$2,520/semester (out-of-state residents)

Part-time (fewer than 12 credit hours): $90 per credit hour + fees associated with student activities, technology, and special nursing needs

FINANCIAL AID
Many scholarships are available to potential nursing students through a large fund supported by the College Foundation office. Contact the admissions or financial aid office for more information. The College utilizes the Free Application for Federal Student Aid (FAFSA) to determine financial aid eligibility. You can apply on-line at www.fafsa.org.

ADMISSION PROCESS
Students must have satisfactorily completed at least high school level algebra, biology, and chemistry for initial entrance into the nursing program. Students who have not met these pre-requisites may still be eligible to attend the College to gain these pre-requisites and apply for admission into nursing upon completing such requirements. Nursing admission may be limited due to demand for spaces. Contact the admissions office at 315-255-1743 for more information.

Find our more about Cayuga Community College by visiting our website at www.cayuga-cc.edu, or contact us at:
197 Franklin St., Auburn, New York 13021
(315) 255-1743

CHARLESTON SOUTHERN UNIVERSITY
Derry Patterson Wingo School of Nursing
Charleston, South Carolina

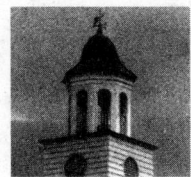

MISSION
Promoting Academic Excellence in a Christian Environment

THE UNIVERSITY
Located on 300 scenic acres near historic Charleston, South Carolina, Charleston Southern University provides an education and an experience that combines the best of the traditional and the contemporary. The Low country's moderate climate allows CSU's 2500 students to take advantage of cultural, historical, and recreational opportunities. As a private, four-year, liberal arts university, Charleston Southern offers thirty undergraduate majors and graduate programs in business administration, education, and criminal justice.

THE SCHOOL OF NURSING
The mission of the Derry Patterson Wingo School of Nursing is to provide excellence in nursing and health care to individuals, groups, families, and society through its program of education and service while respecting cultural, ethnic, religious, and individual differences and commonalties. The school is committed to the undergraduate education of a professional nurse who integrates Christian values into the practice of nursing.

PROGRAMS OF STUDY
The DPW School of Nursing is a baccalaureate nursing program leading to the Bachelor of Science in Nursing. The program prepares graduates for professional practice in a variety of health care settings and for continued professional development and graduate study. Graduates are eligible to take the National Council Licensure Examination for Registered Nurse practice (NCLEX-RN). A RN-BSN option is also offered for registered nurses with associate degrees and diplomas in nursing who desire to return to school to complete the Bachelor of Science in Nursing degree. The program has Full Approval of the Board of Nursing of South Carolina and is designed to meet all standards for accreditation by the National League for Nursing Accrediting Commission.

AFFILIATIONS WITH HEALTH CARE FACILITIES
The DPW School of Nursing affiliates with over thirty area health care agencies in providing clinical learning experiences to meet the objectives of the individual courses and the program.

ACADEMIC RESOURCES AND FACILITIES
Charleston Southern University has a modern library that contains more than 200,000 volumes, a modern chapel-auditorium with impressive fine arts facilities, and a multipurpose gymnasium. Among other facilities on campus are one of the nation's three Earthquake Centers and a distinctive computer center. The Derry Patterson Wingo School of Nursing houses a computer lab and a simulation clinical lab. Tutorial, counseling, and career services are also available.

COSTS
Tuition for the 2003–2004 academic year is $14,426, and room and board are $5,544. A clinical fee is added for nursing students. Tuition and fees are subject to change.

FINANCIAL AID
A comprehensive financial aid program, consisting of scholarships, grants, loans, and employment, has been established at Charleston Southern. Approximately 90% of the student body receive some type of financial assistance.

APPLYING
Since enrollment in the Nursing major is limited, admission is competitive. Students must apply and be accepted by Charleston Southern University. However, admission to the university does not guarantee admission to the School of Nursing. A completed application for admission to the School of Nursing must be submitted by March 15 for fall admission. For the basic/generic program, admission requirements include a GPA of at least 2.5 in 34 semester hours of pre-nursing courses and a cumulative CSU GPA of 2.0. For the RN-BSN option, a minimum GPA of 2.5 on prerequisite courses, a CSU GPA of 2.0, and a current, active license as a Registered Nurse in South Carolina are required. For a complete detailed description of the admission and application requirements, contact the Derry Patterson Wingo School of Nursing at (843) 863-7075.

CORRESPONDENCE AND INFORMATION
Charleston Southern University
Office of Enrollment Services
P.O. Box 118087
Charleston, SC 29423-8087
(843) 863-7050 or (800) 947-7474
Fax: (843) 863-7070
E-Mail: enroll@csuniv.edu
Web: http://www.csuniv.edu

COLLEGE OF EASTERN UTAH
Department of Nursing
Price, Utah

College of Eastern Utah offers students two options in nursing education at two locations:

Certificate of Completion in Practical Nursing
Associate of Applied Science Degree in Nursing leading toward RN Licensure.

At the College of Eastern Utah, nursing theory is correlated with knowledge from the biological, physical, and behavioral sciences. Our nurse educators have extensive experience in the field and guide students in theory, laboratory practice, and a variety of clinical experiences.

WHY CEU?

- Small personal classes
- Culturally diverse experiences
- High success rate on passing boards
- Varied clinical experiences
- Location offers varied scenic and recreational opportunities

Each program is a 2.5 semester curriculum. Completion of the program qualifies the student to take the NCLEX Examination for nursing licensure in the state of Utah. CEU's program is accredited with NLNAC and approved by the Utah State Board of Nursing. The application process starts January 1 and ends February 28 each year.

For more information:
College of Eastern Utah
Nusing Department
451 East 400 North
Price, UT 84501
(435) 613-5262
Web: www.ceu.edu

College of Eastern Utah
Nursing—"It's not a career . . . It's a Profession"

COLLEGE OF MOUNT ST. JOSEPH
Nursing Department
Cincinnati, Ohio

Caring Moments
with Communities
College of Mount St. Joseph
Nursing Department

THE COLLEGE
The College of Mount St. Joseph, located in suburban Cincinnati, is a Catholic college that provides its students with a liberal arts and professional education emphasizing values, integrity, and social responsibility. In addition to small class sizes that encourage individualized learning, the Mount offers its 2,200 students opportunities for leadership development and service learning, as well as a wide range of student activities.

NURSING DEPARTMENT
The outstanding reputation of the Mount's Nursing program is built on 75 years of experience in educating nurses. The innovative primary health care community-focused curriculum has been praised as visionary and on the leading edge of nursing education for preparing competent and confident nurses for the 21st century.

PROGRAMS OF STUDY
There are two tracks leading to the BSN degree. The Day Track (prelicensure) has as its major focus the preparation of students for the initial entry into the professional practice of nursing. The accelerated Weekend Track is specifically designed for registered nurses (RNs), graduates of diploma and associate degree programs, who wish to pursue the BSN degree in an accelerated format. Certifications or licensures in Parish Nursing, Paralegal Studies for Nurses, and School Nursing are also available.

AFFILIATIONS WITH HEALTH CARE FACILITIES
The Nursing Department maintains contractual agreements with more than 20 health care agencies. Students gain valuable clinical experience in agencies such as homeless clinics, schools, health care agencies, acute care hospitals, and long-term care facilities.

ACADEMIC RESOURCES
The Academic Performance Center is a centralized system of support for the enhancement of students' academic skills. The Nursing Department includes a state-of-the-art multimedia and skills lab, which supports competency-based learning.

COSTS AND FINANCIAL AID
The College of Mount St. Joseph offers a variety of financial aid programs that are funded by government and private sources. Nursing students may take advantage of additional programs to make their education more affordable. Tuition is the same for in-state and out-of-state residents: $14,200 per year for full-time study or $363 per credit hour for part-time study.

APPLYING
All applicants must meet with an intake advisor, send high school and official college transcripts (if transferring), and complete an application. To begin the clinical portion of the program, students must have completed all pre-requisites with a C or better, have a cumulative GPA of 2.5 or higher, and have completed at least 28 credits.

CORRESPONDENCE AND INFORMATION:
Chairperson, Department of Nursing
College of Mount St. Joseph
5701 Delhi Road
Cincinnati, OH 45233-1670
(513) 244-4511
Web: www.msj.edu

THE COLLEGE OF STATEN ISLAND
The City University of New York
Staten Island, New York

THE COLLEGE
The College of Staten Island is a senior college of the City University of New York. It is located on a 204-acre campus, the largest site for a college in New York City. The College offers three degree programs in nursing: an AAS, a RN-BS, and an MS in Adult Health Nursing.

ASSOCIATE DEGREE IN NURSING
The department began offering an AAS in nursing in 1965 as the former Staten Island Community College. Students apply for entry into the clinical portion of the program after completing the Pre-Nursing Sequence consisting of Anatomy and Physiology I (4cr.), English Composition (3 cr.), Introduction to Psychology (3 cr.), and Ethics (3 cr.). Admission to the program is competitive; students must earn at least a 2.5 average in those required courses to be considered for admission. The program is 64 credits, and graduates are eligible to take the New York State Registered Professional Nurse Licensure Examination. The College's pass rate on this examination has consistently been among the highest in CUNY.

BACCALAUREATE DEGREE IN NURSING
The College offers an upper division program for students who are graduates of accredited associate degree or diploma nursing programs. A total of 120 credits are required for the degree. Students broaden their liberal arts and science education and expand their professional nursing education. Clinical courses in community health, leadership and management, and critical care nursing are offered with day and evening placements. Nursing courses also include professional development, interpersonal dynamics, nursing research issues, and an elective. Graduates of the BS program are prepared to practice in a variety of health care environments and to continue their education at the graduate level.

MASTER OF SCIENCE IN ADULT HEALTH NURSING
The Adult Health Nursing program leading to the master of science degree is designed to meet health care workforce needs and to provide opportunities for graduate level education to baccalaureate nursing graduates. The program requirements are consistent with the competencies identified by the National Association of Clinical Nurse Specialists. Nurses who successfully complete the program are prepared to meet the needs of culturally diverse patients, families, and communities. In the changing health environment, master's prepared nurses are assuming roles as expert clinician, educator, researcher, and manager. Graduates are eligible for certification as specialists in medical-surgical nursing through the American Nurses Credentialing Center (ANCC) and other certifications offered by the ANCC and other specialty nursing organizations. For further information, please contact Dr. Margaret Lunney, Program Director, at (718) 982-3845.

ADMISSION INFORMATION
Contact the Office of Recruitment and Admissions, 2A-404
(718) 982-2010

COSTS/FINANCIAL AID
Undergraduate Resident Tuition:
$1,600 plus fees per semester, full-time
$135 per credit, part-time

Non-resident Tuition:
$3,400 plus fees per semester, full-time
$285 per credit, part-time

Financial Aid is available, contact (718) 982-2030.

Scholarships are available to eligible students. In particular, Elsie Marcus Scholarships are available for full-time study in the BS and MS programs.

CORRESPONDENCE AND INFORMATION
Professor Linda E. Reese, Chairperson
Department of Nursing
The College of Staten Island
2800 Victory Boulevard
Staten Island, NY 10314
(718) 982-3810
Web: www.csi.cuny.edu

COLUMBIA UNIVERSITY
School of Nursing
New York, New York

THE UNIVERSITY

Columbia University was founded in 1754. It is the oldest institution of higher learning in New York State and the fifth largest in the nation. It is organized into fifteen schools. The Health Science Division includes the Schools of Medicine, Dental and Oral Surgery, Nursing, Public Health and programs in physical therapy, nutrition, and occupational therapy. Total enrollment is close to 2,500 at the Health Science Campus and nearly 17, 500 at the Morningside Campus.

THE SCHOOL OF NURSING

Founded in 1892 as the Presbyterian Hospital School of Nursing, the School first offered the baccalaureate degree when it joined Columbia University. In 1956, it became the first nursing program in the country to award a master's degree in a clinical nursing specialty. Today the focus of the School is to educate the advanced practice nurse: the nurse practitioner, the nurse midwife, the nurse anesthetist, and the clinical nurse specialist. The School also offers a doctoral program (DNSc) that has a research emphasis on supporting advanced practice by either health outcomes or health policy research.

A major strength of the School is that faculty members maintain clinical practices in the advanced practice roles and incorporate students into these settings. One of these practices, Columbia Advanced Practice Nurse Associates (CAPNA), has gained national exposure as an innovative model of primary-care delivery by advanced practice nurses who are on the primary provider panel of several managed-care organizations.

In addition to these programs, the School sponsors five academic centers: the Center for Women and Children at Risk, the Center for AIDS Research, the Center for Health Policy and Health Services Research, the Center for Advanced Practice, and the World Health Organization Collaborating Center for International Nursing Development in Advanced Practice. Columbia was the first nursing school to be awarded this designation, which makes the School an active participant in international exchange and collaborative research in advanced practice and health services research. It also facilitates the development of international study opportunities for its students.

PROGRAMS OF STUDY

The School of Nursing offers four levels of educational programs. The Entry to Practice (ETP) Program is an accelerated BS/MS for non-nurse baccalaureate prepared graduates. Academic studies are closely integrated with clinical experience. Phase I of the Program consists of 60 credits over three semesters with a residency during the fourth semester. Upon completion of the 60 credits, a BS degree is granted and the graduate is eligible to sit for the professional nurse licensure exam in any state. Post-licensure, Phase II, is the MS piece of the Program, which focuses on a clinical specialty.

The Accelerated Master's Program (AMP) is also a combined degree program (BS/MS) designed to further the educational and career goals of RNs with either an Associate Degree in Nursing (ADN) or an ADN and a non-nursing baccalaureate degree. Admission criteria have been revised to be more "user-friendly." Curriculum revisions enable us to offer an individualized curriculum based on entering credentials and nursing experience.

The Master's Program for RNs with BS degrees in Nursing offers clinical majors in anesthesia, acute care, psychiatric-mental health nursing, midwifery, oncology, the primary-care specialties (adult, family, geriatric, and pediatric neonatal), and women's health. Credit requirements range from 45-59 credits and include core,

concentration, and elective courses. Dual degrees are available with The Schools of Public Health and Business.

The Advanced Certificate Program prepares RNs with a master's degree in nursing to pursue an advanced practice program as a nurse practitioner. The credits needed range from 22-34.

The Doctor of Nursing Science Program (DNSc) is designed to prepare clinical nurse scholars to examine, shape, and refine nursing science and nursing practice. The program offers students the choice of focusing in either clinical research or health policy. Currently, a master's degree in nursing is required for admission, and the curriculum consists of a minimum of 45 credits post-master's. A post-baccalaureate direct-entry option with an individualized curriculum is planned for the future.

AFFILIATIONS

The Columbia campus of the New York Presbyterian Hospital, which includes the Neurological Institute, the Eye Institute, Babies Hospital, Sloane Hospital for Women, the Center for Geriatrics and Gerontology, the Organ Transplant Center, and the Center for Health Promotion and Disease Prevention, form a hub of clinical activity. Approximately 150 other sites in the tri-state area are available for clinical education.

ACADEMIC FACILITIES

The Augustus C. Long Library is the fourth largest academic medical library in the country and is part of the Columbia University Library system. It houses more than 400,000 volumes and receives more that 4,500 journals, which can be accessed through online computer search programs. The Media and Computer Center contains an extensive variety of computer applications. The School of Nursing's Technology Learning Center contains seven patient units providing a hands-on environment for developing psychomotor skills, as well as state-of-the-art computer assisted monitoring equipment that simulates a real clinical environment.

LOCATION

The School of Nursing is located on the Health Science Campus's 20-acre site overlooking the Hudson River on Manhattan's Upper West Side. The School's students have access to all of the cultural, recreational, and educational opportunities that make New York City the quintessential metropolis.

COSTS

Tuition costs for the 2002–2003 academic year were $834 per credit for both the BS and MS didactic courses. The MS clinical costs were $1,060 per credit. The DNSc per credit cost was $1,138. Housing costs are variable with the average being $5,940 for a twelve- month period. Other expenses, including health fees, books, personal monies, transportation, and uniforms are estimated at $5,200.

FINANCIAL AID

Financial aid is distributed through a combination of scholarships, grants, work, and loans. Students should be able to meet all expenses for the academic year through a melding of these resources.

APPLYING

Applications are accepted throughout the academic year on a rolling basis. The application deadline for the ETP and anesthesia program is November 15. Admission is based on past academic performance and professional acumen. Admission requirements include the application

COLUMBIA UNIVERSITY
(continued)

form and fee, a considered personal statement detailing professional goals and achievements, three letters of reference, official transcripts from all postsecondary schools, official GRE scores, and a college level course in statistics. Applicants should have a minimum 3.0 cumulative grade point average with ETP applicants required to have 9-12 credits in the sciences. Anatomy and Physiology are required. All RN applicants must also submit a copy of their current license and registration and have a course in physical assessment with a minimum of one year of clinical experience in nursing. Additional requirements for the Doctoral Program are available upon request.

INFORMATION
Columbia University School of Nursing
630 West 168th Street, Box 6
New York, NY 10032
(212) 305-5756
Fax: (212) 305-3680
E-Mail: nursing@columbia.edu
Web: www.nursing.Columbia.edu

COMMUNITY COLLEGE OF PHILADELPHIA
Philadelphia, Pennsylvania

THE COLLEGE
Community College of Philadelphia is an urban community college located near center-city Philadelphia. It is the city's only community college and its third largest institution of higher education. The College is committed to providing an excellent education in a caring environment.

THE NURSING DEPARTMENT
The nursing program is located on the College's main campus. Founded in 1966 to meet the health care needs of Philadelphia, this program prepares graduates for beginning Registered Nurse (RN) positions in acute, long-term or community-based health care.

PROGRAM OF STUDY
The nursing program offers an associate in applied science (AAS) degree and prepares students to write the NCLEX-RN licensing examination. This program is approved by the Pennsylvania Board of Nursing and accredited by the National League for Nursing Accrediting Commission. A highly qualified faculty prepares graduates for work or transfer as juniors to most four-year nursing programs in the region.

AFFILIATIONS WITH HEALTH CARE FACILITIES
The nursing program has contractual agreements with over thirty health care agencies in Philadelphia. Nursing students take classes at the College and complete clinical laboratory learning experiences in medical center hospitals, community hospitals, long term care facilities, and community based agencies.

ACADEMIC RESOURCES
Nursing students benefit from four state-of-the-art nursing laboratories. The College's library includes over 90,000 books, 450 periodicals and newspapers, and an integrated on-line catalog. The College also has computing centers, free tutoring, and a child development center.

COST
Tuition is $83.00 per credit for Philadelphia residents, $166.00 for other Pennsylvanians, and $249.00 for non-Pennsylvanians. Students also pay a $3.00 general college fee and $10.00 technology fee. Other fees or deposits may apply.

FINANCIAL AID
The College participates in federal and state funded programs: Federal Pell Grant, Federal Supplemental Educational Opportunity Grant, Federal Work Study Program, Pennsylvania Higher Education Assistance Agency Grant, and Federal Stafford Loan.

APPLYING
Admission to the nursing program is selective. Students must fulfill all College admissions requirements. All nursing applicants must hold a high school diploma or a GED and have successfully completed one year of high school biology and chemistry and two years of college preparatory high school mathematics within the past ten years with grade of C or better. Equivalent college level courses are acceptable. Students attending the College must have a grade point average of 2.5 or higher to apply to the nursing program. All applicants are required to take the allied health and placement tests offered at the College. Some applicants will be required to attend a non-credit summer workshop prior to admission. Factors considered in admission are allied health test scores and previous academic work. Admission is conditional pending evaluation of the applicant's criminal background check to determine whether there is any conviction or crimes of moral turpitude that may bar the student from the program. Licensed practical nurses, corpsmen, and candidates with one year of successful previous nursing school may apply for advanced placement through credit by examination.

FOR INFORMATION
Community College of Philadelphia
Admissions Office
1700 Spring Garden Street
Philadelphia, PA 19130
(215) 751-8010
Web: www.ccp.cc.pa.us

CONCORDIA UNIVERSITY WISCONSIN
Nursing Division
Mequon, Wisconsin

THE UNIVERSITY

Concordia University was founded in 1881 as a school of The Lutheran Church Missouri Synod and officially became a university on August 27, 1989.

Concordia is one of twelve colleges and seminaries maintained by The Lutheran Church-Missouri Synod. In addition to its traditional focus on teacher-training (teacher supply for Lutheran parochial schools, lay ministry/pre-seminary education), innovative programs in the liberal arts, business, nursing, and adult education have been added. A Master's program was established in 1988.

NURSING DIVISION

Concordia University Wisconsin has offered a baccalaureate degree in nursing since 1982. The National League for Nursing made its initial visit to Concordia and granted NLN accreditation to the nursing program in 1988.

Accreditation was granted in 1996 for eight years. The Bachelor of Science in Nursing track for registered nurses was developed and in May of 1991, the first RN-to-BSN completion students graduated; the first LPN to graduate as a graduate nurse was in the summer of 1995. In the Fall of 1995, Concordia began a Master of Science in Nursing (MSN) degree program. The MSN program graduated its first class in May, 1998, and is accredited by the NLNAC.

The BSN completion track, the LPN-to-RN track, and the traditional generic track of nursing are rooted in the same philosophy. The conceptual framework that is utilized is the Betty Neuman Systems Model. The delivery of the courses differ in that the BSN completion program was designed for the adult learner. Modular courses are delivered over 3 to 7 weeks time during the day and evening hours to facilitate the working adult. The delivery of the traditional course content is typically over a semester's length.

PROGRAMS OF STUDY

The curriculum in nursing prepares individuals for beginning a practice of professional nursing and is built around the core curriculum/ supplemental courses that facilitate the development of a professional nurse. Students will have an opportunity to gain a basis of knowledge from the liberal arts curriculum. The traditional student's nursing experience begins with on-campus instruction in both the classroom and nursing laboratory. The first learning experience with patients begins in the sophomore year. Throughout the program, students are introduced to nursing experiences in both hospitals and community agencies. In their senior year, a nursing student can take a Global Education class during Concordia's Winterim and experience life in another country. During the past 3 Winterims, our students spent 7 days in Costa Rica. Upon graduation, the students are eligible to take the NCLEX-RN exam administered by the State Board of Nursing.

The RN seeking a baccalaureate degree is offered a curriculum focusing on the liberal arts and nursing. Classes are offered emphasizing adult education principles with flexible scheduling in the late afternoons, evenings, and some optional weekends.

The Parish Nurse is the visible symbol of a congregation's pursuit of wellness, which is our faith response to Jesus Christ, driven by the Holy Spirit. This holistic health program is based on the belief that health is growth towards well-being of body, soul, mind, and relationships. The Parish Nurse is available to all age levels of the congregation and becomes part of the ministry team, which also includes the pastor and members of the congregation.

The MSN program is designed for nurses seeking preparation for advanced practice nursing as nurse practitioners, or gerontological family nurse practitioners, as well as a Nurse Educator Program. Nurses from all nationally accredited basic nursing programs are eligible to apply. Both an on-campus and a long distance (50 miles or more away from CUW) course of study are available. The first class graduated in May, 1998. This program's five-year accreditation has been granted.

The program's biggest plus is its emphasis on a Christian response in nursing and a respect for human life. The professional faculty provides individualized attention and emphasizes "Excellence in Christian Education."

ACADEMIC FACILITIES

Clinicals are held in neighboring hospitals and health care facilities. Computer literacy is a must on the Concordia Campus. The new Health Sciences building features state-of-the-art labs for Physical/Occupational Therapy and offices.

LOCATION

Concordia is located just 15 minutes from Milwaukee, which is a modern commercial center with an old European flavor. This metropolitan area of more than 1.5 million people supports an interesting variety of art and culture. Students may choose the world-renowned Milwaukee Symphony, The Great Circus Parade, Ballet, or repertory theater. Art lovers can visit the Milwaukee Art Museum.

COSTS

All students have the initial application fee and tuition deposit of $25 and $100 respectively. Educational fees per semester are $7,795 with room and board at $2,965. Costs for BSN, MSN, LPN, and Parish Nurse Programs vary depending upon where a student is credit-wise in our program based on previous transcripts. Average cost per credit is $300 for BSN Completion and $400 for the Master's Program.

FINANCIAL AID

The amount of financial aid awarded is based mainly on the applicant's financial need. As a general rule, the primary financial responsibility lies with the student and parents. Therefore, in order to help determine student need and make it possible to grant aid fairly, the parents of aid applicants are asked to file a confidential statement of their income, assets, expenses and liabilities. On the basis of this financial information, the University is able to determine the difference between University costs and the amount a student and parents can reasonably be expected to provide. This difference is

CONCORDIA UNIVERSITY WISCONSIN
(continued)

defined as need. If a student is self supporting and not dependent on parents, the student would submit a financial statement without parental information. There are various loans, grants, and scholarships available, as well as veterans educational assistance.

APPLYING

Students must submit evidence of adequate preparation for college from a regionally accredited high school. A minimum of 16 units of secondary school work is required, of which at least 11 should be in basic liberal arts areas. A minimum entrance grade point average of 2.5 is required. When entering other than the traditional program, transcripts from previous colleges/universities attended are required.

CORRESPONDENCE AND INFORMATION

Nursing Division
Concordia University Wisconsin
12800 N. Lake Shore Dr.
Mequon, WI 53097
(262) 243-4374
Fax: (262) 243-4466
E-Mail: grace_peterson@cuw.edu

CONNECTICUT COMMUNITY COLLEGES

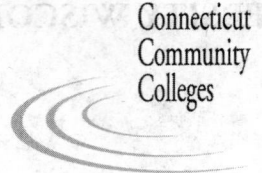

Connecticut
Community
Colleges

THE COLLEGES

The Community Colleges of Connecticut—twelve, public two-year colleges with open admissions—offer associate degree and certificate programs in over 100 career-related areas. Many of these programs are related to the health professions, including Nursing. Five of the colleges—Capital in Hartford, Gateway in New Haven, Housatonic in Bridgeport, Naugatuck Valley in Waterbury, Norwalk in Norwalk, and Three Rivers in Norwich—offer associate degrees in Nursing. The curriculum described below is typical of each program's requirements and was prepared to inform students considering a career as a nurse about the employment opportunities available for well qualified candidates. For more specific information about the program or prerequisites for enrollment please contact each college directly at the numbers listed.

PROGRAM

Graduates of the Associate Degree Registered Nurse program are eligible to sit for the National Council Licensing Examination for Registered Nurses (NCLEX-RN). Graduates are eligible for employment in a variety of health care facilities/agencies, where they function as contributing members of the health team by using the nursing process to meet psychosocial, safety, and physiological needs of family members from diverse cultural groups. Critical thinking and problem-solving skills are utilized to maximize the individual's potential for wellness.

TYPICAL COURSES TO BE STUDIED AT A CONNECTICUT COMMUNITY COLLEGE
(Example from Naugatuck Valley Community College)

General Education Courses	College Credits
Anatomy & Physiology I and Anatomy & Physiology II	8
Microbiology	4
English Composition	3
General Psychology and Developmental Psychology	6
General Sociology	3
Microcomputer as a Productivity Tool	3
Arts & Humanities Course or Social Science Course (Elective)	3

Specialized Program Courses	
Fundamentals of Nursing	6
Concepts of Family Care	6
Physical & Emotional Illness I, II, III, and IV	26
Clinical practice (2 days per week)	

Total College credits	68

SKILLS FOR YOUR JOB

Upon graduation, you will have required job skills. You should be able to:

- Integrate the principles of the physical, biological, and behavioral sciences and nursing theory to provide holistic nursing care to individuals, families, and groups
- Utilize the nursing process to promote the adaptation of individuals, families, and groups toward the achievement of optimal wellness
- Function as a member of an interdisciplinary health team

CONTACT INFORMATION

Call Capital at (860) 520-7835; Gateway at (203) 285-2390; Housatonic at (203) 332-5105, Naugatuck Valley at (203) 575-8057, Norwalk at (203) 857-7060, or Three Rivers at (860) 383-5241. Visit www.commnet.edu for more information about the Community Colleges of Connecticut.

COVENANT SCHOOL OF NURSING
Covenant Health System
Lubbock, Texas

THE SCHOOL
Covenant School of Nursing, founded in 1918, is a hospital-based diploma program that prepares the student for licensure as a Registered Nurse (RN). It is the oldest school of professional nursing on the South Plains and has graduated over 3,000 students. As a member of Covenant Health System, which is a ministry of St. Mary Hospital and Lubbock Methodist Hospital System, Covenant School of Nursing offers exceptional learning opportunities for students. Comprising 6,600 people system-wide, Covenant Health System employees over 4,000 in Lubbock alone, which is a city of approximately 200,000 residents. In addition to three Lubbock hospitals that are licensed for 1,338 beds, the system includes a regional network in Texas and eastern New Mexico of 25 regional hospitals, 55 neighborhood centers, about 250 physicians, 16 home health locations, an air ambulance helicopter service, a school of radiology, and the school of nursing.

PROGRAM OF STUDY
Covenant School of Nursing accepts new students, transfer students, and Licensed Vocational Nurses (LVN)/Licensed Practical Nurses (LPN) who desire to complete the registered nursing program. Nine specific academic pre-requisite courses must be completed before beginning the nursing curriculum. These college courses include the following: Freshman English (2 semesters or one freshman English plus Speech Communications), Chemistry with lab, Human Anatomy & Physiology with lab (2 semesters), Microbiology with lab, Introduction to Psychology, Lifespan Human Growth and Development, and Nutrition. Mathematics is required if pre-entrance testing indicates the need.

NURSING CURRICULUM
The nursing curriculum consists of 80 weeks of lectures, laboratory, and clinical experiences. The first 40 weeks (two 20-week semesters) cover topics in Medical-Surgical Nursing, Pathophysiology, and Pharmacology. The second 40 weeks include specialty courses in Pediatric Nursing, Critical Care Nursing, Maternal-Newborn Nursing, Nursing Leadership and Management, Perioperative Nursing, and Psychiatric/Mental Health Nursing.

ADVANCED CREDIT PROGRAM
A shorter program available for LVNs/LPNs includes a 100-clock hour Transition Course followed by the 40 weeks of specialty nursing courses. The Transition Course is offered twice annually, for eight weeks beginning in June, and during a long 20-week semester that begins the first Monday of August.

ADMISSION DATES
New classes begin on the first Monday of August and the first Monday after January 1.

COST OF PROGRAM
Tuition and fees are $5,000 for the 80-week program and $3,000 for the Advanced Credit Program, which includes the cost of required textbooks and uniforms. (A tuition increase is anticipated effective August 4, 2003.)   Additional costs include the application fee, pre-entrance test fee, graduation fee, testing fees, and state licensing exam fee.

FINANCIAL AID
Covenant School of Nursing participates in the Federal Pell Grant, Federal Supplemental Education Opportunity Grant (FSEOG), Federal Stafford and Federal PLUS loan programs. Additional information and assistance is available through the Financial Aid Office. Covenant Health System offers a contract-based financial assistance program called Health Traxx. For information about Health Traxx, call 806-725-6673.

APPLYING
The Covenant School of Nursing Application Packet provides detailed information regarding admission requirements and application procedures.

APPLICATION REQUIREMENTS
1. High school graduation or completion of General Education Development (GED)
2. Completion of nine specific college pre-requisite courses (with grades of "C" or higher)
3. Informational interview
4. Pre-entrance testing
5. Letters of recommendation

In addition to the above requirements, Advanced Credit Students must meet the following guidelines:
6. Current licensure as an LVN/LPN
7. Graduation from an approved LVN/LPN School of Nursing
8. Completion of one year of LVN/LPN experience, routinely performing basic nursing skills, within the last 3 to 5 years. This requirement is waived if the LVN/LPN graduated from an LVN/LPN program within two years of the start date at Covenant School of Nursing.

APPLICATION PROCESS
1. Submit Application Form, biography, high school transcript or GED certificate, college transcript(s), and application fee
2. Interview with Nursing Careers Counselor
3. Take pre-entrance test
4. Submit letters of recommendation
5. Complete nine pre-requisite college courses
6. Apply for financial aid, if applicable
7. Complete medical requirements and CPR course

APPLICATION DEADLINES
1. February 15 for classes beginning in August. Late applications accepted until April 15 with applicable late fee.
2. September 1 for classes beginning in January.

CORRESPONDENCE AND INFORMATION
Covenant School of Nursing
2002 Miami Avenue
Lubbock, TX 79410-1096
(806) 797-0955
(800) 787-6421
E-Mail: admissionscsn@covhs.org
Web: www.covenantson.com

DELAWARE COUNTY COMMUNITY COLLEGE
College of Nursing
Media, PA

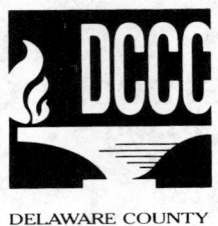

DELAWARE COUNTY
COMMUNITY COLLEGE

ABOUT DELAWARE COUNTY COMMUNITY COLLEGE

Delaware County Community College, the ninth largest college in the Philadelphia metropolitan area, is a public, accredited two-year institution offering more than 60 programs of study. Established in 1967, DCCC has nearly 10,000 students on its wooded, 123-acre main campus and a number of satellite centers in Delaware and Chester counties.

Our competency-based curriculum, rooted in functional skills development, is the basis of our reputation for high-quality education. State-of-the-art information technology is emphasized both in academic programs and the classrooms and labs that house them. DCCC provides a supportive environment focused on students' needs. Our average class size of 24 provides a personal, small-school atmosphere where faculty and staff get to know students by name. Committed to teaching, our award-winning faculty takes our students' success seriously.

University-parallel programs are designed to satisfy the requirements for transfer to a four-year college or university.

THE COLLEGE OF NURSING

The College of Nursing is located on the main campus in Marple Township and was founded in 1968. The College of Nursing awards an Associate in Applied Science degree in nursing. The NLNAC-approved curriculum prepares students for beginning staff positions in health care agencies.

ABOUT THE NURSING PROGRAM

The nursing curriculum prepares students for positions as beginning staff nurses in a variety of settings—acute- and long-term/transitional care facilities and community settings.

Upon successful completion of the curriculum, students receive an associate in applied science (AAS) degree and are eligible to sit for the state licensure examination to become registered nurses (NCLEX-RN).

Most nursing students attend classes at the College and off-campus sites. For residents of Chester County, two sections are available with some classes at The Chester County Hospital.

Selected clinical laboratory learning experiences, under the direct guidance of nursing faculty or clinical preceptors, are provided at a variety of health care agencies. The purpose of these experiences is to provide the student with the opportunity to apply classroom learning in direct patient-care situations.

All nursing applicants are required to submit a "Criminal History Record Information Report" and child abuse clearance. Students who have been convicted of a prohibitive offense contained in Act 13

and/or Act 169 (detailed list available for review in the Admissions and Allied Health offices) may not be able to complete their studies because clinical experiences needed for course/program success may be prohibited. If a student cannot complete their clinical studies, they will not be accepted into the nursing program.

The nursing program is accredited by the National League for Nursing Accrediting Commission, 61 Broadway, New York, NY 10006, 212-363-5555, www.nlnac.org. It is also approved by the Pennsylvania State Board of Nurse Examiners, P.O. Box 2649, Harrisburg, PA 17105-2649, 717-783-7142, www.dos.state.pa.us.

SPECIAL OPTIONS AVAILABLE

1. Licensed Practical Nurses, corpsmen, and candidates who have had one year of successful previous nursing school experience may apply for advanced placement in the curriculum through the Assessment Center.
2. A five-semester evening/weekend option is available. Course sequencing begins in January. Criteria for admission and progression are the same as for the generic curricula.

FINANCIAL AID

Financial aid is available and is based on need.

COSTS

Delaware County residents pay $65 per credit hour, non-residents of Delaware County pay $130 per credit hour, out-of-state students pay $195 per credit hour, and international students pay $238 per credit hour.

APPLICATION PROCESS

Call the DCCC Admissions Office for an application at (610) 359-5050.

CORRESPONDENCE INFORMATION

Director of Admissions
College of Nursing
Delaware County Community College
901 South Media Line Road
Media, PA 19063-1094
(610) 359-5050
Fax: (610) 359-5343
Web: www.dccc.edu

DUKE UNIVERSITY
School of Nursing
Durham, North Carolina

THE UNIVERSITY
Since its founding in 1839 as the Union Institute, and later as Trinity College before incorporating in 1924, the basic principles of Duke University have remained constant. Duke University seeks to engage the mind, elevate the spirit, and stimulate the best effort of all who are associated with the University; to contribute in diverse ways to the local community, the state, the nation, and the world; and to attain and maintain a place of real leadership in all that we do. Today, Duke University enrolls more than 12,000 students, of whom 5,250 are enrolled in the graduate and professional programs and represent nearly every state and many countries.

The School of Medicine, School of Nursing, and Duke Hospital and Health Network are the core institutions of Duke University Health System, which ranks among the outstanding healthcare providers of the world. The opening of Duke Hospital North in 1980 made Duke Hospital, with over 1,000 inpatient beds, one of the most modern patient-care facilities available anywhere. The mission of the Health System is to be a leader in world health care. This involves maintaining superiority in its four primary functions: excellent patient care, dedication to educational programs, national and international distinction in the quality of research, and service to the region.

THE SCHOOL OF NURSING
Since the funding of the School in 1930, Duke has prepared outstanding clinicians, educators, and researchers. Drawing on the intellectual and clinical resources of both Duke University Health System and Duke University, the School offers an Accelerated Bachelor of Science in Nursing degree program, a Master of Science in Nursing degree program and a Post-master's Certificate that balance education, practice, and research.

PROGRAMS OF STUDY
The School of Nursing offers a 58-credit-hour, full-time, Accelerated Bachelor of Science in Nursing (BSN) degree program in a sixteen-month, intensive format.

A Master of Science in Nursing (MSN) degree and Post-master's Certificate are offered in the following areas of study:

Nurse Practitioner:
Adult Acute Care, Adult Cardiovascular, Adult Oncology/HIV, Adult Primary Care, Family, Gerontology, Neonatal, Pediatric, Pediatric Acute/Chronic Care, Combined Neonatal/Pediatric in Rural Health.

Clinical Nurse Specialist:
Adult Critical Care, Adult Cardiovascular, Gerontology, Neonatal, Pediatric and Pediatric Acute/Chronic Care.

Also offered are Nurse Anesthesia, Health and Nursing Ministries, Leadership in Community-based Long-term Care and an MSN MBA Program. Online programs include: Clinical Research Management, Nursing Informatics, Nursing Education, Nursing and Healthcare Leadership, Family Nurse Practitioner, and Gerontological Nurse Practitioner. The graduate curriculum is designed to provide maximum flexibility and most programs offer both full-time and part-time study.

AFFILIATIONS WITH HEALTHCARE FACILITIES
As one of the word's leading academic health systems, Duke University Health System has assembled and integrated a comprehensive range of health care, health education, and clinical research facilities. The clinical faculty members of the Duke University School of Nursing number more than 100 and represent all specialties.

Cooperative teaching and clinical facilities, including health departments, retirement centers, and private practices in both urban and rural settings, are available to students mostly within the state of North Carolina. Occasionally, placements are arranged out-of-state or in other countries to accommodate student needs.

LOCATION
Durham, a city of 218,000, is about 250 miles south of Washington, DC. Durham, and nearby Raleigh and Chapel Hill, constitute the three points of the Research triangle, one of the nation's foremost centers of research-oriented industries and government, research, and regulatory agencies.

THE NURSING STUDENT GROUP
Approximately 90 students are enrolled in the Accelerated BSN program, and 300 students are enrolled in the graduate programs. Of these, about 11% are men and 16% are members of minority groups.

COSTS
Tuition for 2003–2004 was $672 per credit hour for graduate nursing courses and $520 per credit hour for undergraduate nursing courses.

FINANCIAL AID
Merit and need-based scholarships traineeships, and federal/state loan programs are generally available. Approximately 80 percent of School of Nursing students receive some form of financial aid.

APPLYING
Admission requirements for the Accelerated BSN program include a bachelor's degree from an accredited college of university, a minimum 3.0/4.0 GPA, three letters of recommendation, GRE or MAT scores, and completion of prerequisite coursework. Admission requirements for the graduate programs include a BSN degree from an NLNAC- or CCNE-accredited program, an introductory course in descri8ptive and inferential statistics, GRE or MAT scores, three letters of recommendation, and licensure as a registered nurse in North Carolina. Exceptions to any of the above qualifications are considered on an individual basis.

INFORMATION
Office of Admissions and Student Services
Duke University School of Nursing
Box 3322 Medical Center
Durham, North Carolina 27710
Telephone: (919) 684-4248 or (877) 415-3853 (toll-free)
Fax: (919) 681-8899
E-Mail: SONAdmissions@mc.duke.edu
Web: http://www.nursing.duke.edu

DUQUESNE UNIVERSITY
Pittsburgh, Pennsylvania

THE UNIVERSITY
Duquesne University, located in Pittsburgh in southwestern Pennsylvania, is a private coeducational Catholic University that enrolls more than 10,000 students. Named one of the top ten national Catholic universities in the United States, Duquesne has been called one of the "best buys" in higher education.

Complemented by a variety of non-academic activities and programs, the curriculum is designed to prepare men and women with a broad, well-balanced, and fully integrated education.

UNIQUE CHARACTERISTICS
The School of Nursing offers innovative online programs at both the undergraduate and graduate level. The School of Nursing has been a pioneer in using distance education. We currently have students from around the world enrolled in our online programs.

The School of Nursing supports a Center for International Nursing that offers a transcultural perspective on health care in other countries through student/faculty exchanges, practical hands-on experience, and collaborative international research.

Faculty members operate two Nurse-Managed Wellness Centers that focus on health promotion and management of chronic illness. The Centers also offer valuable clinical learning opportunities for students.

The mission of the Center for Health Care Diversity is to address issues of equity and diversity in order to meet the health care needs of minority populations through community-focused research, education and training of nurses, health policy development, and community service.

PROGRAMS OF STUDY
The 4-year undergraduate program (126 credits) leads to the Bachelor of Science in Nursing (BSN) degree. Students are introduced to the nursing profession at the freshman level and begin clinical experience with clients and families during the sophomore year. The nursing curriculum provides students with a strong foundation in the natural, biological, and behavioral sciences, most of which are taken the first two years and include the University core curriculum. World-class medical centers, as well as community sites, are used for student clinical experiences. Faculty members teach all professional courses and direct the clinical learning experiences. Minors are available in business, psychology, sociology, Spanish, and communications. A focus area in music therapy is also offered, as is a business certificate.

The Second Degree – BSN Option is designed for college graduates who hold a bachelor's degree in another field of study and desire to pursue nursing as a second degree. The BSN can be completed in 12 months after the prerequisite courses are met. Upon completion of the BSN, students who have maintained a 3.0 GPA can begin MSN coursework.

The RN-BSN/MSN Option offers online-only courses for registered nurses pursuing the BSN and MSN degrees in nursing. Students will complete 17 credits of graduate coursework while earning the BSN degree. The MSN program can be completed as a part-time student in an additional 2 years.

Students who wish to transfer to Duquesne from another college or university are considered on an individual basis.

The Master of Science in Nursing (MSN) program is consistent with the School's belief that specialization in nursing occurs at the graduate level. All courses for the MSN degree are available only online.

The three MSN tracks are:
MSN with Nursing Education specialization (41-43 credits)
MSN with Nursing Administration specialization (42 credits)
   The four Options are:
    MSN/MBA (73 credits)
    MSN with Basic Business Certificate (47-48 credits)
    MSN with Advanced Business Certificate (51-52 credits)
    MSN with Forensic Nursing specialization (36 credits)
MSN with Family Nurse Practitioner specialization (46 credits)

The Post-Master's Certificates are offered online as a way for nurses to learn specific skills that may not have been offered in their graduate programs and are designed to prepare nurses for certification through the professional organizations.

The Post-Master's Certificates are:
    Nursing Administration (15 credits)
    Nursing Education (12-16 credits)
    Family Nurse Practitioner (34 credits)
    Psychiatric-Mental Health (21 credits)
    Transcultural Nursing (12 credits)
    Forensic Nursing (19 credits)

The Doctor of Philosophy in Nursing (PhD) degree (57 credits) is designed to provide core content in nursing theory development and research, and practical experience in a functional role, clinical specialty, or research activity. The doctoral degree is offered only online.

TUITION AND FINANCIAL AID
Costs for the 2003-2004 academic year:
Undergraduate full-time tuition and fees (12-18 credits) = $19,425.
Undergraduate full-time tuition, fees, room & board = $26,907.
Undergraduate tuition and fees per credit (part-time) = $642.
Graduate tuition and fees per credit (full or part-time) = $688.

University awards, grants, and scholarships are available to undergraduate students of the School of Nursing. Additional financial aid resources include federal and state scholarships, grants, and loans. Undergraduate students should contact the University's Financial Aid Office for additional information.

CONTACT INFORMATION
Duquesne University School of Nursing
600 Forbes Avenue
Pittsburgh, PA 15282
(412) 396-6550
Fax: 412-396-6346
E-Mail: nursing@duq.edu
Web: http://www.nursing.duq.edu

D'YOUVILLE COLLEGE
Department of Nursing
Buffalo, New York

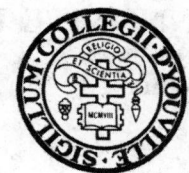

THE COLLEGE

D'Youville College is a private, coeducational, liberal arts and professional college that has offered students an education of high quality since 1908. The College was the first in Western New York to offer baccalaureate degrees to women. Its current enrollment is 1,900 men and women. Students may choose from thirty undergraduate and graduate degree programs that are enhanced by a 14:1 student-faculty ratio. The College is committed to helping its students to grow not only in academics but in the social and personal areas of their college experience as well.

PROGRAMS OF STUDY

The multiple-option Nursing Degree Program is one of the largest four-year private-college nursing programs in the country. Programs offered in the Department of Nursing include: four year Bachelor of Science in Nursing program preparing for the NCLEX professional nursing licensing examination; Bachelor of Science in Nursing completion program for registered nurses; combined Bachelor of Science and Master of Science in Community Health Nursing for new students or registered nurses; Master of Science Family Nurse Practitioner program; Master of Science in Nursing; Master of Science Clinical Nurse Specialist in Community Health Nursing with preparation in management, teaching, or community addictions nursing for nurses, and Certificate Programs in Addictions in the Community and Long Term Care Administration. All the programs are approved by the State Education Department and accredited by the National League for Nursing Accrediting Commission. Clinical affiliations are conducted with a majority of the health care institutions in Western New York.

NEW BACHELOR OF SCIENCE IN NURSING

This is a four year Bachelor of Science in Nursing program preparing for the NCLEX professional nursing licensing examination. The curriculum emphasizes knowledge and skills needed for the 21st century: interdisciplinary introduction to the health system course in the first semester; business and management preparation with 6 credits of undergraduate management courses; collaboration and partnerships with clients, healthcare professionals, and agencies; and a community-based emphasis. Clinical nursing courses start in the second year while students are completing the science prerequisite courses and liberal arts courses. The strong clinical preparation is acquired through 1,320 clinical hours. Multiple options are available to link with our other graduate nursing programs.

RN-BSN PROGRAM

A 2-year (5-semester) program may be completed in 69 credits. Up to 65 credits with grades of C or better may be transferred in from associate degree programs. There is a 50% tuition waiver for the first 135 credits, inclusive of credits transferred in. Classes are offered on one or two day a week schedules, when possible, to meet the needs of RNs with work commitments.

BACHELOR OF SCIENCE/MASTER OF SCIENCE IN NURSING (5 YEARS)

This program combines a BSN/MS in Nursing with a choice of clinical specialization at the master's level. No other school in Western New York or Southern Ontario offers such a comprehensive educational program. This community-based nursing program is designed for high school students, college transfers, career changers, or associate degree RNs. It provides an MS degree in a short period of time, which offers greater potential for advancement and employment.

COSTS

2002–2003: Undergraduate tuition was $6,560 per semester and room and board cost $3,280 per semester. Graduate tuition was $405 per credit hour.

FINANCIAL AID

D'Youville offers institutionally-sponsored non-need grants/scholarships, Federal Nursing Student Loans, Federal Pell Grants, Federal Perkins Loans, Federal Supplemental Educational Opportunity Grants, Federal Work-Study, Federal PLUS loans, Federal Stafford Loans, and state aid.

New instant scholarships worth up to $41,000 also are available. For example, the Honors scholarship gives a student with 1100 SAT or 24 ACT 50% off tuition and 25% off total room and board.

APPLYING

Undergraduate: D'Youville admits students on a rolling admission basis; therefore, applications are reviewed as they are received by the Admissions Office.

BSN program: The SAT or ACT and TOEFL are required for non-native speakers of English, with minimum 900 SAT, 80% high school average, upper 1/2 of class, and transfer minimum GPA 2.5. Three years of high school science (including biology and chemistry) and two years of math are required. RN program: An RN license, associate degree, or Canadian diploma.

MS program: A Baccalaureate degree in Nursing from an NLNAC-accredited undergraduate program, valid state or provincial license, cumulative undergraduate GPA 3.0 or better in the upper half of undergraduate work, interview with the program director, a physical assessment course, statistics course, and computer science course. For enrollment in the Nurse Practitioner program, one year of clinical practice as an RN and references of clinical performance are required.

CORRESPONDENCE AND INFORMATION

D'Youville Office and Admission
Undergraduate or Graduate Nursing Program
320 Porter Ave.
Buffalo, New York 14201
(716) 881-7600
(800) 777-3921
Fax: (716) 515-0679
Web: www. dyc.edu

EASTERN MENNONITE UNIVERSITY
Nursing Department
Harrisonburg, Virginia

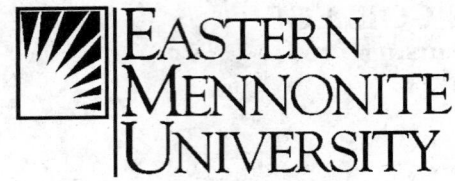

THE UNIVERSITY
Eastern Mennonite University is a religious private liberal arts college in the beautiful Shenandoah Valley of Virginia. EMU seeks to glorify God and serve students, the community of learning, the community of faith, and the world by becoming a university of distinction. The Shenandoah Valley offers advantages of rural life with metropolitan areas, such as Washington, DC, close by. Harrisonburg, one of the most rapidly growing cities in Virginia, has two universities in the city, and another college is located nearby. Shenandoah National Park and other forests are easily accessible.

WHAT NURSING GRADUATES SAY ABOUT EMU
"The main reason I wanted to come to EMU was its faculty. They have a strong relationship with students. I like the fact that the faculty members allow us to be on a first-name basis. It makes the university setting more family oriented. I feel that I can turn to many of my faculty members if I have a problem and they will always be there to listen and try to give support."

"One of the things I love most about a small school, such as EMU, is that the professors know each student on a personal basis, including strengths and weaknesses, and strive to guide the student based on their knowledge of them. I feel that the professors know and respect each student as an individual, and are constantly changing things around to suit the needs of students! I feel that I have a close relationship with my professors, and I noticed they were every bit as excited for me when I received a job as my own friends and family members."

THE NURSING DEPARTMENT
EMU's small nursing program is a mastery-based program that affords students the opportunity to develop a more personalized educational program.
   EMU's nursing program is a flexible nursing program that offers the following tracts:
Bachelor of Science in Nursing
Bachelor of Science in Nursing (RN-BS in day or evening programs)
Accelerated LPN-to-BS
Second Degree Students (BS in Nursing)

AFFILIATIONS WITH HEALTH CARE FACILITIES
The Nursing Department maintains contractual relationships with over 20 agencies including community agencies (schools, public health departments), community hospitals, a psychiatric hospital, and a medical center.

COSTS
Annual full-time tuition/fees: $16,370
Annual room and board: $ 5,350

FINANCIAL AID
EMU uses the Free Application for Federal Student Aid (FAFSA) to determine financial need. Discounts, grants (include Virginia Tuition Assistance Grant, Pennsylvania Higher Education Assistance Authority and others), scholarships, employment opportunities, and loans are among the types of aid available.

FOR ADDITIONAL INFORMATION AND ADMISSION APPLICATION
Director of Admissions
Eastern Mennonite University
Harrisonburg, VA 22802-2462
(800) 368-2665
E-Mail: admiss@emu.edu
Web: www.emu.edu

ELMIRA COLLEGE
Program in Nursing Education
Elmira, New York

THE COLLEGE
Elmira College, founded in 1855, is a selective, private, coeducational college emphasizing quality education in the liberal arts and sciences, nursing, business, and education, located in the beautiful Finger Lakes Region of New York. An enrollment of 1,200, from 35 states and 23 countries, an average class size of 16, and an outstanding faculty combine to provide students with exceptional academic opportunities. Over 80 extracurricular activities, a strong NCAA Division III athletic program, and an unusual emphasis on traditions are all features of Elmira College, and provide an outstanding college experience for its students.

THE PROGRAM IN NURSING EDUCATION
The four-year program of study leads to a baccalaureate degree for the generic student. The program reflects the liberal arts and community orientation of the College. The curriculum provides for the development of nursing knowledge and skills appropriate for practice in a variety of healthcare settings and as the necessary foundation for graduate study in nursing. Advanced placement options are available for Registered Nurses and Licensed Practical Nurses seeking a baccalaureate degree.

DISTINCTIVE FEATURES
- Acceptance into the College ensures acceptance into the Nurse Education Program
- Total integration of students into the College's wide range of activities
- Nursing courses and clinical experiences begin in the sophomore year
- Individualized mentoring by nursing faculty
  - Low student/faculty ratio
  - Small classes and clinical laboratory groups
- Clinical experiences
  - Concentrated clinical experiences in the College's unique Term III
  - In all major clinical areas—medical/surgical, pediatric, orthopedic, obstetrical, psychiatric, community health, home care, rehabilitation
  - 6 week senior capstone internship that provides opportunities to hone clinical skills and serves as a bridge to graduate employment
- Sites for clinical experiences close to the College
- Sites for clinical experiences include
  - State-of-the-art maternity unit that serves a 16-county area for high-risk pregnancy
  - Neonatal Intensive Care Unit
  - Regional rehabilitation center
  - State Psychiatric/Mental Health Hospital with unique children and youth unit
- Provides the framework for education to assume advanced practice roles, such as nurse anesthetist, midwife, and educator
- Advanced placement option for RNs who wish to complete a baccalaureate degree
- No deadline for applications
- Full- and part-time study options

ACADEMIC FACILITIES
- Fully automated campus library with access to world wide resources; recipient of New York State Recognition as an "electronic doorway" library
- Campus nursing learning lab with video tutorials, computer programs, and self-directed learning packets

NURSING ACTIVITIES AVAILABLE
- Active Nursing Club
- Sigma Theta Tau International Honor Society of Nursing Chapter

COSTS
Tuition: $23,990 (academic year 2002–2003). Full-time mandatory fees: $580. Room and board: $7,850. Application fee: $40. Books and supplies: $1,000.

FINANCIAL AID
Institutionally sponsored long-term loans, institutionally sponsored need-based grants/scholarships, Federal Pell Grants, Federal Perkins Loans, Federal Supplemental Educational Opportunity Grants, Federal Work-Study, Federal PLUS Loans, Federal Stafford Loans, and Academic Honors Scholarships are available.
80% of undergraduate nursing students received some form of financial aid in the 2002–2003 academic year.

BACCALAUREATE PROGRAM
Applying required. SAT I or ACT, TCEFL for nonnative speakers of English, letters of recommendation, written essay, high school transcript, and interview recommended.
   Options: Advanced standing available through the following means: Advanced placement exams, credit by exam. Coursework may be accelerated. Students may apply for transfer of up to 90 total credits.
   Application Fee: $40
   Degree Requirements: 120 total credit hours, 44 in nursing.

TO APPLY
Mr. William Neal
Dean of Admissions
(607) 735-1724
E-Mail: admissions@elmira.edu or www.elmira.edu

Or for information contact:
Dr. Lois Schoener
Director Nurse Education
(607) 735-1890
E-Mail: nursing@elmira.edu

EMORY UNIVERSITY
Nell Hodgson Woodruff School of Nursing
Atlanta, Georgia

NELL HODGSON
WOODRUFF
SCHOOL OF
NURSING

THE UNIVERSITY

Emory University, founded by the Methodist Church in 1836, has 11,300 students and 2,500 faculty members who represent all regions of the United States and some 90 foreign nations. Emory has nine academic divisions, numerous centers for advanced study, and a host of prestigious affiliated institutions. The University has a two-year and four-year undergraduate college; a graduate school of arts and sciences; and professional schools of medicine, theology, law, nursing, public health, and business. Located just six miles northeast of downtown Atlanta, Emory University is a top-tier institution in a world-class city.

NELL HODGSON WOODRUFF SCHOOL OF NURSING

The Nell Hodgson Woodruff School of Nursing is part of the Robert W. Woodruff Health Sciences Center. The School offers undergraduate, graduate, and doctoral nursing education to nearly 300 students. The mission of the Nell Hodgson Woodruff School of Nursing is to demonstrate excellence in research, teaching, and practice based on independent scholarship and collaborative interdisciplinary partnerships with university and health care colleagues.

PROGRAMS OF STUDY

Bachelor of Science in Nursing

The first two years of required prerequisite coursework may be taken at Emory College, Oxford College, or any accredited university or liberal arts college. During the second year of prerequisite coursework, students apply for admission to the Nell Hodgson Woodruff School of Nursing. Qualified students are then admitted for the remaining two years of professional study, enrolling in clinical nursing courses and support courses.

MSN, RN-BSN Completion, RN-MSN Bridge, MSN-MPH, Post-Master's

Programs of study leading to the Master of Science in Nursing include the following specialties: acute/critical care, adult medical-surgical, adult immunology/oncology, family nurse-midwife, family nurse practitioner, gerontology, international health nursing, leadership in health care, leadership in public-health nursing, nurse-midwifery, pediatrics, women's health nurse practitioner, and women's health for graduates of Title X programs. Length of the specialty programs ranges from three semesters (one calendar year) to five consecutive semesters of full-time study. Part-time study is available. Minors in teaching and management are available. The RN/MSN bridge program provides an opportunity for associate degree or diploma prepared nurses to obtain the MSN. Also, an MSN/MPH dual degree is available in conjunction with Emory's Rollins School of Public Health. Post-Master's options are available in all graduate specialty areas.

PhD Program

A PhD in nursing focusing on health outcomes, ethics, and health policy is offered. The program is a four-year, full-time program. Students accepted to the program receive an annual stipend plus financial support to cover tuition for a maximum of four years.

AFFILIATIONS WITH HEALTHCARE FACILITIES

As part of The Robert W. Woodruff Health Sciences Center, the School of Nursing maintains close ties with the Centers for Disease Control and Prevention (CDC), the Carter Center, and the American Cancer Society. The School of Nursing at Emory is also the home of the Lillian Carter Center for International Nursing.

ACADEMIC FACILITIES

In January 2001, the School of Nursing opened a state-of-the-art facility for nursing study and research. Designed with tomorrow's technology in mind, the building offers ample space for research and clinical training.

COST

The Emory University School of Nursing is committed to providing a generous package of financial assistance to all who qualify. Currently, 98% of undergraduate nursing students and 95% of graduate nursing students receive financial assistance. Merit-based scholarships and need-based grants are available at both the undergraduate and graduate levels. Tuition for the 2002-2003 academic year was $12,605 per semester.

APPLYING

All applicants to the School of Nursing are considered on an individual basis. Applications and credentials should be submitted as early as possible in the academic year prior to entrance; however, applications will be reviewed as long as class space is available.

The School of Nursing selects those applicants who are best qualified academically and personally. After all application materials are received, the Admissions and Continuance Committee reviews the applicant's credentials and makes the decision to accept, defer, or deny. Final acceptance is contingent upon satisfactory completion of prerequisite coursework.

CORRESPONDENCE AND INFORMATION

Office of Admission
School of Nursing
Emory University
1520 Clifton Road
Atlanta, Georgia 30322
(404) 727-7980
(800) 222-3879
Fax: (404) 727-8509
E-Mail: admit@nursing.emory.edu
Web: www. nursing.emory.edu

EPISCOPAL SCHOOL OF NURSING
Philadelphia, Pennsylvania

THE HOSPITAL
Episcopal Hospital is an accredited, non-profit, non-sectarian teaching hospital. The campus is located in the North Central Philadelphia community. Subway and bus transportation are conveniently located near the hospital.

SCHOOL OF NURSING
Established in 1888, Episcopal Hospital School of Nursing offers applicants a program leading to a Diploma in Nursing and prepares graduates to take the National Council Licensing Examination for Registered Nurses (NCLEX-RN).

The program is approved by the Pennsylvania State Board of Nursing and accredited by the National League for Nursing Accrediting Commission.

PROGRAM OF STUDY
Episcopal School of Nursing offers qualified applicants a Part-Time Evening/Weekend Program.

The Part-Time Evening/ Weekend Program begins each January and is taught over a period of three years. Students attend classes two evenings each week. Clinical experiences are scheduled on two weekends of each month.

Advanced standing is granted to those qualified individuals, once accepted, who successfully complete the Challenge Process. Up to eight of the program's nursing courses may be challenged.

CLINICAL RESOURCES
Class size is limited to 32 students to allow a low student-to-faculty ratio in the classroom and in the clinical setting.

The School's clinical resources are based primarily within the Temple University Health System. Temple University Hospital is located within two miles of the Episcopal Campus.

ACADEMIC RESOURCES
Students benefit from the use of a new Computer Learning Laboratory, a Nursing Arts Laboratory, and the Medical Library.

COSTS
Tuition cost is $170 per credit hour or approximately $15,120. Books and uniforms are additional expenses.

FINANCIAL AID
Episcopal School of Nursing offers Federal Pell Grants, Federal Stafford Loans, and State grants.

A financial aid packet is sent upon acceptance.

APPLYING
Graduation from an accredited secondary school, or completion of the General Educational Development (GED) test, is required for each program.

Applicants must *complete* seven prerequisite courses at an accredited college with a minimum grade of C and a total cumulative average of 2.5 or better.

The prerequisite courses are:

Anatomy & Physiology I	4 credit hours
Anatomy & Physiology II	4 credit hours
English Composition I	3 credit hours
*Introduction to Chemistry	4 credit hours
Introduction to Psychology	3 credit hours
Microbiology	4 credit hours
Normal Nutrition	3 credit hours

*Completion of high school Chemistry with a grade of C or better meets the requirement for this course.

The School has an open admissions policy and early applications are encouraged.

CORRESPONDENCE AND INFORMATION
Admissions Office
Episcopal School of Nursing
100 East Lehigh Avenue
Philadelphia, PA 19125-1000
(215) 707-0010
Web: www.health.temple.edu/episcopalnursing/index.html

ESSEX COUNTY COLLEGE
Department of Nursing
Newark, New Jersey

THE COLLEGE

Essex County College, established in 1966, is committed to providing comprehensive and quality educational programs and life-long learning activities at the most affordable cost. The College is open to students with a wide variety of backgrounds and abilities. It takes pride in the richness of its diversity and its nurturing atmosphere, which encourages people to enroll and excel.

The main campus is located in the University Heights section of the city, adjacent to Rutgers-Newark and the New Jersey Institute of Technology, and near the University of Medicine and Dentistry. Articulation agreements exist with the area four-year institutions that guarantee that all the credits students earn at ECC will transfer for the completion of baccalaureate degree programs. An extension center known as the West Essex Campus located in West Caldwell offers a wide range of credit courses, The college's enrollment exceeds 8,000 students in its degree programs and another 12,000 in its continuing education (credit and non-credit).

DEPARTMENT OF NURSING

The Department of Nursing is located at the Newark campus in the Main Building. The Nursing Program offers a balance of general education and nursing courses to prepare individuals for entry level Registered Nurse positions. The Nursing Program has enjoyed a 97-100% pass rate on the RN licensing exam for the last 6 graduating classes.

PROGRAMS OF STUDY

The Department of Nursing offers a Generic Associate Degree RN program and an LPN-to-RN Option. Nursing courses are offered during the daytime, and non-nursing courses are offered in the evening.

AFFILIATIONS WITH HEALTHCARE FACILITIES

The ECC Department of Nursing maintains contractual agreements with over 15 acute care and community agencies throughout the Essex County area. In addition, students gain experience in primary care in the ECC Day Care Centers, various schools in the area, and participation in county and college-sponsored health fairs.

ACADEMIC RESOURCES

The Department of Nursing has access to the College Learning Resource Center, individualized tutoring, and individualized academic advisement and counseling. The Nursing skills laboratory is a simulated hospital environment with equipment for recreating real hospital experiences. The Nursing Program has a state-of-the-art computer lab with over 175 nursing software programs including CD-ROM and Interactive Video Simulations. Students give nursing care in hospitals and community agencies.

COSTS

Essex County residents pay tuition per credit at a rate of $73.50/credit. Out of county residents pay $147.00/credit. There is an addition of $400.00 for fees and approximately $1,000.00 for books and supplies.

FINANCIAL AID

Various federal and state financial aid programs exist for students who are in need. In addition, various private sector scholarships are available.

APPLYING

Contact the Admissions Office at (973) 877-3100 and obtain an admission packet. Enter as a Pre-Nursing major (code 6000). Take a placement test for Reading, English, and Math or complete a waiver form. If your scores on the placement test are not at College level, complete remedial course work. Current high school students must have a B average and complete high school biology and chemistry. SAT score should be 500 or higher in verbal and math.

The following courses must be completed with a grade of C or better concurrent with admission:

    College Chemistry
    Anatomy and Physiology I
    English Composition I
    College GPA above 2.5
    Passing Score on Nurse Entrance Test

CORRESPONDENCE AND INFORMATION

Chairperson
Department of Nursing
Essex County College
303 University Avenue
Newark, New Jersey 07102
(973) 877-1868
Fax: (973) 877-1930
E-Mail: dey@essex.edu

EXCELSIOR COLLEGE
School of Nursing
Albany, New York

THE COLLEGE
Excelsior College is the nation's only exclusively outcomes-based degree-granting institution. Founded in 1971, it awards undergraduate and graduate degrees through 32 programs in business, liberal arts, nursing, and technology. Believing that "what you know is more important than where or how you learned it," the College has no residency requirement and awards degree credit earned from a variety of accredited sources.

NURSING PROGRAMS
Creator of the first nontraditional distance nursing programs in the United States, Excelsior College offers the largest assessment-based nursing program in the nation with programs that have served as models for other nontraditional programs. The College offers degree programs at the associate, baccalaureate, and master's levels as well as RN-BSN and RN-MSN programs and certificate programs in Home Health Care Nursing and Health Care Informatics.

Associate degree requirements incorporate general education (30 semester hours) and nursing (36 semester hours) components. General education requirements include anatomy, physiology, microbiology, lifespan developmental psychology, sociology, and English composition. The nursing component includes seven Excelsior College theory examinations and one performance examination.

Bachelor's degree requirements incorporate general education (65 semester hours) and nursing (55 semester hours) components. General education requirements include anatomy, physiology, microbiology, psychology, sociology, statistics, English composition, expository writing, and ethics. The nursing component includes six Excelsior College theory examinations and five performance examinations.

The MSN program is designed to prepare students for nurse administrator roles related to clinical systems management. It is also available as an RN-MSN program. Engaging in the study of foundational material for advanced nursing roles, exploration of health care informatics, and in-depth study of the administrative role, master's-level students in the program earn a total of 44 graduate-level credits through online coursework, computer-delivered examinations, and an interactive capstone experience. The Health Care Informatics portion of the program, also offered as a distinct certificate program for health professionals, awards 17 graduate-level credits and includes four online courses with interactive components.

ADMISSION
The School of Nursing degree programs are specifically designed for individuals with significant background or experience in clinically oriented health care disciplines. Undergraduate admission is open to Registered Nurses, Licensed Practical/Vocational Nurses, paramedics, emergency medical technicians, military service corpsmen, certified surgical technologists, individuals with degrees in clinically oriented health care fields in which they have provided direct patient care (i.e., physicians, respiratory therapists, chiropractors, and physicians' assistants), and individuals who have completed at least half of the clinical nursing courses in a registered nursing education program. (Exceptions may be made for individuals who do not meet these qualifications but who can document significant clinical background.) The RN-BSN and RN-MSN programs admit RNs and individuals licensed to practice as RNs in the United States; the MSN program admits BSNs and BSN-equivalent health professionals licensed to practice as RNs in the United States who also meet specific additional requirements.

ACCREDITATION
Excelsior College is accredited by the Commission on Higher Education of the Middle States Association of Colleges and Schools, 3624 Market Street, Philadelphia, Pennsylvania 19104, 215-662-5606. All its academic programs, including the undergraduate and graduate programs in nursing, are registered (i.e., approved) by the New York State Education Department. The associate, baccalaureate, and master's nursing degree programs are accredited by the National League for Nursing Accrediting Commission. The MSN program will be eligible for its first NLNAC accreditation visit when its first students are nearing graduation in 2002.

AFFILIATIONS WITH HEALTH CARE FACILITIES
Excelsior College has developed a national network of Regional Performance Assessment Centers (RPACs) at major hospitals in four regions of the country (California, Georgia, New York, and Wisconsin) at which performance examinations are administered.

COSTS
Costs depend on the degree sought, amount of prior credit accepted, pace of degree requirement completion, credit sources chosen (proficiency examinations are the least expensive mode of earning credit), and other factors. Particular fees and fee structures apply to specific student populations and to students who choose the Tuition Plan. Additional costs include books and other learning materials, travel (if necessary), postage, online resources, and miscellaneous charges and supplies.

CORRESPONDENCE AND INFORMATION
School of Nursing
Excelsior College
7 Columbia Circle
Albany, NY 12203-5159
(888) 647-2388 or
(518) 464-8500
Fax: (518) 464-8777
E-Mail: admissions@excelsior.edu
Web: http://www.excelsior.edu

FAIRFIELD UNIVERSITY
School of Nursing
Fairfield, Connecticut

THE UNIVERSITY
Fairfield University, founded in 1942, is a comprehensive Jesuit university that prepares students for leadership and service in a constantly changing world. The University offers a well-rounded education distinguished by real-world opportunities within and beyond the classroom. One-on-one contact with professors, access to first-rate facilities and technology, and a wide array of co-curricular activities give students many ways to develop new interests and expertise. Approximately 5,000 undergraduate and graduate students from 36 states, 34 countries, the District of Columbia, and Puerto Rico are enrolled. Thirty-two buildings grace the 200-acre campus.

THE SCHOOL OF NURSING
Fairfield nursing students are fully integrated into Fairfield's academic and social life, with opportunities to participate in sports, clubs, and volunteer programs. Nursing faculty are accomplished clinicians, researchers, and professional leaders. Small class sizes and individualized academic counseling provide students with comprehensive experiences in the classroom and clinical setting.

PROGRAMS OF STUDY
The four-year undergraduate BSN program begins with nursing early in the curriculum. Nursing electives are available, and students may study abroad at Harlaxton College in England. Part-time study is available. Individuals with a degree in another field complete the curriculum in an intensive 18-month program. The RN-BSN program individualizes learning experiences for completion of the baccalaureate degree. The Master of Science in Nursing program offers Family Nurse Practitioner and Psychiatric Nurse Practitioner tracks. Full and part-time study and Post-master's Certificates are available. Individualized curriculum plans allow for non-nurses and RNs to study at their own pace. Individualized practicum placements allow students to pursue expertise in areas of interest.

AFFILIATIONS WITH HEALTH CARE FACILITIES
Nursing students at Fairfield have access to a variety of clinical agencies, including major medical centers like Yale-New Haven Hospital. The School has affiliations with over 35 agencies including small Catholic hospitals, nursing homes, major hospitals, community health centers, in-patient psychiatric institutions, and elementary schools. Opportunities are available in urban and suburban settings, servicing both the poor and the affluent, for students to work with people of different cultures, backgrounds, and needs.

THE HEALTH PROMOTION CENTER
Fairfield nursing students gain community health experience through clinical rotations at the School's Health Promotion Center in Bridgeport. The Center, created in 1993 and funded in part by the Southern Connecticut Gas Company, is nationally recognized for its community health outreach program that provides care to the region's underserved population. Students provide services both at the Center and at satellite sites in the community, offering health screenings, education, and immunization programs for children and the elderly. Opportunities exist for volunteering, work-study, and summer internships at the Center.

ACADEMIC RESOURCES
The Nyselius library houses over 265,000 volumes, including a comprehensive selection of nursing and science texts and journals. Computer laboratories, a Writing Center, a Career Planning Center, and a full range of student services, including individualized tutoring, are available. The Nursing building houses multimedia classrooms, faculty offices, a study/reference room for students, conference rooms, and a tiered lecture hall. Its modern, multi-purpose Learning Resource Center is well-equipped with demonstration stations and state-of-the-art technology designed to develop and sharpen students' patient care, critical thinking, and decision-making skills.

COSTS
Expenses for 1999-2000: Tuition—$19,560; Room and board—$7,380; Fees—$435.

FINANCIAL AID
The University is committed to helping students afford a Fairfield education. Institutional resources supplement federal and state loans, grants, and work-study. Two-thirds of the student body qualify for financial aid. Qualified students may receive renewable merit scholarships ranging up to $10,000 per year.

APPLYING
Undergraduate students are accepted directly into the nursing program. SAT or TOEFL scores, high school transcript, and a counselor recommendation are required. An interview is recommended, and advanced standing is available. Part-time and adult students meet with advisors to assess individual options. RN and MSN students require RN license and college transcripts. MSN admission requires 2 letters of recommendation and GRE or MAT scores.

CORRESPONDENCE AND INFORMATION
Fairfield University
School of Nursing
1073 North Benson Road
Fairfield, Connecticut 06824
Web: www.fairfield.edu

Undergraduate students contact admissions: (203) 254-4100. Part-time, adult, accelerated, and RN students contact the School of Continuing Education: (203) 254-4220. MSN students contact the School of Nursing: (203) 254-4150.

FELICIAN COLLEGE
Department of Nursing
Lodi, New Jersey

THE COLLEGE
Felician College is a co-educational, liberal arts, Catholic college founded in the Franciscan tradition by the Felician Sisters in 1942. Enrolling 1500 students in 40 undergraduate and graduate programs in the arts and sciences, health sciences, and teacher education, Felician College is located on two campuses in Lodi and Rutherford, New Jersey. The college's Golden Falcons compete at the NCAA Division II level, fielding teams in basketball, soccer, softball, baseball, cross country, track & field, and cheerleading.

THE NURSING PROGRAM
The Nursing Program at Felician, which began in 1965, is located on the Lodi Campus in the Main College Building. Felician College is accredited by the Middle States Association of Colleges and Schools, and carries program accreditation from the National League for Nursing Accrediting Commission, and the Commission on Collegiate Nursing Education. The Program is approved by the New Jersey Commission on Higher Education and the New Jersey State Board of Nursing.

PROGRAMS OF STUDY
Felician College offers a program in basic nursing education to qualified women and men that prepares them to give safe, effective, direct patient care. Upon satisfactory completion, the student earns an AAS Degree in nursing. The graduate is then eligible to take the examination for licensure given by the NJ Board of Nursing. Graduates who pass this examination will qualify for the title Registered Nurse (RN).

The MSN program has two levels: undergraduate and graduate. Within this program, the BSN degree may be selected as an option at anytime after acceptance into the program. The MSN Program prepares professional nurses for primary care as Family or Adult Nurse Practitioners. The program emphasizes nursing care of families or adults with a specific focus on vulnerable or underserved populations.

ACADEMIC RESOURCES
The Nursing Resource Center (NRC) is available to all nursing students. The setting is conducive for students to practice new skills learned or for those students who wish to improve their present skills. Various workshops such as test taking, nursing care plans, mathematics, and critical thinking are offered to enhance the students' studies. Computer-assisted instructional programs for nursing are accessible to help students in their clinical and professional skills. These include CAI, NCLEX, and interactive videos. The NRC offers flexible scheduling to meet the students' needs.

The College Library offers a broad selection of books, periodicals, and microforms and can help students by providing information, journal articles, and books from sources all over the country. In addition, computer labs, tutorial services, writing labs, and career planning and placement services are available to students.

COSTS
The full-time undergraduate tuition for Fall of 2003 is $7,250 per semester for 12 or more credits. Graduate tuition is $525 per credit. The college offers housing in two residence halls on the Rutherford campus for $3,600 per semester.

FINANCIAL AID
Various federal and state financial aid programs exist for students who are in need. Work-study programs are also available. In addition, qualified students are eligible to apply for a variety of scholarships.

APPLYING
Applications for admission to Felician College are considered for Fall or Spring Semesters. Admission decisions are made on a rolling basis. To receive an admission packet, call the Office of Admission at (201) 559-6131. The Office of Admission or the appropriate department chair can provide information regarding specific admission requirements for the Nursing Programs.

CORRESPONDENCE AND INFORMATION
Felician College Division of Health Sciences
Dr. Muriel Shore, Dean
262 South Main Street
Lodi, NJ 07644
(201) 559-6030
Fax: (201) 559-6188

Department of Associate Nursing
Professor Joann Frazer, Chair
E-Mail: frazerj@inet.felician.edu

Department of Baccalaureate Nursing
Dr. Maureen Ruocco, Chair
E-Mail: ruoccom@inet.felician.edu

Department of Graduate Nursing
Dr. Margo Griffin, Chair
E-Mail: griffinm@inet.felician.edu

FLORIDA A&M UNIVERSITY
School of Nursing
Tallahassee, Florida

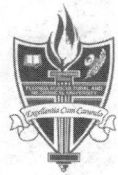

THE UNIVERSITY
Founded in 1887 as the State Normal College for Colored Students, FAMU is one of the three oldest universities in the State University System. Spread over 419 acres in Tallahassee, the University is a four-year public, coeducational and fully accredited institution of higher learning. With a faculty of 620, FAMU offers 110 undergraduate, 40 graduate, and nine PhD degrees.

FAMU has an enrollment of 12,000 and has consistently been one of the national leaders in the recruitment of National Achievement Scholars. In 1992, 1995, and 1997, FAMU was ranked No. 1 in the recruitment of these students, surpassing Harvard, Stanford, and other institutions of higher learning.

In 1997, FAMU was selected as the TIME Magazine/ Princeton Review "College of the Year." Editors cited innovative programs, rising enrollment, surging SAT scores, and the recruitment of National Achievement Scholars as the reasons for the selection. In 2000, *Black Issues in Higher Education* featured FAMU as the no. 1 producer of African-American baccalaureates in the United States.

THE SCHOOL OF NURSING
The Florida A&M University School of Nursing was founded in 1904 and became the first baccalaureate nursing program in the State of Florida in 1936. The School of Nursing offers the baccalaureate and master's degrees in nursing. The undergraduate degree program is approved by the Florida Board of Nursing and is accredited by the National League for Nursing Accrediting Commission. The baccalaureate program is approved by the Florida Board of Nursing. Both the baccalaureate and master's programs are accredited by the National League for Nursing Accrediting Commission. The mission of the Florida A&M University School of Nursing is to (1) educate men and women to function as generalists at the undergraduate level and as specialists at the master's level in professional nursing, (2) provide a supportive environment to foster research activity by faculty and students; (3) be responsive to the service needs of the community.

PROGRAMS OF STUDY
Baccalaureate Degree: The School of Nursing offers an upper division major in nursing that leads to a Bachelor of Science degree.

RN to BSN Program: The School of Nursing offers the graduate of diploma and associate degree nursing programs who are licensed in the State of Florida the opportunity to complete requirements for the baccalaureate degree in nursing.

Masters Degree: The School of Nursing offers the Master of Science in Nursing Program with an emphasis in Adult/Gerontological Nurse Practitioner preparation. The master's program prepares nurses for advanced practice in primary health care with young, middle, and older adults in acute, ambulatory, long-term, and community settings. The graduate of this program is eligible to take the American Nurses Credentialing Center's national certification examination for both Adult and Gerontological Nurse Practitioner and apply for licensure as an Advanced Registered Nurse Practitioner in the state of Florida.

APPLYING FOR ADMISSION
Students may apply for admission to FAMU by submitting a State University System application or by completing the online FAMU application that can be downloaded from the University's website at www.famu.edu.

The selection process includes, but may not be limited to, grades, test scores, educational objectives, pattern of courses completed, past conduct, recommendation, and personal records.

COSTS
	In-State	Out-of-State
Undergraduate	$ 81.96	$344.88
Graduate	$ 164.14	$571.30

FINANCIAL AID
Florida A&M University offers a variety of financial aid programs. Contact the University's Office of Student Financial Aid at (850) 599-3730; E-Mail: finaid@famu.edu.

CONTACT INFORMATION
Baccalaureate Program Information
Mrs. Kathleen Karran-McCoy, M.Ed.
Director, Student Affairs
(850) 599-3458
Fax: (850) 599-3847
E-Mail: kathleen.mccoy@famu.edu

Ms. Kimberly R. Davis, M.Ed.
Coordinator of Recruitment Director, Student Affairs
(850) 412-7066 or (850) 599-3458
Fax: (850) 599-3847 or (850) 599-3508
E-Mail: kimberly.davis@famu.edu

Master's Program Information
Doris Ballard-Ferguson, Ph.D., APN
Associate Dean, Graduate Program
(850) 412-7067
Fax: (850) 599-3847 or (850) 599-3508
E-Mail: doris.ballardferguso@famu.edu

or

Jaibun Earp, Ph.D., APN
Professor
(850) 412-2969
Fax: (850) 599-3847 or (850) 599-3508
E-Mail: jaibun.earp@famu.edu

FLORIDA GULF COAST UNIVERSITY
School of Nursing
Fort Myers, Florida

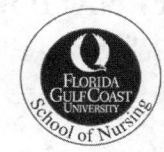

Florida Gulf Coast University School of Nursing is accredited by the National League for Nursing Accrediting Commission (NLNAC), and offers innovative, exemplary, learning-centered, and community-partnered programs. Learners are prepared as caring scholar clinicians for professional nursing practice in contemporary healthcare settings. Interdisciplinary and discipline-specific knowledge, values, competencies, and practice opportunities prepare graduates to assume vital roles within an evolving 21st century healthcare delivery system.

PROGRAMS

Our Bachelor of Science in Nursing program is designed to prepare caring scholar clinicians for professional practice in contemporary health care settings. Graduates are prepared to assume vital roles in the improvement of the health care system. General education and state-mandated common prerequisites for nursing form the foundation of study for the major. The community partnered, learning-centered nursing curriculum is grounded in knowledge of the theory and practice of nursing with integration of critical thinking, communication, health promotion, caring, and cultural connectedness constructs.

In addition to the traditional nursing program, FGCU offers a RN-BSN Accelerated Pathway, developed in accordance with statewide articulation guidelines. This pathway provides Associate of Science in Nursing (ASN) graduates with an expeditious and convenient route to the BSN while maintaining high standards of quality.

The Master of Science in Nursing program prepares advanced practice nurses for career opportunities in a variety of evolving global health care environments. The ability to create innovative roles as well as consolidate existing roles is a hallmark of graduates. Extensive practice experiences enable student-initiated opportunities that promote development of diverse knowledge, values, and competencies essential for advanced practice. Students choose a focal area of study in Primary Health Care (specialty areas within PHC include nurse educator and nurse practitioner) or Nurse Anesthesia.

ADMISSIONS

The School of Nursing has a selective, competitive admission process and all qualified applicants may not be admitted into the program. To learn more about the admission process, or request BSN program information, please contact the Office of Student Alumni Relations at (239) 590-7485. To request MSN program information, please contact the graduate studies office at (239) 590-7454.

You may also visit our web site at www.fgcu.edu/chp/nursing.

FOR MORE INFORMATION

To learn more about Florida Gulf Coast University, or to request a complete 2003-2004 catalog, please contact the Office of Admissions toll free at (888) 889-1095. You may also visit us online at www.fgcu.edu.

FLORIDA INTERNATIONAL UNIVERSITY
College of Health Sciences
School of Nursing
Miami, Florida

SCHOOL OF NURSING
The School of Nursing offers the following programs of study:

BACHELOR OF SCIENCE IN NURSING

- Generic BSN
- RN to BSN
- MD to RN

MASTER OF SCIENCE IN NURSING

- Advanced Adult Health Nursing
- Advanced Child Health Nursing
- Advanced Psychiatric-Mental Health Nursing
- Advanced Family Health Nursing
- Anesthesiology Nursing
- Nursing Administration

The School of Nursing faculty is dedicated to the development of nurse clinicians to deliver high quality care to clients from diverse cultures.

FOR MORE INFORMATION CONTACT
Divina Grossman, PhD, RN, ARNP, FAAN
Director and Professor
Florida International University
School of Nursing
3000 N.E. 151st Street, ACII 230
Miami, FL 33181
(305) 919-5915
Fax: (305) 919-4717

GEORGIA STATE UNIVERSITY
College of Health and Human Sciences
School of Nursing
Atlanta, GA

THE UNIVERSITY
Georgia State University (GSU) is a Research II University located in the heart of downtown Atlanta. As the only Urban Research university in Georgia, GSU offers educational opportunities to nearly 25,000 traditional and non-traditional students at both the graduate and undergraduate levels. GSU educates leaders for Georgia, the nation, and the worldwide community. The university is accredited by the *Southern Association of Colleges and Schools* (SACS).

SCHOOL OF NURSING
The School of Nursing (SON) is located on the downtown campus of the university. Founded in 1969, the SON is fully accredited and has clinical affiliations with over 200 agencies in the city and around the state, offering state-of-the-art, community-focused education to its baccalaureate, masters, and doctoral students. The school is accredited by the National League for Nursing Accrediting Commission and the American Association of Colleges of Nursing. The SON maintains a Web site at www.gsu.edu/nursing.

PROGRAMS OF STUDY
The School of Nursing offers the Generic Baccalaureate (*Bachelor of Science with a Major in Nursing), RN Baccalaureate*, Master of Science with a major in Nursing, RN to MS, and the Doctor of Philosophy with a major in Nursing. The Masters programs include the Family Nurse Practitioner, Pediatric Nurse Practitioner–Clinical Nurse Specialist, Women's Health Practitioner–Clinical Nurse Specialist, Adult Health Clinical Nurse Specialist, and the Psychiatric–Mental Health Clinical Nurse Specialist foci. The focus of the Doctoral program is on health promotion, protection, and restoration with an emphasis on vulnerable populations.

Graduates of the baccalaureate program are eligible to apply for licensure as a Registered Nurse (RN), while graduates of the Masters tracks may sit for certification examinations in their various specialties.

ACADEMIC RESOURCES
The School of Nursing has at its disposal the resources of an urban research university, including open computer labs, and the Pullen Library, which houses more than 1,100,000 volumes, more than 7,000 periodicals, and sophisticated electronic information sources. The SON maintains a state-of-the-art learning resource center and an informatics laboratory.

COSTS

Matriculation	Tuition Per Semester Hour	Amount for 12 or Greater Semester Hours
Resident Undergraduate	$110.00	$1,316.00
Non-Resident Undergraduate	$440.00	$5,264.00
Resident Graduate (MS/PhD)	$141.00	$1,689.00
Non-Resident Graduate	$564.00	$6,756.00

Student Activity fees for all students are $330.00 per semester. Housing per semester is $2,250.00

FINANCIAL AID
The office of Student Financial Aid provides full information on available financial aid. Information on financial aid can also be obtained on the Web site www.gsu.edu under Student Services.

APPLYING
For the BS Program   Students must apply by April 15th of each year. Applications received by February 15 will receive early consideration.

For the MS Program   Students must apply by March 1st for summer or fall semester; by October 1st for spring semester.

For the Doctoral Program   Students must apply by February 15th for summer or fall semester; by September 15th for spring semester.

For information or to obtain an application to the BS, MS, or PhD program, please contact the Office of Academic Assistance in the College of Health and Human Sciences at:

Office of Academic Assistance
College of Health and Human Sciences
Georgia State University
8th Floor Urban Life Building
University Plaza
Atlanta, GA 30303
(404) 651-3064
Fax: (404) 651-4671
Web: www.gsu.edu/nursing

GOSHEN COLLEGE
Department of Nursing
Goshen, Indiana

THE COLLEGE
Goshen College is a four-year liberal arts college dedicated to the development of informed, articulate, sensitive, responsible Christians. As a ministry of the Mennonite Church, we seek to integrate Christian values with educational and professional life. As a community of faith and learning, we strive to foster personal, intellectual, spiritual, and social growth. We view education as a moral activity that produces servant-leaders for the church and the world.

THE DEPARTMENT OF NURSING
Since 1950, when the Goshen College nursing program became the first liberal arts college in Indiana to offer a bachelor of science degree in nursing, 1,300 graduates have established themselves in successful careers as registered nurses. GC's nursing program is highly respected in the United States and abroad; graduates are known by their ethical standards, personal integrity, Christian commitment, caring attitude, and clinical knowledge.

PROGRAMS OF STUDY
The Department of Nursing offers a generic Bachelor of Science in Nursing and a Bachelor of Science in Nursing completion program for Registered Nurses. The mission of the Department of Nursing is to prepare the student upon graduation to function as a beginning practitioner of professional nursing. Graduates of the generic program are eligible to apply for licensure as a Registered Nurse (RN).

CLINICAL EXPERIENCES
Students in the nursing program experience a variety of clinical settings. Clinical experiences include medical, surgical, acute care, pediatrics, and maternal nursing in the hospital setting. Clinical experiences in the community setting include home health care, clinics, school and community health, and long-term care.

LEARNING THROUGH OTHER CULTURES
A unique general education requirement at GC is international education. This can be met with courses on campus, or on Study-Service Term (SST). Most GC students opt for SST because it's a challenging opportunity for an international experience and it typically costs the same as a term on campus. Nursing students see first-hand how health care beliefs and practices are interwoven with culture. Nursing students sometimes serve in rural health clinics of a developing nation.

ADMISSION REQUIREMENTS
Application to the nursing program is made during the first year of study at GC. Applicants should be in the upper half of their high school graduating class. The high school program should have included foreign language, mathematics, algebra, chemistry, and biology. Physics is recommended. A student needs to have a college grade point average of 2.5 or higher to be admitted into the program.

COSTS
For 2003–2004, the estimated comprehensive fee for full-time study was $22,120. This included $16,320 for tuition, $3,000 for room and $2,800 for board. Books and supplies cost approximately $700 and personal expenses approximately $1000.

SCHOLARSHIPS
Institutionally sponsored need-based and non-need-based grants and scholarships, institutionally sponsored long-term loans, the Federal Work-Study Program, Federal Supplemental Educational Opportunity Grants, Federal Direct Loans, Federal Perkins Loans, and Federal Nursing Student Loans are available sources of financial aid. In 2002–2003, 98 percent of undergraduate nursing students received some form of financial aid. Specialized scholarships are available for nursing students who demonstrate leadership abilities, high scholastic standing, financial need, and/or the desire to work in a mission/service setting. All the nursing students who applied for financial aid during the 2002–2003 academic year received it.

CORRESPONDENCE AND INFORMATION
Department of Nursing
Goshen College
1700 South Main Street
Goshen, Indiana 46526
(219) 535-7370
Fax: (219) 535-7609
E-Mail: lindasb@goshen.edu
Web: http://www. goshen.edu

GRAHAM HOSPITAL
School of Nursing
Canton, Illinois

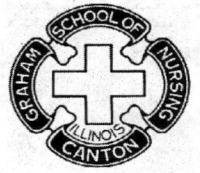

HISTORY OF SCHOOL
Graham Hospital School of Nursing in Canton is located in the western part of central Illinois. The original structure of Graham Hospital was a gift of the Graham sisters and both the hospital and school were formally opened in 1909.

PROGRAM
Graham Hospital School of Nursing is a 3-year diploma program whose mission is to provide educational experiences which nurture growth in professional values, develop competencies in the nursing discipline, and prepare the student to contribute to and live in a changing society.

Graham Hospital is the major clinical facility utilized. Our direct link to a healthcare facility enables us to quickly recognize and respond to changes in the healthcare delivery system. The school has a long history of involvement in the use of community healthcare agencies as clinical sites for our students. Clinical experiences also occur in other area hospitals. Students attend Spoon River college, three miles southwest of the city, for the general education courses in the curriculum.

All nursing courses include both classroom and clinical nursing experiences, which allow students to apply knowledge gained in the classroom.

APPROVAL AND ACCREDITATION
Graham Hospital School of Nursing is approved by the Illinois Department of Professional Regulation and is accredited by the National League for Nursing Accrediting Commission.

FACILITY AND HOUSING
Resident students live in air-conditioned, furnished dormitory rooms. A library with current periodicals and reference texts is available for student use. There are a number of options available to locate material via interlibrary loan through the library's membership in the Resource Sharing Alliance. The library also includes a computer room with Internet access.

FINANCIAL COST INFORMATION
Tuition: $3,000 per semester
Activity Fees: $150 per semester
Room: $850 per semester

Upon receipt of final acceptance, all entering students are required to pay a non-refundable $75.00 enrollment deposit to ensure a place in the entering class. This deposit is applied toward payment of first semester.

FINANCIAL AID
Graham Hospital School of Nursing recognizes that many students need assistance meeting the costs of their education. Students are advised to contact the Coordinator of Admissions, Recruitment and Financial Aid to discuss the many types of financial assistance available.

APPLICATION PROCEDURE
The applicant must submit the following to the Coordinator of Admission, Recruitment and Financial Aid:

1. A completed application form.

2. Official transcripts from all high schools, GED scores, and post-secondary institutions.
3. ACT and/or SAT scores.
4. Three letters of recommendation.

Complete an interview with the Coordinator of Admissions, Recruitment, and Financial Aid.

MINIMUM REQUIREMENTS FOR ADMISSION
1. The applicant must have graduated from a state-approved high school, or GED, have a cumulative GPA of 2.00 on a 4.00 scale, and received a grad of "C" or better in each of the following courses at either high school or college level (1 unit equals 1 year of high school or 1 semester of college):
A. English ....3 units
B. Algebra............................2 units
(2 years of high school algebra or intermediate college algebra.)
C. Geometry...........................1 unit
(1 year high school or college geometry)
D. Biology............................1 unit
(High school biology within past 5 years.)
E. Chemistry.........................1 unit
F. Social Sciences...................2 units

ADVANCED PLACEMENT
Advanced placement of certified nursing assistants and licensed practical nurses is available. Applicants should discuss these options with the Coordinator of Admissions, Recruitment and Financial Aid.

CORRESPONDENCE AND INFORMATION
Coordinator of Admissions, Recruitment and Financial Aid
Graham Hospital School of Nursing
210 West Walnut Street
Canton, Illinois 61520
(309) 647-4086
Fax: (309)649-5127
E-Mail: mkepple@grahamhospital.org
Web: www.grahamschoolofnursing.org

GULF COAST COMMUNITY COLLEGE
Panama City, Florida

THE OPPORTUNITY

Nursing is the practice of caring for individuals, families, and communities, focusing not only on caring for the ill and dying, but on health promotion and illness prevention. Many nurses practice at the bedside in health care institutions or in clients' homes in community health care settings. Because the profession of nursing comprises the largest number of health care providers in the country, numerous opportunities exist in a variety of settings, such as hospital, school, and occupational health nursing; nurse consultants, researchers, educators, and advanced registered nurse practitioners; military nursing; and independent health care businesses.

The opportunity to become a nurse and make a difference in the lives of others begins here, at Gulf Coast Community College.

Located in Panama City, Florida, home of the "The World's Most Beautiful Beaches," Gulf Coast Community College overlooks tranquil St. Andrews Bay. The College campus is only minutes away from the Panama City-Bay County International Airport and the sugar sand beaches of the Gulf of Mexico.

NURSING PROGRAMS AVAILABLE

ADN (Associate in Science Degree in Nursing): A two-year program full time. Successful completion allows the graduate to sit for the national exam to obtain a registered nurse (RN) license.

LPN Articulation: Licensed Practical Nurses, following successful completion of 26 credit hours of general education courses and 3 Regents College Mobility Exams, are admitted and complete the ADN program in 1 year.

RN-BSN: Following completion of the ADN program and pre-nursing (Pre-BSN) requirements, students may obtain a Bachelor of Science Degree in nursing though university programs.

Pre-BSN: This Associate in Arts Degree pre-nursing curriculum is designed to prepare students who desire entry into a university of their choice to obtain a Bachelor of Science Degree in nursing.

To begin the application process:

- Apply for general admission to the College
- Complete the Health Sciences Division Application
- Provide high school (or GED) and previous college transcripts
- Request a transcript evaluation if you have attended another college
- Take the Florida College Entry Level Placement Test (FCELPT)
- Obtain a Nursing Faculty Advisor

The Nursing Program admits two classes of students per year, in the fall and spring semesters. Application deadlines are: February 28th for the following fall term class, and September 30th for the following spring term class. Other requirements that must be fulfilled before consideration for acceptance into the program are identified in the application packet and can be explained to you by the Health Sciences Recruiter.

CORRESPONDENCE AND INFORMATION

For questions, or to obtain an application packet, contact:
Craig Wise, Assistant Coordinator for Health Sciences Admissions
Room 203, George G. Tapper Health Sciences Building
Gulf Coast Community College
5230 West U.S. Highway 98
Panama City, FL 32401
(850) 913-3311 or toll free 1-800-311-3685, ext. 3311
E-Mail: swise@ccmail.gc.cc.fl.us

24 Hour Health Science Information Line: (850) 913-3260 or toll free 1-800-311-3685, ext. 3260

Visit our Web site: http://www.gc.cc.fl.us. Click "Health Sciences" under Department pages, then "Nursing" under Associate in Science Degrees.

HAMPTON UNIVERSITY
School of Nursing
Hampton, Virginia

THE UNIVERSITY

Hampton University, founded in 1868, is located on 254 acres of Virginia's Peninsula. It is a privately endowed, co-educational, nonsectarian institution of higher education. Hampton University is dedicated to the promotion of learning, of building character, and of preparing promising students for positions of leadership and service. The University has an enrollment of 5,700 students drawn from 50 states, territories, and foreign countries. The full time faculty numbers 395. The Undergraduate College has six schools: Business, Engineering and Technology, Liberal Arts and Education, Nursing, Pharmacy, and Science. Within these schools, the bachelor's degree is offered in 45 areas. The Graduate College offers the doctoral degree in physics, pharmacy, physical therapy, and nursing, and the master's degree in 14 fields. The College of Continuing Education also offers programs leading to degrees in a variety of disciplines.

THE SCHOOL OF NURSING

The School of Nursing is an integral unit of Hampton University and shares its goals and ideals of excellence in the teaching-living-learning process. Since 1944, the nursing faculty of Hampton University has provided high-quality professional nursing education at the Bachelor of Science degree level. This undergraduate program has the distinction of being the oldest baccalaureate nursing program in the Commonwealth. In 1976, the nursing faculty instituted a Master of Science degree program, making Hampton University the first historically black college or university to offer a master's degree in nursing. Hampton University School of Nursing implemented a doctor of philosophy program in nursing in 1999, which remains the only such program in a historically black college or university. Post-Master's Family and Gerontological Nurse Practitioner Certificate Programs are offered for graduate level students through the College of Continuing Education. The curriculum in the School of Nursing is community-based and family focused throughout all programs. The School of Nursing is approved by the Virginia Board of Nursing, is fully accredited by the National League for Nursing Accrediting Commission and the Commission on Collegiate Nursing Education.

The Nursing Center and the Health Mobile deliver primary health care services and emphasize the implementation of health promotion and disease prevention for client groups in urban and rural communities including the homeless, and other displaced, underserved, or unserved populations.

PROGRAMS OF STUDY

The School of Nursing offers generic baccalaureate, LPN-BS, and RN-BS programs. The School of Nursing offers a Master of Science degree with three areas of role development: education, administration, and nurse practitioner. There are four nurse practitioner areas of specialization: geriatric, pediatric, women's health, and family. The clinical areas of specialty offered are Community Health, Advanced Adult and Community Mental Health/Psychiatric Nursing. In addition, the School of Nursing offers a Doctor of Philosophy (PhD) degree in nursing with a focus on families and family-related research.

AFFILIATIONS WITH HEALTH CARE FACILITIES

The School of Nursing utilizes approximately thirty health care agencies throughout the Southeast Virginia. They include acute and long-term care facilities, a children's hospital, community health agencies, clinics, and military hospitals.

ACADEMIC RESOURCES

The School of Nursing is located in William Freeman Hall and contains a nursing skills laboratory, computer laboratory, an electronic auditorium, and library. The University Academic Technology Mall offers a variety of high tech services for students, faculty, and staff. The William R. and Norma B. Harvey Library opened in 1992 and has over 363,206 volumes. The Academic Support Center assists students from admission to graduation, providing academic counseling, peer tutoring, and seminars to enrich the students' educational experience.

COSTS

Total cost for the 2003-2004 school year is $18,982 for on-campus and $12,864 for off-campus. The cost per credit hour is $275.

FINANCIAL AID

The University offers a number of grants, loans, scholarships, and work opportunities from federal, state, and private sources. The Free Application for Federal Student Assistance (FAFSA) should be completed as early as possible. The School of Nursing will counsel students regarding available nursing scholarships.

APPLYING

A formal application for admission must be made to the Director of Admissions, Hampton University, Hampton, Virginia 23668. There is no separate application for the School of Nursing. An application may be downloaded by visiting our Web site.

CORRESPONDENCE AND INFORMATION

School of Nursing
Hampton University
Hampton, Virginia 23668
(757) 727-5251
Fax: (757) 727-5423
E-Mail: nursing@hamptonu.edu
Web: http://www.hamptonu.edu

HAWAII PACIFIC UNIVERSITY
College of Nursing
Honolulu, Hawaii

THE UNIVERSITY

Hawaii Pacific University is the largest private postsecondary institution in the state of Hawaii. The University is coeducational, with over 8,300 undergraduate and graduate students, more than 300 faculty, a student-faculty ratio of 20:1, and an average class size of 24. At the heart of the Pacific, Hawaii Pacific University has two campuses ideally located in the city of Honolulu on the island of Oahu. We are a comprehensive university with a global perspective. Programs at HPU provide students with the most up-to-date knowledge available to meet the challenges of this changing world. HPU provides a creative learning environment, where programs integrate theory and practice, and talented faculty bring their expertise and professional backgrounds into the classroom.

NURSING PROGRAM

Hawaii Pacific University offers four pathways to a Baccalaureate Nursing degree: Basic Pathway, 23-Month Pathway, LPN to BSN Pathway, and RN-to-BSN Pathway. Hawaii Pacific University's Master of Science in Nursing program offers the registered nurse the opportunity to advance his or her career as either a Community Clinical Nurse Specialist (CNS) or Family Nurse Practitioner (FNP). The RN-MSN pathway allows registered nurses without baccalaureate degrees in nursing to transition into the MSN program. Students interested in gaining a solid foundation in modern business and management principles may also pursue a joint MSN/MBA degree.

RESEARCH FACILITIES

To support studies, University libraries, with a collection approaching 159,000 volumes, add an average of 2,500 volumes annually. Periodical titles number more than 1,700, and 200,000 pieces of microfiche and 5,200 rolls of microfilm are maintained. Dial-up access to local area databases of public and state university library catalogs is available in the Library. The University's accessible on-campus computer center houses more than 100 IBM-compatible microcomputers, with stand-alone support and networked configurations that support the Nursing Programs' integrated computer applications approach.

AFFILIATIONS WITH HEALTH CARE FACILITIES

The College of Nursing maintains contractual agreements with more than 30 health-care agencies. The school's clinical resources include community hospitals and clinics, military hospitals, a specialized women and children's hospital, psychiatric and mental health facilities, community-based outpatient settings, and acute care inpatient facilities.

COSTS

For the 2002-2003 academic year, graduate tuition was $4,925 per semester for freshman and sophomore students, and $7,100 for junior and senior students. Graduate tuition was $4,925 per semester (12 credits). Books, supplies, and health insurance cost approximately $700.

FINANCIAL AID

The University participates in all federal financial aid programs. These programs provide aid in the form of subsidized (need-based) and unsubsidized (non-need-based) Federal Stafford Student Loans. Through these loans, funds may be available to cover a student's entire cost of education. To apply for aid, students must submit the Free Application for Federal Student Aid (FAFSA) after January 1. Mailing of student award letters usually begins in April.

APPLYING

Hawaii Pacific University seeks students with academic promise, outstanding career potential, and high motivation. Applicants should complete and forward an admissions application, have official transcripts sent from all colleges or universities attended, and forward two letters of recommendation. Admissions decisions are made on a rolling basis, and applicants are notified between one and two weeks after all documents have been submitted.

CORRESPONDENCE AND INFORMATION

Hawaii Pacific University
Graduate Admissions Office
1164 Bishop Street, Suite 911
Honolulu, Hawaii 96813
(808) 544-1120 or (800) 669-4724
Fax: (808) 544-0280
E-Mail: gradservctr@hpu.edu
Web: http://www.hpu.edu

HELENE FULD SCHOOL OF NURSING
With Camden County College
Blackwood, New Jersey

THE SCHOOL
Helene Fuld is a century old, independent school of nursing with an enrollment of approximately 300 students. Its modern facility is located on the 320 wooded acres of Camden County College in Blackwood, NJ. Under a cooperative agreement, Camden County College offers the liberal arts and science courses and confers the Associate in Science degree. Helene Fuld is responsible for the nursing courses and grants the diploma in nursing. The program is fully accredited by the NLNAC.

AFFILIATIONS
The School's two major teaching affiliates are the Virtua Health System, the leading multi-hospital system in New Jersey, and Cooper Health System, a large urban teaching hospital with many specialty services.

ACADEMIC RESOURCES
The School houses state-of-the-art technologies for student learning including a computer laboratory with Internet access, an up-to-date nursing skills laboratory, and a spacious nursing library featuring the largest journal collection in the South Jersey area.

COST, FINANCIAL AID, AND SCHOLARSHIPS
The cost of the three-year nursing program is approximately $17,500. Helene Fuld students are eligible for federal, state, and county funds administered through the financial aid office of Camden County College. Accepted students are provided with scholarship information from a wide variety of resources.

ADMISSIONS
Admissions criteria include a cumulative GPA of 2.50 in college courses; minimum SAT scores of 450 in math and 450 in verbal (if high school was recent) and an NET score in the 50th percentile or better. A rolling admissions policy is in place.

CURRICULUM OPTIONS
Both a day and evening program are offered with January and September entrance for day students and September entrance for evening students. A summer option may be elected to accelerate in the program.

Advanced placement is offered for LPNs and selected applicants with previous nursing education background.

NCLEX PASS RATE
Helene Fuld has an NCLEX pass rate of 86% to 100%, well above the national and state averages.

BSN OPTIONS
Helene Fuld has agreements with seven colleges and universities for accelerating in their BSN programs.

CORRESPONDENCE AND INFORMATION
Coordinator of Student Services
Helene Fuld School of Nursing
in Camden County
PO Box 1669, College Drive
Blackwood, NJ 08012
(856) 374-0100
Fax: (856) 374-0710
Web: www.virtua.org/HeleneFuld.cfm

HOLY FAMILY COLLEGE
Division of Nursing
Philadelphia, Pennsylvania

THE COLLEGE
Holy Family College is a private, Catholic, coeducational commuter college located on two campuses, one in Northeast Philadelphia and one in Bucks County, Pennsylvania.

THE DIVISION OF NURSING
The Division of Nursing was founded in 1971, and is one of the largest of the five academic divisions.

PROGRAMS OF STUDY
Bachelor of Science in Nursing (BSN)
Evening/Weekend BSN
RN-to-BSN (accelerated program)

ACADEMIC RESOURCES
Nursing students will benefit from the 11:1 student-faculty ratio, as well as from a full-time Student Affairs Chair available for counseling and advisement. Within the Nursing Education Building, the School of Nursing provides a computer lab, an audiovisual resources center, an advanced skills lab, classrooms, and faculty offices.

COSTS AND FEES
Tuition at Holy Family College is $13,990 annually for full-time students. This cost includes a technology fee and malpractice insurance for non-licensed students. Application fees are $25.

FINANCIAL AID
Holy Family offers financial aid through Federal Pell Grants, Pennsylvania Higher Education Assistance Agency, and the Nursing Student Loan Program. Also available are private institutionally-funded need- and non-need-based scholarships and grants.

ADMISSIONS
Holy Family has a rolling admissions policy but encourages applicants to apply early. Required for consideration for admission are appropriate transcripts, SAT or GRE/MAT scores, letters of recommendation/references, and current licensure for RN students.

CONTACT INFORMATION
Holy Family College
Grant and Frankford Avenues
Philadelphia, PA 19114-2094
(215) 637-3050
Web: www.hfc.edu

HOLYOKE COMMUNITY COLLEGE
Holyoke, Massachusetts

THE COLLEGE
Holyoke Community College (HCC) is a state-supported public college. First established in 1971, the Nursing Program has graduated over 1,360 students, many of whom have gone on to earn baccalaureate and masters degrees in nursing. The Nursing Program is approved by the Massachusetts Board of Registration for Nursing and is accredited by the National League for Nursing Accrediting Commission.

STUDENTS AND UPWARD MOBILITY
Students range in age from 19–64 and come from varied backgrounds. We are dedicated to the upward mobility of nursing assistants and LPNs, and offer advanced placement for LPNs. We value the diversity of our student population and offer unique and individualized, academic support services through the Nursing Success Program.

THE CURRICULUM
We believe in a strong clinical-based curriculum and place students in a variety of health care settings. The curriculum integrates multiple community experiences throughout the program and utilizes up-to-date computer technology in all course offerings.

General Curriculum Requirements		Semester Hours
ENG 101	Language and Literature	3
ENG 102	Language and Literature	3
BIO 117	Human Anatomy and Physiology	4
BIO 118	Human Anatomy and Physiology II	4
PSY 110	Introduction to Psychology	3
SOC 110	Introduction to Sociology	3

Nursing Curriculum Requirements		Semester Hours
PHM 110	Clinical Pharmacology	3
NTR 101	Introduction to Nutrition	3
BIO 112	Microbiology	4
μ NUR 101	Introduction to Self-Care and Nursing	6
NUR 111	Nursing College Lab I	2
NUR 105	Nursing Issues and Trends I	1
NUR 102	Nursing Care as it Relates to Self Care Across the Life Span	8
NUR 103	Nursing Care as it Relates to Self Care of the Ill or Injured Person	8
NUR 123	Nursing College Lab II	2
§ NUR 106	Transition to Associate Degree Nursing	2
NUR 204	Introduction to the Role of the Nurse Managing Care of Individuals, Families, and Groups	8
NUR 214	Nursing College Lab III	1
NUR 215	Nursing Issues and Trends II	1
	Total credits required for graduation:	**67**

μ Prerequisite: Acceptance to Nursing Major
§ Licensed Practical Nurses (LPNs) may take NUR 106 in the first semester of the program for 2 credits and receive 6 credits for LPN licensure.

APPLYING
Interested persons are advised to contact the Admissions Office for information. Students must achieve a minimum grade of C in all nursing courses, a C- in Biology 117 and 118, and a minimum of a C for previous college work. Applicants are required to take the HCC Assessment/Placement Test, provide proof of high school graduation or a GED, pass a physical examination, be certified in Cardiopulmonary Resuscitation (CPR), and give permission for a Criminal Offender Record Information (CORI) check.

COSTS/FINANCIAL AID
The estimated annual cost is $2,777.00. Financial Aid is available for qualified students. HCC offers Federal Pell Grants, state-funded grants, scholarships, Federal Stafford Loans, and work-study.

CORRESPONDENCE AND INFORMATION
Director of Admissions
Holyoke Community College
303 Homestead Avenue
Holyoke, MA 01040
(413) 552-2850
E-Mail: admissions@hcc.mass.edu

Director of Nursing
Joan Culley
(413) 552-2458 or (413) 552 –2443
E-Mail: jculley@hcc.mass.edu
Web: http://www.hcc.mass.edu

HOUSTON BAPTIST UNIVERSITY
College of Nursing
Houston, Texas

THE UNIVERSITY

Houston Baptist University is a coeducational independent university founded in 1960. It is located in the southwest area of Houston within minutes of the Texas Medical Center, the Galleria, the arenas where Houston's professional sports teams play, museums, great churches, and more.

The campus atmosphere is one that is open to new ideas and traditional academic pursuits, all within a Christian framework that allows for differences and encourages acceptance and inclusion. HBU students come from more than 16 states and 19 foreign countries, and a variety of religious affiliations is represented.

HBU offers a complete curriculum for nursing students.

THE COLLEGE OF NURSING

The College of Nursing is one of five prestigious colleges on campus. The academic program is recognized for its quality. The low student to faculty ratio is designed to promote success as well as development of the whole student.

PROGRAMS OF STUDY

The College of Nursing offers the Bachelor of Science in Nursing (BSN), the Associate Degree in Nursing (ADN), and ADN-to-BSN and LVN-to-ADN/BSN options. The graduate programs include a Master of Science in Nursing (MSN), the Family Nurse Practitioner (FNP), Family Nurse Practitioner-Congregational Care (FNP-CC) and Congregational Care Nurse (CCN).

The mission of the College of Nursing is to prepare the student upon graduation to function in current and future health care settings. Many of the clinical experiences occur in institutions in the world-renowned Texas Medical Center.

Graduates of the ADN and BSN programs are eligible to apply for licensure as a Registered Nurse. The Master of Science degree program leads to advanced nursing practice.

AFFILIATIONS WITH HEALTH CARE FACILITIES

The College of Nursing maintains contractual agreements with health care agencies in the Texas Medical Center as well as numerous community sites and clinics.

FINANCIAL AID

HBU offers institutionally sponsored non-need grants/scholarships, student loans, Federal Pell Grants, Federal Supplemental Educational Opportunity Grants, Federal Work-Study, Federal PLUS Loans, Federal Stafford Loans, and state aid.

COSTS

Estimated expenses for undergraduates per quarter are $3,860 (includes semi-private dorm room with meal plan). Expenses for the MSN-FNP (per 2-year program) are approximately $14,000, for the MSN-FNP-CC (per 2-year program) are approximately $16,250, and for the MSN-CC (per 2-year program) are approximately $11,050.

APPLICATION PROCESS

ADN program—Clear admission to the University, completion of prerequisite courses with no grades below a C with a minimum GPA of 2.25 in required sciences courses and overall GPA of 2.0

BSN program—Clear admission to the University, 3.0 GPA on prerequisite courses with no grade below a C and 3.0 cumulative GPA

MSN program—Clear admission to the University, evidence of an earned baccalaureate degree from a regionally accredited college or university, a GPA of 2.5 or better, and an unencumbered license to practice professional nursing from the Board of Nurse Examiners for the State of Texas

CORRESPONDENCE AND INFORMATION

College of Nursing
Houston Baptist University
7502 Fondren
Houston, Texas 77074-3298
(281) 649-3430
Fax: (281) 649-3340
E-Mail: lcoffman@hbu.edu

HOWARD UNIVERSITY
College of Pharmacy, Nursing and Allied Health Services
Division of Nursing
Washington, DC

THE UNIVERSITY

Howard University was founded in 1867. It has welcomed all serious students—of various ethnic and racial backgrounds, male and female, domestic and international. For generations, Howard has played a singularly pivotal role in African-American culture and life. Howard University is the first truly comprehensive predominantly black institution of higher learning in the world. The almost limitless resources available in the Washington, DC metropolitan area contribute to the total Howard University educational experience.

THE DIVISION OF NURSING

In 1968, a four-year School of Nursing was established, with a program of study leading to a Bachelor of Science degree in nursing. The School of Nursing changed its name to the College of Nursing in 1974. In 1980, the Master of Science degree program in nursing was initiated. In 1993, a post-master's certificate program was added. In 1997, the College of Nursing was merged with two other colleges to form the College of Pharmacy, Nursing and Allied Health Sciences. Both the baccalaureate and master's programs are fully accredited by the National League for Nursing Accrediting Commission and the American Association of Colleges of Nursing.

THE GRADUATE PROGRAM

The Howard University Division of Nursing Graduate Program is designed to prepare baccalaureate-prepared nurses as advanced practice nurses. It offers both the Master of Science in Nursing degree for Family Nurse Practitioners, and a Post-Master's Certificate for Family Nurse Practitioners. In the Graduate Program advanced nursing knowledge is both acquired and generated through the integration of knowledge from the sciences, humanities, nursing theory, and research. Prior experience and future professional goals are considered in designing individualized learning experiences. Students are provided opportunities to implement their roles and assume leadership in a variety of traditional and nontraditional settings utilizing the resources of the healthcare system. In addition to collegial relationships with peers and nursing faculty, the Graduate Program fosters collaborative activities with other disciplines.

AFFILIATIONS WITH HEALTHCARE FACILITIES

The clinical resources available include a wide array of facilities: hospital outpatient clinics, free-standing primary care clinics, HMOs, homeless shelters, senior citizen facilities, Howard University Hospital, and the Howard University ambulatory clinics. Clinical sites are located in Washington, DC and nearby Virginia and Maryland.

ACADEMIC RESOURCES.

The Division of Nursing Learning Resource Center is newly renovated and includes computers with varied software, including computer-assisted instruction. Equipment includes teaching aids for developing nursing expertise—models, examination kits, and audio-visual aids. The Health Science Library provides bibliographic print and non-print informational support to health professionals. Other services and resources provided include assisting with research documentation and computerized literature searches. Inter-library services include other university libraries, the Library of Congress, and the National Library of Medicine. A new state-of-the-art health science library has just been opened.

COSTS

Tuition at Howard University is $11,195 for the 2001–2002 academic year for full-time graduate study. Students taking 9 credit hours or more are classified as full-time students. Part-time tuition is $622 per credit hour. University fees total approximately $350 per semester. Living costs in the Washington, DC, Maryland, and Virginia areas vary depending on location and individual needs. Howard University's housing includes dormitories, and apartments that are available to graduate students as well as faculty members. Specific information on housing can be obtained from the Office of Residence Life.

FINANCIAL AID

Financial assistance includes scholarships, traineeships, and student loans. Although there are many demands on Howard's financial aid resources, the University makes every effort to ensure that all academically qualified students can enjoy the benefits of a Howard University education.

APPLYING

Applicants to the Graduate Program in Nursing must hold a Bachelor of Science in Nursing degree from an accredited college or school, have a cumulative GPA of 3.0 or above, submit three letters of recommendation from persons knowing the applicant professionally or academically, submit a statement of personal goals, and be eligible for RN licensure in the District of Columbia. An interview may be required.

CORRESPONDENCE AND INFORMATION

Howard University
Division of Nursing
Graduate Program
501 Bryant Street, N.W.
Washington, DC 20059
(202) 806-7456
Fax: (202) 806-5958
Web: www.nursing.howard.edu

HURON SCHOOL OF NURSING
Cleveland, Ohio

THE SCHOOL
Huron School of Nursing, located in Cleveland, Ohio, is a quality, progressive program offering dual credentials: a Diploma in Nursing from Huron School of Nursing and an Associate of Science degree from Cuyahoga Community College. Applicants to the school may choose from the 2-year Day or Evening/Weekend program. The School of Nursing places a strong emphasis on the study of nursing in both a classroom and clinical setting. The courses taken in the program include the majority of the support courses required for a Bachelor of Science in Nursing (BSN) completion program. Graduates of Huron School of Nursing are excellently prepared to begin nursing careers in a variety of health care settings.

After more than a century of nursing evolution, Huron School of Nursing continues to be an innovator in nursing education. Originally founded in 1884 as the Cleveland Training School for Nurses, Huron School of Nursing was the first such school of its kind west of the Allegheny Mountains. The establishment of the School of Nursing signaled the beginning of a trend that led to a more rigorous academic and clinical program for the education of registered nurses. Today, as part of the Cleveland Clinic Health System, Huron School of Nursing continues to provide high quality educational resources to meet the needs of the adult learner.

EDUCATIONAL RESOURCES
Huron School of Nursing is committed to providing educational resources to meet the needs of the community that it serves. An outstanding feature of the course of study is a comprehensive liberal arts and science background. The School of Nursing offers the advantage of student clinical experiences at Euclid, Hillcrest, Huron, and South Pointe hospitals, as well as several other respected community health care institutions.

School of Nursing offices and facilities are located at Huron Hospital. The Professional Library offers a wide selection of periodicals and reference material and up-to-date computer technology for the access of nursing and medical information. A Learning Resource Center provides a variety of opportunities for learning via computer and other electronic media, and the Nursing Arts Lab is available for the practice of nursing skills.

Faculty is an important resource in nursing education. The qualified faculty of Huron School of Nursing represents varied backgrounds in education and experience, thus ensuring a learning environment in which the current trends and practices of nursing and patient care are taught.

ADMISSION REQUIREMENTS
To be considered for admission to the School of Nursing, an applicant must be or expect to be a high school graduate. The GED is also accepted. In addition, the following courses at Cuyahoga Community College (or their equivalents at other colleges) must be completed before full acceptance can be granted.

Biology 1100--Introduction to Biological Chemistry OR
Chemistry 1010--Introduction to Inorganic Chemistry (take ONE only)
Biology 2330--Anatomy & Physiology I
English 1010--College Composition I
Psychology 1010--General Psychology
Sociology 1010--Introductory Sociology

A minimum cumulative grade point average of 2.5 is required in the above courses and in all college coursework. In selected instances, an applicant who does not meet admission requirements may be advised to follow a recommended course of study at Cuyahoga Community College. After completion of the recommended coursework, the applicant will be reconsidered for admission.

Applicants to the school must submit a completed School of Nursing application form and a $30 application fee. Official high school and college transcripts and results of the American College Test (ACT), as applicable, are required for admission consideration. Once the school has received the applicant's completed application, an interview will be scheduled with the Coordinator of Student Services. To evaluate written communication skills, applicants will be required to complete a short written exercise at the time of the admission interview. All candidates for admission to the School of Nursing are considered on individual merits without discrimination of the basis of age, creed, national and ethnic origin, race, color, sex, gender/sexual orientation, marital status, or disability.

ADVANCED PLACEMENT FOR LICENSED PRACTICAL NURSES (LPNs) THROUGH ACCESS IN NURSING
Licensed Practical Nurses may seek advanced placement through the ACCESS to Registered Nursing option. Huron School of Nursing was one of the first participants in Access in Nursing, an innovative educational model for nursing advancement in Northeast Ohio. LPNs can achieve advanced placement credit without excessive repetitive coursework and testing. Once the LPN candidate has met admission criteria, eligibility to enroll in the ACCESS to RN transition course will be granted. The transition course, offered at various colleges, validates prior learning and prepares the student for placement into the RN program. For the candidate who is successful in the advanced placement process, it is possible to complete the Day program in 12 months and the Evening/Weekend program in 16 months.

FINANCIAL AID AND SCHOLARSHIP PROGRAMS
Several sources of financial aid, both private and government sponsored, are available to students. Federal and state financial programs include Federal PELL/SEOG grants, Ohio Instructional Grant, Federal Direct Student Loan (subsidized and unsubsidized), Federal Perkins Loan, Nurse Education Assistance Loan Program (NEALP) and Federal College Work Study.

The Florence Mackey Pritchard and P.J. Pritchard Fund, established with the Cleveland Foundation in 1985, awards annual scholarships to qualified students in the second year of the program. The Elizabeth Husni Memorial Scholarship is awarded annually, pending availability of funds, to a qualified East Cleveland resident who is entering Nursing 110. Nursing 110 students residing in East Cleveland (or the surrounding zip codes if there is no qualified East Cleveland resident) are automatically considered for this award. The half tuition scholarship is renewable each semester if the recipient maintains a 3.0 grade point average and earns at least a B in each nursing course. The Cleveland Clinic Health System, Eastern Region offers a generous tuition assistance program for those individuals who are employed by the CCHS, Eastern Region and are enrolled in the Huron School of Nursing.

HURON SCHOOL OF NURSING
(continued)

ACCREDITATIONS AND MEMBERSHIPS

Huron School of Nursing is accredited by the National League for Nursing Accrediting Commission (NLNAC) and approved by the Ohio Board of Nursing. The school is a member of the Council of Diploma Programs of the National League for Nursing and the Ohio Council of Hospital Based Schools of Nursing.

CORRESPONDENCE AND INFORMATION

For an application or more information contact
Barbara Szigeti, MA Coordinator of Student Services or
Kathleen Knittel, RN, MSN, Director
Huron School of Nursing
13951 Terrace Road
Cleveland, Ohio 44112
(216) 761-7996
Fax: (216) 761-7541
Web: www.meridia.com/student.htm

JOHNS HOPKINS UNIVERSITY
School of Nursing
Baltimore, Maryland

THE UNIVERSITY
Since its founding in 1876, the Johns Hopkins University has been in the forefront of higher education. Originally established as an institution oriented toward graduate study and research, it is often called America's first true university. The University has eight academic divisions; Nursing, Medicine, Public Health, Arts and Sciences, Engineering, Professional Studies in Business and Education, Advanced International Studies, and the Peabody Conservatory of Music. With a full-time enrollment of approximately 6,570 students, it is the smallest of the top-ranked universities in the United States and, by its own choice, remains small.

SCHOOL OF NURSING
The School of Nursing attracts a national and international student body of a little over 500. Students become leaders in the nursing profession and are provided a solid foundation on which to base a lifelong career in the ever-growing field of nursing. Students enjoy advantages of an education at an institution with a worldwide reputation and an outstanding network of alumni who serve as mentors. A rigorous academic curriculum, which includes a strong scientific orientation, gives students the background to understand the health-care decisions they will make as professionals. The atmosphere is one where excellence is expected, valued, and reinforced.

PROGRAMS OF STUDY
The School of Nursing offers an upper-division program leading to a BS in nursing. Students with a prior BA/BS degree are eligible to apply to the 13-month Accelerated Program, beginning in June, or to the 2-year Traditional Program. A Direct Entry to a Combined BS to MSN Program is available. The Peace Corps Prep Program integrates academic study followed by volunteer service in the United States Peace Corps. Returned Peace Corps Volunteers are eligible to participate in the Fellows Program, which provides opportunities for clinical education in the Community Outreach Program where human needs of underserved families are met.

Graduate programs leading to the Master of Science in Nursing (MSN) degree are offered. The master's program prepares nurse experts in advanced practice and/or management for leadership in professional nursing practice and patient-centered health-care delivery. Graduate study and research opportunities are available in Adult, Family and Pediatric Primary Care Nurse Practitioner; Adult Acute/Critical Care Nurse Practitioner; Health Systems Management; Clinical Specialist; Community Health; a joint MSN/MBA program with the School of Professional Studies in Business and Education; and a joint MSN/MPH program with the Bloomberg School of Public Health. A 12-credit graduate certificate program, the Business of Nursing, for midlevel career nursing, is offered with the School of Professional Studies in Business and Education. Post-Master's Adult, Family and Pediatric Primary Care Nurse Practitioner Programs, as well as Adult Acute/Critical Care Nurse Practitioner programs are available.

The PhD program prepares nurse scholars to conduct research that advances the theoretical foundation of nursing practice and health-care delivery. Research opportunities are available in selected areas that correspond with the expertise of faculty and University resources.

An MSN/PhD is available. The DNSc program, a summer intensive full-time program offered over four to six consecutive summers, focuses on health outcomes management, health care economics, statistical analysis, and informatics.

ACADEMIC RESOURCES
The School of Nursing is located on the Johns Hopkins Medical Institutions campus, including the School of Medicine, the Bloomberg School of Public Health, Kennedy-Krieger Institute and the Johns Hopkins Hospital. The William H. Welch Medical Library provides the Johns Hopkins Medical Institutions and its affiliates with information services that advance research, teaching, and patient care. The Welch Library Gateway allows access to remote and local online databases. The Carol J. Grey Nursing Information Resources Center (NIRC) is located at the School of Nursing. The Center for Nursing Research provides consultation on research design and conduct. The Nursing Research Laboratory is dedicated to research projects in nursing that incorporate basic biological science methods. There are also three microcomputer, computer/interactive video laboratories, and three nursing Practice Labs are available to provide the student with an opportunity to gain experience and confidence in performing a wide variety of nursing technologies.

COSTS
For the 2001-2002 academic year, undergraduate tuition was $19,022 and graduate tuition was $21,122. The PhD tuition was $25,880 while the DNSc was $15,750. The Business of Nursing tuition was $5,200.

FINANCIAL AID
The School of Nursing attempts to provide financial assistance to all eligible accepted students. Such assistance is usually in the form of loans, grants, scholarships, and work-study programs. Academic and merit based scholarships are also available.

APPLYING
The School of Nursing seeks individuals who will bring to the student body the qualities of scholarship, motivation, and commitment.

Undergraduate program applicants are required to have a completed application form, nonrefundable $50 application fee, three recommendations, official college transcripts, official high school transcript, and SAT/ACT scores (unless holding a college degree or out of high school for over 5 years). Registered nurses must send copy of their Maryland State nursing license. A grade point average of at least 3.0 on a 4.0 scale is recommended. Personal interviews may be requested.

Master's program applicants are required to have a completed application form, nonrefundable $50 application fee, have graduated from a baccalaureate degree program in nursing with a GPA of 3.0 or above on a 4.0 scale, a current nursing license, preferably a year of nursing practice, a score of 1500 or above on the Graduate Record Examinations (GRE) is recommended, three recommendations, and official transcripts from all previous school attended. Personal interviews may be requested.

JOHNS HOPKINS UNIVERSITY
(continued)

PhD applicants are required to submit a completed application form, a nonrefundable $75 application fee, official transcripts from a baccalaureate or master's degree program in nursing (a GPA of 3.5 or above on a 4.0 scale is recommended), official GRE scores not more than 5 years old, a current nursing license, three recommendations, written goal statement and research interests, and research interests that match faculty expertise and School resources.

DNSc applicants are required to have a completed application form, a nonrefundable $75 application fee, have graduated with a GPA of 3.5 or above on a 4.0 scale, a current nursing license, three recommendations, written goal statement, writing samples, and evidence of quantitative expertise.

International students whose native language is not English must submit official test score reports of the Test of English as a Foreign Language (TOEFL). In order to be considered for admission, nonpermanent residents must establish their ability to finance their education and living expenses in the United States. International students must submit official records of all college/university level course work to World Education Service (WES) or to the Commission on Graduates of Foreign Nursing Schools (CGFNS). Students should contact the Office of Admissions and Student Services for additional information regarding the WES and CGFNS evaluation service.

CORRESPONDENCE AND INFORMATION

Johns Hopkins University
School of Nursing
Office of Admissions and Student Services
525 North Wolfe Street
Baltimore, Maryland 21205-2110
(410) 955-7548
Fax: (410) 614-7086
E-Mail: jhuson@son.jhmi.edu
Web: www.son.jhmi.edu

KENNESAW STATE UNIVERSITY
College of Health and Human Services
Kennesaw, Georgia

THE UNIVERSITY
Kennesaw State University (KSU) is a public university in the University System of Georgia. Located in the northwestern side of metropolitan Atlanta, the University offers baccalaureate and professional master's degrees to its 13,000 students in the arts, humanities, sciences, and professional fields of business, social services, and nursing. KSU is located in an ideal position to access the excitement of the urban center as well as the natural beauty and recreational activities of the north Georgia mountains. KSU is a nontraditional, commuter university serving a diverse student body.

THE DEPARTMENTS OF NURSING
The Nursing Programs at KSU are located in a modern building in the center of the main campus. To support their educational experiences, students have both on-campus, state-of-the art learning resources and computer laboratories as well as access to the diverse array of clinical facilities available in metropolitan Atlanta.

PROGRAMS OF STUDY
KSU offers the Baccalaureate Nursing Program to students seeking to be licensed as registered nurses, a bridge option for registered nurses seeking the baccalaureate degree, and a master's program to prepare primary care nurse practitioners. All programs are accredited by the National League for Nursing Accrediting Commission, and the Department of Baccalaureate Degree Nursing has preliminary approval for accreditation by the Commission on Collegiate Nursing Education.

The Department of Primary Care Nursing is a weekends-only program for experienced professionals. The RN-BSN Program is tailored to meet the needs of working nurses and projects online availability of courses in the upcoming year.

AFFILIATIONS WITH HEALTH CARE FACILITIES
The Departments of Nursing maintain contractual agreements with major hospitals, primary care clinics, health departments, and community organizations throughout metropolitan Atlanta. The Department of Primary Care Nursing maintains contracts with a large number of health professionals as preceptors for student learning. Students may also participate in clinical experiences in nursing centers staffed and directed by nursing faculty members.

COSTS
State resident full-time undergraduate tuition is $865 per semester. Nonresident full-time tuition is $3,475 per semester. Additional fees of approximately $200 are added for student services, parking, and technology. The campus does not have dormitories.

FINANCIAL AID
The KSU financial assistance program provides need-based, scholastic and athletic scholarships. The Office of Student Financial Aid processes need-based scholarships and grants, government-guaranteed loans, and work-study programs. In addition, KSU participates in the HOPE scholarship program for superior students. Nursing students are also eligible for Service Cancellable Loans and various targeted scholarships.

APPLICATION
BSN applicants must have full admission to the University, which requires an official transcript from high school and SAT I or ACT scores and/or official transcripts from each university attended, along with a $20 application fee.

Applications are taken during the fall and spring semesters for acceptance into the following spring or fall BSN class. Completion of seven of the twelve prerequisites with a grade point average of at least 2.75 is the minimum requirement for admission. Admission is competitive.

Registered nurses are admitted during the spring semester to begin the one-year completion program in summer. Students must complete sixteen prerequisite courses with a minimum grade point average of 2.75 and include a letter of reference for consideration. All applicants must comply with the requirements of the Georgia RN-BSN Articulation Model and present a current, valid Georgia RN license.

Applicants to the MSN primary-care nurse practitioner program must have a baccalaureate degree in nursing from an NLNAC-accredited institution and a GPA of at least 2.5; a minimum of three years' full-time professional experience within the last five years involving direct patient care; a current license in the state of Georgia; an acceptable score on the GRE; a statement of personal goals for the program; an undergraduate physical assessment course; and full admission into KSU.

CORRESPONDENCE AND INFORMATION
Fran Paul
Administrative Coordinator
College of Health and Human Services
Kennesaw State University
1000 Chastain Road
Kennesaw, GA 30144-5591
(770) 499-3211 or (770) 423-6565
Fax: (770) 423-6627
E-Mail: fpaul@ksumail.kennesaw.edu
Web: www.kennesaw.edu

LAGRANGE COLLEGE
College of Nursing
Lagrange, Georgia

THE COLLEGE
Founded in 1831, LaGrange College is the oldest private college in Georgia. Affiliated with the United Methodist Church, LaGrange College seeks to admit any qualified student. With an enrollment of approximately 1,000 men and women and only 17 students in the average classroom, LaGrange College provides a challenging and supportive academic environment.

PROGRAMS OF STUDY
The Bachelor of Science in Nursing (BSN) curriculum consists of two plans of study. The basic program prepares graduates for entry into professional nursing practice and confers eligibility for initial licensure as a registered professional nurse (RN). A degree-completion option is designed for licensed RNs who wish to earn the BSN degree.

The curriculum provides professional nursing education within a heritage of Christian faith and liberal arts learning. The nursing major, grounded in an ethic of caring, encourages independent thought, appreciation for the discovery of excellence, and commitment to supporting the health of individuals and society. BSN studies establish a sound foundation for professional nursing practice, graduate study, and continuing progress toward personal and professional goals. Faculty and students serve as resources for the College and community in nursing education, service, and research. Opportunities for collaborative study with students of other majors and clinical experience with varied health care providers emphasize the interdisciplinary nature of nursing practice. As professional nurses, graduates will be able to assist individuals, groups, and communities in meeting health care goals.

The BSN program is fully approved by the Georgia Board of Nursing and is accredited by the National League for Nursing Accrediting Commission.

AFFILIATIONS WITH HEALTH CARE FACILITIES
LaGrange College of Nursing clinical resources include West Georgia Health Systems, a comprehensive facility in LaGrange, which provides multiple sites for student learning. Many community-based health care agencies also provide valuable practice opportunities.

ACADEMIC RESOURCES
The William and Evelyn Banks Library is a modern academic learning center that provides volumes of books, periodicals, and multimedia. Students benefit from two computing centers and a Writing Center.

COSTS
Tuition and fees for 2002–2003 were $16,000, and room and board were $5,600 for the year, bringing the total estimated costs for 2002–2003 to $21,600. Estimated book costs range from $800 to $1,200 per year.

FINANCIAL AID
LaGrange College offers institutionally-sponsored non-need grants/scholarship, Federal Nursing Student Loans, Federal Pell Grants, Federal Perkins Loans, Federal Supplemental Educational Opportunity Grants, Federal Work-Study, Federal PLUS Loans, Federal Stafford Loans, and state aid. Scholarships are available.

APPLYING
For the BSN program, application for admission to the upper-division program is made during the sophomore year. Admission requirements are as follows:

1. A completed Application for Admission to Nursing
2. Complete a sufficient number of credits in General Education and other required courses
3. A grade of C or higher is required in anatomy, physiology, microbiology, and English composition courses
4. A cumulative overall GPA of 2.5 or higher

For the BSN Completion Option, application for admission is made to the College and nursing program. Admission requirements are as follows:

1. RN licensure
2. RN students must have completed all General Education Requirements and all required non-nursing courses through the junior level
3. Thirty-eight (38) additional nursing course credits must be earned at the upper division level

CORRESPONDENCE AND INFORMATION
Director of Nursing
Division of Nursing
LaGrange College
601 Broad Street
LaGrange, GA 30240
(706) 812-7220
Fax: (706) 884-6567

LANCASTER INSTITUTE FOR HEALTH EDUCATION
Lancaster, PA

OVERVIEW
The Lancaster Institute for Health Education is a small, private, non-profit institution dedicated to the education of health care workers. The Institute is a division of Lancaster General Hospital, one of the five busiest hospitals in Pennsylvania. The School of Nursing enrollment is 225.

PROGRAM OF STUDY
The School of Nursing curriculum is planned to provide the student with the principles and skills necessary to assume a beginning professional nurse position in hospitals and related institutions. Graduates of the two year program receive a diploma in nursing and are eligible to take the examination for licensure. The School of Nursing is affiliated with Lancaster General College of Nursing and Health Sciences.

The nursing program integrates classroom study with hands-on experience in a variety of clinical settings. A 10:1 student/faculty ratio assures individualized attention from professional and caring instructors.

LEARNING RESOURCE PROGRAM
The Learning Resource Program is a special academic assistance program designed to help all students achieve maximum academic success. The program includes individual tutorial assistance as well as special programs designed to promote students' success. These include computer classes, writing workshops, study skills, special interest seminars, and study groups. Two Computer Learning Laboratories are available to all students to enhance learning, provide remedial assistance, and facilitate completion of student assignments.

CLINICAL LABORATORY
Facilities of the Lancaster Health Alliance comprise the primary clinical settings. Additional experiences are offered to students through agreements with various acute care hospitals, outpatient clinics, home health agencies, long-term care facilities, schools, and community health agencies.

FEES
First year tuition is $8,100; second year tuition is $6,975.

FINANCIAL AID
Students are eligible to apply for grants, Stafford loans, state aid, and veteran's benefits. Students may also apply for private scholarships and loans administered jointly by private agencies, governmental agencies, and the School of Nursing.

ADMISSION REQUIREMENTS
Students applying for admission to the School of Nursing must meet the following requirements:

1. Must qualify or have graduated from an approved secondary school or met the requirements for the GED. A minimum of 16 units must be completed as follows: english-4; chemistry-1, biology-1, algebra-1, other mathematics-1, social studies-3, and electives-5
2. Satisfactory achievement on the Scholastic Aptitude Test or the ACT Assessment Program
3. Satisfactory performance on the pre-nursing assessment test
4. Three references from teachers, guidance counselors, or employers

APPLICATION
The School of Nursing has a rolling admissions policy and usually notifies applicants within a month after completed forms and supporting credentials are received. Classes begin in August and January. An evening program begins each August.

FOR INFORMATION
Lancaster Institute for Health Education
School of Nursing
410 N. Lime St.
Lancaster, PA 17602
(717) 290-4912 or toll-free 1-800-622-5443
Web: www.lha.org

LA SALLE UNIVERSITY
School of Nursing
Philadelphia, PA and Newtown, PA

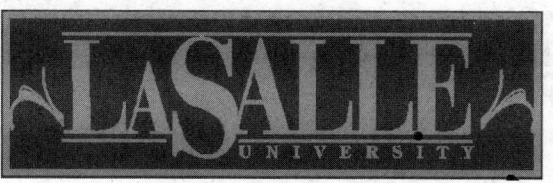

THE UNIVERSITY
La Salle University is a private Roman Catholic University conducted under the auspices of the Christian Brothers. Established in 1863, La Salle is a comprehensive university committed to a liberal education of both general and specialized studies. La Salle offers small classes, numerous academic and non-academic opportunities in the City of Philadelphia and surrounding counties, and the expectation that its students will become involved in service to the community.

SCHOOL OF NURSING
Founded in 1980, the School of Nursing offers programs of study that educate nurses to develop knowledge, values, and basic and advanced skills to enable them to think critically, sharpen esthetic perception, communicate effectively, and intervene therapeutically with individuals and communities. The ultimate aim of the School of Nursing is to continuously affirm the mission of the University in preparing its graduates to live meaningful and productive lives.

PROGRAMS OF STUDY
The School of Nursing offers multiple programs of study for all levels of learners at baccalaureate and graduate level. Baccalaureate programs include generic BSN, LPN-BSN, and RN-BSN. A part time evening and weekend generic BSN program is offered. An RN-MSN option and MSN Bridge Program for nurses with a non-nursing baccalaureate degree are also available. Graduate level programs include six specialization tracks: Adult Clinical Nurse Specialist, Adult Nurse Practitioner, Family Nurse Practitioner, MSN in Nursing Administration/MBA (dual degree), Nurse Anesthesia, and Public Health Nursing.

Certificate Programs offering graduate credits include: Clinical Research Operations (drug trials), Nursing Informatics, School Nurse, and Wound, Ostomy, Continence Nursing Education Program (WOCNEP) (Enterostomal Therapy).

COSTS
Tuition costs are $550 per credit for graduate level courses. Application fees are $35. Semester fees are $75 per semester. Nursing students may also have physical examination and other miscellaneous fees.

FINANCIAL AID
La Salle University offers a variety of financial aid programs that are funded by government and private sources. Graduate students are eligible for federal traineeship grants and University-based graduate assistantships.

APPLYING
All applicants must complete the appropriate application. Graduate Nursing Program applicants are expected to have a minimum GPA of 3.0 and acceptable scores in the Graduate Record Examination (GRE), Miller Analogies Test (MAT), or Graduate Management Test (GMAT). All applicants must have graduated from an NLNAC- or CCNE-accredited School of Nursing or completed an MSN-Bridge Program. Courses in undergraduate research and statistics are prerequisite.

INFORMATION
Director of Graduate Program
or
Director of Undergraduate Program

La Salle University
School of Nursing
1900 W. Olney Avenue
Philadelphia, PA 19141
(215) 951-1430
Fax: (215) 951-1896
Web: www.lasalle.edu

LAWRENCE MEMORIAL/REGIS COLLEGE
Collaborative ASN Program
Medford, Massachusetts

THE SCHOOL
The school, established in 1924, continues to prepare graduates for RN licensure. The strengths of the original diploma program are incorporated into the new associate degree of science in nursing offered in collaboration with Regis College, which was incorporated in 1927. Two campuses in the Boston suburbs offer many cultural, educational, and social opportunities. On the Medford campus, located eight miles north of Boston, the School shares 16 acres with Lawrence Memorial Hospital of Medford, a 150-bed acute care facility, and the Courtyard Nursing Care Center, a 224-bed state-of-the-art nursing home. The Weston campus of Regis College, 12 miles west of Boston, provides a beautiful New England residential campus of 168 acres.

THE NURSING PROGRAM
Students may choose full-time study in the two-year day division or part-time study in the three-year day or evening/weekend division. Small instructor to student ratios (1:32 in class and 1:6–8 in clinical experiences) provide individualized instruction. Previous education is recognized through the transfer of college credits for comparable courses. Advanced placement options are available for LPNs and transferring nursing students. Students have varied backgrounds; some come directly from high school, others have post-secondary education, some have college degrees in other fields.

The 72 credits earned within the curriculum facilitate admission to a baccalaureate and master's degree program in nursing. The school offers dual admission at the time of acceptance for qualified candidates to the BSN/MSN program for graduates who wish to pursue further degrees. Completion of the MSN degree takes three years on a full-time basis; part-time study is available.

VARIETY OF CLINICAL AFFILIATIONS
Students' learning experiences are maximized through early involvement with patients. Clinical learning opportunities are provided in local suburban hospitals, major Boston teaching hospitals, long-term care facilities, and community, home care, and social service agencies.

SCHOOL FACILITIES
The facilities include state-of-the-art computer and audio-visual laboratories. A fully equipped nursing arts lab allows students to become proficient in nursing skills in the safety of a laboratory environment. The library and laboratories on the Medford campus are available to students 24 hours a day, seven days a week, allowing for unlimited learning and practice opportunities. A new renovated residence is available.

COSTS AND FINANCIAL AID
Tuition cost for the entire program is $22,165 (2 years full-time study or 3 years part-time). Room costs are $1,750 per semester for single rooms, $1,500 for double rooms.

The school administers Federal Pell Grants, Federal Supplemental Educational Opportunity Grants, Federal Perkins Loans, Federal Stafford Loans, Federal Parents' Loan to Undergraduate Students, Federal Nursing Student Loans, Massachusetts state grants and loans, and institutional grants and private scholarships.

APPLICATION
The school uses a rolling admissions program with one-month admission notification after all materials are received. Requirements include: high school diploma (B average) or GED (scores of 45 in each of 5 test areas); high school algebra, biology and chemistry (C- or better); SAT for high school graduates within past 5 years. For international applicants, TOEFL is required.

FURTHER INFORMATION
Admission Coordinator
Lawrence Memorial/Regis College Collaborative ASN Program
Lawrence Memorial Hospital
170 Governors Avenue
Medford, MA 02155
(781) 306-6657
Fax: (781) 306-6142
Web: www.lmregisnurse.org

LOMA LINDA UNIVERSITY
School of Nursing
Loma Linda, CA

THE UNIVERSITY
Loma Linda University, an academic health sciences center supported by the Seventh-day Adventist Church, was founded in 1905. It is located in the San Bernardino valley, part of inland Southern California. The original School of Nursing and School of Medicine have been joined by the School of Allied Health Professions, School of Dentistry, School of Pharmacy, School of Public Health, Graduate School, and the Faculty of Religion.

THE SCHOOL OF NURSING
The mission of the School of Nursing is to train individuals from diverse ethnic and cultural communities to become professional nurses who are dedicated to excellence in nursing science. Baccalaureate and graduate nursing programs contribute to the development of expert clinicians, educators, administrators, and researchers who contribute to society by providing and improving delivery of whole-person care to clients. Committed to Christian service and distinctive Seventh-day Adventist ideals, the School seeks to reflect God's love through its teaching and healing ministry.

The School of Nursing is accredited by the California Board of Registered Nursing, the National League for Nursing Accrediting Commission, and the Commission of Collegiate Nursing Education.

ADMISSION TO THE NURSING MAJOR
The School accepts applicants who have successfully completed all prerequisite courses at an accredited college. Because Loma Linda University is a health sciences campus, it does not offer general education courses. The following options are available:

Undergraduate program in nursing

1. BS in nursing—3 year program for students who have completed prerequisite courses.
2. BS/BA—2 year program for students with a four-year degree in another major.
3. RN/BS—1 year program for nurses with an associate degree.
4. LVN/BS—3 year program for nurses with an LVN license.
5. AS to MS—3 year program for nurses with an AS degree who have at least three years of experience.

Graduate program in nursing

1. MS degree for clinical nurse specialists (6 to 7 quarter program for nurses with a BS degree) in nursing with specializations in:

   Adult and Aging Family
   Growing Family
   School Nursing

2. MS degree for nurse practitioners—(8 quarter program for nurses with a BS degree in nursing, and at least one year of experience) with specialization in:

   Adult nurse practitioner
   Family nurse practitioner
   Neonatal critical care nursing
   Pediatric nurse practitioner

FINANCIAL AID
Loma Linda University recognizes that financing a college education is a concern for many families. Scholarships and loans are available. We encourage all students to contact the office of financial aid at (909) 558-4509.

APPLYING
Application forms may be obtained by calling (800) 422-4558, option 2 for an undergraduate nursing program application, and option 6 for a graduate nursing program application. Students wishing to contact the undergraduate nursing program may write the Loma Linda University School of Nursing admissions office. The graduate nursing program may be reached by calling the School of Nursing or the Graduate School. You may also access our Web site.

CORRESPONDENCE
Loma Linda University
School of Nursing
Loma Linda, CA 92350
(909) 558-4923 or (800) 422-4558
Web: www.llu.edu/llu/nursing/

dsalinas@sn.llu.edu—undergraduate nursing program
jbates@sn.llu.edu—graduate nursing program

LONG ISLAND UNIVERSITY
Brooklyn Campus
School of Nursing
Brooklyn, New York

GENERAL INFORMATION
Long Island University has grown to be one of the largest multi-campus institutions of higher learning in the U.S., with a total enrollment of 23,500 students and a complement of more than 600 full-time faculty. Coeducational and nonsectarian, Long Island University is accredited by the Middle States Association of Colleges and Secondary Schools, and is a member of the College Board and Association of American Colleges and the Middle Atlantic Association of Colleges of Business Administration.

CAMPUS BACKGROUND
The Brooklyn Campus, founded in 1926, is the original unit of Long Island University and the only one located in New York City. It occupies a 10-acre site in downtown Brooklyn, convenient to all subway lines, many bus lines, and the Long Island Rail Road. Serving an enrollment of 6,300 undergraduate and 1,800 graduate students, it includes the following administrative units: Richard L. Conolly College of Liberal Arts and Sciences; the School of Business, Public Administration, and Information Sciences; the School of Education; the School of Health Professions; the Arnold & Marie Schwartz College of Pharmacy and Health Sciences; and the School of Nursing, which is housed in the new William Zeckendorf Health Sciences Center.

ACADEMIC PROGRAMS
BS in Nursing: The program, leading to a Bachelor of Science with a major in Nursing, is accredited by the National League for Nursing Accrediting Commission and holds preliminary approval from the Commission on Collegiate Nursing Education. The Program is designed to prepare the student to develop the competencies essential for beginning professional nursing practice and to build a foundation for graduate study.

RN-BS Connection Program (Program for Registered Nurses): The BS in Nursing is also available to registered nurses seeking the baccalaureate degree through the RN-BS Connection Program. Registered nurses admitted into the program may transfer up to 64 credits, including required core curriculum, pre-requisite and distribution credits. Transferred credits may also include up to 31 credits in previously completed nursing courses. Flexible course schedules are available for the working professional.

MS in Nursing for Adult, Geriatric, and Family Nurse Practitioners, and Advanced Certificate Program: The Adult, Geriatric, and Family Nurse Practitioner Programs are designed for the development of refined analytical skills, the ability to connect theory to practice, and the acquisition of advanced practitioner skills to provide primary care to an adult population. The Post Master's Certificate program is available to nurses who have an earned master's degree and are seeking clinical expertise in the advanced practice role for the care of adult, geriatric, and family clients.

MS in Nursing—Executive Program for Nursing and Health Care Management: The Executive Program for Nursing and Health Care Management provides advanced nursing content and understanding of complex nursing issues through courses taught by both Nursing and Business faculty. It prepares nurses for leadership positions in hospitals, nursing homes, community health centers, HMOs, home care agencies, consulting firms, and entrepreneurial ventures.

Graduate programs are fully accredited by the Commission on Collegiate Nursing Education.

BS/MS Accelerated Program: The Bachelor of Science/Master of Science Program is designed for the registered nurse with an associate degree who wishes to fulfill career goals by pursuing the baccalaureate and the Master's degrees in nursing with preparation as an Adult Nurse Practitioner or Nurse Executive.

FACULTY AND ADMINISTRATION
Composed of the Dean and eighteen full-time faculty. Five hold doctorates and twelve hold Master's degrees. Many faculty are certified nurse practitioners or hold other advanced clinical credentials. Thirty-three adjunct faculty provide didactic instruction and supervision at clinical sites. A full-time Laboratory Resource Instructor and two full-time Academic Advisors provide additional student support.

SPECIAL FEATURES OF THE SCHOOL AND PROGRAMS

- Multicultural student body with high minority enrollment
- Individual support and advisement to facilitate academic success on the pre-professional and professional levels
- Pathways for access to baccalaureate entry-level and advanced graduate nursing education leading to upward professional mobility
- Flexibility in course of study for non-traditional students

LOURDES COLLEGE
Sylvania, OH

THE COLLEGE
Lourdes College is an independent, coeducational liberal arts college sponsored by the Sylvania Franciscans. In the tradition of fine liberal arts schools, Lourdes focuses on helping every student reach his or her potential as an educated person and as a well-rounded human being.

DEPARTMENT OF NURSING
The Lourdes College Bachelor of Science in Nursing Program prepares professional nursing practitioners who can perform as generalists within a variety of settings. Students learn in "an atmosphere that nurtures an holistic approach to learning within a caring, supportive, faith community." The curriculum provides a general education with a foundation for lifelong learning and post-graduate education in nursing.

The course work is based on a foundation in liberal arts and seven major components or organizers: adaptive nursing process, health, professional leadership, client, scholarship/critical thinking, communication, and management. The curriculum is flexible to meet the changing needs of students and society. Full and part-time study and some evening classes are available.

PROGRAMS OF STUDY
Lourdes College accepts freshman applicants, transfer students, and RNs who are graduates of associate degree and diploma programs.

ADMISSION FOR RN STUDENTS
Graduates of diploma and associate degree programs in nursing may apply as matriculated candidates for the BSN degree. Registered nurses who have college credits should apply as transfer students.

ADMISSION TO THE NURSING MAJOR
Applicants are considered for the Nursing Major on a competitive basis. Admission decisions are based on the following criteria: completion of formal admission at Lourdes College, completion of formal application to the Nursing Major, completion of specified prerequisite courses, Lourdes College GPA of 2.5 or better, and "C" or better in all natural science courses.

AFFILIATIONS WITH HEALTH CARE FACILITIES
The Department of Nursing maintains contractual agreements with more than 47 health care agencies. Clinical settings provide a variety of direct practice sites in hospitals, extended care facilities, clinics, schools, homes, and other community venues.

ACADEMIC RESOURCES
Resources include the Duns Scotus Library, as well as the Nursing Learning Resource Center. The WIN Center offers workshops and tutoring.
Degrees
-BSN Basic
-RN-BSN Completion

ACCREDITATION
The Lourdes College BSN Program is accredited by the National League for Nursing Accrediting Commission (NLNAC, 61 Broadway, New York, NY 10006, 800-669-1656). The program has preliminary approval by the Commission on Collegiate Nursing Education, is Ohio Board of Regents authorized, and is Ohio Board of Nursing approved.

COSTS
Full-time students: $6,850 per semester (12+ credit hours)
Part-time students: $315 per credit hour per semester.
Additional general fees also apply.

FINANCIAL AID
Lourdes College administers financial aid programs that provide assistance to eligible students. All financial aid applicants are required to file the Free Application for Federal Student Aid (FAFSA) and the Lourdes College Financial Aid Application.

CONTACT INFORMATION
Lourdes College
6832 Convent Blvd.
Sylvania, OH 43560
Admissions: (419) 885-5291
1-800-878-3210, ext. 1299
E-Mail: LCADMITS@lourdes.edu
Web: www.lourdes.edu

For more information, contact
Department of Nursing
Susan Bernheisel, MSN, RN
800-878-3210, ext. 3793
E-Mail: SBERNHEI@lourdes.edu

LUTHERAN MEDICAL CENTER SCHOOL OF NURSING
South Point Hospital
St. Louis, Missouri

THE SCHOOL OF NURSING

Mrs. Louise Krauss-Ament organized the training program for nurses and accepted its first six students in 1896. The two-year program graduated its inaugural class in 1900, and since that time more than 3,500 graduate nurses have joined the ranks of professional nursing. The program has, for more than a century, dedicated itself to the training of nurses who have earned their diplomas and translated them into a legacy of caring. Lutheran Medical Center School of Nursing is the only diploma school in the state of Missouri and is accredited by the National League for Nursing Accrediting Commission and the Missouri State Board of Nursing Approval.

PROGRAMS OF STUDY

The Lutheran Medical Center School of Nursing offers a Registered Nurse diploma program, which is 22 months in duration. A Licensed Professional Nurse-to Registered Nurse bridge program is also offered and is 14 months (full-time) or 26 months (part-time) in duration. Both courses provide the eligibility for application for licensure as a Registered Nurse.

CLINICAL AFFILIATIONS

The school of nursing holds contractual agreements with over 15 health care agencies. Students are trained in a wide variety of clinical settings including community hospitals, home health agencies, school health, day care facilities, and clinics. The student trains in the full gamut of experience from acute care learned in emergency and intensive care units to community ambulatory care. Clinical experience begins the fourth week of enrollment in the program.

COSTS

Tuition is based on $180 per credit hour for nursing and non-nursing courses. Each student incurs uniform, book, fees, physical examination, and other miscellaneous expenses. (A full description of the fee and tuition structure is available through the admissions office and the school brochure, which is available upon request.)

FINANCIAL AID

Financial aid opportunities exist for the Lutheran Medical Center School of Nursing student. Institutional work-study programs, federal student loans, grants, and the Tenet Future Nurse program are but a few offered. For information and a pre-application interview with the Financial Aid Director, call (314) 577-5878 or contact by E-Mail at: debatinm@hotmail.com.

APPLICATIONS

Applications are accepted for Fall and Spring enrollment. The following are requirements for consideration for admission:

- Admission application form with the $20 application fee
- Autobiographical statement (1-2 typed pages)
- Official High School transcript with a GPA of 2.3 or above on a 4.0 scale or a GED equivalency certificate
- ACT score of 20 or SAT total score of 830
- ACT/SAT requirement may be waived if applicant has 20 or more college level credit hours
- Official transcripts from all institutions of higher learning with a college GPA of 2.3 or above on a 4.0 scale in English Comp 1, Intro to Sociology, and General Psychology
- College Level Examination for Proficiency (CLEP) scores can be accepted for the three prerequisite courses if the student scores five points above the passing score recommended by the American Council of Education, and the student has a high school GPA of 2.3 or higher, an ACT score of 20 or higher, or has completed 20 or more college-level credits
- Finally, three letters of suitability must be provided from persons other than family members knowing the student six (6) months or more.

LPNs must take and pass the LPN-GAP test if required. The student must take and pass the Lutheran Medical Center School of Nursing Role Transition LPN to RN courses with a "C" or better. All other prerequisites for nursing program apply for the LPN-RN bridge program.

CORRESPONDENCE AND INFORMATION

Enrollment Coordinator
Lutheran Medical Center School of Nursing
3547 South Jefferson Avenue
St. Louis, Missouri 03118
(314) 750-6567
Web: www.nursingschoolmc.com

MASSACHUSETTS BAY COMMUNITY COLLEGE
Framingham, Massachusetts

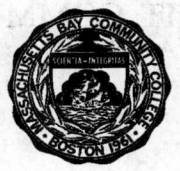

THE COLLEGE
Massachusetts Bay Community College is a publicly supported associate degree- and certificate-granting institution. The College was founded in 1961 and operates two campuses. The Wellesley Hills Campus is located on a scenic 84-acre site ten miles west of Boston. The Framingham Campus is twenty miles west of Boston. It is home to over 5,000 full- and part-time students and 199 faculty and staff. The primary programmatic focus is Advanced Technologies and the Health Sciences, with strong transfer programs in Liberal Arts and Business.

NURSING PROGRAMS OF STUDY
The Nursing Program offers an Associate of Science in Nursing Degree, a LPN to RN Transition Program, and a Practical Nursing Certificate (Day and Evening Options). Graduates are eligible to apply for licensure as a Registered Nurse (RN) or a Licensed Practical Nurse (LPN) respectively. The mission of the Nursing Program is to prepare the student upon graduation to function as a beginning practitioner of nursing. The nursing programs are both located on the Framingham campus.

AFFILIATIONS WITH CLINICAL FACILITIES
Mass Bay Community College's Health Professions Division maintains contractual agreements with more than 250 health care agencies. The school's clinical resources include inpatient and outpatient community hospitals/facilities, Boston area teaching hospitals, skilled nursing facilities, mental health facilities, and community nursing placements.

ACADEMIC RESOURCES
Students have state-of-the-art lab facilities, a Learning Resource Center, a Writing Center, Computer Centers, Tutoring Services, and Library facilities on both campuses.

COSTS
State resident tuition is $63 per credit, and non-resident is $269 per credit. In addition, the nursing program fee is $68 per credit for ADN and $30 per credit for PNs. The ADN program is 77 credits, with 44 nursing credits, for a total cost of $7,843 for residents. The LPN program is 48 credits, with 32 nursing credits, for a total cost of $3,984 for residents.

FINANCIAL AID
Financial aid is available to all qualified students for basic college expenses. The aid may be in the form of a grant, scholarship, loan, a form of employment, or any combination of these. The College's resources are obtained from federal, state, local, or private sources. Applicant eligibility is defined by the funding source.

APPLYING
Enrollment in the nursing programs is limited, and may not accommodate all qualified applicants. Priority is given to MBCC students.
Prerequisites for the ADN program include:

- Completion of college level chemistry with lab with a grade of C or better
- Proficiency in reading, writing, and mathematics as determined by the College placement testing.

Prerequisites for LPN to RN Transition program:

- LPN licensure
- Testing is required for some advanced placement options.

Prerequisites for the LPN Program include:

- High school diploma or GED
- Proficiency in reading, writing, and mathematics as determined by the College placement testing.

Transfer Students for ADN or LPN:

- Submit course syllabi to the department chairperson. A maximum of one semester of nursing is accepted in transfer.

International Students:
Evidence of proficiency in English such as:

- Test of English as a Foreign Language
- Michigan Test Scores
- Success in English course work at the secondary or college level

CORRESPONDENCE AND INFORMATION
Office of Enrollment Services
Massachusetts Bay Community College
50 Oakland Street
Wellesley, MA 02481
(781) 239-2511 Health Professions Recruiter
(781) 239-3000 main number
Web: www.massbay.edu

MASSASOIT COMMUNITY COLLEGE
Brockton, MA

THE COLLEGE
Massasoit Community College, founded in 1966, is a state supported, comprehensive two year college that offers a quality education leading to Associate Degree in Arts, Sciences, and Applied Sciences, as well as one-year certificate programs. Our career and transfer programs provide students with a wide variety of educational opportunities that prepare them for life, leadership, and work. With two campus settings in Brockton and Blue Hills/Canton, the college allows for limitless options in a variety of Liberal Arts, Allied Health, Engineering Technologies, and Business fields of study. The college also offers continuing education day and evening credit and non-credit courses as well as community service programs at both the Brockton and Blue Hills/Canton campuses.

The Brockton Campus is a 100-acre facility that offers students a Fine Arts Building with two theaters, a TV studio and a radio station; a Field House, which houses an Olympic-sized swimming pool, racquetball courts, and weight room; and modern classroom buildings and laboratory facilities.

THE NURSE EDUCATION DEPARTMENT
Massasoit Community College, through its Nurse Education Department, offers a two year program leading to an Associate in Science Degree in Nursing. Graduates of the program are eligible to take the NCLEX Exam for licensure as Registered Nurses. Massasoit is approved by all state and federal agencies including the Veteran's Administration and the Department of Health and Education. It is an Associate member of the American Association of Community and Junior Colleges, and an accredited member of the New England Association of Schools and Colleges. The Nursing program is also fully accredited by the National League for Nursing Accrediting Commission. Full approval status is granted by the Massachusetts Board of Registration in Nursing.

CLINICAL AFFILIATIONS
All nursing students have clinical experience in acute, long-term, and community-based settings. Clinical areas are gerontology, maternity, medical-surgical, pediatrics, and psychiatric nursing.

ACADEMIC RESOURCES
The Academic Resource Center offers a full range of tutoring and academic support services. Individual and small group tutoring is available in most subject areas, and students can work with certified special needs or learning disabilities tutors. The focus of most tutoring is on helping the student become a more effective, more independent learner. In addition, students are encouraged to come to the ARC to study, either individually or with a classmate. Walk-in tutoring is available in several subject areas, and there are a number of study groups, some with tutors and some without, running out of the ARC.

In addition to tutorial services, students can utilize the ARC for access to computers for word processing and tutorials in certain subject areas.

COSTS
In-state, full-time tuition and fees—$2,070 per semester. Per credit cost is $69. Nursing students pay an additional $20 per credit for nursing courses.

FINANCIAL AID
Massasoit Community College participates in a number of financial aid programs in order to assist in financing the cost of your education. Financial Aid assistance includes scholarships, grants, loans and employment awards. Awards are made when personal and family resources are not sufficient to pay educational expenses.

Students who wish to be considered for all forms of financial aid must file an FAFSA (Free Application for Federal Student Aid) and a Massasoit Community College Financial Aid Application. The priority deadline is April 10th for the Fall Semester and November 1st for the Spring Semester. Applications received after the priority deadline will be considered based on available funding.

ADMISSION REQUIREMENTS
Application Deadline: February 1

1. Complete the application process for the Nursing Program through the Admissions Office by deadline date: February 1.
2. High School graduate or equivalent.
3. Recommended high school biology or chemistry.
4. Biological Principles course as a prerequisite for Anatomy & Physiology or challenge of Biological Principles examination arranged by the Testing & Assessment Office (508) 588-9100, ext. 1991.
5. All candidates will be required to take the Entrance Examination for Schools of Nursing developed by the Psychological Corporation (Call the Testing/Assessment Office at the College—x1991).
6. Submit one letter of reference and one letter written in your own behalf stating why you would be a good candidate for the Nursing program.
7. Upper 1/2 of class upon graduation from high school or demonstrated college level performance with a GPA of 3.0, based on 15 credits.

CONTACT PERSON
Roberta Noodell
Director of Admissions
Massasoit Community College
One Massasoit Blvd.
Brockton, MA 02302
(508) 588-9100, ext. 1410

MEDCENTER ONE
COLLEGE OF NURSING
Bismarck, North Dakota

EXCELLENCE, SERVICE, RESPECT, AND CARING
These are the hallmarks of nursing education at Medcenter One College of Nursing. If you are seeking a college that nurtures excellence through continuous improvement, service to students, respect for the individual, and a deep commitment to caring, then Medcenter One College of Nursing is the right choice.

ABOUT THE COLLEGE
Medcenter One College of Nursing (MOCN) is an accredited, coeducational institution in Bismarck, the capital of North Dakota. An upper division college, the class size is small. The student/faculty ratio is eight to one, helping students acquire individual education in a caring environment.

The mission of the college is to prepare a knowledgeable and caring professional nurse who is conscious of and sensitive to the health needs of individuals, families, and communities. We believe that humans are integrated holistic beings having dignity and worth. In holistic nursing, human compassion is blended with technical skills to treat both the mind and body of the individual.

We require a liberal education as the basis for professional nursing education. Prerequisite requirements include the natural, behavioral, and social sciences, and the arts and humanities.

HISTORY
In 1909, Bismarck Hospital, the predecessor of Medcenter One, established a school of nursing. During the ensuing years, the school changed to keep pace with trends in professional nursing education and practice. Medcenter One College of Nursing was authorized to operate as a college in 1988. More than 2,000 nurses have graduated from the former school of nursing and the college of nursing.

PROGRAMS OF STUDY
Completion of the curriculum leads to a bachelor of science in nursing degree (BSN). The college offers programs of study for generic students, RNs seeking a Baccalaureate degree, and LPN to RN students.

The MOCN evidence-based curriculum uses science and research to confirm the methods of nursing. Students learn more than technical and clinical skills. They study wellness and illness through the life cycle, read and report on research in professional journals, and participate in community activities and agencies dealing with issues of well being.

AFFILIATIONS WITH HEALTH CARE FACILITIES
The college utilizes a major referral health center to provide experiences in pediatrics, intensive care, nursery, emergency care, telemetry, oncology, maternity care, and many other areas of the hospital. MOCN works closely with allied health agencies to provide students additional healthcare experience in clinics, schools, rural areas, and community settings.

ACADEMIC RESOURCES
The Medcenter One College of Nursing building houses classrooms, faculty and administration offices, two clinical learning labs, a computer lab, conference rooms, and study areas. The Medcenter One/Q&R Clinic Health Science Library consists of 15,000 books and 350 periodicals on which to base your nursing research experiences.

COSTS
Full-time tuition is $8,000 per year. Dormitory suites are available at $900 per semester for a single room and $450 per semester for double occupancy.

FINANCIAL AID
MOCN participates in all federal Title IV financial aid programs. The college also offers many nursing scholarship and loan options.

APPLYING
Applicants are considered on the basis of scholastic ability and achievement, maturity, and integrity. To be considered for admission, an applicant must demonstrate satisfactory completion of general education work with a minimum GPA of 2.5 and science minimum GPA of 2.5. Students are encouraged to apply after completion of three prerequisite sciences. Once this prerequisite course work is complete, applications will be accepted until classes are filled.

RNs and LPNs must provide evidence of a current/unencumbered license from any USA jurisdiction and/or proof of eligibility of licensure in North Dakota.

CORRESPONDENCE AND INFORMATION
Mary Smith, Director of Student Services
Medcenter One College of Nursing
512 N. 7th Street
Bismarck, ND 58501
(701) 323-6271
E-Mail: dschwe@mohs.org
Web: www.medcenterone.com/nursing/nursing.htm

MEDCENTRAL COLLEGE OF NURSING
Mansfield, Ohio

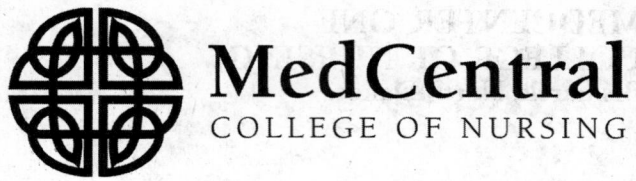

THE COLLEGE
MedCentral College of Nursing is an independently incorporated academic institution that awards a Bachelor of Science degree in Nursing (BSN) to candidates who successfully complete a four-year course of study. Located in Mansfield,Ohio, the college collaborates with The Ohio State University–Mansfield Campus and MedCentral Health Care System, the largest health care provider between Cleveland and Columbus.

The faculty of MedCentral College of Nursing is committed to fostering an environment supportive of academic excellence and the personal and professional growth of its students. The unique experiences, talents, and capabilities of each student are respected as both faculty and students work to promote an educational environment conducive to learning.

MedCentral College's curriculum is designed to offer rigorous classroom instruction combined with a wide range of clinical experiences to prepare the graduate for career opportunities in a variety of health care settings. The low faculty to student ratio supports this educational process.

The faculty of MedCentral College is comprised of individuals with a breadth of expertise in the scholarship, practice, and leadership in nursing that supports their commitment to excellence in the education of the next generation of nurses. Like the OSU-M faculty, they come to Mansfield from the nation's most respected universities. Contracts with affiliating agencies within the region support the faculty's efforts to provide clinical experiences in acute and long term care, hospice, public health departments, social service agencies, and local schools in both urban and rural communities. Students are supported in achieving their educational objectives by access to the Learning Center, the Clinical Resource Center, and library facilities of OSU-M.

AFFILIATIONS WITH OTHER UNIVERSITIES
For non-nursing courses, we have established an exciting partnership with The Ohio State University–Mansfield (OSU-M). OSU-M provides the benefits of fulfilling the General Education Curriculum in the Liberal Arts, Humanities, and Physical and Social Sciences at a widely respected academic institution just minutes away from our campus. Both institutions have committed to an institutional relationship that supports a seamless experience for the student.

CONTACT INFORMATION
For more information regarding preparation for a nursing career at MedCentral College of Nursing, contact the Admissions Office: E-Mail: admissions@medcentral.edu, or call toll-free: (877) 656-4360.

Information and assistance with financial aid is available by contacting: Robert Carlisle, Director of Financial Aid & Student Services
335 Glessner Avenue
Mansfield, Ohio 44903
(419) 520-2512
E-Mail: rcarlisle@medcentral.edu
Web: www.medcentral.edu

Candidate–The Higher Learning Commission of the North Central Association of Colleges & Schools

MEDICAL COLLEGE OF GEORGIA
School of Nursing
Augusta, Georgia

THE UNIVERSITY
The Medical College of Georgia, Georgia's Health Sciences University, is located at Georgia's eastern border on the Savannah River and is the state's primary institution to educate health care professionals. It is the third-largest of the 32 colleges and universities in the state-assisted University System of Georgia, with approximately 2,500 students, interns, and residents and more than 700 faculty and staff members.

THE SCHOOL OF NURSING
In response to the wartime need for additional nurses, the University System of Georgia voted August 11, 1943 to offer courses in nursing education. This participation in the U.S. Cadet Nurse Corps paved the way to establish a department of nursing at the University of Georgia the following Fall. The program moved from Athens, Georgia to Augusta in 1956 and became a part of the Medical College of Georgia. The School of Nursing, with a strong commitment to research, moved forward in its development as a university-based nursing program. In 1974, to meet Georgia's growing need for baccalaureate-prepared nurses, a free-standing, self-contained satellite campus was opened in Athens, Georgia. This campus, for more than 20 years, has prepared one-third of the graduates of the baccalaureate program each year. To assist faculty research, an essential component in graduate education, the Center for Nursing Research was established in 1987. In 1994, the Board of Regents approved more than $1.5 million to renovate the historic Stoney Building, where the school moved in January 1995. In 1996, a second satellite campus was created in cooperation with Gordon College to offer an RN to BSN Program using distance-learning technology. In 1999, a third satellite campus began in cooperation with Columbus State University to offer the Family Nurse Practitioner Program and the Adult Critical/Acute Care Program using distance-learning technology.

The School of Nursing faculty has approximately 50 full-time and 11 part-time members representing many areas of teaching and research. More than 50 percent of the faculty members hold doctoral degrees in nursing or related fields.

PROGRAMS OF STUDY
The School of Nursing is accredited by the National League for Nursing Accrediting Commission. In addition, the School of Nursing has preliminary approval from the Commission on Collegiate Nursing Education. Degrees offered are the Bachelor of Science in Nursing (BSN), Master of Science in Nursing (MSN) (clinical nurse specialist program), Master of Nursing (MN) (nurse practitioner program and nursing anesthesia), and the Doctor of Philosophy in nursing (PhD). The baccalaureate program has a community-based curriculum that incorporates a wide variety of clinical experiences in inpatient, outpatient and community settings. As part of the baccalaureate program, a BSN completion program for registered nurses is offered.

The Master of Science in Nursing program offers specialties in adult nursing, parent-child nursing, mental health-psychiatric nursing, and community nursing. The Master of Nursing program offers specialties in nursing anesthesia, family nurse practitioner, pediatric nurse practitioner, and neonatal nurse practitioner.

The doctoral program specialties are in health care along the life span and nursing administration.

ACADEMIC FACILITIES
The present five-school campus consists of more than 90 buildings, including a 540-bed teaching hospital, on approximately 90 acres of land. The university operates community outreach clinics in 28 counties. Telemedicine sites are located across the state. The institution also occupies space in the Georgia cities of Athens and Rome and delivers distance learning to students in Atlanta, Dalton, Barnesville, and Columbus. The university houses a large multimedia library that participates in the state library system, GALILEO, with MERLIN. GALILEO provides access to more than 50 databases and services.

STUDENT LIFE
The Medical College of Georgia offers many learning experiences in a variety of settings. Organizations are available to enhance the student's career including the Georgia Association of Nursing Students; the IMHOTEP-Leadership Honor Society; MCG Student Government Association; Sigma Theta Tau International, Beta Omicron Chapter; and Phi Chi Beta of Chi Eta Phi Sorority.

CORRESPONDENCE AND INFORMATION
Office of Academic Admissions
170 Kelly Building-Administration
Medical College of Georgia
1120 Fifteenth Street
Augusta, GA 30912
(706) 721-2725 or (800) 519-3388
Web: www.mcg.edu/son

MGH INSTITUTE OF HEALTH PROFESSIONS
Graduate Program in Nursing
Boston, MA

THE INSTITUTE
The MGH Institute of Health Professions is affiliated with hospitals such as Massachusetts General Hospital and the Partners HealthCare System, Inc., which includes the Brigham and Women's, McLean, and Spaulding Rehabilitation Hospitals and a large network of hospitals, primary care organizations, and practices.

THE NURSING PROGRAM
The Graduate Program in Nursing is based on the philosophy that nursing is both an art and science of caring for the body, mind, and spirit of persons in relation to their environment at every level of human existence and connection: individuals, families, groups, and communities. From this framework, nursing addresses the potential for promotion, maintenance, and restoration of health, underscoring the importance of examining the political, economic, and social forces that impact a person. The program is fully accredited by the National League for Nursing Accrediting Commission, and has an enrollment of over 200 students. The twenty-nine nursing faculty members combine extensive expertise with a broad range of clinical experience to provide a singular learning experience for the Institute nursing students.

PROGRAMS OF STUDY

- Master of Science in Nursing Degree for non-nurse college graduates (Entry-level program)
- Master of Science in Nursing Degree for Registered Nurses with a Bachelor's Degree in Nursing or other discipline
- Associate Degree or Diploma
- Certificate of Advanced Study in Primary Care for Registered Nurses with a Master of Science in Nursing Degree

ACADEMIC RESOURCES
Nursing students have a learning resource lab, computer lab, interactive nursing skill videos, and nursing audiovisuals on-site. Also available to nursing students a short distance away, the MGH Treadwell Library houses over 53,000 volumes, over 2,000 of which

are in nursing. Students also have the opportunity to work in hospitals, homeless shelters, clinics, and schools. The Institute has recently relocated to a new site within the historic Charlestown Navy Yard. The newly renovated historic building on the waterfront offers state of the art classrooms, laboratories, and other academic resources.

COSTS
Tuition is $635 per credit. Audited courses are $318 per credit.

FINANCIAL AID
Federal Student Nursing Loans are available to MGH nursing students, as well as need- and performance-based scholarships, nurse traineeships, and graduate assistantships.

ADMISSIONS
All applicants except Master's prepared nurses must provide GRE scores, all appropriate college transcripts, 3 letters of recommendation, an essay, and a $50 application fee.

CONTACT INFORMATION
Office of Enrollment Management and Student Affairs
MGH Institute of Health Professions
Charlestown Navy Yard
36 First Avenue
Boston, MA 02129
(617) 726-3140
Web: www.mghihp.edu

MIAMI UNIVERSITY
Department of Nursing
Hamilton and Middletown, OH

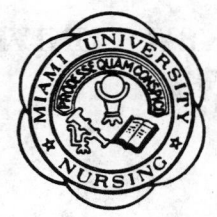

THE UNIVERSITY
Miami University is a state-assisted comprehensive university located in southwestern Ohio. Established in 1809, Miami has developed into a selective public university with a highly recognized tradition of dedication to teaching excellence and undergraduate liberal arts education and with an increasingly strong record of scholarly achievements. *U.S. News & World Report* ranked Miami among the nation's top public universities in 2002. *Fiske Guide to Colleges for 1998* listed Miami as a "Best Buy." *Kaplan-Newsweek* "College Catalogue 2002" rated Miami as one of 27 "hidden treasures."

THE DEPARTMENT OF NURSING
The Department of Nursing has programs on the Hamilton and Middletown campuses. The campuses are located in Butler County in southwest Ohio. The Associate Degree program was founded in 1968, and the BSN completion program was founded in 1976. State-of-the-art Nursing Resource Centers are maintained for our students.

PROGRAMS OF STUDY
The Department of Nursing offers an Associate Degree in Applied Science in Nursing (ADN) and a Bachelor of Science Degree (BSN) for RNs. Both programs are accredited by the National League for Nursing Accrediting Commission. The ADN curriculum provides courses in liberal arts, sciences, and nursing. Classroom instructions are correlated with clinical experiences in area health care agencies, and the program prepares the student to provide nursing care to people of all ages. Graduates are qualified to take the NCLEX-RN® exam that allows them to practice as a registered nurse. They may continue their education toward the BSN degree.

The BSN program is for registered nurse graduates of diploma and associate degree programs. RN students will build on previous learning and add depth and breadth to their nursing knowledge. Emphasis is on liberal education and nursing process for health promotion, prevention, restoration, and maintenance with clients, families, and client groups in the community as well as leadership and management. Students are prepared for functioning as a practitioner of professional nursing and/or graduate education.

COSTS
Miami University offers many financial aid packages and scholarships. There are several scholarships specific to nursing students. Ohio resident full-time undergraduate tuition for 2003-2004 is $4,962.

APPLICATION INFORMATION
Application must be made to Miami University and the nursing program. For the ADN program, students need a minimum ACT score of 21 or SAT score of 970, completed high school chemistry and math, and a high school or college GPA of 2.5 or higher. BSN applicants must hold an Ohio RN license, diploma, or associate degree in nursing, and a GPA of 2.5.

CORRESPONDENCE AND INFORMATION
Department of Nursing
1601 Peck Blvd
Hamilton, OH 45011
(513) 785-3282

Department of Nursing
4200 E. University Blvd
Middletown, OH 45042
(513) 727-3266
Web: www.ham.muohio.edu/nursing

MICHIGAN STATE UNIVERSITY
College of Nursing
East Lansing, MI

THE UNIVERSITY

Founded in 1855 as the nation's first land-grant university, MSU served as the prototype for 69 land-grant institutions established under the Morrill Act of 1862, and was the first institution of higher learning in the nation to teach scientific agriculture. Today, MSU has grown into a comprehensive research university with over 4,244 faculty and academic staff, 33,966 undergraduates, and 9,072 graduate and professional students. The total enrollment is the largest single campus student body of any Michigan university and among the largest in the country. MSU is a leader in scientific and technological advancement and has been a member of the prestigious Association of American Universities, which represents the nation's leading graduate research institutions since 1964. MSU's research program now includes more than 3,000 projects. Federal agencies provide the largest proportion of research funds; the Department of Health and Human Services and the National Science Foundation are the largest sponsors.

COLLEGE OF NURSING

The Nursing program at Michigan State University began in 1950 as a generic baccalaureate program and has grown to include a baccalaureate completion program, a Master's degree with tracks in primary care focusing on family and gerontology, as well as a doctoral program; post-Master's and post-doctoral opportunities also exist within the College. The College of Nursing was one of the MSU campus pioneers, through the Virtual University, in the use of the Internet for education delivery. Currently the College offers four graduate courses totally on the Web (one elective, and three required courses) and additional Web-based courses are under development. Nursing was also one of the first colleges at MSU to use two-way interactive television for distance learning. Community based outreach degree programs are offered at the baccalaureate and master's level. Outreach programs are offered in collaboration with local community colleges and health care agencies. Community based clinical experience is an essential component of nursing education at MSU. Over 300 clinical preceptors and adjunct faculty provide clinical instruction in more than 150 health care agencies throughout Michigan.

PROGRAMS OF STUDY

The College of Nursing offers an undergraduate program leading to the Bachelor of Science degree with a major in Nursing and graduate programs leading to the Master of Science in Nursing degree and a Doctor of Philosophy degree with a major in Nursing. The focus of the undergraduate program is basic professional education, the Master's program is the education of advanced practice nurses, while the PhD program prepares nurse researchers.

The undergraduate nursing program provides a foundation for professional practice based on the biological, physical, and behavioral sciences and the humanities. The program is designed to prepare the student for nursing practice with individuals, families, and aggregates of persons in a variety of health states and health care settings, including hospitals and community health agencies. With professional experience, the graduate may progress to beginning-level leadership positions. The program, which has been approved by the Michigan Board of Nursing and accredited by the National League for Nursing Accrediting Commission, also provides a foundation for graduate study in nursing.

The Master of Science degree program consists of five academic semesters, and focuses on the preparation of advanced practice nurses. There are two areas of concentration in the program: gerontology and family. Students who are enrolled in the Master of Science in Nursing degree program may elect specializations in infant studies. The program prepares students for leadership positions in advanced nursing practice in primary care. Completion of a thesis is an optional component of the degree.

The Doctor of Philosophy degree program with a major in Nursing is designed with a major emphasis in health status and health outcomes research related to individuals and families within the context of community-based primary care. The focus of the PhD program is to prepare clinical researchers. Graduates will conduct and facilitate research in a variety of academic, clinical, and community-based settings.

ACADEMIC FACILITIES

The MSU Libraries have an extensive research collection of more than 4,000,000 volumes housed in the main library and 14 branch libraries serving classroom buildings across campus. The collection includes more than 28,000 periodicals, 200,000 maps, 40,000 sound recordings, Michigan and U.S. government documents, and publications of the United Nations and other international organizations. MSU is the nation's only university with three on-campus medical schools, graduating medical doctors, veterinarians, and osteopathic physicians. The College of Nursing is housed in the Life Sciences Building and includes a Media Laboratory, a Demonstration Laboratory for clinical skills, as well as a recently established technology classroom.

COSTS

Tuition costs per credit hour are: In-State: Lower Division Tuition is $147.25 (average tuition, fees, and taxes for one academic year $5,043.50). Upper Division Tuition is $164 (average total costs, including fees for one academic year $5,546.00). Graduate Tuition is $229.25. Out-of-State: Lower Division Tuition is $394.00 (average annual total costs $12,446.00) and Upper Division Tuition is $408.00 (average annual total costs $12,873.50). Out-of-state Graduate tuition is $463.50 per credit.

FINANCIAL AID

Financial aid is available for direct educational costs and for personal living expenses. Undergraduates are eligible for scholarships and grants from numerous sources, loans, and jobs. Graduate assistantships, private scholarships, Professional Nurse Traineeships, and MSU Fellowships are available through the College of Nursing. Graduate and research assistantships, which offer tuition waivers and pay monthly stipends, are also available. College scholarships from private donors of the College are available to students at all levels.

APPLYING

Applicants must submit their applications to the College of Nursing by April 1 of the year that admission is sought for the undergraduate program and by February 1 for all graduate programs. Undergraduate applicants must complete the required prerequisite courses and have a minimum grade point averages of 2.50 (cumulatively, and 2.20 in the sciences).

Applicants to the Master of Science in Nursing program must have: a minimum grade-point average of 3.00 (4.0 scale) in last two years of the baccalaureate degree, one year of full-time clinical work experience as a RN, and 3.0 GPA in an approved statistics course within five years of the planned date of enrollment. RNs with a bachelors degree in other fields are eligible to apply.

Applicants to the PhD program must have: minimum GPA 3.0 for all previous academic work, GRE (Verbal, Quantitative, and Analytic) within last five years, an MSN degree, and three references. Admission to both the MSN and PhD programs also includes an interview with faculty.

CORRESPONDENCE AND INFORMATION
College of Nursing
A230 Life Sciences Building
East Lansing, MI 48824
(517) 353-4827; (800) 605-6424
Fax: (517) 353-9553
E-Mail: nurse@msu.edu
Web: http//:nursing.msu.edu

MINNESOTA STATE UNIVERSITY, MANKATO
School of Nursing
Mankato, Minnesota

THE UNIVERSITY

Minnesota State University, Mankato, located in south central Minnesota on a bluff above the Minnesota River, is a comprehensive, multipurpose regional university with an enrollment of approximately 13,000 students. The University has the second largest graduate studies program in Minnesota. The College of Allied Health and Nursing is a leading institution in health care within the Minnesota State College and Universities (MnSCU) system.

THE SCHOOL OF NURSING

The School of Nursing is committed to excellence, and recently received top national honors for an exceptional and innovative curriculum in Gerontologic Nursing by the Hartford Foundation Institute for Geriatric Nursing in collaboration with the AACN. Classrooms, laboratories, and offices for the School of Nursing are located in the Leichsenring Nursing Center, third floor of Wissink Building in the center of the campus. The latest in educational technology is available. Entire courses or segments of courses are either online over the Internet or via ITV to several sites in southern Minnesota for students in the RN Option and the graduate program. The School of Nursing is actively involved in several grant funded collaborative initiatives in Minnesota that provide opportunities for interdisciplinary work within rural and underserved areas. Nursing faculty are committed to excellence in learning within an environment of caring. Faculty are actively involved in a variety of research projects and community endeavors. Recent faculty honors include the prestigious MN Association of Colleges of Nursing (MACN) Nurse Educator of the Year Award for 1998 and the prestigious MN Nurses Association (MNA) Nurse Researcher of the Year award for 1998.

PROGRAMS OF STUDY

Since 1953, the School of Nursing has offered a program leading to a bachelor of science degree with a major in nursing. Two options exist: basic option and RN option. The program is approved by the Minnesota Board of Nursing, which authorizes graduates to take NCLEX-RN®. Graduates are qualified for Public Health Nurse certification and School Nurse licensure. The School of Nursing also offers a graduate program designed to prepare advanced practice nurses. Graduate students earn a Master of Science in Nursing (MSN) degree. The program emphasis is Family Nursing with options for the advanced nursing roles of Clinical Nurse Specialist (CNS) and Family Nurse Practitioner (FNP). A post-Master's FNP option is also available. Both the undergraduate and graduate programs are accredited by the NLNAC.

HEALTH CARE AFFILIATIONS

Students have a variety of clinical experiences in rural and metro/urban settings. The clinical resources include hospitals in Mankato and the Twin Cities area, long-term care facilities, a regional mental health center, and various public health and home care agencies.

ACADEMIC RESOURCES

Besides School of Nursing resources, students have access to a state of the art Academic Computer Center, Counseling Center, and Learning Center. The Memorial Library has nearly 1 million print volumes and 3,200 current periodical subscriptions.

COSTS

2002-2003 tuition for resident undergraduate students is $159.90 per credit hour with a flat rate of $1,990.60 for 12-18 credits. Tuition for nonresident undergraduate students is $307.90 per credit hour. Tuition for graduate students is $199.15 for residents and $298.50 for nonresidents. Residence hall costs vary according to the type of room and meal plan.

FINANCIAL AID

The University offers financial aid in the form of scholarships, grants, loans, or part-time employment. Nursing also has several scholarships available to students in the program.

APPLYING

For admission, undergraduate students in both options must have completed the prerequisite courses with a grade of C or better, completed 30 semester credits and have a cumulative GPA of at least 2.5. Students in the RN option must provide proof of active unrestricted licensure and validation of clinical competence. For admission to the MSN program, a BS/BA degree from an NLNAC-accredited school of nursing is preferred. A baccalaureate degree in another field is acceptable with equivalency demonstrated in leadership/management, research, and public health nursing theory and clinical. Other requirements include current RN licensure, a minimum cumulative GPA of 3.0, and a minimum of two years of work experience as an RN.

CORRESPONDENCE AND INFORMATION

School of Nursing
Minnesota State University, Mankato
360 Wissink Hall
Mankato, MN 56001
(507) 389-6022
Fax: (507) 389-6516
E-Mail: brenda.garbers@mnsu.edu
Web: www.mankato.msus.edu/dept/nursing/welcome.html

MISSISSIPPI COUNTY COMMUNITY COLLEGE
Department of Nursing
Blytheville, Arkansas

Mississippi County Community College in Blytheville is committed to educating students for promising futures. Their very successful nursing program is a testimony to that fact. For over twenty-five years, MCCC has been educating students both in the classroom and healthcare facilities to become registered nurses through its two-year degree plan.

"In regard to their potential in finding employment upon graduation, this is a very positive time for individuals considering careers in the health industry," stated Sharon Fulling, MCCC Director of Nursing. Fulling added that MCCC offers a very comprehensive nursing program, which allow students a great deal of time "out in the field" training in a clinical setting. "Our students have a very stringent regimen in this program, but it has to be that way because we're dealing, in many instances, with life and death situations. My staff and I are going to make sure that we prepare these students beyond the best of their abilities."

In doing so, the MCCC Nursing Program maintains a high degree of performance procedures—keeping it in line with and accredited by the National League for Nursing Accrediting Commission and the Arkansas State Board of Nursing. In addition, the program enlists the newest of technologies in instruction and individual student preparation. "All of our students have access to our computer lab, which includes health-related software for them to use in studying and practicing for the NCLEX-RN® exam," said Fulling, who added that instructors are encouraged to team-teach and provide lots of individual, hands-on assistance.

The MCCC Department of Nursing offers an Associate in Applied Science Degree in Nursing. One class is admitted each fall semester. Throughout the program, general education courses and nursing courses are combined with client care in clinical settings in hospitals and healthcare agencies in the area. The nursing courses integrate application of the nursing process, communication skills, nutrition, pharmacology, and drug administration in the care of patients. Once students are accepted into the program, they begin very specific coursework in the nursing field, and by their second year, they spend twelve hours a week in local hospitals gaining actual, supervised, clinical experience.

"I believe our program has a reputation among health organizations in the area as being a very successful program—one that adequately prepares its graduates for the workforce. Our graduates are sought out for employment," stated Fulling.

The MCCC Nursing Department is doing its part in providing area students the opportunity to become involved with one of the most sought-after professions today. "In a time of economic strife, it's nice to know that we can help our students in their desires to become caregivers and that their services will be needed and appreciated," stated Fulling.

For more information about the MCCC Nursing Program, contact the department at 870-762-1020 extension 1511 or the MCCC Admissions Office at extension 1114.

- Low Tuition
- Financial Aid Available
- Many Scholarship Opportunities
- Hands-On Learning
- High Rate of Job Placement
- Low Student to Teacher Ratio

Mississippi County Community College
P.O. Box 1109
Blytheville, AR 72316-1109
Web: www.mccc.cc.ar.us

MONMOUTH UNIVERSITY
Marjorie K. Unterberg School of Nursing and Health Studies
West Long Branch, New Jersey

THE UNIVERSITY

Monmouth University is a private, co-educational, teaching university dedicated to educating undergraduate and graduate students for full participation in their professions and in society. A faculty of teacher-scholars is at the heart of Monmouth's academic programs. In contrast to students attending large universities, Monmouth's students have the opportunity to work closely with senior faculty. Monmouth offers more than 45 undergraduate and graduate degree programs and concentrations, which are delivered through seven schools.

SCHOOL OF NURSING AND HEALTH STUDIES

The Marjorie K. Unterberg School of Nursing and Health Studies reflects in its philosophy the mission of Monmouth University: to provide a learning process and the environment that enable students to realize their full potential and enhance the quality of life for individuals, families, groups, and the community.

PROGRAMS OF STUDY

The School of Nursing and Health Studies offers the following programs:

• Designed for graduate nurses from associate degree programs and/or diploma schools of nursing, the BSN program focuses on the promotion, restoration, and maintenance of health for individuals and groups. An integrated BSN/MSN program allows qualified BSN students to take up to 6 graduate credits (2 courses) during their senior year and apply them to both the BSN and the MSN degrees. Designed to meet the new requirements for certified school nurses to act as health advocates for school-age children, the Post-Baccalaureate School Nurse Certificate program prepares registered nurses for NJ School Nurse Certification. A Post-Baccalaureate Forensic Nursing Certificate program is also available.

• The MSN program provides the foundation necessary for advanced nursing practice, an advanced practice nursing concentration to develop the skills necessary for positive healthcare delivery, and a detailed study and clinical practice of common and complex problems in primary healthcare practice. Specializations include adult nurse practitioner, family nurse practitioner, nursing administration, school nursing, nursing education, and forensic nursing. A "bridge" program for students with non-nursing bachelor's degrees is also offered.

• Designed for nurses who have already completed a master's degree in nursing, the post-master's certificate combines a broad knowledge base with a concentration in a selected area of specialization. Specializations include adult nurse practitioner, family nurse practitioner, nursing administration, and nursing education.

ACADEMIC RESOURCES

The Guggenheim Memorial Library houses some 249,000 volumes and nearly 1,300 periodicals. The Library provides online campus access to the book catalog over the Internet, Web-based databases of scholarly journal articles and book titles, full-text databases from newspapers and general periodicals, E-Mail delivery of interlibrary loan articles, government and legislation information, and business information and full-text images of articles on the Web.

COSTS

Undergraduate tuition is $502/credit. Graduate tuition is $549/credit. The comprehensive fee for less than 9 credits is $142/semester; for 9 or more credits the fee is $284/semester.

FINANCIAL AID

The staff of the Financial Aid Office assists students in developing a comprehensive educational financial plan, which may include scholarships, grants, loans, fellowships, assistantships, or payment plans. A number of sponsored and endowed nursing scholarships are available.

ADMISSION REQUIREMENTS

In addition to general admission requirements, applicants to the School of Nursing and Health Studies must meet these requirements:

• For the BSN program, applicants must have sat for or be eligible to sit for the NCLEX examination and must have achieved a GPA of at least 2.0 in lower-division college work.

• The School Nurse and Forensic Nursing Certificate programs require a nursing license and a baccalaureate degree from an accredited program with an undergraduate GPA of 2.75. Students holding a BSN may receive a waiver for some or all of the foundation courses.

• The MSN program requires candidates to have a BSN from an accredited program, with a minimum undergraduate GPA of 2.75 and a course in health assessment. The GRE is waived for students who achieve a B or better in each of the first 12 credits of the program; students who do not maintain a B in each course will have to submit GRE scores after completing 12 credits. Registered nurse students without a baccalaureate degree in nursing may be admitted into the "bridge" program, which allows students to take 11 undergraduate BSN credits and then proceed directly into the MSN program. Two letters of recommendation, a resume, and a personal statement of 150 to 300 words are also required. Students are expected to have at least one year of clinical experience prior to their clinical specialty courses.

• The post-master's certificate requires that applicants hold a master's degree in nursing and have at least a year of experience as a registered nurse. Two letters of recommendation, a resume, and a personal statement of 150 to 300 words are also required for admission.

• Candidates for all programs must have a current New Jersey registered nurse license and the ability to produce a photocopy of a current $1,000,000/$3,000,000 liability and malpractice policy. All full-time students are required to have a physical examination prior to registration; part-time students are not required to have a physical examination until they begin the clinical component of the program. Students in the Nurse Practitioner or Advanced Practice Nursing concentrations are required to have successfully completed a college-level course in health assessment.

MONMOUTH UNIVERSITY
(continued)

CORRESPONDENCE AND INFORMATION
Office of Graduate Admission
Monmouth University
400 Cedar Avenue
West Long Branch, NJ 07764-1898
(800) 320-7754
Fax: (732) 263-5123
E-Mail: gradadm@monmouth.edu
Web: www.monmouth.edu

MOUNT CARMEL COLLEGE OF NURSING
Columbus, Ohio

THE COLLEGE

Mount Carmel College of Nursing (MCCN) is a small, private, Catholic, specialized institution of higher education offering a Bachelor of Science Degree in Nursing, an RN to BSN Program, a Dietetic Internship Program, a Surgical Technician Program, and a division of Continuing Education.

The college is accredited by the North Central Association of Colleges and Schools and the nursing program is accredited by the National League for Nursing Accrediting Commission.

MCCN boasts one of the largest undergraduate nursing programs among all Ohio private colleges. MCCN is a subsidiary of Mount Carmel Health, an integrated delivery network, which includes three acute care hospitals, community outreach programs, hospice, home health and ambulatory care centers.

Founded in 1903 by the Congregation of the Sisters of the Holy Cross, Mount Carmel offered a diploma program until 1993. In 1993, MCCN was established.

OUR NURSING PROGRAMS OF STUDY

- The Prelicensure Program, leading to a Bachelor of Science degree in nursing. This four–year program is designed for students without previous nursing experience. The first two years of study focus on completing general education requirements. Nursing studies begin in the sophomore year when the curriculum combines both "hands-on" clinical experiences with classroom theory. Nursing coursework emphasizes clinical practice in a variety of acute-care hospitals and community based centers.
- The Advanced Placement Program allows students to transfer in all non-nursing courses from their first two years of study at other institutions of higher learning. When degree requirements (prerequisite courses completed) are met, a degree may be obtained in 5 semesters. All transfer students must complete a summer 12-week Advanced Placement tract at the college prior to fall semester start-up.
- The RN/ BSN Tract is designed for registered nurses who want to earn a Bachelor of Science degree in nursing. The registered nurse can complete degree requirements in four semesters of full-time study. Classes are small, scheduled one full day per week so that RNs may work full time if necessary, and designed to meet individual student needs.
- New in Fall 2002: A Master's in Nursing Program

AFFILIATIONS WITH HEALTHCARE FACILITIES

Clinical learning experiences are offered:

- At several hospitals, including those within the Mount Carmel network and at Children's' Hospital in Columbus.
- In conjunction with numerous community health agencies

ACADEMIC FACILITIES

Students at MCCN have access to:

- A full professional library
- A Learning Resource Center with a fully equipped computer lab and a multimedia area

LOCATION

MCCN is located on the near West Side of Columbus, Ohio on the hospital campus of Mount Carmel West.

STUDENT SERVICES AND ACTIVITIES

MCCN has a full range of services to meet students needs including:

- A Student Union with kitchen, vending machines, and numerous sitting and reading areas
- A gymnasium and exercise room
- Mount Carmel Intramural sports
- SNAM, the student nursing organization
- On-campus full-service dormitories

FOR OUR NURSING STUDENTS

Faculty and staff are committed to fostering personal and academic growth. MCCN graduation and retention rates are among the highest in Ohio and surpass national averages.

Mount Carmel's cultural environment embraces diversity. The successful "Learning Trails Program" assists students of various cultural backgrounds by nurturing academic, personal, and professional growth through one-on-on consultation.

Job placement services are available both during college and upon graduation. Many opportunities exist within the Mount Carmel Health network.

FINANCIAL AID

Numerous financial aid options are available. Students may find assistance through the College's own financial aid programs and through federal programs. MCCN financial aid representatives can assist students in exploring various options.

APPLYING

Applicants with College Credit: Students within this category must meet MCCN general admission requirements and must have earned a college GPA of 2.0 or higher. ACT/ SAT scores need not be submitted if 30 hours of college credit have been successfully completed. Please submit official transcripts from all colleges and universities attended.

Admission Criteria: The following admission criteria are used for admission:

- High school graduation (or GED) with a minimum cumulative grade point (GPA) of 2.25 is required. A GPA of 3.0 is preferred. The applicant may submit evidence of a college GPA of 2.0 or higher in lieu of the high school GPA.
- High School course requirements/ successful completion of the following high school courses:

English	4 courses
College Preparatory Math	2 courses (3 recommended)
Laboratory Science	2 courses (Biology and Chemistry)
Social Science	2 courses
Foreign Language	2 courses (Sign language is an option)
Visual or Performing Arts	1 course (2 recommended)

MOUNT CARMEL OF NURSING
(continued)

If any of the above courses are not passed in high school, the applicant is required to take theses classes at the college level and earn a minimum grade of C (+/ -). The courses must be completed prior to the applicant attending Mount Carmel College of Nursing. (All applicants must submit a transcript from high school.)

- All applicants must provide ACT or SAT scores. However, applicants who have been out of high school over five years or have at least 30 college/ university credits do not have to provide ACT/ SAT scores.
- Essay
- Interview

CORRESPONDENCE AND INFORMATION

For information, call (614) 234-5800 or toll free, (800) 556-6942.
Mount Carmel College of Nursing
127 South Davis Avenue
Columbus, Ohio 43222
Web: www.mccn.edu

MOUNTAIN STATE UNIVERSITY
Beckley, WV

⚑ Mountain State University™

THE UNIVERSITY
Mountain State University prepares students to succeed. A philosophy of responsiveness to student needs and a student-faculty ratio of 14 to 1 ensure that each student is treated as an individual, while more than 3,000 students from 43 states and every continent except Antarctica provide the diversity of a larger institution. The University offers associate, bachelor's, and master's degree programs in approximately 75 fields, and a location in the mountain playground of southern West Virginia provides a relaxed atmosphere that lends itself to both learning and fun.

Formerly The College of West Virginia, Mountain State University is a private, independent, not-for-profit university. It is accredited by the Higher Learning Commission and is a member of the North Central Association (800.621.7440, www.ncahigherlearning commission.org). Nursing programs are accredited by the West Virginia State Board of Examiners for Registered Professional Nurses and by the National League for Nursing Accrediting Commission (61 Broadway, New York NY 10006, tel. 212-363-5555).

UNDERGRADUATE NURSING PROGRAM
The School of Health Sciences offers a traditional BSN program and, in collaboration with the School of Distance and Extended Learning, accelerated LPN-to-BSN and RN-to-BSN programs. The undergraduate nursing program consists of general studies, including humanities and the natural and social sciences, along with a concentration in nursing science. A clinical practice component places students in such settings as hospitals, health departments, clinics, nursing homes, and doctors' offices, providing them with an opportunity to improve their application of nursing theory and skills. Graduates are eligible to apply for the National Council Licensure Examination (NCLEX-RN®) and are prepared for beginning nursing positions with the potential for movement into leadership positions or graduate study.

Students are admitted to the nursing program as freshmen, although program admission is limited and competitive. Criteria for acceptance include an ACT cumulative score of at least 20; high school GPA of at least 2.5 on a 4.0 scale; and high school courses in algebra, one laboratory science, and biology with a minimum grade of C. Applicants who do not meet the above requirements may be accepted on a provisional basis.

Transfer applicants must have a grade of C or better in all mathematics, natural sciences, and psychology courses, as well as in two terms of English composition. Transfer students must complete a minimum of 16 credit hours in nursing at Mountain State University, including at least two clinical laboratory courses.

Eligibility for Fast Track program admission requires an active, unencumbered LPN license and a score in at least the 50th percentile on the NLN Mobility I Test. Eligibility for the Pathway program requires graduation from a state-approved associate or diploma program in nursing and a current, unrestricted RN license.

The nursing program begins in the fall semester. The recommended application deadline is January 10, although applications will be considered as long as openings remain.

GRADUATE NURSING PROGRAM
An MSN program, offered at the Beckley campus and via distance learning in Martinsburg, WV, includes tracks in administration/ education and in family nurse practitioner. The MSN program combines state-of-the-art theoretical knowledge and the reality of current practice—a combination that will carry graduate students successfully into a competitive job market or into continued professional education. Because most MSN students continue to work full- or part-time during their studies, classes are offered in a variety of formats.

Admission to graduate study at Mountain State University requires a bachelor's degree from an accredited college or university with a minimum overall GPA of 3.0 on a 4.0 scale, although applicants with a GPA of 2.5 may be eligible for provisional admission. Those whose native language is not English must also have a minimum score of 500 on the Test of English as a Foreign Language (TOEFL). Admission to graduate study in nursing further requires a BSN from an NLNAC–accredited program; current unrestricted RN licensure in a U.S. jurisdiction; 12 clock hours of community service over the past year; and coursework including 3 hours of basic statistics, 3 hours of pharmacology, 4 hours of anatomy and physiology, and 2 hours of basic research.

LEARNING RESOURCES
The University's learning resource center includes a library with 90,000 volumes as well as a wealth of electronic databases and networks. Spacious computer labs are equipped with current hardware and software. Additional resources range from multimedia classrooms to teleconferencing facilities.

STUDENT LIFE
Campus life amenities include a three-year-old residence hall, a new coffeehouse, and a student union with a dining hall, weekend cinema, and game tables. The University's "Great Dates" program features campus events as well as trips to regional attractions. All students receive a complimentary membership to the Beckley-Raleigh County YMCA, with facilities for workouts, swimming, basketball, and racquetball within walking distance of campus. The Cougars compete in NAIA Division I men's basketball and women's volleyball and softball, and intramural sports include volleyball, three-on-three basketball, and soccer.

COST OF ATTENDANCE / FINANCIAL AID
In 2000-01, undergraduate nursing courses followed the University's overall price schedule of $140/hour, with a $30 general fee. Additional program costs add $855 to the first year of study and $1,335 to each following semester for full-time undergraduate students. Most undergraduates receive some form of federal, state, or institutional financial aid. Graduate nursing courses in 2000–01 were $280/hour.

ADDITIONAL INFORMATION
Mountain State University Office of Admissions
Box 9003
Beckley, WV 25802-9003
(304) 253.7351 / (800) 766.6067
Web: www.mountainstate.edu

MUHLENBERG REGIONAL MEDICAL CENTER
Schools of Nursing, Medical Imaging and Therapeutic Sciences
Plainfield, New Jersey

MUHLENBERG REGIONAL MEDICAL CENTER
Muhlenberg Hospital was founded in 1877. It moved to its present location in 1903, and has grown to become one of the largest voluntary, non-profit hospitals in the state of New Jersey.

SCHOOL OF NURSING
The School of Nursing was established in 1894. In 1971, the School of Nursing established an affiliation with Union County College in Cranford, New Jersey. This affiliation is known as Muhlenberg Regional Medical Center School of Nursing/Union County College Cooperative Nursing Program and leads to a diploma in nursing from Muhlenberg and an Associate in Science (AS) degree from Union County College.

PROGRAM OF STUDY
A. REGISTERED NURSING
The School of Nursing offers 3 tracks toward registered nurse licensure.

1. GENERIC
   A day or evening, full- or part-time program that requires a high school diploma or a GED/Adult Diploma.
2. ACCELERATED
   A full-time day program requiring a baccalaureate degree; the degree may be in any discipline.
3. LPN-to-RN TRANSITION
   This bi-annual 3-week full-time day transition course bridges the LPN's experience and Nursing I. Successful students are then given the opportunity to challenge Nursing II. The student will then have the choice of day or evening for Nursing III and Nursing IV.

All three tracks include 75(76) credits: 41(42) general education credits and 34 nursing (clinical) credits. The general education credits are taken at Union County College – Cranford, Elizabeth, or Plainfield campuses.

Up to 32 transfer credits are available for comparable courses (40 transfer credits for holders of baccalaureate degrees). A cumulative grade point average of 2.5 or higher is required in these comparable courses.

Nursing courses are taught at Muhlenberg and JFK Medical Centers and various other clinical sites and affiliations.

B. ADVANCED NURSING PROGRAMS

1. RN RESIDENCY – a 16-week post graduate program providing focused experience in medical/surgical, home care, operating room, labor and delivery, or behavioral health.
2. CRITICAL CARE RESIDENCY – A 16-week post-graduate program providing focused experience in intensive and cardiac care, emergency room, or telemetry.

COSTS
A. REGISTERED NURSING
Tuition costs will vary with individual student requirements, courses selected each semester, and the number of transfer credits accepted. A current tuition and fee sheet is included with each application. Resident facilities are available. The estimated cost is $850 per semester. Out-of-county residents (non-Union county residents) will pay additional charges for the general education courses, but not for the nursing courses.

B. ADVANCED NURSING PROGRAMS
1. RN RESIDENCY – The entire cost is $2,000.
2. CRITICAL CARE RESIDENCY – The entire cost is $2,500.

FINANCIAL AID
The Muhlenberg Regional Medical Center Schools of Nursing, Medical Imaging and Therapeutic Sciences are approved for Title IV Financial Aid Programs as well as Veterans Programs for eligible students. Institutionally sponsored non-need grants/scholarships are also available.

INFORMATION AND APPLICATION
Information, specific program applications and general correspondence may be directed to:

Director of Admissions and Recruitment Services
Muhlenberg Regional Medical Center
Schools of Nursing, Medical Imaging and Therapeutic Sciences
Park Avenue and Randolph Road
Plainfield, New Jersey 07061
(908) 668-2400
Fax: (908) 226-4568
E-Mail: SSONMITS@solarishs.org

NEUMANN COLLEGE
Aston, PA

THE COLLEGE
Neumann College, founded in 1965 and sponsored by the Sisters of St. Francis of Philadelphia, is a Catholic co-education institution of higher education in the liberal arts and Franciscan traditions located in the suburbs southwest of Philadelphia. Neumann provides innovative programs of excellence and maintains a community defined by values that shape lives and relationships.

BACHELOR OF SCIENCE DEGREE WITH A MAJOR IN NURSING
DAY PROGRAM

- The Neuman Systems Model is the foundation of the Nursing curriculum, providing a holistic approach to Nursing.
- Students must have a minimum 2.5 GPA to enter the major and maintain a grade of C or better in all Nursing courses.

NURSING
An exciting new Nursing curriculum prepares professional nurses who will be able to:

- Anticipate and respond to change that affects continuing and new health needs of individuals, groups, and communities.
- Provide nursing care to people of all ages and diverse cultures in varying circumstances and settings.

EVENING PROGRAM

- Upon completion of core and allied prerequisites, the Nursing major courses can be completed in two and a half years.
- Course content and clinical settings are essentially the same as in the day program.
- Second degree students welcome.

PROGRAMS OF STUDY

BACCALAUREATE PROGRAM
- Day Program
- Evening Option
- Master of Science in Nursing Program
- Gerontologic Nurse Practitioner track
- Clinical Nurse Specialist in long-term care
- Post-Master's GNP Certificate
- RN to MSN Program for RNs seeking a baccalaureate or BSN and MSN degrees

MASTER OF SCIENCE IN NURSING
Gerontological Nurse Practitioner

- Primary care provider for diverse older population
- Can be completed in 4 full-time semesters
- 46 credits
- Excellent clinical sites over a wide geographic area

Clinical Nurse Specialist in Long-term Care

- Expert clinician with chronically ill populations
- Can be completed in 3 full-time semesters
- 40 credits

RN-TO-MSN PROGRAM

- Accelerated program designed for RNs with either a diploma or AD
- Express route to a graduate degree
- 13 credits that meet BSN and MSN requirements
- Core nursing courses designed for the non-traditional student

COSTS
Undergraduate:

Tuition per semester (12-18 credits)	$7,230
General Fee per semester	$ 250
Part-Time (1-11 credits, per credit)	$ 350
Graduate:	
Tuition per credit	$ 440

Financial aid is available.

ADMISSION
Applicants to each program are evaluated on an individual basis. Please see the College Catalogues for details or call (610) 558-5561.

AFFILIATIONS
Neumann College has contractual agreements with hospitals, facilities, and preceptors in Pennsylvania, New Jersey, and Delaware.

CONTACT INFORMATION
Neumann College
One Neumann Drive
Aston, PA 19014-1298
Phone: 1-800-9-Neuman
E-Mail: nursdiv@neumann.edu

NEW YORK UNIVERSITY
New York, New York

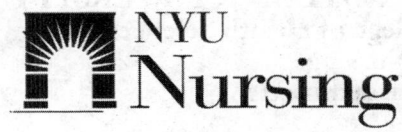

THE UNIVERSITY AND THE SCHOOL
New York University, the largest private university in the country, was founded in 1831. The Steinhardt School of Education, established in 1890 as the first university-based school of pedagogy in the country, enrolls 6,700 undergraduate and graduate students in degree programs in education, health, nursing, communications, and the arts.

THE DIVISION OF NURSING
NYU's Division of Nursing ranks among the nation's top nursing programs. The intellectual energies of the faculty and students, the quality of academic resources, and the rich interaction with a vibrant city provide a learning experience that is unique in its rigor and diversity. All programs provide a balance between nursing theory and practice. All programs are accredited by the NLNAC.

PROGRAMS OF STUDY
The NYU Division of Nursing offers a four-year BS program; a BS program for college graduates; a study option for Registered Nurses; a dual-degree BS/MA program; MA programs in teaching and nursing administration; an MA program and advanced certificates in nursing informatics, nurse midwifery, advance practice nursing: adult acute care, adult primary care, geriatrics, pediatrics, mental health, holistic, and palliative care; a joint degree program with the Wagner Graduate School of Public Service; and a PhD program in research and theory development in nursing science.

AFFILIATIONS WITH HEALTH CARE FACILITIES
The Division of Nursing offers clinical and practicum experiences at many hospitals in the New York metropolitan area, including the Mount Sinai-NYU Medical Center/Health System, Bellevue Hospital Center, St. Vincent's Hospital, and Beth Israel Medical Center. Students also gain significant experience in community settings, including the division's health clinics at public schools and community courts.

ACADEMIC RESOURCES
Students have access to all of the libraries within NYU including the Bobst Library, one of the largest open-stack libraries in the world, and the Ehrman Medical Library. The entire holdings of the libraries are accessed free electronically for all NYU students. The full texts of over 100 health and science journals and the Core Biomedical Collection are available through library Web sites. All enrolled students have free access to the Internet and E-mail both on campus and at home.

COSTS
Tuition and fees per term for 12 to 18 points in 2002–2003 were $12,475 (plus nonreturnable registration and services fee) for full-time undergraduates or $729 per point for fewer than 12 credits per term. Graduate students paid $834 per point (plus nonreturnable registration and services fee).

FINANCIAL AID
NYU offers aid that may include scholarships, grants, loans, or work study programs. Nursing students may qualify for Federal Nursing Student Loans, Phi Theta Kappa Scholarships, and scholarships for part-time study. For master's and doctoral candidates, a number of fellowships, assistantships, and federal nurse traineeships are available.

APPLYING
Baccalaureate program requirements differ for the four year, RN, college graduate, and dual BS/MA programs. Contact the nursing recruitment coordinator for details. The MA program requires a baccalaureate degree from a nursing program accredited by the National League for Nursing Accrediting Commission. A strong academic record, RN licensure, two professional letters of reference, a goal statement, and an interview may also be required. TOEFL scores are required for nonnative speakers of English.

CORRESPONDENCE AND INFORMATION
Nursing Recruitment Coordinator
Division of Nursing
The Steinhardt School of Education
New York University
246 Greene St., 4th Floor
New York, NY 10003-6677
(212) 998-5317
E-Mail: nursing.programs@nyu.edu
Web: www.nyu.edu/education/nursing

New York University is an affirmative action/equal opportunity institution.

NORTHEASTERN UNIVERSITY
Bouvé College of Health Sciences
School of Nursing
Boston, Massachusetts

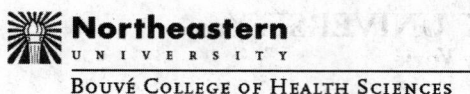

THE UNIVERSITY
Northeastern University is a private urban university and a world leader in cooperative education. With distinguished faculty, researchers, and scholars, the University is committed to providing high quality instruction in liberal and professional curricula.

THE SCHOOL OF NURSING
The primary mission of the School of Nursing is to prepare nursing leaders for basic and advanced nursing practice that contributes to the health of the nation.

The School of Nursing supports a community-based partnership with neighborhood health centers. This partnership enables students to develop skills for nursing practice in community based settings.

Students and faculty at the School of Nursing represent a wide variety of academic, professional, geographic, and cultural backgrounds from all over the world. Men comprise twelve percent of the student body.

PROGRAMS OF STUDY
Courses are scheduled on a quarterly basis in fall, winter, spring, and summer. The School of Nursing offers a Bachelor of Science degree program and a two-year, nine-month transfer-track BSN program. In the baccalaureate program, students alternate between academic quarters and co-op work assignments.

The Graduate School of Nursing offers a Master of Science degree program with clinical specializations in administration, anesthesia, community health, critical care, neonatal care, primary care, and psychiatric-mental health nursing. Additionally, the MS/MBA program prepares nurses for executive-level management in health care.

The Certificate of Advanced Study is a post-master's program designed for nurses with a master's degree in nursing who seek further academic preparation to learn advanced practice skills in another specialization area, or to qualify for national certification.

The RN to BS/MS program is designed for diploma/associate degree nurses with five years of nursing experience who seek an advanced degree. Opportunities for specialization in an area of practice lead to the Master of Science degree.

AFFILIATIONS WITH HEALTH CARE FACILITIES
The University's location in Boston enables the School of Nursing to assign students to supervised clinical experiences in renowned teaching hospitals. The School of Nursing has a partnership with the City of Boston's Commission on Public Health, which oversees all city public health initiatives and its system of neighborhood health centers.

ACADEMIC RESOURCES
University libraries contain more than 855,000 bound volumes, 1.7 million microforms, 150,000 documents, 5,500 periodical subscriptions, and 18,491 audio, video, and software titles. The Division of Academic Computing provides students with Internet access via the campus network to resources around the world. A central library contains technologically sophisticated services, including online catalog and circulation systems.

COSTS
The School of Nursing undergraduate tuition ranges from $16,450 to $19,590 for three-quarters depending on the year of study. Graduate tuition is $480 per quarter hour. (Mandatory fees are additional for both undergraduate and graduate students.)

FINANCIAL AID
Information about undergraduate financial aid is available from Northeastern University's Office of Financial Aid, (617) 373-3190.

The University offers financial aid to graduate students through several loan programs. There is also a limited number of teaching assistantships that provide a stipend and/or tuition remission.

CORRESPONDENCE AND INFORMATION
Northeastern University
Bouvé College of Health Sciences
School of Nursing (102RB)
Boston, MA 02115-5096
(617) 373-2200 Undergraduate Admissions
(617) 373-3125 Graduate School of Nursing

NORTHERN KENTUCKY UNIVERSITY
Highland Heights, KY

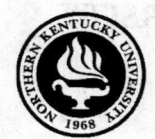

THE DEPARTMENT OF NURSING

The Department of Nursing at Northern Kentucky University (NKU) offers three programs in nursing: Bachelor of Science in Nursing (BSN), RN-BSN Program, and Graduate Program (MSN)—offering two tracks: 1) Administration and 2) Primary Care Nurse Practitioner.

CONTACT INFORMATION

For additional information please contact:
Northern Kentucky University
Department of Nursing
Nunn Drive
Highland Heights, KY 41099
(859) 572-5248
Fax: (859) 572-6098
E-Mail: andersonm@nku.edu
Web: www.nku.edu/nursing

OLD DOMINION UNIVERSITY
School of Nursing
Norfolk, VA

THE UNIVERSITY
Old Dominion University is a coed, state-supported university that currently boasts an enrollment of almost 19,000. The university was founded in 1930, and is situated on 172 acres in downtown Norfolk.

THE SCHOOL OF NURSING
The Old Dominion University School of Nursing was founded in 1963, and currently has 22 faculty members. Of these, 36% have doctorates. There are almost 600 students enrolled in the undergraduate program and almost 200 in the graduate program. The nursing school offers the opportunity to join the student nurses association and Sigma Theta Tau.

PROGRAMS OF STUDY
Nursing students at Old Dominion can achieve a generic Baccalaureate through a traditional or weekend program. The RN Baccalaureate is offered at more than 30 sites across the US and enrolls more than 550 students. Graduate courses are also offered via distance learning. Currently the Family Nurse Practitioner program is offered at 5 rural sites in Virginia.

ACADEMIC RESOURCES
The School of Nursing provides nursing audiovisuals, a learning resource lab, a computer lab, and CAI. Of the 851,194 volumes housed in the campus library, 40,598 are in health; the library also has 6,789 periodical subscriptions.

COSTS
Old Dominion University School of Nursing's current tuition costs are in-state $4,121 full-time, $134/credit, and out-of-state $10,640 full-time, $346/credit. Housing fees range from $3,000-$5,000.

FINANCIAL AID
Students can apply for direct loans, federal loans, and need- and/or performance-based scholarships. There are also Federal Work Study opportunities available.

ADMISSIONS
For undergraduates nursing applicants, ODU requires the SAT I, minimum college GPA of 2.0, all applicable transcripts, and 22 college credits for admission to the nursing program. For graduate school applicants, an RN license, diploma, or AD in nursing, transcripts, 29 prerequisite credits, and a minimum GPA of 2.0 are required. The application deadline for all programs is February 1.

CONTACT INFORMATION
M. Phyllis Barham, Chief Academic Adviser
358 Technology Building
School of Nursing
Old Dominion University
Norfolk, VA 23529-0500
(757) 683-5245
E-Mail: pbarham@odu.edu

DISTANCE RN INFORMATION:
Dr. Rob Curry
1-800-YOUR-BSN

PENNSYLVANIA COLLEGE OF TECHNOLOGY
Nursing, School of Health Sciences
Williamsport, Pennsylvania

Pennsylvania College of Technology

PENNSTATE

THE COLLEGE
An affiliate of The Pennsylvania State University (Penn State), Pennsylvania College of Technology (Penn College) is Pennsylvania's premier technical college and a respected leader in health sciences education. Located in beautiful northcentral Pennsylvania, the College has an 85-year history of education and service, and is renowned for its ongoing partnerships with industry and workforce development initiatives. Approximately 5,000 students attend credit classes and many more enjoy continuing education and lifelong learning in noncredit classes.

THE SCHOOL OF HEALTH SCIENCES
The School of Health Sciences is located in the Robert L. Breuder Advanced Technology and Health Sciences Center on Penn College's Main Campus in Williamsport. State-of-the-art facilities and associated clinical and practicum work in area hospitals provide students excellent learning opportunities in the following majors: applied health studies (BS), dental hygiene (BS and AAS), nursing (BS and AAS), physician assistant (BS), health arts (AAS), occupational therapy assistant (AAS), paramedic (AAS), physical fitness specialist (AAS), medical radiography (AAS), and practical nursing (certificate). BS degrees in Dental Hygiene and Applied Health Studies are available via Distance Learning.

PROGRAMS OF STUDY
Within the nursing curriculum, students may choose a variety of options. The BS degree option in Nursing is a degree-completion major, designed for the registered nurse who wishes to earn a degree on a full-time or part-time basis. It offers a core of nursing and general education courses, to be completed in four semesters. The AAS in Nursing prepares graduates for beginning staff nurse positions. Upon completion, graduates are eligible to take the registered nurse licensing examination (NCLEX-RN). It also is a foundation for the BS degree major. The certificate in Practical Nursing is designed as a three-semester curriculum to prepare graduates to take the practical nurse licensing exam (NCLEX-PN) and enter the field or to continue their education at the associate or bachelor degree level. Other related majors include: an associate degree in Health Arts major or BS Applied Health Studies major, both designed for licensed, certified, or registered health care workers who are looking for advancement opportunities (open to individuals with a college degree) and a BS degree in Physician Assistant major open to both freshmen and transfer students who wish to join the ranks of health professionals licensed to practice medicine with physician supervision.

AFFILIATIONS WITH HEALTH CARE FACILITIES
The School of Health Sciences maintains partnerships with hospitals and health care organizations in the region and provides a variety of opportunities for students to benefit from the clinical resources of these facilities. Students participate in clinical practice and gain experience in direct patient care during their program of study.

ACADEMIC RESOURCES
In addition to the modern laboratories of the Advanced Technology and Health Sciences Center and the experience of working in area hospitals and health care facilities, students enjoy the benefit of the Penn College Library on the Main Campus and open computer laboratories, which provide convenient access to computers for studying. Academic support services and free tutoring also are available to all students.

COSTS
On average, in-state students will pay approximately $7,500 in tuition and fees; out-of-state residents will pay an average of $10,000 per year. In addition, students in the nursing majors will pay $2,500-3,000 for tools, uniforms, and supplies. On-campus residence fees are approximately $1,600 per semester. Other costs may include laboratory instruction fees.

FINANCIAL AID
Financial aid, including loans, grants, scholarships, and work-study assistance, is available to eligible students. Students are encouraged to explore each option and to contact the Financial Aid Office for details. The College uses the Free Application for Federal Student Aid (FAFSA) for need analysis purposes. The form can be obtained from Penn College or high schools.

APPLYING
Admission to any Health Science major is competitive. Acceptances are granted twice a year, in January and May. Completion of minimum requirements does not guarantee acceptance into the program. Penn College reserves the right to accept only the most qualified applicants. A point system is used to help determine acceptance. Influencing factors in the point system include grade point average, SAT/ACT scores, high school rank, grades, and an interview process. All students must complete medical, dental, and eye exams prior to beginning the clinical/pre-clinical/laboratory portion of their curriculum. Students are responsible for related costs including health insurance, malpractice/liability insurance, travel, CPR certification, inoculations, and exam fees.

The BSN completion program is open only to RNs who have graduated from diploma and associate degree nursing programs.

CORRESPONDENCE AND INFORMATION
Director of Nursing
School of Health Sciences
Pennsylvania College of Technology
One College Avenue
Williamsport, PA 17701
(570) 327-4525

Office of Admissions
1-800-367-9222
healthsciences@pct.edu
admissions@pct.edu

POTTSVILLE HOSPITAL SCHOOL OF NURSING
Pottsville, PA

THE UNIVERSITY
Type of School: Private
Campus Setting: Suburban
Total Enrollment: 104

PROGRAM INFORMATION
Programs Offered: Diploma
Options: Continuing Education
Articulations: Diploma to BSN
NLNAC Accredited

NURSING STUDENT PROFILE
First-Year Undergraduate Enrollment: 45
Total Graduates: 26
Total Enrollment: 104

ACADEMICS
Academic Calendar: Semesters
Semester Start Date(s): September
Number of Faculty: 12
Nursing School Resources: Skills Lab; Separate Computer
Lab/Nursing Resources Center; CAI, Multimedia, Video, Access to
Internet

STUDENT LIFE
On-Campus Housing Facilities: No
Services Available: Health Clinic, Personal Counseling, Volunteer
Services, Campus Safety Program, Special Assistance for Disabled
Students, Tutoring, Counseling
Nursing Student Activities: NSNA Chapter

ADMISSIONS
Application Fee: $25
Preadmission Test: Yes
Transcript: Yes
Other Requirements: Letter(s) of recommendation, personal
interview, written essay, health exam, immunizations, advanced
standing available.

FINANCES
Grants: Federal Pell Grants
Scholarships: Institutionally-Sponsored Need-Based and Non Need-
Based Scholarships
Loans: Institutionally-Sponsored Loans, Federal PLUS Loans, Federal
Stafford Loans
Percentage of Students Receiving Some Type of Aid: 92%
Financial Aid Application Deadline: May 1
Financial Aid Office Phone: (570) 621-5027

CONTACT INFORMATION
Mrs. Angela Pasco, Director
Pottsville Hospital School of Nursing
Washington and Jackson Streets
Pottsville, PA 17901
(570) 621-5035
Web: www.pottsville.koz.com/randhsite/phnursing

THE READING HOSPITAL SCHOOL OF NURSING
Reading, Pennsylvania

The Reading Hospital
School of Nursing

The Reading Hospital School of Nursing is accredited by the National League for Nursing Accrediting Commission (NLNAC), and offers an exceptional educational program of both classroom and clinical experience in preparation for an exciting career in nursing.

For more than 100 years, our School has educated women and men who have gone on to serve in every field of nursing, both here at The Reading Hospital and Medical Center and in locations around the globe.

THREE WAYS TO LEARN MORE
The School of Nursing offers three great ways for prospective students to learn more about its nursing program and the student life: Open Houses, the Student Nurse for a Day and the Discover Nursing programs.

Open House: Our Open House Schedule runs from October through April. For the complete schedule, visit our Web site at www.readinghospital.org. Click on Allied Health Schools, then School of Nursing.

Student Nurse for a Day Program: Open to qualified high school juniors and seniors, this program takes you into the Hospital to experience the daily work of professional nurses. The Reading Hospital School of Nursing is pleased to offer a one-day program, which will match you with a member of the student body or faculty, and allow you to experience the life of a student nurse. The day is filled with valuable information and guided tours through key areas of the campus. If you're thinking about a career in nursing, don't miss this opportunity!

Discover Nursing Program: This four-day program runs through the summer and is open to qualified students who are entering either their junior or senior year in high school. The program allows the participant the opportunity to work with nurses in various positions within the Hospital, such as maternity, pediatrics, medical-surgical, and emergency-care nursing.

PROGRAMS
Our diploma programs include our Day Program (24 months) and our Evening/Weekend Program (36 months), and are based upon theoretical knowledge and hands-on application of that knowledge. Supervised clinical practice begins early in the freshman year, assisting students in gaining nursing skills, confidence, and critical thinking ability. After completion of the program, graduates are eligible to take the licensure examination for professional registered nurses.

ADMISSIONS
All applicants to the School of Nursing are considered on the basis of academic ability, personal qualities, and potential to meet the academic standards of the School. Admission decisions are based on the applicant's complete academic and personal profile, which includes current and previous academic work, standardized test scores (SAT or ACT), work or life experience, professional references, and, in some cases, an interview. The Admission office accepts applications on a rolling basis.

COSTS
Tuition for full time students living on campus ranges from $8,109 - $9,081. For a complete listing of tuition and fees for each program (day or evening/weekend), visit our Web site at www.readinghospital.org. Click on Allied Health Schools, then School of Nursing.

FINANCIAL AID
The Financial Aid Office is designed to help qualified students pursue a nursing education regardless of financial circumstances. Counseling and assistance are provided to make it financially possible for admitted students to attend the Reading Hospital School of Nursing. Financial Aid packages include The Reading Hospital Tuition Incentive Program, Federal Pell Grant, Federal Plus Loan, PHEAA State Grant, Employer Tuition Assistance, Federal Subsidized Stafford Loan, Federal Unsubsidized Stafford Loan, Veterans Funding, and Sheetz Scholarships.

FOR MORE INFORMATION
To learn more about The Reading Hospital School of Nursing, or request a complete catalog, please contact the program coordinator at (610) 988-8336, or E-Mail rhsn@readinghospital.org.
You may also visit us online at: www.readinghospital.org.

REGIS COLLEGE
Division of Nursing
Weston, Massachusetts

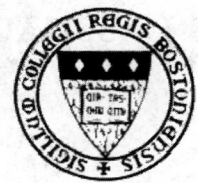

THE COLLEGE

Regis College is a small, Catholic, liberal arts and sciences college for undergraduate women and graduate-level men and women. Founded in 1927 by the Congregation of the Sisters of Saint Joseph of Boston, their members desired to put their resources to use for the good of society through education. The College is consistently rated among the top small liberal arts colleges in the North in "America's Best Colleges" by *U.S. News & World Report.* Regis College offers bachelor's degrees in a wide variety of majors and master's degrees in Nursing, Education, Leadership and Organizational Change, Communications, and Health Product and Policy Regulation.

PROGRAMS OF STUDY

The undergraduate program offers a BSN, a four-year course of study that prepares individuals for professional practice as registered nurses. Students gain diverse clinical experiences within the greater Boston area and develop skills that prepare them to provide care to clients in a wide variety of healthcare settings.

The graduate program offers a Master of Science with a focus in nursing administration for diverse healthcare systems, or nurse practitioner. The nurse practitioner track offers three primary care options: pediatric, family, and psychiatric mental health nurse practitioner. An accelerated curriculum track is designed for non-nurses who hold a baccalaureate degree in a field other than nursing. This track requires the completion of certain prerequisite courses and requires three years, including two summers of study. Students take the NCLEX-RN exam after the second year, and a BSN is awarded. At the completion of the third year, the MS is awarded, and students are eligible to take nurse practitioner certification examinations.

The RN to BS to MS Upward Mobility track allows students with an associate degree or diploma in nursing to earn both the BS and MS within one curriculum. Students have the option of exiting the program with the BSN. Registered nurses who have a baccalaureate degree in a discipline other than nursing may enter this accelerated pathway as well. Classes are offered during the day, in the evening, on weekends, and during the summer.

AFFILIATIONS WITH HEALTH-CARE FACILITIES

The Division of Nursing at Regis College offers a wide variety of health-care settings in which students may obtain clinical experiences appropriate for their educational and professional goals. Students are placed in acute-, subacute-, and long-term-care facilities; nurse-managed clinics in homeless shelters; elementary and secondary schools; and elderly and low-income housing in both urban and suburban settings. Qualified nurse practitioner students have the opportunity to complete a portion of the clinical requirement in approved national or international settings. The Division of Nursing also offers two workplace satellite programs for registered nurses employed in the Boston area, one at the Lahey Clinic and the other at Hallmark Health Systems.

COSTS

Tuition for 2002–03 was $365 per credit for undergraduate nursing courses, $970 per course for non-nursing undergraduate courses, and $480 per credit for graduate courses. Full-time tuition for undergraduate and graduate students was $9,500 per semester. Regis offers a 30% discount for the first two courses taken at the graduate

level and a 20% discount to Regis graduates and students from non-profit organizations. Summer tuition depends on the number of credits carried. VISA, MasterCard, or Discover may be used for tuition payment. A tuition payment plan is also available. For further information, students should contact the Controller's Office at (781) 768-7200. The total cost of the program varies depending upon the number of credits transferred or granted by examination or articulation.

FINANCIAL AID

The Regis College Office of Financial Aid is located in College Hall, Room 121. Students interested in applying for financial aid may request information by calling (781) 768-7180. Prospective students should investigate any possible sources of financial assistance, including loans, employer tuition remission, and scholarships.

ADMISSIONS

All nursing applicants are processed through the Regis College Office of Admission and are considered on a rolling basis. Applicants must submit a complete application, including a resume, a signed personal statement, three confidential letters of recommendation, and official transcripts from the nursing program and/or colleges attended. Scores from the Graduate Record Examinations (GRE) or Miller Analogies Test (taken within the past five years) are required for admission to the graduate program. Prospective students should inquire about exceptions. GREs may be waived in certain circumstances. There is a $30 application fee. A minimum GPA of 3.0 from undergraduate, diploma, associate degree, and prerequisite courses is advised. A personal interview is required of all applicants. RN applicants must be graduates of accredited diploma, associate degree, or baccalaureate programs in nursing. Documentation of individual malpractice insurance and current Massachusetts license to practice as a registered nurse must be provided four weeks prior to clinical courses. Regis College offers the registered nurse the opportunity for advanced placement through CLEP and other Advanced Placement examinations. For further information, prospective students should contact the Division of Nursing.

CORRESPONDENCE AND INFORMATION

Lisa Krug
Assistant Director of Admission
Box 49
Regis College
235 Wellesley Street
Weston, Massachusetts 02493-1571
(781) 768-7188
800-456-1820 (toll-free)
Fax: 781-768-7089
E-Mail: nursing@regiscollege.edu
Web: www.regiscollege.edu

REGIS UNIVERSITY SCHOOL FOR HEALTH CARE PROFESSIONS
Denver, Colorado

Regis University is accredited by the North Central Association of Colleges and Secondary Schools. The Department of Nursing is accredited by the American Association of Colleges of Nursing-Commission on Collegiate Nursing Education (AACN-CCNE). The Department of Nursing offers exceptional educational programs to prepare students for an exciting career in nursing.

Programs offered include:

- Bachelor of Science in Nursing—traditional and accelerated options (campus-based)
- Bachelor of Science in Nursing—RN to BSN Completion Option (campus-based and online)
- Master of Science, Nursing—Family Nurse Practitioner Emphasis (campus-based)
- Master of Science, Nursing—Leadership in Health Care Systems, Education and Management Emphasis (campus-based and online)

WAYS TO LEARN MORE
To learn more about the nursing programs offered at Regis University, you can attend one of our information sessions or check out our Web site.

Information Sessions: Information sessions for the Traditional and the Accelerated program are held the second Tuesday of each month at noon and the fourth Tuesday of each month at 5:30 P.M. Please call the Office of Admissions for details at 1-800-388-2366 ext. 4344.

Internet: Our Web site gives valuable information, such as a brief description of the program, admission process, tuition, program requirements, and course descriptions. Go to www.regis.edu for more information.

PROGRAMS
BSN Traditional Option
The program is offered in a traditional college schedule, covering 57 semester hours over four semesters and two calendar years.

- Strong clinical practice component
- You are eligible to take the Licensed Practical Nurse exam after successful completion of your Junior year.
- Prerequisite coursework can be taken via Regis College or transferred in from other schools.

BSN Accelerated Option
Regis University's Accelerated Option is designed to provide fast-paced, quality nursing education for students with previous bachelors degrees and appropriate prerequisite coursework.

- One-year program of study, starting twice yearly, in January and May
- Colorado's most rapid option for students with prior bachelors degrees and required prerequisites, seeking a Bachelor of Science in Nursing
- The program is complemented by more than 700 clinical practice hours.

RN to BSN Option
Regis University offers convenient and flexible campus-based, online, and worksite options for Registered Nurses seeking a Bachelor of Science in Nursing.

- Convenient Internet-based or one-evening-per-week campus-based formats for Diploma or Associate Degree-level Registered Nurses
- Flexible pace for returning adult students

Master of Science, Nursing
Only 10 percent of nurses nationwide are Master's-prepared. You can take your nursing career to the next level with a graduate degree from Regis University.

The Family Nurse Practitioner program prepares you to deliver primary care services to families across the life span. It is five semesters in length and meets in a convenient every-other-weekend format.

The Leadership in Health Care Systems program prepares you for leadership, management, and education positions throughout the health care system. The program is seven semesters in length and meets one night per week. This program is offered in an online format as well.

ADMISSIONS
Applications are evaluated on a rolling admission basis, meaning it is to your advantage to submit your materials as soon as they are completed. Your application is reviewed and an enrollment decision made once all required application materials are submitted. Course size is limited.

COSTS
Tuition for each program varies. For a complete listing of tuition and fees for each program, visit our Web site at www.regis.edu.

FINANCIAL AID
Financial aid information is available through the Office of Financial Aid at Regis University. Please contact the office directly at 1-800-388-2633 ext. 4066 or visit their Web site at www.regis.edu/financialaid.

FOR MORE INFORMATION
To learn more about Regis University's School for Health Care Professions Department of Nursing, or request an information packet, please contact the Admissions Office at 1-800-388-2366 x4344, or E-Mail shcp@regis.edu. You may also visit us online at www.regis.edu.

RIVERSIDE SCHOOL OF PROFESSIONAL NURSING
Newport News, Virginia

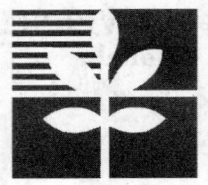

RIVERSIDE REGIONAL MEDICAL CENTER

Riverside Regional Medical Center (RRMC), is a 576-bed tertiary medical center located in Newport News, Virginia. Since its beginning in 1916, RRMC has continually expanded patient care facilities and programs, and has become a major referral center for the Peninsula and Middle Peninsula regions of Virginia. Riverside's Cardiovascular Program has been recognized by HCIA Sachs as one of the top 100 cardiovascular hospitals in the nation. The Riverside Cancer Treatment Center is affiliated with dozens of leading academic centers across the continent and has been recognized by the Commission on Cancer of the American College of Surgeons as offering high-quality cancer care. Our Level II Emergency/Trauma Center provides comprehensive emergency services. Planning for every possible medical need, Riverside Regional Medical Center provides a host of specialized services and units, including the Centers of Excellence in Diabetes, Geriatrics, Dialysis, Orthopedics, and Women's Services.

RIVERSIDE SCHOOL OF PROFESSIONAL NURSING

The Riverside School of Professional Nursing (RSPN) has been a leader in providing quality nursing education since its beginning in the early 1900's. The Riverside Regional Medical Center-based school offers a diversified curriculum that includes advanced placement for practical nurses and medical corpsman that are interested in a nursing career. An Evening/Weekend program as well as a Day program is offered. The school's program leads to a diploma in nursing. The curriculum, well known for the strong clinical component, begins with closely supervised clinical experience early in the first course. RSPN requires specific college courses to supplement the clinical experience and classes offered. RSPN is approved by The Virginia State Board of Nursing and accredited by the National League for Nursing Accrediting Commission.

ADMISSION REQUIREMENTS

- Applicants must be a graduate of an accredited high school or have earned a high school equivalency (GED) certificate.
- A minimum of 12 academic units (grade level 9-12) Required units: 4 units of English; 1 unit of Biology; 1 unit of Chemistry; 2 units of Mathematics. Overall GPA of 2.5 on 4.0 system and 2.5 in required academic subjects. Students with prior college credits will be considered on an individual basis.
- College Entrance Examination board required. Post high school academic courses may be substituted.
- Four satisfactory Personal Evaluation Forms
- Satisfactory score on Nurse Entrance Test (NET)
- Must be able to meet the essential requirements of the program.
- Test of English as a Foreign Language (TOEFL) with a minimum score of 550 is required for students with English as a second language.
- Immigration card required for resident aliens.
- Satisfactory Personal Interview
- Essay

APPLICATION PROCESS

Applications are accepted on an ongoing basis. A completed application packet includes the following:

- Completed signed application for admission
- Four completed evaluation forms
- Pre-Admission Examination completed
- TOEFL Scores and Immigration Card
- Recommendation from Dean/Director, Nursing course syllabi, if you are a transfer student
- College transcripts, if applicable
- High school transcript or GED
- Satisfactory interview
- Current State License if you are an LPN

The School of Professional Nursing reserves the right to select those applicants who seem best qualified for the study of nursing.

Applications for Admission may be obtained by writing to the address listed below.

SERVICES/RESOURCES AVAILABLE

- Financial Assistance Program including Power-Of-One Scholarships (free tuition)
- Grant/Scholarship Assistance
- Health Sciences Library
- Health Services
- Parking Facilities
- National Student Nurses' Association
- Hospital Publications
- Student Employment Opportunities

TUITION & FEES

Application Fee:	$ 25
Registration Fee:	$ 100
Challenge Fee:	$ 400
Transfer Fee:	$ 50

Fixed Tuition Expenses:
First Level:

First Trimester/Semester	$1,465
Second Trimester/Semester:	$1,000
Third Trimester/Semester:	$1,000

Second Level:

First Trimester/Semester	$1,490
Second Trimester/Semester:	$1,000
Third Trimester/Semester:	$1,000

Variable Expenses Include:

- Prerequisite college courses
- Textbooks
- Uniforms
- Dormitory fees, if applicable
- Meal Tickets, if desired

CORRESPONDENCE AND INFORMATION

Student Personnel Coordinator
Riverside School of Professional Nursing
500 J. Clyde Morris Blvd.
Newport News, VA 23601
(757) 594-2705

ROCKFORD COLLEGE
Rockford, Illinois

PROGRAM DESCRIPTION

Health care is a field with a future—and Rockford College graduates find they are well prepared to be a part of that future!

Meeting and managing society's health care needs requires the skills of many different people; doctors, nurses and other health care practitioners, to be sure, but also educators, administrators, social workers, and other related and well-educated professionals. Whether you are planning on a white coat or a white collar, you'll find that Rockford College offers a widely respected program in nursing as well as pre-professional programs for those interested in medicine, dentistry, physical therapy, or other health careers. In addition, a program in Athletic Training is offered as well. You will also find a full slate of liberal arts degrees and programs—excellent preparation for graduate school or a future in health care! By integrating professional preparation with a liberal arts-oriented course of study for those going into health care, Rockford College helps you gain an appreciation for different people and perspectives, lets you develop confidence in your own abilities, and offers you the skills you will need to work in tandem with other health care providers. The liberal arts context of a Rockford College education gives you the opportunity to focus on decision-making and communication skills, analytical thinking, and ethical concerns – abilities you will need in any health care field. "Rockford College was the best thing that ever happened to me," said Dr. Marc Pfeffer '69, who now teaches at Harvard Medical School. "I could hold my head high when I went to my graduate classes."

A small average class size and a dedicated faculty mean that you will receive personal attention and have the opportunity to develop close working relationships with your faculty. Alice Zwangstra '84, a clinical nurse specialist at Rockford Memorial Hospital, appreciated the "special interest" that professors took in students. "My education at Rockford College was excellent preparation for graduate school," she says. Rockford College graduates do wind up in some of the nation's best medical schools and graduate health care programs — as well as in great jobs.

Located in the second largest city in Illinois, Rockford College places you close to excellent internship and practicum sites, from hospitals and clinics, to social service agencies and homeless shelters, to research laboratories. Recently, for example, Rockford College students have completed internships and practicums at Rockford Memorial Hospital, St. Anthony Medical Center, and Swedish American Hospital.

The Rockford College nursing program is fully accredited by the National League for Nursing Accrediting Commission and approved by the State of Illinois Department of Professional Regulation. The Athletic Training Education Program (ATEP) has been admitted to "Candidacy" by CAAHEP (Commission on Accrediting Allied Health Education Programs) for accreditation.

PROGRAMS OF STUDY

Nursing -- BSN and BSN completion
Athletic Training
Health Sciences/Pre-professional Programs
Dentistry
Medicine
Medical Technology
Occupational Therapy
Optometry
Pharmacy
Physical Therapy
Veterinary Medicine

CONTACT INFORMATION

For more information about the Rockford College nursing program, athletic training program, or any other health-related course of study, call the Office of Admission toll-free at (800) 892-2984, fax us at (815) 226-2822, or visit our Web site at www.rockford.edu.

Rockford College
5050 East State Street
Rockford, Illinois 61108-2393
Web: www.rockford.edu

ROCKLAND COMMUNITY COLLEGE
Department of Nursing
Suffern, NY

THE COLLEGE
Rockland Community College, a division of the State University of New York, opened in September of 1959. It is a comprehensive Community College offering transfer programs, career entry programs, and continuing education programs in a wide variety of areas. SUNY Rockland's 6000+ students have the opportunity to participate in an array of campus-based clubs, sports, and cultural events. They are also lucky enough to be able to experience the cultural and educational benefits of Manhattan, only 30 miles away, while enjoying the rural life of Rockland County.

THE NURSING PROGRAM
The Nursing Program, which began in 1961, leads to an Associate of Science Degree in nursing. The goals of the program are to 1) meet the needs of the community for individuals who are both informed citizens and registered nurses, and 2) provide access into practice as a Registered Nurse and the basis for baccalaureate and higher education in nursing for all who desire it. The program is registered by the new York State Education Department and has been accredited by the National League for Nursing Accrediting Commission (formerly the National League for Nursing) since its inception. It maintains a direct articulation agreement for baccalaureate study with SUNY New Paltz and with New York University.

PROGRAMS OF STUDY
The nursing program may be completed on a full- or part-time basis and as a day and/or evening student. The curriculum consists of a four-level sequence of Nursing Process courses, a course in Calculations for Pharmacology, and related courses in the arts and sciences. Each Nursing Process level includes two courses with lecture, college laboratory, and clinical laboratory components. The courses in each level may be taken concurrently or successively dependent on students' needs.

Licensed Practical Nurses may qualify for advanced placement through the LPN to RN Express track. The LPN to RN Express was designed to prepare Licensed Practical Nurses to become Registered Nurses in a time efficient manner by providing credit for existing knowledge and skills. LPNs in this track receive credit for the first Nursing Process level and are eligible to challenge Nursing Process courses in Levels II and III.

A special offering of the Department of Nursing is a seminar of Transcultural Nursing offered for two weeks each January in London, England. This is a 3 credit course which may be used to meet degree requirements or may be taken for continuing education credits. Cost of the course, which includes airfare from New York, hotel, tuition, and all scheduled course activities abroad varies with the exchange rate but has been in the vicinity of $1,800.

ACADEMIC RESOURCES
The Library Media Arts Center provides over 140,000 volumes, as well as over 1,000 periodicals and multimedia resources. Study centers are available in three different off-campus locations. Students are able to take advantage of extensive career development and placement resources as well as academic support services. Within the Department of Nursing, students have access to a Support Module, which provides reinforcement of the major concepts taught in each clinical course. Selected courses are also available online.

COSTS
Tuition at Rockland Community College for full-time, in-state students is $2,325 per year.

FINANCIAL AID
Work-Study is available at RCC, as well as many federal aid packages. The Rockland Community College Foundation also awards over $80,000/year at the annual Honors Convocation.

ADMISSIONS
SUNY Rockland is an open-admission institution. To enroll in a Nursing Process course, students must be admitted to the college, take the English and Mathematics Assessments, complete any required English or Mathematics remediation, and fill out an application for Nursing. Students who have fulfilled these requirements and attached required health documents are admitted into the first Nursing Process course on a first come-first served basis. Reentering and transfer students are placed on a space available basis.

CONTACT INFORMATION
For detailed information on the Nursing Program, request the Nursing Program Guide by writing or calling:
Dr. Frances D. Monahan
Director, Department of Nursing
SUNY Rockland Community College
145 College Road
Suffern, NY 10901
(914) 574-4222

ROXBOROUGH MEMORIAL HOSPITAL
School of Nursing
Philadelphia, PA

THE HOSPITAL
Roxborough Memorial Hospital's history dates back to 1890 when a community of clergy and laymen founded St. Timothy's Memorial Hospital and House of Mercy of Roxborough. The hospital has grown from its 11-bed capacity to a 187-bed modern medical facility. The Mission of the Hospital remains unchanged. It continues to provide quality health care services to the community by promoting health, preventing disease, and treating illness.

THE SCHOOL
The School of Nursing was founded in 1898 and graduated five women in 1901. Since that time, the school has graduated over 1,000 men and women. Many of our graduates hold distinguished positions in Nursing Education and Nursing Service. The School of Nursing is a 21-month hospital-based program providing a unique blend of nursing theory, a strong clinical component, and college credits.

THE COMMUNITY
Roxborough is a northwestern neighborhood within the city limits of Philadelphia. Although conveniently located to downtown Philadelphia, Roxborough is a close knit community with a small town atmosphere. In recent years the community has been recognized as the home of "The Wall," a steep winding street that challenges world class cyclists each year during the First Union Bicycle Race. Located "down the hill" from Roxborough is Manayunk, once a center of manufacturing, which in recent years has seen a rebirth, and has become the home to fine dining, unique shops, and exciting night life.

ACCREDITATION
School of Nursing
Accredited by: The National League for Nursing Accrediting Commission (NLNAC)
Approved by: The Pennsylvania State Board of Nursing
For information regarding accreditation contact:
National League for Nursing Accrediting Commission
61 Broadway
New York, NY 10006
(212) 363-5555
Hospital
Accredited by: The Joint Commission on Accreditation of Health Care Organizations
Member of: The Hospital Association of Pennsylvania and the Delaware Valley Hospital Council

THE EDUCATIONAL PROGRAM
The Educational Program has been developed from the philosophy and objectives of the School of Nursing. It extends over a period of 21 months and prepares the graduate to take the National Council Licensure Examination to practice as a registered nurse. The major objective of the first year's curriculum is that the student be able to provide for the changing needs of patients by assessing altered needs, identifying plans of nursing action, and implementing the plans of nursing action for selected patients and families. This is accomplished because the student has a knowledge base of the biopsychosocial influences on health throughout the human life cycle. In addition, students can recognize the pathophysiologic and compensatory responses of the patient to stress during the human life cycle.

Students' effectiveness of learning is evaluated through observation and testing. Specific standardized tests are administered to the students near the completion of their educational program. The Mosby Assess Test and National League for Nursing tests in Medical-Surgical Nursing, Maternal Child Health, Pharmacology, and Psychiatric Nursing are administered. The ultimate goal of education is the growth of the student into a professional capable of making sound decisions in the provision of nursing care.

AFFILIATIONS WITH HEALTH CARE FACILITIES
The Roxborough Memorial Hospital School of Nursing maintains contractual agreements with many health care facilities. The School's educational resources include community hospitals and clinics, a specialized children's hospital, psychiatric and mental health agencies, community-based outpatient settings, and acute care inpatient facilities.

TUITION
The approximate tuition for the program is estimated at $7,918 for Year I and $8,027 for Year II. Additional costs include fees, books, uniforms, transportation, and personal living expenses.

FINANCIAL AID
FFELP Federal Family Education Loan Program (Stafford)
Federal Pell Grant
PHEAA State Grant
Institutional Awards
Institutional Financial Aid deadline is April 30

APPLICATION & ADMISSION
Applicants must have a high school diploma or a GED (General Education Diploma). They must have completed 16 high school units or equivalents of Biology, Chemistry, Algebra, Geometry, Social Studies, and English. SAT scores of 400 in each area, taken in the last 5 years, will be considered. An NLN pre-nursing exam or pre-admission exam may be required. If college courses are taken prior to starting the nursing program, a GPA of 2.5 is required. Along with an application, official high school, college, and financial aid transcripts (if applicable) are required.

CORRESPONDENCE AND INFORMATION
Roxborough Memorial Hospital
School of Nursing
Director, Admissions and Recruitment
5800 Ridge Avenue
Philadelphia, PA 19128
(215) 487-4344
Fax: (215) 487-4591

SACRED HEART UNIVERSITY
Department of Nursing
Fairfield, CT

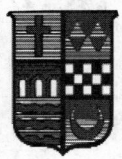

THE UNIVERSITY

Sacred Heart University, established in 1963, is a coeducational independent institution of higher learning in the Catholic intellectual tradition whose primary objective is to prepare men and women to live in and make their contributions to the human community. Sacred Heart University is committed to combining education for life with preparation for professional excellence. Ideally located in beautiful Fairfield County in southwestern Connecticut, more than half of the 56-acre campus is surrounded by a thirty-six hole golf course. The campus location promotes easy accessibility to shopping, dining, cultural, and leisure activities.

THE DEPARTMENT OF NURSING

Nursing at Sacred Heart University is an integral part of the overall University, whose aim is to assist in the development of people who are knowledgeable of self, rooted in faith, educated in mind, compassionate in heart, responsive to social and civic obligations, and prepared to contribute to an ever-changing world. The Nursing Faculty believes that Nursing is an evolving professional discipline, grounded in the liberal arts, sciences, and humanities. These disciplines support the science and art of nursing, providing the framework for practice, development of new knowledge, and nursing education.

The nursing curriculum at Sacred Heart University incorporates both traditional hospital and community practice settings to assure that students have access to state-of-the-art practice and the opportunity to develop the essential skills of clinical practice. With dramatic change occurring within the healthcare environment, nurses play an increasingly important role in improving the delivery of care through their critical thinking skills and holistic perspective, while ensuring that patients receive the care and services required.

Hallmarks of the Sacred Heart University Nursing Programs include strong emphasis on the spiritual and ethical implications of healthcare, the impact of diversity on patients and caregivers, the health of individuals within communities, and special consideration of the needs of the growing population of older people. The Sacred Heart Nursing Program was recently recognized by the American Association of Colleges of Nursing and the Hartford Institute for Geriatric Nursing for implementation of an innovative curriculum in geriatric nursing.

The Nursing Faculty is comprised of highly experienced professionals recognized as experts among their peers, representing the major clinical specialties within nursing. The full-time faculty works closely with selectively recruited adjunct faculty who provide special skills and focus areas.

PROGRAMS OF STUDY

The following programs of undergraduate and graduate study are offered:

- BSN for beginning and transfer students
- RN-BSN with the option of Web-based courses
- MSN in Family Nurse Practitioner and Patient Care Services Administration
- MSN/MBA
- RN-MSN in Patient Care Services Administration
- Post-master's Certificate option in Family Nurse Practitioner

The BSN plan of study introduces core nursing courses in the sophomore year, including foundations of practice and health assessment, medical/surgical nursing, and obstetrics and pediatric content. The junior and senior years build upon that knowledge, increasing the complexity and number of patients cared for while developing the expected leadership, communication, evaluation, and critical thinking skills. Service learning activities are planned in several courses, coupling real world experience with learning objectives.

The RN-BSN program is a highly flexible course of study that is influenced by individual professional goals and experiences. Students may elect traditional classroom experiences, a Web-based curriculum, or a combination of both to fulfill the requirements of the BSN.

The Family Nurse Practitioner major prepares graduates for advanced practice across the life span. This rigorous curriculum incorporates traditional and interactive classroom activities, case study analysis, demonstration, clinical laboratory and supervised clinical practice with an expert preceptor. Completion results in an MSN, or for nurses already prepared at the Master's level, a certificate, qualifying graduates to take a national certification examination.

The Patient Care Services program prepares RNs for positions of administrative responsibility within healthcare organizations. Contemporary leadership theory and practice are examined within the context of the dramatically changing healthcare environment to ensure graduates are prepared to lead the next generation of healthcare providers. Students have the option to enroll for a dual MSN-MBA degree if they meet entry requirements.

AFFILIATIONS

More than eight acute-care hospitals and a large variety of healthcare facilities and organizations are located within 30 minutes of the main campus, providing a rich resource of learning experiences in virtually every major clinical practice area. Opportunities for internships and other types of experiential programs are in place and are increasing due to employer demand and a growing nursing shortage.

ACADEMIC FACILITIES

The University's library contains more than 164,000 volumes, 2157 periodical titles, and 110,000 nonprint items such as videotapes, audiocassettes, etc. It also provides online database searching services. There are 4,823 volumes for the health sciences as well as 106 periodicals in nursing.

Sacred Heart University is in the sixth year of its Student Mobile Computing Program. Full-time students receive an IBM ThinkPad computer. The campus has been transformed into a fully networked environment that uses state-of-the-art multimedia educational technology to enhance learning.

The Nursing Laboratory is a large multipurpose location containing 5 computers with programs on nutrition, NCLEX success, comprehensive reviews for NCLEX, and full access to the University Library and the Internet. The clinical laboratory component includes inpatient stations and related equipment as well as examining tables and instruments appropriate for outpatient settings.

SACRED HEART UNIVERSITY
(continued)

STUDENT SERVICES

A five-year Strategic Plan calls for the construction of new facilities as well as the implementation of new academic, athletic, and social programs. Seven new residence halls have opened in the last four years. A $17 million health and recreation complex opened in 1997.

Sacred Heart University is committed to providing students with extensive services to complement their education, offering a large and diverse array of student activities and services, including tutoring, study skills support, clubs and learning, social, and athletic events.

There is an active Student Nurses Association, a significant number of loyal alumni involved in numerous program efforts, and a strong chapter of Sigma Theta Tau, the honor society for nursing. Faculty are committed to individualized advisement, and a low faculty to student ratio is designed to provide meaningful educational experiences.

SAINT LOUIS UNIVERSITY
School of Nursing
St. Louis, Missouri

THE UNIVERSITY
Saint Louis University, a private Catholic university, was founded in 1832, and is the oldest institution of higher learning west of the Mississippi River. With two campuses in the heart of St. Louis, Missouri and one campus in Madrid, Spain, the University has a combined enrollment of 11,000. Saint Louis University has been named a Research II facility by the Carnegie Foundation for the Advancement of Teaching.

THE SCHOOL OF NURSING
Since it was founded in 1928, the School of Nursing has been a national leader in nursing education. The School was the first nursing school in Missouri to offer a doctoral program in nursing and the first nursing school in the U.S. to develop and offer a second-degree accelerated baccalaureate program. Recently, the School became the first to offer complete nurse practitioner master's degree programs online through the World Wide Web. The Gorman Report ranks the School in the top 3 percent of nursing schools in the United States.

The School of Nursing is located on the prestigious Health Sciences Center campus of Saint Louis University. Located directly across from the campus are the Saint Louis University Hospital complex and research center and Cardinal Glennon Children's Hospital, just two of the facilities where nursing students complete clinical experiences. The School of Nursing also offers clinical opportunities at a large number of area hospitals and clinics and community health, mental health, and long-term care facilities.

BACCALAUREATE DEGREE PROGRAMS
Four-Year BSN: Four-year, eight-semester BSN program. Students accepted as freshmen or college transfer. *Admission requirements:* ACT, minimum cumulative GPA of 2.5, one year of high school biology and chemistry. *Application deadline:* rolling.
One-Year Second-Degree Accelerated BSN: Full-time, three-semester BSN program that begins during the summer session each year. *Admission requirements:* BA, BS or higher degree in another area, minimum cumulative GPA of 2.5, completion of nursing prerequisites. *Recommended application deadline:* January 1.
RN to MSN: BSN completion program for RNs that provides direct matriculation into the master's program. Part- and full-time study plans. Transfer of nursing and non-nursing courses credit hours. No testing required. *Admission requirements:* Current RN licensure, minimum cumulative GPA of 2.5. *Application deadline:* rolling.

MASTER'S DEGREE PROGRAMS
MSN and MSN(Research): 36 to 50 credit-hour curriculum programs in Adult, Family and Community Health, Gerontological, Informatics, Pediatric, Perinatal, and Psychiatric/Mental Health Nursing. Part- and full-time study plans. *Nurse practitioner programs:* Adult, Family, Gerontological and Pediatric. *Joint MSN degree programs available with MPH. Admission requirements:* baccalaureate degree in nursing, minimum cumulative GPA of 3.0, current RN licensure. *Application deadline:* July 1 for fall, Nov. 1 for spring, April 1 for summer.

POST-MASTER'S CERTIFICATES
Post-master's certificates are available in all master's specialty areas and role preparations. Minimum of 15 credit hours required for completion. *Admission requirements:* master's degree in nursing, minimum cumulative GPA of 3.0, current professional nurse licensure, current CPR certification. *Application deadline:* July 1 for fall, Nov. 1 for spring, April 1 for summer.

DOCTORAL PROGRAM
The PhD program is a 72-credit hour program that includes 60 credit hours of course work and 12 credit hours of dissertation research. Up to 18 credit hours accepted from master's program in nursing. *Admission requirements:* master's degree in nursing, minimum cumulative GPA of 3.25, GRE, current professional nurse licensure. *Application deadline:* July 1 for fall.

DISTANCE LEARNING
Complete master's degree programs are offered online through the World Wide Web for the nurse practitioner role in Adult, Family, Gerontological and Pediatric nursing and for the clinical nurse specialist role in adult and gerontological nursing. Students must meet MSN admission requirements.

FINANCIAL AID
Saint Louis University offers academic scholarships, need-based tuition assistance, and loans for undergraduate students. For graduate students, graduate assistantships, traineeships, and loans are available. The School of Nursing provides a limited number of need-based tuition awards for undergraduate and graduate students.

ACCREDITATION
Saint Louis University is accredited by the North Central Association of Colleges and Secondary Schools. The School of Nursing is fully accredited by the National League for Nursing Accrediting Commission and the Missouri State Board of Nursing.

FOR MORE INFORMATION
Director of Marketing and Recruitment
Saint Louis University School of Nursing
3525 Caroline Mall
St. Louis, MO 63104
(314) 577-8995
Fax: (314) 577-8949
E-Mail: slunurse@slu.edu
Web: www.slu.edu/colleges/NR

SAN DIEGO CITY COLLEGE
Nursing Education Department
San Diego, California

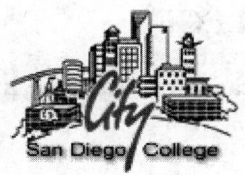

THE COLLEGE
San Diego City College, founded in 1914, is a public, comprehensive community college offering a wide variety of occupational and academic programs. It is a multicultural institution committed to providing open access to all and preparing students for transfer to a four year college or university. City College is in the beautiful community of downtown San Diego near the San Diego Zoo, Sea Port Village, Gas Lamp Quarter, the Harbor, beaches, and more. The college is conveniently situated near bus and trolley stops, three major freeways, and major city and county services and facilities. San Diego City College is accredited by the Western Association of Schools and Colleges.

THE DEPARTMENT OF NURSING EDUCATION
The San Diego City College Nursing program prepares its graduates to function in today's evolving health care market. Graduates receive an Associate of Science Degree in Nursing and are eligible to take the NCLEX-RN® for licensure as a Registered Nurse. The City College Nursing program has an excellent reputation in the community providing graduates with multiple employment opportunities. The nursing program is accredited by the California Board of Registered Nursing and the National League for Nursing Accrediting Commission.

AFFILIATIONS WITH HEALTH CARE FACILITIES
The Nursing Education Department affiliates with many health care agencies in San Diego County. These clinical settings provide a variety of experiences for students in acute, long term, and community health care.

ACADEMIC RESOURCES
Resources include the San Diego City College Library and the Nursing Resource Center and Computer Lab. A new Learning Resource Center, including Library, Independent Learning Center, and Audiovisual/Multimedia Center, opened in 2002. The Center for Reading, Writing, English as a Second Language, and Critical Thinking offers peer tutoring in reading, writing, and critical thinking assignments in classes across the curriculum.

COSTS
Resident Tuition is: $11 per unit
Nonresident Tuition is: $120 per unit
Additional expenses for books, uniforms, standardized examinations, Health Services, liability insurance, parking, and instructional supplies make the estimated costs of attendance in the Nursing Program at San Diego City College approximately $1,500 per year.

FINANCIAL AID
San Diego City College recognizes that many students may need assistance in meeting the costs of education. Students are encouraged to seek advice and assistance through the Financial Aid Office at (619) 388-3501.

APPLICATION
Students may apply to San Diego City College online at www.sdccd.net.

ADMISSION TO THE NURSING PROGRAM
All students who complete the academic prerequisites are eligible for admission.

BASIC ENTRANCE REQUIREMENTS:
Completion of the following prerequisites with a minimum grade of "C" or better and a combined grade point average of 2.5 or higher is required.

a.	Biology 230	Human Anatomy	4 semester units or equivalent
* b.	Biology 235	Human Physiology	4 semester units or equivalent
* c.	Biology 205	Microbiology	5 semester units or equivalent

* Must be completed within a 7-year period preceding qualifying date of eligibility.

Students may also be admitted by transfer or challenge having met all basic entrance requirements and other designated criteria.

FOR MORE INFORMATION
Contact the Nursing Admissions Office at (619) 388-3471 or see the City College Web site at www.city.sdccd.net.

SANFORD-BROWN COLLEGE
Nursing and Allied Health Programs
Fenton, Hazelwood, North Kansas City, and St. Charles, MO
Granite City, IL

- Associate Degree in Nursing
- Practical Nursing
- Radiography
- Respiratory Therapy
- Medical Assistant

THE COLLEGE
Sanford-Brown College is a system of five campuses offering programs in nursing, business, information technology, and allied health care. Campuses are located in Fenton, Missouri; North Kansas City, Missouri; Hazelwood, Missouri; St. Charles Missouri; and Granite City, Illinois.

MISSION
Sanford-Brown College is a private, proprietary, nonsectarian, coeducational institution founded in 1866. The College offers highly focused, high quality, short-term, degree and non-degree career-oriented programs.

NON-DISCRIMINATION
Sanford-Brown College is a private, proprietary college and a wholly owned subsidiary of a publicly-held corporation, Whitman Education Group, Inc. The College offers equal opportunity without distinction or discrimination on the basis of race, color, gender, religion, age, marital status, national origin, sexual orientation, or disability in any of its programs, activities, or employment practices.

ACCREDITATION
SBC's Missouri campuses are accredited by the Accrediting Council for Independent Colleges and Schools (ACICS) to award diplomas and associates degrees. ACICS is listed as a nationally recognized accrediting agency by the United States Department of Education. Its accreditation of degree-granting institutions also is recognized by the Council for Higher Education Accreditation. ACICS is located at 750 First Street N.E., Suite 980, Washington, DC 20002-4241; phone (202) 336-6780.

The Practical Nursing and Associate Degree Nursing programs offered at the Fenton, St. Charles, and North Kansas City campuses are accredited by the Missouri State Board of Nursing.

The Radiography programs offered at the Fenton and North Kansas City campuses are accredited by the Joint Review Committee on Education in Radiologic Technology (JRCERT). The JRCERT is recognized by the U.S. Department of Education as an independent accrediting agency with offices at 20 North Wacker Drive, Suite 900, Chicago, IL 60606-8901, phone (312) 704-5300.

The Medical Assistant programs offered at the Hazelwood and North Kansas City campuses are accredited by the Accrediting Bureau of Health Education Schools (ABHES), 803 West Broad Street, Suite 730, Falls Church, VA 22046, phone (703) 533-2082.

The Respiratory Therapy program at the Fenton campus is accredited by Commission on Accreditation of Allied Health Education Programs (CAAHEP).

CERTIFICATION
Upon completion of the specified curriculum for each health career program and several business and information technology programs, the SBC graduate will have met educational requirements to apply to take appropriate licensure/certification examinations.

Completion of the curriculum does not guarantee eligibility to sit for or pass the examination(s) leading to licensure or certification. Each regulatory organization may refuse to license an applicant for violation of its standards.

GENERAL ADMISSION REQUIREMENTS
Sanford-Brown College is open to all applicants without discrimination on the basis of race, color, gender, religion, age, national origin, disability, sexual orientation, or marital status.

Applications for admission are processed in the order received, on a rolling admission basis. Unless an applicant indicates otherwise, his/her application will be considered for the earliest academic term for which the applications are being received for the program specified. Specific admissions requirements for programs related to nursing are available by calling the SBC admissions department at (888) 434-3980.

FINANCIAL AID
Sanford-Brown College believes that students and their families have primary responsibility for a student's educational costs. However, many families are unable to fund immediately the entire cost of education. To that end, SBC participates in several federal Title IV financial assistance programs that are available to students who qualify. In addition, SBC offers a limited number of institutional scholarships and grants, as well as tuition payment plans.

APPROVALS
Sanford-Brown College is approved or recognized by the following agencies/funding sources:

- U.S. Department of Education
- U.S. Department of Justice (INS)
- Vocational Rehabilitation Departments of Missouri and Illinois
- Missouri State Approving Agency (Veterans Education Benefits)
- Job Training Partnership Act
- The Missouri Coordinating Board for Higher Education
- Missouri State Board of Nursing

CORRESPONDENCE
For more information about tuition and fees, and to set up a tour of the college, please contact one of the following locations:

St. Charles, Missouri Campus
3555 Franks Drive
St. Charles, MO 63301
(636) 949-2620 or (888) 434-3980

North Kansas City, Missouri Campus
520 E. 19th Avenue
North Kansas City, MO 64116
(816) 472-0275 or (888) 434-3986

Web: www.sanford-brown.edu

SANTA ANA COLLEGE
Santa Ana, CA

THE COLLEGE
Santa Ana College was opened in 1915 and is the largest college in the Rancho Santiago Community College District. It is located in the heart of Santa Ana on approximately 60 acres of land. The college is accredited by the Western Association of Schools and Colleges.

THE NURSING PROGRAM
The Nursing Program was established in 1979, and is accredited by the National League for Nursing Accrediting Commission and the California Board of Registered Nurses.

PROGRAMS OF STUDY
Students can pursue their Associate Degree of Nursing at Santa Ana College in either a weekday or evening/weekend format.

ACADEMIC RESOURCES
Students at Santa Ana are provided with complete career counseling and assessment and job placement services.

COSTS
Enrollment fee is $11 per unit (subject to change for Fall semester, 2003); non-resident tuition is $157 per credit unit. There is a Health Fee of $12, and various fees for student services, parking, and course materials.

FINANCIAL AID
Students can apply for federal loans as well as for private institutionally sponsored grants and scholarships.

ADMISSIONS
An application to the Santa Ana College Nursing Program may be submitted upon completion of achievement testing and pre-requisite courses.

CONTACT INFORMATION
Mary Crook
Director of Nursing/Health Sciences
Santa Ana College Nursing Department
1520 W. 17th St.
Santa Ana, CA 92706
(714) 564-6825

SEATTLE UNIVERSITY
School of Nursing
Seattle, Washington

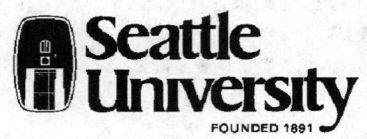

THE UNIVERSITY
Seattle University (SU) is a Jesuit university located in the heart of one of the country's most interesting and livable cities, and the center for the medical, legal, business, and high-tech industries in the Northwest. Established in 1891, SU has become a comprehensive regional university that embraces people from all faith traditions, economic and social backgrounds, and walks of life. It offers a values-oriented education that encourages students to think critically, develop a sense of responsibility for themselves and their community, and make ethical choices. Some 6,500 students are enrolled in 44 undergraduate degree programs, 22 graduate degree programs, and 18 certificate programs.

THE SCHOOL OF NURSING
The Seattle University School of Nursing has a history of more than 60 years of educating nursing professionals, with an equally long tradition of community outreach and service. The mission of the school is to ensure quality nursing care for the community by educating professional nurses who seek excellence through scholarship, leadership, service, and personal growth.

THE BACHELOR OF SCIENCE IN NURSING PROGRAM
The Bachelor of Science in Nursing Program (BSN) is designed for students with no previous education in nursing seeking a BSN degree. The program prepares students for professional practice as generalists.

THE MASTER OF SCIENCE IN NURSING PROGRAM
Seattle University's Master of Science in Nursing Program offers several graduate study options to students with or without a nursing background. Professional nurses with a Bachelor of Science in Nursing, or a bachelor's degree in another field and an associate degree in nursing, are eligible to apply for the traditional MSN program. The Advanced Practice Nursing Immersion program (APNI) is an innovative offering for people who are not nurses but who hold a bachelor's degree in another field. Students from either background choose from two major study options: Primary Care Nurse Practitioner (PCNP) and Leadership in Community Nursing (LCN). The PCNP track offers two specializations: Family Nurse Practitioner, and Psychiatric/Mental Health Nurse Practitioner with an addictions focus. Specializations in the LCN track are Program Development, and Spirituality and Health.

COSTS
Information regarding tuition, fees, and length of programs may be obtained from the Seattle University School of Nursing or from The National League for Nursing Accrediting Commission (NLNAC), 61 Broadway, New York, NY 10006; 1-800-669-1656.

FINANCIAL AID
Seattle University offers a variety of strategies and resources aimed at helping eligible undergraduate and graduate students meet the costs of education, including grants and/or scholarships, work-study opportunities, and low-interest loans.

ADMISSION REQUIREMENTS—BSN PROGRAM
The BSN Program is designed for high school graduates, college transfers, and second-degree students. All qualified students are admitted to Seattle University and the School of Nursing simultaneously. A cumulative and major prerequisite course GPA of 2.75 or above is required to enroll in nursing courses.

ADMISSIONS REQUIREMENTS—MSN PROGRAM
Applicants to the traditional MSN program for registered nurses must have a bachelor's degree in nursing recognized by a national nursing accreditation agency. Registered nurses with an Associate Degree in Nursing (ADN) and a non-nursing bachelor's degree are also eligible for admission. Applicants to the APNI program must hold a baccalaureate degree from a regionally accredited college or university. A minimum undergraduate cumulative GPA of 3.0 is required. Individuals who have less than a 3.0 may be given consideration, with evidence of other accomplishments. Applicants must have taken the Graduate Record Exam (GRE) within the past five years. Applicants who do not meet all of the admission requirements will be considered on an individual basis.

CORRESPONDENCE AND INFORMATION
School of Nursing
Seattle University
900 Broadway
Seattle, WA 98122-4340
(206) 296-5660
Toll Free: 1-800-426-7123
E-Mail: nurse@seattleu.edu
Web: www.seattleu.edu/nurs

ST. ELIZABETH COLLEGE OF NURSING
Utica, NY

THE COLLEGE
St. Elizabeth College of Nursing, founded in 1904, is located in the foothills of the Adirondack Mountains. Located in a pleasant residential area, it is adjacent to St. Elizabeth Medical Center, an acute care facility that is accredited by J.C.A.H.O. The college is registered by the New York State Education Department, Office of Higher Education and the Professions.

The weekday or evening/weekend program at St. Elizabeth College of Nursing attracts both the recent high school graduate and the older, returning student. Our graduates qualify for nursing positions in public and private institutions as well as in community agencies.

PROGRAM OF STUDY
The mission of the College of Nursing is to prepare the student to function as a beginning practitioner of professional nursing. Emphasis is placed on continuing education to the BSN level. Graduates of the AAS program are eligible to apply for licensure as a Registered Nurse (RN).

AFFILIATION
St. Elizabeth College of Nursing has contractual agreements with Mohawk Valley Community College, SUNY Institute of Technology–Utica, and many healthcare agencies.

ACADEMIC RESOURCES
The college's resources are housed within its educational building and include a state-of-the-art nursing skills laboratory, a science laboratory, an on-line computer center, and a library equipped with computers.

TUITION & FEES
The total cost for either weekday or evening/weekend programs, which includes Mohawk Valley Community College tuition, fees, and books, is approximately $12,000. Dormitory room charge is $1,200 for a single room. Meal charge is $800 per semester for resident students. Financial aid is available through St. Elizabeth's for the Tuition Assistance Program (TAP), Pell and Guaranteed Student Loan.

APPLYING
The College of Nursing admits eligible students of any age, race, color, creed, national or ethnic origin, sex, marital status, handicapping condition, or sexual orientation, to all the rights, privileges, programs, and activities available at the college, if they meet the criteria.

The applicant must be a graduate of an accredited high school or its equivalent, that is acceptable to the New York State Education Department and the College of Nursing. He/she must also meet the admission requirements of Mohawk Valley Community College.

High School courses must include:

English	4 units
Social Studies	3 units
Biology or Human Life Science	1 unit
Chemistry (or essentials of Chem)	1 unit
Algebra or Equiv. (Course I)	1 unit

Application forms and information can be obtained by writing to the College of Nursing or may be submitted online via the College of Nursing Web page. An articulation agreement is in effect with Herkimer County Community College for transfer credits. Students are eligible to take the LPN exam after the first year. Advanced placement for LPNs is in effect for those who qualify.

CORRESPONDENCE AND INFORMATION
Additional and updated information is available through the College of Nursing during the hours of 7:00 a.m.–3:00 p.m.

Admissions Coordinator and Registrar
St. Elizabeth College of Nursing
2215 Genesee Street
Utica, NY 13501
(315) 798-8253
Fax: (315) 798-8271
Web: www.stemc.org/college/schools.htm

ST. ELIZABETH SCHOOL OF NURSING
Lafayette, IN

THE SCHOOL
St. Elizabeth School of Nursing offers a rich heritage to guide you in developing the personal qualities you'll need in nursing. The Sisters of St. Francis traveled from Germany to the United States in 1875 to establish St. Elizabeth Hospital. In 1897, St. Elizabeth School of Nursing was opened as a training school for members of their order. From our humble beginnings a century ago, many lives have been touched by the light and hope carried by graduates of St. Elizabeth School of Nursing. We invite you to master the knowledge you will need as a nurse, to discover your own inner light, and to help us carry light and hope into the 21st century. Remember, you are the light of the world.

PROGRAM OF STUDY
The curriculum offered by the St. Elizabeth School of Nursing leads to a diploma in professional nursing. Graduates of the program are eligible to take the National Council Licensure Examination for Registered Nurse (NCLEX-RN). The program covers 28 months (3 academic years with 6 semesters or a minimum of 118 semester credit hours). It is based on the integration of case management with the problem-solving approach of the nursing process. The concepts of learning, nursing, man, environment, society, and health are woven throughout the curriculum. The program prepares the student in a community-based, community-focused healthcare system. Health promotion and disease prevention are stressed.

AFFILIATE COLLEGE
St. Elizabeth School of Nursing is affiliated with Saint Joseph's College in Rensselaer, IN, a four-year catholic liberal arts institution approximately 40 miles and 45 minutes north of Lafayette off of Interstate 65. The Core Curriculum is utilized integrating liberal arts education each semester throughout the course of study.

AFFILIATIONS WITH HEALTHCARE FACILITIES
The St. Elizabeth School of Nursing maintains contractual agreements with more than twenty-five healthcare agencies. The school's clinical resources include both campuses of Greater Lafayette Health Care Services, area community hospitals, two behavioral management facilities, and community-based clinics and agencies.

ACADEMIC RESOURCES
The school's resources are housed in the St. Elizabeth School of Nursing library. On the campus of Saint Joseph's College the library, writing clinic, two computer centers, and a tutorial center are available. On both campuses are nursing skills laboratories.

COSTS
Full-time (12 or more credit hours) tuition is $10,440.00/year. Room and board $5,940.00/year.

FINANCIAL AID
St. Elizabeth School of Nursing offers Federal Nursing Student Loans, Federal Pell Grants, Federal Supplemental Educational Opportunity Grants, Federal Work-Study, Federal PLUS Loans, Federal Stafford Loans, and state aid, and Greater Lafayette Health Services Incentive Scholarship program.

APPLYING
Applicants must be a United States citizen or have proper international student credentials. A Graduate of a state-approved high school, with a grade point average of C or better in the upper half of their graduating class, or its equivalent, the completion of the General Educational Development Test (GED) with an overall standard score of 50. Required high school courses are at least 2 semesters of high school Algebra, Biology, and Chemistry; and 8 semesters of English. Applicants who have completed high school within three years prior to making application are required to take the SAT I achieving a 920 or above combined or the ACT with a composite score of 19 or above. Two letters of reference are required, as is an entrance test for nursing. Students may begin in the nursing program in either Fall (application deadline is June 1) or Winter (application deadline is November 1).

CORRESPONDENCE
Coordinator of Admissions
St. Elizabeth School of Nursing
1508 Tippecanoe Street
Lafayette, IN 47904-2918
(765) 423-6400
Fax: (765) 423-6385
Web: www.ste.org/newson

ST. LUKE'S SCHOOL OF NURSING AT MORAVIAN COLLEGE
Bethlehem, Pennsylvania

AN INNOVATIVE PARTNERSHIP
St. Luke's Hospital School of Nursing and Moravian College, the nation's sixth-oldest college, have joined resources to establish an innovative nursing major leading to a BS degree. Through the partnership between St. Luke's and Moravian, the nursing major has access to resources of St. Luke's Hospital, including the advanced facilities of the Priscilla Payne Hurd Education Center.

THE COLLEGE
Moravian College is a private, coeducational, selective liberal arts college that traces its origins to 1742. Conveniently located in the city of Bethlehem, Moravian College is approximately 90 miles west of New York City and 60 miles north of Philadelphia. Committed to liberal arts as a foundation for personal and professional growth, Moravian aims to give students a foundation for careers or graduate/professional school, for continued lifelong learning, and for a values-oriented approach to society.

THE SCHOOL OF NURSING
The St. Luke's School of Nursing at Moravian College offers an integrated, holistic nursing curriculum that emphasizes health promotion, maintenance, and restoration for individuals, families, and their communities. Committed to the core curricular components of community, holism, inquiry, and professionalism, the nursing major enjoys more than 1,000 hours of clinical practice with which to apply and test theoretical concepts in a range of health care settings.

THE BACHELOR OF SCIENCE DEGREE IN NURSING PROGRAM
The Bachelor of Science Degree (BS) in Nursing program is designed for students with no previous education in nursing and for registered nurse students who seek the BS degree. The program prepares students for professional practice in acute and community-focused health care settings and for pursuit of graduate study in nursing.

AFFILIATIONS WITH HEALTH CARE FACILITIES
The student is guaranteed broad-based clinical practice experiences through the partnership with St. Luke's Health Network and regional service programs across Eastern Pennsylvania. St. Luke's Health Network encompasses comprehensive acute care services across the life continuum, as well as community-focused health services through the Bethlehem Partnership, the community arm of the network.

COSTS 2002-2003
Tuition and fees - $21,285. Room and board costs average $6,835 but can vary slightly depending on residence hall.

FINANCIAL AID
Moravian College offers a variety of resources aimed at assisting the undergraduate student meet the costs of education, including scholarships and specialized awards in specific disciplines. For more information, contact the Financial Aid Office at (610) 861-1330.

ADMISSION REQUIREMENTS
The baccalaureate program is designed for high school graduates and college transfers, including RNs and second degree students. All qualified students are admitted to Moravian College and the School of Nursing simultaneously.

CORRESPONDENCE AND INFORMATION
Moravian College
Department of Nursing
1200 Main Street
Bethlehem, PA 18018
(610) 861-1607
E-Mail: sipplej@moravian.edu
Web: www.moravian.edu
School of Nursing Homepage: http://home.moravian.edu/public/nursing

ST. PETERSBURG COLLEGE
Department of Nursing
Pinellas County, Florida

ABOUT ST. PETERSBURG COLLEGE
In 1927, a private college opened in downtown St. Petersburg. One hundred students enrolled in the fledgling institution, taught by 14 faculty. In 1948, this private college became public as a countywide community college—St. Petersburg Junior College. In early 2001, the Florida Legislature changed the college's name and granted it the authority to award baccalaureate degrees in selected programs including Nursing. St. Petersburg College is now a public, four-year institution with nearly 58,000 students annually across 10 sites in Pinellas County.

The BSN program is a degree-completion program for nurses who want to further their education. Nurses are awarded full credit for their pre-licensure program based on a valid and current state registered nursing license. The college also offers an associate degree in Nursing that fully articulates into the BSN program. Both programs have state-of-the-art technology used in developing skills and computer-based competencies.

NURSING DEPARTMENT
The Nursing program was founded in 1954 to meet the need for nurses in Pinellas County, Florida. The program incorporates the use of human patient simulators to build skills and develop critical-thinking competencies. Additionally, the program boasts a computer lab housing nearly 30 computers to help students build computer-based testing skills, and participate in interactive learning. The program is nationally recognized for the annual number of graduates completing the program.

PROGRAM OF STUDY
St. Petersburg College offers an Associate of Science degree in Nursing and transitional programs for LPN/LVN, respiratory therapist, and paramedic applicants. The programs are offered full-time and part-time, as well as partially online (within state guidelines). In August 2002, the RN-BSN program began. It can be completed in 18-20 months while maintaining a work schedule. The Nursing program is approved by the Florida Board of Nursing, with accreditation for the ADN program by the National League for Nursing Accrediting Commission. As a new baccalaureate program, accreditation for the RN-BSN is currently being sought from the National League for Nursing Accrediting Commission.

AFFILIATIONS WITH HEALTH CARE FACILITIES
The Nursing program maintains contractual agreements with a variety of health care agencies. The program's clinical resources include BayCare Medical Care, Bayfront Medical Center, All Children's Hospital, Morton Plant Hospital, St. Anthony's Hospital, and Edward White Hospital.

ACADEMIC RESOURCES
The program's learning resources are comprised of a newly-built Information Commons that houses the latest computer equipment, as well as the most current holdings of health-care journals. The online library resources contain several comprehensive databases that provide access to full-text articles, books, and Web resources.

COSTS AND FINANCIAL AID
St. Petersburg College and the Nursing program offer access to federal financial assistance, as well as local grants and scholarships. The Office of Scholarships and Student Financial Assistance is readily available to assist students in this process.

FOR ADDITIONAL INFORMATION & ADMISSION APPLICATION:
St. Petersburg College
Nursing Program
PO Box 13489
St. Petersburg, FL 33733
(727) 345-7752
Web: www.spjc.edu

STATE FAIR COMMUNITY COLLEGE
Associate Degree Nursing Program
Sedalia, Missouri

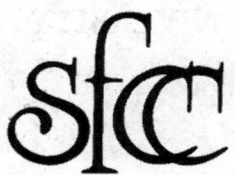

THE COLLEGE
State Fair Community College is a publicly supported institution that grants associate of arts and associate of applied science degrees and professional certificates. Founded in 1968 in historic Sedalia, Missouri, SFCC is located in the heart of the Midwest on a 120-acre campus. SFCC's current enrollment is over 3,200 and continues to grow. Our teaching staff includes 70 full-time and 117 part-time instructors, making the student to faculty ratio a comfortable 18:1.

ACCREDITED PROGRAMS
At SFCC, Allied Health programs include Practical Nursing (PN), Associate of Applied Science Degree (ADN), and a wide variety of adult health courses.

The career ladder AAS degree in Nursing requires LPN licensure and specific prerequisites, which may be transferred from previous colleges or may be taken anytime prior to the start of the Nursing curriculum. General education courses may be taken prior to or during the sophomore year. Graduates of this program are eligible to apply to take the State Board Examination for Registered Nurse. The practical nursing program and the AAS degree program in nursing are accredited by the State Department of Education and approved by the Missouri State Board of Nursing. SFCC is also accredited by the North Central Association of Colleges and Schools, Chicago, Illinois.

AFFILIATIONS WITH CLINICAL FACILITIES
State Fair Community College's Associate Degree Nursing Program offers learning experiences in classes and labs at SFCC, Bothwell Regional Health Center, Golden Valley Memorial Hospital, and a wide variety of community agencies and sites.

ACADEMIC RESOURCES
Small class and clinic sizes offer individualized instruction opportunities. Caring and experienced faculty work hard to ensure the success of all students. Students have access to state-of-the-art lab facilities, computer lab, library, and of course, open access to all faculty
at all times.

COSTS
Tuition for residents of the SFCC district is $49 per credit hour; Missouri resident tuition is $76 per credit hour; and out-of-state tuition is $129 per credit hour. The ADN program requires 72 credits with 38.5 nursing credits for a total cost of $3,020, including fees, for district residents. This total does not include prerequisites or general education courses.

FINANCIAL AID
If financial assistance is needed in order to attend SFCC, the College offers a comprehensive financial aid program funded by Federal and state agencies and private organizations. The aid programs include grants, loans, part-time employment, and scholarships. For more information about Financial Aid, please call 660-530-5800 ext. 298 or ext. 295.

APPLYING AND ADMISSIONS
The application deadline for the ADN program is April 1 for the January class.

Prerequisites for ADN program:
  High School or GED, NET score;
  LPN-GAP score;
  attendance at the Career Mobility Nursing
    Workshop;
  three references;
  completed work from an accredited school of
    practical nursing with a current state license
    to practice;
  and an application on file by the April 1 deadline.

CORRESPONDENCE AND INFORMATION
State Fair Community College
Associate Degree Nursing Program
Sandy Whitehead, Program Director
3201 W. 16th Street
Sedalia, Missouri 65301
(660) 530-5800 ext. 330
Fax: (660) 530-5827
E-Mail: whitehea@sfcc.cc.mo.us
Web: www.sfcc.cc.mo.us

SYRACUSE UNIVERSITY
College of Nursing
Syracuse, New York

THE UNIVERSITY
Syracuse University is a major research university ranked among the country's top 50 universities and is recognized worldwide. Founded in 1870, Syracuse University is a private residential institution. SU's size assures students have an abundance of resources—from over three hundred extracurricular offerings to wonderful on-campus libraries and athletic facilities.

THE COLLEGE OF NURSING
Founded in 1943, the College of Nursing educates competent, ethical, and caring nurses through graduate and undergraduate studies. The mission is to meet the educational needs of regional, national, and international students to prepare nurses who improve health in a complex global society. This is accomplished by faculty developing partnerships among a diverse community of scholars that promote innovation in teaching, research, practice, and service. The nursing program is noted for its individualized approach to the variety of interdisciplinary studies available.

AFFILIATIONS WITH HEALTH-CARE FACILITIES
Syracuse University partners with innovative high-tech hospitals and health agencies, providing unparalleled clinical experiences and a full scope of professional nursing practice. Many sites are within a few blocks of campus. Placements are available locally and in nationally recognized facilities.

PROGRAMS OF STUDY
The BS in Nursing (BSN) curriculum combines a study of arts and science courses with professional nursing courses throughout the program. Freshman and transfer applicants are admitted directly to the College. Nursing courses begin the first semester.

Special options available to undergraduate students include the semester away experience, honors program, study abroad, ROTC, and hundreds of professional, social, athletic, and recreational activities available on campus. Students can elect to immediately continue their education in the accelerated MS program.

An accelerated two-year BS in Nursing program is available to students who already have a BS or BA in another discipline. Students immediately enter a concentrated curriculum of nursing theory and clinical studies and are eligible for special grant incentives and an accelerated MS, which is completed in one additional year of study.

An accelerated RN-BSN with MS option program provides opportunity for RNs to continue their education at the baccalaureate and graduate levels in an accelerated pathway.

The 45-credit community-based graduate program gives the student the opportunity to design an individualized plan of study based on career goals in an environment that facilitates and supports personal growth. The program specialties reflect new options available to nurses in a rapidly changing health-care environment. Certification requirements are fulfilled for all specialties. Clinical specialties can be supplemented with a second specialty area or with functional practice options in teaching, administration, or nursing informatics. Also available is the innovative Summer Limited Residency Independent Study Master's program. A culminating experience of a clinical project is required.

Advanced (post-master's) certificate programs in nurse practitioner studies, nursing administration, teaching, and nursing informatics are programs that qualify students for certification in their chosen focus area.

All programs are NLNAC accredited and are offered full-time and part-time.

ACADEMIC FACILITIES
The SU library system is a major academic resource for the region, state, and nation. The collections contain more than 2.7 million volumes, 16,000 current serials and periodicals, more than 3.7 million microforms, and 1,700 computer-readable disks, tapes, and CD-ROMs. There are fourteen public and 20 departmental computing clusters.

LOCATION
Syracuse is located in the geographic center of the state and has a population of 600,000. It is large enough to deliver the latest in health care to diverse population, yet small enough for individual efforts to be recognized.

COSTS
Tuition costs for the 2003–2004 academic year are $24,170 for full-time undergraduates, $437 per credit for part-time undergraduates, and $742 per credit for graduate and postgraduate students. Rates are the same for in-state and out-of-state students. The undergraduate activity fee and health fees are $560, and books are estimated at $1,104 per year. Room and board are $9,130. Personal expenses are estimated as $1,030 and transportation expenses as $508.

FINANCIAL AID
Approximately 83 percent of all SU students receive financial aid. This may be in the form of loan programs and college work-study. Graduate students may receive merit-based awards and appointments, including fellowships, scholarships, and assistantships. State and federal awards are also available. Nursing employment opportunities are available in the community. Many agencies offer tuition support.

APPLYING
For admission to the BSN program, SAT I or ACT scores and 3 years of science are required. High school seniors must apply by January 15th. Transfer and second-degree applications are reviewed on a rolling basis. Transfer applicants should have a minimum GPA of 2.5. Second-degree applicants should have a minimum GPA of 2.8.

For the RN-BS-MS program, a minimum GPA of 2.5 from the AD or diploma program is required. The master's and post-master's programs require a BSN or an MS in Nursing, respectively, from an NLNAC-accredited institution. The MS requires competence in basic statistics and basic health assessment. The GRE is required. International students must submit TOEFL scores and licensure as an RN. Contact the nursing office for complete information about admission requirements.

CORRESPONDENCE AND INFORMATION
Director of Admissions
College of Nursing
Syracuse University
426 Ostrom Avenue
Syracuse, New York 13244-3240
(315) 443-4266
Fax: (315) 443-9807
Web: http://www.syracuse.syr.edu

TEMPLE UNIVERSITY
College of Allied Health Professions
Department of Nursing
Philadelphia, PA

THE UNIVERSITY
Temple University was founded in 1884 by Dr. Russell Conwell, who wanted to make higher education available to all capable and motivated students regardless of their backgrounds and finances. From its roots in the historical and cultural richness of Philadelphia, it now has five regional campuses, as well as foreign campuses in Tokyo, Japan and Rome, Italy. Temple attracts 28,000 students from across the nation and around the world.

COLLEGE OF ALLIED HEALTH PROFESSIONS
Founded in 1969, the College of Allied Health Professions offers undergraduate programs in Communication Sciences, Health Information Management, Nursing, and Occupational Therapy. Graduate programs are offered in Nursing, Occupational Therapy, Physical Therapy, Public Health, and Therapeutic Recreation.

PROGRAMS OF STUDY
The Department of Nursing offers Generic Baccalaureate, RN-BSN Baccalaureate, and MSN in Psychiatric/Mental Health Nursing degrees. It also offers the MSN degree and a Post-Master's Certificate in Adult Nurse Practitioner and Pediatric Nurse Practitioner, as well as a 45-credit Nurse Anesthesia program in collaboration with Pennsylvania Hospital. With the exception of the full-time Generic Baccalaureate program, all other programs can be completed part-time, some in the evening on city and suburban Temple campuses. Graduates of the Generic Baccalaureate program are eligible to apply for licensure in the Commonwealth of Pennsylvania as a Registered Nurse (RN). Post-Master's and Nurse Anesthesia graduates are eligible for state certification.

HEALTH-CARE AFFILIATIONS
The Department of Nursing maintains contractual agreements with more than 100 health-care agencies in Philadelphia and surrounding counties, including Temple University Hospital.

ACADEMIC RESOURCES
The Health Sciences Center libraries house a total of 62,603 volumes, 1,239 journals, nearly 200 AV titles, microcomputer software titles, and CD/ROM data files. Students also have access to the Paley Library on Main Campus, housing more than a million volumes, and a Learning Resource Center in the Department of Nursing.

COSTS
2002–2003 Schedule: State-resident, full-time undergraduate tuition for prenursing studies is $7,602; non-resident tuition is $13,856. State-resident, undergraduate tuition for the Department of Nursing is $9,186; non-resident tuition is $16,304. Part-time tuition for Health Science programs is $344 (in-state) and $566 (out-of-state). Part-time graduate nursing tuition is $418 per credit (in-state) and $607 (out-of-state). Fees range from $50 to $175.

FINANCIAL AID
Temple University administers a variety of federal, state, and institutional aid programs.

APPLYING
BSN program: The application period is November 1 through January 31 for a September-only admission. Minimum GPA of 3.0 required.

RN-BSN program: Applicants must have RN licensure in the Commonwealth of Pennsylvania and have graduated from an accredited nursing school. Rolling admission applies to RNs only.

MSN, Post-Master's, and Anesthesia programs: Applicants must have a BSN degree from an accredited nursing program, be licensed in the Commonwealth, taken the GRE examination, and have cumulative GPA of 3.0.

Nurse Practitioner programs: One year in clinical practice as an RN is required.

CORRESPONDENCE AND INFORMATION
Director of Nursing Student Services
College of Allied Health Professions
Temple University
3307 North Broad Street
Philadelphia, PA 19140
(215) 707-4688
Fax: (215) 707-1599
Web: http://www.temple.edu/nursing

TENNESSEE TECHNOLOGICAL UNIVERSITY
School of Nursing
Cookeville, Tennessee

THE UNIVERSITY
Tennessee Technological University is located in Cookeville, TN, a city of 26,000, midway between Nashville and Knoxville, TN. The University was established in 1915 and enrolls approximately 8,500 students, awarding bachelors degrees in more than 50 fields of study, master's degrees in 22 fields of study, a Specialist in Education Degree, and Doctor of Philosophy Degrees in Engineering and Environmental Science. The major component of the academic mission is high quality instruction in the University's undergraduate, master's, specialist, and doctoral degree-granting programs. The University is also engaged in scholarly activity, creative endeavors, and public service. Tennessee Tech serves students from throughout the state, nation, and many other countries, but retains a special commitment to serve the Upper Cumberland region of Tennessee.

THE SCHOOL OF NURSING
Founded in 1980, the School of Nursing baccalaureate degree program (BSN) is accredited by the National League for Nursing Accrediting Commission, the Southern Association of Colleges and Schools, and maintains full approval by the Tennessee Board of Nursing. Approximately two hundred students are enrolled in pre-nursing, Lower Division Nursing. Upper Division Nursing consists of generic BSN students and RN/BSN completion students averaging 40 graduates per year. The BSN program is designed for high school graduates and college transfers, including RNs and second-degree students. The prerequisite nursing core courses are completed during the freshman and sophomore years. During the first two years of study, students receive an introduction to nursing and acquire a basic foundation in the physical and social sciences, the humanities, nutrition, and computer technology. General education core courses include writing and related skills, American History, math, and physical education. Clinical experiences in Upper Division Nursing are in local community hospitals, health departments, schools, community mental health centers, and other community agencies. Opportunities exist for both rural and urban experiences.

ADMISSION
All School of Nursing students begin the admission process by applying directly to the University Office of Admissions. Any student meeting University requirements for admission will be admitted to Lower Division Nursing. Acceptance into the Upper Division Nursing, junior and senior years, is not automatic. Consideration for admission is contingent on a required 2.5 quality point average in previous course work. Emphasis is on success in the sciences. In addition, all prerequisites must be successfully completed prior to beginning the junior level nursing courses. The School of Nursing welcomes applications from students who have completed two years of the required course work at other colleges and universities.

   Application for Upper Division Nursing is made during the fall semester of the sophomore year. See the School of Nursing Handbook for additional requirements (www2.tntech.edu/nursing/handbook.html).

COSTS
Fees for the academic year 2003-2004 are $3,778 for a full-time undergraduate in-state student. For fewer than twelve credits per semester, the fee is $178 per credit hour. The current year fee schedule is available by contacting the school. There are additional cost for textbooks, fees for standardized testing, liability insurance, etc.

FINANCIAL AID
Tennessee Technological University and the School of Nursing offer aid that may include scholarships, grants, loans, or work study programs to assist eligible undergraduate students to meet the costs of education.

CORRESPONDENCE AND INFORMATION
School of Nursing
Tennessee Technological University
P.O. Box 5001
Cookeville, TN 38505-0001
(931) 372-3203
1-800-255-8881
E-Mail: nursing@tntech.edu
Web: www2.tntech.edu/nursing/handbook/html

TEXAS TECH UNIVERSITY HEALTH SCIENCES CENTER
School of Nursing
Lubbock, Texas

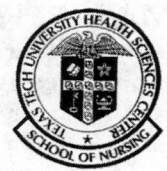

TEXAS TECH UNIVERSITY HEALTH SCIENCES CENTER
This Research I institution is home to the Schools of Allied Health, Graduate Biomedical Sciences, Medicine, Nursing, and Pharmacy. Located on the South Plains of West Texas at 3,250 feet, the dry crisp air and sunny days provide a healthful and invigorating climate for the 250,000 people residing in Lubbock.

SCHOOL OF NURSING
The School of Nursing was founded in 1981 to meet the need for nursing professionals in the West Texas area. The first students were admitted to the undergraduate degree program in the Fall of 1981. In Fall 1988, a graduate program was initiated to meet the increasing demands for nurses prepared at the graduate level. The School of Nursing has been and continues to be fully accredited by the National League for Nursing Accrediting Commission (NLNAC) and The Board of Nurses Examiners for the State of Texas. In addition, the Southern Association of Colleges and Schools also accredits TTUHSC.

UNDERGRADUATE PROGRAM
The undergraduate program is designed with two entry levels, allowing students to begin the program as a college transfer student or as an RN returning for a BSN.

GRADUATE PROGRAM
The graduate program (Masters of Science in Nursing and Post-Master's Family Nurse Practitioner) is designed to produce a nursing leader who is prepared with specific functional abilities to practice with a specified patient/client population. Students can choose from Community Health or Gerontics Clinical tracks with an Education, Administration, or Family Nurse Practitioner functional track. A collaborative program has been created with The University of Texas-Tyler, allowing their students to obtain a Master of Science in Nursing with a Family Nurse Practitioner Certificate from TTUHSC. There is also a PhD collaborative program with Texas Women's University.

CLINICAL SIMULATION CENTER
The Clinical Simulation Center (CSC) is an invaluable part of the learning experience at TTUHSC School of Nursing, and is recognized as a leader in technological applications in nursing. The CSC provides a hands-on environment for students to rehearse health assessment and clinical applications. Our unique facility is designed to prepare students for patient care in hospital, clinical, home, and emergency settings.

FINANCIAL AID
TTUHSC offers institutionally sponsored non-need based grants/scholarships, Federal Nursing Student Loans, Federal Pell Grants, and Federal Perkins Loans. In addition, the School of Nursing offers numerous need and non-need based scholarships.

COSTS
The approximate cost for in-state, full time, undergraduate tuition, books, and fees for a 12-month period is $6,000 (out-of-state $13,000). The approximate cost for in-state, full time, graduate tuition, books, and fees for a 12-month period is $8,000 (out-of-state $15,000).

APPLICATION AND ADMISSIONS INFORMATION
Applicants are selected on the basis of past academic achievement and the ability to perform capably in positions of responsibility for self and others. A minimum cumulative GPA of 2.0 for the undergraduate program (3.0 for the graduate program) is required for admissions consideration.

CORRESPONDENCE & INFORMATION
Texas Tech University Health Sciences Center
School of Nursing-Undergraduate Program
3601 4th Street, Room 3BC100
Lubbock, TX 79430
(806) 743-2737
E-Mail: Heather.Morris@ttuhsc.edu
or
School of Nursing-Graduate Program
3601 4th Street, M/S 6264
Lubbock, Texas 79430
(806) 443-3055
E-Mail: Barbara.Johnston@ttuhsc.edu
Web: www.ttuhsc.edu

THOMAS JEFFERSON UNIVERSITY
Department of Nursing
Philadelphia, Pennsylvania

PROGRAMS OF STUDY

Thomas Jefferson University is a private, nonsectarian academic health center. The Department of Nursing prepares students for the Bachelor of Science in Nursing (BSN) and the Master of Science in Nursing (MSN). The National League for Nursing Accrediting Commission accredits both programs. The curriculum includes interdisciplinary learning experiences among students in the health professions. The Department currently enrolls approximately 350 undergraduate and 125 graduate students.

The BSN program is an upper-division curriculum. Students transfer to Jefferson after completing 59 lower-division credits in the sciences and humanities. Full-time, part-time, day, and evening options are available. The Generic BSN program prepares graduates to practice professional nursing as generalists in a variety of health care settings. The RN-BSN program prepares graduates of diploma or associate degree nursing programs for an increased leadership role in nursing. The Department offers the unique opportunity for RN students to earn 30 upper-division credits for previous nursing knowledge and as many as 12 additional credits in nursing leadership or community health nursing through Portfolio Assessment. This enables RN students to begin the program in their senior year and complete the program in two semesters of full-time study or two years of part-time study.

The Department also offers an Accelerated Pathway to the MSN program for highly motivated, academically talented students who hold a bachelor's degree in a field other than nursing. Generic students may complete the Accelerated Pathway to the MSN program in seven semesters of full-time study; registered nurses in five semesters.

The RN-BSN/MSN is an accelerated option that enables RN students to qualify for admission to graduate nursing education through a combined BSN/MSN program. The goal is to provide a mechanism for RN students to earn the BSN and MSN degrees in a seamless integrated curriculum.

The MSN program prepares nurses for advanced and sophisticated clinical practice. Specialty courses are available in adult health with concentrations available in a wide range of specialty areas, community systems administration, and family nurse practitioner (FNP) studies. The FNP program offers a post-master's certification option. All specialty areas require 36 credits.

LOCATION

Thomas Jefferson University is located in historic Center City Philadelphia, the fourth-largest city in the United States. It is within walking distance of many places of historic and cultural interest. Convenient bus, rail, and subway lines offer transportation to Jefferson, as well as to a variety of interesting attractions.

STUDENT SERVICES

The University has many resources and services available to meet the needs of students. These include academic advising, counseling, housing and dining, student health, tutoring, day care, fitness facilities, computing services, student organizations, and career services.

FINANCIAL AID

Jefferson is committed to meeting the financial needs of its students. More than 82% of the current students receive financial assistance. Aid can include Pell Grants, National Direct Student Loans, College Work-Study Program, Air Force ROTC scholarships, nursing scholarships, nursing loans, state grants, work scholarships, state-guaranteed loans, and academic scholarships. Completed applications must be received by the Financial Aid Office no later than May 1 to ensure the maximum award.

APPLICATION

Applications to the BSN program are accepted and evaluated on an ongoing basis. Candidates are encouraged to apply after September 1 for the following fall. Along with a completed application, applicants must submit transcripts for all college work, a personal statement of academic and professional intent, and two letters of recommendation. A high school transcript is required for applicants who do not have a bachelor's degree. Applicants to the Accelerated Pathway to the MSN Program and the RN-BSN/MSN Program must submit an additional letter of recommendation, a resume, and GRE or MAT scores.

Applications to the MSN Program are accepted on an ongoing basis. Admission requirements include competitive scores on the GRE or MAT, undergraduate statistics, nursing research, physical assessment, computer literacy, three letters of reference, a resume, and a personal statement addressing professional goals.

CORRESPONDENCE AND INFORMATION

Office of Admissions and Enrollment Management
Thomas Jefferson University
130 S. 9th Street
Edison Building, Suite 1610
Philadelphia, PA 19107
1-877-JEFFCHP (533-3247)
Fax: (215) 503-7241
Web: www.tju.edu/chp

TRINITAS HEALTH
School of Nursing
Elizabeth, New Jersey

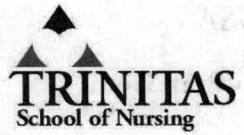

TRINITAS
School of Nursing

SCHOOL OF NURSING

The School of Nursing was conceived under the auspices of the Ladies' Aid Society in 1891. Growth in enrollment from the first year's admission of six students to a student body of more than 480 students in 2001 attests to the community's recognition of the School's high quality standards of education over the past century.

The School of Nursing and Union County College, Cranford, New Jersey, jointly conduct a Cooperative Nursing Program. The Program grants students a Diploma in Nursing from the School of Nursing and an Associate in Science Degree from Union County College. General education, science and humanities courses may be taken at the Cranford, Elizabeth, or Plainfield campuses of Union County College, while nursing courses are offered at the School of Nursing. For the past 54 years, the School has enjoyed an educationally advantageous association with Union County College. The association has enhanced the School's ability to keep abreast of educational and scientific advancements, and has strengthened the student's base of knowledge and intellectual skills.

PROGRAM OF STUDY

Fully accredited by the National League for Nursing Accrediting Commission and the New Jersey State Board of Nursing, the Program offers a basic course of study in nursing. It provides a sound theoretical base of knowledge in nursing, biological, behavioral, and social sciences, and integrates this knowledge into academic and practical experiences within the health and illness continuum of client care.

The curriculum has many options from which to select in order to complete the program of study. Students may enroll in the Day, Evening, or the LPN to RN Completion division on either a full-time or part-time basis. Upon graduation, students are eligible to apply for the National Council Licensing Examination (NCLEX) for Registered Nurse licensure. A total of 75 credits in nursing and general education courses are designed to be completed over a 2-year period. The RN Completion division is specifically designed for Licensed Practical Nurses who wish to further their nursing education within a realistic time frame, without undue repetition of previous learning, and while continuing their employment and/or family responsibilities.

CLINICAL AFFILIATIONS

In addition to Trinitas Hospital, the School of Nursing has established contractual agreements with other acute care institutions, specialized rehabilitation facilities, and community agencies in order to provide students with optimum clinical experiences. Students have opportunities to provide direct care and interact with clients of all ages and backgrounds in medical/surgical, maternal/child, psychiatric, and geriatric settings.

RESOURCES

The School offers a variety of resources and services to facilitate students' achievement of school and curriculum objectives. Being able to provide such a rich collection of resources in the environment of a modern facility has infused much strength into the program, and has aided and supported the School's many educational innovations throughout the years.

Students are strongly encouraged to utilize all available resources at the School of Nursing and Union County College. These resources include academic counseling, a Student Support Program for students and their families, state-of-the-art Computer and Skills Laboratories, and Health Science Library. These services are generally available during the day, evening, and weekend hours.

COSTS

In-county tuition for Union County College courses is $73 per credit, and $146 per credit for out-of-county residents. The primary cost of each clinical nursing course is the tuition at $73 per credit and clinical fees at $400 per credit.

FINANCIAL AID

Financial aid is available to eligible students through the Union County College Financial Aid Office. Students may call or visit any one of the three campuses to receive additional information on Financial Aid Workshops, the application process, or student aid eligibility.

In addition to federal and state funded aid, scholarships are available to assist qualified students to meet their educational expenses. Scholarships are applied for and administered through the School of Nursing and/or Union County College.

ADMISSIONS

Admissions to the School of Nursing are processed through the Admissions Office at Union County College. An Open Admissions policy is maintained in accordance with the College. Students seeking advanced standing or course waivers need to provide official high school and college transcripts for a review of the credits completed. Applicants who have completed college level courses in an accredited college and/or university will be evaluated for advanced standing for up to 22 credits. Advanced standing in nursing is available to qualified applicants for Fundamentals of Nursing courses. Applicants who hold an Associate Degree or higher in another area of study may elect the "Diploma only" in Nursing option.

Students without collegiate experience are required to take a College Placement Test at Union County College. If students' test results indicate the need for developmental course work, the recommended non-credit courses must be completed satisfactorily before nursing courses may be taken. Students requiring English as a Second Language courses will be deferred admission to the nursing program until they have completed their requirements.

Admission to the LPN to RN Completion division requires applicants to have a current Licensed Practical Nurse license.

FURTHER INFORMATION

Admissions Office
Union County College
1033 Springfield Avenue
Cranford, New Jersey 07016
(908) 709-7518
E-Mail: castaldi@ucc.edu
Visit our Web site at: www.ucc.edu/nursing

Trinitas School of Nursing
925 E. Jersey Street
Elizabeth, New Jersey 07201
(908) 994-8144
Fax: (908) 994-8404

UNIVERSITY OF ARKANSAS
Eleanor Mann School of Nursing
College of Education and Health Professions
Fayetteville, AR

THE UNIVERSITY
The University of Arkansas is located in Fayetteville, a city of nearly 60,000 residents. The University of Arkansas main campus comprises 345 acres and is situated on a hilltop that overlooks the Ozark Mountains. Since the University's founding in 1871, over 112,000 students have graduated. Each of their names is etched in the much-loved Senior Walk, with more than five miles of campus sidewalks that contain graduates' names arranged by their year of graduation. The University is a mainly residential campus, currently serving over 15,000 students. There are 864 faculty, of which 94 percent are full time and 90 percent hold either the doctorate or the terminal degree in their field. Sixty-three percent of the faculty is tenured. The student–faculty ratio of 16 to 1 reflects the University's commitment to teaching and faculty–student interaction. For the past two years, the University has been named to *The Princeton Review's The Best 331 Colleges and Universities* and the quality of teaching and strength of instructional environment was ranked third highest among the 12 southeastern Conference universities.

THE SCHOOL OF NURSING
The Eleanor Mann School of Nursing was initially established as an Associate Degree Program in 1969, became a Department of Nursing in the College of Education and Health Professions in 1987, launched the baccalaureate nursing program in 1992, and was named the Eleanor Mann School of Nursing in 1998. The School offers the Bachelor of Science in Nursing (BSN) with accelerated tracks for RNs, LPNs, and LPTNs.

The School of Nursing provides students with extensive knowledge and hands-on experience in a wide variety of settings, offering small class sizes, excellent faculty–student ratios and one-on-one support from professors.

CORRESPONDENCE
To receive information on the Eleanor Mann School of Nursing, please send an E-mail with your name, address, and phone number to nursing@uark.edu.

Or contact us by mail:

The Eleanor Mann School of Nursing
University of Arkansas
217 Ozark Hall
Fayetteville, AR 72701
(501) 575-3904
Web: www.uark.edu/depts/coehp/NURS.htm

UNIVERSITY OF CHARLESTON
Department of Nursing
Charleston, West Virginia

THE UNIVERSITY
The University of Charleston strives to educate each student for a life of productive work, enlightened living, and community involvement. Therefore, the University takes very seriously its responsibility to provide students with the knowledge, abilities, and character necessary for them to have successful careers and to be active citizens.

Founded in 1888 and formerly known as Morris Harvey College, the University acquired its new name in 1979 when it began offering several graduate degrees. Today, 1,500 students representing 29 states and 30 other countries enjoy the University's 40-acre riverfront campus overlooking the State Capitol Complex and the beautiful City of Charleston.

THE DEPARTMENT OF NURSING
The Department of Nursing is one of four health care programs in the Bert Bradford Division of Health Sciences. Nursing education has been offered at the University of Charleston since the inception of the associate degree program in 1964. Beginning in 1987, students were admitted to a baccalaureate program in nursing. The Department utilizes newly completed state-of-the-art laboratories, numerous excellent clinical agencies, and an innovative nursing and interdisciplinary health science curriculum to prepare graduates for the dynamic future of health care.

PROGRAMS OF STUDY
The Department of Nursing offers Generic Baccalaureate, RN Baccalaureate, and Associate Degree Nursing Programs. As a part of the Division of Health Sciences, the Baccalaureate Program participates in a core of interdisciplinary health science courses designed to prepare the graduate to function as a beginning practitioner of professional nursing. Graduates of the AD and BS programs are eligible to apply for licensure as a Registered Nurse.

AFFILIATIONS WITH HEALTH CARE FACILITIES
UC's location in the capitol of WV affords access to a wide variety of acute care and community based agencies. The Department of Nursing maintains contractual agreements with more than twenty-five healthcare agencies, including a multi-campus medical center, a specialized women and children's hospital, psychiatric and mental health facilities, home care, community-based clinics and outpatient settings, schools, and public and private community agencies, as well as general and rehabilitation hospitals.

ACADEMIC RESOURCES
The school's resources are housed in newly renovated areas of Riggleman Hall. Students benefit from state-of-the-art skill and assessment labs, simulating patient units and examination cubicles, with supporting audio-visual and computing resources. The Clay Tower Building, completed in 1998, houses the natural sciences, computer laboratories, and the Schoenbaum Library. The library provides access to its online catalog, commercial databases, and other Internet resources. Current library holdings include print volumes, microforms, audio-visual items, and electronic journal subscriptions with full text access.

COSTS
For the academic year 2003-2004, tuition costs $16,500, room (double-occupancy) costs $3,180, and board costs $2,800 for a total of $22,480. This does not include the cost of books, insurance, transportation, or laboratory fees.

FINANCIAL AID
The University of Charleston provides financial assistance that may include a combination of scholarships, grants, loans, and work-study. In 2002–2003, approximately 75 percent of students received financial aid. Special academic scholarships and grants are awarded to outstanding full-time students. The University also offers grants to qualified athletes and to students who are involved in leadership, community service, or vocal music.

NURSING PROGRAM ADMISSION
Students wishing to enroll in a nursing program must complete the appropriate application process by January 15 of the academic year previous to the desired starting term to receive priority consideration. Because of the highly competitive nature of the health sciences programs, initial admission decisions are made in late February for the fall academic term. Applications received after the January 15 deadline will be considered only if space is available. A complete application consists of the Application for Admission, plus official copies of all college and high school transcripts and official test scores.

Only those students who are admitted to the University by the Office of Admissions will be qualified for consideration for the nursing programs. Admission to the University does not guarantee admission to a Nursing program. If a Nursing program is filled, and the applicant qualifies for admission to the University but not to the program, admission to the preparatory curriculum will be offered. Qualified applicants will be reviewed for admission to individual programs utilizing a point scale. Points will be awarded for cumulative academic grade point average, composite ACT/SAT scores, and successful cumulative college hours. All qualified applicants will be reviewed for admission to their program during the last week in January each year.

CORRESPONDENCE AND INFORMATION
Associate Degree Nursing Program Coordinator or
Baccalaureate Nursing Program Coordinator
Department of Nursing
University of Charleston
2300 MacCorkle Ave., S.E.
Charleston, WV 25304
(304) 357-4840
Fax: (304) 357-4965

Office of Admissions
2300 MacCorkle Ave., S.E.
Charleston, WV 25304
(304) 357-4750
Fax: (304) 357-4781
E-Mail: admissions@uchaswv.edu

UNIVERSITY OF CONNECTICUT (UCONN)
School of Nursing
Storrs, Connecticut

THE UNIVERSITY OF CONNECTICUT

UCONN is a state-supported coed university founded in 1881, and has a total enrollment of 21,298 students. The University is the land-grant institution in the state and is the only public institution in New England to be designated as a Research I institution by the Carnegie Foundation. The main campus encompasses 3,100 acres in a quiet rural atmosphere 35 miles east of Hartford, approximately mid-way between New York and Boston. The School of Nursing is located on the main campus of the University in Storrs, Connecticut. There are five regional campuses in other parts of the state. The University sponsors numerous theater and musical activities throughout the year and the cultural activities available in Hartford, New Haven, Boston, and New York City are close enough to attend on a regular basis. Multiple social and support services are available to meet students' needs. Active sports enthusiasts use state-of-the-art recreation facilities and sports fans enjoy the competitive spirit of the Big East.

THE SCHOOL OF NURSING

Founded in 1942, the programs are accredited by the Connecticut State Board of Nurse Examiners and the National League for Nursing Accrediting Commission. The baccalaureate and master's programs have preliminary approval by the Commission on Collegiate Nursing Education. The programs are supported by 23 full-time and 23 part-time faculty members, all of whom have at least a master's degree in a clinical specialty. Ninety-five percent of the full-time faculty members are prepared at the doctoral level. The School has access to more than 100 adjunct clinical faculty members from a wide variety of agencies in the state to serve as preceptors, and is affiliated with approximately forty health-care agencies within Connecticut as well as many other nationally.

ACADEMIC FACILITIES

Specialized services and resources for students are provided in modern facilities, multimedia classrooms, and newly built academic centers. Homer Babbidge Library is a rich storehouse of valuable information. Ranked among the country's top thirty for research resources, it has a strong book collection in nursing and the physical and social sciences. The University Computer Center provides access to the mainframe system nearly 24 hours a day from terminals throughout the campus, from PCs attached to the campus network, or via modem. Nursing laboratories provide undergraduate students a location to transfer knowledge from theory to actual practice. The School has a Center for Nursing Research to facilitate student and faculty research.

PROGRAMS OF STUDY

Undergraduate Bachelor of Science: Provides an opportunity to combine a general education with professional preparation in nursing. The curriculum requires four academic years. Courses in the social, behavioral, and biological sciences and humanities serve as a foundation for the nursing major. Upon successful completion of the 131-credit program, students receive the Bachelor of Science degree and are eligible for examination for licensure as registered nurses.

Master of Science: Graduates of a baccalaureate program with a major in nursing may prepare for professional careers in the various specialty tracks. Nurse Practitioner: Acute Care, Neonatal, Gerontological, Primary Care; Clinical Nurse Specialist: Community Health, Neonatal, Patient Care System Administration, Critical Care, Perioperative; Dual Degree Programs: Business Administration in combination with the Patient Care System Administration (MS/MBA), Public health in combination with the community health nursing program (MS/MPH).

Other Options: RN/MS program for RNs who graduated from NLNAC-accredited diploma or associate degree programs and those who have a baccalaureate degree in a non-nursing field; BS/PhD option for students dedicated to a research career; Advanced Graduate Study (AGS) for those with master's degrees in nursing who are interested in pursuing study in a graduate specialty track. Under Development: Master's Entry in Nursing (MEIN) for non-nurses with baccalaureate degrees in other fields.

Doctor of Philosophy (PhD): The PhD program in nursing prepares nurse leaders who will advance the scientific body of knowledge that is unique to professional nursing practice. Educational experiences are offered in philosophy of nursing science, nursing theory development, qualitative and quantitative research, and advanced statistics.

APPLICATION AND INFORMATION

Potential applicants can seek application material from the
Academic Advisory Center
University of Connecticut School of Nursing
231 Glenbrook Rd. Unit -2026
Storrs, CT 06269-2026
(860) 486-4730 (24 hour message center).
E-Mail: Eva.Gorbants@Uconn.edu.
Web: www.nursing.uconn.edu.

UNIVERSITY OF ILLINOIS AT CHICAGO
College of Nursing
Chicago, Illinois

THE COLLEGE OF NURSING
The College of Nursing at UIC is consistently recognized as one of the top ten nursing programs in the United States. The mission of the College includes the triad of university functions—teaching, research, and service—providing a university education in nursing to meet the present and future needs of society. In 2001, the College was third in total NIH research and research training dollars, and was ranked third out of 142 schools of nursing in *U.S. News & World Report.* Fully accredited by the Commission on Collegiate Nursing Education (CCNE), the College offers programs leading to the degrees of Bachelor of Science in Nursing, Master of Science in nursing sciences, and Doctor of Philosophy in nursing sciences. The College, which has provided high-quality education since 1951, is currently designated as a WHO Collaborating Centre for Nursing and Midwifery. The faculty includes 16 members of the American Academy of Nursing. Worldwide, alumni are a source of leadership in academic, health system, corporate, and political arenas.

PROGRAMS OF STUDY
GENERAL BSN: Transfer students are admitted to the generic baccalaureate program in Chicago and Urbana-Champaign. The program, which prepares beginning nurses to function in a variety of settings, requires 57 liberal arts and sciences semester hours and 63 nursing semester hours for graduation. Students must complete the 57 semester hours of liberal arts credit before entering the nursing curriculum.

RN-BSN: RN-BSN students applying to the program offered in Chicago, Quad Cities, and Urbana-Champaign must meet the transfer admission requirements, which include 57 semester hours of liberal arts and sciences course work and a cumulative GPA of at least 3.5 (A=5.0). Completion of three NLN Mobility Profile II examinations and three transition courses determines credit by exemption for up to 33 semester hours of nursing course work, leaving 30 semester hours of nursing course work, which may be completed in two semesters.

MASTER'S: The master's program prepares nurses for advanced practice roles with an emphasis on basic, clinical, and nursing sciences; knowledge of health systems and environment; and understanding of professional issues of advanced practice roles, while a research focus is maintained. The College offers both clinical nurse specialist and nurse practitioner roles with the following concentrations: administrative studies in nursing (alone or combined as a dual-degree option with an MBA), medical-surgical nursing (critical care, cardiopulmonary, neurocognitive, geriatric), maternal-child nursing (nurse midwifery, women's health, pediatric [including PNP], perinatal), public health nursing (dual-degree option with an MPH, school health, community nurse specialist, family nurse practitioner, occupational health nursing), and psychiatric–mental health nursing.

The 36 required semester hours include statistics, nursing inquiry I & II, health environment and systems, and issues of advanced practice in nursing (10 semester hours); advanced nursing courses (23–36 semester hours); electives (2–3 semester hours); a thesis (5 semester hours) or research project (3 semester hours); and a final examination. More than 36 semester hours are required to complete most of the specialty concentrations.

Post-master's programs are available in the women's health and nurse midwifery, pediatric, and family and critical-care nurse practitioner study options, which prepare individuals to sit for examinations for certification in these fields.

DOCTORAL: The PhD program develops leaders in nursing who influence the provision of health care through systematic investigation, education, policy development and implementation, and expert professional practice. The PhD degree requires 96 semester hours, including nursing theory (6 semester hours), statistics (6 semester hours), research methods (6 semester hours), advanced nursing and nonnursing courses (15 semester hours), independent research (31 semester hours), and a previously completed MS program (32 semester hours). A preliminary oral examination, dissertation, and final oral examination are required to earn the PhD in nursing sciences.

The new BSN to PhD program allows the exceptional student to proceed directly from the BSN to simultaneously meet the requirements for the MS in nursing and PhD in nursing science degrees.

APPLYING
Prospective applicants should contact the College of Nursing Office of Academic Programs for specific application requirements, deadlines, and priority application dates. Applications for the BSN, selected MS, and the PhD programs are accepted for fall only. Admission to several of the MS options is for any term.

CORRESPONDENCE AND INFORMATION
Office of Academic Programs
College of Nursing (M/C 802)
University of Illinois at Chicago
845 South Damen Avenue
Chicago, Illinois 60612-7350
(312) 996-7800
Fax: (312) 996-8066
E-Mail: con@uic.edu
Web: http://www.uic.edu/nursing

UNIVERSITY OF THE INCARNATE WORD
Nursing Program
San Antonio, Texas

THE UNIVERSITY
The University of the Incarnate Word is a private institution founded by the Sisters of Charity of the Incarnate Word in 1881. The campus is 100-plus acres of oak shaded parkland at the headwaters of the San Antonio River. The university provides liberal arts and professional education grounded in the Catholic tradition. Incarnate Word offers 44 undergraduate and 24 graduate fields of study. The overall student-to-faculty classroom ratio is 14:1.

THE NURSING PROGRAM
The mission of the nursing program is to extend the healing ministry of Jesus Christ , the Incarnate Word, through the educational preparation of professional nurses, and to serve as a center for leadership development. The Nursing program offers both undergraduate and graduate degrees. Within the undergraduate program there are two pathways, one designed for students without previous preparation in nursing, the Generic Pathway, and the other designed for registered nurses, the Alternate Pathway (RN-BSN). The graduate program offers concentrations in advanced pratice (clinical specialist role), education, and administration. The nursing program at UIW is fully accredited by the Commission on Collegiate Nursing Education.

APPLICATION PROCESS
Students wishing to study nursing must first be accepted for admission to the University. Students must complete approximately 57 semester hours of prerequisite and general education courses prior to admission to the nursing program. Applicants then apply to the nursing program and must be accepted prior to the semester when the first nursing courses will be taken. Applications must be received in the nursing department by March 1 for Fall admission and October 1 for Spring admission. Students who plan to follow the Alternate Pathway (RN-BSN) should apply directly to the School of Extended Studies at (201) 829-3889.

Applicants are required to submit:

1. A completed application form (obtain from the School of Nursing)
2. Official transcripts from all colleges attended

The Alternate Pathway (RN-BSN) applicant must also submit evidence of current licensure to practice professional nursing in Texas and have at least six months of experience as a registered nurse. Military personnel may submit evidence of current licensure in the United States.

The student's overall academic record is considered for admission, including the following criteria:

1. Completion of all prerequisite courses with a minimum grade of C
2. A minimum cumulative GPA of 2.5 in all course work to date
3. Overall achievement in science courses

Students applying to transfer from another baccalaureate nursing program must satisfy the same prerequisite course work as do all other applicants. Nursing course work will be evaluated for equivalency with the UIW curriculum. The decision for admission and placement in the program will be considered on an individual basis. Graduate students apply directly to the School of Graduate Studies at (210) 829-3157.

AFFILIATIONS WITH HEALTH CARE FACILITIES
The Department of Nursing has contracts with more than 500 agencies in the San Antonio metropolitan area.

FINANCIAL AID
Financial assistance is awarded on a first come, first serve basis; therefore, it is important to begin the application process as early as possible. Copies of the Free Application for the Federal Student Aid (FAFSA) and a UIW Student Information Form must be completed each year and are available in the Office of Financial Assistance. (Note: There is an April 1 priority deadline.)

CONTACT INFORMATION
University of the Incarnate Word
Office of Admissions
4301 Broadway
San Antonio, Texas 78209
1-800-749-WORD
(210) 829-6005
Fax: (210) 829-3921
E-Mail: admis@universe.uiwtx.edu
Web: http://www.uiw.edu

UNIVERSITY OF KANSAS
School of Nursing
Kansas City, Kansas

THE UNIVERSITY
The University of Kansas is a major educational and research institution with more than 28,000 students and 2,200 faculty members dedicated to serving the state of Kansas and the nation.

THE SCHOOL OF NURSING
KU School of Nursing students are prepared for an exciting career in health care and technology. Ranked as one of the top 36 graduate public university schools of nursing in the nation, KU is proud of the academic opportunities available to undergraduate and graduate students. In 2000, the School of Nursing moved into a new multi-million dollar, state-of-the-art building. This new 103,000 square-foot facility enhances the ability to provide an integrated education that crosses multiple disciplines and introduces students to the very latest in medical and information technology.

PROGRAMS OF STUDY
The educational components of the School of Nursing undergraduate program are a broad foundation in the liberal arts and sciences and a focus in the nursing major. Students enter the nursing program after two years (62 semester credit hours) of preparatory work in an accredited liberal arts college. Registered nurses also can enter an RN-BSN degree completion program to complete their Bachelor of Science degree in nursing.

The Master of Science in Nursing program enlarges the focus of nursing, using as its foundation the basic baccalaureate nursing program. The program's goals are directed toward educating the Advanced Practice Nurse and the Nursing Administrator. Advanced Practice specialty tracks are: Adult/Gerontological Clinical Nurse Specialist and Community Health Clinical Nurse Specialist; Family Nurse Practitioner, Adult/Gerontological Nurse Practitioner, and Psychiatric/Mental Health Nurse Practitioner; and Nurse Midwife.

The Advanced Practice major prepares nurses to perform in an expanded role caring for a particular kind of patient or client, or for functioning in a particular kind of setting. The Nursing Administration major is directed toward preparing the nurse to assume management positions in hospitals and other health agencies.

The purpose of the PhD program is to prepare graduates to conduct research that contributes to nursing; to generate and expand the theoretical, empirical, and philosophical bases for nursing practice; to function in faculty positions in college and university settings; and to provide leadership to the profession and interpret nursing to society.

The KU School of Nursing also features a Virtual Classroom program. The Virtual Classroom is an Internet Web site on the University of Kansas Medical Center computer network that houses courses, supplemental material, and study aids. Complete degree programs available through the Virtual Classroom include a Master of Science in nursing for BSN, certificate-prepared nurse practitioners (Family, Adult, Gerontological, and Nurse Midwife) and the RN-to-BSN degree completion program. Many of the courses for other master's specialty tracks also are available online or are Web-enhanced.

AFFILIATIONS WITH HEALTH CARE FACILITIES
The University of Kansas Medical Center in Kansas City, Kansas offers educational programs through its Schools of Medicine, Nursing and Allied Health, and a division of the Graduate School. Clinical services include a full-service, tertiary-care hospital that serves a wide region including Kansas, Missouri, Oklahoma, Arkansas, and Nebraska.

COSTS
The cost to attend the KU School of Nursing will vary from student to student. The average tuition rate for undergraduate students on a 12 month schedule is approximately $3,564. The average tuition rate for graduate students on a 12 month schedule is approximately $4,576. Room, board, meals, out-of-state tuition, and extra expenses are not figured into these costs.

FINANCIAL AID
Students may receive financial assistance through scholarships, loans, work-study, traineeships, and research and teaching assistantships. Federal loans and traineeships are awarded to the school annually. Applications for research and teaching assistantships should be directed to the Office of Student Affairs, School of Nursing. Students enrolling at the Medical Center should contact the Office of Student Financial Aid for information about other types of financial aid. The deadline for aid applications is February 14.

The University Of Kansas Medical Center
Office of Student Financial Aid
3901 Rainbow Boulevard
4008 Student Center
Kansas City, KS 66160-7192
(913) 588-5170

APPLYING
Correspondence and information can be received by contacting:
Office of Student Affairs
KU School of Nursing
3901 Rainbow Boulevard
Kansas City, Kansas 66160-7501
(913) 588-1619
1-888-588-1619
TDD (888) 766-3777
Web: www2.kumc.edu/son/

KUMC is an AA/EO/Title IX Institution.

UNIVERSITY OF MARYLAND
School of Nursing
Baltimore, Maryland

THE UNIVERSITY
The School of Nursing is part of the Baltimore campus of the University of Maryland. The campus includes six professional schools: nursing, medicine, dentistry, pharmacy, social work, and law; the Graduate School; the Maryland Institute for Emergency Medical Systems; the University of Maryland Medical Center; and the Baltimore VA Medical Center. The Baltimore campus of the University of Maryland enrolls nearly 5,500 students and has more than 1,600 faculty members.

The Baltimore campus of the University of Maryland, one of the fastest growing biomedical research centers in the United States, received more than $300 million in extramural support in fiscal year 2003. The unique composition of the campus enables health professionals to address health care, public policy, and social issues through multidisciplinary research, scholarship, and community action. Its location in the Baltimore-Washington-Annapolis triangle maximizes opportunities for student placements and collaboration with government agencies, healthcare institutions, and life science industries.

THE SCHOOL OF NURSING
The University of Maryland School of Nursing was established in 1889 under the direction of Louisa Parsons, a graduate of Florence Nightingale's Nursing School in London. The School offers a bachelor's, master's, and doctoral degrees. The School is consistently ranked among the top ten schools of nursing in the nation and currently enrolls more than 1,400 students.

Consistent with its mission, the School of Nursing is dedicated to creating a research-intensive environment that will advance the science of nursing through research, practice, and scholarship of the highest quality.

The School of Nursing has pioneered a variety of innovative educational programs, including the first nursing informatics program in the world, and the nation's first nursing health policy program. Nineteen specialties are offered at the graduate level. The School of Nursing is the only school in Maryland to offer a midwifery program.

A variety of flexible and combined programs are offered to accelerate degree completion. These include the second bachelor's degree option, the RN-to-BSN online program, the RN-to-MS program, the post-baccalaureate entry option into the PhD program, and the MS/MBA and PhD/MBA programs offered in conjunction with the University of Baltimore; Frostburg State University; and the Robert H. Smith School of Business, University of Maryland College Park.

The School of Nursing offers a range of courses at several off-campus locations, including the Shady Grove Education Center in Rockville, Maryland. Linking regional, national, and international audiences, the School incorporates the most advanced classroom and laboratory design, as well as modern distance learning communications technology, to provide a state-of-the-art educational experience.

To provide clinical programs for students, the School of Nursing maintains affiliations with more than 300 hospitals and healthcare agencies throughout Maryland. In addition, within the 154,000 square-foot School of Nursing building, which offers the latest in research, instructional, and patient-care facilities, are state-of-the-art clinical simulation laboratories, which also afford our students extensive hands-on-training in a real-life setting. These innovative clinical practice sites enhance the School's instructional programs, as well as provide much-needed services to Maryland residents.

LOCATION AND HOUSING
In addition to professional opportunities, the city of Baltimore offers a stimulating environment in which to live and study. Baltimore boasts lively entertainment, world-class museums, such as the Walters Art Gallery and the Baltimore Museum of Art, fine music and professional theater at the Lyric Opera House, Joseph Meyerhoff Symphony Hall (home of the Baltimore Symphony Orchestra), the Morris A. Mechanic Theatre, and small theater and repertory companies. For sports fans, Baltimore features Orioles baseball and Ravens NFL football, with both stadiums located a few short blocks from the campus.

Educational and research opportunities abound in greater Baltimore, home to 12 public and private universities. The School's strategic location in the Baltimore-Washington corridor, including its proximity to the nation's capital, and to Annapolis, the capital of Maryland, provides unparalleled opportunities for student participation in governmental, cultural, and policy-related activities.

Baltimore has many affordable and convenient housing options. On-campus living options include furnished, University-owned apartments. Many students choose to live in neighborhoods surrounding the campus. Room, apartments, and home rentals are available through the Metropolitan area.

CONTACTS
For information and application visit our Web site at www.nursing.umaryland.edu or E-Mail to admissions@son.umaryland/edu or call (410) 706-0501. An online catalogue and applications are available at the Web site.

UNIVERSITY OF MASSACHUSETTS DARTMOUTH
College of Nursing
North Dartmouth, MA

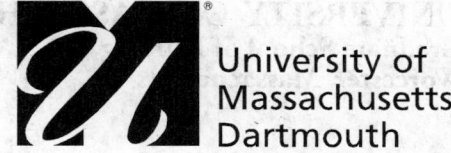

THE UNIVERSITY
Founded in 1863, UMass Dartmouth is now part of a 5-campus University system including campuses in Amherst, Boston, Dartmouth, and Lowell and a Medical School in Worcester. The 710-acre campus, located part way between New Bedford and Fall River, is the home to over 6,000 students, 2,000 of whom live on campus. It offers 40 undergraduate majors and 16 graduate programs, and has more than 300 full-time faculty. UMass Dartmouth offers a broad range of baccalaureate and master's degrees vital to the economic and cultural well being of the region and the Commonwealth.

THE COLLEGE OF NURSING
The College of Nursing at UMass Dartmouth offers the only baccalaureate and graduate degree programs in southeastern Massachusetts and is accredited by the National League for Nursing Accrediting Commission. Our mission is to provide visionary leadership to advance the practice of nursing in a dynamic environment. The college is committed to generating collaborative and consultative relationships with professional colleagues and consumers to enhance the health of the region and beyond. The college actualizes this mission by providing excellent nursing education, meaningful service, and challenging scholarship opportunities to diverse populations.

PROGRAMS OF STUDY
Students are admitted to one of two baccalaureate options: (1) Students with no prior nursing education and LPNs and (2) RN students who are graduates of associate degree and/or diploma schools. The College of Nursing also offers the Master of Science Degree for Advanced Practice nursing, with tracks for Adult Advanced Practice, Adult Nurse Practitioner, and Community Advanced Practice Nursing.

AFFILIATIONS WITH HEALTH CARE FACILITIES
UMass Dartmouth College of Nursing maintains contractual agreements with regional hospitals and health care agencies where a student develops skills in assessment, caring for acutely ill adults, caring for childbearing and childrearing families in the hospital and community, caring for populations at risk, and interacting with individuals in social and welfare agencies that impact the distribution of health care.

ACADEMIC RESOURCES
Located in the Dion Building, the College of Nursing maintains three nursing laboratories for learning: a therapeutics laboratory, a media center, and an interactive assessment area. A junior or senior nursing student whose cumulative grade point average is at least 3.0 may apply for membership in the Theta Kappa Chapter of Sigma Theta Tau, a Nursing Honor Society. All students are invited to join the Massachusetts Student Nurses' Association, a Local Chapter of the National Student Nurses' Association. The University houses an Academic Advising Center, an Alcohol and Drug Education Program, a Career Resource Center, an Academic Resource Center, a Health Office, a Library Communications Center, Multicultural/Retention Support Services, a Religious Resource Center, a Student Activities Center, and a Women's Resource Center.

COSTS
State resident full-time undergraduate tuition is $1,574 and fees are $2,195. New England regional plan tuition is $2,361 and fees are $2,788. Other states' residents tuition is $7,250 and fees are $3,381. Room and board ranges between $4,734 and $5,142. There is a Health Campus Center fee of $402 and, depending on their courses, students will have additional costs. Students will also spend at least $700 for books and supplies every year. Also, all students not covered by their family's health insurance are charged between $450 and $500 annually for insurance.

FINANCIAL AID
UMass Dartmouth awards financial aid based upon federal, state, and institutional guidelines and determines eligibility by using the Free Application for Federal Student Aid (FAFSA). In addition to financial aid based on demonstrated need, the university also makes awards for academic merit, such as the University Commonwealth Scholarships, the University Scholars Program, the Chancellor's Merit Scholarships, the Chancellor's Transfer Merit Scholarship, and Talent Scholarships.

APPLYING
The university is interested in attracting students whose achievements, aptitude, interests, character, and motivation indicate promise of success in the academic subjects they plan to study. Along with the university application, academic records and SAT or ACT results are considered, as well as recommendation letters and personal statements explaining work experiences and other significant interests. Applications for admission can be obtained by contacting the Admissions Office.

CORRESPONDENCE AND INFORMATION
UMass Dartmouth
College of Nursing
285 Old Westport Road
North Dartmouth, MA 02747-2300
College of Nursing: (508) 999-8586
College of Nursing Fax: (508) 999-9127
Admissions: (508) 999-8605
Admissions Fax: (508) 999-8755
University E-Mail address: www.umassd.edu
College of Nursing E-Mail address: psimmons@umassd.edu

UNIVERSITY OF MASSACHUSETTS WORCESTER
Graduate School of Nursing
Worcester, Massachusetts

PROGRAMS
• PhD • Master's • Post-Master's • BS to Master's

THE UNIVERSITY
State-supported graduate institution includes Medical School, Graduate School of Biomedical Sciences and Graduate School of Nursing. Founded in 1962. Primary accreditation: specialized. Total enrollment 665.

THE GRADUATE SCHOOL OF NURSING
Founded in 1985. Faculty: 10 (75% with doctorates). Accredited by NLNAC.

GRADUATE PROGRAMS
The Graduate School of Nursing offers master's and doctoral degrees. The collaborative doctoral program between the University of Massachusetts Amherst and Worcester campuses prepares nurse scientists for faculty, research, and other nursing leadership positions. Located on the University of Massachusetts Worcester campus, the school offers excellent practitioners, clinical resources, library, computer, and research facilities.

The Master's program educates advance practice nurses within two specialties: Adult Acute/Critical Care-Nurse Practitioner/Clinical Specialist and Adult Ambulatory/Community Care-Nurse Practitioner. Subspecialties in the areas of HIV, Cardiac, Cancer Prevention/Control, Geriatric NP, and Correctional/Institutional care are also available.

BS to Master's and Post-Master's options are also available.

APPLYING
PhD Program
GRE General Test, master's degree in nursing, 2 scholarly papers, 2 letters of recommendation, vitae, competitive review by faculty committee

Master's Program (MS)
GRE General Test, TOEFL for non-native speakers of English, bachelor's degree in nursing, minimum GPA of 3.0, RN license, 1 year clinical experience, physical assessment course, statistics course

Post-Master's Program (PMC)
MS in nursing degree from a school accredited by a nationally recognized accrediting agency, minimum GPA of 3.0, RN license, 1 year clinical experience, physical assessment course, statistics course

COSTS
PhD Program State resident tuition; $5,940 full-time, $104.50 per credit hour part-time. Non-resident: $20,142 full-time, $373 per credit hour part-time. Full-time mandatory fees: $675. Books and supplies per academic year range from $500 - $600.

MS Program State resident tuition: $1,254 full-time, $104.50 per credit hour part-time. Non-resident tuition: $4,509 full-time, $375.75 per credit hour part-time. Full-time mandatory fees: $1,914.50 for 9 or more credits for 2 semesters.

FINANCIAL AID
Graduate assistantships, Nurse Traineeships, Federal Family Education Loans, institutionally sponsored loans, and opportunities for employment. Application deadline March 22.

ACADEMIC FACILITIES
Campus library: 258,800 volumes, 1659 periodical subscriptions. Nursing school resources: CAI, computer lab, nursing audiovisuals. Student Services Health clinic, child-care facilities, career and personal counseling, job placement, campus safety program, special assistance for disabled students. International student services: counseling/support. Nursing student activities: Sigma Theta Tau.

CORRESPONDENCE AND INFORMATION
PhD Program
Dr. James Fain
Director, Collaborative PhD Program and Associate Professor
Graduate School of Nursing
(508) 856-5661
Fax: (508) 856-6552
E-Mail: james.fain@umassmed.edu

Master's and Post-Master's Programs
Kathleen Trumpaitis
Coordinator, Student Affairs
Graduate School of Nursing
(508) 856-5801
Fax: (508) 856-6552
Web: www.umassmed.edu/gsn

UNIVERSITY OF MICHIGAN
School of Nursing
Ann Arbor, MI

THE UNIVERSITY

The University of Michigan, located in Ann Arbor, Michigan, has more than 510,000 alumni worldwide. Graduates of the University have made substantial contributions to intellectual, scientific, and cultural growth. Its internationally ranked faculty, supported by the most advanced research programs, prepares students to teach, lead, heal, and innovate in the global society of the twenty-first century. The University of Michigan is consistently ranked among the nation's top ten universities.

THE SCHOOL OF NURSING

The University of Michigan School of Nursing has held an unsurpassed reputation of excellence for more than 100 years because it has kept pace with advances in knowledge and technology and trends in health care. The School of Nursing is also unparalleled in terms of its distinguished faculty, with over 90 percent of all tenure-track faculty members doctorally prepared. The caliber of faculty preparation enhances the balance between clinical and theoretical experiences for students.

PROGRAMS OF STUDY

The baccalaureate degree program is the basis for a career in nursing. The School of Nursing baccalaureate programs include: (1) a four-year BSN Program that offers applicants direct admission as freshmen; (2) a Second Career Nursing Program for persons with bachelor's degrees in other fields; and (3) an RN-BSN Completion Program.

At the master's level, the School of Nursing, through the University's Horace H. Rackham School of Graduate Studies, offers advanced practice certification and clinical nurse specialist programs: Nursing Informatics, Nursing and Health Care Policy, and Entrepreneurial Nursing. Program offerings include: Management of Patient Care Services (combined weekend/web-based format); Dual Degree – Nursing Administration (MS/MBA); Medical-Surgical Nursing; Adult or Pediatric Acute Care Nurse Practitioner; Psychiatric-Mental Health Nursing; Psychiatric-Mental Health Nurse Practitioner; Gerontological Nursing; Gerontological Nurse Practitioner; Community Health Nursing; Home Health Care; Occupational Health Nursing; Adult Primary Care Nurse Practitioner with a Women's Health/Childbearing Families Concentration Option; Family Nurse Practitioner; Infant, Child & Adolescent Health Pediatric Nurse Practitioner; and Nurse-Midwifery. An RN-MS is available in any of the specialties. Some programs offer post-master's options, and some programs are available through On Job/On Campus.

The School of Nursing also offers a doctoral program and post-doctoral study opportunities. Currently, post-doctoral training is offered in health promotion and risk reduction, neurobehavior, and in Women's Health Disparities.

ACADEMIC RESOURCES

There are more than six million volumes in the twenty-three libraries on the University's campus. Also on campus are nine museums, several hospitals, hundreds of laboratories and institutes, and thousands of microcomputers.

LOCATION

The University of Michigan is located in Ann Arbor, a city well-known for its parks, rivers, and historical heritage. Ann Arbor's designation as an "All-American City" complements its well-earned title, "Research Center of the Midwest."

FINANCIAL AID

Financial aid is available through the Office of Financial Aid. It may consist of a combination of grants, scholarships, and loans, including nursing student loans and work-study opportunities. Graduate assistance can be obtained from various sources. Some Graduate Student Teaching and Graduate Student Research Assistantships are available within the School of Nursing. Fellowships and scholarships are available through the Horace H. Rackham School of Graduate Studies.

APPLYING

The deadline for applications to the Second Career, BSN, RN/BSN, and master's nursing programs is February 1. Specific master's programs may have extended application deadlines. The deadline for applications to the PhD program is December 1. To request additional information about School of Nursing Programs or to inquire about an application deadline, please call 1-800-458-8689.

CORRESPONDENCE AND INFORMATION

University of Michigan
School of Nursing
Office of Academic Affairs
400 North Ingalls
Ann Arbor, MI 48109-0482
1-800-458-8689
E-Mail: umnursing@umich.edu
Web: www.nursing.umich.edu

THE UNIVERSITY OF NEW ENGLAND
Westbrook College Campus
Portland, Maine

COLLEGE OF HEALTH PROFESSIONS
The University of New England's College of Health Professions is widely recognized for offering some of the nation's strongest health-care programs. Located on our Westbrook College Campus in Portland, Maine's largest city, the College offers unparalleled opportunities for internships, clinical work, career placement, and personal growth. At the historic Westbrook College Campus, a committed group of undergraduate and graduate students share the benefits of a close-knit campus community, state-of-the-art teaching and research facilities, and a faculty that is dedicated to the success of each and every student. In addition, the College's revolutionary new model of integrated, interdisciplinary health and healing education, known as I2H2, gives UNE's College of Health Professions' graduates a unique ability to thrive in today's fast-changing health-care environments.

I2H2—THE FUTURE OF HEALTH-CARE EDUCATION
In 1999, the College of Health Professions at the University of New England launched a revolutionary initiative that promises to transform health-care education in the United States. Known as I2H2, this new model offers integrated, interdisciplinary instruction in health and healing. Combining classroom instruction, research, and clinical practice, I2H2 brings together faculty members, graduate students, and undergraduates from the College's programs of study. I2H2 will prepare you to play a leading role in today's increasingly collaborative health and healing professions.

I2H2 enables students across the spectrum of health-care disciplines to share clinical learning experiences. For example, in the College's geriatrics practicum, a team of six or seven students from different programs such as Physical Therapy, Occupational Therapy, Nursing, Social Work, and Dental Hygiene, works together at an off-campus geriatric facility. Drawing upon each team member's area of expertise, they work collaboratively to assess a patient's overall health and health-care needs.

Team members share observations and exchange ideas for further treatment. Over the course of the geriatrics practicum, students become increasingly adept at pooling their knowledge and skills to promote the best possible health outcome for every patient. What's more, they learn how to view each patient as a complex individual whose well-being depends upon the interplay of many diverse factors, and every member of the team.

THE NURSING PROGRAM
The Nursing Program at the University of New England is uniquely designed to facilitate student growth and entry into the profession of nursing.

The freshman and sophomore years provide a course of study, which is heavily concentrated in the Nursing major. Extensive nursing classroom and clinical experiences define these first two years. Upon completion of the sophomore year, the student has fulfilled adequate study in the major to be awarded an Associate of Science Degree in Nursing (ADN). This enables the student to sit for the Registered Nurse (RN) license examination.

The junior and senior years are designed for practicing registered nurses who embrace the opportunity to broaden and enhance current knowledge and skills, acquire knowledge in the theory and practice of nursing, increase career opportunities and provide the credentials necessary for graduate education. During this time, nursing course work is delivered in a compressed schedule, generally one day per week. This format allows the student to continue practicing as a registered nurse and encourages the individual to apply concepts presented in the classroom to actual clinical practice.

This curriculum design accommodates the student who is entering the nursing profession as well as those nursing professionals wishing to complete a bachelor's degree in nursing.

Graduates of the University of New England BSN program are offered direct entry into our Master of Science in Nurse Anesthesia degree program.

ADMISSIONS
All applicants to the Nursing Program are considered on the basis of their academic ability, personal qualities, and potential to meet the academic standards of the program. Candidates for admission must file a completed application that will include the application, copies of all academic work (high school and/or college), standardized test scores (SAT or ACT), and an interview with the Nursing Department. Registered nurses applying to complete a Bachelor's Degree in Nursing must have graduated from an NLNAC accredited associate degree or diploma program, and be a licensed registered nurse.

COSTS
Tuition for a full time student during the 2003-2004 academic year is $18,990, room and board is $7,560. The per-credit hour rate for a part time student is $680.

FINANCIAL AID
The University of New England offers a very competitive financial aid program. UNE has the University Scholarship Program, awarded based on academic performance; the UNE Incentive Grant Program, which is based on financial need; as well as all the federal programs—Pell Grants, Perkins Loans, Stafford Loans both subsidized and unsubsidized, and Plus Loans.

FOR MORE INFORMATION
To learn more about the University of New England call 800-477-4863 or E-Mail admissions@une.edu. You may also visit UNE online at www.une.edu.

UNIVERSITY OF PENNSYLVANIA
School of Nursing
Philadelphia, Pennsylvania

THE UNIVERSITY
The University of Pennsylvania offers an outstanding array of resources for both undergraduate and graduate students. The excellence of its many schools offers students the opportunity to take courses across the campus, making it a major center for learning and research. This framework fosters student/faculty collaboration throughout the University, enhancing opportunities for a diversified approach to education and research.

LOCATION
Philadelphia is the fourth-largest city in the United States. The four undergraduate schools and twelve graduate schools of the University are located on a 260-acre tract. Unified by pedestrian walkways and almost entirely closed off to traffic, the campus contributes to the sense of community that is characteristic of Penn. Situated in a major urban setting less than two miles from the center of Philadelphia, the University is surrounded by a largely residential community known as University City.

THE SCHOOL OF NURSING
The University of Pennsylvania is the only Ivy League institution offering a baccalaureate nursing program that begins day one, over 20 master's programs in nursing, and doctoral nursing study. Penn Nursing is consistently ranked among the nation's top graduate schools of nursing in a major survey conducted by *U.S. News & World Report*. The undergraduate nursing program is listed in *Ruggs Book of Colleges* as high school guidance counselors' first choice for nursing.

Nursing students have matchless opportunities for clinical experience at the world-renowned University of Pennsylvania Medical Center, the Children's Hospital of Philadelphia, Children's Seashore House, and many other clinical agencies in Philadelphia and the tri-state area.

At Penn, nursing students are taught and mentored by nationally and internationally recognized faculty known for their leadership in education, practice, and research. Undergraduate and graduate students often take advantage of the opportunity to participate in faculty research.

PROGRAM OF STUDY
The School of Nursing offers a Bachelor of Science in Nursing (BSN) degree with a program that balances the liberal arts, science, and professional nursing preparation. Special opportunities include nursing-specific study abroad programs; joint degree programs and minors with Penn's Wharton School, College of Arts and Sciences, School of Engineering, and Annenberg School for Communication; submatriculation (initiating pursuit of a graduate degree while working toward the BSN) into Penn's School of Law or one of nursing's MSN specialties; and a direct entry BSN/PhD option.

Penn offers a program allowing students with a baccalaureate degree in another field or a RN to apply to either the BSN completion program or an accelerated BSN/MSN program, which enables students to complete their BSN as well as a master's. Previous college and university courses are evaluated for transfer credit, and many clinical courses may be challenged by taking the Regents College examination.

The School of Nursing offers the Master of Science in Nursing (MSN) degree in more than twenty different areas including: Adult Acute Care Nurse Practitioner (NP); Oncology Advanced Practice Nurse (APN); Adult-Gerontological NP with a Home Care option; Health Care of Women NP; Nurse Midwifery; Perinatal NP & Clinical Nurse Specialist (CNS); Neonatal NP; Pediatric and Family Primary Care; Pediatric Acute/Chronic Care NP; Pediatric Oncology NP; Pediatric Critical Care NP; Occupational Health Nursing, Nursing and Health Care Administration; Health Leadership; and Psychiatric/Mental Health APN with a Forensics option. Penn offers a Midwifery distance learning option that allows students in rural areas in Pennsylvania and surrounding states to complete the program within their own communities. An MSN in Nursing Administration/MBA is also offered in conjunction with the Wharton School.

The School of Nursing recognizes the evolving nature of health care and the desire of many nurses to expand or alter current roles and responsibilities. It is possible to pursue post-master's work, designed for those with a MSN and interested in either extending their knowledge and skill in their current area or changing to a new area of practice.

The Doctor of Philosophy program provides learning opportunities emphasizing scholarship and research. The program can be constructed from either the baccalaureate or the master's degree. The program is flexibly structured into four parts: clinical field, required core, related field, and doctoral dissertation. The curriculum provides a general structure within which students participate in developing their own programs of study based on their nursing backgrounds and research interests. The opportunity also exists to pursue a PhD in the School of Nursing with an MBA from the Wharton School.

ACADEMIC FACILITIES
The University of Pennsylvania libraries house more than 4,672,777 bound volumes and 34,276 periodical subscriptions. The Biomedical Library, adjacent to the School of Nursing, houses more than 185,787 books and journals in the nursing, medical, and biological sciences. Students may access CD-ROM databases and nine other major information databases, including MEDLINE and nursing databases.

The School of Nursing has, for student use, a computer lab, TV facilities, a multimedia production center, photography services, learning laboratories, and Pennet with access to the Internet.

COSTS
Tuition for full-time BSN students for the 1999-2000 academic year was $21,746. Part-time tuition was $2,777 per course. Tuition for full-time MSN students was $21,812; $2,750 per course. PhD tuition was $17,982 for full-time students and $2,997 per course.

UNIVERSITY OF PENNSYLVANIA
(continued)

FINANCIAL AID

The University strives to meet the financial needs of all of students. Many different sources of aid are available. Scholarships, grants, low-interest student loans, and teaching and research assistantships are awarded appropriately, based on a student's need and level of study. Students are encouraged to work directly with Nursing's financial aid counselors to help develop the means to support their education.

APPLYING

Freshmen apply (online or hard copy) under one of two admissions plans. The Early Decision Plan is for those applicants who have decided that the University of Pennsylvania School of Nursing is their first-choice and agree to attend if accepted. Applications are due by November 1, with decisions mailed in mid-December. Regular decision applicants are reviewed on a rolling admissions basis. Applications are due by January 1, and students are notified beginning in the middle of February.

Transfer and second degree students are admitted in both the fall and spring semesters. The application deadline is October 15 with notification in December for spring semester and March 15 for fall semester, with notification beginning end of April.

BSN/MSN applicants apply by December 1 for September admission and will hear by late February.

An early consideration program for BSN/MSN applicants allows students who apply by October 15 to receive notification by mid-December. Early applicants must be approved by the BSN/MSN Program Director before filing an application.

MSN and PhD students can access an online application from the School's Web site or use a hard copy application. The deadline for fall entrance is January 1 for doctoral programs and February 15 for master's programs, although specific programs should be contacted for flexibility in submitting an application.

CORRESPONDENCE AND INFORMATION

School of Nursing
University of Pennsylvania
Nursing Education Building
Philadelphia, Pennsylvania 19104-6096
(215) 898-4271
Fax: (215) 573-8439
E-Mail: susansz@pobox.upenn.edu
Web: http://www.upenn.edu

UNIVERSITY OF PHOENIX
College of Health Sciences and Nursing
Campuses Nationwide

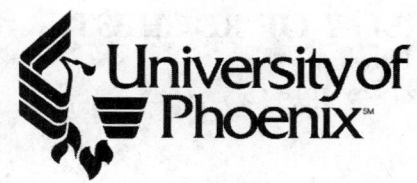

THE UNIVERSITY
Founded in Phoenix, Arizona, the University of Phoenix is the largest, private, higher education institution whose mission is to provide quality education to working adults. Our innovative educational model is offered at more than 100 campuses and learning centers with cluster groups in 22 states.

The University of Phoenix provides nursing programs for students attending in a ground-based environment as well as an Online/Internet environment. Nursing campuses are located in 1) Phoenix and Tucson, Arizona, 2) San Jose, Los Angeles, San Diego, and Sacramento, California, 3) Denver and Colorado Springs, Colorado, 4) Jacksonville, Orlando, and Tampa, Florida, 5) Honolulu, Hawaii, 6) Metairie, Louisiana, 7) Detroit and Grand Rapids, Michigan, 8) Albuquerque and Santa Teresa, New Mexico, 9) Salt Lake City, Utah, 10) Oklahoma City and Tulsa, Oklahoma, and 11) Atlanta, Georgia. The Online Campus distance learning programs enables us to teach students around the globe in a virtual classroom using asynchronous interactive learning environments. Accredited in 1978, the University of Phoenix enrolls some 90,000 working adult students with approximately 4,500 students in nursing and health care programs.

THE COLLEGE OF HEALTH SCIENCES AND NURSING
The College responds to the educational and professional needs of registered nurses and other health care professions. Degree programs are specifically designed to give nurses and health care professionals the skills necessary to effectively respond to today's dynamic and challenging health care environment. With over 1,400 alumni, student, faculty, and community leaders, the College supports its Sigma Theta Tau chapter, Omicron Delta.

PROGRAMS OF STUDY
The College offers the following National League of Nursing Accrediting Commission accredited degree programs: RN to Bachelor of Science in Nursing (BSN) with an LPN to BSN track, Master of Science in Nursing (MSN), and Master of Science Nursing /Family Nurse Practitioner (MSN/FNP). Additional programs include Bachelor of Science in Health Care Services (BSHCS) and Master of Science in Nursing/ Masters of Business Administration/ Health Care Management (MSN/MBA/HCM) dual degree. A blend of theory and practice, each program offers a learning environment that allows students to build knowledge, and apply what they learn.

ACADEMIC RESOURCES
The University of Phoenix is home to an extensive electronic library housing more than 9,000 journals and over 17,000,000 full text articles. Encyclopedias, directories, dissertations, and other reference materials add to the depth and scope of the collection. Students and faculty members make extensive use of the Online Collection, which receives over 6,000 visitors on a typical day. Open 24 hours a day, seven days a week, the University Library provides students with access to thousands of journals and millions of citations on business, management, technology, education, counseling, health care administration, and nursing.

COSTS
Costs vary by campus, by degree program, and by delivery format. Inquire with specific campuses.

FINANCIAL AID
The University of Phoenix offers Federal Stafford Student Loans, Federal PLUS Loan, Federal Pell Grants, Comprehensive Assistance in Student Lending Alternative Loans, and Comprehensive Assistance in Student Lending Line of Credit.

APPLYING
BSN program: Associate degree or diploma in Nursing, 2.0 GPA; valid, unrestricted, unencumbered RN license; must be currently employed as an RN and have a minimum of one year of health care; English or score of 550 or higher on TOEFL.

LPN to BSN track: Completed LPN program, unencumbered LPN license, 2 years LPN experience

MSN program: Undergraduate degree in nursing with an upper division major in nursing; 2.5 GPA; valid, unrestricted, unencumbered, RN license; minimum three years full-time RN work experience; English or score of 550 or higher on the TOEFL. The RN student who has a undergraduate degree in a field other than nursing may be admitted under the Bridge Program.

MSN/ Nurse Practitioner program: Undergraduate degree in nursing; 3.0 GPA; valid, unrestricted, unencumbered RN license; minimum three years full-time RN work experience; two letters of recommendation; additional health status documentation required; advanced practice role essay; English or score of 550 or higher on the TOEFL.

MSN/MBA/HCM program: Undergraduate degree in nursing; 2.5 GPA; valid, unrestricted, unencumbered RN license; three years work experience; current employment in health care; English or score of 550 or higher on the TOEFL.

BSHCS program: High school graduate; minimum age of 23; current employment (preferably in health care); English or score of 550 or higher on the TOEFL.

ACCREDITATION
Higher Learning Commission
North Central Association
30 North LaSalle Street, Suite 2400
Chicago, IL 06002
(312) 263-0456

National League for Nursing Accrediting Commission (NLNAC)
61 Broadway, New York, NY 10006
(212) 363-5555

CORRESPONDENCE AND INFORMATION
University of Phoenix
College of Health Sciences and Nursing
4615 East Elwood Street
Phoenix, AZ 85040
Attn: Prospective Student
(800) 228-7240 or (480) 557-1140
Fax: (480) 929-7164

UNIVERSITY OF ROCHESTER
School of Nursing
Rochester, New York

ROCHESTER

The University of Rochester is a private, nationally ranked research university offering a variety of majors for both undergraduates and graduate students. The city of Rochester is the third largest metropolitan area in New York, recognized by *American Demographics Magazine* as the kindest, most helpful city in the United States. One million Rochester residents enjoy the beauty of upstate New York, including the Finger Lakes region, Lake Erie, Niagara Falls, and 11,000 acres of park land locally.

THE SCHOOL OF NURSING

Founded in 1925, the School of Nursing today ranks 18th in the nation (*US News & World Report*) and some of the specific nurse practitioner programs rank in the top 10! About 375 students are matriculated in the undergraduate and graduate programs. Exciting changes are part of the strategic plan for the next decade and emphasize the Unification Model, integrating nursing practice, education, and research. Nationally, the School of Nursing is one of the few programs committed to the unification philosophy. Students have the benefit of instruction and practice supervision by leading practitioners and researchers in an integrated delivery system.

PROGRAMS

The baccalaureate program is offered exclusively for students who are registered nurses. The revised RN completion program includes the option of transferring up to 96 credits, evening hours and block scheduling, and self-study for arts and sciences courses. An RN/BS/MS program is also available.

The clinically focused master's and post-master's programs include Acute Care Nurse Practitioner, Care of Children and Families (pediatric nurse practitioner with a neonatal nurse practitioner option), Adult Nurse Practitioner, Family Nurse Practitioner, and Psychiatric/ Mental Health Nurse Practitioner. An accelerated RN/MS program and post-master's certificate programs are also available.

The PhD program is designed to prepare nurse scholars for academic and research leadership roles within health care and educational settings. Doctoral students may pursue study in a variety of areas of scientific interest, with emphasis placed on Aging and Vulnerable Children and Youth, the school's two Centers of Excellence.

RESOURCES

The School of Nursing is part of the University of Rochester Medical Center, which includes the School of Medicine and Dentistry, the 700-bed Strong Memorial Hospital, a tertiary care hospital, and the region's Trauma Center. The school also sits within Strong Health, the largest integrated delivery system in Rochester, which includes Strong Memorial Hospital, Highland Hospital, the Visiting Nurse Service, and sub-acute and long-term care services. Students also have opportunities to work as members of a community based research study team. Resources include a Teaching Learning Center, skills lab, and computer lab. Students have access to three million volumes and 10,000 periodicals in the university's libraries.

COSTS

Full-time undergraduate tuition is $22,300. Part-time and graduate student cost is $697 per credit hour. Generous tuition benefits are available to University of Rochester and Strong Health employees.

APPLICATIONS

For the RN completion baccalaureate program, a 2.5 GPA is preferred. A copy of the nursing license/registration is also required. Applications are accepted on a rolling basis.

For the MS programs, requirements include a BS (3.0 minimum GPA) from an accredited undergraduate nursing program, RN licensure, two favorable references, a personal statement, and a statistics course (grade C or above).

Applicants must declare a specialty area. Deadlines are February 15 for fall admission and September 15 for January admission; applications received after that will be considered if space is available. An interview may be required. GRE or MAT is optional. Some specialties require a year of clinical experience.

For the PhD program, requirements include a master's degree (3.5 GPA) from an accredited nursing program, Graduate Record Examination (general test only), interview, statement of goals, sample of writing, and three letters of recommendation from academicians.

CORRESPONDENCE AND INFORMATION

Elaine Andolina, MS, RN
Director of Admissions
601 Elmwood Avenue, Box SON
Rochester, New York 14642
(716) 275-2375
Fax: (716) 756-8299
Web: http://www.urmc.rochester.edu/son/programs.htm

UNIVERSITY OF SOUTH FLORIDA
College of Nursing
Tampa, FL

THE COLLEGE

The College of Nursing at the University of South Florida enjoys its highly regarded reputation in baccalaureate, master's, and doctoral nursing education in part because of the faculty's commitment to outstanding teaching, scholarly research, and service to the profession and community. This distinctive group of highly motivated members is leading USF in its mission to become the premier institution for those striving to achieve leadership in nursing. Faculty members of the College of Nursing prepare their students in the full spectrum of healthcare settings and clinical specialties available in one of the countries finest and most diverse metropolitan areas.

Tampa-St. Petersburg-Clearwater is the second largest metropolitan area in the fourth largest state. The Tampa Bay area provides USF faculty and students with unlimited leadership, academic, employment, social, and cultural opportunities beyond the classroom. Strategically located in the Tampa Bay metro area, this multicultural metropolis offers a wealth of arts and leisure activities—a professional orchestra, Broadway theatrical productions, world-class concert halls, art museums, big-city nightlife, bountiful ethnic restaurants, and professional baseball, football, hockey, and soccer teams. From the historic charm of Ybor City to the booming downtown riverfront, the Tampa Bay area is poised to become one of the great American cities of the 21st century. One of the largest and richest regions in Florida, Tampa Bay is expected to lead the state in new jobs well into the 21st century.

USF is one of the 20 largest universities in the nation, offering roughly 200 programs at the undergraduate, master's, specialty, and doctoral levels to more than 35,000 students. Since its establishment as a single-campus baccalaureate institution, USF has become a vibrant, comprehensive, multicampus research university serving the higher education needs of the rapidly growing west coast of Florida. More than three million people in a ten-county region of west central Florida reside within convenient commuter access to one of the four USF regional campuses and teaching sites spread across the Tampa Bay area. The USF Tampa campus is located in north Tampa near the expanding community of "New Tampa" and forms the hub of major medical facilities for the area. The main campus in Tampa offers the most comprehensive choice of degree programs and draws faculty and students from many different countries and cultures. The USF College of Nursing is a dynamic player in this University Community.

"USF's College of Nursing has been quick to respond to new demands. We've increased public service initiatives, developed community partnerships with health care product manufacturers, added multidisciplinary health care training and forged a partnership with Sarasota Memorial Hospital to create a national model for nursing education in managed care. But we're not stopping there! With support from community and educational leaders, we plan to expand current education classroom and support facilities, establish a nursing research department, develop a virtual learning center and build a distance learning center to support the existing program for the growing number of regional campuses." Patricia A. Burns, PhD, RN, FAAN

CORRESPONDENCE AND INFORMATION

Patricia A. Burns, PhD, RN, FAAN
Dean and Professor
USF College of Nursing
12901 Bruce B. Downs Boulevard, MDC Box 22
Tampa, FL 33612-4766

UNIVERSITY OF ST. FRANCIS
College of Nursing and Allied Health
Joliet, IL

THE UNIVERSITY

Today's dynamic health care environment has created the need for nursing professionals who can apply a broad range of knowledge and skills. At the University of St. Francis, you will be prepared not only for the imminent changes in the nursing field, but also to be a competent clinician and a sensitive, caring advocate for your patients.

A national leader in offering educational opportunities to health care professionals, the University of St. Francis offers the BSN degree in three formats: the traditional four-year program, a transfer program, and a Fast Track program for registered nurses with an ADN or diploma. The University's MSN degree in Adult Health offers three tracks of study: nurse practitioner, clinical specialist, and family nurse practitioner (Albuquerque campus).

USF's challenging programs emphasize experiential learning, critical thinking skills, patient advocacy, and cultural awareness. The university's relationship with nearby Provena Saint Joseph Medical Center offers educational opportunities rich in practical application. USF students participate in health care on a daily basis as they are learning.

The university strives to prepare nurses to assume leadership roles in health care. Upon graduating from the university's Saint Joseph College of Nursing and Allied Health, you will be ready for the professional demands of nursing.

BSN

Preparation to become a nursing professional will begin with a strong liberal arts component of general education and science courses during the first two years. This enhances the critical thinking skills necessary for the scientific inquiry portion of nursing studies.

Once in the nursing program, coursework will be intensive and focused. The many areas of health care—hospitals, home health, managed care, primary care clinics, public health, hospice care, long-term care (nursing homes) and mental health—are addressed in the curriculum and made available to students through clinical experiences. Clinical experiences can be with any of the more than 100 health care organizations with which the university has a working relationship. Supervisors at these organizations tell us that USF students are among the best prepared, most enthusiastic, and most inquiring of the nursing students they work with.

BSN FAST TRACK

At the University of St. Francis, we recognize that educational and work experiences have formed an important base of knowledge. The Fast Track option will expand on that knowledge, helping registered nurses pursue an even higher level of professional excellence.

Students in the Fast Track program (for registered nurses with an ADN or diploma) take upper-division BSN courses, with 32 hours of nursing coursework required. Successful completion of a prior learning assessment portfolio detailing professional experience or challenge examinations may reduce the number of actual classes that must be taken.

Clinical courses are designed to fit the individual's goals and schedule. Courses may be completed online or on-site. On-site courses meet one evening a week for eight week terms. The program can be completed in two years or less.

MSN

The University of St. Francis offers three tracks in the Master of Science in Nursing program. The nurse practitioner tracks prepare nurses to provide primary health care in community settings. The clinical nurse specialist track prepares nurses to perform a lead role in improving care through education and consultation as well as to serve as a role model for professional practice.

The MSN program can be completed on a part-time basis in three years. Courses may be completed for the nurse practitioner or clinical nurse specialist programs online or at a classroom site in Joliet. The family nurse practitioner program can also be complete online or at USF's Albuquerque campus. A minimal on-site clinical component will be required.

CONTACT INFORMATION

For application or financial aid information, contact:
University of St. Francis
500 Wilcox Street
Joliet, IL 60435
(800) 735-7500
Fax: (815) 740-4285
E-Mail: admissions@stfrancis.edu

THE UNIVERSITY OF TOLEDO
Associate Degree Nursing Program
Toledo, OH

THE UNIVERSITY

The University of Toledo Associate Degree Nursing Program is located in one of the eight colleges within the University known as the College of Health and Human Services. This College contains various specialties including Nursing, Physical Therapy, Social Work, Criminal Justice, Kinesiology, Public Health, Nurse Paralegal, Respiratory Therapy, and Emergency Medical Technology. The Nursing Program, housed in the Department of Health Professions, is in a consortium with the Medical College of Ohio to provide Bachelors Completion coursework for students who might be interested in furthering their education. Students interested in continuing their education can apply for a Master's (MCO) or Doctoral (UT-non-nursing major) program within this college.

THE NURSING PROGRAM

The Nursing Program Curriculum is a community-based focus that utilizes Dorthea Orem's self-care deficit model as a theoretical framework. The program is four semesters in length with summers off and includes rotations to clinical sites, both acute and community-based, in each of the four semesters. Students are given hands-on experience at a rate of five hours per credit hour of clinical time, which is one of the highest ratios in the State of Ohio. The curriculum is set up to include 15 week classes with matching clinical during the semester.

ACADEMIC RESOURCES

The Nursing Program Resource Center is an experiential, laboratory-based center that is student-friendly and allows for study, interaction with peers, consultation, and programming for at-risk nursing students. The Nursing Resource Center is focused on support for students and their needs, which includes ability to congregate, eat more than a lunch, interact regarding coursework with friends or faculty, and participate in skills check-off's or computer assisted programs. The nursing program utilizes a computerized testing package throughout the course of studies, which is centered on test taking skills and NCLEX exam prep.

ADMISSION CRITERIA

Admission Criteria for the Nursing Program requires all students to have a GPA higher than 2.5, "C" or better in pre-requisite sciences, less than two failures in pre-requisite sciences, and entrance scores above the 50th percentile.

LPN students or transfer students must begin the program with incoming freshman. Inquiries are welcome; please contact Dr. Celeste Baldwin, RN, CNS at cbaldwi@utnet.utoledo.edu for a personal interview.

CONTACT INFORMATION

The University of Toledo
Associate Degree Nursing Program
2801 Bancroft Sreet, #400
Toledo, OH 43606-3390
(419) 530-3372
Fax: (419) 530-3096

THE UNIVERSITY OF TULSA
School of Nursing
Tulsa, Oklahoma

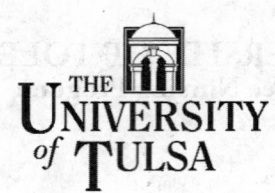

THE UNIVERSITY
The University of Tulsa is a comprehensive, independent, doctoral-degree institution, with historic ties to the Presbyterian Church (USA). The university has an undergraduate enrollment of 3,000 and a graduate and law enrollment of about 1,200. It is located about two miles from the heart of downtown Tulsa, a vigorous southwestern city in a metropolitan area of over three-quarter million people.

THE SCHOOL OF NURSING
The School of Nursing offers an undergraduate curriculum leading to the Bachelor of Science degree in nursing. The curriculum is designed to provide a broad general education and a solid professional program based on a nursing model (the Roy Adaptation Model) rich in content and applicability. Our goal is an educated individual who is a professional nurse.

The School of Nursing's program is approved by the Oklahoma Board of Nursing and is accredited by the National League for Nursing Accrediting Commission, 61 Broadway, New York, NY 10006 (1-800-669-1656). The school is a member of the National League for Nursing and the American Association of Colleges of Nursing.

PROGRAMS OF STUDY
The School of Nursing offers Generic Baccalaureate, RN to Baccalaureate, LPN to RN Baccalaureate, BS in Athletic Training, and BS in Exercise and Sport Sciences. For the RN program, an RN license, diploma, or ADN in nursing is required. Advanced standing is available. For the LPN to RN baccalaureate, an LPN license is required. Advanced standing is available through credit by exam and proficiency examination of transcripts, clinical experiences, and licensure.

NURSING CURRICULUM AND UNIQUE FEATURES
"Nursing is a service profession. We deal with lives at a point when they are most fragile," says Susan Gaston, Director of the School of Nursing. "There is an art and science to nursing. We impart both at TU. At the same time, health care is a business, and nursing is responsible for the management of patient care. The School of Nursing's position within the College of Business Administration is a distinct advantage for our students. Nursing majors are required to take three business courses." The TU nursing curriculum is an integrated program, with common threads running from the sophomore to senior years. In addition to intensive clinical and classroom work, students are taught the communication skills, cultural diversity, and information technology knowledge that have become so vital to nursing in a changing world. The School of Nursing employs the Roy Adaptation Model. Developed by Sister Callista Roy, the model helps students understand the stimuli affecting patients and their various behaviors.

Students also have the opportunity for study abroad nursing courses, such as International Nursing and Technology (http://www.cba.utulsa.edu/gastonsk/international00.asp). These courses are offered with international travel during spring break or as a summer session.

FACILITIES
In the School of Nursing, there is no substitute for an academically nurturing environment. Our students find our remarkable student-teacher ratio a decided advantage that promotes interaction among students and faculty. The personal learning experience in the School of Nursing is enhanced further by an on-campus 12-bed skills laboratory. Located in Chapman Hall, the skills lab affords students opportunities to practice what they have learned in the classroom in a setting that simulates the health care problems they will face in the real world. The skill laboratory also includes a computer lab. Theory classes are held in technology classrooms with computer projection systems and World Wide Web connections.

After students are thoroughly educated in basic skills, they continue their clinical experience in Tulsa's local hospitals and community health agencies. These hospitals have bed capacities ranging from 100 to 500.

COST
Undergraduate tuition per semester is $7,455 for both in-state and out-of-state students. Room and board is estimated at $4,700 for the year.

FINANCIAL AID
The University of Tulsa recognizes that financing a quality college education is often difficult, and we are dedicated to providing equal access to all qualified students. Grants, loans, and work-study opportunities are available through the University's Offices of Student Financial Services. A scholarship fund, with no requirement for repayment, has been established for the School of Nursing that can pay up to one-half of tuition for those who have made exceptional grades in high school or college and who have financial need. To apply for a nursing scholarship, a student must be admitted to The University of Tulsa, complete the FAFSA financial aid form, and have the results sent to this university each spring semester. All university scholarships are awarded by the Office of Student Financial Services (http://www.utulsa.edu/financial/aid.html).

APPLICATION
Students can apply to The University of Tulsa online at its Web site at http://www.utulsa.edu. Once admitted to the University, students apply to the School of Nursing for progression in the nursing program. As clinical spaces are limited, a competitive selection process occurs during the spring semester for students who wish to enroll in fall sophomore level nursing courses. For first consideration, submit the application by February 1 for sophomore nursing classes beginning the next fall. The School of Nursing continues to accept applications until the beginning of the fall semester. The School of Nursing application form can be downloaded from the nursing Web site at http://www.cba.utulsa.edu/nsg/.

Students must earn at least a "C" in all major core courses before entering courses for which the core course is a prerequisite. Students must have earned "C" or better in Biol 1023—Anatomy and Physiology, Biol 1021—Anatomy and Physiology Lab, Psy 3063—Human Development over the Life Span, and AHS 2122—Normal Nutrition prior to the spring sophomore courses. The student must have a University of Tulsa cumulative grade point average of 2.5 before entering the Level I sophomore nursing courses.

CORRESPONDANCE AND INFORMATION
Susan Gaston, PhD, RN
Director, School of Nursing
University of Tulsa
600 S. College
Tulsa, OK 74104
(918) 631-3116
Fax: (918) 631-2068
E-Mail: susan-gaston@utulsa.edu
Web: www.cba.utulsa.edu/nsg

UNIVERSITY OF VERMONT
School of Nursing
Burlington, Vermont

PROGRAMS
Generic Baccalaureate, RN-BS-MS, MS, Master's for Nurses with Non-nursing degrees, Post-Master's

THE UNIVERSITY
Chartered in 1791, the same year that Vermont became the fourteenth state in the union, The University of Vermont was established as the fifth college in New England. The campus of The University of Vermont is located in the State's largest city and enjoys magnificent views of Lake Champlain and the Adirondack Mountains to the west and Vermont's Green Mountains to the east. The University of Vermont is a state-supported co-ed university with a total enrollment of 8,900.

THE SCHOOL OF NURSING
The University of Vermont School of Nursing creates the feeling of a small college, yet offers the best of life at a prestigious university. The School of Nursing, founded in 1943, provides the best of the two worlds. Because the total enrollment is only about 300 students, you receive personal attention from your professors. They are committed to your academic and personal success and have time to make your education as complete as possible. In addition to teaching and advising, faculty members are involved in service, scholarly work, and research. They provide expertise on local, state, regional, and national health issues in both public and professional forums. This exchange of new ideas and methods promotes an innovative and dynamic quality of instruction. The research interests of the faculty are diverse and include major themes related to health needs arising from rural living.

BACCALAUREATE DEGREE PROGRAM
The baccalaureate degree program prepares students for beginning positions in professional nursing practice. Graduates are able to provide nursing care to individuals of all ages and families from diverse cultural backgrounds in any setting offering health care services. While health maintenance, disease prevention, and teaching are emphasized, careful attention is paid to the skills needed in the treatment of the acutely ill.

The baccalaureate program curriculum provides students with a balance between professional nursing courses and those in the liberal arts and sciences. Courses in the natural and behavioral sciences and humanities serve as a foundation for the nursing courses. Nursing courses begin during the sophomore year and continue with increasing emphasis through the junior and senior years. Clinical preparation begins in the second year of study.

RN-BS-MS PROGRAM
The program for registered nurses has been designed in light of the current and future changes in the health care delivery system. The program is an RN-BS-MS accelerated program, with an option for students to "step-out" after completion of the baccalaureate requirements with a BS degree.

The nursing courses for the baccalaureate portion of the program are offered online through the "Learning by Degrees" program. The focus of the baccalaureate program is on the nurse's role in health promotion for individuals, families, and communities and the factors that influence delivery of health care services. Online learning combines the benefits of the classroom with consideration for the individual learners' personal needs. Upon completion of the baccalaureate degree, students may choose to pursue a master's degree.

MASTER OF SCIENCE PROGRAM
The graduate program offered by the School of Nursing prepares professional nurses to assume leadership roles within the discipline of nursing in a variety of settings, to expand knowledge of nursing, to develop expertise in a specialized area of nursing, and acquire the foundation for doctoral study and continued professional development.

The tracks offered are: Adult Health Nursing, Advanced Population Focused Nursing (community focus) and Primary Health Care Nursing (adult or family nurse practitioner or nurse midwifery focus). Upon completion of the Adult Health Nursing or Advanced Population Focused Nursing, graduates are eligible to take the American Nurses Credentialing Center certification examination for Clinical Nurse Specialist. Upon completion of the Primary Health Care Nursing track (family or adult nurse practitioner), graduates are eligible to take the American Nurses Credentialing Center or American Academy of Nurse Practitioners certification examination. Students who complete the primary care track with a nurse midwifery focus are eligible to take the American College of Nurse Midwives certification examination.

FINANCIAL AID
Scholarship and loan funds are available through the University of Vermont Financial Aid Office. In addition to awards based on demonstrated financial need, scholarships based on leadership, community service, character, and academic excellence are also available. For information please contact:

Office of Financial Aid
330 Waterman Building
University of Vermont
Burlington, VT 05405-0160
(802) 656-3156

CORRESPONDENCE AND INFORMATION
School of Nursing
Rowell Building, Room 216
Burlington, Vermont 05405
(802) 656-3830
Web: http://nursing.uvm.edu

UNIVERSITY OF WISCONSIN–MILWAUKEE
College of Nursing
Milwaukee, Wisconsin

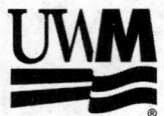

THE UNIVERSITY

The University of Wisconsin–Milwaukee (UWM) was established in 1956 with the merger of the University of Wisconsin Extension center in Milwaukee and Wisconsin State College. Since then, UWM has flourished into a major part of the intellectual, cultural, and economic life of southeastern Wisconsin. Ranked by the Carnegie Foundation as a research II institution, UWM supports a dynamic academic community of nearly 26,000 students, 1,350 faculty and instructional staff, and 1,900 staff members. As Wisconsin's premier urban research university, UWM offers more than 100 undergraduate majors and sub-majors, 48 master's programs, and 18 doctoral programs, in 11 schools and colleges.

THE COLLEGE OF NURSING

Since its inception in 1965, the College of Nursing has been dedicated to providing academic programs of the highest quality that are at the forefront of nursing. The programs are nationally ranked and the faculty is widely recognized for achievements and innovations.

Reflective of its commitment to the urban community, the College operates the Institute for Urban Health Partnerships. The Institute oversees four Community Nursing Centers, which offer the unique ability to integrate the multiple missions of an urban university through outstanding opportunities for student learning, faculty practice, research, and community service.

ACADEMIC RESOURCES AND FACILITIES

The College maintains state-of-the-art resources to support a rich academic environment. The Nursing Learning Resource Center, serving students, faculty, and the community, is an integral component of both the undergraduate and graduate curricula. This college laboratory is a mediated and simulated learning environment in which students perform skills foundational to safe nursing practice. Used as a resource in the development and evaluation of media, the Center also houses a modern, well-equipped computer laboratory.

In the Center for Nursing Research and Evaluation, staff work to develop the research potential of faculty, students, and the greater nursing community. Personnel offer consultation in design, methodology, data analysis, computer programming, grant proposal writing, and writing for publication.

The Center for Cultural Diversity and Health houses a collection of comprehensive health behavior information for culturally diverse groups in the Milwaukee community. The Center provides for students, faculty, and health professionals stimulating learning opportunities in health care for culturally diverse groups through continuing education seminars, clinical practice models, and research in meeting the health needs of culturally diverse groups.

The College's Center for Nursing History includes the Inez G. Hinsvark Historical Gallery, a unique learning resource located on the ground floor of Frances Cunningham Hall. The significant role of nurses in history is brought to life by artifacts, mementos, and photographs, as well as borrowed collections.

ACADEMIC PROGRAMS

BACCALAUREATE PROGRAM

Degree: BS; Tracks offered:

1. Traditional option 4-year Undergraduate Curriculum; also available at UW–Parkside
2. Accelerated options for individuals who already hold a bachelor's degree.
3. Completion option for graduates of diploma and associate degree programs in nursing.

Program Entrance Requirements: Students who seek to enter the nursing major in September must submit applications by the preceding January 15; for January entrance the deadline is the preceding July 15. Students who have completed 15 credits of required courses with a cumulative GPA of 3.5 or higher may be eligible for earlier admission. Individuals may be considered for admission as prenursing students in the fall and spring as beginning freshmen or transfer students.

Admission to the prenursing classification is no guarantee of admission to the nursing professional program.

EXPENSES (2003-04)

Full-time tuition and fees for resident undergraduate students were $5,107, and $17,858 for non-residents. Room and Board: $4,352 per academic year.

Financial Aid: The Campus Financial Aid Office awards financial aid based on need. Financial aid packages consist of loans, grants, and work-study assistance. The College of Nursing administers a number of scholarships to qualified students. Scholarships in varying amounts are awarded annually.

MASTER'S DEGREE PROGRAM

Degree: MS

Clinical Nurse Specialist with concentrations in community health, adult health, maternal/child health, psychiatric/mental health, or systems management.

Family Nurse Practitioner with additional options in Post Nurse Practitioner, Post Master's FNP, RN to Master's.

Health Professional Educational Certificate

Master's applications are due to the UWM Graduate School by January 1 and to the College of Nursing by February 1 for fall enrollment, and to the UWM Graduate School by September 1 and to the College of Nursing by October 1 for spring semester enrollment.

DOCTORAL DEGREE PROGRAM

Degree: PhD

Nursing Research with individualized areas of study. Students may elect to pursue their programs of study in a traditional (on-site) format or through online study (web-based instruction). A BSN to PhD option is also offered to nurses who want to pursue research and scholarship goals consistent with doctoral level education.

Applications are due to the UWM Graduate School and to the College of Nursing by February 1 for fall enrollment. Applications received after these dates will be reviewed on a rolling basis.

UNIVERSITY OF WISCONSIN–MILWAUKEE
(continued)

EXPENSES (2003-04)
Full-time tuition and fees for resident graduate students were $7,402 and $21,768 for non-residents.
Room and Board: $5,412 per academic year.
Financial Aid: Financial aid available to graduate students includes traineeships, fellowships, scholarships, research and teaching assistantships, and loans. Aid is available to part-time students.

CORRESPONDENCE AND INFORMATION
UWM College of Nursing
Student Affairs Office
P.O. Box 413
Milwaukee WI 53201-0413
(414) 229-5482
Fax: (414) 229-5554
E-Mail: asknursing@uwm.edu
Web: http://www.nursing.uwm.edu

URSULINE COLLEGE
The Breen School of Nursing
Pepper Pike, Ohio

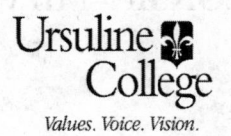

THE COLLEGE
Ursuline College offers undergraduate and graduate education within a Catholic tradition marked by the Ursuline legacy of educating women. Values-based curricula provide the foundation for liberal arts and professional programs. Respecting a diverse student population, we offer varied approaches to learning for growth of the whole person. We prepare students for further education, careers, and service to society while encouraging the search for wisdom, academic excellence, and leadership.

THE SCHOOL OF NURSING
The Breen School of Nursing, the largest academic program on campus, offers professional programs within Ursuline's values-based learning environment. An individualized approach enables students to enjoy personal instruction, learn material in greater depth, and gain experience in a wide variety of health care environments. The Breen School's graduates are sought by employers who find them to be well prepared and flexible in adapting to new settings.

PROGRAM OF STUDY
The Breen School offers programs that prepare nurses for the health care marketplace of the future at both the basic (BSN) and advanced practice (MSN) levels. In addition to a highly qualified full-time faculty, the MSN program has visiting professors who are nationally recognized leaders in nursing.

The BSN program provides a broad foundation by combining Ursuline's liberal studies core with an intensive three-year sequence in the nursing major. Qualified students are admitted directly into nursing. Unique classroom and clinical assignments at renowned health care institutions enable students to develop critical thinking, communication, technical, and leadership skills. The School's holistic and values-based nursing program provides a framework for students to learn about the caring and ethical side of healthcare, pass the NCLEX licensing exam (100% pass rate in 1998), and adapt to practice in the 21st century. There are accelerated RN/BSN and LPN/BSN tracks.

The MSN program prepares advanced practice nurses (CNS & NP) in four clinical areas: case management, palliative care, plus adult and family nurse practitioner. All tracks are presented within Ursuline's values-based framework and emphasize the clinical components of advanced practice nursing. The MSN degree can be completed in two years on a part-time basis. Post-master's certificate programs are also offered.

AFFILIATIONS
The Breen School of Nursing is affiliated with numerous internationally renowned and community-based healthcare agencies throughout the greater Cleveland area. MSN students may elect to do their practicum in another state or country.

ACADEMIC FACILITIES
The new Pilla Student Learning Center houses a state-of-the-art-nursing laboratory. Ursuline's library houses over 110,000 volumes and 600 periodicals. Membership in OhioLINK and a comprehensive media collection provide access to thousands of additional resources. Other campus resources include media and computer centers.

STUDENT SERVICES
The College provides sports, a fitness center, personal and career counseling, mentoring and cooperative education programs, campus ministry, and an Office for Multicultural Affairs. The Learning Resource Center provides academic support for all students, including assistance with study, testing, and writing skills. Tutoring is available in reading, writing, math, and science. The Program for Academic Success (PAS) was designed to help students not prepared for college level work, especially math and science.

COSTS
For 2002-2003, undergraduate tuition was $570 per credit hour. Full-time students usually carry 12 to 16 credits. Graduate tuition was $620 per credit hour.

FINANCIAL AID
The Office of Financial Aid administers a number of institutional, state, and federal programs. Financial assistance may include a combination of scholarships, loans, grants, and work-study opportunities.

APPLYING
Undergraduate and graduate applications are accepted on a rolling basis. Admission to the BSN program is through the Office of Admission. In addition to criteria for clear admission to the college, BSN applicants need to have successfully completed algebra, biology (with lab), and chemistry (with lab), each with a grade of 2.5.

Admission to the MSN program is through The Breen School of Nursing. Admission criteria include an official transcript verifying completion of an accredited BSN program with a GPA of 3.0. The MAT or GRE may be required of applicants whose GPA is less than 3.0.

CORRESPONDENCE AND INFORMATION
Ursuline College
2550 Lander Road
Pepper Pike, OH 44124
1-888-URSULINE (toll-free)
Web: http://www.ursuline.edu

For the Undergraduate Program:
Director of Admission
(440) 449-4203
Fax: (440) 684-6138

For the Graduate Program:
Carol H. Waggoner, PhD, RN
Director, Graduate Program, The Breen School of Nursing
(440) 449-3425
Fax: (440) 449-4267
E-Mail: cwaggoner@ursuline.edu

VANDERBILT UNIVERSITY
School of Nursing
Nashville, TN

THE UNIVERSITY
When Commodore Cornelius Vanderbilt gave a million dollars to build and endow a university in 1873, he did so with the wish that it "contribute to strengthening the ties which should exist between all sections of our common country." Today, that dream has been realized in Vanderbilt University, a comprehensive research university in Nashville, Tennessee, providing innovative programs, state-of-the-art facilities and a supportive environment for interdisciplinary inquiry.

THE SCHOOL OF NURSING
Founded in 1908 as a diploma program, in 1925 we were one of five schools funded by the Rockefeller Foundation to establish a University School of Nursing. As a leader, Vanderbilt University School of Nursing has pioneered nursing's move into an institution of higher learning. Today, we prepare individuals to become advanced practice nurses through our Master of Science in Nursing degree programs and our PhD in Nursing Science program.

MULTIPLE ENTRY OPTIONS
Applicants who already have a Bachelor's of Science in Nursing may earn their MSN in as little as one full calendar year (3 semesters).

Applicants who are Associate Degree or Diploma RNs with 78 semester hours of college coursework may earn their MSN in as little as two years (5 semesters).

Applicants who are college graduates in another field or who have 78 semester hours of college coursework may earn their MSN in as little as two full calendar years (6 semesters).

PROGRAMS OF STUDY
Vanderbilt University offers the following programs:
Acute Care Nurse Practitioner
Adult Nurse Practitioner* with concentrations in:
- correctional health
- the prevention and management of cardiovascular disease and its associated symptoms.

Adult/Gerontological Nurse Practitioner
Family Nurse Practitioner
Health Systems Management* with concentrations in:
- case management
- clinical research management
- practice management

MSN/MBA Joint Degree
Neonatal Nurse Practitioner*
Nurse Midwifery

Nurse Midwifery/FNP dual program
Pediatric Nurse Practitioner
Nursing Informatics
Psychiatric-Mental Health Nurse Practitioner*
Women's Health Nurse Practitioner
PhD in Nursing Science

*Programs offered in modified format for students who live at a distance

FOR ADDITIONAL INFORMATION CONTACT
Vanderbilt University School of Nursing
226 Godchaux Hall
Nashville, Tennessee 37240
(615) 322-3800
Fax: (615) 343-0333
E-Mail: VUSN-Admissions@mcmail.vanderbilt.edu
Web: http://www.mc.vanderbilt.edu/nursing/

VILLANOVA UNIVERSITY
College of Nursing
Villanova, PA

THE NURSING PROGRAM

The health care of a complex and technologically advanced society requires professional nurses who are liberally educated, clinically competent, compassionate, and ethically motivated. In responding to these objectives, the College of Nursing is a tangible expression of Villanova's mission, values, and commitment to human service.

Villanova University first responded to society's need for baccalaureate-prepared nurses in 1932 when it offered a program of study leading to a Bachelor of Science degree in Nursing Education. This commitment was expanded in 1953 to create a College of Nursing that now offers a generic BSN program, a BSN completion program for registered nurses, an MSN program, and a Continuing Education Program.

The College of Nursing is a tangible expression of Villanova University's mission, tradition, and commitment to human service. As a major school of nursing under Catholic auspices, it carries responsibility for the education of nurses within the framework of Christian beliefs, values, ethical principles, and the heritage of the Order of St. Augustine. The academic programs in the College of Nursing are directed to the interpretation of nursing as a healing ministry and demonstrated through service and the care of others. As a healing art as well as an applied science and practice discipline, nursing emphasizes the concern for spiritual health as well as that of mind and body. Curricula reflect the integration of these elements and their application in clinical practice and concern for others regardless of race, ethnicity, or religion.

The practice of nursing within a Christian environment requires that those who nurse recognize and respect the needs of each person, and that they teach while they nurse in order to assist their patients and the community to achieve the highest possible level of wellness of body, mind and spirit.

The College of Nursing is committed to providing high quality education in the liberal arts and sciences, and expert preparation in the knowledge and clinical skills of professional nursing to qualified individuals who must be prepared and empowered to confront the health care demands of a complex and technologically advanced society.

DEGREES AND PROGRAMS

The College awards the baccalaureate degree in nursing (BSN) and provides basic preparation in nursing to those who are studying for the first professional degree in the field. Such students include high school graduates with no prior college experience, registered nurses who were prepared in hospital or junior college programs and who have not yet attained the baccalaureate, college graduates with degrees in other disciplines who have made a late decision to study nursing, and mature adults who are studying for their first college degree.

The Graduate Program awards the master's degree (MSN) and provides preparation and leadership development in selected areas of advanced nursing practice, development of research skills, and knowledge of health policy. In addition, graduate concentrations prepare individuals for positions as health care administrators, case managers, educators, nurse practitioners, and nurse anesthetists. The Graduate Nursing Program is ranked among the "top 60" graduate nursing programs in the country by *U.S. News and World Report*.

Through the Continuing Education Program, the College of Nursing recognizes its responsibility to the profession and the public by providing short courses, conferences, workshops, and symposia for nurses and other health professionals on topics related to health care and the development of professional roles. This Program is nationally accredited by the American Nurses Credentialing Center (ANCC) Commission on Accreditation. The approval is reciprocal in all states and for all specialty organizations that recognize the ANCC approval mechanism.

The College of Nursing is approved by the State Board of Nursing of the Commonwealth of Pennsylvania. Upon completion of the undergraduate program, graduates are eligible to take the licensing examination (NCLEX) for professional registered nurses. This license is transferable within the United States nationally by state. The undergraduate and graduate programs are both fully accredited by the National League for Nursing Accreditation Commission and the Commission on Collegiate Nursing Education. The Nurse Anesthesia concentration in the Graduate Program is accredited by the Council on Accreditation of Nurse Anesthesia Educational Programs. The Continuing Education Program is accredited as a provider of Continuing Education in Nursing by the American Nurses Credentialing Center, Commission on Accreditation.

CONTACT INFORMATION

You are invited to visit our campus or call to speak with someone from our admissions office at (610) 519-4911. You are also invited to visit our Web site at www.nursing.villanova.edu.

VIRGINIA COMMONWEALTH UNIVERSITY
School of Nursing
Richmond, Virginia

THE UNIVERSITY
A public, urban university located in the state capitol, Virginia Commonwealth University was founded in 1838. VCU is ranked by the Carnegie Foundation as one of the nation's top research universities and is one of only three such universities in the state. VCU is composed of two campuses, the Academic Campus and the Medical College of Virginia Campus. More than 23,000 students attend VCU with thirty percent of students representing minority groups.

MEDICAL COLLEGE OF VIRGINIA CAMPUS
VCU's Medical College of Virginia Campus is home to the Schools of Nursing, Allied Health, Pharmacy, Dentistry, and Medicine. The campus' affiliated Medical College of Virginia Hospitals is one of the most comprehensive teaching hospitals in the country. In 1998, it was ranked in the annual study, 100 Top Hospitals: Benchmarks for Success, which identifies U.S. hospitals that deliver the highest quality and most cost-efficient health care.

THE SCHOOL OF NURSING
The School of Nursing originated in 1893 and has evolved from a basic diploma program to a school of over 700 students with multiple programs at the baccalaureate, master's, and doctoral degree levels. Additionally, the School of Nursing offers post-master's certificate programs. In 2001, the School awarded degrees to 211 candidates. The School of Nursing takes pride in its long history of service to the profession of nursing and continues to be a leader in nursing education in Virginia and the country. In 1999, the Virginia Nurses Association recognized 26 VCU nurses for their contributions to the profession. The School's program in Nursing Administration was ranked by *U.S. News and World Report* as one of the top ten programs in the country in 2000. The School of Nursing is accredited by the National League for Nursing Accrediting Commission and approved by the Virginia State Board of Nursing.

PROGRAMS OF STUDY
Undergraduate Program
Traditional Program
Individuals seeking their first professional nursing education program may be admitted to the VCU School of Nursing as freshman, sophomores, or juniors. Junior entry is limited and requires attending a 10-week summer session prior to the junior year.

RN-BS Completion Program
This program is designed for individuals with an associate degree in nursing or a diploma in nursing, who wish to earn a bachelor of science degree with a major in nursing. Classes meet once a month, Friday evening and all day Saturday. The program is offered at multiple sites across the state.

Graduate Program
Accelerated Second-degree Program
In response to the growing number of individuals with bachelor's degrees in other disciplines who are seeking a career in nursing, the school offers this graduate program where an individual can earn both a bachelor's degree and a master's degree in nursing. Students in the Accelerated Second-Degree program take courses in the undergraduate and master's program until licensure as an RN is

obtained. The master's degree is awarded after two to four semesters of additional study depending on the area of concentration.

Master's Program
The master's program is designed to offer general core content requisite for advanced practice in nursing and content aimed at preparation in a speciality concentration. Additionally, the program prepares individuals for certification as nurse practitioners and/or clinical nurse specialists.

Post-Master's Certificate Program
The Post-Master's Certificate program is offered in all MS speciality areas for Master's-prepared individuals seeking additional certification.

PhD Program
The goal of the doctoral program in nursing is the preparation of scholars to develop knowledge in the discipline of nursing. Areas of inquiry are: Healing, Health Systems; Immunocompetence; Risk and Resilience. A comprehensive program, it remains flexible, bearing in mind full-time professional nurses who cannot leave their positions for full-time doctoral study.

COSTS AND FINANCIAL AID
In-state resident full-time undergraduate tuition and fees are $10,480, and $19,409 for those out-of-state. Financial aid is available through the University's Financial Aid Office. The School of Nursing offers scholarships for full-time study.

APPLICATION PROCESS
All programs use a self-managed application process and require standardized test scores of all applicants. Suggested application deadlines are as follows: Entry Level Master's program – December 15, Traditional Undergraduate – January 15, Traditional Master's – February 1, RN-BS Weekend – February 15, Doctoral – April 1.

CONTACT INFORMATION
Office of Enrollment & Student Services
School of Nursing
Virginia Commonwealth University
P.O. Box 980567
Richmond, VA 23298-0567
(804) 828-5171
Fax: (804) 828-7743
Web: www.nursing.vcu.edu
Monthly information sessions offered.

WALSH UNIVERSITY
Nursing Division
North Canton, OH

THE UNIVERSITY
Walsh University is an independent, coeducational Catholic, liberal arts institution. Founded by the Brothers of Christian Instruction, Walsh University is dedicated to a values-based education with an international perspective in the Judeo-Christian tradition. Walsh University believes in the desirability of a small university that promotes academic excellence, a diverse community, and close student-teacher interaction. The University provides an education that fosters critical thinking, effective communication, spiritual growth, and personal, professional, and cultural development. Walsh University encourages individuals to act in accordance with reason guided by the example of Jesus Christ.

NURSING DIVISION
The mission of the Walsh University Nursing Division is to provide excellence in nursing education grounded in human experience. The Nursing Division prepares the graduate to think critically, communicate effectively, and act compassionately, responsibly, and maturely as a contributing member of the profession and society. The BSN curricula prepare students to function in the role of caregiver, manager and coordinator of care, and leader in a variety of settings with diverse populations.

PROGRAMS OF STUDY
The Bachelor of Science in Nursing (BSN) degree can be obtained through two curriculum options. The first option is a four-year pre-licensure curriculum that is designed to prepare the graduate to become licensed as a registered nurse. The second option is a non-sequenced RN-BSN curriculum for the registered nurse that is designed to build upon the student's current knowledge and experience in order to meet the changing career needs within an evolving health care system.

AFFILIATIONS
The Nursing Division maintains contractual agreements with 15 health care agencies that include community hospitals, home health agencies, clinics, and health centers.

ACADEMIC RESOURCES
The Nursing Division has a state-of-the-art nursing skills laboratory to serve both BSN programs.

COSTS
The cost per credit hour is $430 for a non-resident. There are additional residence fees for students who choose to live on campus. There is an additional laboratory and testing fee for nursing students in addition to uniform expenses.

FINANCIAL AID
Walsh University offers a competitively priced liberal arts education. The Office of Financial Aid provides assistance in three basic forms: scholarships/grants, loans, and employment. Scholarships are available to new and returning students, made possible by donations from supporters of Walsh University, and are awarded primarily on the basis of academic ability and need. The Walsh University Application for Financial Aid, the results of the FAFSA, and the student's academic record are used to distribute scholarships and may be renewed annually if a recipient maintains the required criteria.

APPLICATION PROCESS
Walsh University applicants are required to have a minimum GPA of 2.0, and an ACT score of 17 or SAT score of 830 must be attained to be considered for admission. To facilitate student success, enrolling students are required to take mathematics, English, and foreign language placement tests. Students who have been enrolled in another institution of higher education and are seeking admission to Walsh University must have a cumulative grade point average of 2.0 and be in good academic and social standing. Credit to be transferred must be graded a C or better and must apply towards the student's intended course of study.

The Division of Nursing considers advanced placement for the registered nurse (RN) in the Bachelor of Science in Nursing Program. The registered nurse is admitted to the baccalaureate nursing program upon successful completion of the admission criteria.

CORRESPONDENCE AND INFORMATION
Chair, Nursing Division
Walsh Unviersity
2020 Easton Street, N.W.
North Canton, OH 44720
(330) 490-7250
Fax: (330) 490-7206
Web: www.walsh.edu

WATTS SCHOOL OF NURSING
The School of Nursing
Durham, North Carolina

THE UNIVERSITY
Founded in 1895, Watts School of Nursing is distinguished as the oldest nursing program in North Carolina, as well as the first diploma program in the state to achieve National League for Nursing accreditation. With over 2,700 graduates, it is renowned for its excellence in nursing education and for the accomplishments and recognized leadership of its graduates and faculty. Located in the "City of Medicine," Watts is housed on the campus of Durham Regional Hospital as part of the Duke University Health System.

PROGRAM OF STUDY
A two-year hospital-based diploma program, Watts concentrates solely on nursing, providing a strong theoretical knowledge coupled with closely correlated clinical experiences. Five prerequisite courses in biological, social, and physical sciences must be completed at a community college or other accredited college prior to enrollment. The nursing curriculum at Watts comprises four semesters, and students may begin their program either in January or August. Graduates of the program are eligible to apply for licensure as a Registered Nurse (RN). Watts has historically maintained an excellent record on the state board licensure examination, with a 100% passing rate in 2001.

HEALTH CARE FACILITIES
Durham's unexcelled spectrum of medical facilities, health care services, and highly trained medical personnel provides Watts with a wealth of clinical opportunities for student learning. Facilities of Durham Regional Hospital comprise the School's primary clinical settings, with additional clinical experiences occurring in other area hospitals, home health agencies, physicians' offices, clinic settings, and community skilled nursing facilities. Together, these clinical opportunities provide a broad base for professional practice.

ACADEMIC RESOURCES
The School maintains a well-equipped simulated clinical practice lab for instructor guided learning and independent practice. Access is available to the Medical Library at Durham Regional Hospital, which offers a wide variety of print, non-print, and electronic resources. Students also have access to a national interlibrary loan program. In addition, the library is the site of a computer center reserved for use by Watts students.

COSTS
The cost for the two year program is $6,070. This includes tuition, fees, and liability insurance. Students should allow $730 for books during the first year and $360 for the second year. Other costs will be incurred for uniforms and equipment kits.

FINANCIAL AID
Watts School of Nursing offers a variety of financial aid resources—Pell Grant, Stafford Loan, in-house loans, North Carolina Scholars Program, Crain Scholarships, Watts Alumni Scholarships, and Friends of Watts Scholarships.

ADMISSION REQUIREMENTS
An applicant must be a graduate of an approved high school or hold a high school equivalency certificate (GED). If high school diploma or GED is received within 5 years of the date of application, an SAT or ACT score is required. All applicants must pass a school-administered pre-admission test to continue with the application process. A personal interview with a member of the Student Affairs Committee is required, as well as five written personal references.

ADMISSIONS OFFICE
Watts School of Nursing
3643 N. Roxboro Road
Durham, NC 27704
(919) 470-7348
Web: http://wattsschoolofnursing.org

WEBER STATE UNIVERSITY
Nursing Program
Ogden, UT

THE NURSING PROGRAM
Founded in 1953, nursing at Weber State University offers students career progression from Practical Nursing (PN) to Associate of Science/Associate of Applied Science Degree Nursing (AS/AAS) to progression through various preparation levels in accordance with individual ability, aspirations, career goals, and changing life circumstances. The program trains entry level practitioners by providing a foundation from the physical, biological, behavioral, and nursing sciences for application in caring for clients in a variety of nursing environments.

The Nursing Program is a part of the Dr. Ezekiel R. Dumke College of Health Professions located in the Marriot Allied Health Building.

The Program embraces three levels of preparation for nursing practice: PN, AS/AAS, and BSN. Educational offerings provide distinctive purposes and expectations for each level of nursing preparation while recognizing common areas of achievement within each level. Competency standards define graduate characteristics at each preparation level.

Four entry options are available for students. Three of these lead to licensure by examination at the PN and AS/AAS levels. The remaining option is based on the AS/AAS curriculum and requires valid RN licensure prior to entry.

ENTRY OPTIONS
Practical Nursing: The first year of the nursing program constitutes the practical nursing curriculum. Students selecting this option are awarded an Institutional Certificate by WSU following one year of study. For licensure as a practical nurse, graduates are required to sit for the National Council of Licensure Examination (NCLEX-PN).

Straight AS/AAS: Two years are required for students entering this option. Students selected for an Associate of Science/Associate of Applied Science degree in nursing may write the NCLEX-PN through equivalency clause in the Utah Nurse Practice Act at completion of the first year. An additional year of course work entitles graduates to write the National Examination for licensure as a registered nurse (NCLEX-RN).

PN to AAS (Advanced Placement): This entry option is open only to LPNs and other qualified health care workers. Entering students enroll for the second year of the nursing program. Graduates write the NCLEX-RN at completion of this curricular year.

RN to BSN: Entry options for achieving the baccalaureate degree are only open to RNs. Students may directly enter baccalaureate nursing after graduating from the associate degree level, provided they meet admission criteria. Additionally, RNs from other associate degree or diploma programs, or those who have been out of school for an unspecified period of time, can enter the RN to BSN option. A two year upper division curriculum rounds out the nursing program at this level.

LICENSURE
Applicants who have been convicted of a felony or treated for mental illness or substance abuse should discuss their eligibility status with the Utah Board of Nursing. Acceptance to the nursing program should not assure eligibility to write the PN or RN licensing examination. The Utah Board of Nursing makes final decisions on issue of license.

ACCREDITATION
The nursing program (PN, AS/AAS, and BSN) is fully accredited by the National League for Nursing Accrediting Commission (61 Broadway, New York, NY 10006, Phone: (212) 363-5555 ext. 153, Fax: (212) 812-0309, www.nlnac.org).

ADMISSION PROCESS FOR ENTRY OPTIONS
Telephone Contact: Robert Holt (801) 626-6128
PN/ADN:
Applicants must first apply for admission to Weber State University. Applicants must also apply for admission to the Nursing option they choose (PN, ADN). Admission selections are made once per year for the PN and ADN, twice for PN to AS/AAS, and twice for RN to BSN. Applications may be obtained from the Admission Counselor, ROOM MH108B, Dr. Ezekiel R. Dumke College of Health Professions.

Applications must be completed and on file by February 1 each year for PN and ADN. A $10 application fee must be paid at the time the application is submitted. Admission applications are reviewed by the Nursing Admission and Advancement Committee. Applicants are notified of committee decision by mail.

WEST SUBURBAN COLLEGE OF NURSING
Oak Park, IL

WEST SUBURBAN COLLEGE OF NURSING
The College of Nursing is located in historic Oak Park, IL. West Suburban College of Nursing offers a Bachelor of Science degree with a major in nursing, an RN-BS completion option program, and a fast-track program for second degree students.

FACILITIES
The College of Nursing campus, on-site in the West Suburban Hospital Medical Center, includes classrooms, a 4,000 volume health science library, a nursing skills laboratory, a student-faculty center, and clinical sites.

ACCREDITATION
The joint program is accredited by the National League for Nursing Accrediting Commission and approved by the Illinois Department of Professional Regulation.

ADMISSION CRITERIA
Freshman Applicants:

1. Earned 11 high school units in a college preparatory curriculum, which must include one unit of biology, one unit of chemistry and two units of college preparatory math;
2. A minimum 2.5 high school grade point average in a college preparatory curriculum;
3. Ranked in the top third of your high school graduating class;
4. A composite score of at least 20 on the ACT or equivalent on the SAT.
5. One written recommendation from a guidance counselor, teacher, or employer;
6. An official high school transcript (with final transcript to be submitted after graduation) or official GED Certificate.

Transfer Applicant:

1. Official transcripts of all college work;
2. Earned minimum cumulative college grade point average of 2.5 (4.0 scale); and a minimum cumulative college grade point average of 2.5 (4.0) scale in the following sciences (if taken): Anatomy & Physiology, Chemistry, and Microbiology;
3. In good academic standing at the last college attended;
4. If you have earned less than 30 semester hours (45 credit hours) of college work, see freshman admission criteria;
5. One written letter of recommendation from an advisor, employer, or professor;
6. An essay using the following guidelines
   - Must be typewritten
   - Double spaced
   - Maximum of 2 pages

Choose one of the following topics for your essay:

a. The College of Nursing holds four values: respect all persons; advocate for the pursuit of personal and academic excellence; show concern and kindness towards others; practice personal and academic integrity. Select one of the values and discuss how it plays into your own life.
b. Discuss your personal and professional goals as related to becoming a part of the nursing profession and how West Suburban College of Nursing can help you achieve these.
c. Share a story about yourself that will help us get to know you better and tell us something that we wouldn't otherwise know from your application.

CORRESPONDENCE AND INFORMATION
West Suburban College of Nursing
Office of Admission
3 Erie Ct.
Oak Park, IL 60302
(708) 763-6530
Fax: (708) 763-1531
Web: www.wscn.edu

WEST VIRGINIA WESLEYAN COLLEGE
The Nursing Program
Buckhannon, WV

THE COLLEGE
With a strong commitment to a rich tradition and state-of-the-art technology, West Virginia Wesleyan College offers a unique, total-life educational experience. Complementing an exceptional academic curriculum, Wesleyan supplies IBM ThinkPad laptop computers to all full-time students. The laptop is a tool that allows students access to information 24 hours a day, 7 days a week, 52 weeks a year. The College has a long-standing reputation as a distinctive liberal arts institution, and mobile computing has allowed the College to enhance its strong liberal arts foundation with the widespread integration of technology. Information technology has created a culture of learning that includes information access, processing and management in the classroom, student employment opportunities, internships, and permeates all aspects of living and learning in the 21st century. Wesleyan offers over 35 majors with more than 50 programs of study and eight pre-professional programs. With a student-faculty ratio of 14:1, students can be sure that every class they take will be taught with a personal touch. The College's contract major allows individuals to custom-design a program to achieve their goals. At Wesleyan, students can be involved in any number of 70 clubs and organizations. Greek life, student government, intramurals, and 17 NCAA Division II athletic teams add to an already dynamic student life program. The College provides an opportunity for students to participate in a rich campus life program, enabling them to strike an important balance between academic and social interests.

THE NURSING PROGRAM
Students who complete the Wesleyan Nursing program are awarded a bachelor of science in nursing degree (BSN). This degree qualifies individuals to take their professional licensure examination to practice as registered nurses. Students take support courses in natural and behavioral sciences and learn modern methods of client care in the context of humanistic service and respect. All participants receive extensive clinical experience at a variety of healthcare facilities, including community agencies, local and regional hospitals, and a tertiary medical center. The Wesleyan Nursing Department goal is to prepare graduates to enter the profession of nursing as competent practitioners, thoroughly familiar with the nursing process, who also possess a sound foundation for graduate study and advance practice in nursing.

RN/BSN PATHWAY
Within the Wesleyan Nursing program, Wesleyan offers an RN/BSN Pathway. This plan allows a registered nurse with a diploma or associate degree to complete the bachelor of science in nursing degree from home. We offer a flexible program through Distance Education so you can accomplish your educational goals while meeting the other demands placed on your time.

ACCREDITATION
West Virginia Wesleyan College is accredited by the Commission on Institutions of Higher Education of the North Central Association of Colleges and Schools, (30 North La Salle St., Suite 2400, Chicago, IL 60602-2504, telephone 1-800-621-7440). The Nursing Program is accredited by the National League for Nursing Accrediting Commission (61 Broadway, New York, NY 10006, telephone 1-800-669-1656) and approved by the West Virginia Board of Examiners for Registered Nurses.

FINANCIAL AID
- Tuition management
- Student loans
- Outside grants and scholarships may be applied
- Veterans administration programs
- Must file FAFSA to qualify

COSTS
The tuition per hour for an RN/BSN course is $250. Twenty-five hours of nursing are required as part of the BSN and are available **ONLINE**. Other fees are associated with this plan. Fee schedules are available online and from the institution.

CORRESPONDENCE AND INFORMATION
Assistant Director of Distance Education
West Virginia Wesleyan College
59 College Avenue
Buckhannon, WV 26201
(888) 340-7574
Web: www.wvwc.edu/nursing/rnbsn

WESTERN MICHIGAN UNIVERSITY
Bronson School of Nursing
Kalamazoo, Michigan

WESTERN MICHIGAN UNIVERSITY
Western Michigan University is one of Michigan's five graduate-intensive universities and has reached Doctoral/Research Universities-Extensive classification by the Carneigie Foundation. It enrolls almost 30,000 students, 21 percent at the graduate level. More than eight hundred faculty offer a wide variety of doctoral and master's programs along with 165 baccalaureate programs in six academic colleges: arts and science, business, education, engineering and applied sciences, fine arts, and health and human services. Five regional centers serve over two thousand off-campus students.

COLLEGE OF HEALTH AND HUMAN SERVICES
In 1976, Western Michigan University created its College of Health and Human Services, bringing together a number of related programs previously scattered throughout the university's administrative structure. Today, the college consists of the departments of blind rehabilitation, occupational therapy, physician assistance, and speech pathology and audiology; and the schools of nursing, social work, and community health services (including certificate programs in alcohol and drug abuse, gerontology, and holistic health). A graduate healthcare administration concentration is offered through the School of Public Administration.

WMU BRONSON SCHOOL OF NURSING
The nursing school was established in 1994 as a unit of the College of Health and Human Services. The Michigan Board of Nursing initially approved the School with commendation for being a model program for the future. The National League for Nursing Accrediting Commission accredited the School in its fourth year for its innovative approach to education emphasizing community-based and holistic nursing care. The School is also endorsed by the American Holistic Nurses' Certification Corporation.

The WMU Bronson School of Nursing offers a Bachelor of Science (BS) degree with a major in nursing. The pre-licensure track provides the nursing degree for individuals who are entering the nursing profession, while the Registered Nurse (RN) progression track offers an avenue to the BS degree for the licensed nurse who graduated from a diploma or associate degree program in nursing. Planning of a master's degree program is being initiated.

PROGRAM ENTRANCE REQUIREMENTS
Minimum overall college and minimum overall GPA in nursing pre-requisites of 2.5 and a written essay. Standardized Tests Required: TOEFL for international students and ACT. Application Deadline: rolling (freshman), October 1st/March1st (transfer). Notification: continuous (freshman). Application fee: $25.

ADVANCED PLACEMENT
Credit is given for nursing courses completed elsewhere dependent upon specific evaluations.

EXPENSES (2002-2003)
State Resident Tuition: lower level $129.91/credit hour, upper level $145.32/credit hour; Nonresident and International Tuition: lower level $321.78/credit hour, room and board $6,128.00, room only $2,722.00/academic year; Required Fees: full-time $539.00/semester, part-time $370.00/semester.

CONTACT INFORMATION
Dr. Marie F. Gates, Professor and Director
Ms. Marsha Mahan, Student Advisor
WMU Bronson School of Nursing
Western Michigan University
1903 West Michigan Avenue
Kalamazoo, Michigan 49008-5345
(616) 387-8150
Fax: (616) 387-8170
E-Mail: marie.gates@wmich.edu or marsha.mahan@wmich.edu
Web: http://www.wmich.edu/hhs/nurs/index.html

THE WESTERN PENNSYLVANIA HOSPITAL
School of Nursing
Pittsburgh, PA

SCHOOL OF NURSING

Today, health care is changing at an exciting and rapid rate. The Western Pennsylvania Hospital's School of Nursing has a rich tradition of preparing nurses with the academic and clinical background to match this pace. No matter where they practice, "West Penn grads" find they have a solid foundation for meeting the challenges of a career in professional nursing.

THE PROGRAM

Highlights of The Western Pennsylvania Hospital School of Nursing program, founded in 1892 and one of the first to be accredited by the National League for Nursing, include:

- A 22-month curriculum
- Small classes and low student/faculty ratio
- Articulation with Clarion University of Pennsylvania for BSN degree
- Financial aid and daycare available
- Only Pittsburgh hospital-based program with on-site housing

CLINICAL SETTINGS

The primary clinical setting for the School of Nursing is The Western Pennsylvania Hospital, a 532-bed regional referral and teaching institution with these regionally or nationally recognized programs:

- The Burn Trauma Center has gained international acclaim for its innovative approaches in treating burn injures. The largest burn care center in the tri-state area, the Burn Trauma Center is the first and only burn center in Pittsburgh to receive verification honors by the Committee on Trauma of the American College of Surgeons and the American Burn Association.
- West Penn's Cardiovascular Institute is a regional leader in heart procedures, performing more than 4,000 cardiac catheterizations and 1,000 open-heart surgical procedures each year, and is one of the first in the area to offer coronary brachytherapy, a leading-edge procedure to re-open clogged coronary stents.
- The Cancer Institute draws patients from other states and countries for its specialized services. The Institute provides the most advanced diagnostic and treatment services for all types of cancer, and has earned national recognition for its bone marrow transplant program, the largest in Pennsylvania.
- West Penn is a tertiary care provider of obstetrical, neonatal, and gynecological services, treating patients from throughout the tri-state area. The NICU is one of the region's largest referral resources for sick newborns.
- The Institute for Computer-Assisted Orthopaedic Surgery is the only comprehensive center in the region that combines computer-assisted orthopaedic research for total joint replacement with patient-focused clinical programs and a clinical outcomes program based on a Total Joint Registry.

ACADEMIC RESOURCES

Faculty of The Western Pennsylvania Hospital School of Nursing update the curriculum to include breakthroughs in nursing as they happen and work closely with students to provide the best possible learning opportunities.

School of Nursing classrooms and administrative and faculty offices are located in the School of Nursing adjacent to West Penn Hospital. The new Richard M. Johnston Health Sciences Library includes the collections and resources of the School of Nursing Library and offers the latest technology for accessing online information.

ADMISSION REQUIREMENTS

Acceptance into the School of Nursing is based on academic, personal and health requirements, as well as availability of class openings. Academic requirements include:

- graduation from an approved high school, preferably in the top two-fifths of the class, or a General Equivalency Diploma (GED), with 4 units in English, 2 units in science (one course must be chemistry with a grade of "C" or better; both courses must include a laboratory), 3 units in social studies, 2 units in mathematics (one course must be algebra with a grade of "C" or better), and 5 units in electives (preferably academic courses).
- minimum SAT scores of 800 total with 350+ Verbal and 350+ Math (before April 1, 1995) or 920 total with 430+ Verbal and 400+ Math (after April 1, 1995).

COSTS AND FINANCIAL AID

Tuition and fees for the class of 2003 were estimated at $8,009 for the first year and $6,395 for the second year. The School of Nursing's Financial Aid Office is committed to helping students and their families explore all available forms of assistance to offset the costs of education.

FOR FURTHER INFORMATION

Develop learning skills for a lifetime at the School of Nursing at The Western Pennsylvania Hospital:

Call: 1-877-33NURSE
Write: Admissions Office
        The Western Pennsylvania Hospital School of Nursing
        4900 Friendship Avenue
        Pittsburgh, PA 15224

Visit our Web site:
http://www.wpahs.org/education/undergraduate/nursing.html
E-Mail us: sonadmissions@wpahs.org

WILKES UNIVERSITY
Department of Nursing
Wilkes-Barre, Pennsylvania

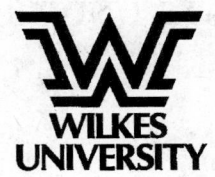

THE UNIVERSITY

Wilkes University was founded as Bucknell University Junior College in 1933 in order to provide educational opportunities comparable to those offered in other leading communities. On June 26, 1947, Wilkes College received its charter as a four-year liberal arts college. Its character had already been established during the years in which its trustees and faculty had worked to achieve an independent status. From its beginning, the College had been non-sectarian; its purpose was and is to serve all students equally in harmonious and effective thinking. Cognizant that group differences endanger progress, alienate people, and discourage the formation of campus organizations that were open to all students, the College concentrated its efforts on the cultivation of a unity of spirit among its students from the onset. In January 1990, Wilkes College became Wilkes University, an institutional change capping nearly sixty years of growth and development.

THE DEPARTMENT OF NURSING

Wilkes College offered a Bachelor of Science Degree in Nursing Education from 1954 until 1974. In 1972, in response to trends in nursing education, a decision was made to phase out this program and to offer, instead, the Bachelor of Science Degree with a major in Nursing. Currently the University offers both Bachelor of Science and Master of Science Degrees with majors in nursing.

The Department is located in Pearsall Hall. The Nursing Learning Resource Center (NLRC) is located on the first floor of this building. The NLRC is a state-of-the-art laboratory. The physical layout includes simulated patient units, which are used to illustrate acute, subacute, and home care situations. This facility is available to students for study, tutoring by faculty and peers, and student meetings. The NLRC also provides a computer lab, variety of self-paced programs, and Internet access and other multimedia resources.

PROGRAMS OF STUDY

The Department supports the comprehensive role of the University by offering both bachelor's and master's degree programs, which have direct relevance to the region's development in the area of health care. The Department of Nursing offers a Generic Baccalaureate program with a major in nursing, Licensed Practical Nurse (LPN)-BS, RN-Baccalaureate, RN-Master's and a Master of Science Degree with a major in nursing with a Clinical Nurse Specialist (CNS). There are two concentrations available for the CNS: Psychiatric/Mental Health or Gerontological Nursing. A Post-Master's certificate is also available in either of these concentrations.

AFFILIATIONS WITH HEALTH CARE AGENCIES

The Department of Nursing maintains contractual agreements with more than 60 health-care agencies. These facilities include community hospitals and clinics, psychiatric and mental health facilities, and community-based outpatient settings.

ACADEMIC RESOURCES

Academic support is available to students from several places. The Writing Center is available to help with written work. Additional services from the University's Learning Center include supplemental instruction and professional tutoring, workshops on study skills, test taking and time management, and weekly study sessions.

The E. S. Farley Library holds approximately 220,000 volumes of books and bound journals. 13,000 current journal units of microfilm are available. Online searches are also available from the library, in offices, dormitories, and open computer labs. The Thomas P. Shelburne Telecommunications Center houses two full-size production studios and capabilities for distance learning. The University also has several state-of-the-art computer labs.

COSTS 2003–2004

Full-time undergraduate tuition $9,815/semester, Room and Board $4,215/semester, Part-time $476/credit, Graduate tuition $596/credit.

FINANCIAL AID

Wilkes University maintains an extensive program of financial assistance for its students in the form of scholarships, grants, loans, and part-time employment. To assist qualified students, the University receives substantial gifts each year from friends and alumni. These funds, combined with those furnished by the federal and state governments, are offered to students in financial aid packages. All applicants should also apply for financial assistance, both need-based and achievement-based. Students with questions about financial aid or students seeking applications for financial aid should contact the Financial Aid Office. More detailed information regarding the financial aid programs and requirements is included in the *Consumer's Guide to Financial Aid, Costs, and Charges at Wilkes University*, which is also available at the Financial Aid Office.

ADMISSION REQUIREMENTS

Students majoring in Nursing are required to have completed courses in English (four units), Social Studies (three units), Mathematics (two units including algebra) and Science (two units including biology and chemistry) during their secondary school programs.

Applications for admission and instructions regarding secondary school records, recommendations, and entrance examinations may be obtained from the Office of Admissions.

The Scholastic Aptitude Test (SAT) of the College Entrance Examination Board or the Achievement College Test (ACT) is required of all applicants.

International students must also submit official results of the TOEFL (Test of English as a Foreign Language) or evidence of successful completion of an accredited intensive English language program.

Transfer students who have earned 30 credits or more need only submit a formal application and an official transcript from each post-secondary institution attended. Transfer students must have a minimum grade point average of 2.0 at the beginning of the semester they first enroll at Wilkes.

CORRESPONDENCE AND INFORMATION

For further information contact:
Dr. Mary Ann Merrigan, Chairperson
Department of Nursing
Wilkes University
109 South Franklin Street
Wilkes-Barre, PA 18766
(570) 408-4074
1-800-Wilkes U ext. 4074
Fax: (570) 408-7807
E-Mail: merrigan@wilkes.edu
Web: www.wilkes.edu

WRIGHT STATE UNIVERSITY-MIAMI VALLEY
College of Nursing and Health
Dayton, OH

Wright State University-Miami Valley College of Nursing and Health is accredited by the National League for Nursing (NLN), and offers an exceptional educational program for pre-licensure students, an RN/BSN completion program for registered nurses, and a Master of Science degree with eight concentrations.

Wright State University is dedicated to teaching, research, and service. The university serves nearly 16,000 students with programs leading to more than 100 undergraduate and 40 graduate and professional degrees through six colleges and three schools.

Wright State University's 557 acre campus is located approximately 10 miles east of Dayton, Ohio, a city with a metropolitan population of over nine hundred thousand. To take a virtual tour of the campus, log onto www.wright.edu.vr.

The College of Nursing and Health is located in WSU's newest building, University Hall—a state-of-the-art educational facility. Clinical instructional facilities are abundant and varied. The college has contracts with over 200 agencies in the area including hospitals, rehabilitation centers, county health departments, nursing homes, school systems, senior citizen centers, and day care centers, which can be used for clinical experiences and/or research.

PROGRAMS
The undergraduate pre-licensure program is a four-year program leading to the Bachelor of Science in Nursing degree (BSN). Professional nurses provide care for patients of diverse and multicultural backgrounds, and should represent those backgrounds. The admission process will seek applicants with evidence of intellectual ability, maturity, motivation, ability to interact with diverse populations, dedication to human concerns, ability to independently learn, ability to perform functions required in the practice of nursing, and potential for providing nursing services to underserved areas of Ohio. Graduates are eligible to sit for the National Council Licensure Examination for Registered Nurses (NCLEX-RN).

The RN/BSN Program offered through WSU includes two options for registered nurses to earn a baccalaureate degree in nursing. Both options are fully accredited by the National League for Nursing Accrediting Commission.

1. The distance classroom option is offered one day per week by teleconferencing on the WSU main campus with several outreach campuses. The program is scheduled for the same day each week throughout the program of study to accommodate work schedules.
2. The online instruction option offers registered nurses the opportunity to complete the Bachelor of Science in Nursing degree via an innovative Web-based instructional program. Nursing courses can be accessed any time or any place with the aid of a computer and Internet access.

The College of Nursing and Health offers a graduate program leading to a Master of Science degree with a major in nursing, and a dual degree program leading to a Master of Science and a Master of Business Administration in administration of nursing and health care systems. The graduate program prepares nurses for advanced leadership roles in practice and administration, as well as for doctoral study in nursing. The curriculum offers students the opportunity to individualize the nursing major by selecting from areas of clinical specialization and roles (clinical specialist, nurse practitioner, nurse administrator, or school nurse). The programs accommodate both full-time and part-time students, with most classes offered in the late afternoon and evening. The sequence of course offerings is flexible.

ADMISSIONS
Applications for both undergraduate programs are accepted for fall quarter and spring quarter. The graduate program has rolling admissions. All applicants are reviewed on their academic qualifications. Some graduate concentrations require a personal interview.

COSTS
Tuition for full-time undergraduate students is $1,787. Tuition for full-time graduate students is $2,387. Non-Ohio residents pay a higher fee.

FOR MORE INFORMATION
To learn more about Wright State University-Miami Valley College of Nursing and Health, please contact us at (937) 775-3132 or visit us online at www.nursing.wright.edu.

Section 5

SPECIALTY INDEX

Nurse Anesthetist

Bradley University, IL
California State University–Fullerton, CA
Case Western Reserve, OH
Columbia University, NY
Florida Gulf Coast University, FL
Gannon University, PA
Georgetown University, DC
La Salle University, PA
MCP Hahnemann University, PA
Medical College of Georgia, GA
Murray State University, KY
Northeastern University, MA
Oakland University, MI
Old Dominion University, VA
Rush University, IL
Samuel Merritt College, CA
Southern Illinois University–Edwardsville, IL
State University of New York at Buffalo, NY
SUNY Health Science Center–Brooklyn, NY
Temple University, PA
Uniformed Services University, MD
The University of Akron, OH
University of Cincinnati, OH
University of Iowa, IA
University of Medical Dentistry of New Jersey, NJ
University of North Carolina–Charlotte, NC
University of North Dakota, ND
University of Pittsburgh, PA
University of Scranton, PA
University of Southern California, CA
The University of Tennessee–Chattanooga, TN
The University of Tennessee College of Nursing, TN
University of Texas Health Science Center at
    Houston, TX
Villanova University, PA

Nurse Anesthetist/Post-Masters

Bradley University, IL
Florida Gulf Coast University, FL
Gannon University, PA
Medical College of Georgia, GA
Old Dominion University, VA
Rush University, IL
Villanova University, PA

Case Management

Gannon University, PA
Millersville University, PA
Saint Peter's College, NJ
University of Alabama, AL
University of North Carolina–Chapel Hill, NC
Villanova University, PA

CLINICAL NURSE SPECIALIST

Acute Care
California State University–Los Angeles, CA
Gonzaga University, WA

Ida V. Moffett School–Samford University, AL
Rutgers The State University of New Jersey, NJ
University of California, Los Angeles, CA
University of Delaware, DE
University of Illinois–Chicago, IL
University of Michigan, MI
University of Missouri–St. Louis, MO
University of Oklahoma, OK
University of Texas Health Science Center at
    Houston, TX
University of Texas Health Science Center at
    San Antonio, TX
University of Utah, UT
University of Virginia, VA
Widener University, PA
Winona State University, MN

Adult
Adelphi University, NY
Andrews University, MI
Angelo State University, TX
Arkansas State University, AR
Armstrong Atlantic State University, GA
Azusa Pacific University, CA
Bellarmine College, KY
Bloomsburg University, PA
Clemson University, SC
College Misericordia, PA
College of Mount St. Vincent, NY
College of Saint Scholastica, MN
Creighton University, NE
East Carolina University, NC
George Mason University, VA
Georgia College and State University, GA
Georgia State University, GA
Indiana University–Purdue University, IN
Johns Hopkins University, MD
La Salle University, PA
Loma Linda University, CA
Long Island University, NY
Louisiana State University, LA
Loyola University–Chicago, IL
Madonna University, MI
McNeese State University, LA
Medical College of Georgia, GA
Medical College of Ohio, OH
Medical University of South Carolina, SC
Mount Saint Mary College, NY
Murray State University, KY
Northern Illinois University, IL
Oakland University, MI
Oregon Health Sciences University, OR
Otterbein College, OH
Pennsylvania State University, PA
Pontifical Catholic University of Puerto Rico, PR
Purdue University–Calumet Campus, IN
Radford University, VA
Rush University, IL
Saint Louis University, MO
Saint Xavier University, IL
South Dakota State University, SD
State University of New York at Buffalo, NY
SUNY Health Science Center–Brooklyn, NY

Syracuse University, NY
Tri-College University Nursing Consortium, ND
Troy State University, AL
The University of Akron, OH
University of Central Arkansas, AR
University of Central Florida, FL
University of Colorado–Colorado Springs–Beth-El
   College of Nursing, CO
University of Colorado–Denver, CO
University of Colorado Health Sciences Center, CO
University of Iowa, IA
University of Kentucky, KY
University of Louisville, KY
University of Massachusetts–Dartmouth, MA
University of Minnesota–Minneapolis, MN
University of Missouri–Columbia, MO
University of Missouri–Kansas City, MO
University of Nevada–Las Vegas, NV
University of Nevada–Reno, NV
University of New Hampshire, NH
University of New Mexico, NM
University of North Carolina–Charlotte, NC
University of North Dakota, ND
University of Scranton, PA
University of Southern Indiana, IN
University of Southern Maine, ME
The University of Southern Mississippi, MS
The University of Tennessee–Knoxville, TN
University of Texas at Austin, TX
University of Texas–El Paso, TX
University of Texas–Pan American, TN
University of the Incarnate Word, TX
University of Vermont, VT
University of Virginia, VA
University of Washington, WA
University of Wisconsin–Milwaukee, WI
Valparaiso University, IN
Wichita State University, KS
Widener University, PA
Wright State University, OH

Community/Home Health

Albany State University, GA
Bloomsburg University, PA
California State University–San Bernadino, CA
Capital University, OH
Case Western Reserve, OH
The Catholic University of America, DC
D'Youville College, NY
East Carolina University, NC
Eastern Michigan University, MI
Emory University–Nell Hodgson Woodruff School of
   Nursing, GA
Hawaii Pacific University, HI
Holy Family College, PA
Ida V. Moffett School–Samford University, AL
Indiana University–Purdue University, IN
Jacksonville State University, AL
Johns Hopkins University, MD
La Roche College, PA
La Salle University, PA
Medical College of Georgia, GA
Northeastern University, MA

The Ohio State University, OH
Pennsylvania State University, PA
Rutgers The State University of New Jersey, NJ
Salisbury State University, MD
San Diego State University, CA
Southern Illinois University–Edwardsville, IL
Thomas Jefferson University, PA
University of Alaska–Anchorage, AK
University of California, San Francisco, CA
University of Central Arkansas
University of Cincinnati, OH
University of Colorado–Colorado Springs–Beth-El
   College of Nursing, CO
University of Colorado–Denver, CO
University of Connecticut, CT
University of Hartford, CT
University of Illinois–Chicago, IL
University of Iowa, IA
University of Kansas, KS
University of Kentucky, KY
University of Massachusetts–Dartmouth, MA
University of Michigan, MI
University of Minnesota–Minneapolis, MN
University of Nebraska Medical Center, NE
University of New Mexico, NM
University of North Dakota, ND
University of South Carolina–Columbia, SC
The University of Southern Mississippi, MS
University of Utah, UT
University of Vermont, VT
University of Virginia, VA
University of Washington, WA
University of Wisconsin–Milwaukee, WI
University of Wyoming, WY
Valparaiso University, IN
Viterbo College, WI
Washington State University, WA
West Chester University, PA
Widener University, PA
Worcester State College, MA
Wright State University, OH

Critical Care

Case Western Reserve, OH
La Roche College, PA
Loyola University–Chicago, IL
Purdue University–Calumet Campus, IN
Rush University, IL
University of California, San Francisco, CA
University of Colorado–Denver, CO
University of Colorado Health Sciences Center, CO
University of Massachusetts–Boston, MA
University of Virginia, VA
University of Wisconsin–Milwaukee, WI
Widener University, PA
Yale University, CT

Family

Capital University, OH
Minnesota State University–Mankato, MN
Niagara University, NY
San Diego State University, CA
Southeast Missouri State University, MO

Southern University and A&M College, LA
University of Massachusetts–Boston, MA
University of Wisconsin–Milwaukee, WI
Webster University, MO

Gerontology
California State University–Dominquez Hills, CA
Creighton University, NE
Duke University, NC
Gwynedd-Mercy College, PA
La Roche College, PA
Marquette University, WI
Medical University of South Carolina, SC
Oregon Health Sciences University, OR
Rush University, IL
Saint Louis University, MO
University of California, San Francisco, CA
University of Delaware, DE
University of Illinois–Chicago, IL
University of Iowa, IA
University of Kentucky, KY
University of Massachusetts–Boston, MA
University of Michigan, MI
University of Minnesota–Minneapolis, MN
University of Oklahoma, OK
University of Rhode Island, RI
University of Texas Health Science Center at Houston,
   TX
Viterbo College, WI
Wilkes University, PA

Neonatology
University of Texas Health Science Center at Houston,
   TX

Oncology
George Mason University, VA
Loyola University–Chicago, IL
University of Colorado–Denver, CO
University of Colorado Health Sciences Center, CO
University of Pennsylvania, PA
University of Texas Health Science Center at Houston,
   TX

Pediatrics
Azusa Pacific University, CA
Duke University, NC
Gwynedd-Mercy College, PA
Indiana University–Purdue University, IN
Loma Linda University, CA
Medical University of South Carolina, SC
Rush University, IL
Rutgers The State University of New Jersey, NJ
Temple University, PA
University of Delaware, DE
University of Illinois–Chicago, IL
University of Iowa, IA
University of Kentucky, KY
University of Minnesota–Minneapolis, MN
University of Missouri–St. Louis, MO
University of New Mexico, NM
University of Washington, WA
University of Wisconsin–Milwaukee, WI

Valparaiso University, IN
Wichita State University, KS

Perinatology
University of California, San Francisco, CA
University of Kentucky, KY
University of Washington, WA

Psychiatric/Mental Health
Albany State University, GA
Boston College, MA
California State University–Los Angeles, CA
The Catholic University of America, DC
College of Saint Scholastica, MN
Florida State University, FL
Georgia College and State University, GA
Georgia State University, GA
Gonzaga University, WA
Grand Valley State University, MI
Husson College, ME
Indiana University–Purdue University, IN
Medical College of Ohio, OH
Medical University of South Carolina, SC
Monmouth University, NJ
The Ohio State University, OH
Pontifical Catholic University of Puerto Rico, PR
Rutgers The State University of New Jersey, NJ
Saginaw Valley State University, MI
Saint Louis University, MO
Saint Xavier University, IL
Southern Illinois University–Edwardsville, IL
Temple University, PA
University of Alaska–Anchorage, AK
University of California, San Francisco, CA
University of Central Arkansas, AR
University of Cincinnati, OH
University of Colorado–Denver, CO
University of Connecticut, CT
University of Hawaii at Manoa, HI
University of Illinois–Chicago, IL
University of Iowa, IA
University of Kansas, KS
University of Kentucky, KY
University of Louisville, KY
University of Michigan, MI
University of Minnesota–Minneapolis, MN
University of North Carolina–Chapel Hill, NC
University of North Carolina–Charlotte, NC
University of Oklahoma, OK
University of Rhode Island, RI
The University of Southern Mississippi, MS
The University of Tennessee–Knoxville, TN
University of Texas at Austin, TX
University of Texas–El Paso, TX
University of Texas Health Science Center at Houston,
   TX
University of Utah, UT
University of Washington, WA
University of Wisconsin–Milwaukee, WI
Valparaiso University, IN
Virginia Commonwealth University, VA
Wichita State University, KS
Widener University, PA

Wilkes University, PA
Yale University, CT

School Nursing
Bethel College, MN
Bloomsburg University, PA
Capital University, OH
East Carolina University, NC
Loma Linda University, CA
San Diego State University, CA
San Jose State University, CA
University of Illinois–Chicago, IL
University of Missouri–Columbia, MO
Wright State University, OH

Women's Health
University of Delaware, DE
University of Kentucky, KY

Other
Azusa Pacific University, CA
Capital University, OH
Clemson University, SC
College Misericordia, PA
College of New Rochelle, NY
Creighton University, NE
Daemen College, NY
D'Youville College, NY
Gannon University, PA
Gonzaga University, WA
Gwynedd-Mercy College, PA
Harding University, AR
Johns Hopkins University, MD
Loma Linda University, CA
Louisiana State University, LA
Loyola University–Chicago, IL
Marquette University, WI
Medical College of Georgia, GA
Medical College of Ohio, OH
Neumann College, PA
New Mexico State University, NM
Rush University, IL
Saint John Fisher College, NY
Saint Louis University, MO
Saint Xavier University, IL
Salem State College, MA
Southeastern Louisiana University, LA
Southern Illinois University–Edwardsville, IL
SUNY Health Science Center–Brooklyn, NY
Tennessee State University, TN
Troy State University, AL
University of California, Los Angeles, CA
University of California, San Francisco, CA
University of Colorado–Colorado Springs–Beth-El
    College of Nursing, CO
University of Connecticut, CT
University of Delaware, DE
University of Illinois–Chicago, IL
University of Kansas, KS
University of Louisiana–Lafayette, LA
University of Maryland–Baltimore, MD
University of Michigan, MI
University of Minnesota–Minneapolis, MN

University of Nebraska Medical Center, NE
University of North Carolina–Charlotte, NC
University of North Carolina–Greensboro, NC
University of Northern Colorado, CO
University of Oklahoma, OK
University of Southern California, CA
University of Texas at Austin, TX
University of Texas–El Paso, TX
University of Texas Health Science Center at Houston,
    TX
University of Wisconsin–Milwaukee, WI
Ursuline College, OH
Virginia Commonwealth University, VA
Wesley College, DE
Yale University, CT
Youngstown State University, OH

CLINICAL NURSE SPECIALIST/POST-MASTERS

Acute Care
University of Illinois–Chicago, IL
University of Utah, UT

Adult
Arkansas State University, AR
College of Saint Scholastica, MN
Georgia College and State University, GA
Georgia State University, GA
Loma Linda University, CA
Medical College of Georgia, GA
Rush University, IL
Saint Xavier University, IL
University of Southern Indiana, IN

Community/Home Health
Emory University–Nell Hodgson Woodruff School of
    Nursing, GA
Medical College of Georgia, GA
Rutgers The State University of New Jersey, NJ
University of Illinois–Chicago, IL
University of Kentucky, KY

Critical Care
Rush University, IL

Gerontology
Rush University, IL
University of Illinois–Chicago, IL

Pediatrics
Loma Linda University, CA
Rush University, IL
University of Illinois–Chicago, IL
University of Maryland–Baltimore, MD

Psychiatric/Mental Health
Albany State University, GA
Duquesne University, PA
Georgia College and State University, GA
Georgia State University, GA
Husson College, ME
Medical University of South Carolina, SC
Rutgers The State University of New Jersey, NJ

Saint Xavier University, IL
Temple University, PA
University of Colorado Health Sciences Center, CO
University of Hawaii at Manoa, HI
University of Illinois–Chicago, IL
University of Kansas, KS
University of North Carolina–Chapel Hill, NC
University of Rhode Island, RI
University of Utah, UT

School Nursing
Loma Linda University, CA
San Jose State University, CA
University of Illinois–Chicago, IL

Other
College of New Rochelle, NY
Duquesne University, PA
Harding University, AR
Rush University, IL
Saint Xavier University, IL
University of Illinois–Chicago, IL

CNS-NP

Armstrong Atlantic State University, GA
Augustana College, SD
California State University–Dominquez Hills, CA
Carlow College, PA
College of Saint Scholastica, MN
Fitchburg State College, MA
Harding University, AR
Illinois State University, IL
Loma Linda University, CA
Marquette University, WI
New Mexico State University, NM
Northeastern University, MA
South Dakota State University, SD
Thomas Jefferson University, PA
University of Cincinnati, OH
University of Colorado–Colorado Springs–Beth-El
   College of Nursing, CO
University of Delaware, DE
University of Virginia, VA
University of Washington, WA
Widener University, PA
Yale University, CT

CNS-NP/Post-Masters

Carlow College, PA
Harding University, AR
Illinois State University, IL
Marquette University, WI
New Mexico State University, NM
University of Cincinnati, OH
University of Delaware, DE
University of Maryland–Baltimore, MD

Health Policy

University of Colorado Health Sciences Center, CO
University of Maryland–Baltimore, MD

NURSE PRACTITIONER PROGRAM

Acute Care
California State University–Los Angeles, CA
Case Western Reserve, OH
College of New Rochelle, NY
Columbia University, NY
Duke University, NC
Emory University–Nell Hodgson Woodruff School of
   Nursing, GA
Georgetown University, DC
Indiana University–Purdue University, IN
Johns Hopkins University, MD
Marquette University, WI
MCP Hahnemann University, PA
Monmouth University, NJ
New York University, NY
Northeastern University, MA
Northwestern State University of Louisiana, LA
Otterbein College, OH
Rush University, IL
Rutgers The State University of New Jersey, NJ
Saint Louis University, MO
San Diego State University, CA
Seton Hall University, NJ
Texas A&M University–Corpus Christi, TX
University of Alabama, Huntsville, AL
University of California, San Francisco, CA
University of Colorado–Denver, CO
University of Connecticut, CT
University of Illinois–Chicago, IL
University of Kentucky, KY
University of Maryland–Baltimore, MD
University of Massachusetts–Worcester, MA
University of Michigan, MI
University of Minnesota–Minneapolis, MN
University of Mississippi Medical Center, MS
University of Nebraska Medical Center, NE
University of New Mexico, NM
University of Pennsylvania, PA
University of Pittsburgh, PA
University of Rochester, NY
University of South Alabama, AL
University of South Carolina–Columbia, SC
University of Southern Indiana, IN
University of Texas Health Science Center at Houston,
   TX
University of Texas Medical Branch–Galveston, TX
University of Utah, UT

Adult
Adelphi University, NY
Andrews University, MI
Armstrong Atlantic State University, GA
Ball State University, IN
Bloomsburg University, PA
Boston College, MA
California State University–Los Angeles, CA
Case Western Reserve, OH
The Catholic University of America, DC
College of Mount St. Vincent, NY
College of Saint Catherine, MN
College of Saint Scholastica, MN

Columbia University, NY
Creighton University, NE
Daemen College, NY
East Tennessee State University, TN
Emory University–Nell Hodgson Woodruff School of Nursing, GA
Fairleigh Dickinson University, NJ
Felician College, NJ
Florida Atlantic University, FL
George Mason University, VA
Grand Valley State University, MI
Gwynedd-Mercy College, PA
Indiana University–Purdue University, IN
Indiana Wesleyan University, IN
Jewish Hospital, MO
Johns Hopkins University, MD
Kennesaw State University, GA
La Salle University, PA
Loma Linda University, CA
Long Island University–Brooklyn, NY
Loyola University–Chicago, IL
Madonna University, MI
Marquette University, WI
McNeese State University, LA
Medical University of South Carolina, SC
Metropolitan State University, MN
Monmouth University, NJ
Mount Saint Mary College, NY
New York University, NY
North Park University, IL
Northeastern University, MA
Northern Kentucky University, KY
The Ohio State University, OH
Oregon Health Sciences University, OR
Quinipiac University, CT
Richard Stockton College of New Jersey, NJ
Rush University, IL
Rutgers The State University of New Jersey, NJ
Saint Louis University, MO
Saint Peter's College, NJ
Seton Hall University, NJ
Simmons College, MA
South Dakota State University, SD
Southeastern Louisiana University, LA
Southern Adventist University, TN
Spalding University, KY
State University of New York at Buffalo, NY
State University of New York at Stony Brook, NY
State University of New York at Syracuse, NY
State University of New York at Utica/Rome, NY
Syracuse University, NY
Temple University, PA
Texas Woman's University, TX
The University of Akron, OH
University of Arizona, AZ
University of California, Los Angeles, CA
University of California, San Francisco, CA
University of Central Arkansas, AR
University of Central Florida, FL
University of Colorado–Colorado Springs–Beth-El College of Nursing, CO
University of Colorado Health Sciences Center, CO
University of Connecticut, CT

University of Florida, FL
University of Hawaii at Manoa, HI
University of Kentucky, KY
University of Louisville, KY
University of Maryland–Baltimore, MD
University of Massachusetts–Dartmouth, MA
University of Massachusetts–Worcester, MA
University of Medical Dentistry of New Jersey, NJ
University of Michigan, MI
University of Mississippi Medical Center, MS
University of Missouri–Kansas City, MO
University of Missouri–St. Louis, MO
University of Nebraska Medical Center, NE
University of New Hampshire, NH
University of North Carolina–Chapel Hill, NC
University of Pennsylvania, PA
University of Rochester, NY
University of Saint Francis–Joliet, IL
University of Southern Maine, ME
University of Tampa, FL
University of Texas Medical Branch–Galveston, TX
University of Utah, UT
University of Vermont, VT
University of Virginia, VA
University of Washington, WA
University of Wisconsin–Eau Claire, WI
University of Wisconsin–Oshkosh, WI
Valdosta State University, GA
Vanderbilt University, TN
Villanova University, PA
Virginia Commonwealth University, VA
Wichita State University, KS
William Patterson University, NJ
Wilmington College, DE
Winona State University, MN
Wright State University, OH
Yale University, CT

Critical Care
Emory University–Nell Hodgson Woodruff School of Nursing, GA
Georgia Southern University, GA
Loyola University–Chicago, IL
San Diego State University, CA
University of Colorado–Denver, CO
University of Nebraska Medical Center, NE
University of Pittsburgh, PA
The University of Tennessee College of Nursing

Family
ACU–HSU–MCM Consortium, TX
Albany State University, GA
Alcorn State University, MS
Allen College, IA
Andrews University, MI
Arkansas State University, AR
Azusa Pacific University, CA
Ball State University, IN
Barry University, FL
Baylor University, TX
Belmont University, TN
Boston College, MA
Brenau University, GA

Brigham Young University, UT
California State University–Bakersfield, CA
California State University–Dominquez Hills, CA
Carson Newman College, TN
Case Western Reserve, OH
The Catholic University of America, DC
Clarion University, PA
Clarke College, IA
Clarkson College, NE
Clemson University, SC
College Misericordia, PA
College of Mount St. Vincent, NY
The College of New Jersey, NJ
College of New Rochelle, NY
College of Saint Scholastica, MN
Columbia University, NY
Concordia University Wisconsin (LCMS), WI
Creighton University, NE
Delta State University, MS
Drake University, IA
Duke University, NC
Duquesne University, PA
D'Youville College, NY
East Carolina University, NC
East Tennessee State University, TN
Edinboro University of Pennsylvania, PA
Emory University–Nell Hodgson Woodruff School of
    Nursing, GA
Fairfield University, CT
Felician College, NJ
Florida Atlantic University, FL
Florida State University, FL
Franciscan University–Steubenville, OH
Gannon University, PA
George Mason University, VA
Georgetown University, DC
Georgia College and State University, GA
Georgia State University, GA
Gonzaga University, WA
Grambling State University, LA
Grand Valley State University, MI
Hampton University, VA
Hawaii Pacific University, HI
Holy Names College, CA
Houston Baptist University, TX
Husson College, ME
Ida V. Moffett School–Samford University, AL
Indiana State University, IN
Indiana University–Purdue University, IN
Indiana Wesleyan University, IN
Johns Hopkins University, MD
Kennesaw State University, GA
La Roche College, PA
La Salle University, PA
Lawrence Memorial/Regis College, MA
Loma Linda University, CA
Long Island University, NY
Louisiana State University, LA
Loyola University–Chicago, IL
Loyola University–New Orleans, LA
Marshall University, WV
Marymount University, VA

Massachusetts College of Pharmacy, MA
McNeese State University, LA
MCP Hahnemann University, PA
Medical College of Georgia, GA
Medical College of Ohio, OH
Medical University of South Carolina, SC
Metropolitan State University, MN
Michigan State University, MI
Millersville University, PA
Minnesota State University–Mankato, MN
Monmouth University, NJ
Montana State University–Bozeman, MT
Murray State University, KY
Northeastern University, MA
Northern Illinois University, IL
Northern Kentucky University, KY
Northwestern State University of Louisiana, LA
Oakland University, MI
The Ohio State University, OH
Old Dominion University, VA
Oregon Health Sciences University, OR
Otterbein College, OH
Pace University, NY
Pacific Lutheran University, WA
Pennsylvania State University, PA
Purdue University–Calumet Campus, IN
Radford University, VA
Regis College, MA
Regis University, CO
Rivier College, NH
Rutgers The State University of New Jersey, NJ
Sacred Heart University, CT
Saginaw Valley State University, MI
Saint John Fisher College, NY
Saint Louis University, MO
Saint Xavier University, IL
Salisbury State University, MD
Samuel Merritt College, CA
San Jose State University, CA
Seattle University, WA
Shenandoah University, VA
Simmons College, MA
Sonoma State University, CA
South Dakota State University, SD
Southeast Missouri State University, MO
Southern Adventist University, TN
Southern Connecticut State University, CT
Southern Illinois University–Edwardsville, IL
Southern University and A&M College, LA
Southwest Missouri State University–Springfield, MO
Spalding University, KY
State University of New York at Buffalo, NY
State University of New York at Stony Brook, NY
State University of New York at Syracuse, NY
SUNY Health Science Center–Brooklyn, NY
Syracuse University, NY
Tennessee State University, TN
Texas A&M University–Corpus Christi, TX
Texas Tech University Health Sciences Center, TX
Texas Woman's University, TX
Thomas Jefferson University, PA
Tri-College University Nursing Consortium, ND

Gerontology

San Jose State University, CA
Seton Hall University, NJ
Simmons College, MA
South Dakota State University, SD
State University of New York at Syracuse, NY
University of Arizona, AZ
University of California, Los Angeles, CA
University of California, San Francisco, CA
University of Colorado–Colorado Springs–Beth-El
    College of Nursing, CO
University of Colorado–Denver, CO
University of Connecticut, CT
University of Florida, FL
University of Hawaii at Manoa, HI
University of Illinois–Chicago, IL
University of Louisville, KY
University of Maryland–Baltimore, MD
University of Massachusetts–Boston, MA
University of Michigan, MI
University of Minnesota–Minneapolis, MN
University of Nebraska Medical Center, NE
University of Pennsylvania, PA
University of South Alabama, AL
The University of Tennessee–Knoxville, TN
University of Texas Health Science Center at Houston,
    TX
University of Texas Medical Branch–Galveston, TX
University of Utah, UT
Vanderbilt University, TN
Villanova University, PA
Viterbo College, WI
Winona State University, MN
Yale University, CT

Neonatology

Baylor University, TX
Case Western Reserve, OH
College of Saint Catherine, MN
Creighton University, NE
Duke University, NC
East Carolina University, NC
Emory University–Nell Hodgson Woodruff School of
    Nursing, GA
Jewish Hospital, MO
Louisiana State University, LA
Medical University of South Carolina, SC
Northeastern University, MA
Northwestern State University of Louisiana, LA
Old Dominion University, VA
Pennsylvania State University, PA
Rush University, IL
State University of New York at Stony Brook, NY
University of California, Los Angeles, CA
University of California, San Francisco, CA
University of Cincinnati, OH
University of Colorado–Colorado Springs–Beth-El
    College of Nursing, CO
University of Connecticut, CT
University of Florida, FL
University of Kansas, KS
University of Louisville, KY
University of Maryland–Baltimore, MD
University of Mississippi Medical Center, MS

University of Missouri–Kansas City, MO
University of Missouri–St. Louis, MO
University of Nebraska Medical Center, NE
University of Pennsylvania, PA
University of Rochester, NY
University of South Alabama, AL
The University of Tennessee College of Nursing, TN
The University of Tennessee–Knoxville, TN
University of Texas Health Science Center at Houston,
    TX
University of Utah, UT
University of Washington, WA
Vanderbilt University, TN
Wichita State University, KS

Pediatrics

Adelphi University, NY
Bellarmine College, KY
Boston College, MA
California State University–Los Angeles, CA
Case Western Reserve, OH
The Catholic University of America, DC
College of Saint Catherine, MN
Columbia University, NY
Duke University, NC
Emory University–Nell Hodgson Woodruff School of
    Nursing, GA
Georgia State University, GA
Grand Valley State University, MI
Gwynedd-Mercy College, PA
Hampton University, VA
Indiana University–Purdue University, IN
Johns Hopkins University, MD
Lawrence Memorial/Regis College, MA
Loma Linda University, CA
Loyola University–Chicago, IL
MCP Hahnemann University, PA
Medical College of Georgia, GA
Medical University of South Carolina, SC
New York University, NY
Northeastern University, MA
Northern Kentucky University, KY
Northwestern State University of Louisiana, LA
The Ohio State University, OH
Old Dominion University, VA
Oregon Health Sciences University, OR
Regis College, MA
Rush University, IL
Rutgers The State University of New Jersey, NJ
Saint Louis University, MO
Seton Hall University, NJ
Simmons College, MA
South Dakota State University, SD
Spalding University, KY
State University of New York at Buffalo, NY
State University of New York at Stony Brook, NY
State University of New York at Syracuse, NY
Syracuse University, NY
Texas Woman's University, TX
The University of Akron, OH
University of California, Los Angeles, CA
University of California, San Francisco, CA
University of Cincinnati, OH

University of Colorado–Denver, CO
University of Colorado Health Sciences Center, CO
University of Florida, FL
University of Illinois–Chicago, IL
University of Iowa, IA
University of Kentucky, KY
University of Maryland–Baltimore, MD
University of Massachusetts–Amherst, MA
University of Michigan, MI
University of Minnesota–Minneapolis, MN
University of Missouri–Columbia, MO
University of Missouri–Kansas City, MO
University of Missouri–St. Louis, MO
University of Nebraska Medical Center, NE
University of North Carolina–Chapel Hill, NC
University of Oklahoma, OK
University of Pennsylvania, PA
University of Pittsburgh, PA
University of Rochester, NY
University of South Alabama, AL
University of South Carolina–Columbia, SC
The University of Tennessee–Knoxville, TN
University of Texas at Austin, TX
University of Texas Health Science Center at Houston, TX
University of Texas Health Science Center at San Antonio, TX
University of Texas Medical Branch–Galveston, TX
University of Texas–Pan American, TN
University of Utah, UT
University of Virginia, VA
University of Washington, WA
Vanderbilt University, TN
Villanova University, PA
Virginia Commonwealth University, VA
West Virginia University, WV
Wichita State University, KS
Wright State University, OH
Yale University, CT

Perinatology
Old Dominion University, VA
Regis University, CO
University of Colorado–Denver, CO
University of Pennsylvania, PA
University of Texas Health Science Center at Houston, TX

Psychiatric/Mental Health
Adelphi University, NY
Case Western Reserve, OH
College of Saint Scholastica, MN
Columbia University, NY
Creighton University, NE
Emory University–Nell Hodgson Woodruff School of Nursing, GA
Fairfield University, CT
Grand Valley State University, MI
MCP Hahnemann University, PA
New York University, NY
Northeastern University, MA
The Ohio State University, OH
Oregon Health Sciences University, OR

Pace University, NY
Rush University, IL
South Dakota State University, SD
State University of New York at Stony Brook, NY
The University of Akron, OH
University of Arizona, AZ
University of California, San Francisco, CA
University of Colorado Health Sciences Center, CO
University of Massachusetts–Amherst, MA
University of Medical Dentistry of New Jersey, NJ
University of Missouri–Columbia, MO
University of Nebraska Medical Center, NE
University of Pittsburgh, PA
University of Rochester, NY
University of South Alabama, AL
University of South Carolina–Columbia, SC
University of Southern Maine, ME
University of Texas Health Science Center at Houston, TX
University of Virginia, VA
University of Washington, WA
Vanderbilt University, TN
Washington State University, WA
Yale University, CT

Women's Health
Adelphi University, NY
Boston College, MA
Case Western Reserve, OH
Columbia University, NY
Emory University–Nell Hodgson Woodruff School of Nursing, GA
Georgia Southern University, GA
Georgia State University, GA
Hampton University, VA
Indiana University–Purdue University, IN
Loyola University–Chicago, IL
MCP Hahnemann University, PA
Northwestern State University of Louisiana, LA
The Ohio State University, OH
Oregon Health Sciences University, OR
Rutgers The State University of New Jersey, NJ
Seton Hall University, NJ
Simmons College, MA
State University of New York at Buffalo, NY
State University of New York at Stony Brook, NY
SUNY Health Science Center–Brooklyn, NY
Texas Woman's University, TX
University of Cincinnati, OH
University of Colorado–Denver, CO
University of Colorado Health Sciences Center, CO
University of Florida, FL
University of Illinois–Chicago, IL
University of Louisville, KY
University of Maine, ME
University of Maryland–Baltimore, MD
University of Michigan, MI
University of Minnesota–Minneapolis, MN
University of Missouri–Kansas City, MO
University of Missouri–St. Louis, MO
University of Nebraska Medical Center, NE
University of North Carolina–Chapel Hill, NC
University of Pennsylvania, PA

University of Pittsburgh, PA
University of South Alabama, AL
University of South Carolina–Columbia, SC
The University of Tennessee–Knoxville, TN
University of Texas–El Paso, TX
University of Texas Health Science Center at Houston, TX
University of Utah, UT
University of Washington, WA
University of Wisconsin–Milwaukee, WI
Vanderbilt University, TN
Virginia Commonwealth University, VA
Wilmington College, DE
Yale University, CT

Other
Clarke College, IA
Columbia University, NY
Duke University, NC
East Carolina University, NC
Florida Gulf Coast University, FL
Florida State University, FL
Monmouth University, NJ
Northern Illinois University, IL
Oregon Health Sciences University, OR
Rush University, IL
Rutgers The State University of New Jersey, NJ
Samuel Merritt College, CA
Simmons College, MA
Southern Connecticut State University, CT
Spalding University, KY
State University of New York at Stony Brook, NY
University of Arizona, AZ
University of California, Los Angeles, CA
University of California, San Francisco, CA
University of Central Arkansas, AR
University of Florida, FL
University of Hartford, CT
University of Hawaii at Manoa, HI
University of Illinois–Chicago, IL
University of Kansas, KS
University of Maryland–Baltimore, MD
University of Medical Dentistry of New Jersey, NJ
University of Missouri–Columbia, MO
University of North Carolina–Chapel Hill, NC
University of North Carolina–Greensboro, NC
University of Pennsylvania, PA
University of Texas Health Science Center at Houston, TX
University of Texas Medical Branch–Galveston, TX
University of Utah, UT
University of Washington, WA
Western Kentucky University, KY
Wichita State University, KS
Yale University, CT

NURSE PRACTITIONER/POST-MASTER'S PROGRAM

Acute Care
California State University–Los Angeles, CA
College of New Rochelle, NY

Columbia University, NY
Duke University, NC
Georgetown University, DC
Johns Hopkins University, MD
Marquette University, WI
Monmouth University, NJ
New York University, NY
Rush University, IL
Saint Louis University, MO
University of Connecticut, CT
University of Illinois–Chicago, IL
University of Maryland–Baltimore, MD
University of Massachusetts–Worcester, MA
University of Michigan, MI
University of Nebraska Medical Center, NE
University of New Mexico, NM
University of Pennsylvania, PA
University of Rochester, NY
University of South Alabama, AL
University of Southern Indiana, IN
University of Texas Health Science Center at Houston, TX
University of Texas Medical Branch–Galveston, TX
University of Virginia, VA
Wichita State University, KS
Wright State University, OH
Yale University, CT

Adult
Adelphi University, NY
Andrews University, MI
Ball State University, IN
Bloomsburg University, PA
Boston College, MA
California State University–Los Angeles, CA
Case Western Reserve, OH
College of Saint Catherine, MN
College of Saint Scholastica, MN
Columbia University, NY
Creighton University, NE
East Tennessee State University, TN
Emory University–Nell Hodgson Woodruff School of Nursing, GA
Fairleigh Dickinson University, NJ
Florida Atlantic University, FL
Gwynedd-Mercy College, PA
Indiana University–Purdue University, IN
Jewish Hospital, MO
Johns Hopkins University, MD
Loma Linda University, CA
Long Island University–Brooklyn, NY
Loyola University–Chicago, IL
Madonna University, MI
Marquette University, WI
McNeese State University, LA
Medical University of South Carolina, SC
New York University, NY
North Park University, IL
Northern Kentucky University, KY
The Ohio State University, OH
Oregon Health Sciences University, OR
Quinipiac University, CT

Southeast Missouri State University, MO
Southern University and A&M College, LA
Spalding University, KY
State University of New York at Stony Brook, NY
State University of New York at Syracuse, NY
SUNY Health Science Center–Brooklyn, NY
Syracuse University, NY
Texas Tech University Health Sciences Center, TX
Texas Woman's University, TX
Thomas Jefferson University, PA
Troy State University, AL
Uniformed Services University, MD
University of Alabama–Huntsville, AL
University of Alaska–Anchorage, AK
University of Central Arkansas, AR
University of Central Florida, FL
University of Colorado Health Sciences Center, CO
University of Detroit Mercy, MI
University of Florida, FL
University of Hawaii at Manoa, HI
University of Illinois–Chicago, IL
University of Kansas, KS
University of Kentucky, KY
University of Louisiana–Lafayette, LA
University of Louisville, KY
University of Maine, ME
University of Maryland–Baltimore, MD
University of Massachusetts–Amherst, MA
University of Missouri–Columbia, MO
University of Missouri–Kansas City, MO
University of Missouri–St. Louis, MO
University of Nebraska Medical Center, NE
University of Nevada–Las Vegas, NV
University of New Hampshire, NH
University of New Mexico, NM
University of North Carolina–Chapel Hill, NC
University of North Dakota, ND
University of Northern Colorado, CO
University of Oklahoma, OK
University of Phoenix, AZ
University of Portland, OR
University of Rhode Island, RI
University of Rochester, NY
University of South Alabama, AL
University of South Carolina–Columbia, SC
University of Southern Indiana, IN
The University of Southern Mississippi, MS
University of Tampa, FL
University of Texas–El Paso, TX
University of Texas Health Science Center at Houston, TX
University of Texas Medical Branch–Galveston, TX
University of Texas–Pan American, TN
University of Utah, UT
University of Vermont, VT
University of Virginia, VA
University of Washington, WA
University of Wisconsin–Milwaukee, WI
University of Wyoming, WY
Valparaiso University, IN
Virginia Commonwealth University, VA
Washington State University, WA

West Texas A&M University, TX
West Virginia University, WV
Wichita State University, KS
Widener University, PA
Wright State University, OH

Gerontology
California State University–Hayward, CA
Duke University, NC
Emory University–Nell Hodgson Woodruff School of Nursing, GA
Florida Atlantic University, FL
Howard University, DC
Idaho State University, ID
Marquette University, WI
Midwestern State University, TX
Neumann College, PA
New York University, NY
Northern Kentucky University, KY
Rush University, IL
Saint Louis University, MO
Seton Hall University, NJ
University of California, Los Angeles, CA
University of Colorado–Colorado Springs–Beth-El College of Nursing, CO
University of Connecticut, CT
University of Florida, FL
University of Illinois–Chicago, IL
University of Michigan, MI
University of Nebraska Medical Center, NE
University of Pennsylvania, PA
University of South Alabama, AL
University of Texas Health Science Center at Houston, TX
University of Texas Medical Branch–Galveston, TX
University of Utah, UT
Winona State University, MN

Neonatology
Baylor University, TX
Duke University, NC
Emory University–Nell Hodgson Woodruff School of Nursing, GA
Northwestern State University of Louisiana, LA
Old Dominion University, VA
Rush University, IL
State University of New York at Stony Brook, NY
University of California, Los Angeles, CA
University of Connecticut, CT
University of Florida, FL
University of Nebraska Medical Center, NE
University of South Alabama, AL
University of Texas Health Science Center at Houston, TX

Pediatrics
California State University–Los Angeles, CA
The Catholic University of America, DC
College of Saint Catherine, MN
Columbia University, NY
Duke University, NC

Emory University–Nell Hodgson Woodruff School of Nursing, GA
Georgia State University, GA
Gwynedd-Mercy College, PA
Indiana University–Purdue University, IN
Lawrence Memorial/Regis College, MA
Loma Linda University, CA
Loyola University–Chicago, IL
Medical College of Georgia, GA
Northwestern State University of Louisiana, LA
Old Dominion University, VA
Oregon Health Sciences University, OR
Regis College, MA
Rush University, IL
Saint Louis University, MO
Seton Hall University, NJ
Simmons College, MA
South Dakota State University, SD
State University of New York at Stony Brook, NY
State University of New York at Syracuse, NY
Syracuse University, NY
Texas Woman's University, TX
The University of Akron, OH
University of California, Los Angeles, CA
University of Colorado Health Sciences Center, CO
University of Florida, FL
University of Illinois–Chicago, IL
University of Maryland–Baltimore, MD
University of Missouri–Kansas City, MO
University of North Carolina–Chapel Hill, NC
University of Pennsylvania, PA
University of South Alabama, AL
University of Texas at Austin, TX
University of Texas Health Science Center at Houston, TX
University of Texas Medical Branch–Galveston, TX
University of Utah, UT
University of Virginia, VA
Villanova University, PA
Virginia Commonwealth University, VA
Western Kentucky University, KY
Wright State University, OH

Psychiatric/Mental Health
College of Saint Scholastica, MN
Emory University–Nell Hodgson Woodruff School of Nursing, GA
Fairfield University, CT
New York University, NY
Oregon Health Sciences University, OR
Pace University, NY
Rush University, IL
State University of New York at Buffalo, NY
State University of New York at Stony Brook, NY
The University of Akron, OH
University of Michigan, MI
University of Missouri–Columbia, MO
University of Nebraska Medical Center, NE
University of Rochester, NY
University of South Alabama, AL
University of Southern Maine, ME

University of Texas Health Science Center at Houston, TX
University of Virginia, VA
Washington State University, WA
Yale University, CT

Women's Health
Emory University–Nell Hodgson Woodruff School of Nursing, GA
Georgia State University, GA
Indiana University–Purdue University, IN
Loyola University–Chicago, IL
State University of New York at Buffalo, NY
University of Florida, FL
University of Illinois–Chicago, IL
University of Louisville, KY
University of Maine, ME
University of Maryland–Baltimore, MD
University of Nebraska Medical Center, NE
University of North Carolina–Chapel Hill, NC
University of South Alabama, AL
University of South Carolina–Columbia, SC
University of Texas Health Science Center at Houston, TX
University of Utah, UT

Other
Duke University, NC
Florida Gulf Coast University, FL
Rush University, IL
University of Illinois–Chicago, IL
University of Kansas, KS
University of Maryland–Baltimore, MD
University of Pennsylvania, PA
University of Texas Health Science Center at Houston, TX
University of Utah, UT
Yale University, CT

NURSING ADMINISTRATION/MANAGEMENT

Administration/Executive-Community Health
Delta State University, MS
Loyola University–Chicago, IL
Northern Illinois University, IL
Northern Kentucky University, KY
Old Dominion University, VA
Oregon Health Sciences University, OR
Rush University, IL
Saint Xavier University, IL
Salem State College, MA
Seattle University, WA
Southeastern Louisiana University, LA
University of Colorado Health Sciences Center, CO
University of Iowa, IA
University of Kentucky, KY
University of Michigan, MI
University of North Carolina–Charlotte, NC
University of North Carolina–Greensboro, NC
University of South Alabama, AL
University of Southern California, CA

University of Tampa, FL
William Patterson University, NJ

Administration/Executive-General
Albany State University, GA
Ball State University, IN
Barry University, FL
Baylor University, TX
Brigham Young University, UT
California State University–Fullerton, CA
The Catholic University of America, DC
College Misericordia, PA
Duquesne University, PA
East Carolina University, NC
East Tennessee State University, TN
Emory University–Nell Hodgson Woodruff School of
    Nursing, GA
Gannon University, PA
George Mason University, VA
Gonzaga University, WA
Hampton University, VA
Ida V. Moffett School–Samford University, AL
Indiana University–Purdue University, IN
Indiana University–Purdue University –Fort Wayne,
    IN
Loma Linda University, CA
Louisiana State University, LA
Loyola University–Chicago, IL
Madonna University, MI
Marquette University, WI
Marshall University, WV
Marymount University, VA
McNeese State University, LA
MCP Hahnemann University, PA
Medical College of Ohio, OH
Monmouth University, NJ
New York University, NY
Northwestern State University of Louisiana, LA
Oregon Health Sciences University, OR
Queens College, NC
Sacred Heart University, CT
Saint Louis University, MO
Salisbury State University, MD
Seton Hall University, NJ
Southern Adventist University, TN
Southern Illinois University–Edwardsville, IL
Texas Tech University Health Sciences Center, TX
University of California, San Francisco, CA
University of Central Florida, FL
University of Colorado Health Sciences Center, CO
University of Hartford, CT
University of Hawaii at Manoa, HI
University of Illinois–Chicago, IL
University of Maryland–Baltimore, MD
University of Massachusetts–Boston, MA
University of Missouri–Columbia, MO
University of New Mexico, NM
University of North Carolina–Chapel Hill, NC
University of Pennsylvania, PA
University of Rhode Island, RI
University of South Carolina–Columbia, SC
University of Southern Indiana, IN

The University of Southern Mississippi, MS
University of Texas–Tyler, TX
West Texas A&M University, TX
Wheeling Jesuit University, WV
Wichita State University, KS
Wright State University, OH

Management/Administrative/Executive-Other
Andrews University, MI
Armstrong Atlantic State University, GA
Bellarmine College, KY
Bradley University, IL
California State University–Bakersfield, CA
California State University–Dominquez Hills, CA
Capital University, OH
Clarke College, IA
Clarkson College, NE
Clemson University, SC
College of New Rochelle, NY
College of Saint Scholastica, MN
Drake University, IA
Duke University, NC
Edgewood College, WI
Excelsior College, NY
Florida Atlantic University, FL
Georgia College and State University, GA
Grand Valley State University, MI
Indiana University of Pennsylvania, PA
Johns Hopkins University, MD
La Roche College, PA
Lawrence Memorial/Regis College, MA
Lewis University, IL
Long Island University–Brooklyn, NY
Medical University of South Carolina, SC
Montana State University–Bozeman, MT
New Mexico State University, NM
New York University, NY
Newman University, KS
Northeastern University, MA
Otterbein College, OH
Regis College, MA
Regis University, CO
Saginaw Valley State University, MI
Saint John Fisher College, NY
Saint Joseph's College, ME
San Diego State University, CA
San Francisco State University, CA
San Jose State University, CA
Spalding University, KY
Texas A&M University–Corpus Christi, TX
The University of Akron, OH
University of Alaska–Anchorage, AK
University of California, Los Angeles, CA
University of Central Florida, FL
University of Cincinnati, OH
University of Colorado–Denver, CO
University of Colorado Health Sciences Center, CO
University of Connecticut, CT
University of Delaware, DE
University of Florida, FL
University of Kansas, KS
University of Kentucky, KY

University of Missouri–Kansas City, MO
University of Missouri–St. Louis, MO
University of New Hampshire, NH
University of North Dakota, ND
University of Oklahoma, OK
University of Pittsburgh, PA
University of Saint Francis–Fort Wayne, IN
University of Southern Maine, ME
The University of Tennessee–Chattanooga, TN
The University of Tennessee–Knoxville, TN
University of Texas at Austin, TX
University of Texas–El Paso, TX
University of Texas Health Science Center at Houston,
  TX
University of Texas Health Science Center at San
  Antonio, TX
University of the Incarnate Word, TX
University of Utah, UT
University of Virginia, VA
University of Washington, WA
Valdosta State University, GA
Valparaiso University, IN
Vanderbilt University, TN
Villanova University, PA
Virginia Commonwealth University, VA
Wilmington College, DE
Winona State University, MN
Xavier University, OH

Mid-level Nursing Management
Adelphi University, NY
University of Wisconsin–Eau Claire, WI

MSN/MBA
Adelphi University, NY
Barry University, FL
Bellarmine College, KY
Bloomsburg University, PA
Capital University, OH
Case Western Reserve, OH
Gannon University, PA
Grand Valley State University, MI
Hawaii Pacific University, HI
Ida V. Moffett School–Samford University, AL
Johns Hopkins University, MD
La Salle University, PA
Lewis University, IL
Loyola University–Chicago, IL
Madonna University, MI
New York University, NY
North Park University, IL
Northeastern University, MA
Sacred Heart University, CT
Saint Xavier University, IL
Salem State College, MA
Samuel Merritt College, CA
Southern Adventist University, TN
University of Cincinnati, OH
University of Colorado Health Sciences Center, CO
University of Connecticut, CT
University of Illinois–Chicago, IL
University of Indianapolis, IN

University of Iowa, IA
University of Maryland–Baltimore, MD
University of Phoenix, CA
University of Tampa, FL
University of Texas–Tyler, TX
Wichita State University, KS
Wright State University, OH
Xavier University, OH

NURSING ADMINISTRATION/MANAGEMENT/
   POST-MASTERS

Administration/Executive-Community Health
Rush University, IL
Saint Xavier University, IL
University of Tampa, FL

Administration/Executive-General
Barry University, FL
Duquesne University, PA
Emory University–Nell Hodgson Woodruff School of
  Nursing, GA
Loma Linda University, CA
Marshall University, WV
University of Illinois–Chicago, IL

Management/Administrative/Executive-Other
Bradley University, IL
Georgia College and State University, GA
New York University, NY
University of Kentucky, KY

MSN/MBA
Barry University, FL
Georgia College and State University, GA
Saint Xavier University, IL
University of Illinois–Chicago, IL
University of Southern California, CA

NURSING EDUCATION

Academic Role
Bellarmine College, KY
California State University–Bakersfield, CA
Cardinal Stritch University, WI
Clarke College, IA
Drake University, IA
Florida Atlantic University, FL
Georgia College and State University, GA
Gonzaga University, WA
Hampton University, VA
Ida V. Moffett School–Samford University, AL
Indiana University of Pennsylvania, PA
Jewish Hospital, MO
MCP Hahnemann University, PA
New York University, NY
Northwestern State University of Louisiana, LA
South Dakota State University, SD
Southeastern Louisiana University, LA
Southern Adventist University, TN
Southern Connecticut State University, CT
Southern Illinois University–Edwardsville, IL

Southern University and A&M College, LA
Southwest Missouri State University, MO
Southwest Missouri State University–Springfield, MO
Texas Tech University Health Sciences Center, TX
Tri-College University Nursing Consortium, ND
University of California, San Francisco, CA
University of Hartford, CT
University of Louisiana–Lafayette, LA
University of Maine, ME
University of Massachusetts–Boston, MA
University of Minnesota–Minneapolis, MN
University of Mississippi Medical Center, MS
University of Missouri–St. Louis, MO
University of North Carolina–Greensboro, NC
University of Oklahoma, OK
University of Pittsburgh, PA
University of Rhode Island, RI
University of Southern Indiana, IN
The University of Tennessee–Chattanooga, TN
University of Texas–Tyler, TX
University of the Incarnate Word, TX
University of Utah, UT
University of Wisconsin–Eau Claire, WI
University of Wyoming, WY
Villanova University, PA
West Texas A&M University, TX
Western Kentucky University, KY
Winona State University, MN
Wright State University, OH

General

Albany State University, GA
Alcorn State University, MS
Allen College, IA
Ball State University, IN
Barry University, FL
Bethel College, MN
California State University–Chico, CA
Cardinal Stritch University, WI
The Catholic University of America, DC
Duquesne University, VA
Florida Gulf Coast University, FL

Staff Development

Cardinal Stritch University, WI
Gonzaga University, WA
Grand Valley State University, MI
Saginaw Valley State University, MI
San Jose State University, CA
University of Maine, ME
University of Missouri–St. Louis, MO
University of Oklahoma, OK
University of Rhode Island, RI

NURSING EDUCATION/POST-MASTERS

Academic Role
Georgia College and State University, GA

General
Barry University, FL
Florida Gulf Coast University, FL

University of Maryland–Baltimore, MD

Nurse-Midwifery

Case Western Reserve, OH
Columbia University, NY
East Carolina University, NC
Emory University–Nell Hodgson Woodruff School of
    Nursing, GA
Georgetown University, DC
Marquette University, WI
New York University, NY
The Ohio State University, OH
Oregon Health Sciences University, OR
Pontifical Catholic University of Puerto Rico, PR
San Diego State University, CA
Shenandoah University, VA
State University of New York at Stony Brook, NY
SUNY Health Science Center–Brooklyn, NY
University of California, Los Angeles, CA
University of Cincinnati, OH
University of Colorado Health Sciences Center, CO
University of Florida, FL
University of Illinois–Chicago, IL
University of Kansas, KS
University of Maryland–Baltimore, MD
University of Michigan, MI
University of Minnesota–Minneapolis, MN
University of Missouri–Columbia, MO
University of New Mexico, NM
University of Pennsylvania, PA
University of Rhode Island, RI
University of Southern California, CA
University of Texas–El Paso, TX
University of Texas Medical Branch–Galveston, TX
University of Utah, UT
University of Vermont, VT
University of Washington, WA
Vanderbilt University, TN
Wichita State University, KS
Yale University, CT

Nurse-Midwifery/Post-Masters

Columbia University, NY
East Carolina University, NC
Emory University–Nell Hodgson Woodruff School of
    Nursing, GA
Georgetown University, DC
State University of New York at Stony Brook, NY
University of Colorado Health Sciences Center, CO
University of Florida, FL
University of Illinois–Chicago, IL
University of Kansas, KS
University of Michigan, MI
University of New Mexico, NM
University of Pennsylvania, PA
University of Rhode Island, RI
University of Southern California, CA
University of Texas Medical Branch–Galveston, TX
University of Utah, UT

ALPHABETIC INDEX

*Page numbers in **bold** refer to in-depth profiles*

*Page numbers in **bold** refer to in-depth profiles*

Page numbers in **bold** *refer to in-depth profiles*

*Page numbers in **bold** refer to in-depth profiles*